Managing Drug Supply

Managing Drug Supply

The Selection, Procurement, Distribution, and Use of Pharmaceuticals

SECOND EDITION, REVISED AND EXPANDED

MANAGEMENT SCIENCES FOR HEALTH

IN COLLABORATION WITH THE
WORLD HEALTH ORGANIZATION
ACTION PROGRAMME ON ESSENTIAL DRUGS

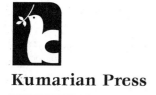

Kumarian Press

Managing Drug Supply: The Selection, Procurement,
Distribution, and Use of Pharmaceuticals
Second Edition, Revised and Expanded

Published 1997 in the United States of America by Kumarian
Press, Inc., 14 Oakwood Avenue, West Hartford, Connecticut
06119-2127 USA.

Production supervised by Jenna Dixon
Copyedited by Linda Lotz
Text design by Jenna Dixon
Typeset by Sarah Albert
Proofread by Beth Richards
Index by Alan M. Greenberg

Printed in the United States of America on acid-free paper
by Edwards Brothers, Inc. Text printed with soy-based ink.

 PRINTED WITH
SOY INK™

Library of Congress Cataloging-in-Publication Data
Managing drug supply : the selection, procurement, distribution, and use of pharmaceuticals. — 2nd ed., rev. and
expanded
         p.   cm. — (Kumarian Press books on
international development)
  "Management Sciences for Health in collaboration with
the World Health Organization."
    Editors: Jonathan D. Quick and others.
    Includes bibliographical references and index.
    ISBN 1-56549-047-9 (paper : alk. paper)
    1. Pharmaceutical policy—Developing countries.
I. Quick, Jonathan D. II. Management Sciences for
Health (Firm). III. World Health Organization.
IV. Series.
    [DNLM: 1. Drugs, Essential—supply & distribution.
2. Economics, Pharmaceutical. QV 736 M2667 1997]
RA401.D44M36   1997
362.1'782—dc20
DNLM/DLC
for Library of Congress
96-42268

06 05 04 03 02 01 00 99 98 97   10 9 8 7 6 5 4 3 2 1
1st Printing 1997

Editors

JONATHAN D. QUICK
Management Sciences for Health

JAMES R. RANKIN
Management Sciences for Health

RICHARD O. LAING
Management Sciences for Health

RONALD W. O'CONNOR
Management Sciences for Health

HANS V. HOGERZEIL
Action Programme on Essential Drugs,
World Health Organization

M. N. G. DUKES
Euro Health Group

ANDREW GARNETT
Feilden Battersby Health Systems Analysts

Contributors

CHRISTEL ALBERT
Cologne, Germany

WILBERT BANNENBERG
Amsterdam, The Netherlands

ANTHONY BATTERSBY
Feilden Battersby Health Systems Analysts,
Bath, England

ELVIRA BERACOCHEA
Management Sciences for Health, Arlington, Va.

CARL F. BROWNE
Ministry of Health and the Environment,
Kingstown, St. Vincent and Grenadines

PASCALE BRUDON
Action Programme on Essential Drugs,
World Health Organization, Geneva, Switzerland

MIGUEL M. DE CLERCK
Médecins sans Frontières, Brussels, Belgium

DAVID H. COLLINS
Management Sciences for Health, Boston, Mass.

GABRIEL DANIEL
Africare, Washington, D.C.

VIMAL S. DIAS
Management Sciences for Health, Panadura, Sri Lanka

JAN F. DIK
Euro Health Group, Copenhagen, Denmark

JOHN ELLERY
Greenshields Cowie, Sutton, Surrey, England

ENRIQUE FEFER
Pan American Health Organization, Washington, D.C.

CHRIS FORSHAW
Malawi Essential Drugs Programme,
World Health Organization, Lilongwe, Malawi

JOHN FOX
Intermedia, Nairobi, Kenya

DAPHNE A. FRESLE
Action Programme on Essential Drugs,
World Health Organization, Geneva, Switzerland

AIDA GIRMA
Bamako Initiative Management Project,
UNICEF, New York, N.Y.

PETER J. GRAAFF
Malawi Essential Drugs Programme,
World Health Organization, Lilongwe, Malawi

SHERITA GREGOIRE
Goodwill, Dominica

AGNES B. GUYON
UNICEF, Dhaka, Bangladesh

KARA HANSON
Harvard School of Public Health, Boston, Mass.

JOHAN VAN HAPEREN
Danida, Entebbe, Uganda

MYRIAM HENKENS
Médecins sans Frontières, Brussels, Belgium

DAVID HENRY
University of Newcastle, Australia

JOHN HOLLEY
Integral Development Associates, Washington, D.C.

MARGARET HUME
Management Sciences for Health, Boston, Mass.

KEITH W. JOHNSON
US Pharmacopeia, Rockville, Md.

O. M. J. KASILO
University of Zimbabwe Medical School,
Harare, Zimbabwe

IRENE KLINGER
Pan American Health Organization, Washington, D.C.

PAUL KRYSTALL
Data Dynamics, Nairobi, Kenya

JEAN-PIERRE DE LAMALLE
Médecins sans Frontières, Brussels, Belgium

PAUL J. N. LAMBERTS
Deventer Hospital Pharmacy, Deventer, Netherlands

DAVID LEE
Management Sciences for Health, Arlington, Va.

Affiliations listed are those at the time contributions were made.

JENNIE I. LITVACK
World Bank, Washington, D.C.

JULIE E. MCFADYEN
Management Sciences for Health, Arlington, Va.

SAM MUZIKI
Action Programme on Essential Drugs,
World Health Organization, Geneva, Switzerland

KIRSTEN MYHR
Department of Pharmacy, University Hospital
of Trondheim, Trondheim, Norway

HANIF S. NAZERALI
Pharmaceuticals Consultant, Harare, Zimbabwe

WILLIAM NEWBRANDER
Management Sciences for Health, Boston, Mass.

DAVID OFORI-ADJEI
Centre for Tropical Clinical Pharmacology and
Therapeutics, University of Ghana Medical School,
Accra, Ghana

CHRIS B. OLSON
Management Sciences for Health,
San Diego, Calif.

IGNACIO J. PACKER
Médecins sans Frontières, Brussels, Belgium

THERESE EDERA-PIECH
Design Development, Nairobi, Kenya

CANDACE ROOSEVELT
Management Sciences for Health, Boston, Mass.

DENNIS ROSS-DEGNAN
Drug Policy Group, Harvard University,
Cambridge, Mass.

JEAN-PIERRE SALLET
Management Sciences for Health, Arlington, Va.

BUDIONO SANTOSO
Department of Clinical Pharmacology,
Gadjah Mada University, Yogyakarta, Indonesia

ANTHONY SAVELLI
Management Sciences for Health, Arlington, Va.

PAUL D. SPIVEY
Robert Gordon University, Aberdeen, Scotland

JOHN C. TURNBULL
Willowdale, Ontario, Canada

HILARY VAUGHAN
Crown Agents, Sutton, Surrey, England

GERMÁN VELÁSQUEZ
Action Programme on Essential Drugs,
World Health Organization, Geneva, Switzerland

MARCELO VERNENGO
Universidad de Belgrano, Buenos Aires, Argentina

CATRIONA WADDINGTON
Overseas Development Administration, Accra, Ghana

ROBERT L. WATT
Coatesville, Penn.

DAVID R. WILSON
Management Sciences for Health,
Antananarivo, Madagascar

Illustrators

EUSTACE GITHONGA
Nairobi, Kenya

UTO HOGERZEIL
Newtownmountkennedy,
County Wicklow, Ireland

TONY NAMATE
Harare, Zimbabwe

Contributors to the First Edition

JAMES BATES
Management Sciences for Health, Haiti

HENK DEN BESTEN
International Dispensary Association,
Amsterdam, The Netherlands

PETER N. CROSS
Management Sciences for Health, Bolivia

A. FREDERICK HARTMAN
Management Sciences for Health,
Boston, Mass.

M. LEE MORSE
Health Information Designs,
Washington, D.C.

WILLIAM HEWITT
Pharmaceutical Production Consultancy, Ltd.,
Spetchley, Worcester, England

PETER J. HUFF-ROUSSELLE
Management Sciences for Health,
Boston, Mass.

AIDA A. LEROY
Health Information Designs,
Washington, D.C.

To Halfdan Mahler and Ernst Lauridsen,
whose vision and energy brought
the essential drugs concept to life,
and to the decision-makers throughout
the world who are putting it into action

Contents

Preface

The worst tragedies in public health are the avoidable ones: those problems for which solutions are known and that local resources are available to deal with on a sustainable basis, but which remain inadequately addressed. We see evidence of these tragedies in the media every day: children dying of preventable illnesses, adults suffering from major but treatable diseases, and women bearing unwanted babies in circumstances that foretell generations of suffering. Such tragedies define the mission of Management Sciences for Health: to help decision-makers make the best use of limited resources to narrow the gap between what is known about and what is done to solve the most pressing problems of public health. To pursue that goal, there is no more promising field than drug supply management.

The three reasons for this manual remain essentially unchanged from the first edition, as underscored by the many positive achievements of health policy-makers and managers in the intervening fifteen years:

1. *Essential drugs are critical to the success of health programs.** Drugs are part of the final link between patients and health services, a link that determines whether the vast societal investment in training providers, building facilities, and buying equipment will succeed or fail. That final link to a positive impact on health often depends on whether an essential drug is available and is used appropriately: when it is not, for that patient, much of the entire health-sector investment is wasted.

2. *Improving the management of drug supply is a high-leverage opportunity to improve health services.* Years of experience from health policy-makers and decision-makers throughout the world confirm that major improvements are possible and affordable and can save money.

3. *Knowledge and experience concerning effective drug management are spreading rapidly worldwide, but they remain disparate, unsynthesized, and frequently unavailable to decision-makers.* This is so because they cross the boundaries between clinical medicine, pharmacology, management, finance, and economics.

For these reasons, this manual is organized to serve two closely related and interdependent audiences: health policy-makers and the staff who manage drug systems and the drug use process.

Health policy-makers are not specialists in drug management and will never have the time to be, yet they regularly face important decisions about selection, procurement, distribution, and use of pharmaceuticals: What are the likely health effects, costs, and benefits of policy choices? How much effort and resources are involved in each, and how quickly will various strategies to improve essential drug management start to repay these investments? The introductory chapters of each section in this manual put these kinds of issues into perspective to support policy-makers' choices for action.

Operational managers must analyze drug management systems and problems to select and implement changes. In the chapters that follow the overview chapters of each section, *Managing Drug Supply* provides detailed information on effective and efficient ways to solve problems.

This manual focuses on management of essential drugs and the problems faced by policy-makers and managers operating with scarce resources, but the tools and ideas discussed are based on those used in the most developed countries. Today, rapid advances in information-sharing technology and the use of computers worldwide offer decision-makers everywhere the benefits of these proven modern management techniques.

The challenge for policy-makers in public health revolves around making choices: deciding which problems to address and organizing the resources to solve them. For those who are striving to eliminate the unnecessary tragedies that result from lack of essential drugs, *Managing Drug Supply* was created to ensure that they have the tools at hand.

Ronald W. O'Connor, MD
President, Management Sciences for Health

*In this manual, *drug, drug product, pharmaceutical, medicine,* and *medication* are used interchangeably to refer to any drug product used in the prevention or treatment of health problems, including vaccines, oral rehydration sachets, tablets, capsules, injectables, and galenicals.

Acknowledgments

Fifteen years ago, the first edition of *Managing Drug Supply* emerged from a dozen collaborators and reviewers in a relatively brief process that, in part, reflected the underdeveloped state of discourse on essential drugs programs. Although we planned to produce a second edition after ten years, an additional five years have elapsed on the way to press. This extra time has allowed us to involve more than sixty authors from all parts of the world and even more reviewers, at the cost (even in this era of the Internet) of extending the editorial exchange and the production process. Today, a rapidly expanding international community of colleagues is contributing to the dialog on management of essential drugs, and it is they who have collectively created this revised and expanded edition.

Seven editors collaborated to develop the outline, identify potential contributors, take responsibility for management of the major sections, and review draft chapters. Individual authors' contributions (see the list of authors at the end of the book) were coordinated by the section editors: Ronald W. O'Connor, Introduction; M. N. G. Dukes, Policy and Legal Framework; Hans V. Hogerzeil, Selection; James R. Rankin, Procurement; Andrew Garnett, Distribution; Richard O. Laing, Use; and Jonathan D. Quick, Management Support Systems.

Each chapter was reviewed by at least three other experts (see the list of reviewers at the end of the book). People who were particularly active in reviewing chapters include Henk den Besten, International Dispensary Association, Amsterdam; Denis Broun, World Bank, Washington, D.C.; Ernst Lauridsen, Euro Health Group, Copenhagen; Maria Miralles, Management Sciences for Health (MSH), Arlington, Va.; Mogens Munck, Zimbabwe Essential Drugs Programme, Harare; Judith B. Seltzer, MSH, Boston; Gerrit Weeda, Government Medical Stores, Harare; and the staff pharmacists from the Mission for Essential Drugs (MEDS), Nairobi. Several authors were particularly helpful in the review and revision process: James Bates, Vimal S. Dias, Daphne A. Fresle, Paul J. N. Lamberts, David Lee, Chris B. Olson, Jean-Pierre Sallet, Paul D. Spivey, and Robert L. Watt.

Finally, senior editors Quick and Rankin edited the combined manuscript for accuracy and consistency, with input from the other editors. Any errors or lack of clarity are the editors' responsibility.

Country studies and figures adapted from published sources are acknowledged at the end of each item. When no source is listed, the item is based on the knowledge of the chapter author, another contributor, or the editors.

Ernst Lauridsen, of the Euro Health Group in Denmark and former director of the Action Programme on Essential Drugs (DAP) of the World Health Organization (WHO) in Geneva, was instrumental in generating support for this second edition. Margaretha Helling-Borda, director of WHO/DAP, Geneva, was supportive in providing access to the DAP Documentation Center, which was helpful in preparing country studies, and in sharing the expertise of DAP staff members as authors, reviewers, and section editors.

Penelope Caponigro, Christopher Welch, Jennifer Teig von Hoffman, and Herb Wang assembled the manuscript with unending energy and dedication, and Barbara Timmons's able management of the final editing process has served MSH well. The artistic contributions of Eustace Githonga, Uto Hogerzeil, and Tony Namate were critical to convey information clearly, concisely, and in a user-friendly way.

The development of this edition was supported by grants from the Pew Charitable Trusts, Danida, the Swedish International Development Agency (SIDA), the Stubbs Memorial Fund of MSH, WHO/DAP, and the Overseas Development Administration of the British government. Additionally, the US Agency for International Development (USAID) Rational Pharmaceutical Management (RPM) Project facilitated input by MSH/ RPM staff.

We are grateful for the commitment of all to narrowing the gap between what is known and what is done to improve the management of drug supply. ■

How to Use This Manual

This manual may seem formidable, but it need not be read from cover to cover. Instead, it is organized to provide a sequential overview of major topics and, within each section, detailed explanations of fundamental concepts, definitions of basic terms, and practical ideas for designing and implementing effective changes in drug management.

The following features are included to make the material accessible to those looking for information in specific areas.

Overview Chapters. After the introductory and policy and legal background sections (Parts I and II), overview chapters introduce each element in the drug management cycle: selection (Chapter 10), procurement (Chapter 13), distribution (Chapter 21), rational use (Chapter 28), and managing drug programs (Chapter 34). These chapters provide background information for policy-makers and lead into more detailed discussions in the following chapters for those who operate aspects of essential drug supply systems.

Chapter Summaries. Each chapter begins with a summary of the chapter's contents. Those interested in a rapid overview of an area or of all aspects of drug supply can read the summaries for that area or for all the chapters.

Country Studies. Reports of drug managers' experiences in different countries illustrate points in the text. Even though conditions in some countries may have changed since these country studies were written, they provide useful examples of the ways in which the drug management process can operate and, in some cases, how it should not operate.

Boxes. Boxes are used in several chapters to make information such as the steps of a process easy to locate and use.

Assessment Guides. Most of the chapters close with assessment guides, structured as a series of questions to help readers appraise their systems in light of the issues covered in the chapter. These assessment guides can be used in training programs and to stimulate policy discussions or guide evaluations of supply activities. Many of the assessment guides contain objective indicators—to use in documenting needs, planning drug management improvements, and measuring progress—that are based on work by Management Sciences for Health and the World Health Organization (see Chapters 4 and 36).

Glossaries. Terms are defined and grouped within the section of the manual in which they first appear and with which they are most closely associated. Individual glossaries are included for selection (Chapter 10), procurement (Chapter 13), distribution (Chapter 21), use (Chapter 28), management (Chapter 34), financing (Chapter 40), and computers for drug management (Chapter 46).

References and Further Readings. Each chapter contains a list of references on topics covered in the chapter; particularly useful ones are marked with a star.

Chapter Annexes. Annexes provide sources of further information and samples of drug management forms currently used in different parts of the world, which may be used as they are or modified to suit local circumstances. ∎

Abbreviations

ABPI	Association of British Pharmaceutical Industries	DDP	delivered duty paid
ADR	adverse drug reaction	DDU	delivered duty unpaid
AHFS	American Hospital Formulary Service	DEA	Drug Enforcement Administration (US)
AHRTAG	Appropriate Health Resources and Technologies Action Group, Ltd.	DEQ	delivered ex quay
		DIC	Drug Information Center
		DICP	*Drug Intelligence and Clinical Pharmacy*
AIDS	acquired immune deficiency syndrome	DMIS	drug management information system
AIM	Action in International Medicine	DPI	dots per inch
AIS	Acción Internacional para la Salud	DPT	diphtheria, pertussis, tetanus
AMA	American Medical Association	DRA	drug regulatory authority
AMA–DE	American Medical Association–Drug Evaluations	DT	diphtheria, tetanus
		DTC	drug and therapeutics committee
APUA	Alliance for the Prudent Use of Antibiotics	DUE	drug utilization evaluation
ARI	acute respiratory infection	DUR	drug utilization review
ASEAN	Association of Southeast Asian Nations	ECCB	Eastern Caribbean Central Bank
ASHP	American Society of Health-System Pharmacists	ECDS	Eastern Caribbean Drug Service
ATC	anatomical therapeutic classification	ECHO	Equipment for Charitable Hospitals Overseas
ATV	all-terrain vehicle	EDL	essential drugs list
BCG	bacillus Calmette-Guérin (tuberculosis vaccine)	EDLIZ	essential drugs list of Zimbabwe
BFAD	Bureau of Food and Drugs (Philippines)	EDP	essential drugs program
BHU	basic health unit	EFTA	European Free Trade Association
BNF	*British National Formulary*	EHG	Euro Health Group
BNMT	Britain Nepal Medical Trust	EIS	executive information system
BP	British Pharmacopoeia	EPI	Expanded Programme on Immunization
C&F	costs and freight	ESAMI	Eastern and Southern African Management Institute
CARICOM	Caribbean Community		
CCSS	Social Security Fund (Costa Rica)	EXW	ex works
CDC	Centers for Disease Control and Prevention (US)	FAS	free alongside ship
		FCA	free carrier
CDHSH	Commonwealth Department of Human Services and Health (Australia)	FDA	Food and Drug Administration (US)
		FEFO	first expiry/first out
CFR	cost and freight	FIFO	first in/first out
CHC	community health center	FIP	Fédération Internationale Pharmaceutique
CHW	community health worker	FIS	financial information system
CIF	cost, insurance, and freight	FOB	free on board
CIP	carriage and insurance paid	FP	family planning
CMC	Christian Medical Commission–Churches' Action for Health	FPI	fee per item
		FPS	fee per script
CMS	central medical stores	GMPs	good manufacturing practices
COT	course of therapy	GNP	gross national product
CPA	Commonwealth Pharmaceutical Association	GPL	Government Pharmaceutical Laboratory (Malaysia)
CPM	critical path method		
CPS	characters per second	GPO	Government Pharmaceutical Organization (Thailand)
CPT	carriage paid to		
DAF	delivered at frontier	HAI	Health Action International
DALY	disability-adjusted life-year	HDI	human development index
DAP	Action Programme on Essential Drugs	HIS	health information system
DDD	defined daily dose	HIV	human immunodeficiency virus
DES	delivered ex ship		

HMO	health maintenance organization	PBAC	pharmaceutical benefits advisory committee (Australia)
IBRD	International Bank for Reconstruction and Development	PBM	pharmaceutical benefits management
ICB	international competitive bidding	PC	personal computer
ICD	international classification of diseases	PDCA	plan-do-check-act
ICDRA	International Conference of Drug Regulatory Authorities	PDR	*Physicians' Desk Reference*
		PER	product evaluation report scheme
IDA	International Dispensary Association	PERT	project evaluation and review technique
IE&C	information, education, and communication	PHC	primary health care
IFPMA	International Federation of Pharmaceutical Manufacturers' Associations	PhRMA	Pharmaceutical Research and Manufacturers of America (US)
IMT	intermediate form of transport	PIC	pharmaceutical inspection convention
INN	international nonproprietary name	PPM	pages per minute
INRUD	International Network for Rational Use of Drugs	PPO	private provider organization
		PSD	Pharmaceutical Services Division (Papua New Guinea)
IOCU	International Organization of Consumer Unions	QALY	quality-adjusted life-year
IQC	indefinite quantity contract	QC	quality control
ISCP	International Society of Clinical Pharmacology	RAM	random-access memory
		RAP	rapid assessment procedure
ISDB	International Society of Drug Bulletins	RCT	randomized control trial
ISPE	International Society of Pharmaco-Epidemiology	RIMS	rapid inventory monitoring system
ITC	International Trade Center	RMA	rural medical aide
LAN	local area network	SPC	State Pharmaceutical Corporation (Sri Lanka)
LCB	local competitive bidding	STD	sexually transmitted disease
LICB	limited international competitive bidding	STG	standard treatment guideline
LIFO	last in/first out	TAC	technical advisory committee
MA	medical assistant	TACHC	Texas Association of Community Health Centers
MAC	maximum allowable cost		
MaLAM	Medical Lobby for Appropriate Marketing	TALC	Teaching Aids at Low Cost
MAR	medication administration record	TBA	traditional birth attendant
MBO	management by objectives	TCAC	technical cooperation among countries
MBWA	management by wandering about	TQM	total quality management
MCH	maternal and child health	TT	tetanus toxoid
MEDS	Mission for Essential Drugs and Supplies (Kenya)	UNCTAD	United Nations Conference on Trade and Development
MIMS	*Monthly Index of Medical Specialties*	UNDP	United Nations Development Programme
MIS	management information system	UNHCR	United Nations High Commissioner for Refugees
MOF	ministry of finance		
MOH	ministry of health	UNICEF	United Nations Children's Fund
MRP	maximum reimbursement price	UNIDO	United Nations Industrial Development Organization
MSH	Management Sciences for Health		
NDL	national drug law	UNIPAC	United Nations International Packing and Assembling Centre
NDP	national drug policy		
NDTPAC	National Drug and Therapeutics Policy Advisory Committee	UPS	uninterruptible power supply
		USAID	United States Agency for International Development
NEDL	national essential drugs list		
NGO	nongovernmental organization	USP	United States Pharmacopeia
NLEMSE	national list of essential medical supplies and equipment	USP–DI	*United States Pharmacopeia–Drug Information*
		USPHS	United States Public Health Service
ODA	Overseas Development Administration (UK)	VAT	value-added tax
OECD	Organization for Economic Cooperation and Development	VEN	vital, essential, nonessential
		VHV	village health volunteer
OECS	Organization of Eastern Caribbean States	WFI	water for injection
OPD	outpatient department	WFPPM	World Federation of Proprietary Medicine Manufacturers
OPV	oral polio vaccine		
ORS	oral rehydration salts (or solution)	WHO	World Health Organization
OTC	over-the-counter	WISN	workload indicator of staffing need
OXFAM	Oxford Committee for Famine Relief	WMA	World Medical Association
P&T	pharmacy and therapeutics (committee)	WYSIWYG	what you see is what you get
PAHO	Pan American Health Organization	ZEDAP	Zimbabwe Essential Drugs Action Programme
PASS	Prescription Analysis Software System		

Part I
Introduction

Part I Introduction	Part II Policy and Legal Framework	Part III Drug Management Cycle	Part IV Management Support Systems

1 **Toward Sustainable Supply and Rational Use of Drugs**
2 Historical and Institutional Perspectives
3 Economics for Drug Management
4 Pharmaceutical Supply System Assessment

Chapter 1

Toward Sustainable Supply and Rational Use of Drugs

≡ Summary

Most leading causes of death and disability in developing countries can be prevented, treated, or at least alleviated with cost-effective essential drugs. Despite this fact, literally hundreds of millions of people do not have regular access to essential drugs. Many of those who do have access are given the wrong treatment, receive too little medicine for their illness, or do not use the drug correctly.

Managing Drug Supply is concerned with practical ways in which government policy-makers, essential drugs program managers, nongovernmental organizations (NGOs), donors, and others can work to ensure that high-quality essential drugs are available, affordable, and used rationally. Drugs are of particular importance because they can save lives and improve health, and they promote trust and participation in health services. They are costly, and there are special concerns that make drugs different from other consumer products. In addition, substantive improvements in the supply and use of drugs are possible.

Within a decade after the first modern pharmaceuticals became available, efforts began to ensure their widespread availability. From the mid-1950s to the mid-1970s, basic drug management concepts began to evolve in countries as diverse as Norway, Papua New Guinea, Sri Lanka, Cuba, and Peru.

In 1975, the World Health Organization (WHO) defined essential drugs as those drugs that meet the health needs of the majority of the population. Over the last twenty years, countries have acquired considerable experience in managing drug supply. Broad lessons that have emerged from this experience include:

- *National drug policy provides a sound foundation for managing drug supply.*
- *Wise drug selection underlies all other improvements.*
- *Effective management saves money and improves performance.*
- *Rational drug use requires more than drug information.*
- *Systematic assessment and monitoring are essential.*

Although much has been achieved over the last two decades, many challenges remain:

- *Achieving financial sustainability through greater efficiency and financing mechanisms that increase avail-ability while ensuring equity (financing options include public financing, user charges, health insurance, voluntary and other local financing, and donor financing);*
- *Improving efficiency in public drug supply through strategies that build on public-sector strengths while incorporating greater flexibility and competitiveness;*
- *Changing the behavior of providers, patients, and the public to promote effective, safe, and economical prescribing, dispensing, and patient use of drugs;*
- *Reorienting the role of government to improve the availability, affordability, and rational use of drugs in the private sector, which supplies 60 to 80 percent of the drugs consumed in developing countries;*
- *Regulating safety, efficacy, and quality through legislation and regulations that ensure that all drugs meet basic quality standards.*

Managing Drug Supply is organized around the four basic functions of the drug management cycle:

- *selection*
- *procurement*
- *distribution*
- *use*

At the center of the drug management cycle is a core of management support systems:

- *organization*
- *financing and sustainability*
- *information management*
- *human resources management*

The entire cycle rests on a policy and legal framework that establishes and supports the public commitment to essential drug supply (Part II of this manual). Other major sections of the manual are devoted to each of the main functions of the drug management cycle (Part III) and management support (Part IV).

This manual provides concepts and approaches that can produce measurable health improvements through greater access to and more rational use of drugs. Governments, private organizations, donors, and others who use this manual must provide the will and the resources to put these concepts and approaches into action.

≡ Interest in human health and illness is as old as humanity. Scientific study of human anatomy and human diseases can be traced to the Greek physician Hippocrates and earlier. Yet as recently as 100 years ago, the best that medicine could offer was a handful of demonstrably effective preparations. Penicillin, the first antibiotic, and chloroquine, the first modern antimalarial, are scarcely fifty years old. Drugs for common conditions such as diabetes are only forty years old. And oral contraceptives have been generally available for only thirty years.

In industrialized countries, the age of modern pharmaceuticals has eliminated or dramatically reduced mortality from most common infections, allowed families to plan their growth, extended the lives of millions of people suffering from chronic illnesses, and provided relief from pain and suffering for hundreds of millions more people. From the simple discovery of penicillin in 1941 has grown a $200 billion-a-year pharmaceutical industry. The research efforts of that industry continually provide safer, more effective products. The industry's distribution networks ensure ready access to thousands of products for people throughout the industrialized world.

But for people in many parts of the world, it is as if penicillin had never been discovered and the age of modern pharmaceuticals had never dawned. In the late 1970s, it was estimated that 60 to 80 percent of people in the developing countries lacked regular access to even the most essential drugs. By the early 1990s, it was estimated that half the world's population—over 2 billion people—still lacked regular access to essential drugs (WHO 1992). Perhaps only one-third of the 435 million people in sub-Saharan Africa had access to essential drugs as of 1990 (Foster 1991).

It constitutes a fundamental failure of health and pharmaceutical supply systems that such a large share of the world's population still cannot benefit from simple, safe, effective pharmaceuticals and that literally millions of children and adults die each year from acute respiratory infections, diarrheal diseases, malaria, pregnancy-related anemia, and other common conditions that can be prevented or treated with modern drugs.

For those who do have access to essential drugs, many receive the wrong drug, the wrong dosage, or a quantity insufficient for their needs. In some countries, over half of all potent modern medicines are dispensed without prescription by untrained and unlicensed drug sellers. Even when patients and consumers receive the correct drug, between one-third and two-thirds do not consume it correctly.

Managing Drug Supply is concerned with practical ways in which government policy-makers, essential drugs program managers, nongovernmental organizations, donors, and others can work to close the huge gap between the need for essential drugs and public access to them—between the vast number of people who could benefit from modern pharmaceuticals and the much smaller number of people who actually do benefit. This manual is also concerned with closing the gap between the availability of drugs and their rational use.

This chapter focuses on the role of drugs in health care and health policy. It describes the essential drugs concept, reviews major lessons in drug management from the last twenty years, and summarizes major challenges still facing the pharmaceutical sector.

≡ 1.1 Why Worry about Drugs?

To clinicians facing the sick and injured on a daily basis, the importance of drugs is obvious. But it is useful to consider the reasons that ministers of health, directors of health programs, donors, and others involved in the health sector should be concerned with drugs. Accessible health services and qualified staff are necessary components of any health care system, but drugs have special importance for at least five reasons:

- ▶ Drugs save lives and improve health.
- ▶ Drugs promote trust and participation in health services.
- ▶ Drugs are costly.
- ▶ Drugs are different from other consumer products.
- ▶ Substantive improvements in the supply and use of drugs are possible.

These observations were the primary motivation for the preparation of this manual. The richness and diversity of opportunities for practical, effective improvements in drug supply and use are the focus of most of the following chapters.

Drugs Save Lives and Improve Health

Most leading causes of discomfort, disability, and premature death can be prevented, treated, or at least alleviated with cost-effective essential drugs. Although the relative frequencies of specific conditions vary among countries, outpatient services throughout the world are presented with a fairly common set of health problems for which essential drugs have an important role: acute infections, skin diseases, gastrointestinal complaints, musculoskeletal conditions, and injuries.

Mortality figures across developing regions (see Figure 1.1) reflect a huge burden of illness that can be substantially reduced if carefully selected, low-cost pharmaceuticals are available and appropriately used. Essential drugs have a major impact on common causes of morbidity and mortality, including acute respiratory infections (ARIs), diarrheal diseases, measles, malaria, maternal and perinatal mortality, sexually transmitted diseases (STDs), tuberculosis, and cardiovascular and other chronic diseases (see Box 1.1).

Figure 1.1 Mortality from Infectious, Chronic, and Other Conditions in Developing Countries, 1990

| | Number of Deaths (in thousands) | | | | | | | | |
| | By Age Group | | By Region | | | | | |
Condition	All Ages	0–4 Years	5 Years and Above	India	China	Asia	Africa	Latin America	Middle East
Infectious and parasitic diseases									
Respiratory infections	3,984	2,710	1,274	1,096	411	691	1,029	211	546
Diarrheal diseases	2,866	2,474	392	825	95	432	887	171	455
Tuberculosis	1,978	72	1,906	452	356	353	536	112	170
Other infections and parasites	1,027	443	584	278	94	97	331	98	131
Measles	1,006	863	144	276	9	123	473	11	115
Malaria	926	632	294	28	—	74	805	12	7
Tetanus	505	450	54	160	22	65	175	8	76
Pertussis	321	277	44	82	13	33	134	18	42
HIV	248	56	192	—	—	—	218	29	—
Meningitis	232	121	111	62	22	40	50	21	37
Syphilis	192	77	115	26	2	—	153	12	—
Chronic and other noninfectious diseases									
Cerebrovascular disease	3,181	14	3,168	619	1,271	350	389	224	327
Ischemic heart disease	2,469	2	2,467	783	442	589	109	269	277
Chronic obstructive lung disease	1,714	20	1,694	141	1,320	76	47	67	62
Inflammatory cardiac disease	1,229	68	1,161	528	92	130	234	122	123
Diabetes	483	0	483	145	60	87	25	85	82
Rheumatic heart disease	440	2	438	141	163	34	65	8	30
Asthma	147	9	138	33	56	18	15	12	14
Malignant neoplasms	3,698	43	3,655	776	1,408	541	305	341	327
Maternal and perinatal causes	2,830	2,402	428	795	319	398	627	265	447
Other causes	9,611	1,709	7,902	2,146	2,731	1,389	1,333	897	1,117
All deaths	39,088	12,443	26,645	9,371	8,885	5,519	7,937	2,992	4,384

Source: Murray and López 1994.

Not only are essential drugs *effective* against common health problems, they are also *cost effective*. It is undeniable that long-term health gains can be made by investing in prevention through health education and other programs to improve nutrition, sanitation, water supply, housing, environment, and personal health habits. At the same time, essential drugs provide a direct, low-cost response for many diseases.

Drugs Promote Trust and Participation in Health Services

The credibility of health workers depends on their ability to save a dying village elder with a course of penicillin, to restore life to a limp child with oral rehydration, or to relieve an irritating skin infection with a simple ointment. Aside from their direct health impact, however, the availability of essential drugs attracts patients, who can then also receive preventive and public health messages. It has been observed that provision of essential drugs is one element of primary health care that families everywhere take an interest in and that brings them to health facilities.

Household and patient surveys in Africa, Asia, and Latin America find that drug availability is a major determinant of where patients go for health care and how satisfied they are with that care. A rural health survey in one Asian country revealed that the villagers valued drugs more than they did the health workers or the clinic. In Africa, more expensive mission health facilities are preferred by many patients, in part because their drug supply is reliable.

Availability of drugs and supplies also affects the productivity of health staff. When drug supplies fail to arrive, patient volume drops, and health workers are left idle. In many settings, irregular drug supply is a greater constraint on program effectiveness than inadequate numbers or inadequate training of health workers.

Drugs Are Costly

Although drugs are cost effective, they can still be quite costly for an individual, a household, a government health system, or a country.

At the individual and household levels, drugs represent the major out-of-pocket health expenditure. A survey from Mali found that 80 percent of household health expenditures were for modern drugs, 13 percent for traditional medicine, 5 percent for provider fees, and 2 percent for transportation costs (Diarra and Coulibaly 1990). In

Pakistan and Côte d'Ivoire, more than 90 percent of household health expenditures was related to drugs (World Bank 1993).

Of importance from a health perspective is the fact that household expenditures on drugs are closely tied with household income. In Ghana, for example, annual per capita drug expenditures varied from US$1.45 per person in the lowest-income households to $3.32 in middle-income households to $8.50 in the highest-income households (World Bank 1994).

For ministries of health in most developing countries, drugs expenditures are second only to staff salaries and benefits, accounting for perhaps 50 to 90 percent of non-personnel costs. Payment of personnel costs is standardized and largely unavoidable as long as staff are employed. Drug expenditures, therefore, represent the largest expenditure over which ministries have year-to-year discretionary control. This makes drug expenditures both extremely important and extremely vulnerable—vulnerable to fluctuations in the availability of public funding as well as to various political pressures.

At the national level, pharmaceuticals represent 10 to 20 percent of health expenditures for leading industrialized countries. But for most developing countries, they may represent one-third to two-thirds of *total public and private health expenditures* (WHO/DAP 1996). In the Mali survey, drugs not only accounted for most household health expenditures but also represented 66 percent of total recurrent health expenditures (Diarra and Coulibaly 1990).

In absolute figures, the amounts that countries spend on drugs vary tremendously. For most developing countries, the figure was under US$20 per capita in 1990 (see Figure 1.2); for industrialized countries in the same year, the figure ranged from $89 in Norway and $97 in the United Kingdom to $222 in Germany and $412 in Japan (Ballance et al. 1992). In general, drug expenditures increase with gross national product (GNP), such that a 10 percent rise in per capita GNP is associated with an 11 to 13 percent increase in per capita drug expenditures (World Bank 1994).

Drugs Are Different from Other Consumer Products

Since pharmaceuticals are produced by a competitive industry that responds to demand, it might be expected that their production and sale could be left almost wholly to the play of market forces. In that case, politicians and lawmakers would have only the same sorts of concerns that apply to other forms of trade—prevention of fraud, protection of trademarks, and so forth. But drugs are different and require special attention, because

Box 1.1 Impact of Essential Drugs on Common Causes of Morbidity and Mortality

Respiratory infections, which accounted for nearly 4 million deaths in 1990 (10 percent of all developing country deaths) are usually cured readily with inexpensive oral antibiotics.

Diarrheal diseases, the second leading cause of childhood mortality, can be prevented through improved water and sanitation. They can be treated in the home with simple fluid preparations. Mortality would be greatly reduced with widespread availability of simple glucose-electrolyte solutions and selective use of antimicrobial drugs.

Measles, another leading cause of childhood mortality, is preventable through immunization. But when immunization is missed, much of the resulting mortality can still be eliminated through the treatment of respiratory, diarrheal, and other potentially fatal complications.

Malaria, once on the decline, is responsible for nearly 1 million deaths each year; nearly 90 percent of fatal cases are in Africa, and almost half are among children. Prompt treatment with antimalarial drugs, especially for the very young, is lifesaving.

Maternal and perinatal mortality can be reduced through antenatal care and nondrug interventions such as high-risk case management. But maternal anemia, a major contributing factor to maternal and perinatal morbidity and mortality, can be reduced with preventive doses of iron-folate preparations. In addition, child spacing through family planning (using largely oral, injectable, and implanted contraceptives) improves both maternal and neonatal outcomes.

Sexually transmitted diseases (STDs) are epidemic in many areas, and drug resistance is increasingly common. Yet proper diagnosis and treatment of STDs are possible, besides being a cost-effective measure to reduce transmission of the human immunodeficiency virus (HIV). In addition, although a cure for AIDS does not yet exist, AIDS patients benefit from treatment of tuberculosis, respiratory infections, diarrhea, and other common illnesses that are frequently seen in AIDS patients in developing countries.

Tuberculosis (TB), once on the decline, is now on the increase. Although TB drugs are costly and resistance is growing, short-course chemotherapy is curative, and the investment is highly cost effective.

Cardiovascular and other chronic diseases are rapidly increasing in developing countries as socioeconomic development, immunization, and other improvements increase life expectancy. Health services are facing a growing demand for essential drugs to treat hypertension, ischemic heart disease, diabetes, and other chronic diseases.

► the consumer (patient or parent) often does not choose the drug—it is prescribed by a clinician or recommended by pharmacy staff;

► even when the consumer chooses the drug, he or she is not trained to judge its appropriateness, safety, quality, or value for money;

► neither the average medical practitioner nor the average pharmacist is equipped to independently assess

Figure 1.2 Per Capita Drug and Health Expenditures in Selected Developing Countries, 1990

| | —— Per Capita Expenditures (US$) —— | |
Country	Drugs	Health
Bangladesh	2	6
Brazil	16	146
Chile	30	100
China	7	11
Costa Rica	37	132
Ghana	10	15
India	3	21
Indonesia	5	12
Kenya	4	16
Mexico	28	89
Morocco	17	26
Mozambique	2	5
Pakistan	7	12
Philippines	11	16
Turkey	21	76

Note: Drug costs based on producer prices. Adjusted to 1990 prices.
Sources: Drug expenditures from Ballance et al. 1992; health expenditures from Murray and López 1994.

the quality, safety, or efficacy of each new drug;

► fear of illness can lead patients to demand from health workers, or to buy for themselves, costly drugs when cheaper drugs—or no drugs—would achieve the same result;

► the consumer often cannot judge the likely consequences of *not* obtaining a needed drug. This problem is most troublesome when the decision-maker is a parent and the patient is a child.

These knowledge gaps, anxieties, and uncertainties associated with both acute and chronic illnesses create special concerns about the supply and use of drugs.

Substantive Improvements Are Possible
Substantive improvements in the supply and use of pharmaceuticals are possible. In most health systems, the potential for improving the supply process is tremendous, reflecting in part the magnitude of current inefficiencies and waste.

Figure 1.3 shows a hypothetical example of a program in which a US$1 million annual expenditure on drug supply results in only $300,000 worth of therapeutic benefit to the patient. Lack of careful selection, incorrect quantification, high prices, poor quality, theft, improper storage, expiration of drugs, irrational prescribing, and incorrect drug use by patients result in losses totaling 70 percent of the original expenditure.

However, much can be accomplished with a great deal of effort, a moderate amount of know-how, and relatively little additional funding. Examples of significant improve-

ments in specific areas of drug management are cited later in Section 1.3.

Some drug management improvements require an initial investment in systems development, training, physical infrastructure, and other development initiatives. But the potential cost reductions and therapeutic improvements are dramatic. Even small improvements, when made in a number of related areas of drug management, can yield substantial overall savings.

≡ 1.2 Public Health Objectives and the Essential Drugs Concept
Public health is concerned with using available resources to achieve maximum health improvements for the population. The perspective is not that of the individual patient, who may well benefit from a costly drug, but of the entire community or population, which will benefit most if safe, effective drugs are accessible to all who need them.

Within a decade after the first modern pharmaceuticals became available, efforts began to ensure their widespread availability. From the mid-1950s to the mid-1970s, basic drug management concepts began to evolve in countries as diverse as Norway, Papua New Guinea, Sri Lanka, Cuba, and Peru. In 1975, WHO defined essential drugs as "indispensable and necessary for the health needs of the population. They should be available at all times, in the proper dosage forms, to all segments of society." And in 1978, the WHO Conference at Alma Ata recognized essential drugs as one of the eight elements of primary health care. (See Chapter 2 for additional historical background.)

The first WHO *Model List of Essential Drugs,* containing about 200 products and a description of the essential drugs concept, was published in 1977. Since 1977, the WHO model list has been revised every two to three years, and over 120 countries have adopted essential drugs lists.

Consistent with a public health perspective, the essential drugs concept embraces the following guiding principles:

► The vast majority of health problems for most members of the population can be treated with a small, carefully selected number of drugs.

► In practice, most doctors and other health professionals routinely use fewer than 200 drugs. Training and clinical experience should focus on the proper use of these few drugs.

► Procurement, distribution, and other supply activities can be carried out most economically and most efficiently for a limited number of pharmaceutical products.

Figure 1.3 Waste in Drug Management and Potential for Improvement

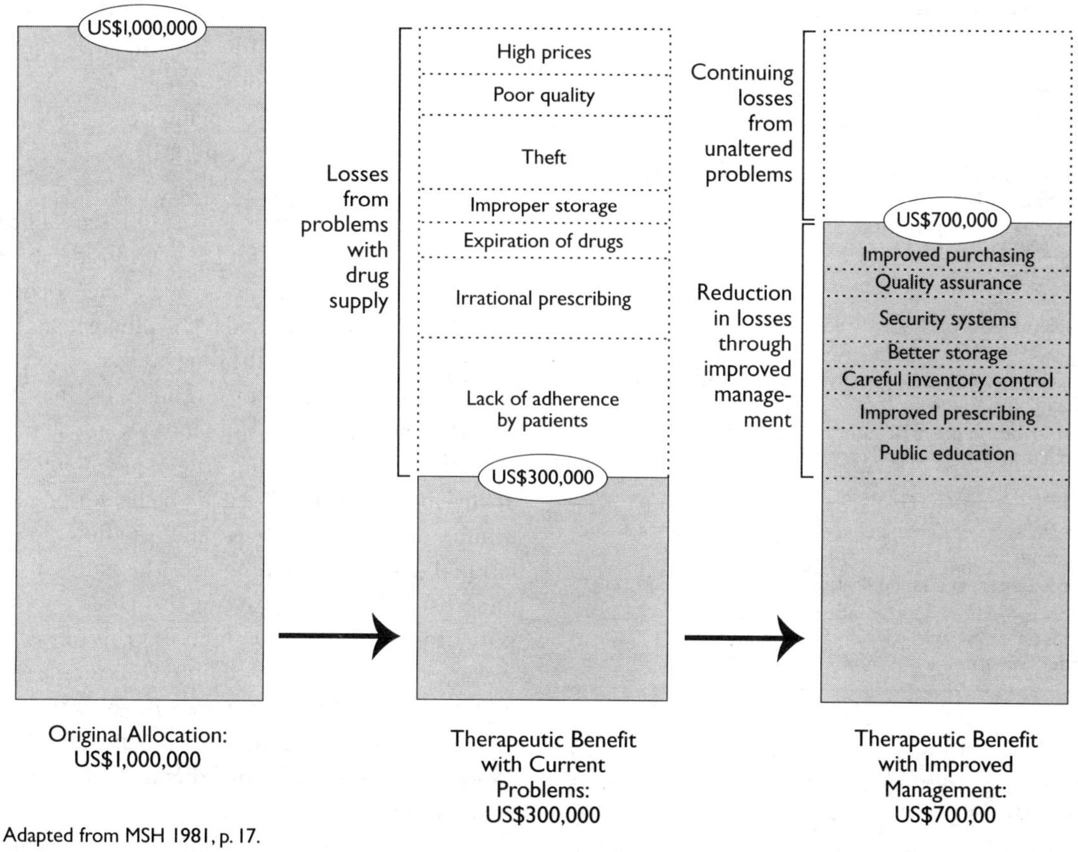

Losses from problems with drug supply:
High prices
Poor quality
Theft
Improper storage
Expiration of drugs
Irrational prescribing
Lack of adherence by patients

Continuing losses from unaltered problems

Reduction in losses through improved management:
Improved purchasing
Quality assurance
Security systems
Better storage
Careful inventory control
Improved prescribing
Public education

US$1,000,000
US$300,000
US$700,000

Original Allocation:
US$1,000,000

Therapeutic Benefit with Current Problems:
US$300,000

Therapeutic Benefit with Improved Management:
US$700,00

Source: Adapted from MSH 1981, p. 17.

► Patients can be better informed about the effective use of drugs when the number of drugs they are confronted with is limited.

Implementation of these principles occurs through the adoption of national drug policies and through practical drug management improvements. The major goals of such initiatives are outlined in Figure 1.4.

≡ **1.3 Lessons in Drug Management**

Over the last twenty years, countries have acquired considerable experience in managing drug supply. Although many important lessons have emerged from this experience, five broad themes capture the most important insights:

1. National drug policy provides a sound foundation for managing drug supply.
2. Wise drug selection underlies all other improvements.
3. Effective management saves money and improves performance.
4. Rational drug use requires more than drug information.
5. Systematic assessment and monitoring are essential.

Within these five broad areas are many specific lessons, some of which are referred to below, and most of which are covered in detail in the chapters that follow.

National Drug Policy Provides a Sound Foundation for Managing Drug Supply

A national drug policy (NDP) is a guide for action; it is generally a document containing the goals set by the government for the pharmaceutical sector and the main strategies for reaching those goals. It provides a framework to coordinate activities by the various actors in the pharmaceutical sector: the public sector, NGOs, the private sector, donors, and other interested parties.

The NDP concept began receiving support during the 1980s, when piecemeal approaches were leaving important problems unsolved. A focused NDP, suited to the needs of the particular country and with clear priorities, was found to have a significant impact on the availability and use of pharmaceuticals in such countries as Australia, Bangladesh, Colombia, and the Philippines.

Comprehensive, officially adopted policies can focus efforts to improve access to drugs, drug use, and drug quality. At the same time, the policy formulation process

Figure 1.4 Goals for National Drug Policies and Drug Management Improvements

Health-Related Goals
► Make essential drugs available to the entire population.
► Ensure the safety, efficacy, and quality of medicines manufactured and distributed in the country.
► Increase attendance at health facilities by increasing the credibility and acceptance of the health system.
► Promote rational prescription, dispensing, and patient use of medicines.

Economic Goals
► Lower the cost of drugs to the government, other health care providers, and the public.
► Reduce foreign exchange expenditures for drugs without reducing the supply.
► Provide jobs in pharmaceutical supply and possibly production.

National Development Goals
► Increase skills of personnel in management, pharmacy, and medicine.
► Improve internal communication systems.
► Encourage, where appropriate, the evolution of industrial competence in packaging, formulation, and other production areas.

sometimes engenders such strong opposition that all energy becomes focused on the policy, effectively stalling other useful but less controversial efforts to improve the availability and use of drugs.

Some countries have been successful by having a clear strategy without an official policy. Papua New Guinea in the 1960s, Peru and Malaysia in the 1970s, and Kenya and the eastern Caribbean states in the 1980s are all examples of countries that achieved some notable successes with strategies that addressed specific needs but did not have formal NDPs.

Formal NDPs provide a sound foundation for managing essential drugs programs. Of equal or greater importance, however, is the underlying strategic planning process: What are the long-term goals of the pharmaceutical sector? What strategies should be involved? How can key stakeholders be engaged in the process? The experiences of the last two decades suggest that governments and programs with clear objectives and strategies can make progress in the pharmaceutical sector.

Wise Drug Selection Underlies All Other Improvements
Establishing and using a limited list of carefully selected essential drugs is perhaps the single most cost-effective action that any health care system or health care provider can take to promote regular supply and rational use of drugs.

By 1995, over 120 countries had adopted national essential drugs lists. In contrast, in the mid-1970s, few countries had selective drug lists organized by generic name. Many of the national formularies that did exist were unselective and often contained over 1,000 products. Ministry of health procurement lists were commonly dominated by brand-name drugs.

Studies of the economic impact of essential drugs lists and formulary lists demonstrate that considerable savings can be achieved, primarily through careful choices for those few high-unit-cost and high-volume items that consume the major share of the drug budget.

An essential drugs list or formulary list that identifies drugs by level of care becomes the basis for all training in therapeutics; for estimating drug requirements; for competitive procurement by generic name; for planning distribution to health facilities; and for efforts to promote rational, cost-effective drug use. The national essential drugs list or formulary list can also guide public education efforts, local production, and private-sector drug management. The list, based on WHO criteria, should be updated regularly (usually every two to three years), divided by level of care, and accompanied by a clear policy on its application for procurement, distribution, and use of drugs.

Effective Management Saves Money and Improves Performance
Effective management makes a vital difference in all aspects of drug supply. This is especially true with respect to the procurement and distribution of essential drugs. The basic principles of efficient procurement and distribution have been known for several decades. Over the last fifteen years, the benefits of applying these principles have been demonstrated in individual essential drugs programs in Africa, Asia, the Caribbean, Latin America, and the western Pacific.

Examples of the positive consequences of good management include savings of 40 to 60 percent in drug costs through competitive procurement in Brazil, the eastern Caribbean, Mozambique, and Thailand; improved drug availability as a result of better quantification in Belize, Bhutan, and Zimbabwe; and more reliable delivery as a result of redesigned distribution systems in Indonesia, Peru, and South Africa.

Good pharmaceutical procurement practices include restriction of purchases to the essential drugs list (national formulary list), determination of order quantities based on reliable needs estimation, competitive tendering from qualified suppliers, separation of key functions, prompt payment, regular audits, and a formal system of supplier qualification and monitoring.

Effective distribution management is achieved by designing an efficient network of storage facilities with the fewest number of levels appropriate to the country's geography, selecting the appropriate strategy for delivery, keeping reliable records of drug stocks and consumption, allocating supplies based on actual workload and treatment needs, maintaining accountability procedures and secure storage at each level of the system, constructing or renovating facilities appropriate for storing drugs, managing storage facilities to maintain drug quality and efficiently serve health units, making reliable transport arrangements, and reinforcing reporting and supervision arrangements. Kit system distribution has both benefits and costs; it should be used only when necessary to ensure that supplies reach lower levels of the system.

Rational Drug Use Requires More Than Drug Information

Although 50 percent or more of drug expenditures may be wasted through irrational prescribing, dispensing, and patient use of drugs, most methods for promoting rational drug use have never been scientifically evaluated. Among those methods that have been properly studied, most have been found to have little, if any, measurable effect on drug use.

The actual use of pharmaceuticals is influenced by a wide range of factors, including drug availability, provider experience, economic influences, cultural factors, community belief systems, and the complex interactions among these factors. Drug use patterns reflect human behavior and must be viewed from a social science perspective rather than a biomedical perspective.

Drug companies succeed in changing the habits of doctors and patients because they understand what influences these habits. Interventions to promote rational drug use often fail because they are based on the notion that simply improving knowledge will improve drug use. Examples of interventions that are likely to fail include lifeless drug bulletins that dryly present "the facts," standard treatment manuals distributed to health staff without an active orientation, withdrawal of dangerous or ineffective products with no advice for prescribers on what to prescribe instead, and campaigns to discourage injection use that do not address the reasons that many patients prefer injections.

Fortunately, much has been learned during the 1980s and 1990s about principles for promoting rational drug use. These principles involve informed, focused, active, engaging approaches for changing drug use practices by prescribers, dispensers, and patients. Examples of specific interventions that have been effective include standard treatment guidelines (provided they are actively implemented); training linked to improved drug supply, as in Yemen and other countries; and guided discussions among mothers and providers, which in Indonesia led to a persistent decrease in the use of injections.

Systematic Assessment and Monitoring Are Essential

One of the most basic, yet most significant, advances in drug management has been the introduction of objective standard *indicators* for assessing, comparing, and monitoring drug policies and management effectiveness. Since their introduction in the early 1990s, drug use indicators have been developed for the assessment of virtually all key aspects of drug management and NDPs. Examples of standard indicators include the percentage of government drug purchases conforming to the national essential drugs list, the ratio of local drug prices to world market prices, the number of drugs per patient prescription, and the percentage of key drugs available at health facilities.

Measured at one point in time, such indicators allow a program to compare itself to a target level of performance, to identify areas of relative strength and weakness, and to make comparisons with other programs for which data are available. Measured over time, such indicators can be used to set and monitor performance targets for pharmaceutical sector improvements.

Systematic assessment and monitoring based on standard indicators are becoming a routine part of planning, program management, and donor evaluation in the field of essential drugs and drug management. Each country and program needs to select, develop, and adapt indicators to suit local circumstances and needs, but the basic concept of objective indicators should be considered in any essential drugs program.

≡ 1.4 Challenges for Drug Management

Although much has been achieved over the last two decades, huge gaps remain between the need for drugs and the supply of drugs, especially among poorer, less urbanized populations. A gap also remains between the availability of drugs and their rational use.

Major challenges for policy-makers and managers include achieving financial sustainability; improving efficiency in public drug supply; changing the perceptions and behaviors of providers, patients, and the public; reorienting the role of government; and regulating safety, efficacy, and quality.

Achieving Financial Sustainability

Financial sustainability is achieved only when expenditures and financial resources balance and are sufficient to support a given level of demand. If demand for drugs exceeds the available resources, the health system is left with only four options: improve efficiency, increase financial resources, reduce demand, or accept a decline in quality of care. When the components of financial sustainability are not in balance, it simply defies economic reality to promise constant availability of high-quality essential drugs without improving efficiency, increasing financing, or limiting demand.

Efficiency means getting the most benefit from available resources. Much of this manual is devoted to improving therapeutic efficiency through better selection and drug use and improving operational efficiency through better organization, procurement, and distribution of drugs.

To achieve financial sustainability, policy-makers and essential drugs program managers must become familiar with economic concepts and methods related to cost containment, efficiency, cost-effectiveness analysis, public expenditure decisions, the roles of the public and private sectors, and the economics of regulation. High-income countries have become increasingly reliant on economic methods and perspectives. Countries with more limited resources must also make maximum use of the insights offered by the field of economics.

Health-sector reform is concerned with improving efficiency through changes in the organization and allocation of health care resources. It is also concerned with health care financing.

People pay for health care in different ways: collectively, through national health insurance or through the taxes they pay on goods, services, or income; in groups, through premiums paid for voluntary health insurance; or individually, through user fees at government facilities or private out-of-pocket health expenditures. Local funding for recurrent health expenditures may be supplemented by external development assistance. In fact, it is sometimes impossible for the poorest countries to provide certain basic health services, including essential drugs, without some external assistance. But in most countries, the primary burden for health financing falls directly or indirectly on the people of the country.

Public financing provides an essential foundation for a country's health system and, in particular, for health promotion and preventive services. But providing free drugs through public resources has proved unsustainable in many developing as well as developed countries. Government budgets are squeezed, and donor funds are directed to a variety of other worthy causes. The policy of free drugs is often, in practice, a policy of shortages.

Full or partial cost recovery through user fees is one way to supplement public financing. Revolving drug funds and community drug schemes linked to strengthening primary health care (such as the Bamako Initiative) are operating in scores of countries in Africa, Asia, and Latin America. Some programs have led to a serious decline in utilization, with no visible improvement in drug availability. Yet other user fee programs have increased both equity of access and quality. Exemptions and other protection mechanisms, good management, community supervision, and phased implementation are important for success.

Social health insurance (compulsory health insurance or social security), private health insurance, and community health insurance schemes finance drug supply for a small but growing portion of the population in developing countries.

In the face of changing epidemiologic patterns, increasing demand for modern health care, and growing populations, the challenge for countries is to implement those drug financing strategies that best ensure equity of access and a continuous supply of drugs. For many countries, this means taking a pluralistic approach—one that uses different approaches to serve different needs and different groups and that combines the benefits of public financing, user fees, health insurance, voluntary financing mechanisms, and (in some cases) donor support.

Improving Efficiency in Public Drug Supply

The twenty-year history of the essential drugs concept has witnessed a mixture of successes and failures in public drug supply. As of 1988, countries as diverse as Algeria, Costa Rica, Cyprus, Indonesia, Kenya, Malaysia, Papua New Guinea, and Sri Lanka were all judged to have achieved reasonable success in selection, procurement, distribution, and coverage for essential drugs. Other countries had achieved fair to poor results in these areas, including Cameroon, Côte d'Ivoire, El Salvador, Haiti, Honduras, Madagascar, Niger, and Tunisia (WHO 1988).

Since 1988, some countries have continued to progress, but others have experienced setbacks. Aside from the problem of financing, public-sector drug supply in many countries continues to be plagued by ineffective management systems, lack of staff incentives, inability to control fraud and abuse, political pressures that channel drug supplies to better-off areas, and inefficient drug selection and use. There are examples of successful central supply systems, but there are also numerous examples in which the conventional central medical stores (CMS) approach to drug procurement and distribution continues to result in chronic drug shortages—even after considerable investment in training, management systems, and physical infrastructure.

Sustainability is the extent to which a program will continue to achieve its policy and drug supply objectives without additional outside financial or technical support. Key factors for program sustainability are motivated, capable staff; effective management systems; and political support. Low pay, inadequate training, lack of incentives, inappropriate recruitment, and ineffective disciplinary measures undermine staff performance. Civil service reform, which is being considered or initiated in a number of countries, may help address these constraints.

At the same time, alternative strategies for public drug supply are attracting interest. These include formation of an autonomous supply agency, direct delivery, the prime vendor system, various privatized models, and mixed systems. Alternative strategies for public drug supply have been implemented in Benin, Indonesia, South Africa, and Uganda.

With an autonomous supply system, bulk procurement, storage, and distribution are managed by an autonomous or semi-autonomous agency. With the direct delivery (non-CMS) system, the government tenders to establish prices and suppliers for essential drugs, which are then delivered directly by suppliers to districts and major health facilities. With the prime vendor system (another non-CMS system), the government drug procurement office establishes a contract with a single prime vendor as well as separate contracts with drug suppliers. The prime vendor is contracted to manage drug distribution by receiving drugs from the suppliers and then storing and distributing them to districts and major facilities. In private models, public administration of drug supply is minimized, with drugs being provided by independent pharmacies within government facilities or through other mechanisms; various financing and reimbursement arrangements can be used.

Selection, procurement, and distribution can each be carried out in centralized, partially decentralized, or fully decentralized systems. Decentralization aims to improve the responsiveness, quality, and efficiency of health services. Improvements are far from certain, however. Problems with attempts to decentralize drug management functions have included lack of local management capacity, increased costs (due to loss of savings from bulk purchasing), lack of local staff trained in drug management, inadequate financial resources, self-interested interference by local officials, and poor drug quality (due to difficulty in selecting and monitoring suppliers).

For managing drug supply, it may be useful to think in terms of a task-specific approach to decentralization. Examples of tasks that may be better performed centrally include development of essential drugs lists, preparation of standard treatment guidelines, management of competitive tenders, selection and monitoring of suppliers, quality assurance, and development of training programs in rational drug use.

Tasks that can be decentralized include those that do not require uncommon technical skills. Decentralization is advisable when local information is required, local circumstances are important and variable throughout the country, and local interests favor improved performance. Examples of such tasks include adapting drug lists or standard treatments to local needs, quantifying drug requirements, coordinating local distribution, conducting training in rational drug use, and monitoring drug use at health facilities.

The effectiveness of the drug supply system in achieving a reliable supply of essential drugs must be continually and objectively assessed. Fundamental restructuring of drug supply arrangements challenges the status quo and may threaten a variety of interests. But continuing to support an ineffective supply system wastes precious resources and denies patients access to lifesaving essential drugs.

Changing the Perceptions and Behaviors of Providers, Patients, and the Public

One of the greatest challenges is to change the way in which providers, patients, and the public view and use pharmaceuticals. Major problems, noted earlier, include prescribing and dispensing incorrect, harmful, or unnecessary drugs; failure by patients to use needed medications correctly; and wasteful or harmful self-medication practices.

The basic methods and alternatives for improving selection, procurement, and distribution have been well understood for some time. The difficulty has been in implementation. In contrast, there are few demonstrably effective—and cost-effective—methods for improving drug use. Examples of apparently effective methods are discussed above in Section 1.3.

Given the huge share of public and private drug expenditures that may be wasted through irrational drug use, it is essential that governments, NGOs, and others continue to explore effective, sustainable ways of improving drug use patterns.

Reorienting the Role of Government

Access to health care, including essential drugs, is a fundamental human right. Realization of this right may involve various combinations of public and private financing and provision of services. In high-income countries, public financing of pharmaceuticals predominates. In low- and middle-income countries, the public-private mix varies remarkably, from 90 percent public provision of drugs in Papua New Guinea and Bhutan to roughly 90 percent private market supply and financing of drugs in Nepal and the Philippines. Typically, however, 60 to 80 percent of drugs are obtained on the private market, even among low-income households.

Overprescription by health care providers is common, as is self-medication, which in some countries accounts for the majority of "prescription" drug consumption. Although even the poorest are willing to pay for drugs, the combination of high prices and lack of information may delay treatment and too often results in the purchase of subtherapeutic doses. Pharmacy surveys in some countries have found that most antibiotics are purchased in quantities sufficient for only one to three days' treatment—insufficient for most conditions requiring an antibiotic. Studies of self-administration of antimalarials show similar underdosing. When purchasing power is concentrated in urban areas and the number of pharmacists is limited, the availability and range of drugs may decline significantly in remote areas.

From a public health perspective, therefore, the main concerns with the private pharmaceutical market are availability (geographic access), affordability (economic access), and rational use of drugs. Measures to improve availability include certification and training of pharmacy aides and other drug sellers; licensing provisions and incentives for wholesalers, pharmacies, and other drug outlets; dispensing by doctors and other clinicians in selected areas; and community drug schemes. Affordability can be improved with greater insurance coverage, better price information, price competition through generic substitution, regulation of producer prices, and modification of retail sales margins. Finally, rational drug use can be promoted through regulation of drug information and marketing; inclusion of essential drugs concepts in basic medical education; focused continuing education for health professionals; enforcement of licensing requirements for doctors, pharmacists, and other health professionals; and active public and patient education.

The public health challenge is to work with the private sector and NGOs to achieve universal access to essential drugs and rational use of drugs. This involves mutual understanding, constructive partnerships, and the right incentives. Among other things, greater coverage of essential drug needs through the private sector means that public

resources can be focused on prevention, on control of communicable diseases, and on the poorest segments of the population.

Regulating Safety, Efficacy, and Quality

Regulatory control, often neglected in the pharmaceutical sector, is an indispensable foundation for ensuring the safety, efficacy, and quality of drugs in a country. With increasing private-sector supply, it is incumbent upon governments to ensure that all drugs meet basic standards. And the same quality standards applied to the open market must also apply to drugs procured through the public sector. Drug legislation and regulation also establish basic professional standards in both the public and the private sectors.

In industrialized countries, regulatory capacity has developed in phases over many decades. It is reasonable to expect that most developing countries also will require time to develop effective regulatory capacity. Such capacity requires a firm legislative basis, trained personnel, specific technical resources, adequate funding, and—perhaps most important—public commitment to establishing and maintaining basic standards.

≡ 1.5 The Drug Management Cycle

Drug management involves four basic functions: selection, procurement, distribution, and use (Figure 1.5). Selection involves reviewing the prevalent health problems, identifying treatments of choice, choosing individual drugs and dosage forms, and deciding which drugs will be available at each level of health care. Procurement includes quantifying drug requirements, selecting procurement methods, managing tenders, establishing contract terms, assuring drug quality, and ensuring adherence to contract terms. Distribution includes clearing customs, stock control, stores management, and delivery to drug depots and health facilities. Use includes diagnosing, prescribing, dispensing, and proper consumption by the patient.

The drug management cycle is truly a cycle: each major function builds on the previous function and leads logically to the next. Selection should be based on actual experience with health needs and drug use, procurement requirements follow from selection decisions, and so forth. Costs rise, shortages become common, and patients suffer when the separate tasks are performed not as part of a system but independently and disjointedly.

At the center of the drug management cycle is a core of management support systems: organization, financing and sustainability, information management, and human resources management. These management support systems

Figure 1.5 Drug Management Cycle

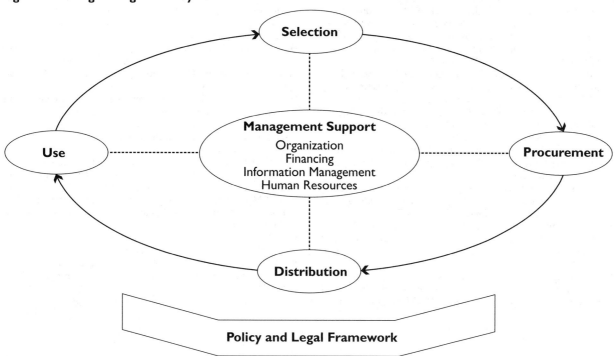

hold the drug management cycle together. Although individual parts of the cycle may function independently for a short time, the cycle as a whole will soon cease to operate and patient care will suffer without a functional organizational structure, adequate financing, reliable management information, and motivated staff.

Finally, the entire cycle rests on a policy and legal framework that establishes and supports the public commitment to essential drug supply.

≡ 1.6 Managing Pharmaceutical Sector Improvements

This manual is meant to provide policy-makers and managers with practical, accessible advice on a wide range of topics relevant to managing drug supply. The basic functions of management are planning, implementation, and monitoring.

Effective planning requires thoughtful reflection on basic goals, systematic assessment of the current situation, creative consideration of all reasonable strategies for improvement, and selection of strategies based on defined criteria.

Implementation is an interactive process that involves organizing people, finances, and other resources to achieve the desired results. The test of any policy or plan is in its implementation. Gradual phasing-in of new initiatives can help build management systems, which can then support full-scale implementation. Active decision-making and problem-solving are fundamental to the implementation process.

Finally, ongoing monitoring and periodic evaluation are needed to measure progress, to adjust implementation plans, and to assess the impact of drug management improvements. Objective indicators and specific program targets provide concrete measures against which actual performance can be compared. Without such indicators, it is difficult to judge the success and, therefore, the value of human and financial investments in pharmaceutical sector improvements.

The experiences of countless countries and programs demonstrate that substantive, sustainable improvements in the supply and use of drugs are possible. But an equal or greater number of negative experiences demonstrate that success is by no means assured. Clear goals, sound plans, effective implementation, and systematic monitoring of performance are essential ingredients in pharmaceutical sector development. ∎

≡ References and Further Readings

Ballance, R., J. Pogány, and H. Forstner. 1992. *The world's pharmaceutical industries: United Nations Industrial Development Organization document*. Brookfield, Vt.: Ashgate Publishers.

Diarra, K., and S. Coulibaly. 1990. Financing of recurrent health costs in Mali. *Health Policy* 5(2):126–38.

Dumoulin, J., M. Kaddar, and G. Velásquez. 1991. Access to drugs and finance: Basic economic and financial analysis. WHO/DAP/91.5. Geneva: World Health Organization.

Foster, S. D. 1991. Supply and use of essential drugs in sub-Saharan Africa: Some issues and possible solutions. *Social Science and Medicine* 32(11):1201–18.

Hogerzeil, H. V., G. J. Walker, A. O. Sallami, and G. Fernando. 1989. Impact of an essential drugs program on availability and rational use of drugs. *Lancet* 1:141–42.

MSH (Management Sciences for Health). 1981. *Managing drug supply: The selection, procurement, distribution, and use of pharmaceuticals in primary health care*. Boston: MSH.

MSH (Management Sciences for Health/Rational Pharmaceutical Management Project). 1995. *Rapid pharmaceutical management assessment. An indicator-based approach*. Washington, D.C.: MSH/RPM.

Murray, C. J. L., and A. D. López, eds. 1994. *Global comparative assessments in the health sector: Disease burden, expenditures, and intervention packages*. Geneva: World Health Organization.

Wang'ombe, J. K., and G. M. Mwabu. 1987. Economics of essential drugs schemes: The perspectives of the developing countries. *Social Science and Medicine* 25:625–30.

WHO (World Health Organization). 1977. *The selection of essential drugs*. Technical report series no. 615. Geneva: WHO.

WHO (World Health Organization). 1988. *The world drug situation*. Geneva: WHO.

WHO (World Health Organization). 1992. How essential is an essential drugs policy? *World Health* March–April: 3.

WHO (World Health Organization). 1995. *Privatization in health*. WHO Task Force on Health Economics. WHO/THFE/TBN/95.1. Geneva: WHO.

WHO/DAP (World Health Organization/Action Programme on Essential Drugs). 1994. *Selected annotated bibliography on essential drugs*. WHO/DAP/94/5. Geneva: WHO/DAP.

WHO/DAP (World Health Organization/Action Programme on Essential Drugs). 1996. *Global comparative pharmaceutical expenditures*. Geneva: WHO/DAP.

World Bank. 1993. *World development report 1993: Investing in health*. New York: Oxford University Press.

World Bank. 1994. *Better health in Africa: Experience and lessons learned*. World Bank report no. 12577-Afr. Washington, D.C.: World Bank.

Part I **Introduction**	Part II Policy and Legal Framework	Part III Drug Management Cycle	Part IV Management Support Systems

1 Toward Sustainable Supply and
  Rational Use of Drugs

**2 Historical and Institutional
  Perspectives**

3 Economics for Drug Management
4 Pharmaceutical Supply System Assessment

Chapter 2
Historical and Institutional Perspectives

≡ Summary

Concerns about medicines can be traced back for centuries. The discovery of "wonder drugs" about the time of World War II, however, was a milestone in drug management. The obvious effectiveness of some new pharmaceuticals and intensive marketing combined to catalyze widespread use of modern medicines. A rapidly growing and profitable industry, together with an enthusiastic but largely uninformed audience and an unregulated marketplace, resulted in excesses of promotion and consumption, along with substantial levels of expenditure. Despite the advent of wonder drugs, by the 1970s, it had become clear that the least-advantaged nations were not even meeting the basic needs of their people for essential lifesaving and health-promoting drugs.

Through the 1970s and 1980s, governments and international organizations such as the World Health Organization (WHO) began to redress this imbalance, with support from nongovernmental organizations (NGOs) for the promotion of essential drugs programs.

Rapid shifts in the relationships between pharmaceutical producers and their major clients are creating an environment where most countries are using some of the same strategies for dealing with essential drugs. More and more, the approaches covered in this book are being applied throughout the world to obtain and use the right medicines for the right reasons.

≡ 2.1 The Discovery of Miracle Drugs

During and soon after World War II, new and powerful drugs began to emerge in rapid succession from laboratories around the world (Dowling 1977). Penicillin was isolated and first used clinically in 1941; chloroquine, first investigated in the mid-1930s, was released for trial against malaria in 1943, and streptomycin followed in 1944 as the first effective drug for tuberculosis. Adding to the earlier impact of smallpox and typhoid immunizations, diphtheria and tetanus toxoid vaccines were first adopted during the war for large military populations. Tetracycline and chloramphenicol were introduced in 1948, isoniazid in 1951, and erythromycin in 1952. Chlorpromazine signaled a new era of mental health drug therapy in the same year. In 1954, the sulfonylureas became the first oral diabetic preparations, and nystatin emerged as an antifungal agent. In 1955, field trials of oral contraceptives occurred in Puerto Rico, leading to a virtual revolution that enabled women and their spouses to begin to effectively control family size, and hence their future.

In just over a decade, the whole field of therapeutics had been revolutionized, putting into the hands of practitioners and the public drug compounds that could cure or control problems in ways largely unknown in earlier times. As both scientific and anecdotal evidence spread, practitioners and patients demanded, and were willing to pay for, the exciting and powerful products that the drug industry was patenting and producing.

≡ 2.2 The Increasing Gap in Access to Drugs

In this exciting period around the middle of the twentieth century, many authors of popular books on drugs wrote of the revolution in medical care that modern drugs had made possible: antibiotics seemed on the verge of eradicating killing infections such as pneumonia and septicemia; cortisone had arrived to suppress painful inflammation; asthma was yielding to isoprenaline; one vaccine after another was appearing to stop fatal epidemics. *Miracle* was the word most authors used.

Looked at globally, however, these were miracles for the few. The affluent countries stood in stark contrast to the rest of the world, where entire populations had little access to drugs or were struggling to cope with a maze of competitive products, many of which were obscure, overpriced, outdated, ineffective, or dangerous. In many countries, two problems existed side by side: no drugs at all in the countryside, but hundreds or thousands of drugs competing for customers' attention in the cities. Medical and nursing staff in some areas worked without the medicines they needed, while practitioners in other areas faced a flood of expensive products about which they had no reliable information or that their patients could not afford. The age of miracles had arrived in some places, but much of the world was still suffering in the midst of plenty.

≡ 2.3 The Rise of the Essential Drugs Concept

An idea gradually emerged: why not concentrate first on a basic list of reliable drugs to meet the most vital needs—understanding them, finding ways to pay for them, supplying them to the people? The idea of working with a limited range of drugs had long been in use in places where there was no alternative; doctors had learned to carry 20 vital drugs in their bags, and oceangoing liners commonly carried 100 or fewer.

Before World War II, while it was still a poor country, Norway started extending the basic list idea to whole populations, supplying its people with a limited range of affordable drugs to meet basic needs. The idea slowly developed. Papua New Guinea had a policy based on "essential drugs" by the early 1950s; Sri Lanka followed in 1959, and Cuba had a list of essential drugs by 1963.

How many drugs were needed? Sri Lanka chose 500, a number similar to that on Norway's original list. Whatever choice was made, it provided a starting point; one day, there might be money for more. Newly independent countries, committed to providing universal health care yet desperately short of resources, saw an essential drugs policy as a means of moving ahead in spite of the obstacles.

It became clear that an essential drugs list could also make better use of limited financial resources. For many purposes, a low-cost drug was as good as a more recent product at ten or fifty times the price; saving money by buying drugs at lower cost and by avoiding worthless or fraudulent products would release funds to supply a much greater part of the population. The essential drugs concept was growing into a practical policy.

At the same time, developing countries became increasingly appreciated as a market for modern drugs. By the mid-1970s, some of these countries were spending large percentages of their public health budgets on medicines (for example, 30 percent in Thailand, 60 percent in Bangladesh), although health services reached only a minority of the urban and wealthier segments of the population. The majority of the population remained underserved. Many producers and sources of raw materials remained abroad, requiring scarce foreign exchange to pay for imports, often at high prices compounded by substantial in-country distributor markups. In addition, thousands of brand-name combination products, often of questionable efficacy and safety, were flooding private markets.

The pharmaceutical industry grew rapidly in the postwar era. Substances that cured, prevented, or ameliorated many problems were formulated into products that were protected by patents, giving producers a long period in which to establish a dominant market presence and accumulate profits. Sophisticated production and testing methods allowed the formation of efficient, largely automated high-volume manufacturing processes, resulting in large profits that could be plowed back into new product research and the acquisition of smaller firms. All these forces created an increasingly concentrated multinational industry.

The market also produced a series of disasters. Inadequately tested or misused drugs resulted in many cases of serious or fatal drug-induced diseases before sufficient evidence accumulated in the public eye to mandate change. The use of thalidomide resulted in thousands of deformed children in Europe; clioquinol produced widespread neurologic disease in Japan; and chloramphenicol, widely misused in Latin America, produced dysentery deaths from resistant shigella as well as aplastic anemia. These examples generated a growing recognition that pharmaceuticals often brought problems as well as great promise.

Many countries began to examine drug expenditures, noting both the rapid and unsustainable cost increases and the fact that a large portion of expenditures was for products that had little direct effect on their major health problems. At the same time, many important products such as antibiotics began to enter the generic market as their patent protection expired, and countries found that they could obtain much more favorable prices as competition among producers developed. All these trends created momentum among countries to act individually and to call publicly for concerted action by international agencies.

Toward Sustainable Supply and Rational Use

By the 1970s, countries were urging international agencies to take up the problems of imbalances in growth, inequities, and redistribution of resources in developing countries. In 1974, the International Labor Office adopted the idea of defining and meeting "basic needs" in the developing world; at the same time, the WHO director general proclaimed a new policy aimed at improving the health of rural and periurban populations. In 1975, he defined essential drugs as "those considered to be of utmost importance and hence basic, indispensable, and necessary for the health needs of the population. They should be available at all times, in the proper dosage forms, to all segments of society."

A year later, WHO prepared its first *Model List of Essential Drugs*, listing 224 drugs and vaccines. In Alma Ata in 1978, the WHO/UNICEF Conference on Primary Health Care adopted the essential drugs concept as one of its basic tools. In Geneva, the Division of Drug Policy and Management came into being to develop the concept as part of national drug policy for member states. There was also important backing from an interagency task force set up by the United Nations (UN), which by 1979 recommended the adoption of national drug lists using generic names.

By the mid-1970s, other UN agencies were also focusing on drugs. The UN Conference on Trade and Development (UNCTAD) supported generic names, competitive procurement, and cooperative purchasing arrangements. The

UN International Development Organization (UNIDO) emphasized local and regional cooperative production. The UN Children's Fund (UNICEF), long active in direct provision of drugs through its Supply Division, embraced the essential drugs idea with WHO in the late 1970s. The involvement of UN agencies became more visible, and eventually more coherent, as a series of conferences and task forces created a rough division of labor: UNICEF concentrated on supply, WHO on health policy, UNCTAD on trade, and UNIDO on industrial development.

The Movement Accelerates

WHO's Action Programme on Essential Drugs (DAP) grew vigorously in the early 1980s. By 1984, large amounts of extrabudgetary funds from European donors were provided specifically to support projects in each region of the world for developing drug selection, procurement, and distribution. Issues of drug financing were tackled, and standards were set for drug information and training. In 1985, a WHO Conference of Experts in Nairobi broadened the approach with a new emphasis on the need to use drugs rationally. That same year, the *Essential Drugs Monitor*, an international newsletter advocating an essential drugs policy in all its forms, began publication. Such initiatives were heavily backed by voluntary efforts from the outside, notably by Health Action International, an international coalition of NGOs from some fifty countries with a special interest in pharmaceuticals.

The Emergence of Generic Drugs

The development of essential drugs policies worldwide coincided with another vitally important development: the expiration of many of the patents on drugs that had revolutionized medical care in the decade after World War II. At the same time, drug manufacturing industries were established in countries that did not recognize international drug patents. New manufacturers started producing generic versions of drugs at much lower prices with high levels of quality, allaying fears that their products were low-quality and unreliable imitations of the originals. Increasingly, essential drugs programs with limited budgets were able to provide an adequate selection of modern generic drugs, which supplanted older remedies.

The Industry's Reaction

As they gained momentum, these dramatic developments produced mixed reactions from the international pharmaceutical industry. The major multinational corporations had reaped substantial profits from selling their new products in the industrialized world. The rest of the globe was a potentially lucrative market, with promise for the future. In many countries, drugs from the multinationals reached only a small fraction of the population, but prices were high and users uncritical. As Western countries introduced stricter systems of drug regulation and were forced by the economic recession of the 1970s to look critically at their drug costs, the largely unregulated countries of the rest of the world provided a new prospect for profitability. The fact that the UN and WHO were encouraging restrictive policies and ethical criteria for drug marketing in the developing world seemed to threaten multinationals' future prospects. At the same time, other industry segments, particularly the generic manufacturers and distributors, were also growing rapidly and saw opportunities where the multinationals saw threats. The issue of international patents on pharmaceuticals became increasingly controversial, as major multinational firms pushed for tighter and more universally applicable patent laws and countries that had large local industries resisted such efforts. This issue was still unresolved in many countries in 1995 (see Chapter 8).

The pharmaceutical industry's early reactions to essential drugs policies varied from hostile to mixed, with representatives declaring on occasion that the essential drugs concept was completely unacceptable. The Geneva-based International Federation of Pharmaceutical Manufacturers Associations (IFPMA) suggested that the adoption of an essential drugs list "would result in substandard rather than improved medical care and might well reduce health standards already attained." The IFPMA was heavily backed in its protests by the US Pharmaceutical Manufacturers Association (PhRMA), which by 1985 was arguing that the imposition of additional and arbitrary criteria involving "essentiality" or "medical interest" would clearly be contrary to the public interest. In retrospect, one major problem was the failure to communicate to the industry and practitioners what "essential drugs" really meant.

Subsequently, having accepted that for poorer countries the essential drugs approach might be "practical, even if regrettable," the research-based segment of the pharmaceutical industry turned to limiting its application, insisting that the concept applied only in the public sectors of the least-developed countries. This segment of the industry discouraged WHO's initiatives relating to advertising standards and continued to foster the view that generic drugs were substandard and even dangerous.

Since 1985, the industry has largely come around to the view that a fair income can be earned by providing low-cost drugs—whether brand-name or generic—on a large scale to essential drugs programs, with the volume of sales compensating for low profit margins. On some fronts, the IFPMA has collaborated with essential drugs programs, with WHO, and with donors. The relationship between manufacturers and international organizations will never be entirely free of tension, but the sharp conflict of earlier years has subsided.

The Campaign for Rational Use of Drugs

Once access to essential drugs is assured, proper use remains a challenge, since waste by both prescribers and users is common. The notion that if one drug is good, two are better (and three ideal) dies hard, and both prescribers and users are prone to overuse. The quantities of drugs prescribed for a given illness are often far more than what is reasonably needed. Drugs are often prescribed when no drug is needed at all, because patients expect or demand a pill or an injection, or because physicians or medical assistants are anxious to be seen as doing something. In some cases, half of drugs reaching the periphery are wasted by irrational prescribing and by irrational use by patients, who fail to follow the instructions given by prescribers.

The notion that all drug policies need to include "rational use of drugs" was only slowly accepted. Drug policies had always centered on drugs, not on patients. Drug policies had been the concern largely of pharmacists, whereas drug use was largely in the hands of physicians and paramedical staff. The medical profession in particular resented any suggestion that it might be acting irrationally as a group or that it might be in need of guidance or control. Medical personnel often insisted on the "right" to prescribe the drug of their choice, although no such right exists in most legal codes.

Rational use of drugs took the stage after WHO's 1985 Nairobi Conference of Experts used it as its central theme. The conference emphasized the need for the public to understand and use drugs better, particularly in view of all that was known about nonadherence to treatment. In many cases, neither the prescriber nor the patient was to blame for irrational use; it often resulted from lack of proper information and training, compounded in some cases by fear, carelessness, or misleading persuasion from the seller or others. With half the world's drugs probably being wasted because of irrational use, the effort to promote proper use, although time consuming, is vital to any effective policy and any well-managed economy.

Basic data on how drugs are actually being used in a particular country and situation, why errors are made, and the types of intervention that may improve the situation are important aids to understanding drug use. WHO's European Drug Utilization Research Group has developed methods for studying these matters, some of which can be applied simply and quickly.

In 1989, the International Network for Rational Use of Drugs (INRUD) was formed to bring together developing-country teams composed of ministry of health decision-makers, researchers, social scientists, and support groups. INRUD continues to grow as a forum for joint country-level efforts to investigate drug use problems, test strategies to change providers' and consumers' behavior with regard to specific problems, implement large-scale behavior change efforts, and share the experiences internationally with colleagues.

≡ 2.4 Current Organizational Roles in Essential Drugs

Organizations that are active in the essential drugs field may be useful points of contact, particularly if their interest, mission, and experience are relevant. Figure 2.1 lists these organizations, several of which are discussed briefly below. Those listed in Annex 2.1 offer a range of experience in advocacy for the public and private sectors, in public policy development, and in education and technical assistance. Organizations that primarily finance development projects (such as the World Bank, the regional development banks, and aid agencies in Europe and the United States) are discussed separately in Chapter 43.

WHO and Other UN Organizations

The WHO Action Programme on Essential Drugs (DAP) has played a leading role in promoting the essential drugs concept. DAP publishes documents on practices and methods as well as the *Essential Drugs Monitor* newsletter on current developments around the world. It convenes expert committees, holds workshops and training sessions worldwide, and has supported some country-specific drug management programs, largely with funds provided by interested donors.

Also based at WHO headquarters in Geneva, the Division of Drug Management and Policies (DMP) is responsible for assuring drug quality, providing information on safety and efficacy, and convening an expert committee that revises the *Model List of Essential Drugs* every two to three years. DMP is also responsible for the quality certification scheme and good manufacturing practices (GMPs) standards.

Other WHO offices dealing with specific disease areas, such as diarrhea, immunizations, and AIDS, have interests in essential drugs. The WHO regional offices and individual country programs may have additional technical staff in advisory positions.

Figure 2.1 Some International Organizations in the Drug Field

United Nations Organizations

ILO	International Labour Organization
ITC	International Trade Centre
UNCTAD	United National Conference on Trade and Development
UNDCP	United Nations International Drug Control Programme
UNDP	United Nations Development Programme
UNFPA	United Nations Population Fund
UNHCR	United Nations High Commissioner for Refugees
UNICEF	United Nations Children's Fund
UNIDO	United Nations Industrial Development Organization
WB	World Bank
WHO	World Health Organizaton
	■ DAP: Action Programme on Essential Drugs
	■ DMP: Drug Management and Policies
	■ Disease-specific programs

Nongovernmental Organizations and Private Foundations

APUA	Alliance for Prudent Use of Antiobiotics, Boston
CMC	Churches' Action for Health/Christian Medical Commission, Geneva
HAI	Health Action International
INRUD	International Network for Rational Use of Drugs
	International Federation of Red Cross and Red Crescent Societies, Geneva
IOCU	International Organization of Consumer Unions
MaLAM	Medical Lobby for Appropriate Marketing
MSH	Management Sciences for Health, Boston
OXFAM	Oxford Committee for Famine Relief
USP	United States Pharmacopeia

Professional Associations

ASEAN	Association of Southeast Asian Nations (pharmaceutical association)
CPA	Commonwealth Pharmaceutical Association
FIP	International Pharmaceutical Federation
ISCP	International Society of Clinical Pharmacology
ISDB	International Society of Drug Bulletins
ISPE	International Society of Pharmaco-Epidemiology
WMA	World Medical Association (national associations of physicians)

Meetings of Regulatory Bodies

ICDRA	International Conference of Drug Regulatory Authorities
ICH	International Conference on Harmonization
PIC	Pharmaceutical Inspectorate Convention

Industry Organizations

ABPI	Association of British Pharmaceutical Industries, England
IFPMA	International Federation of Pharmaceutical Manufacturers Associations
IFPW	International Federation of Pharmaceutical Wholesalers
PhRMA	Pharmaceutical Research and Manufacturers of America
WFPPM	World Federation of Proprietary Medicine Manufacturers (national associations of manufacturers of drugs for self-medication)

The Pan American Health Organization (PAHO) is WHO's regional office for the Americas. Its technical drug management staff collaborates with ministries of health, social security agencies, and other governmental and nongovernmental institutions to strengthen national and local health systems. Other regional offices contribute to supporting and managing essential drugs activities in their regions.

UNICEF is actively involved in program and project development internationally and at the country level. Headquarters activities include technical supervision, design, and support of country-level programs ranging from large-scale procurement (through its Supply Division based in Copenhagen) to strategies for the purchase, distribution, and use of medical supplies. In some countries, UNICEF teams formulate and obtain funding for essential drugs activities, particularly under the banner of the Bamako Initiative, which focuses on community participation, local funding, and procurement of essential drugs.

Nongovernmental Organizations and Private Foundations

Health Action International (HAI) is an association of NGOs founded in 1982 "to further the safe, rational, and economic use of pharmaceuticals worldwide, to promote full implementation of the WHO Action Programme on Essential Drugs." HAI, and local and regional affiliates such as Acción Internacional para la Salud (AIS), are focal points for campaigns on essential drugs action by governments and UN agencies and against industry products and practices that counter the concept.

The International Network for Rational Use of Drugs (INRUD) works through national groups representing individuals from ministries of health, universities, NGOs, and private-sector institutions to understand local drug use problems and create reproducible activities that improve drug use. INRUD's interdisciplinary focus links clinical and social sciences and emphasizes the behavioral aspects of drug use, particularly as they concern providers and consumers; the promotion of well-designed research studies; and the sharing of experiences and technical expertise among participating individuals. INRUD also promotes cooperation among donors interested in funding activities that contribute to these objectives. The INRUD secretariat, a coordinating body for the support groups and country core groups, publishes a semiannual newsletter, *INRUD News*, and can provide further information.

The International Organization of Consumer Unions (IOCU), as a principal partner in HAI, remains in the forefront of lobbying efforts to promote essential drugs policies and to encourage the drug industry to alter detrimental practices. It and its member associations are actively engaged at the international level to promote DAP and at the national level to influence local practices.

The Medical Lobby for Appropriate Marketing (MaLAM) was formed in 1983 in Australia, and by 1993, it had approximately 800 members in forty different countries. MaLAM uses the influence of doctors to encourage drug companies to provide accurate and consistent information so that correct decisions can be made about prescribing and dispensing drugs. The organization works by targeting an example of misleading advertising each month. MaLAM has been a stimulus for other groups to monitor advertising of pharmaceuticals and other medical products. It has also influenced multinational corporations to modify their promotional practices.

Through its Drug Management Program, Management Sciences for Health (MSH) is involved in research, technical assistance, training, and publications to improve health through the rational use of medicines. MSH staff work with international agencies and other NGOs, as well as directly with the public and private sectors in many countries. MSH produces training materials, software for pharmaceutical management, and publications such as this manual.

The United States Pharmacopeia (USP) is involved in developing drug information materials such as USP–DI and translating them into multiple languages. USP plays a leading role in groups working toward harmonizing international pharmacopeial standards. It provides fellowships, information, and support and participates in international meetings related to pharmacopeial and drug information issues.

As noted in Chapter 6, missions and other NGOs provide a substantial portion of health care and pharmaceutical service in many countries. In several of these countries, there is a Churches' Action for Health/Christian Medical Commission (CMC) drug distribution service. At the international level, the CMC acts as a coordinating body and clearinghouse for information.

Professional Associations

The International Pharmaceutical Federation (FIP) maintains an interest section on pharmaceutical issues in developing countries.

The International Society of Drug Bulletins (ISDB) is an association of independent and official drug information bulletins, providing the medical community with the most current information on individual drugs.

Regulatory Bodies

The International Conference of Drug Regulatory Authorities (ICDRA) is a biennial forum of officials from national regulatory authorities. Their principal concerns include mechanisms to guard against substandard, counterfeit, and dangerous products. They also support WHO's certification scheme and guiding principles for small regulatory authorities.

Industry Organizations

Most countries have individual national associations that represent manufacturers, distributors, and private pharmacies. These associations are intended primarily to protect members' interests, but they provide support to selected activities such as training, local publications, and community drug outlets in some countries. The International Federation of Pharmaceutical Manufacturers Associations (IFPMA) is an international advocacy group formed of several national pharmaceutical manufacturers' associations; it prepares position papers for the industry, testifies before international organizations, acts as a public-relations focus for the industry, and occasionally undertakes demonstration projects, such as quality control training for developing-country staff. The International Federation of Pharmaceutical Wholesalers (IFPW) plays a similar role with respect to pharmaceutical distributors.

≡ 2.5 Clients, Governments, Producers, and Beyond: A Time of Rapid Changes in the Pharmaceutical Field

In the early 1990s, the pharmaceutical industry began to make major changes in response to forces in its important markets in high-income countries. In a very short period, the multinational, traditionally research-based firms reversed their hostility to rational drug management issues and generic drugs. This shift in industry strategy has come about because of two major trends. First, the number of essential drugs available in generic form is expanding as patent protection expires and as relatively few significant new drugs are being developed. Second, health care is rapidly being reorganized in some of the economically advantaged countries, with organizations rather than individual practitioners becoming the major clients of pharmaceutical producers. The manufacturers, whose representatives used to promote drugs to individual physicians, must now convince the therapeutics committees that decide which drugs will be used (and, in turn, paid for) in large population-based health programs. These programs, called managed-care organizations, focus on keeping costs down so that they can compete with similar groups. Industry is now forming alliances with managed-care organizations and pharmacy benefits managers, and in many cases, pharmaceutical companies are purchasing such managed-care programs (or setting up new companies).

These trends suggest that the future of rational drug management, and the tools and ideas outlined in this manual, will become increasingly similar among countries in many stages of development. The ideas and experience reflected in *Managing Drug Supply* should become increasingly common ground for solving important drug management issues.

Although death and disability are always tragic, the rationale for national concern and action on essential drugs is driven by the large gap remaining between what we know and what we do. We know how drugs can help eliminate unnecessary and preventable deaths and disability, yet millions still die of tuberculosis, which is essentially curable with medical therapy. Malaria, pneumonia, diarrhea, and hypertension are manageable with basic medicines, yet they still kill millions. Children are born unwanted and without hope of a future when family planning supplies are unavailable.

This clear public health challenge is leading public policy-makers and managers toward a consistent approach to essential drugs. The first step is to identify and attack the major problems that are amenable to solution with available resources. The strategies of many national drug programs in less advantaged nations, and increasingly among decision-makers in more advantaged settings, are converging: first to ensure that the basic drugs that save lives and improve health are available, and then to deal with the drugs that do not fit those criteria. ■

≡ References and Further Readings

★ = *Key readings.*

Ahmad, S. R. 1990. *Bitter facts about drugs.* Karachi, Pakistan: Health Action International.

Dowling, H. F. 1977. *Fighting infection: Conquests of the twentieth century.* Cambridge, Mass.: Harvard University Press.

★ Dukes, M. N. G., ed. 1993. *Drug utilization studies: Methods and uses.* WHO regional publications, European series no. 45. Copenhagen: World Health Organization.

Foster, S. D. 1991. Supply and use of essential drugs in sub-Saharan Africa: Some issues and possible solutions. *Social Science and Medicine* 32:1201–18.

★ Kanji, N., A. Hardon, J. W. Harnmeijer, M. Mamdani, and G. Walt. 1992. *Drugs policy in developing countries.* London: Zed Books (with support from Danida).

London School of Hygiene and Tropical Medicine and Royal Tropical Institute (LSHTM/RTI). 1989. *An evaluation of WHO's Action Programme on Essential Drugs.* London and Amsterdam: LSHTM/RTI.

★ Reich, M. R. 1987. Essential drugs: Economics and politics in international health. *Health Policy and Planning* 8:39–57.

★ Silverman, M., M. Lydecker, and P. R. Lee. 1992. *Bad medicine: The prescription drug industry in the third world.* Stanford, Calif.: Stanford University Press.

Tognoni, G., and J.-R. Laporte. 1993. From clinical trials to drug utilization studies. In *Drug utilization studies: Methods and uses,* ed. M. N. G. Dukes. WHO regional publications, European series no. 45. Copenhagen: World Health Organization.

★ WHO (World Health Organization). 1988. *The world drug situation.* Geneva: WHO.

★ WHO (World Health Organization). 1995. *The use of essential drugs.* Technical report series no. 850. Geneva: WHO.

Annex 2.1 Useful Addresses

Action in International Medicine
Windeyer Building
46 Cleveland Street
London W1P 6DB, England

Action Programme on Essential Drugs
World Health Organization
1211 Geneva 27, Switzerland
Telephone: 41-22-791 2111 Fax: 41-22-791 0746

Alliance for the Prudent Use of Antibiotics
PO Box 1372
Boston, Mass. 02117-1372, US

Appropriate Health Resources and Technologies
   Action Group
Farringdon Point
29-35 Farringdon Road
London EC1M 3JB, England

Churches' Action for Health/Christian Medical Commission
150 Route de Ferney
CH-1211 Geneva 2, Switzerland

Department of International Health Care Research
Karolinska Institute
S-17177 Stockholm, Sweden
Telephone: 46 8 30 08 63 Fax: 46 8 31 15 90

Euro Health Group
Tinghojvej 77
2860 Soborg, Denmark
Telephone and fax: 45 39 696888

Health Action International–Acción Internacional
   para la Salud Coordinator
Acción para la Salud
Avda. Palermo 531, Dpto. 104, Lima, Peru

Health Action International–Europe
Jacob van Lennepkade 334 T
1053 NJ Amsterdam, The Netherlands
Telephone: 31-20-683 3684 Fax: 31-20-685 5002

International Network for Rational Use of Drugs
Management Sciences for Health
1655 North Fort Myer Drive, Suite 920
Arlington, Va. 22209, US
Telephone: 703-524-6575 Fax: 703-524-7898

International Organization of Consumer Unions
PO Box 1045
10830 Penang, Malaysia

International Society of Drug Bulletins
103 Hertford Road
London N2 9BX, England

Management Sciences for Health
165 Allandale Road
Boston, Mass. 02130, US

Medical Lobby for Appropriate Marketing
PO Box 172
Daw Park, SA 5041, Australia
or
MaLAM Canada
PO Box 158, Station D
Toronto, Ont., Canada M6P 3J8

Medicus Mundi International Organization for Cooperation
   in Health Care
Unterer Rheinweg 54
CH-4057 Basel, Switzerland

Pan American Health Organization
WHO Regional Office for the Americas
525 23rd Street, NW
Washington, D.C. 20037, US

UNICEF
UNICEF House, Essential Drugs Unit
Three United Nations Plaza
New York, N.Y. 10017, US

United States Pharmacopeia
12601 Twinbrook Parkway
Rockville, Md. 20852, US

World Health Organization
WHO Regional Office for Africa
PO Box No. 6
Brazzaville, Congo

World Health Organization
WHO Regional Office for the Eastern Mediterranean
PO Box 1517
Alexandria 21511, Egypt

World Health Organization
WHO Regional Office for Europe
8, Scherfigsvej
DK-2100 Copenhagen 0, Denmark

World Health Organization
WHO Regional Office for Southeast Asia
World Health House, Indraprastha Estate
Mahatma Gandhi Road
New Delhi 110002, India

World Health Organization
WHO Regional Office for the Western Pacific
PO Box 2932
1099 Manila, Philippines

Chapter 3
Economics for Drug Management

≡ Summary

Economics helps managers make difficult resource allocation decisions by providing a set of concepts and tools for evaluating alternatives in terms of their costs and benefits. Key economic concepts include

scarcity: *the fact that resources are always limited;*

opportunity cost: *benefits that are given up in choosing one option over another;*

marginal costs and benefits: *additional costs incurred and additional benefits gained by spending "a little more";*

incentives: *factors that influence the behavior of individuals or organizations.*

There is considerable debate about the appropriate role of government in the health sector. The social welfare perspective argues for broad government involvement, whereas the market economy perspective holds that government should become involved only when the market system fails. There is general support for government provision of public goods, goods and services with positive externalities, and merit goods, which tend not to be provided in sufficient quantities by private markets.

Policy-makers must also be concerned with distribution issues—who pays for, and who benefits from, publicly supported services. Through the use of subsidies, governments can encourage the consumption of health services beyond what individuals would pay for on their own.

The private sector is actively involved and often predominant in the health and pharmaceutical sector. Government involvement with the private sector is often seen as a means of correcting market failure, which may result from equity considerations, failure of competition, information failure, and externalities.

Efficiency means getting the most output for a given quantity of resources. The tools of pharmacoeconomic evaluation can help managers identify the most efficient options. Different methods include cost-minimization analysis, cost-effectiveness analysis, cost-utility analysis, and cost-benefit analysis.

Finally, an understanding of patients as consumers can help explain their health-seeking behavior and decision-making.

≡ 3.1 Economics as a Tool for Making Choices

Health economics is about making resource allocation decisions under conditions of scarcity. Because budgets are never large enough, health managers must constantly decide which of several courses of action to follow. These may be choices among programs, among program goals or objectives, or among strategies or activities for achieving specific goals.

Economics provides methods for evaluating choices in terms of their costs and benefits. Figure 3.1 lists examples of resource allocation decisions for which economic tools may offer useful insights.

Although resource allocation can be a highly political process, the tools of economic analysis encourage better decision-making by providing information. This chapter provides an overview of some basic economic concepts applied to public expenditure decisions, understanding the private sector, government interactions with the private sector, efficiency concepts, pharmacoeconomic evaluation, and understanding the patient as consumer.

≡ 3.2 Some Basic Economic Concepts

Economic concepts that are critical issues in public health include scarcity, opportunity cost, marginal benefits and costs, and incentives.

Figure 3.1 Examples of Resource Allocation Decisions at Different Levels of Government

Central Government
- ► How much should the public sector spend for all recurrent budgets?
- ► How much should be allocated to the different ministries?

Central Ministry of Health
- ► How much should be allocated to primary, secondary, and tertiary care?
- ► How much should be allocated to different program activities?
- ► How much should be spent on drugs, personnel, and other operating costs?

Drug Program Managers
- ► How much should be spent on drugs, training, and storage?
- ► What methods can be used to plan for international drug purchases when the value of local currency is falling?
- ► Which drug distribution strategy will deliver drugs to health facilities most efficiently?
- ► Which drugs should be purchased and used?

Scarcity. There are never enough resources to do everything. Choices have to be made about the best ways to use those resources that are available. Resources are not limited to money; time is a scarce resource as well, as every busy program manager knows.

Opportunity Cost. Opportunity cost decisions go beyond

money. They take into account potential benefits that are given up in order to follow a chosen course of action—benefits that could be derived from using resources in another way. For example, if running a training course in stock management means that another course in rational drug use cannot be conducted, the lost rational drug use course is the opportunity cost of running the stock management course. The concept of opportunity cost helps evaluate alternatives by looking explicitly at the tradeoffs they involve.

Marginal Benefits and Costs. When resource allocation decisions are made, the question is often not whether to allocate all or nothing to a particular activity but whether to spend a little more or a little less. The additional costs of doing a little more are called marginal costs, and the additional benefits are called marginal benefits. For example, ministries are rarely faced with decisions about whether or not to provide vaccinations; however, a program manager might have to decide whether to keep the clinic open for another hour at the end of the day. To make this decision, the manager would estimate the marginal cost of keeping the facility open (in terms of extra salaries, utilities, and so forth) and compare this to the marginal benefit of doing so (in terms of numbers of additional children who would be vaccinated during the extra hour). The opportunity cost of keeping the clinic open for another hour would be the activities forgone as a result: for example, there may no longer be sufficient resources to conduct an outreach session.

Incentives. An incentive is some kind of compensation (monetary or otherwise) that influences the behavior of individuals or organizations. For example, governments may have an incentive to provide preventive health care because it reduces the demand for, and thus the cost of, providing, more expensive curative care. Governments can also create incentives to influence the behavior of individuals or organizations. In charging fees, for example, they can discourage individuals from making unnecessary visits to health facilities for minor complaints; through variable fee schedules, they can make it more costly for individuals to seek care at tertiary facilities.

By assessing fines for the distribution of substandard products, governments can encourage pharmaceutical producers to maintain the quality of output. By establishing certain kinds of controls and incentives, government can influence consumers and providers to choose lower-priced drugs.

≡ 3.3 Economics of the Public Sector

The appropriate role of the government in the health sector, as well as in the broader economy, has been debated for centuries by philosophers, economic theorists, and political thinkers. Since the 1980s, the debate has been heightened by a two-pronged dilemma. On the one hand, centrally planned economies have failed to ensure economic security for their populations; on the other hand, some market economies have shown notable inability to ensure universal access to basic social services such as health care.

In appraising the role of government, it is useful to consider the two extreme positions in this debate. The social welfare perspective supports the vision of an active central government that provides virtually all social services and participates actively in the production of goods and services throughout the economy. This perspective assumes without question that education, health, and other social services will be fully provided by the government. The market economy perspective, at the other extreme, holds that the government should intervene only if and when the market system performs imperfectly. The economist's perspective on the appropriate degree of government involvement is to weigh benefits against costs.

Goals of Public Expenditure

For certain activities, the role of the public sector is undisputed. These areas include maintenance of law and order; investment in infrastructure such as roads, electricity, and communications networks; and the provision of certain types of goods and services, called public goods, externalities, and merit goods.

Public Goods. Services that are widely agreed to be essential and that are consumed collectively (for example, national defense and policing), certain types of utilities (such as street lighting and sewerage systems), and public health services (such as aerial spraying for vector control), are termed public goods. Because the benefits of public goods cannot be provided to some and withheld from others, they are often not sold in the market, and it may be impractical to rely on the private sector to provide them.

Externalities. External effects, sometimes called social costs or benefits, extend beyond the party directly involved in the production or use of a good or service. Examples of goods with positive externalities are immunization and communicable disease control: all members of the community enjoy the benefits of immunization or treatment because their chances of contracting these diseases are reduced as a result. Goods with positive externalities also tend to be underprovided by private markets; hence it falls to the government to provide them.

Merit Goods. Merit goods are things that are good in themselves and include, for example, providing health services for the poor. Populations want these services to be provided, but private markets tend not to take care of this group.

Government activity often extends beyond these three types of goods and services. Many people look to government to create a supportive environment for the private sector by encouraging stability and ensuring the availability of basic infrastructure. Arguments for a more active public sector are often most forcefully made in developing countries, where levels of private investment may be low and the private sector is consequently less well developed. The roles that governments can play in the pharmaceutical sector are discussed in Chapter 6 and range from total control and provision of all pharmaceutical services (increasingly rare) to minimal government intervention, with pharmacy services provided mostly by the private sector, without government support or interference.

The Financing of Public Expenditure

Broadly speaking, governments have three options for financing public expenditure: they can raise revenue through taxes (income, sales, and property taxes; producer taxes; import duties), they can sell goods or services to the private sector (or to other governments), or they can borrow from development banks. Each of these options involves a cost in the form of increased current levels of taxation, increased capital and operating costs to provide commercial goods or services, or an increase in future commitments for loan repayment. Costs must be weighed against the benefits of government expenditures and compared with the costs and benefits of the alternative, which is to leave the provision of services to the private sector.

Governments go through a process of resource allocation, allocating funds first among competing ministries and then among different programs or activities within each ministry. At least four factors may influence these decisions:

1. *Historical precedent:* Decisions are based on the previous year's allocations and involve incremental changes.
2. *Political forces:* Powerful groups may carry out explicit lobbying activities, which can influence resource allocation decisions.
3. *External forces:* Donors' and other external agendas may influence public expenditure patterns, especially in countries that depend on external grants and loans.
4. *Program planning:* Program planning, or a "technocratic" approach, involves defining a set of policy

objectives and then using systematic economic analysis to choose the most cost-effective combination of strategies to achieve those objectives.

Political pressure is one explanation for the persistence of resource allocation patterns that are skewed in favor of urban hospital care (urban bias). Urban populations are more likely to be vocal in expressing support or disapproval for government policies and represent a concentrated block of votes. Thus, urban areas are often a relatively more important political force compared with dispersed, poor, and relatively uneducated rural populations.

External pressure from donors may be particularly influential when donor agencies are able to put "conditions" on expenditures; these may include guarantees of funding for specific activities or facilities. Allocation of recurrent expenditures may also be driven by previous donor-funded capital investments.

The program planning or technocratic approach does not rule out a role for political influence, since even the act of choosing policy priorities has a political basis. However, the technocratic approach and the use of economic analysis are increasingly advocated by agencies such as the World Bank.

Since many resource allocation decisions are based on assessments of marginal benefits and costs, carefully documented and well-argued cases for additional resources are likely to be met with greater success than ad hoc requests. Requests for additional resources that are accompanied by evidence that existing resources are being used efficiently are likely to carry more weight.

When developing budgets to provide realistic cost estimates for program options, it is important for public-sector managers to budget in "real" terms. They need to take into account changes in the price level due to inflation and, for imported goods, fluctuations in exchange rates. This is critical in the development of drug budgets, since drugs are procured largely at world market prices. Even locally produced drugs include 60 to 70 percent imported raw materials. Without adjustments for changes in the price level, it is impossible to compare different program options accurately. Moreover, drug budgets that appear to be increasing over time may actually be decreasing in real terms. Issues of public financing and budgeting are discussed in more detail in Chapters 40 and 42.

Distribution Issues and the Use of Subsidies

Besides being concerned with determining what goods and services will be provided with public funds and ensuring the availability of resources to pay for them, policy-makers and public-sector managers must also consider equity in the utilization of services. How will these goods be distributed among the population, and who will benefit from the publicly provided services? Patterns of utilization are often examined along dimensions of income or of rural-urban residence.

Subsidies. From an economic perspective, there are three broad alternatives in the distribution of health services: they can be provided free of charge to all persons (traditional public model), they can be distributed in accordance with consumers' willingness and ability to pay (traditional private model), or they can be provided at reduced or subsidized prices in order to increase consumption beyond what consumers would pay for on their own (government intervention to achieve public goals).

Two main arguments support the use of public funds to subsidize health services. First, a certain level of consumption (for example, use of immunization or other preventive health services) confers positive benefits on society (externalities). Second, health services need to be provided for those who cannot pay (a merit good).

Subsidized services may not be limited to public-sector facilities; sometimes governments or donor agencies provide grants in cash or in kind to other organizations (for example, nongovernmental organizations [NGOs]) to support service delivery, a method used in many African countries. In many industrialized countries, subsidized services are provided by the private sector, which is reimbursed from public funds. Whatever the approach, it is important to recognize that subsidies have an opportunity cost: the funds used to subsidize health services are not available for other activities.

Who Benefits? Policy-makers must also be concerned with ensuring that subsidies reach the intended beneficiaries. To ensure access for the neediest groups, the subsidy may need to be explicitly targeted. For example, beneficiaries can be selected through an identification procedure such as means testing, which usually involves setting an income level below which individuals receive services at a lower rate (or free). Sometimes this is done informally, with certificates of indigence issued by local authorities to individuals deemed unable to afford to pay for services.

An alternative method of targeting subsidies is to focus on services that are disproportionately consumed by the poor, such as primary care in rural areas. This reduces the "capture" of subsidies by nonneedy groups, which is often a problem in large urban areas. Due in part to the urban bias mentioned earlier, hospital-based health services continue to represent large proportions of government spending in many countries.

Who Pays? Distribution issues also arise with regard to the burden of paying for health services. Patterns of financing (through taxes, borrowing, or fees for service) raise equity considerations in relation to income groups, rural versus urban residence, and even generations (because borrowing for present consumption must be repaid by future generations).

When the financing of public services is predominantly through income taxes and the tax system is progressive, the financial burden tends to fall more heavily on higher-income groups who pay a relatively greater share of their income in taxes. If sales taxes or value-added taxes are primarily used, the burden falls relatively more on low-income groups, unless most basic goods and services are exempted from the tax. Loan financing places the burden on future generations by transferring repayment obligations to them. When services are financed by user fees, the burden of paying for services falls on the sick. If fees are fixed, the poor have a relatively greater burden, as they are required to spend a higher proportion of their incomes to pay for services.

≡ 3.4 Understanding the Private Sector

In contrast to the public sector, private-sector resource allocation decisions are determined largely by the interaction of buyers and sellers in the marketplace. Health program managers sometimes think of the private sector as greedy, unscrupulous, unethical, and concerned only with profit at the expense of equity and quality. They see consumers as unable to judge the quality of health services and therefore vulnerable to manipulation by the private sector. In many countries, this negative view of the private sector has been an important factor underlying the bias toward public-sector health service delivery.

The private sector usually plays a significant role in the health sector, however, both in the production, distribution, and sale of pharmaceuticals and in the direct provision of a large proportion of health services through private practices and private hospitals. This fact alone is an important reason for better understanding the private sector, which has advantages over the public sector in certain circumstances and for certain activities. Appreciating both the strengths and the weaknesses of the private sector is essential to good public-sector decision-making.

Markets and Competition

The private sector is characterized by buyers and sellers in the marketplace negotiating the exchange of goods and services. In the pharmaceutical sector, the sellers of drugs may be manufacturers, wholesalers, pharmacies, or drug peddlers. Purchasers may be government, private, and nongovernmental health facilities and individual consumers. When there are many suppliers and many purchasers, markets are described as "competitive." Through the use of prices as signals, competitive markets are able to allocate resources efficiently, making sure that resources get to the people who most value them.

Suppliers enter the market when they see an opportunity to make a profit, that is, to earn revenues in excess of costs. With this incentive, they are willing to invest their own money and take a risk as they engage in new activities, expand into new markets, and respond to consumer demand. Under competitive conditions, suppliers can be expected to earn a reasonable level of profit; if they try to increase their profits above this level, another supplier will likely offer a lower price and take away their business. In this way, the price system functions as a control or discipline mechanism. Suppliers do not compete only on the basis of price; they may compete on quality (providing a higher quality for the same price), reliability, service, or capacity.

Economies of Scale. In competitive markets, suppliers have an incentive to produce goods and services as efficiently as possible, using the least-cost combination of inputs. In some cases, the private sector is able to generate efficiency gains because of the size and diversity of its operations. Economies of scale occur when the production of larger quantities leads to lower average costs. For example, a plant that produces 40,000 tablets a day is likely to do so at a lower cost per tablet than one that produces only 10,000 a day. Beyond some level of output, however, additional machinery or equipment may need to be bought, or more resources may need to be spent in supervising production, which may increase average costs.

Economies of Scope. Economies of scope result when combining a number of different activities permits them to be done at lower average cost. Private distribution networks may benefit from economies of scope by combining the delivery of pharmaceuticals with the delivery of other goods and services.

Ethics and Business

As mentioned above, both NGOs and public-sector groups have tended to attribute unethical and unscrupulous motives to the private sector. Although there are examples of suppliers that brazenly cheat by, for example, providing substandard drugs, it is clearly not in the long-term interests of private providers to engage in this type of activity. As long as there is the prospect of a continued, profitable relationship with a purchaser, the supplier has an incentive to retain customers by providing good-quality services.

≡ 3.5 Government Interaction with the Private Sector

Governments interact with the private sector in many different ways. In its simplest form, this interaction consists of government purchases of drugs and supplies from private pharmaceutical companies. The public and private sectors may also compete by providing similar services. The introduction of community pharmacies in the context of Bamako Initiative projects in some countries, for example, has provoked negative reactions from the pharmaceutical sector because of fears of competition from lower-priced drugs.

Other forms of government involvement are motivated by a desire to correct "imperfect" private markets. "Market failures" in the health sector provide an important rationale for government intervention.

Market Failure

Market failure in the health sector may result from equity considerations, failure of competition, lack of information, and externalities.

Equity Considerations. Because private-sector decision-making is driven more by profit than by equity considerations, equity is often the first motivation for government involvement in essential drugs programs. The relatively high cost of drugs compared with other goods suggests that without government involvement the poor would be denied access to lifesaving pharmaceuticals. This is especially true in remote areas, where cash incomes are usually lower and delivery costs higher.

Failure of Competition. Competitive markets require the presence of many sellers or the threat of entry by sellers, which tends to promote competitive behavior. In the pharmaceutical sector, however, suppliers are sometimes few and the costs of entry are high, both of which tend to limit competition. Makers of individual drugs may establish a virtual monopoly and maintain high prices because they hold the patents or, through marketing, have established their brands as the standard ones. Suppliers may form cartels, setting prices collectively and coordinating their bids on contracts to achieve higher profits.

Lack of Information. Competition increases when purchasers have good information about the price and quality of goods and services, but this is difficult to achieve with pharmaceuticals. Patients are unable to assess the quality, safety, or efficacy of drug products and often rely on clinicians and drug sellers to prescribe them. Ultimately, they depend on pharmaceutical producers to maintain production quality standards. Consumers' inability to assess quality, safety, and efficacy leads governments to intervene:

inspection of drugs, registration and licensing of pharmacists, and drug registration processes are all ways in which governments attempt to protect consumers from dangerous, ineffective, and poor-quality drugs (see Chapters 7 and 18).

Externalities. Some health services (such as treatment of contagious tuberculosis or immunization against measles) have benefits both for the individuals who receive the services and for others, who are consequently protected from exposure to the illness. Since private markets tend to underprovide public goods with positive externalities, governments usually take responsibility for providing them.

Economics of Regulation

The term *regulation* refers to the tools that governments use to ensure that private-sector actions are consistent with the broader welfare of society. The objectives of regulation are usually improvements in quality, efficiency, or equity.

In pharmaceuticals, the instruments used to regulate the private sector (for example, manufacturers, distributors, pharmacies) include controls on drug quality through mandatory inspection programs; controls on imports (restricting imports of dangerous products or permitting the import of only essential drugs), and registration and licensure of pharmacists. Restrictions on the prices at which pharmaceuticals can be sold have also been widely imposed. (Pharmaceutical legislation and regulation are discussed in Chapter 7.)

A number of issues should be considered in evaluating the impact of regulation: the extent of coverage (for example, does it include both public and private sectors?), the capacity of government to monitor compliance, the extent of enforcement and exemptions, and the extent to which the private sector can circumvent or evade regulations (for example, through the emergence of an uncontrolled parallel market for nonessential or banned drugs).

Regulation may provide opportunities for regulator capture—illegal payments or other arrangements between the private-sector companies being regulated and the officials responsible for enforcement. "Who will guard the guardians?" is a common question reflecting the possibility that regulators may be co-opted by those being regulated, which undermines the intended benefits of regulation.

The "law of unintended consequences" reflects the problems that can arise if regulation is initiated without full consideration of the broader effects that it may have. One example of a negative unintended consequence was the increase in imports and the use of metronidazole that accompanied the banning of antidiarrheals in Bangla-

desh: instead of eliminating inappropriate treatment of childhood diarrhea, the ban on antidiarrheals led to an increase in other forms of inappropriate treatment, with accompanying cost implications.

The capacity required to implement and monitor the effects of regulations and the costs of monitoring them need to be carefully weighed against the proposed benefits.

Threats to Government Effectiveness

Arguments in favor of government involvement often contrast private market failure with "perfect" government intervention, but this is only rarely achieved. The private market may fail, but government intervention also fails—spectacularly so at times. Governments in all countries at all levels of development are subject to threats to their effectiveness. Informed decisions about public involvement in essential drugs programs must acknowledge these sources of government ineffectiveness, including inefficiency in service delivery, inequities in revenue collection, interest-group pressures, and lack of good governance.

Inefficiency in service delivery arises from a lack of individual incentives for good performance, bureaucratic inflexibility, and political pressure to create employment. Overexpenditure on staff and underexpenditure on drugs result in idle staff who are unable to meet the needs of patients. Inefficiencies in government accounting systems that cause lengthy delays in payments may result in suppliers raising their prices or deciding not to bid at all on government contracts.

Inequities in revenue collection can result in a reduction in health services, which is felt most acutely by the lower-income groups who are most dependent on them. If the more affluent members of society succeed in avoiding taxes and other government levies, the financial burden for government activity falls on those with fewer means and options.

Even honest, well-meaning politicians and officials are subject to interest-group pressures. Political supporters, age-mates, members of the same ethnic group, and concerned business organizations can influence bureaucrats to allocate services and resources in ways that do not promote equity. It is generally the more affluent who are able to exert such pressures; ironically, the less well-off may lose both directly and indirectly—by paying more in taxes as well as by receiving fewer services.

Finally, lack of good governance can be revealed in self-interested manipulation of the drug selection process, corruption in the award of tenders, nepotism in the appointment of key staff, health staff selling drugs on the outside, and other destructive practices.

≡ 3.6 Efficiency Concepts

Whereas effectiveness has to do with the degree to which services are provided or outputs produced, efficiency can be understood as getting the most output for a given quantity of resources or, alternatively, achieving a given level of output at minimum cost. Efficiency is sometimes referred to as cost effectiveness.

Two broad types of efficiency can be distinguished. The first is technical efficiency, which involves determining the right quantities of different inputs, and the least expensive combination of inputs, to achieve a given outcome. The second is allocative efficiency, which is the broader concept of undertaking the best combination of activities to achieve the greatest net benefit.

Technical efficiency issues arise throughout the drug supply system. In drug selection, decisions about both the number and types of drugs on the list have efficiency implications. For example, in some countries, 20 to 30 percent of drug expenditure is for products that have no relevance to the main health problems of the population—clearly an inefficient use of scarce resources. The use of more expensive brand-name drugs when generic substitutes exist is usually inefficient, since the same health outcome could be achieved at a lower cost.

In procurement, the use of competitive international tendering has indisputable economic advantages: a call for tenders by the Eastern Caribbean Drug Service in 1986–87 produced a 44 percent average price reduction for drugs. Determination of appropriate quantities also has efficiency implications: overstocking brings risks of expiry, and stockouts reduce program output and lead to expensive emergency orders. Efficiency gains can be achieved through consideration of drug packaging as well. The prices of individual drug packs in Mali in 1988 were found to be 400 percent higher than for hospital packs, an unnecessary expenditure where individual packs were not needed.

In drug distribution, when there is not enough transportation or vehicles are often inoperative, personnel may be underutilized. The same output could be achieved with fewer personnel, or output could be dramatically increased with a slightly greater expenditure on vehicle maintenance. A program manager might consider the costs and benefits of changing from using a fleet of program vehicles to contracting delivery to a commercial transportation firm, in an effort to increase efficiency.

In drug use, efficiency implications arise with choice of drug and length of course of therapy. Excessive courses of antibiotics are inefficient, because the same outcome could be achieved using less. Similarly, a subtherapeutic drug dose fails to achieve the desired clinical outcome and wastes resources, since the patient is likely to return for further treatment. Polypharmacy leads to lower rates of adherence to treatment and is inefficient; resources are consumed, but the desired clinical outcome is not achieved.

Decisions affecting allocative efficiency are most often made at the policy level, for example, deciding whether to allocate additional funds to the ministry of health (MOH) or the ministry of education. Within the MOH, decisions involve how much to spend on primary, secondary, and tertiary care, or whether to spend additional program funds on control of tuberculosis or treatment of sexually transmitted diseases. Other policy-level decisions can influence technical efficiency. A decision to reduce spending on drugs and supplies in order to pay salaries, for example, could lead to technical inefficiency if staff are then underutilized because of shortages of complementary inputs. (Think of a surgeon who cannot perform operations because the operating-room equipment has not been maintained, or because anesthetics are in short supply.)

Program managers can control only some of the factors that affect efficiency. For example, program managers may not have control over the allocation of funds among different line items, such as personnel and fuel, making it difficult to use inputs in the most efficient combinations. Incentives and management structures are important: If a more efficient use of resources leads to tangible benefits to health workers, they are more likely to make more efficient choices. If they are penalized (for example, if underspending a budget leads to less money being allocated next year with no offsetting incentives), health workers are unlikely to behave in an efficient and cost-saving manner.

Information is important in increasing efficiency: managers and health care providers who have information about the costs of alternatives are more likely to make efficient use of their resources than those without. Formulary manuals, standard treatments, and therapeutic guidelines are intended to provide such information to health workers and can be one kind of input in a strategy to combat inefficient prescribing of multiple drugs in subtherapeutic doses.

Efficiency is an important economic concept, since demonstrating that existing resources are being used efficiently provides powerful support to requests for additional resources. But demonstrating efficiency requires basic cost information. Relatively simple performance indicators have been developed, using information that should be available to most supply system managers; such indicators can be used to monitor supply system efficiency on a routine basis (see Chapter 36).

≡ 3.7 Economic Evaluation

The term *economic evaluation* refers to a set of analytical tools that can help identify which of several alternatives offers the greatest benefit compared with its cost. Four methods of economic analysis are commonly distinguished and are described here in increasing order of methodological and practical difficulty.

1. *Cost-minimization analysis*: calculating the cost of two or more alternatives that have the same outcome to identify the lowest-cost option;
2. *Cost-effectiveness analysis*: measuring both costs and benefits of alternatives to find the strategy with the best ratio of benefits, measured in therapeutic or program effects, per money unit;
3. *Cost-utility analysis*: same as cost-effectiveness analysis, except that benefits are measured in "utility" units (which are often controversial);
4. *Cost-benefit analysis*: comparison of the costs and benefits of an intervention by translating the health benefits into a money value, so that both costs and benefits are measured in the same unit.

The distinctions among these four methods have mainly to do with the treatment of the benefits of intervention. In cost-minimization analysis, the benefits have to be measured in the same units, and all the alternatives considered need to produce the same quantity of benefits. The choice is merely to identify the lowest-cost alternative, and the analysis is limited to calculation of the costs. For example, if two drugs have the same therapeutic benefits, have the same safety profile, and are of equivalent quality, the drug with the lower cost would be selected.

In cost-effectiveness analysis, the unit of output of the alternatives is the same, but the quantities of output, or effectiveness of the strategy, can differ. The challenge is to identify the option with the lowest cost per unit of benefit. For example, different vaccination strategies (fixed point, outreach, campaign) may reach different numbers of children and have different levels of effectiveness, but cost-effectiveness analysis can help identify the one that has the lowest cost per fully immunized child. Output or benefits can be measured as intermediate outputs (such as cost per child vaccinated, cost per course of therapy delivered, cost per health worker trained) or final outputs (such as cost per death averted).

The disability-adjusted life-year (DALY) is a recently developed measure of health outcome that is increasingly being used in cost-effectiveness analysis to compare interventions with different types of output. DALYs combine mortality and morbidity (or disability) into a single mea-sure by weighting the life-years saved by the amount of disability associated with a specific outcome. The 1993 *World Development Report* (World Bank 1993) presents measures of the cost effectiveness of a number of interventions in terms of cost per DALY saved. For example, vitamin A supplementation costs $1 per DALY saved, chemotherapy for tuberculosis $1 to $3 per DALY saved, and measles vaccination $15 to $20 per DALY saved. In contrast, interventions such as treatment of leukemia and environmental control of dengue fever both cost in excess of $1,000 per DALY saved.

Cost-utility analysis is simply cost-effectiveness analysis conducted with program outcome measured in utility units. The most common utility measure is the quality-adjusted life-year (QALY). QALYs are similar to DALYs in that they calculate program benefits in terms of life-years saved, except that in the case of QALYs, the years are weighted by the "quality" of those years when they are lived in less-than-perfect health. QALYs also allow comparison of interventions with different outputs. QALYs are controversial because it is difficult to compare individual qualities of life and preferences. Further, quality-of-life scales are not perfect measures, nor are they easily translated into QALYs.

Cost-benefit analysis is rarely undertaken in the health sector because of the difficulty of assigning a monetary value to life-years saved. Its main advantage is that it allows the comparison of programs with different outcomes—for example, investment in health versus investment in education.

Figure 3.2 shows how each of these tools can be applied to make choices between alternative drug therapies or alternative transportation schemes.

The description and analysis of the costs of drug therapy to health care systems and society have been defined as *pharmacoeconomics*. Pharmacoeconomic analysis employs the tools described above for examining the impact (desirable and undesirable) of alternative drug therapies and other medical interventions. Pharmacoeconomic analysis can help address questions such as: What drugs should be included on the formulary? What are the patient outcomes of various treatment modalities? How do two options for providing pharmacy services compare? Country Study 3.1 describes the use of cost-effectiveness analysis in Australia.

Steps for Conducting a Cost-Effectiveness Evaluation

There are six key steps in conducting a cost-effectiveness evaluation.

Figure 3.2 Using Economic Analysis Methods to Make Choices

Type of Analysis	Drug Therapy Choice: Antibiotic A versus Antibiotic B for Treating Childhood Pneumonia	Transportation Scheme Choice: Program Fleet versus Contracted Private Firm
Cost minimization	Of two drugs with equal effectiveness, which is the least expensive?	Assuming that both options are identically effective, which is the least expensive?
Cost effectiveness	Two drugs have different degrees of effectiveness: what is the cost per child cured of antibiotic A versus antibiotic B (allowing for different efficacy of drugs A and B)?	The two options have different performances with respect to on-time delivery: what is the cost per drug kit delivered using program transport versus a contracted firm? (Perpetually late deliveries are factored in as a smaller level of desired output.)
Cost utility	What is the cost per QALY saved of treating childhood pneumonia with drug A versus treating tuberculosis with short-course chemotherapy? (Note: method is controversial for comparing drug therapies.)	Since the outcome of interest is the same in both cases (that is, drugs delivered on time), there is no need to use a specially constructed measure of output.
Cost benefit	What is the cost-benefit ratio (value of costs per value of life saved) for treating childhood pneumonia versus the cost-benefit ratio for saving lives through improved road lighting? (Note: method is normally not used to compare alternative therapies.)	As above.

Step 1. Define the Objective. For example, in terms of program output:

▸ Which drug regimen should be the therapy of choice for the treatment of childhood pneumonia?

▸ What is the best approach to transporting essential drugs to health facilities?

Step 2. Enumerate the Different Ways to Achieve the Objective. For example,

▸ short-course chemotherapy with more expensive drugs (option 1), versus traditional long-course chemotherapy with cheaper drugs (option 2);

▸ purchase of program vehicles for delivery of drugs to health facilities (option 1), versus a contract with a private transport firm for delivery of drugs (option 2).

Step 3. Identify and Measure the Costs of Each Option. All the inputs required for each option should be identified and the costs determined. Capital as well as recurrent costs should be included. When there are joint inputs and outputs, cost allocation methods must be used to determine the share of costs of the relevant options. Figure 3.3 lists different types of costs that should be considered (see also Chapter 42).

Step 4. Identify and Measure the Benefits of Each Option. In the drug choice example, benefits could be measured in DALYs, as described earlier. Measures of drug effectiveness will be needed, as well as epidemiological information on the course of illness without treatment. For the transport example, an indicator of performance, such as drug consignments delivered on

Figure 3.3 Types of Costs

Recurrent cost: The cost of goods that are consumed or used up over the course of a year (for example, staff, drugs, fuel).

Capital cost: The cost of goods that are intended to last for longer than a year (such as buildings, vehicles, medical equipment).

Annualized capital cost: Capital cost per year of useful life for a building, vehicle, or other capital item.

Fixed cost: Cost that does not change with the level of output (for example, building, equipment, salaries to a certain extent).

Variable cost: Cost that changes, depending on the amount of services delivered (for instance, drugs and supplies).

Total cost: The sum of recurrent costs and annualized capital costs.

Average cost per unit: Total cost divided by the number of units produced (for example, cost per patient treated, per immunization given, per cure dispensed).

Marginal cost: The cost of producing of providing one additional unit.

time to a health facility, could be used.

Step 5. Calculate and Interpret the Cost Effectiveness of Each Option. The cost-effectiveness ratio is total cost divided by number of units of output. Better overall efficiency is indicated by a lower cost per unit of output.

Step 6. Perform Sensitivity Analysis on the Conclusions. Sensitivity analysis measures how different assumptions made in the course of estimating costs and outputs affect the conclusions. Sensitivity analysis deals with uncertainty in assumptions that underlie the analysis, or with problems of imprecise measurement. In practice, sensitivity analysis identifies the values or assumptions about which there is uncertainty, determines their likely range

Country Study 3.1 Pharmacoeconomics in Formulary Decisions in Australia

One application of pharmacoeconomic analysis is to help make decisions about whether new drugs should be included in a drug formulary list. Decisions are made based on the principle that if a drug is no better than a comparable product, it should not cost more. If it is superior to existing therapies but more expensive (a common situation), and funds are available, any extra expenditure should represent "value for money."

In Australia, the federal government subsidizes the use of pharmaceuticals through the maintenance of a "positive" formulary, called the Pharmaceutical Benefits Schedule (PBS). Recommendations to list new drugs on the PBS are made by a Pharmaceutical Benefits Advisory Committee (PBAC) to the health minister. In making these recommendations, the PBAC considers the importance of the drug, the need for it in the community, its cost effectiveness, and the financial implications of adding it to the formulary.

The PBAC generally does not consider listing a new drug unless the request is accompanied by an economic analysis. Relative clinical performances and costs of both the potential new drug and comparable drugs already listed in the PBS are presented. Costs are not limited to each drug's acquisition cost and can include savings in other areas—for instance, lower use of other drugs or fewer consultations, tests, and hospital admissions. Cost-effectiveness ratios for the new drug and comparable drugs are then developed—for example, the cost of achieving a bacterial cure in the case of an antibiotic, or the cost of achieving a 50 percent reduction in seizure frequency in the case of an anticonvulsant drug.

Once the data have been evaluated, the PBAC must determine whether the cost-effectiveness ratios represent value for money. If the new drug represents modest or significant advances over existing therapies, the committee, in a sense, has to make a judgment about how much society is willing to pay for the extra benefits: what is it worth to gain an additional year of life (a final outcome indicator) or to achieve an extra bacterial cure, a night free of asthmatic wheezing, or a night free of pain (intermediate outcome indicators)? When the benefits have been calculated in the form of years of life saved or quality-adjusted life-years (QALYs), that judgment is possible, although controversial. Valuation of intermediate outcome indicators, such as a night free of wheezing, is more difficult and demands more community input.

Once the committee has made a judgment about value for money, a recommendation is made to a pricing authority, which uses the drug cost as a basis for price negotiations with the sponsoring company.

As pressures increase to reduce the size of the drug budget in Australia, economic analysis will be used increasingly as a means of selecting from a much more restricted range of medications. The effort to improve the management of existing pharmaceutical resources will rely more on the views and practices of prescribers than on national formulary decisions.

Source: Gafni and Birch 1993; Henry 1992; Laupacis et al. 1992.

of values, and recalculates study results based on a combination of the "best guess," most conservative, and least conservative estimates of these key values. The question of interest is whether the conclusions of the analysis would be changed with these extreme values.

Even though certain costs or benefits cannot be measured accurately, it may be possible to show that the results of the analysis do not change over any reasonable range of cost or benefit. Alternatively, the difficulties in measurement may indicate that the results are very sensitive to error in measurement and that caution should be used in interpreting the results of the study. Sensitivity analysis is easy to do and is essential for the proper use and defense of study results (for a good explanation of how to do a sensitivity analysis, see WHO 1994).

≡ 3.8 Understanding the Patient as a Consumer

Other economic concepts relate to patients and their demand for health care. A person who feels ill can be thought of as making two choices: first, whether to seek care outside the home, and second, which health care provider to consult. Implicitly, the individual is thinking of the opportunity cost of seeking care—that is, the cost of using time and resources for health care rather than for something else. The choice clearly depends on how severe the individual thinks the illness is, as well as a host of other factors.

The concepts of *demand* and *need* are often distinguished. Demand refers to individuals' willingness and ability to pay for health services. This can be quite independent of need: people may be ill or require medical services but not have enough money to pay for them, or they may not even be aware of the need, particularly for preventive services. A child will benefit from childhood vaccinations, but the parents may be unwilling to pay for this service because they do not perceive the need.

With infectious diseases such as tuberculosis or sexually transmitted diseases, the benefits of early treatment extend beyond the infected patient to the community. However, people may not demand enough medical care because the benefits to the individual are less than the benefits to society. In such situations, there may be an important role for public funding of treatment. Similar arguments can be made for family planning and immunization services.

The role of quality in the demand for health care and the relationship between quality and willingness to pay are not well understood. It seems clear, however, that people are willing to pay more for care that they perceive to be of adequate quality.

The extent to which medical treatment decisions are affected by the price charged depends on the *elasticity* of demand for health care. Elasticity refers to the responsiveness of demand to price: if the price increases, how much will that affect the quantity of health care demanded? Health care consumption is thought to be relatively insensitive to price, as a sick individual is likely to make other sacrifices in order to get health care. However, there is evidence that there is greater sensitivity to price among lower-income groups, which is cause for particular concern when considering fees for health services; it provides a rationale for subsidy or exemption programs for low-income groups.

The cost of health care borne by patients does not include just the fees charged for consultation and drugs. There may be transport costs and opportunity costs in time spent traveling and waiting for services. For hospital care, the full cost may also include having a relative stay to provide meals and other care. These unmeasured costs may be much larger than the visible cost. Although not health care costs in themselves, they are clearly costs from the point of view of society (and of the individual patients affected). ∎

≡ **References and Further Readings**

★ = *Key readings.*

Beeson, P. 1983. Doctors must learn economics. *World Health Forum* 4:215–16.

★ Bennett, S. 1991. *The mystique of markets: Public and private health care in developing countries.* PHP departmental publication no. 4. London: London School of Hygiene and Tropical Medicine.

★ Bootman, J. L., R. J. Townsend, and W. F. McGhan. 1996. *Principles of pharmacoeconomics,* 2d ed. Cincinnati, Ohio: Harvey Whitney Books.

Catsambas, T., and S. D. Foster. 1986. Spending money sensibly: The case of essential drugs. *Finance and Development* 23:29–32.

★ Drummond, M. F., G. L. Stoddart, and G. W. Torrance. 1987. *Methods for the economic evaluation of health care programmes.* Oxford: Oxford Medical Publications.

Gafni, A., and S. Birch. 1993. Guidelines for the adoption of new technologies: A prescription for uncontrolled growth in expenditures and how to avoid the problem. *Canadian Medical Association Journal* 148:913–17.

Haaijer-Ruskamp, F. M., and M. N. G. Dukes. 1990. *Drugs and money: The problem of cost containment.* Copenhagen: World Health Organization and University of Groningen.

★ Hanson, K., and L. Gilson. 1992. *Cost, resource use, and financing methodology: A practical manual.* New York: UNICEF Bamako Initiative Management Unit.

Hanushek, E. A., and W. S. Comanor. 1986. The political economy of the pharmaceutical industry. *Journal of Economic Literature* 24:1178–1217.

Henry, D. 1992. Economic analysis as an aid to subsidisation decisions: The development of Australian guidelines for pharmaceuticals. *PharmacoEconomics* 1:54–67.

★ Jamison, D. T. 1993. Disease control priorities in developing countries: An overview. In *Disease control priorities in developing countries,* ed. D. T. Jamison, W. H. Mosley, A. R. Measham, and J. L. Bobadilla. New York: Oxford University Press.

Kinnon, C. M., G. Velásquez, and Y.-A. Flori. 1994. *Health economics: A guide to selected WHO literature.* WHO/TFHE/94.1. Geneva: World Health Organization.

Laupacis, A., D. Feeny, A. S. Detsky, and P. X. Tugwell. 1992. How attractive does a new technology have to be to warrant adoption and utilisation? Tentative guidelines for using clinical and economic evaluations. *Canadian Medical Association Journal* 146:473–81.

MSH (Management Sciences for Health). 1992. Systematic cost reduction (trainer's and participant's guides). In *Managing drug supply training series.* Part 1. *Policy issues in managing drug supply.* Boston: MSH.

Phelps, C. E. 1992. *Health economics.* New York: HarperCollins.

WHO (World Health Organization). 1988. *Health economics: A programme for action.* Geneva: WHO.

★ WHO (World Health Organization). 1994. *Cost analysis in primary health care: A training manual for programme managers.* Geneva: WHO.

World Bank. 1993. *World development report 1993: Investing in health.* New York: Oxford University Press.

Part I **Introduction**	Part II Policy and Legal Framework	Part III Drug Management Cycle	Part IV Management Support Systems

1 Toward Sustainable Supply and
   Rational Use of Drugs

2 Historical and Institutional Perspectives

3 Economics for Drug Management

**4 Pharmaceutical Supply System
   Assessment**

Chapter 4
Pharmaceutical Supply System Assessment

≡ Summary

Pharmaceutical system assessments are useful to diagnose problems, plan major projects and interventions, monitor progress, and compare the performance of one system with another.

To produce useful results, all assessments should be structured. Two approaches may be useful:

1. *Comprehensive structured assessment, which generally involves a full-time, dedicated team using structured survey instruments to gather data through site visits, but may be done as a self-assessment exercise by managers;*
2. *Limited assessment, which uses interviews and document reviews.*

Three major categories of issues should be addressed:

1. *The functionality of the public-sector system;*
2. *The capacity and interest of the private sector;*
3. *"Political mapping" to understand the important actors and their attitudes and the feasibility of successfully implementing changes in the pharmaceutical system.*

Specific information objectives should be set in advance, incorporating quantitative as well as qualitative data, performance indicators, and special-purpose analyses.

The most important methods for collecting information are likely to be document review, key informant interviews, collection of data from existing records, and prospective observation.

Key issues in planning and managing the assessment are listed in this chapter, but readers should obtain one or more of the starred manuals listed in "References and Further Readings" for full details on organizing and conducting an assessment. Once the data are in hand, it is necessary to analyze the data efficiently and produce a user-friendly report, supplemented by presentations using graphic aids to help key decision-makers absorb the findings. The assessment results must be used in developing new policies and procedures for the pharmaceutical system; otherwise, the process is a waste of resources.

≡ 4.1 Reasons for Assessing Pharmaceutical Systems

Sustainable improvements in the pharmaceutical sector depend on high-level national commitment to improvement, technically sound plans based on an accurate situation assessment, and the technical and financial resources to implement proposed changes.

High-level commitment to pharmaceutical sector improvements can be stimulated by discontent among health staff and the public about drug shortages, concern in the ministry of finance about rising drug expenditures, or publicity about poor drug quality. Too often, however, the pressure resulting from this commitment leads to hasty assessments and inadequately developed plans for change.

Accurate systematic assessment is a prerequisite for planning changes in the pharmaceutical sector and, in particular, in the drug supply system. Pharmaceutical sector assessments can serve any of four main purposes:

1. Diagnosing emergent problems in the system;
2. Planning a project;
3. Monitoring change in the supply system;
4. Comparing the performance of the supply system with that of other systems.

Diagnosing Emergent Problems
Accurate diagnosis and action are urgently needed when there are major problems: drugs are out of stock in the rural health facilities, patients and politicians are complaining, and money is short. The assessment in such cases must be done quickly, but it still needs to yield a thorough understanding of where the various subcomponents in the pharmaceutical system are functioning and where they are not, what factors are involved, and what sorts of interventions might be feasible and effective.

Planning Pharmaceutical Management Projects
Systematic assessments should be done before all major pharmaceutical management projects and certainly as part of the process of developing a national drug policy (or making any significant legal or policy changes related to pharmaceuticals). When a project is being planned, the preproject assessment should define precisely the problems to be addressed, the interventions and expected outcomes, and the resource requirements in terms of capital, equipment, infrastructure improvements, recurrent expenditures, and technical assistance.

Monitoring Changes
Once an intervention is undertaken, it should be assessed periodically to measure progress and determine whether

strategy changes are warranted. At the end of the project, another assessment should look at process and outcome to determine the extent of change in the system, whether the reforms appear to be sustainable, and whether additional inputs are needed.

Comparing the Performance of Different Systems

An assessment may be needed to compare the effectiveness of one pharmaceutical management system with that of others. For example, an assessment might address two vertical distribution systems (such as drugs and contraceptives in the Ministry of Health [MOH], or MOH and social security) to ascertain how well each is functioning and whether opportunities exist for integrating them. Or the goal might be to compare the strengths and weaknesses of the public and private pharmaceutical sectors to determine what potential exists for collaboration.

Comprehensive Structured Assessments

This chapter proposes comprehensive structured assessments for accurately diagnosing problems in the drug supply system, identifying their causes, prioritizing the problems, developing short- and long-term action plans, and providing indicators for monitoring progress. When a comprehensive structured assessment is carried out with full government commitment by an appropriate expert team (local or international), it enables the government to formulate a sound strategy for improving access, rational drug use, and drug quality. It also provides government officials with a basis for coordinating donor involvement (see Chapter 43). Country Study 4.1 is an example from Russia.

Proposals for pharmaceutical sector assessments sometimes meet with resistance. Decision-makers may believe that action is needed instead of another study. Managers may think that they already know the nature and causes of problems. Government officials responsible for donor coordination may be weary from the seemingly innumerable visits from representatives of donors and technical assistance organizations who ask the same questions but leave little behind. And some donors may prefer action to research.

In such situations, the general nature of the problems may be evident, but the true causes are often not so clearly known, and the full range of solutions that could produce sustainable improvements has not been considered. An assessment *is* needed, but an assessment of a different nature from those previously experienced.

A comprehensive assessment can be an invaluable input into the development of a national drug policy (Chapter 5) or a strategic plan for pharmaceutical sector development

---

Country Study 4.1 Collaborative Study in Russia

A US Agency for International Development project received funding to work with Russian oblasts (states) in 1993 to improve pharmaceutical availability. The initial Russian reaction was that no assessment should be done, because local managers knew everything about the system—the only problem was a shortage of funds. However, the project paper mandated an assessment prior to any assistance, so the oblast chosen for initial assistance grudgingly agreed to a structured field visit assessment. Counterparts from the state pharmacy committee and the primary state hospital worked with external project staff to develop and field-test a survey instrument, based on earlier assessment documents used in Africa, Latin America, the eastern Caribbean, and other regions. The assessment was carried out cooperatively by external and local staff, who also worked together to produce the report.

Russian officials consider the report to be the most comprehensive report ever done on pharmaceutical systems in the country. The results of the assessment ended up being a big hit with local managers, as they reviewed the assembled data and learned how funds were really being spent for drug purchases, how many different drugs were being purchased, how price controls affected pharmacy viability, and where resource gaps were most urgent. Perhaps most importantly, the process brought political managers and health system managers together in an effort to understand the real situation and their options for solving the problems. The oblast has now become a leader in the country in implementing institutional formulary lists, developing a viable strategy for price controls, and licensing and regulating private pharmacies.

(Chapter 35). The assessments discussed in this chapter do not take the place of an ongoing monitoring program (Chapter 36) or a management information system that tracks and reports on performance (Chapter 45). When good management information systems and monitoring programs are in place, the need for special-purpose assessment decreases, as does the effort and expense required to carry out an assessment when it is indicated.

≡ 4.2 Structure of the Assessment

Every pharmaceutical system assessment should have a formal structure; otherwise, any observations, conclusions, and recommendations are wholly subjective, and the opinion of one expert (or assessment team) may be radically different from that of another expert or team that has visited the same offices and talked to the same people. García-Núñez (1992, 49) stresses the need for structure in assessment and project evaluation: "A person who visits a project and conducts a casual assessment of project activities is not conducting an evaluation. He/she is merely making observations. Individual unsubstantiated assessments should not be used as tools for decision making. Evaluations have to be conducted according to specific guidelines and procedures. Without a recognized framework from which to draw conclusions, evaluation results are not credible."

Country Study 4.2 gives an example of an assessment using unstructured methods that failed to produce the necessary results; there are many others from recent history around the world.

The primary questions to be answered when structuring a pharmaceutical system assessment are:

► What issues should be addressed in the assessment?
► What potential information sources exist?
► What information should be collected?
► What methods will be used to collect the information?
► What sort of team will do the assessment?
► What is the time frame and cost for the assessment?
► How will the study be managed?
► How will the results be presented for use by decision-makers?

In order to fit the structure of the assessment to a specific purpose, many different combinations of answers might be appropriate. The rest of the chapter explores options that can be considered.

Prerequisites for Assessment

Assessment approaches range from self-assessment by health system managers to assessment by a team of local experts to assessment by a full-time team of local and external experts doing extensive site visits. The approach should be tailored to the scope of the assessment and the quantity of data and quality of analysis needed for decision support. There are four prerequisites for success with any of the approaches discussed in this section:

1. Government commitment to the process;
2. A qualified assessment team;
3. A clear definition of objectives and procedures;
4. An unbiased approach.

Government Commitment. For a systematic assessment to be successful in public-sector programs, government commitment and active involvement are essential. If the study team is denied access to essential data or if key informants are never available, it will be difficult to produce useful results. Even if a report is produced, the likelihood of fruitful follow-up is greatly reduced without active senior-level commitment to improvements.

Country Study 4.2 Unstructured Assessments

In one African country, several teams of international experts were given the responsibility of assessing the status of the public drug supply system and quantifying resource needs for a World Bank loan. All the teams were experienced in the drug management field, but none of the teams used a structured assessment approach—each team leader was free to develop his or her own methodology. The team responsible for identifying needs for equipment and infrastructure forgot to consider cold-chain equipment. Thus, the budget allocated for cold-chain equipment in the eventual project was a pure guess. The team assigned to evaluate treatment patterns and develop algorithms for morbidity-based quantification developed a treatment manual that was useless for quantification. Another team was assigned to look at the potential for private-sector collaboration in the public system; the team prepared a nice report on the issues that might be assessed but did not actually do the assessment. When decisions had to be made concerning what type of logistics system would be supported, there were no data on private-sector capacity. This gap was still in evidence five years later, when the country and the World Bank were again trying to figure out a way to salvage a viable pharmaceutical system.

Top management support must be translated into making sure that operations staff cooperate with the assessment and that health system staff assigned to the assessment actually participate fully in the process.

Qualified Assessment Team. The team doing the assessment must be familiar with the intricacies of pharmaceutical systems in general and the local pharmaceutical sector in particular. The team also must be familiar with national administrative structures, the national health system, and local development experience. The team principals must be motivated and qualified to collect and analyze data and present the results in an organized fashion. Outside experts are not always essential, but they can supplement local expertise by offering experience in comparable countries, a broader view, and an independent perspective.

Clearly Defined Objectives and Procedures. Various assessment approaches and methods are discussed below; all have their place, but no matter which combination of methods is used, the goals, procedures, data to be collected, scope of the study, participants, and time frame should be clearly defined before the assessment begins. Once established, the structure should be followed within the bounds of normal constraints.

The assessment should be tailored to fit the purpose. The assessment may be broad in scope, in order to design a major essential drugs project, or it might have a limited focus, such as determining how many vehicles are needed for drug distribution in a single region. Even in the latter example, the assessment should be structured broadly enough so that all potential options are identified (including contracts with the private sector).

Unbiased Approach. The assessment should be undertaken without preconceived notions as to what the findings will or should be. When a total lack of bias is not possible, all parties to the study should clearly understand what preconceptions exist.

A biased assessment may not identify the real causes of problems or consider all options for solution. For example, if an assessment is begun with the premise that all pharmaceutical services in the health system must be provided by government, it will probably overlook or downplay the potential for private-sector and nongovernmental organization (NGO) participation.

Assessment Approaches

The two most common approaches to pharmaceutical system assessment are comprehensive structured assessment and limited assessment.

Comprehensive Structured Assessment. A comprehensive structured assessment gathers information from all levels of the pharmaceutical system. A specific team is responsible for making field visits to offices, warehouses, and health facilities and gathering multiple types of information through document review, interviews, data collection from records, and prospective observation. Preprinted survey instruments are used to collect data, which helps ensure that a standard set of information is collected at each field site.

The survey instruments are structured questionnaires and data collection forms; they may be designed for a specific assessment or adapted from manuals (see MSH/RPM 1995; WHO/DAP 1994). This type of assessment is often done as a rapid, intensive exercise by a full-time, dedicated team in cooperation with pharmaceutical system counterparts, but it can also be done as a self-assessment exercise by managers in the health system. The self-assessment option requires less incremental funding but is likely to take more time, and the usefulness of the results will depend on the willingness of officials to document and report problems.

Limited Assessment. Limited assessments rely primarily on interviews and document review, with limited field visits and little if any primary data collection from records or prospective observation. The assessment may be done by a small dedicated team or by a working group from the pharmaceutical system. The assessment normally has a scope of work and should follow a predefined assessment plan, but this approach does not usually use preprinted survey instruments and data collection forms. Because the scope is limited and time is not needed to prepare and validate survey instruments, a limited assessment can usually be completed more quickly and less expensively than a comprehensive structured assessment.

In some cases, a limited assessment obtains a great deal of information; the constraint is that the information tends to be whatever is provided by the officials interviewed. When a structured survey instrument is not used, the quantity and type of data obtained may not be consistent from site to site, which may hamper efforts to compile a valid picture of the whole system.

Time Frame and Assessment Costs

The financial and human resources required for an assessment obviously depend primarily on the assessment approach. A locally managed self-assessment can be done in two or three months at low incremental cost, although a few thousand dollars (or the equivalent) would probably be needed to cover travel costs, meeting expenses, forms, and communication costs.

A typical limited assessment involves two to six person-weeks for site visits, plus another person-week or so to develop a report. Costs depend on whether one or two experts are involved, but an average might be $25,000 to $50,000 to cover all costs.

Time requirements and costs for a comprehensive structured assessment vary considerably, according to the number of levels in the pharmaceutical system and the size of the country. An experienced two-person team of experts might be able to manage a structured field visit survey of public-sector pharmaceutical programs in a small country with three weeks on site, one week before for preparation, and two to three weeks after for analysis and report writing. This assumes that local officials and counterparts are active supporters and participants and that the health system has no more than three levels to be covered: central, provincial, and district. In the same country, one more experienced person plus a counterpart would be needed to cover the private sector in detail, and an additional person would be needed if there were more levels in the public-sector system.

Larger countries and more complex pharmaceutical systems require more effort for a thorough assessment; this can be managed by adding more team members or more field time for existing members, but in any case, costs will increase. If the principal assessment team members are all international consultants, the total cost of a comprehensive structured assessment for a public pharmaceutical system in a medium-sized country may vary between US$50,000 and US$150,000 (as of 1996). These are large sums, but it must be remembered that a project or development loan to be based on the assessment might be worth US$100 million.

If only government budgetary resources are available, it may not be practical to mount a comprehensive structured assessment with external consultants. However, multilateral or bilateral agencies may be prepared to support the assessment (and possibly provide experts). Even if no donors are prepared to provide financial support or experts, advice and information may be available from international agencies such as the World Health Organization (WHO) and the United Nations Children's Fund (UNICEF).

≡ 4.3 Defining the Scope of the Assessment

The issues that *should* be addressed in an assessment depend on its purpose; the issues that *can* be addressed depend on the availability of information, the capacities of the assessment team, and the time frame allowed to collect information (discussed in the previous section). Issues of importance to the pharmaceutical system fall into one of three general categories:

1. Functionality of the public-sector pharmaceutical system;
2. Private-sector capacity;
3. Political situation and attitudes of major players and interest groups in the pharmaceutical sector.

To understand and solve widespread problems in a pharmaceutical system, a broad assessment covering all three categories is needed. If the assessment is looking at only one vertical program or one aspect of the system (for example, drug use in rural health facilities), the scope will be narrower, but many of the issues discussed in this section still need to be considered, if on a smaller scale.

Functionality of the Public Pharmaceutical System

A comprehensive pharmaceutical system assessment needs to look at several subcategories of functions. There are many ways to categorize the functions of a public pharmaceutical system; the following list is drawn mainly from the indicator manuals discussed in Section 4.4:

Policy, legislation, and regulation: Are policies, laws and regulations consistent, comprehensive, and current? Are they enforced?

Budget and finance: What sources of funds are available? Are the funds adequate to purchase all necessary drugs and to manage the pharmaceutical system effectively?

Are the funds that are available effectively managed?

Drug selection: How are drugs selected for use in the system? Are there consistent policies and procedures, or is the choice up to each purchaser and prescriber?

Pharmaceutical procurement: Is there an effective procurement system that gets good prices and manages to purchase drugs in the quantities and time frame needed?

Pharmaceutical logistics: Are drugs well managed at storage facilities and available at the points where they are needed? Are there major losses due to expiration or theft?

Drug utilization: Do prescribers, dispensers, and patients use drugs rationally, or are there major problems with irrational use?

Product quality assurance: Are the products that are purchased and used in the supply system of good quality? Are quality assurance programs adequate to ensure good product quality?

System management: Are there adequate quantities of well-trained managers and operations-level staff at each level of the system? Are modern personnel management and training programs in place? Are salaries adequate to promote good performance?

Monitoring and management information: Are there effective monitoring programs in place at each level of the system? Is there an effective management information system that lets managers track supplies and funds throughout the pharmaceutical system?

Assessment guides at the end of each chapter in Parts II, III, and IV of this manual contain suggestions about the information needed to answer these types of questions and, more importantly, to understand why problems exist and what can be done about them.

When defining the scope of a particular assessment, it is necessary to determine what information will likely be available in that pharmaceutical system from government documents, records, and reports; from interviews with system managers and staff; and from officials in related government offices and ministries. Information access varies from country to country; access largely determines how detailed an assessment is feasible and sensible.

Private-Sector Capacity

Interest is growing in many countries about the potential for incorporating private-sector services into the public pharmaceutical system, particularly when problems in the public system seem intractable. Any assessment that is done in the context of major problems in the public pharmaceutical system should investigate private-sector capacity and the potential for public-private collaboration of the sort outlined in Chapter 6. Note that such investigations should encompass the nonprofit private sector (NGOs) as well as the for-profit private sector.

If the assessment is to address the private sector in a meaningful way, a method is needed to obtain information about the current state of the private pharmaceutical sector—the current types and levels of service provided to clients in various parts of the country, the capacity for providing services to the public sector, the attitude toward public-private collaboration, and the constraints that would need to be resolved to establish a working relationship.

The public sector may not have much reliable information on hand about the private sector, and it may be difficult to establish communication if there is a history of mutual suspicion and hostility between the private and public sectors. For some countries, it is possible to obtain reports compiled by international companies that specialize in selling industry information, but this information is expensive, not always detailed and current, and available for only a limited number of nonindustrialized countries. Most countries have associations that represent manufacturers, distributors, and pharmacies, but getting more than general information from these sources about the market and the member companies may be difficult.

In most situations, the best option for assessing private-sector capacity is a special survey of the various components of the sector (including associations and their member companies). One survey instrument that has proved successful in learning about the public and private pharmaceutical sectors in Latin America can be used in a comprehensive structured assessment (MSH/RPM 1994).

Political Mapping

An assessment aimed at making significant changes in the pharmaceutical system needs to define the consequences of potential changes. The assessment should also determine which politically powerful individuals and interest groups are likely to support potential changes, which will be actively opposed to change, and which will be basically indifferent. This process, called *political mapping*, is also useful in evaluating the feasibility of successfully implementing options for change.

Defining the best sources of information to map interest groups, political feasibility, and attitudes is not always simple; in most countries, the assessment team will be able to assemble at least a rudimentary map of political issues; likely consequences of various options for change; supporters and opponents of change; and individuals, organizations, companies, and interest groups that are prominent in pharmaceutical management (public or private). Truly reliable political mapping requires the active cooperation of senior managers (or ex-managers) in the government who are knowledgeable about the various political issues and interest groups but who have no personal stake in the outcome of the assessment.

Political mapping is an essential component of pharmaceutical system assessment; for example, in most countries, the private pharmaceutical sector is hardly a monolith—there are often important differences in attitudes and interests between local and international manufacturers, manufacturers and distributors, chain and independent pharmacies, and so forth. As noted above, NGOs are another part of the private sector that involves people with unique views, and there are likely to be differences in interests and attitudes among the various NGOs that are active in the country.

The mapping process, if done accurately, helps define the causes of problems in the pharmaceutical system, examine the likely consequences of various changes and interventions, and determine which options are feasible and sustainable. Reich and Cooper (1995) describe political mapping in more detail and offer computer software to assist with the organization and interpretation of information.

≡ 4.4 Defining the Information Targets

Once the issues to be addressed and the assessment approach and time frame have been determined, the next step is to define the specific set of qualitative and quantitative data targeted for collection. In many cases, these data are collected in the form of standard performance indicators and are later organized into tables that provide insight into the pharmaceutical system.

Quantitative and Qualitative Data

Quantitative data describe *what* the situation is—for example, the percentage of a list of essential drugs that is available in a sample of health facilities. *Qualitative data* provide insights into *why* the situation is as it is—for example, why key informants believe that essential drugs are not more widely available.

Because collecting a valid sample of quantitative data can be more time consuming and involve more work than conducting a series of qualitative informant interviews, many reports on country pharmaceutical systems contain very little quantitative data and many unsubstantiated observations from informants. When an assessment does not gather quantitative data for analysis and comparison, it is difficult to know the magnitude of problems or to know how much a situation has changed over time. At the same time, qualitative information is essential to understanding quantitative data, the reasons that specific weaknesses and constraints exist, and what strategies might be effective in overcoming the problem.

As noted, a properly structured assessment gathers and interprets both quantitative and qualitative information; problems with imbalance usually result when there is no formal structure for an assessment. Chapter 29 discusses issues related to quantitative and qualitative data; for more information, see the starred entries in "References and Further Readings."

Performance Indicators

Performance indicators are standardized measurements that theoretically mean the same thing in every country; for that reason, they are widely used to compare the performance of different businesses, economies, and societies. Perhaps the best known set of indicators in international development is published annually by the World Bank in the *World Development Report*; the 1993 edition focused on health issues (World Bank 1993).

Performance indicators should be the foundation for ongoing monitoring in the pharmaceutical system (see Chapter 36) and should also be a fundamental part of any pharmaceutical system assessment. Indicators to assess and monitor public pharmaceutical systems are a relatively recent development, and the optimal indicators to measure system performance have not been fully determined. Several sets of proposed performance indicators for pharmaceutical management systems have been developed; three of them are discussed in Box 4.1.

Defining Information Targets for a Specific Assessment

There are three guiding principles for setting information targets for a specific assessment:

1. Get all the information needed for the purpose, within time limitations, but do not gather data that are unnecessary (doing so wastes time and effort in two phases of the process—collection and analysis).
2. Make sure that the data used in producing analyses and recommendations are as reliable as possible, and know which data are reliable and which are not.
3. Define information targets based on what is available, and do not try to collect information that is nonexistent or impossible to retrieve.

Country Study 4.3 shows some of the information targets for a pharmaceutical system assessment done in Ecuador in 1994.

≡ 4.5 Methods for Collecting Information

The basic methods of obtaining information in a pharmaceutical system assessment are:

- ► document review;
- ► key informant interviews;
- ► collection of data from existing records;
- ► prospective studies.

This chapter summarizes these methods (see also Chapter 29 and INRUD 1995; WHO/DAP 1993; MSH/RPM 1995).

Document Review

Most countries have conducted studies of problems in the pharmaceutical sector and have made attempts to correct them. When donors have been involved in improving pharmaceutical services, there are likely to be many relevant reports. Government agencies can provide budget reports and, in many cases, files of technical reports by various agencies on the pharmaceutical sector. It is also useful to contact international agencies such as WHO, UNICEF, or the World Bank; bilateral donors; and technical assistance organizations to obtain copies of relevant documents.

A review of the literature should be one of the first steps in any assessment. Failure to include this important step inevitably results in a waste of time and money for regathering data that are already available and reinventing analyses and recommendations that duplicate those already made. Worse, interventions that have been unsuccessful in the past may be tried again, with similar lack of success.

Key Informant Interviews

Interviews are the quickest way to learn about urgent problems, if the assessment team is able to identify the people who are most knowledgeable about the situation and if these people are prepared to discuss the situation frankly.

Interviews may be misleading, however, if the informants are not fully frank due to fear of retribution or if they have some vested interest in hiding or distorting information. Nevertheless, interviews are essential for insight into the political and administrative processes, which are major determinants of whether assessments will lead to real action.

Interviews may be conducted with or without structure. In the unstructured format, the interviewer relies on personal experience to ask relevant questions and to make sure that important issues are not overlooked. In the structured approach, the interviewer uses a written survey form

Box 4.1 Examples of Indicators in Drug Management

Working in collaboration with USAID, the International Network for Rational Use of Drugs (INRUD), the Harvard Drug Policy Research Group, and the Pan American Health Organization (PAHO) Essential Drugs Program, the Management Sciences for Health (MSH) Drug Management Program developed and field-tested an initial list of thirty-three indicators plus methods for data collection in 1993. Under the auspices of the USAID-supported Rational Pharmaceutical Management Project, this indicator set and manual have been further tested and revised to include forty-six indicators for the rapid assessment of pharmaceutical systems.

Results from field tests and use in pharmaceutical assessments are shown in the accompanying figure; comparative data are shown for only thirty-five indicators, because the last expansion to forty-six indicators occurred after many of these studies were done. The manual that documents this rapid assessment method also provides practical guidelines for organizing and completing a structured field visit assessment (MSH/RPM 1995).

The *World Drug Situation* (WHO 1988) presented a substantial amount of quantitative data on drug availability and consumption and qualitative ratings as to country status and performance. This publication stimulated widespread interest in pharmaceutical management indicators.

In 1994, the WHO Action Programme on Essential Drugs published a manual that proposed a set of thirty-one background information indicators, fifty structural indicators, thirty-eight process indicators, and ten outcome indicators, primarily for self-assessment by countries (WHO/DAP 1994). Field-testing was in progress as this book went to print.

The Australian Commonwealth Department of Human Services and Health recently adapted the WHO indicator format to develop drug policy indicators focused on drug use (CDHSH 1994). This set has forty-one process indicators, twenty-seven impact indicators, and six outcome indicators. The indicators are used to monitor the services of the Pharmaceutical Benefits Scheme and the effects of the national drug policy.

Pharmaceutical Sector Data for Eight Countries and One Region

	Mozambique 1993	Ghana 1993	Ecuador 1994	El Salvador 1993	Guatemala 1992	Nicaragua[a] 1994	Jamaica 1992	OECS[b] 1993	Nepal 1993
Policy, Legislation, and Regulation									
1. Existence of a government-approved national drug policy	No	No	Yes	No	Yes	No	Yes	No	No
2. Existence of drug control legislation, regulations, and enforcement agencies	No	Yes	Yes	No	Yes		Yes	No	Yes
3. % of unregistered drugs in private-sector sales outlets	N/A	N/A	N/A	23%	7.3%		21%	100%	
4. Type of drug registration system	None	Manual	Mixed	Manual	Computerized		Manual	None	Manual
5. Law regarding generic substitution	N/A	No	No	No	No	No	No	No	No
Formulary/National Essential Drugs List and Drug Information									
1. Number of unique drug products on national drug formulary list (NDFL)	383	222	438	284	428	234	1,010	388	261
2. Existence of an official manual, based on the NDFL, providing basic therapeutic information (revised within last 5 years)	No	No	Yes	Yes	Yes	No	Yes	Yes	Yes
3. % of visited ministry of health (MOH) facilities with the most current edition of an official manual based on the NDFL	100%	45%	70%	0%	0%	7%	N/A	100%	N/A
4. Existence of MOH-approved drug information center	No	No	No	Yes	Yes	Yes		No	No

MOH Budget and Finance									
1. MOH pharmaceutical budget/expenditure per capita	$.62	$0.46c	$.25	$4.96	$3.93	$1.13	$1.98	$5.50	
2. % of total government recurrent budget used for MOH budget	6%	14%		15%	15%	16%	3%	12%	
3. % of total MOH recurrent budget allocated to pharmaceuticals	2%	No budget		4%	26%		8%	6%	4%
MOH Pharmaceutical Procurement									
1. Existence of policy limiting MOH pharmaceutical procurement to drugs on NDFL/NEDL	Yes	Yes	Yes	Yes	Yes	Yes	Yes	Yes	Yes
2. % by value of MOH drugs purchased through a central procurement system	100%	N/A	<50%	80%	27%		80%	100%	N/A
3. % of average international price paid for last regular procurement of a set of indicator drugs	76–205%	79%		114%	164–371%		145%	147%	63%
4. % of MOH drugs centrally purchased through competitive tender	91%	45%d	28%	80%	10%		95%	100%	50%
MOH Pharmaceutical Logistics									
1. Weighted average % of inventory variation in stock record-keeping system at central medical stores (CMS), regional medical stores (RMS), and health facilities (HF) — Tally: CMS	124%	0%	5%	0%	5%	8%	48%	19%	
RMS		3%				8%			
HF		11%	38%						
Ledger: CMS	159%	15%							
RMS		5%							
HF		16%							
2. % of a set of unexpired indicator drugs available in MOH health facilities — CMS	67%	100%		94%	93%	89%	100%	79%	
RMS	80%	87%	72%	81%		72%	95%	58%	
HF	59%	60%	46%	78%	60%				
3. Average % of time out of stock for indicator drugs — CMS		8%		23%	32%	21%	27%	15%	
RMS		7%				13%			
HF		11%	12%						
Patient Access and Drug Utilization									
1. Population per MOH health facility that dispenses drugs	13,798	35,253	6,307	14,430	8,529	8,622	5,855	3,945	15,600
2. Average number of drugs prescribed per curative outpatient encounter in MOH health facilities	2.4	4.3	2.0	2.2	1.4	2.1	2.4	2.0	2.1
3. % of drugs prescribed by generic name in MOH health facilities	99%	59%	39%	72%	71%	86%	40%	49%	44%
4. % of outpatients prescribed injections in MOH health facilities	20%	56%	19%	7%	13%	10%	4%	2%	5%

(cont.)

Box 4.1 Examples of Indicators in Drug Management (cont.)

	Mozambique 1993	Ghana 1993	Ecuador 1994	El Salvador 1993	Guatemala 1992	Nicaragua[a] 1994	Jamaica 1992	OECS[b] 1993	Nepal 1993
Patient Access and Drug Utilization (cont.)									
5. % of outpatients prescribed antibiotics in MOH health facilities	52%	47%	42%	32%	27%	34%	30%	39%	43%
6. % of drugs prescribed that are actually dispensed in MOH health facilities	77%	86%				61%	92%	84%	83%
Product Quality Assurance									
1. MOH drug product quality checks during the past year									
a. Number of drug products tested	N/A	<10	N/A	N/A	0			43	N/A
b. Total number of drug product quality tests performed	N/A	N/A	N/A	3,042	0			N/A	960
2. Use of WHO certification scheme	Limited	Limited	Yes	No	Limited	No	Limited	Limited	Limited
3. Existence of a formal system for reporting product quality complaints	None	None	None	None	Limited	None	None	Functional	None
Private-Sector Pharmaceutical Activity									
1. Population per licensed private-sector drug sales outlet	285,156	3,438	3,569	4,835	4,805		9,720	8,178	
2. Number of licensed drug outlets per government drug inspector	19	262		No inspectors	947		63	One Grenada inspector[e]	
3. Total value of private-sector retail pharmaceutical sales per capita	$.08	N/A	$18.98	$11.09	$10.98		$10.29	N/A	
4. Value of MOH pharmaceutical expenditures and private-sector retail sales per capita	$.70	N/A	$19.23	$16.05	$14.91		$12.27	N/A	
5. % of products on NDFL that are manufactured or co-manufactured within the country	1%	70%		50%	71%		15–20%	0%	7%
6. Existence of price controls for drugs in the private sector	No	Yes	Yes			Yes		No	
7. % of licensed retail drug outlets where an antibiotic was available without a prescription		85%	95%	100%	100%			N/A	

Source: Management Sciences for Health, Rational Pharmaceutical Management Project.

Notes: All dollar amounts are in US dollars. N/A indicates that information was not available despite attempts to collect it. Blanks indicate that these indicators were not part of the original study.

[a] Nicaragua results are based on two regional/intermediate medical stores and twenty health facilities, which may not represent the country as a whole.

[b] OECS is the Organization of Eastern Caribbean States. The countries studied included Dominica, Grenada, Montserrat, St. Kitts and Nevis, St. Lucia, and St. Vincent and the Grenadines.

[c] Ghana CMS purchases only; there were also substantial direct purchases by regional stores and health facilities.

[d] Eighty-seven percent of the Ghana central procurement was done competitively; about 52% of the drugs purchased by regional stores came through the central agency. Thus, about 45% of the MOH drugs were purchased competitively.

[e] The other OECS countries do not have any inspectors.

listing the important questions and the qualitative and quantitative information to be solicited.

There are advantages and disadvantages with both formats. The unstructured interview allows a free flow of conversation and may promote a more revealing interview. It is easy to overlook important issues, however, and it is difficult to collate and analyze responses from a series of such interviews, particularly if different interviewers are involved. The structured interview is usually more formal but is more likely to ensure that all important issues are addressed by each interviewer and that the responses are ordered in a manner that facilitates analysis.

Data Collection from Records

This is a critical step in all structured assessments and should be done at each site where reasonably well-organized, complete, and current records exist. Where records are totally disorganized and badly out-of-date, the information gained may not be worth the effort, and other methods will be needed.

Relevant records include government publications on budgets and expenditures, patient medical records, pharmacy dispensing records, records of procurement and accounts payable to suppliers, warehouse ledgers, bin cards and computer records, and accounting and finance records.

Data Collection by Prospective Field Observation

When needed information cannot be obtained from a retrospective review of records, it may be possible to use prospective observation to obtain the information. For example, one method of reviewing prescribing practices in a health facility is to examine clinical charts and dispensing records. If these records are not available, the team can observe patient encounters directly and record the prescribing in that manner (a patient exit survey).

Some types of data are best obtained by prospective methods. For example, to determine whether private pharmacies are selling prescription-only drugs without a prescription, the best method is a simulated purchase survey, where local data collectors visit a sample of pharmacies and actually attempt to purchase prescription drugs.

Other Methods for Collecting Qualitative Information

Other common methods for obtaining useful data include focus groups and household surveys. These techniques can be important tools in determining why attitudes and practices exist in one group or another (see Chapter 29).

Country Study 4.3 Information Targets for an Assessment in Ecuador

The following list is an excerpt of information targets set for a structured field-visit assessment of public and private pharmaceutical systems in Ecuador in 1994; the assessment surveyed both public- and private-sector systems and capacities and was designed to assist the Ministry of Health (MOH) in considering options for reforming and decentralizing the procurement and distribution of drugs. The complete set of information targets (and the structured survey instruments used to collect the data) can be obtained from the MSH Drug Management Program.

► Total health budget and expenditures for procurement of drugs for the MOH, social security system, and armed forces. Current year and previous two years if possible. Size of private-sector market (wholesale or retail) in same years. Public-sector markets as a percentage of total market. Debts owed to the private sector for public drug purchases.

► Description of the private pharmaceutical market, with tables showing the number of firms at each level and the areas of the country covered. Tables should show the number of products and estimated annual sales for major firms.

► List of suppliers that distribute directly to private pharmacies in each province, with number of health areas served. Estimated service level from private pharmacy survey.

► Table of private companies that could manage public storage and/or transport, with areas of country served, storage and transport capacity, and constraints on providing services to the public. Estimated service level from survey.

► Based on survey of private firms, attitude toward providing service to public sector, constraints reported, and estimation of the likely percentage impact on tender prices of estimated quantity contracts, therapeutic category tendering, central versus decentralized ordering and payment, increasing or decreasing procurement volume, or special packaging for MOH purchases.

► Description of the system by which private firms set prices and provide discounts and payment terms to clients. Description of the official system for price control, and efforts to enforce the system.

► For a sample of indicator drugs:

  —official controlled price

  —average actual price from distributors

  —average retail price

  —average sale price in sample of public pharmacies

  —average sale price in community drug sales program

  —tender price obtained by parastatal

  —sales price from parastatal to public pharmacies

  —average international price

≡ 4.6 Planning and Managing the Assessment

The key issues in planning most assessments are

- defining the assessment approach;
- defining and locating financial resources;
- defining management and technical responsibilities;
- developing a draft workplan.

Once these issues are resolved, a management plan is developed by the leader of the assessment team. The issues that must be covered in the plan are

- making logistics arrangements;
- preparing a system overview;
- selecting sites to be visited;
- selecting indicator drugs;
- defining data collection methods;
- developing and refining data collection forms;
- selecting and training data collectors;
- revising the workplan to its final form.

These issues are relevant to most comprehensive structured assessments, and they are covered in great detail in MSH/RPM 1995 and WHO/DAP 1994, which are available without charge. Any country or supply system that is planning a pharmaceutical assessment should get these manuals to aid in its planning and execution.

Given proper preparation, the actual data collection process may go relatively smoothly and produce reliable data for evaluation. However, it is safe to assume that the assessment will not proceed entirely according to the workplan, no matter how well it was thought out. There will be minor frustrations, such as the unavailability of some key team members, weather-related delays for some site visits, and the unexpected absence of key informants. These can be worked around, as long as the assessment team maintains its flexibility and sense of humor. Major problems such as widespread work stoppages can shut down the entire public health system and make it necessary to postpone the assessment, if it has not started, or interrupt the study until the facilities reopen.

Data Analysis

When a large amount of quantitative data is available on costs, purchases, drug consumption, and utilization patterns, it must be organized to facilitate analysis. Chapter 41 is devoted to the issue of analyzing data to understand and control costs in the drug supply system; most of the analytical techniques in that chapter can and should be incorporated into assessment information targets, if necessary data are available. Several other chapters offer suggestions for organizing data to facilitate analysis during an assessment (see Chapters 29, 36, 42, and 45).

To avoid confusion and haste at the end of an assessment, it is advisable to collate and prepare assessment data for analysis as they are collected (see Chapter 45). If a computerized program such as Epi Info (see Chapter 46) is used for collating survey results, data should be entered at night by team members or a local data-entry person. Both team members and counterparts should play an active role in examining data that are recovered and considering what sorts of additional analyses may be appropriate beyond those prescribed in the assessment workplan.

Preparing the Assessment Report

Chapter 45 discusses how to interpret data from a pharmaceutical management information system. The issues are similar for interpreting results from assessments. No matter how well the assessment was designed, planned, and executed, the data obtained may not be totally reliable. Part of the job of the study team is to determine what sorts of biases, inaccuracies, or inconsistencies may exist and what precautions are necessary in interpreting the data. The report itself must be presented in a way that helps the decision-makers who need to use the information; a clear outline and executive summary of not more than two pages, which includes a statement of the next steps, are important. The methodology and detailed results can be referred to in the text and appended to keep the document concise for interested but nonspecialist readers.

Presentations and Seminars

Many key decision-makers may not have the time to read the whole report. Presentations and seminars are excellent ways to convey important results directly and may be useful before the final report is written, providing feedback for clarification. Charts and graphs are important visual aids to organize the presentation and ensure that key points are covered.

Country Study 4.4 shows how a presentation might be structured for one aspect of the assessment. Actual examples of graphic presentations of findings from a drug use assessment are found in Chapter 29.

Using the Assessment Results

An assessment should be seen as only one of several steps involved in planning and implementing pharmaceutical system changes. The assessment may be part of the development process for a donor project proposal, a national

---

Country Study 4.4 Using Graphics to Present Findings

A study of district-level pharmaceutical management was done in Ecuador in 1995 by a collaborative team representing a USAID–financed project (RPM), a World Bank–financed project (FASBASE), and MOH counterparts. The study was intended to build on the results of a larger 1994 pharmaceutical system assessment carried out jointly by the same collaborators. The following is a partial list of graphs used to present data from the assessment to assist decision-makers in absorbing the findings.

Availability of Tracer (Indicator) Drugs

- ► Bar graph: percentage of a list of tracer drugs available at area warehouses and clinical facilities (presented by site and by area);
- ► Table: percentage of time out of stock over a twelve-month period for a list of tracer drugs at area warehouses and clinical facilities (by site and area);
- ► Bar graph: percentage of facilities in each area with drugs available to treat specific health problems;
- ► Bar graph: percentage of time over a twelve-month period during which drugs were available to treat specific health problems (by site and area);
- ► Table: numbers and percentages of clinical facilities by area with a copy of standard treatment guidelines.

---

pharmaceutical sector restructuring exercise, or a national five-year development plan.

If the assessment is leading to a donor project proposal, the assessment team should be aware of this from the outset. If possible, the prospective donor should contribute to the assessment design. To encourage a sense of involvement, the prospective donor might also be given an opportunity to participate at various points in the assessment and report-writing process. The assessment team should be sure to collect all background information that may be needed. The content and format of the assessment should be compatible with what is needed for a project proposal. Depending on donor requirements, the assessment report may serve as a project proposal with little or no editing.

If the assessment is part of a national restructuring or planning exercise, it is essential to involve key government officials from the beginning. People are much more committed to implementing solutions that they have helped develop.

The whole assessment process will have been wasted if the report goes on a shelf and is not used to effect changes in policies and procedures. Follow-up may be tied to the development of national drug policies, revisions in legis-

---

Country Study 4.5 Using Assessment Results

In one African country, a ten-year project was supported in the 1980s by a consortium of bilateral donors. Cumulative funding of tens of millions of dollars was used to purchase essential drugs and to develop a system of primary care health centers served by a vertical kit distribution system. Training was done in every district of the country, focusing on proper supply management and clinical treatment. During the ten years, at least seven teams of international consultants prepared interim assessment reports on the project and its progress. None of the interim assessment teams used a structured approach to collect data; the reports provided little detail on program operations, but each provided general recommendations such as "improve procurement transparency." None of the reports had quantitative data on how actual kit distribution compared with annual plans, how well the management systems were working, or what impact the training was having.

Most recommendations from these interim assessments were apparently ignored—the same general recommendations appeared in most of the assessment reports, but without substantial documentation to justify the suggestions or the analyses of the recommendations' impact. There was no apparent follow-up on the reports. The final evaluation team, which did use a structured approach, found that kits were not reliably reaching health facilities in the districts studied. The countrywide training had not successfully instilled knowledge of good supply management or treatment practices; management information systems did not produce accurate information; and information that was available at the facility level was not effectively used in decision-making. The system was deemed unsustainable without massive additional donor support.

In contrast, in another African country, a structured assessment was done in the early 1990s with support from multiple donors and agencies. The assessment resulted in a report that documented the depth and nature of the problems, with both quantitative and qualitative analyses. The recommendations were based on the analyses and carefully justified. Both the government and the donors were convinced of the need for action and, more importantly, of the possibility of success. The result was a ten-year project aimed at reforming the pharmaceutical system, with financial support from several donors.

---

lation and regulation, and consideration of public-private collaboration. The assessment results may suggest revised policies and procedures in drug selection, procurement, distribution, and use. The assessment should guide the development of strategic plans for pharmaceutical systems (see Chapter 35) and monitoring programs, program planning, and management information systems. Country Study 4.5 looks at two examples of how assessment results were used (or not used). ∎

≡ References and Further Readings

★ = *Key readings.*

Battersby, A. 1985. How to assess health services logistics with particular reference to peripheral health facilities. WHO/SHS/85.9. Geneva: World Health Organization.

CDHSH (Commonwealth Department of Human Services and Health). 1994. *Manual of indicators to measure the effect of initiatives under quality use of medicines arm of the national medicinal drug policy.* Canberra: Australian Government Publishing Service.

García-Núñez, J. 1992. *Improving family planning evaluation.* West Hartford, Conn.: Kumarian Press.

★ INRUD (International Network for Rational Use of Drugs). 1995. *Field methods for designing drug use interventions* (working draft). INRUD secretariat. Washington, D.C.: Management Sciences for Health.

MSH/RPM (Management Sciences for Health/Rational Pharmaceutical Management Project). 1994. *Country assessment survey documents.* Washington, D.C.: MSH/RPM.

★ MSH/RPM (Management Sciences for Health/Rational Pharmaceutical Management Project). 1995. *Rapid pharmaceutical management assessment: An indicator-based approach.* Washington, D.C.: MSH/RPM.

★ Reich, M. R., and D. M. Cooper. 1995. *Political mapping: Computer assisted political analysis.* Newton, Mass.: PoliMap.

Smith, P. G., and R. H. Morrow. 1991. *Methods for field trials of interventions against tropical disease: A toolbox.* New York: Oxford University Press.

WHO (World Health Organization). 1988. *The world drug situation.* Geneva: WHO.

★ WHO/DAP (World Health Organization/Action Programme on Essential Drugs). 1993. *How to investigate drug use in health facilities: Selected drug use indicators.* Geneva: WHO/DAP.

★ WHO/DAP (World Health Organization/Action Programme on Essential Drugs). 1994. *Indicators for monitoring national drug policies.* Geneva: WHO/DAP.

World Bank. 1993. *World development report 1993: Investing in health.* New York: Oxford University Press.

Part II
Policy and Legal Framework

Part I	Part II	Part III	Part IV
Introduction	**Policy and Legal Framework**	Drug Management Cycle	Management Support Systems

5 National Drug Policies
6   Drug Supply Strategies
7   Pharmaceutical Legislation and Regulation
8   Legal Aspects of Drug Management
9   Pharmaceutical Production Policy

Chapter 5
National Drug Policies

≡ Summary

A national drug policy (NDP) is a guide for action, containing the goals set by the government for the pharmaceutical sector and the main strategies and approaches for attaining them. It provides a framework to coordinate activities of pharmaceutical sector participants: the public and private sectors, nongovernmental organizations (NGOs), donors, and other interested parties.

A nation's drug policy, although similar in many ways to those of other countries, may differ in its objectives, strategies, and approaches. National governments are the principal agency in the formulation and implementation of drug policies, leading a partnership among the government, drug prescribers, drug dispensers, drug consumers, and those who make, market, distribute, and sell drugs.

This chapter analyzes the components of an NDP. Although most of them are common to any country, priorities often need to be set. Countries must choose the components most necessary to their situation, in relation to their human and financial resources. Priority should be given to policy elements that are likely to solve key problems, such as appropriate legislation and regulation, choice of drugs, supply, financing, costs and pricing policies, and rational drug use.

This chapter reviews the main steps in NDP formulation, including

▸ *organizing the process*
▸ *identifying and analyzing problems*
▸ *setting goals and objectives*
▸ *drafting the policy*
▸ *circulating and revising the document*
▸ *obtaining formal endorsement of the policy*
▸ *launching the policy*

Formulating a policy is one thing; implementing it is another. There is no best way to implement an NDP, but this chapter presents approaches used by several countries and methods of monitoring effects of the policy as it evolves.

Experience shows that success in terms of public health is linked to an emphasis on a list of essential drugs for the public sector. An NDP should prioritize essential drugs and include comprehensive strategies to achieve their rational use. Finally, the success of an NDP depends on political commitment from the government and support from doctors and other health professionals.

≡ The second half of the twentieth century has seen the idea of a national drug policy (NDP) emerge as a positive concept. It is now widely accepted that every country should try to achieve optimal availability and use of drugs for patients and consumers. For these efforts to be coordinated and to support one another, well-designed overall drug policies need to be developed and implemented.

The NDP idea arose largely because piecemeal solutions failed in some countries. In the 1970s, efforts were made to solve problems in drug procurement and distribution without looking at drug use. The effort and resources spent on these specific issues had limited impact on the rational use of drugs. In the same way, many essential drugs programs covered only the public sector, but the private sector plays a large role in supplying essential drugs in most countries. Therefore, many of these programs had only a limited impact on drug use in the country as a whole.

These experiences suggested that drug problems might be better tackled within a common framework. The World Health Organization (WHO) has been active in developing and promoting the NDP idea, based on the essential drugs concept (see Chapter 2). As of 1995, over fifty countries had formulated NDPs, two-thirds of which had been officially adopted.

≡ 5.1 What Is a National Drug Policy?

An NDP is a guide for action. It is a document specifying the goals set by the government for the pharmaceutical sector, their relative importance, and the main strategies for attaining them. It provides a framework to coordinate activities of the pharmaceutical sector: the public and private sectors, NGOs, donors, and other interested parties.

In the developed world, many countries do not have written NDPs yet are successful in pursuing pharmaceutical sector goals. However, even in these countries, some experts advocate having a document that clearly outlines the objectives of an NDP, such as the one recently formulated in Australia.

In countries where resources are severely limited, an integrated approach to solving problems is valuable to encourage the best use of limited resources. Without a formal policy document, there may be no overall view of what is needed or how to proceed. Policies may be in conflict with one another: for example, in some East African countries, difficulties in collecting direct taxes have led to a heavier reliance on import duties and manufacturing taxes, including those from drugs. This makes imported drugs more expensive and discourages local production, so low-cost drugs are less likely to reach the people.

What Should a Drug Policy Accomplish?

The overall goal of an NDP in most cases is very general. For instance, in Malawi, the aim of the drug policy is "to develop within the available resources, the potential that drugs have to control common diseases and alleviate suffering." In Tanzania, the drug policy states that the goal is "to make available to all Tanzanians at all times the essential pharmaceutical products which are of quality, proven effectiveness, and acceptable safety at a price that the individual and the community can afford, when these are needed to prevent, cure, or reduce illness and suffering."

Although specific objectives differ according to the priorities set by the government, the most common are

- ► to make essential drugs available and affordable to those who need them;
- ► to ensure the safety, efficacy, and quality of all medicines provided to the public;
- ► to improve prescribing and dispensing practices and to promote the correct use of medicines by health workers and the public.

In addition to basic health-related goals, there may be others, including economic goals (for example, to reduce the use of foreign exchange for drug imports or to provide jobs in areas such as dispensing, prepackaging, or production of drugs) and national development goals (for example, to improve internal transportation and communication systems, develop national pharmaceutical production, or protect intellectual property rights or avoid establishing them). Regardless of a country's specific circumstances, comprehensive NDPs should clearly specify the roles of both the public and the private sectors. In addition, the policy should be concerned with *efficiency* (delivery of the maximum level of services given a certain level of resources), *equity* (fairness in access), and *sustainability* (the ability to provide benefits into the future without external support).

What Approaches Should Be Used?

A good policy presents approaches or strategies for achieving the goals of the policy; for each objective, strategic decisions need to be made about how to attain it. For instance, the supply of essential drugs can be improved through the public sector by increasing the drug budget, introducing cost-sharing mechanisms, and allocating more resources to underserved populations and areas. Drug supplies can also be increased through the private sector by introducing economic incentives for drug manufacturing and transportation. The optimal solution will likely involve applying different policies to the private and public sectors. This combination of different approaches and strategies forms the core of an NDP.

Why Do Drug Policies Differ by Country?

Objectives and strategies may differ from country to country due to differences in the structure of the health care system, the number of trained pharmacists and physicians, the capacity of the drug regulatory agency, features of the pharmaceutical distribution system, and the level of funding for pharmaceuticals.

In most industrialized countries, health care coverage is broad, and access to drugs per se is not a prominent issue (although cost is likely to be a concern). The role of the government is to set up rules for the operations of the private sector without becoming directly involved in the provision of drugs or in the pharmaceutical industry. This model requires the existence of an active private sector that is capable of developing, manufacturing, marketing, and distributing drugs to the entire population. In these settings, pharmaceutical policies are oriented toward containing costs without decreasing access and equity.

In the least-developed countries, total spending on pharmaceuticals is very low (less than US$10 per person per year). The private sector has traditionally failed to supply drugs to more than a fraction of the population (the most affluent sector). Consequently, governments have attempted to supply and distribute essential drugs through the public sector, often with donor support. In addition, more attention is given to such matters as ensuring the proper use of medicines and encouraging the private sector to play a more constructive role in supplying essential drugs.

Who Are the Main Participants in a National Drug Policy?

National governments are the principal agency and driving force in drug policies. The state hopes to guarantee availability and access to effective, high-quality essential drugs for the population and to ensure that they are properly used. This holds true whether the government is directly involved in procurement and distribution of drugs, empowers a parastatal institution to carry out this function, or is mainly a regulatory authority for a largely private pharmaceutical market.

The government is not, however, the only actor involved with the NDP. A partnership is required, involving government ministries of health, finance, and industry; health professionals, including doctors and other prescribers and pharmacists; public and private wholesalers and retailers; consumers; and the pharmaceutical industry (national and multinational). With such diverse groups and conflicting interests, development of a sustainable NDP is not easy. With patience and goodwill, however, an environment conducive to success can be created.

≡ 5.2 Components of a National Drug Policy

The main components of an NDP are legislation and regulation, choice of drugs, supply and financing policies, and rational drug use. Local production is also a key issue in some settings.

These components are widely recognized as the most important for ensuring that essential drugs are available to the whole population and are used rationally; they form the basic framework, with other components added according to local conditions. Figure 5.1 summarizes the basic components of a national drug policy, which are discussed further below.

Legislative and Regulatory Framework

The formulation of a drug policy should be followed by the enactment of appropriate legislation and the introduction of regulations to provide a legal basis for the policy and make it enforceable. An NDP is usually not a law, so the strategies proposed in the policy may need to be legally supported. For instance, in the Philippines, one policy objective was to extend the use of generic drugs, and many activities related to that objective were backed up by a new law (the Generics Act of 1988).

Legislation should define the actors in the system and their responsibilities: who can produce or import pharmaceuticals, who can prescribe which type of products, who can store and sell drugs, and which institution is responsible for monitoring and enforcing regulations. Legislation should provide the basis for ensuring that pharmaceutical products are of acceptable quality, safety, and efficacy.

Several legislative models and structures have been devised for the regulation of drugs, as discussed in Chapter 7. Often, laws and regulations are not enforced, and the penalties and sanctions the law provides are not used. A review of the main regulations applying to the pharmaceutical sector may lead to proposals to amend them so that they are better adapted to local realities and can be better enforced.

Figure 5.1 Components of a National Drug Policy

Legislative and Regulatory Framework
- ► legislation and regulations
- ► drug regulatory authority
- ► drug registration and licensing
- ► pharmaceutical quality assurance
- ► postmarketing surveillance
- ► regulation of prescription and distribution

Choice of Drugs
- ► principles of drug selection
- ► selection process
- ► selection criteria
- ► use of essential drugs lists
- ► traditional medicines

Supply
- ► local production
- ► supply system strategies and alternatives
- ► procurement mechanisms
- ► distribution and storage

Rational Use of Drugs
- ► objective drug information
- ► rational use of drugs by health personnel
- ► rational use of drugs by consumers
- ► promotional activities

Economic Strategies for Drugs
- ► role of government in the pharmaceutical market
- ► measures to encourage competition
- ► public drug financing mechanisms (public financing, user charges, health insurance, external assistance)
- ► measures to improve efficiency and cost effectiveness

Human Resources Development
- ► role of health professions
- ► human resources development plan
- ► education, training, and courses
- ► national collaborating networks
- ► motivation and continuing education

Monitoring and Evaluation
- ► responsibilities
- ► indicators for monitoring
- ► periodic evaluation

Research
- ► operational research
- ► drug research and development

Technical Cooperation among Countries

Source: Adapted from WHO 1995a.

Appropriate legislation and regulation should be accompanied by a functioning quality assurance system; pharmaceuticals of low quality, either imported or locally produced, should never reach the patient. This calls for a well-organized and trained inspection administration that is independent from commercial pressures and a system of quality control (see Chapter 18).

Choice of Drugs

The selection of essential drugs to meet the health needs of the population and the registration of safe, high-quality, and effective drugs are important features of an NDP.

Essential drugs are those considered most vital for saving lives and alleviating serious and common diseases in the majority of the population. The national essential drugs list has become the foundation of public drug supply in many countries. Hospital and outpatient practice formularies commonly guide prescribing in both the private and the public sectors. The principles, criteria, and process for drug selection are described in Chapter 10.

Drug registration or licensing is an important tool. It involves a series of procedures to examine the quality, safety, and efficacy of drugs and the information to be provided to health care providers and patients. In addition to quality, safety, and efficacy, drugs may be selected by other criteria, such as a restrictive attitude toward fixed-combination products or a requirement that the price be competitive with that of similar drugs already on the market. The addition of medical need as a registration criterion is controversial and is likely to provoke broad opposition.

Supply

In many developing countries, universal access to essential drugs is the most pressing NDP concern. To achieve availability of effective, good-quality drugs, governments need to define policies in production, procurement, and distribution. Such policies should take into account what is feasible in the short term and what is necessary for sustainable systems in the long term.

Existing drug supply arrangements vary greatly with respect to public and private roles in financing, distributing, and dispensing drugs. Many developing countries have maintained state systems for procuring and importing drugs for decades, in part because private-sector activities were concentrated in urban areas and there were no health insurance systems. Although the need for many of these state-supported systems persists, they often require improvements in organization, management, and financing.

Government and NGO health services can be supplied through a variety of alternative arrangements that combine components of private-sector flexibility and efficiency (see Chapter 6).

Pharmaceutical production policy (see Chapter 9) is an important aspect of drug supply. For many years, countries have been interested in developing local manufacturing capacity and a degree of national self-sufficiency. Unfortunately, the difficulties of local production have frequently been underestimated. Many factors influence the feasibility of local production, and a range of policy options exists regarding local production (see Chapter 9). When formulating a policy, the most important objective should be to get good-quality, therapeutically useful drugs to the people who need them, at prices they can afford.

Rational Drug Use

Drugs should be used appropriately, safely, and only when needed. Irrational drug use includes overuse, underuse, and inappropriate use because of such factors as lack of adequate regulatory systems; shortages of essential drugs and availability of nonessential drugs; lack of sound, objective drug information; and the considerable influence of drug promotion on both prescribers and consumers.

An NDP should specify major activities and responsibilities for promoting rational prescribing, dispensing, and patient drug use. A wide variety of approaches have been developed in an effort to promote rational prescribing and dispensing (Chapters 31 and 32). Drug prescribing and use have been improved in certain institutional settings. Although not yet widely implemented, focused programs on rational drug use can help improve drug use in the public and private sectors.

Inadequate training of health professionals, lack of control of drug promotion, and dispensing of drugs by untrained persons all promote irrational use of drugs (see Chapter 33). Strategies for public drug education should provide individuals and communities with the information, skills, and confidence necessary to use medicines in an appropriate, safe, and judicious way.

Economic Strategies for Drugs

Ensuring stable and adequate financing for drugs is a major challenge. Public financing of drugs for government health services is accepted as a legitimate policy in most countries and by most institutions (World Bank 1993). In addition, financing mechanisms such as user fees are becoming common in the least-developed countries to increase financial resources. Financing policies should be designed to maximize resources for drugs and to keep prices as low as possible in the public sector. These issues are discussed in Chapters 40–44.

Possible mechanisms to increase economic access to essential drugs in all sectors include increased insurance coverage, price information, price competition through generic substitution, regulation of producer prices, and regulation of retail margins (Chapter 6).

Human Resources, Monitoring, Evaluation, and Research

Implementing an NDP and achieving its objectives depend on people. Human resources development is therefore an important element of the policy. The role of different health

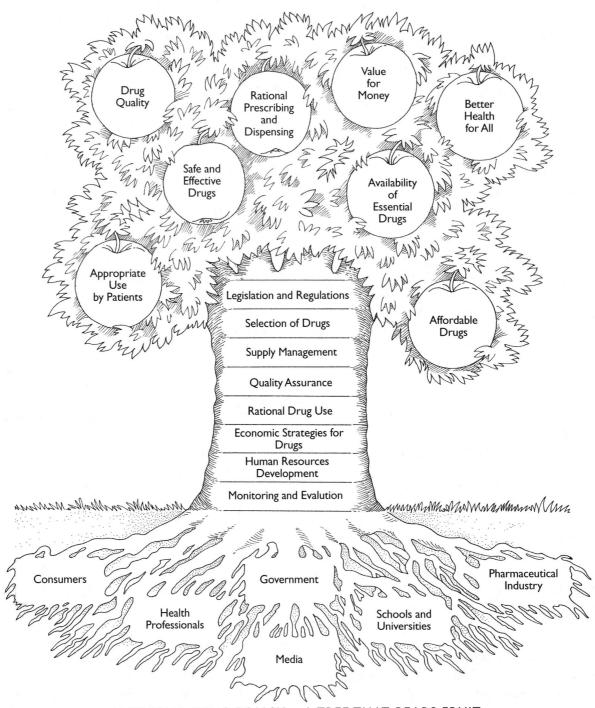

Drug Quality

Rational Prescribing and Dispensing

Value for Money

Better Health for All

Safe and Effective Drugs

Availability of Essential Drugs

Appropriate Use by Patients

Legislation and Regulations

Selection of Drugs

Supply Management

Quality Assurance

Rational Drug Use

Economic Strategies for Drugs

Human Resources Development

Monitoring and Evalution

Affordable Drugs

Consumers

Government

Pharmaceutical Industry

Health Professionals

Schools and Universities

Media

NATIONAL DRUG POLICY— A TREE THAT BEARS FRUIT

professions should be clear. The policy should lead to a human resources development plan that identifies education, training, and continuing education requirements.

The implementation of an NDP should be routinely monitored, and its impact should be thoroughly evaluated at regular intervals.

Research is essential for health service and health care improvements. NDPs are concerned with operational research aimed at improving selection, procurement, distribution, and use of existing drugs. NDPs may also include specific provisions for drug research and the development of new drugs.

Finally, many NDPs address the issue of technical cooperation among countries. Cooperation among countries within the same geographic region and the same economic area has become increasingly common. There are examples of cooperation in virtually every aspect of drug policy and management.

≡ 5.3 Setting Priorities

Once the basic components of a policy have been identified, choices must be made about the most appropriate strategies and activities for each level of the system. For example, to improve the supply system for essential drugs, many possible solutions exist: improve the central medical stores (CMS) or transform the CMS into a parastatal (as in Tanzania); decentralize drug procurement (as in Cameroon); or stimulate the private sector with appropriate incentives. Activities can then be undertaken to implement the approaches selected—for example, using restrictive or competitive tenders, buying only from the essential drugs list, negotiating contracts with the private sector, and so forth.

In another example, various interventions can be undertaken to improve rational prescribing and use of essential drugs. Depending on the country, however, some strategies are more cost effective than others. Choices could involve training medical students, providing independent drug information to all prescribers, or active drug use review programs.

The range of strategies and activities that can be successfully implemented depends on the pharmaceutical situation and the socioeconomic conditions of the country. However, a useful starting point is to consider the following questions:

- ► Is this approach based on scientific evidence, and has it proved to be effective in other countries?
- ► Is this approach or activity really needed to improve the situation in a particular area?
- ► Does it address the greatest needs?
- ► Are there other approaches or activities that might be more effective?

It may be necessary to set aside policy elements that, however successful they may have been in another country, would be no more than expensive luxuries or would not work because there are too few technical and financial resources.

The combination of pharmaceutical policies that can be successfully implemented in a particular country over the short to medium term is closely linked to the structure of the pharmaceutical distribution systems, pharmaceutical spending levels, presence of health insurance schemes, number of trained people, and capacity of the drug regulatory agency. Figure 5.2 shows approaches selected during a 1987 national workshop in Uganda.

Figure 5.2 Selected Approaches to National Drug Policy in Uganda

I. Make essential drugs available in the health care system.
- ► Review the list of essential drugs and the estimation of drug needs.
- ► Restructure central medical stores.
- ► Reorganize procurement.
- ► Improve drug management at peripheral levels.

2. Make drugs affordable to the whole population.
- ► Guarantee the drug budget.
- ► Improve the efficiency of procurement practices.
- ► Introduce drugs under their generic names.
- ► Review registration criteria.
- ► Motivate the private sector.
- ► Review financing mechanisms to ensure equity (patient contribution).

3. Improve drug use.
- ► Develop materials for prescribers and dispensers (national formulary, therapeutic guidelines, and so forth).
- ► Improve prescribing practices (training, supervision).
- ► Improve use of drugs by the public (education campaigns, involvement of nongovernmental and consumer organizations).

4. Improve regulatory and administration structures.
- ► Develop legislation and regulations.
- ► Improve the registration and inspection functions of the drug regulatory authority.

Source: Government of Uganda 1993.

≡ 5.4 Formulating a National Drug Policy

Designing or revising an NDP requires complex negotiations with the interests involved: the national and international pharmaceutical industry, the medical profession, drug sellers, NGOs, the government bureaucracy, and international donors. The challenge involves identifying the substance of an appropriate pharmaceutical policy and constructing a process that will bring the diverse groups together.

Given the various interests in the pharmaceutical sector, resistance and legal confrontations must be expected. Steps must be taken to resolve disputes. Differences may be resolved through effective communications, a collaborative approach, and careful monitoring of the policy formulation process. Nothing can be left to chance, particularly if the proposed policy seeks to change structures, historical practices, or the behavior of people in an important way. The more significant the proposed changes, the more the process of policy formulation should involve all groups. There is no simple recipe, but political will and effective communication are the main ingredients for success.

Step 1. Organize the Policy Process

The ministry of health (MOH) is usually the most appropriate agency to take the lead in developing an NDP. The first step is to decide how the formulation of the policy will be achieved, who will be involved at the various stages, and how the needed financial resources will be obtained. A plan outlining the process and the final output can be drawn up by the pharmaceutical department in the ministry, with the support of a small committee. The more changes the policy seeks to produce, the more people will need to be involved. This should be taken into consideration from the beginning, as it has an impact on the resources needed. The need for external assistance from WHO or other countries with experience in developing an NDP should also be assessed at this stage.

Step 2. Identify and Analyze Problems

The second task when formulating a policy is a thorough analysis of the main problems, in order to set attainable objectives (see Chapter 4). The best way to undertake this analysis is to bring together a small team of experts, including some who have performed similar studies in other countries. Their function is to examine the situation systematically, identify problems, and recommend what must and can be done and what approaches might be taken. The experts should not come only from the MOH; they may be from the health professions, from trade and industry, and from other agencies of government (particularly the treasury). Recommendations can be formulated and discussed in a multidisciplinary workshop to prepare advice for the government. This was done in Uganda in 1987 and led to the passage of an NDP six years later. A similar process was followed in Tanzania and led to the drafting of an NDP by a small team of national and international experts.

However ambitious it may sound in the early stages of drug policy development, the situation in the country as a whole needs to be systematically reviewed to identify viable reforms. In countries where a poor national economic situation is a major factor leading to unsatisfactory drug supply, it makes no sense to base reforms on demands for more government money, since that is not available. The ultimate solution must take these structural constraints into account.

Step 3. Set Goals and Objectives

Once high-priority problems and related goals have been defined, primary objectives can be identified. For instance, if one of the priority problems is the availability of poor-quality drugs, one of the primary objectives should be to decrease the amount of poor-quality drugs on the market. The selection of the strategies or approaches is more complex and should come from the situation analysis in step 2,

perhaps in a workshop with key people from the MOH. Once objectives and strategies are outlined, they can be discussed in a larger workshop to get consensus from all the main participants, as was done in Cambodia and Guinea.

Most likely, there will not be full agreement among all the parties. Members of the pharmaceutical industry may be suspicious; doctors and pharmacists may have different points of view; any party that feels secure in the status quo may feel threatened by change. Not uncommonly, one government agency disagrees with another on objectives, approaches, or timetables. The important thing is to establish as much trust as possible, to identify matters on which consensus and compromise are possible, and to use those matters as the basis on which to proceed.

Step 4. Draft the Policy

Once a thorough analysis of the situation and an outline of the main goals, objectives, and approaches have been completed, a draft of the NDP should be written. It should state the general goal of the policy; in most countries, this will be to ensure that high-quality drugs are accessible and affordable to the entire population and that they are used rationally. Then the specific objectives and the strategy or strategies to be adopted for each should be described. For example, to ensure that essential drugs are available in health facilities (objective), the policy might propose the creation of an autonomous procurement unit and the strengthening of drug management in health facilities (strategies).

This drafting of the policy can be done by the small committee set up in step 2, with the support of the people who performed the situation analysis. The group should remain small, as a big group is difficult to manage and will have problems drafting a coherent text.

Step 5. Circulate and Revise the Policy

To get full support from all sectors, the document should be widely circulated for comments, first within the MOH and then in other government departments and agencies. Endorsement by ministries or departments such as planning, finance, education, and commerce is of particular importance, since the success of decisions regarding registration, foreign exchange allocations, and human resources development depends on the support of government officials outside the health sector. Once this wide consultation is done, the document can be finalized. Although the formulation of the policy should reflect broad participation by the community, health workers, the pharmaceutical industry, and universities, ultimate responsibility for producing the policy remains with the MOH and the government.

Country Study 5.1 The Philippines National Drug Policy: A Carefully Designed Formulation Process

The Philippines National Drug Policy (PNDP), outlined by President Corazón Aquino in 1987, was aimed at improved drug safety, vigorous promotion of rational drug use, self-reliance in drug production, and improved procurement. It had two distinct phases: development and implementation. During the development phase, six key strategies were used to overcome the main problems and create a consensus among the partners.

Strategy 1: Use Democratic Broad Consultation and Participation. The intent was to generate broad involvement so that the positions of the major affected sectors would be understood. Although consensus building was sought and a democratic process was followed, the government took a leadership role in policy formulation and tried to solve any bottlenecks expeditiously. The process of consultation involved three main groups: the top management of the Department of Health (the secretary and the two undersecretaries, who initiated the activities); the Task Force on Pharmaceuticals (including representatives from the drug industry, academia, private medical practice, professional societies, other government agencies, and NGOs), which had to produce a framework for the policy; and a third group composed of organizations, associations, companies, and individuals who felt that they had a stake in the policy. In the course of a one-year development process, two national workshops were held, twenty-five position papers were submitted, and ninety-nine individuals representing sixty-one organizations were involved. This first strategy created a sense of "ownership" of the proposed reforms among those involved and increased their willingness to defend the policy.

Strategy 2: Institutionalize the Policy through Laws and Regulations. The most important legislation was the Generics Act of 1988, passed unanimously in congress and signed into law by the president eighteen months after the PNDP was declared. The act contained straightforward guidelines (on generics, informed consumers, supply, national drug formulary, and so forth) and gave the PNDP a legal basis that ensured its long-term sustainability.

Strategy 3: Formulate as Comprehensive and Practical a Policy as Possible. The group assigned to formulate the PNDP relied on experiences of other countries and developed a comprehensive framework to cover both the supply and demand sides of the pharmaceutical system. The goal was simple: the provision of essential drugs. To achieve this, the PNDP depended on four "pillars" to be built simultaneously: quality assurance, rational use, self-reliance, and tailored procurement.

Strategy 4: Involve the Best-Qualified People. The policy needed to be promoted by high-level officials convinced of its worth, including the secretary, some of the undersecretaries, the assistant secretary responsible for the NDP, and members of the task force selected for their competence and dedication.

Strategy 5: Gather Adequate and Scientifically Sound Data. Data gathered by the task force on pharmaceutical systems and NDP guidelines provided support in the debates on the scientific soundness and social relevance of the PNDP.

Strategy 6: Harness and Mobilize International Support. From the beginning, international support was sought from WHO, members of the Association of Southeast Asian Nations (ASEAN), Japan, and Australia. This support was important when the policy was under strong attack both within and outside the country.

Careful and comprehensive development was absolutely necessary, since the policy aimed to transform the pharmaceutical sector. Such changes require political will and public involvement of the main initiators, with the widest possible consultation and participation of all sectors affected by the policy.

Source: Philippine Centre for Investigative Journalism 1992.

Step 6. Obtain Formal Endorsement for the Policy

In some countries, the document can then go to the cabinet or parliament. In others, it can be an administrative document that serves as a basis for the implementation plans and for changes in pharmaceutical laws, which are often needed. In certain cases—for example, in Uganda—the NDP document became a law and was called the National Drug Policy and Authority Statute. Although a law can demonstrate strong commitment on the part of the government, it is not always advantageous, because it is difficult to change once it is enacted. It may be more useful to have only certain components of the NDP incorporated into a law, such as the Generics Act in the Philippines.

Step 7. Launch the Policy

Introducing an NDP is a political rather than merely a technical task. It needs as much attention as any other political campaign. Promotion should rely on good information, top-level political support, mobilization of highly qualified people, and the securing of international support (see Country Study 5.1). The policy needs to be explained in a way that allows the media and the public to become involved in discussions.

≡ 5.5 Implementing a National Drug Policy

Policy implementation, the execution of approaches included in the policy through specific plans and programs, is a critical step. Given the multisectoral nature of pharmaceutical issues, the MOH should develop, as early as possible, a consensus with other government agencies on action plans dealing with economics and finance (including foreign exchange), commerce, industry, and education.

Once the policy has been designed, countries take different approaches to implementation (see Country Study 5.2 for Australia's approach). Some, like Tanzania, develop

a five-year master plan for the pharmaceutical sector that
outlines the approaches and activities in detail, including
budgets and responsible agencies. Such a plan allows for
coordination of donor inputs and facilitates follow-up
and supervision of the progress made in implementing
the policy. Other countries break down the various strategies into different plans for the agencies involved. In all
cases, if the policy is to succeed, government officials need
to be proactive and committed. A number of strategies are
outlined below.

*Use Appropriate Timing, and a Combination of Approaches
and Methods of Implementation.* Not everything can be
done at the same time. In the Philippines, the rules of
generic labeling and promotion had to be put in place
before generic prescribing and dispensing could be
implemented. In practice, it proved necessary to have a
one-year interval between the issuance of the rules on
generic labeling and the issuance of those on dispensing.
In this way, by the time doctors and pharmacists were
required to switch to generics, the products in the pharmacies had already been generically labeled.

*Start Implementation in Relatively Easy Areas to Ensure
Initial High-Visibility Success.* Perception of success is an
important consideration; if the policy is perceived to have
yielded significant positive results, it is likely to continue
to receive support from important sectors.

Adopt a Flexible Policy. In certain cases, it may be necessary to postpone an activity to promote future cooperation. For example, when developing a policy on pricing, it
may be useful to spend more time convincing pharmacists
rather than imposing measures that will be met with resistance. However, consensus building should always be balanced against compromising too much on key points.

Use Experts to Vouch for the Policy's Technical Soundness.
It is important that the most qualified people in the medical and pharmaceutical fields support the policy (for
example, clinical pharmacologists or specialists in the
main hospitals and universities). These experts are more
likely to support the policy if they have been involved in
developing it.

Mobilize Consumers, the Media, or Other Key Groups.
Although such mobilizations have worked in the Philippines and Australia, they have rarely been used in Africa,
due to the lack of a consumers' movement there.

*Create Constituencies that Support the Policy Both Inside
and Outside the Government.* Such constituencies are critical to the success of the implementation and the long-
term sustainability of the policy.

There is no single best way to implement an NDP. In
most countries, the implementation process is launched

and supported directly from the pharmacy department in
the MOH, as in Guinea, Tanzania, and Zimbabwe. The
pharmacy department is generally supported by committees that deal with different aspects of the policy. The
problem with this approach is the policy's lack of visibility; often, the limited human and financial resources of
these departments make it difficult for them to be proactive and to coordinate all the actors. In addition, the
focus may be too much on the pharmacological rather
than the broad public health aspects that should inform
the NDP.

In the Philippines, the NDP is highly visible. The NDP
office was originally attached to the secretary of health and
was headed by one of the assistant secretaries, who was
also the director of the Bureau of Food and Drugs (BFAD).
He was assisted by the NDP management committee,
which oversaw the implementation of the policy. A
Generics Act implementation program manager was
responsible for supervising several monitoring units and
communicating to the public, NGOs, and other organizations. A national drug committee was responsible for the
preparation of the national formulary and for recommending the drugs to be delisted. The structure has
recently changed and is more institutionalized in the
Department of Health. The national drug committee is
still active, but an advisory committee has been created to
deal with overall issues in the drug field. Four program
managers have been nominated for the four pillars of the
policy (quality assurance, rational use, self-reliance, tailored procurement), and a budget has been allocated to
the NDP office.

≡ 5.6 Monitoring a National Drug Policy

Whenever a national drug policy is implemented, tools
need to be developed for monitoring the effects of the
policy as it evolves. Senior managers need to assess the
progress toward achieving defined targets in each policy
area and adjust strategies accordingly. Indicators for monitoring national drug policies have been developed by
WHO and are discussed in Chapters 4 and 36.

Indicators may need to be developed, adapted, or
deleted to match particular national contexts. For example,
countries may have additional objectives beyond those
included in the WHO manual, such as development of
national drug production. In any case, a monitoring system
needs to be set up; ideally, this would be integrated with
the health information system. This institution-building
process requires the commitment of senior policy-makers
but can be done even in countries with limited monitoring
infrastructure.

Country Study 5.2 Innovative Approaches to National Drug Policy Formulation and Implementation in Australia

By 1992, Australia had three elements of a drug policy in place:

1. A system for regulating the marketing of high-quality, safe, and efficacious products;
2. An equitable system of drug access that ensures supply and controls price;
3. An industry development program.

What was missing, however, was a rational drug use component that would firmly link these three activities to health outcomes.

The minister of health was committed to the issue, and the government began to fund educational programs. After two years, however, it became clear that an overall strategy was needed. Attempts to introduce policy or action that did not adequately involve doctors and pharmacists were likely to fail. Consumers had not traditionally been involved in the decision-making process. Lessons from the past suggested that communication with and involvement of all interested parties were crucial.

In 1990, the minister formed two advisory groups. The first was a council of representatives from the major organizations involved, which would raise issues and make recommendations across the gamut of drug policy. The second was the Pharmaceutical Health and Rational Use of Medicines (PHARM) working party, to advise the ministry on a policy for the use of medicines and a strategy for its implementation. PHARM drew on the best available knowledge and relevant concepts to establish a coherent framework for tackling the complex set of problems involved in the way medicines are used. The group also drew on research in behavioral change and health education; espoused principles of community ownership, participation, and consultation; and acknowledged the importance of media advocacy.

In 1992, this collaborative approach led to the adoption of an NDP. The approach was to

▸ use consumer and professional education as a primary tool;
▸ stimulate partnerships among the major players;
▸ identify
  – what will empower consumers to use drugs well and encourage health professionals to help them do this?
  – what constitutes effective education?
  – what combination of information, skills, and motivation will be effective for different groups?
  – what will work in practice?
  – what standards should apply, and who should set them?

Through various mechanisms of encouragement—including proactive consultation, targeted grants, and support for further development of existing programs—actions were stimulated, and new ideas from various groups were identified, including:

Objective information: The preparation of national prescribing guidelines, a national formulary, consumer information, and independent monitoring of drug advertising have been supported.

Education and training: A school kit for young children was funded.

Consumer services: Medication record cards and innovative consumer education programs have been provided to encourage consumers to ask their health professionals more questions about medicines and to support them in running local campaigns on drug use.

Provider services: Several types of academic detailing programs were developed.

Education campaigns: National education campaigns took place in 1992, including one aimed at educating health professionals and the community about the safety of using nonsteroidal anti-inflammatory drugs.

The "Be wise with medicines" campaign: This major national community awareness campaign used the principles of community development and involved all players. Three hundred fifty local community groups were given small grants to design activities aimed at stimulating discussion and educating their members about medicines. Groups came up with a wide range of activities, including health fairs, discussion groups, talks by local doctors or pharmacists, and shopping center displays. A range of ages, many multicultural groups, and aboriginal groups in metropolitan, rural, and remote settings were represented.

A strong principle underlying the approach to optimizing the use of medicines is to stimulate new programs and ideas whenever possible while supporting existing effective initiatives within local communities or professional and consumer groups. A sustainable infrastructure is needed to facilitate, coordinate, and support initiatives at the state, regional, and local levels in a way that honors this principle.

So far, the partnership developed among groups is fragile. There are signs, however, that continued dialog and experience working jointly on projects are significantly improving the understanding of others' responsibilities and constraints.

Source: Adapted from Hodge 1993.

≡ 5.7 Constraints and Facilitating Factors

Formulating and implementing an NDP seems manageable, yet few countries have succeeded in implementing all aspects of their NDPs. Why? Some of the main reasons are clear:

Lack of political will: Many governments are wary of creating policies that might antagonize industry and other groups, particularly if there is known opposition.

Lack of resources: Often, the true problems and solutions in the drug field are not sufficiently understood or documented to persuade governments to devote scarce resources to building and implementing NDPs.

Opposition: Frank opposition to drug policies often comes from those who benefit from a laissez-faire approach. Doctors fear interference with their freedom to prescribe. Importers and manufacturers are commonly earning large profits on precisely the drugs or drug practices that would be threatened by policy changes. Retail pharmacists may oppose policy initiatives that would threaten their earnings.

Corruption: Corruption can be an issue in the pharmaceutical sector, where there is a great deal of money flowing and where demand greatly exceeds supply.

None of these impediments is easily overcome, but there are also a number of factors that can facilitate the policy process:

Support of domestic and international interest groups: Domestic interest groups include political parties, industry groups, physicians and other health care professionals, consumers, and consumer activist groups. International interest groups include foreign governments, multilateral organizations, multinational corporations, and international lending agencies. Their support is required for successful policy formulation, but to obtain that support, it is sometimes necessary to enter into bargains and tradeoffs. The consequences of each tradeoff in the formulation and implementation of pharmaceutical policies should be carefully considered.

Shared values: The extent to which there is a congruence of interests among groups is another important predictor of the success of an NDP. The interests of a politically weak group (for example, poor consumers) can often be protected if their goals coincide, at least partially, with those of more powerful interest groups (for example, retail pharmacists who want to sell more drugs and are willing to handle generic products because the higher volume of sales compensates for lower unit earnings).

The macroeconomic situation: Improvements in the efficiency of the pharmaceutical system may help countries cope with the consequences of macroeconomic shocks. For instance, the devaluation of the franc in West Africa pushed countries in the region to strengthen their essential drugs policies in the public sector and to introduce mechanisms to promote drugs under generic names in the private sector.

Technical expertise: The existence of technical expertise and capabilities within ministries of health, as well as access to data on patent-related issues and pharmacological, legal, and economic policy (including the policies of other countries), is key to the formulation of a sound and implementable policy.

The presence of committed people in the MOH: In the United Kingdom in 1968, Bangladesh in 1982, the Philippines in 1988, Guinea in 1992, and Uganda in 1993, the development of a drug policy was sustained by individuals and institutions that were persuaded of the need for it and worked toward its realization. In Uganda, a national workshop laid the foundations of what was to become law six years later. The workshop established consensus among the health professions and governmental services, recipients of development aid, voluntary services, and elsewhere. In many such countries, a single person played a role in persuading others through writing, public speaking, and other forms of personal influence. Bilateral donors and international organizations can support the emergence of drug policies in developing countries through planning and technical assistance.

Each country must shape its own NDP in accordance with its needs and resources. The goals outlined at the beginning of the chapter provide a policy focus. Experiences from countries such as Norway and Sri Lanka show that success in terms of public health is linked to the essential drugs concept, with an emphasis on a list of essential drugs. Strategies vary among countries, and in the end, the impact of a country's NDP depends on political commitment from the government and the support of doctors and other health professionals. ■

≡ Assessment Guide

NDP Development and Content

- ► Is there an official NDP document? Has it been updated in the past ten years?
- ► Does the document contain objectives and strategies based on priority problems?
- ► Does it cover issues such as legislation, essential drugs list, registration of drugs, supply of essential drugs, financing and pricing policies, and rational use of drugs?
- ► If no official NDP document exists, are there any unofficial documents that set objectives and strategies for the pharmaceutical sector?

NDP Implementation

- ► Is the NDP used as a guide for action by policymakers and senior management officers in the ministry of health?
- ► Does the drug legislation provide a legal basis for enforcement of the NDP?
- ► Is there a mechanism to put the policy into practice?
- ► Is the policy monitored regularly? If so, how is it monitored?
- ► Is there any report on the performance and outcome of the NDP in terms of attaining its objectives?
- ► Is the NDP highly visible in the ministry of health and the government?

≡ References and Further Readings

★ = *Key readings.*

General

Bannenberg, W. 1994. National drug policies. In *Health and disease in developing countries*, ed. K. S. Lankinen, S. Bergstrom, P. H. Makela, and M. Peltomaa. London: Macmillan.

★ Brudon-Jakobowicz, P., J.-D. Rainhorn, and M. R. Reich. 1995. *Indicators for monitoring national drug policies.* Geneva: World Health Organization.

★ Dag Hammarskjöld Foundation. 1995. Making national drug policies a development priority: A strategy paper and six country studies (Norway, Sri Lanka, Bangladesh, Australia, India, Mexico). *Development Dialogue* 1:1–240.

Dukes, M. N. G., and D. Broun. 1994. *Pharmaceutical policies: Rationale and design.* HRO working paper no. 35. Washington, D.C.: World Bank.

Government of Uganda. 1993. *National drug policy and authority statute.* Kampala, Uganda: Government Printers.

Hodge, M. M. 1993. Australia focuses on the quality use of medicines: Policy and action. *Essential Drugs Monitor* 15:12–13.

★ Kanji, N., A. Hardon, J. W. Harnmeijer, M. Mamdani, and G. Walt. 1992. *Drugs policy in developing countries.* London: Zed Books (with support from Danida).

MSH (Management Sciences for Health). 1992. National drug policy (trainer's and participant's guides). In *Managing drug supply training series.* Part 1. *Policy issues in managing drug supply.* Boston: MSH.

Philippine Centre for Investigative Journalism. 1992. *Prescription for change: National drug policies, social transformation, and the media.* Uppsala, Sweden: Dag Hammarskjöld Foundation.

Rainhorn, J.-D., P. Brudon-Jakobowicz, and M. R. Reich. 1994. Priorities for pharmaceutical policies in developing countries: Results of a Delphi survey. *Bulletin of the World Health Organization* 72:257–64.

Reich, M. R. 1987. Essential drugs: Economics and politics in international health. *Health Policy and Planning* 8:39–57.

Reich, M. R. 1993. *Political mapping of health policy: A guide for managing the political dimensions of health policy.* Boston: Harvard School of Public Health, Data for Decision Making Project.

Saxenian, H. 1994. *Getting the most out of pharmaceutical expenditures.* HRO working paper no. 37. Washington, D.C.: World Bank.

★ WHO (World Health Organization). 1988. *Guidelines for developing national drug policies.* Geneva: WHO.

WHO (World Health Organization). 1995a. *Report of the WHO Expert Committee on National Drug Policies.* Geneva: WHO.

WHO (World Health Organization). 1995b. *The use of essential drugs.* Technical report series no. 850. Geneva: WHO.

World Bank. 1993. *World development report 1993: Investing in health.* New York: Oxford University Press.

World Bank. 1994. *Better health in Africa: Experience and lessons learned.* Report no. 12577-AFR. Washington, D.C.: World Bank.

Reports on Individual National Policies

Ali, H. M., M. M. A. Homeida, A. R. E. Rasheed, and A. Beckele. 1986. Sudan's new drug policy proves its worth. *World Health Forum* 7:256–60.

Islam, N. 1985. Drugs policy in the third world. *Lancet* 1(8436): 1044.

Islam, N. 1989. Bangladesh national drug policy: An assessment. *Tropical Doctor* 19:18–20.

Laporte, J., and G. Tognoni. 1985. Drug policy in Nicaragua: Between need-oriented activities and aggression. *Development Dialogue* 2:121–29.

Paphassarang, C., G. Tomson, C. Choprapawon, and K. Weerasuriya. 1995. The Lao national drug policy: Lessons along the journey. *Lancet* 345:433–35.

Prudencio, I., and G. Tognoni. 1987. Essential drugs policy in Bolivia. *Health Policy and Planning* 2:301–8.

| Part I | Part II | Part III | Part IV |
| Introduction | **Policy and Legal Framework** | Drug Management Cycle | Management Support Systems |

5 National Drug Policies
6 Drug Supply Strategies
7 Pharmaceutical Legislation and Regulation
8 Legal Aspects of Drug Management
9 Pharmaceutical Production Policy

Chapter 6
Drug Supply Strategies

≡ Summary

Access to pharmaceuticals and, in particular, to essential drugs can be achieved through various strategies. National systems vary with respect to public and private roles in financing, distribution, and dispensing of drugs, ranging from fully public to fully private systems.

At least five alternatives exist for supplying drugs to governmental and nongovernmental health services:

1. Central medical stores (CMS): *Conventional drug supply system, in which drugs are procured and distributed by a centralized government unit.*

2. Autonomous supply agency: *An alternative to the CMS system, managed by an autonomous or semi-autonomous drug supply agency.*

3. Direct delivery system: *A decentralized, non-CMS approach in which drugs are delivered directly by suppliers to districts and major facilities. The government drug procurement office tenders to establish the supplier and price for each item, but the government does not store and distribute drugs.*

4. Prime vendor system: *Another non-CMS system in which the government drug procurement office establishes a contract with a single prime vendor, as well as separate contracts with drug suppliers. The prime vendor is contracted to manage drug distribution by receiving drugs from the suppliers and then storing and distributing them to districts and major facilities.*

5. Fully private supply: *In some countries, drugs are provided by private pharmacies in or near government health facilities. With such an approach, measures are required to ensure equity of access for the poor, medically needy, and other target populations.*

These systems vary considerably with respect to the role of the government, the role of the private sector, and incentives for efficiency. Mixed systems in which different categories of drugs are supplied through different mechanisms are also possible.

The government has a central role in ensuring that drugs distributed through the private sector are of high quality, safe, and effective. The government also has a responsibility to promote rational use of drugs. In addition, it may be necessary to actively promote drug availability (geographic access) and affordability (economic access) if a large share of low-income and remote populations depend on private-sector drug supply.

In many countries, missions, charities, and other not-for-profit, nongovernmental organizations (NGOs) provide an important share of health care. NGOs in some countries have established not-for-profit essential drug supply agencies to provide high-quality, low-cost drugs for their health facilities.

Perspectives on the role of government in health care vary from a solidarity or social welfare approach (which holds that the state should provide all health and other social services except when it is unable to do so) to a self-help or market economy approach (which holds that the private market should provide most health services). This chapter does not argue for or against either approach but describes strategies for achieving public health objectives within the context of public, private, or mixed systems.

≡ The basic goals of national drug policies and public-sector drug supply systems are to provide access to needed drugs, promote the rational use of drugs, and ensure the quality, safety, and efficacy of drugs. Various strategies exist to achieve these goals through different combinations of public and private involvement in the drug management cycle.

This chapter provides an overview of systems for financing and distributing drugs. It focuses on different strategies for organizing drug supply for government health services and issues related to decentralization of drug management functions. Issues and options related to meeting public health needs through the private pharmaceutical sector are also considered. The potential contribution of private nonprofit essential drug services is discussed. Finally, the chapter summarizes different government roles, including periods of transition from one model of service delivery to another.

≡ 6.1 Systems for Drug Financing and Distribution

How do countries provide their populations with pharmaceuticals? What combinations of financial and distribution systems exist? What is the rationale for different approaches to the pharmaceutical sector?

This section considers the major approaches to drug financing and distribution and discusses perspectives on the role of government in health care. Differences in the organization of health and pharmaceutical services reflect different views concerning the proper roles of the government and the private sector.

Approaches to Drug Financing and Distribution

Approaches to drug supply can be described in terms of public and private roles in financing, wholesale distribution, and retail distribution. The six main approaches range from fully public to fully private, as shown in Figure 6.1:

1. *Fully public*: The classic public system follows a central medical stores (CMS) approach, in which drugs are financed, procured, and distributed by a centralized government unit. The state is the owner, funder, and manager of the entire supply system. This has been the standard approach in many countries in Africa, Asia, Europe, and Latin America.

2. *Private supply to government health services*: Through direct delivery or prime vendor contracts (described later in this chapter), private channels are used to provide publicly funded drugs to government-operated health facilities. Although most common in North America, this approach can be found in Africa, Asia, and Latin America (see Country Study 6.1).

3. *Social health insurance systems*: Public funding from central budgets and social health insurance premiums can be used to reimburse pharmacies or patients themselves for drugs that are provided through private pharmacies. This approach has been followed in recent years in many Western European countries and in North America and Australia.

4. *Private financing/public supply*: Drugs may be supplied by government medical stores or state-owned wholesalers, dispensed by government health facilities, but paid for (in whole or in part) by patient fees. This was the case in many former socialist economies. In the 1990s, this approach is being used by China and by government health services in Asia, Africa, and Latin America that have implemented user fees for drugs but continue to operate government medical stores.

5. *State wholesale monopoly*: At least through the 1980s, in parts of Europe and Africa, drugs were imported and distributed by a state monopoly that supplied private pharmacies as well as government health services in some cases.

6. *Fully private*: Patients pay the entire cost of drugs and purchase them from private retail pharmacies and drug sellers, which now exist in nearly every country in the world and account in some cases for over 90 percent of drug distribution. This fully private approach probably accounts for the majority of non-prescription drug sales. Outside the market economies that have high levels of social and private health insurance, this approach is also the major source of prescription drugs in most countries, including many of those that nominally provide free pharmaceutical services.

Figure 6.1 Systems for Financing and Distributing Drugs

Financing	Distribution	
	Wholesale	Retail
Public		
Fully public	Public	Public
Private supply to government health services	Private	Public
Social health insurance systems	Private	Private
Private		
Private financing/ public supply	Public	Public
State wholesale monopoly	Public	Private
Fully private	Private	Private

In Figure 6.1, public financing includes government budgets (central, regional, and local) and compulsory social health insurance programs. Private financing includes out-of-pocket payments by individuals and households, private health insurance, community drug schemes, cooperatives, employers, and financing through other nongovernmental entities.

Public distribution includes wholesale distribution and retail dispensing by government-managed drug supply and health services as well as distribution through state-owned enterprises (state corporations). Private distribution includes private for-profit wholesalers, retailers, and nonprofit essential drug supply services.

Figure 6.1 does not exhaust all possible combinations of public and private drug financing and distribution, and it omits the dimension of drug production. Another column could be added to Figure 6.1, indicating whether drugs are produced by private companies, state-owned enterprises, or joint ventures. Pharmaceutical manufacturers, particularly research-based multinationals, have an important influence on drug distribution and drug use (see Chapter 9).

Perspectives on the Role of the State in Health Care

Different perspectives on the role of the state in providing health care result in differences in where drug financing and distribution responsibility is placed. The debate over the proper role of government is as old as government itself. Since the 1980s, the debate has been heightened, on the one hand, by the failure of centrally planned economies to ensure economic security for their populations and, on the other hand, by the inability of some market economies to ensure access to basic social services such as health care. Two views of the role of government can be identified:

1. *Social welfare perspective*: the government should provide all health and other social services, except in specific instances when it is unable to do so;
2. *Market economy perspective*: the private market should be left to provide all health and other social services, except when the private market fails to do so and the state can be expected to achieve better outcomes.

The social welfare and market economy perspectives are sometimes referred to as *solidarity* and *self-help* approaches, respectively.

Governments everywhere, regardless of level of economic development, are subject to a common set of constraints. These include

► inefficiency in service delivery, which may result from lack of individual incentives for good performance, bureaucratic inflexibility, and overemployment;
► interest-group pressures from political supporters, age-mates, business partners, members of one's local community, or concerned parties—which may lead to inefficient or inequitable use of public resources;
► lack of good governance, which may manifest itself in self-interested manipulation of the drug selection process, corruption in the award of tenders, nepotism in the appointment of key staff, or theft of drugs by health staff.

Although there are limits on government effectiveness, leaving the financing and supply of drugs entirely to the market economy may also fail to achieve public health objectives. Issues include

equity: Due to the relatively high cost of drugs compared with incomes, without government involvement, the poor and medically needy may be denied access to necessary and often lifesaving drugs.
information failure: Patients and some health professionals do not have full information about the quality, safety, efficacy, value for money, and appropriateness of individual drugs.
failure of competition: Patents and brand names may establish a virtual monopoly for some products, and cumbersome or obstructive registration procedures, combined with the high initial investment required to build manufacturing facilities and develop drugs, may limit the number of new competitors.
externalities: Health services such as vaccination and

treatment of contagious tuberculosis or sexually transmitted diseases (STDs) benefit other people in addition to those who receive the services.

The remaining sections of this chapter discuss major areas of public involvement in drug supply: organizing drug supply for government and NGO health services, decentralization and drug management, use of private channels to meet health needs, and private nonprofit essential drug services. Government action in each of these areas needs to be informed by a realistic assessment of the appropriate role of the state, given the circumstances of the country. Whatever a society's expectations or a government's promises are, there are constraints to government involvement and dangers in an unregulated market approach to drug supply.

≡ 6.2 Organizing Drug Supply for Government and NGO Health Services

Of all the decisions policy-makers and managers face, the most complex and costly often concern the financing and supply of drugs for government health services. In some countries, public-sector drug supply is well financed and administratively efficient. In other countries, the drug supply system is unreliable and shortages are common; such systems suffer from inadequate funding, outdated procedures, interference of various sorts, and a variety of other ills.

How should drugs be financed? How should drugs be supplied for government health services? Financing options include public financing (government budgets), user charges, health insurance, voluntary and other local financing, and donor financing. Part IV, Section B, considers financing issues in detail. Financing options are described and compared in detail in Chapter 40.

The drug management cycle—including all aspects of procurement and distribution—is the subject of Part III of this manual. Before confronting the particulars of the drug management cycle, however, it is necessary to establish the fundamental structure of the supply system. Once the basic system has been selected, the task is to apply professional drug management practices to achieve maximum efficiency.

Although many variations exist, there are five basic approaches for organizing drug supply for government health services (see Figure 6.2):

1. central medical stores
2. autonomous supply agency
3. direct delivery system
4. prime vendor system
5. fully private system

Figure 6.2 Comparison of Supply Systems for Government and Institutional Health Services

Model	Responsibilities			Advantages	Disadvantages
	Contracting Suppliers	Storage and Delivery	Monitoring Drug Quality		
Central medical stores Conventional supply system; drugs procured and distributed by centralized government unit	CMS	CMS	CMS	Maintains government control over entire system Is easy to monitor	High capital cost for offices, storage, transport facilities Recurrent cost of staff, transport, other operating costs Limited incentive for efficiency Open to political and other interference
Autonomous supply agency Bulk procurement, storage, and distribution managed by autonomous or semi-autonomous agency	Autonomous agency	Autonomous agency	DPO and autonomous agency	Maintains advantages of centralized system Flexibility in personnel and management systems may improve efficiency Is less open to interference Separate finances facilitate revolving drug funds	Cost and effort of establishing supply agency May retain some constraints of CMS Limited competitive pressure for efficiency if operated as monopoly
Direct delivery system Decentralized approach; tenders establish the supplier and price for each item; drugs delivered directly by supplier to districts and major facilities	DPO	Suppliers	DPO	Eliminates cost of government-operated storage and distribution Decentralized order quantities and delivery help adjust to variations in seasonal and local demand Maintains price benefits of centralized tendering Reduces inventory costs, expiration for high-cost, low-volume drugs	Coordination and monitoring of deliveries, payments, quality are demanding Feasible only where adequate private infrastructure exists Suppliers limited to those able to ensure local distribution (may reduce competition, increase cost) Direct delivery by multiple suppliers (especially to remote areas) is inefficient, may raise costs
Prime vendor system DPO establishes contracts with drug suppliers and separate contract with a single prime vendor, which warehouses and distributes drugs to districts and major facilities	DPO	Prime vendor	DPO and prime vendor	Maintains advantages of single distribution system Potential prime vendors compete on service level and cost	Monitoring of service level and drug quality is demanding Competition depends on well-developed private distribution system
Fully private supply Private sector manages all aspects of drug supply	Procurement and distribution by private enterprises		National drug regulatory authority	Least demanding and least costly for the government	Does not ensure equity of access for poor, medically needy, other target groups Drug quality is more difficult to monitor

Notes: CMS = central medical stores; DPO = drug procurement office (ministry of health or other government office).

A mixed system is frequently seen in practice, in which different approaches are used for different levels of health facilities or different categories of products.

The direct delivery system, the prime vendor system, and, in some instances, the autonomous supply agency system involve management or service contracts. There are important differences between contracting for drugs and contracting for services. Contract terms are different, and a different approach is needed for contract monitoring. Government officials must develop special skills to prepare and monitor such contracts (see Chapter 17).

This discussion speaks primarily from a government perspective. However, the mechanisms described here are equally relevant to mission and other nonprofit health services, private hospital purchasing groups, for-profit health systems, and other institutional health services. This is particularly true for the autonomous agency, direct delivery, and prime vendor approaches, as illustrated in Country Study 6.3.

Central Medical Stores
The classic approach to public-sector drug supply is the CMS approach, in which drugs are financed, procured, and distributed by the government, which is the owner, funder, and manager of the entire supply system. Selection, procurement, and distribution are all handled by the government—usually by a unit within the ministry of health. Financing is usually from central treasury allocations and/or donors, although this model can be adapted to a revolving drug fund (see Chapter 44).

With the CMS approach, problems with financial management, quantification of requirements, management of tenders, warehouse management, transport, and security of drugs are common. These problems often arise from political or administrative interference, civil service constraints on discipline or dismissal of ill-performing or dishonest staff, overall inadequacy of financial resources, procurement constraints arising from the treasury payment cycle and erratic release of ministry of health funds or foreign exchange, and transport difficulties resulting from the need to maintain a large vehicle fleet.

One way to address some of these constraints is to contract out specific aspects of the supply system. Outside contractors that specialize in certain services may be able to provide them at lower cost and higher quality. Port clearing, warehouse management, and transport (see Chapter 26) are among the services that are sometimes contracted out to the private sector.

Sustained improvements in the performance of some central supply systems have resulted from initiatives to strengthen their management and physical infrastructure (often with substantial donor input). Some have made efforts to contract out services such as transport. (See the country studies in the chapters on procurement and distribution for examples of improvements in specific aspects of CMS management.)

Autonomous Supply Agency
Problems with central supply systems have led some governments to establish systems that place the responsibility for bulk procurement, quality assurance, storage, distribution, and financial management in the hands of an autonomous or semi-autonomous supply agency. This model has been tried in several countries, particularly in Africa and Latin America (see Country Study 6.1).

Autonomous supply agencies are often constituted as parastatals, either under the ministry of health or as independent organizations with a board of directors from several government ministries. They operate like the nonprofit essential drug supply services described later, except that their primary client is government health services.

Autonomous supply services are established to achieve the efficiency and flexibility associated with private management while maintaining sufficient public-sector supervision to ensure that the services provide essential drugs, at reasonable prices, with adequate control of quality. The basic concept is that, under the right conditions, a well-constituted management board or board of directors (sometimes including representatives of NGOs and donor organizations) will appoint qualified senior managers, who will ensure an efficient, accountable supply service. Country Study 6.2 describes such an approach in West Africa.

Pharmaceutical supply agencies may be established in the context of a public-sector revolving drug fund (where fees are used to purchase drugs on a cash-and-carry basis) or in a system in which government institutions purchase drugs with centrally allocated treasury funds.

Experience to date, though limited, suggests that the following features should be sought in establishing autonomous supply agencies (see Figure 6.3):

- Oversight by an independent management board;
- Professional pharmaceutical supply managers;
- Good personnel management and adequate salaries for staff;
- Adequate financing;
- Public accountability and sound financial management;

Country Study 6.1 Autonomous Drug Supply Agencies in Selected Countries

Haiti. In 1984, AGAPCO (Agency for Supply of Community Pharmacies) was formed by presidential decree as a semi-autonomous body under the Ministry of Health. AGAPCO hired its own staff, maintained its own buildings and warehouses, procured drugs on the international market, and supplied drugs to community pharmacies located in government health facilities or in the community. A management board consisting of government officials and representatives of sponsoring donors oversaw AGAPCO activities. The system experienced serious operational and financial constraints in the late 1980s and eventually ceased to function.

Sudan. With the help of a grant, the CMS became autonomous in 1991 and was renamed the Central Medical Stores Public Organization (CMSPO). It has no direct government involvement, although there is close collaboration. The CMSPO procures only in accordance with the Sudan essential drugs list and only for the national health care system. Government hospitals receive central allocations for drugs and must buy from the CMSPO. Such hospitals and other community pharmacies pay a 20 percent markup; private pharmacies pay a 35 percent markup. Some NGOs and donor agencies purchase for hard currency.

Procurement takes place from nonprofit suppliers such as the International Dispensary Association (IDA) and the United Nations Children's Fund (UNICEF), and inventory control has been computerized. The main problems are that local manufacturers, which produce US$96 million worth of pharmaceuticals, need to be paid 60 percent of their billing in advance, and estimates of drug needs are not accurate.

Uganda. The National Medical Stores (NMS) in Uganda was reorganized in 1993 as an autonomous supply system. The board of directors is autonomous, and the bank account is independent. There were financing problems in the beginning, as the government gave the start-up money directly to twenty-seven of the thirty-nine districts that were being decentralized, making it impossible for the NMS to stock an adequate supply of drugs. As a result, some districts were forced to buy drugs from the private sector at high prices. In early 1995, more funds for procurement became available, and problems related to customer invoices were largely overcome by computerizing operations. All districts are now buying from the NMS. The Joint Medical Stores, representing the Catholic and Protestant Medical Bureau, gets drug kits at 20 percent of their cost. The kits are transported by the Ministry of Health to the district stores, where the mission units collect them. Health workers of the mission units are invited to the Ministry of Health's training workshops at no charge.

Zambia. Since 1988, central drug services have been operated as Central Medical Stores, Ltd., an autonomous body under a board of directors chaired by the permanent secretary of the Ministry of Health. Government institutions purchase drugs from CMS, Ltd. The scheme was initially quite successful but later ran into financial difficulty because of nonpayment by government institutions, which were supplied on credit on the authority of the ministry. This has led to CMS debts to suppliers and, subsequently, reduced availability of drugs.

► Continued focus on essential drugs (rather than "profitable" alternatives);
► Focus on quality assurance, in terms of both products and services provided.

An autonomous supply agency may achieve greater value for money and improved drug availability through more efficient management. The two important questions are: Does the agency have the flexibility to be efficient? Does the agency have the incentive to be efficient? Such agencies are likely to improve drug supply only if they are structured to overcome the constraints of the CMS approach. Competitive pressure encourages efficiency.

Difficulties can be anticipated if senior managers are political appointees rather than professional managers appointed by an independent management board; if the government retains the authority to require distribution of drugs without charge or on a credit basis (without ensuring payment); if special interests outside the agency influence drug procurement; if the agency is required to retain staff members regardless of their ability or performance; or if the agency acts as a monopoly, with no pressure to maintain low prices, reliable service, and high quality. Finally, countries considering an autonomous supply agency should recognize that this approach will not solve problems related to lack of funding for drugs.

Direct Delivery System

CMS and autonomous supply services involve bulk procurement and distribution from a central warehouse. The costs and logistical problems associated with central storage and distribution are substantial. An alternative is the direct delivery system.

In this non-CMS model, a government procurement office tenders to establish prices and suppliers for each essential drug, but the suppliers deliver the drugs directly to individual regional stores, district stores, or major health facilities. Variations of direct delivery contracts have been implemented in many countries (see Country Study 6.3). In Indonesia, annual allocations for drugs are made on a per capita basis to each district. Using its budget and the ministry's current price list for essential drugs, each district determines its own drug order (see Country Study 6.4).

Direct delivery contracts may specify fixed quantities with scheduled deliveries (generally the approach in Indonesia) or estimated quantity tenders with orders placed by the local warehouses or health facilities as needed. Financing arrangements can be tricky. Debts can quickly accumulate if drug supplies are not balanced against available funds. This means maintaining separate

Country Study 6.2 A Supply Agency Approach in Benin

The Benin Central Purchasing Office for Essential Drugs and Medical Supplies was established in 1991 to make drugs more accessible to the 5 million people of this small West African country. It was conceived as a single national supply and sales structure for essential drugs and medical supplies for public-sector health facilities and the private nonprofit sector.

Designed to be self-sustaining, the central office uses funds from cash sales to health facilities to procure additional supplies. Its success has been due in large part to the country's community financing policy, which allows health units to replenish their own funds at the community level and thus maintain their purchasing capacity.

Accountability and Efficiency. Originally accountable to the Ministry of Health, the Central Purchasing Office is now legally established as an autonomous body. Its activities and financial operations are monitored by a nine-member management committee, chaired by the director of pharmacies and laboratories, with members from bilateral cooperation agencies, multilateral cooperation agencies, hospitals, and national NGOs involved in health. A steering committee is responsible for ensuring that the agency's objectives are being met. Half its members are from the Ministries of Health, Finance, Justice, and Commerce, and half are development partners involved in health financing.

Certain management approaches have facilitated efficiency in operations. For example, only cash sales are allowed; no credit is extended to clients. Customers collect products themselves, eliminating the problems involved in maintaining regional depots and vehicles. Finally, the operational budget and personnel are kept to a minimum.

Procurement and Stock Management. Purchases are made according to the financial procedures defined by the management committee. There are three types of procurement: direct purchase, negotiated purchase, and selective tender. Stock management is done with a combination of manual and computerized systems, which emphasize maintaining adequate levels of the products with the highest consumption by volume and the twenty-five products that account for 80 percent of the revenue. The quality assurance system includes use of the World Health Organization (WHO) certification scheme, laboratory testing, and inspection of local manufacturers by a WHO consultant pharmacist.

Small Staff and Efficient Teamwork. The staff consists of three pharmacists, one secretary, three accounting staff, three storekeeper staff, three caretakers, one driver/forwarding agent, and one service and maintenance person. Written job descriptions and a management manual specify staff responsibilities and operating procedures. All staff were recruited by competitive examination or by invitation to apply, and they work under contract rather than as permanent civil servants. The central office has developed a continuing education program to strengthen the technical competence of personnel and to increase their motivation. Courses are also run for health center managers, nurses and midwives, and even for pharmacists from other countries.

Success Factors. The achievements of the central office are attributed to its small, flexible structure, which combines social objectives with private-style management. Key factors for success have been financial autonomy, funding from cash sales, a small staff selected for their competence, a realistic operating budget, good management, and effective supervision by outside management and steering committees.

Source: Hessou and Fargier 1994.

accounts for each supply point (if funding is from central allocations) or ensuring that all supplies are paid for at the time of delivery. Like most procurement systems, direct delivery contracts require a sole-source commitment—that is, for the tender drugs, the local warehouses and facilities order from the supplier that holds the tender contract. The local purchasers are free to order drugs that are not on the tender from any supplier. (See Chapters 16 and 17 for details related to preparing and tendering direct delivery contracts).

Direct delivery supply agreements depend on and encourage further development of a private-sector distribution system. In principle, they reduce storage and transport requirements for the government by specifying in procurement contracts that drugs are to be delivered directly to district stores and major health facilities. The government only has to store drugs at the district level and deliver them to health centers and peripheral health units.

Direct delivery contracts preserve the benefits of centralized selection (the essential drugs list), bulk procurement (suppliers offer favorable prices to get all the business for the products they are awarded), and centralized quality control (only reputable suppliers are invited to tender). Hospitals and districts benefit from being able to manage their own funds and determine the exact quantities needed. Finally, the problems of security, central storage, and transport are shifted from the ministry to the private suppliers.

With a direct delivery system, however, district-level and facility-level drug management responsibilities are much greater, since they include ordering, receiving, and paying for drugs. Success depends on adequate financing and management systems and the ability and willingness of staff to undertake the increased responsibilities.

Prime Vendor System

The prime vendor system is a variation of direct delivery in which the public procurement agency tenders for two types of contracts. First, the public procurement agency contracts with any number of suppliers to establish the

Figure 6.3 Checklist for Evaluating an Essential Drugs Supply Agency

Essential Drugs and Public Health Mandate
- ❏ Drugs limited to those on the national essential drugs list or formulary?
- ❏ Dressings, diagnostic agents, and other medical supplies included in range of products?
- ❏ Distribution restricted to government facilities?

Legal Status
- ❏ Operating unit under the ministry of health? Parastatal? Fully private agency?
- ❏ Status established by ministry directive? Legal notice? Act of law? Other measure?
- ❏ For-profit or nonprofit organization?

Management Board (board of directors)
- ❏ Membership: How appointed? How representative? How independent?
- ❏ Role and authority: How broad? How independent?
- ❏ Chairperson: How selected? How independent?

Senior Managers
- ❏ Recruitment: By whom? Approval by board required?
- ❏ Job descriptions and required qualifications clearly spelled out in writing?

Personnel System
- ❏ Civil service system?
- ❏ Parastatal system with some civil service characteristics?
- ❏ Private-sector flexibility, incentive structure, and controls?

Supply Management and Quality Assurance
- ❏ Professional pharmacists involved in management and supervision?
- ❏ Adequate quality assurance procedures in place and enforced?

Capital Financing (working capital for purchase of drugs, payment of suppliers)
- ❏ Source: central government allocation, donor, development bank, commercial bank?
- ❏ Type: grant, "soft" development loan, commercial loan?
- ❏ Adequacy: capital sufficient for current size and anticipated growth of supply demands?

Recurrent Financing (may come from a mix of sources)
- ❏ Drugs financed from district or facility central allocations?
- ❏ Drugs financed through user fees?
- ❏ Drugs financed through insurance?
- ❏ Salary and other recurrent operating costs financed through central allocations? Through markup on drugs distributed by the agency? Through fixed supply fee?

Financial Control and Accountability
- ❏ Able to maintain its own bank accounts?
- ❏ Annual independent public audit required?
- ❏ Annual report to ministry of health and central government required?
- ❏ Protection from decapitalization through unfunded distribution, distribution during emergency situations, credit sales?

source and price for each drug, but the drugs are not delivered by the suppliers directly; instead, a separate contract is negotiated (through tender, if feasible) with a single private-sector distributor, the prime vendor.

The suppliers deliver tender drugs to the prime vendor, which is responsible for maintaining sufficient stocks of drugs to fill orders from regional warehouses, district stores, and/or health facilities. The local warehouses and health facilities order drugs from the prime vendor, and the prime vendor fills the orders from drugs in stock. Prime vendors may maintain their own vehicle fleets or subcontract for transportation.

Like other direct delivery contracts, this system depends on sole-source commitment for the drugs under tender contract, although districts and health facilities may be allowed to purchase nontender drugs from any source. The system also requires the same level of good information and monitoring.

The prime vendor is paid a fee for storage and delivery services. In some industrialized countries, this fee is less than 2 percent of the invoice value at tender price. Prime vendors are able to achieve such low margins by distributing very large volumes of goods and also by generating revenue through money markets or bank interest. This is done through a difference in payment terms: the prime vendor pays the supplier after thirty to sixty days but requires health facilities to pay within fifteen days. This allows the prime vendor access to the equivalent of fifteen to forty-five days' turnover.

The prime vendor system may appear to add an extra middleman and extra costs, but experience has shown that the cost of a prime vendor can be more than offset in some situations by savings due to efficiency. Competitive awarding of prime vendor contracts is important to achieve this efficiency.

Fully Private Supply

National policy, insufficient financing, or management problems have led some countries to avoid taking on the responsibility for providing hospitals and health centers with even essential drugs. Cash-and-carry pharmacies are established within ministry facilities. Such pharmacies may be part of a parastatal pharmaceutical enterprise or they may be independent enterprises. In some countries, patients are left to buy virtually all drugs on their own from the private sector. This situation usually results from complete lack of funds within the government rather than any official drug management plan.

Pharmacies established in government health facilities may operate on a nonprofit or for-profit basis, depending on the arrangement with the government. Often such pharmacies are limited to the sale of essential drugs. In some cases, private pharmacies operate in parallel with government pharmacies. The government services usually provide basic essential drugs (free or for a fee), whereas the pharmacy supplies drugs for inpatients and specialty outpatient clinics on a fee-for-service basis.

Country Study 6.3 Direct Delivery, Prime Vendor, and Mixed Supply Arrangements

India: Combination Approach in Maharashtra State. Government health units in Maharashtra State are supplied through four main channels. First, since the 1960s, a "red-contract" direct delivery system has existed for a core list of about 300 drug products. Annual or two-year contracts are awarded that fix a single price for each product, with up to three suppliers per item. Health units must purchase red-contract items from one of the contract suppliers. Orders are placed with contract suppliers on a quarterly basis and delivered directly to health units. No state or district stores are required for these suppliers. Second, a limited number of vital items from the red-contract list are purchased for health units by the state stores organization. Third, health units have a small budget for direct local purchase of emergency items. Finally, some national disease control programs, such as malaria and tuberculosis control, distribute drugs to health facilities through the state stores organization.

Peru: Early Experience with Direct Delivery System. Established in 1971, Peru's Basic Medicines Program (BMP) was one of the first efforts to establish a direct delivery system for government health services. A national formulary list was established. Every two years, a tender was held using estimated purchase quantities to establish specific suppliers and prices for each item on the list. The fifty-seven Ministry of Health hospital areas would place regular orders through the BMP, which would confirm availability of funds and forward the order to the supplier. Drugs would be delivered directly from the supplier to the area hospital, from which other hospitals, health centers, and health posts in the area would be supplied. With this system, the BMP operated a coordinating office but maintained no warehouses, vehicles, or delivery services of its own. This system operated effectively for at least a decade. Computer technology available at the time had difficulty keeping up with processing orders and coordinating deliveries with suppliers. Inadequacy of financing was a periodic problem. The system of two-year contracts provided a large market base, which contributed to the development of local producers. Since the 1980s, the system has changed as the country has undergone political and economic changes.

South Africa: Prime Vendor System in Northern Transvaal Province. In South Africa, the secretariat of the Coordinating Committee for Medical Supplies (COMED) was established in 1985 to manage procurement, storage, and distribution of drugs and medical supplies for the public sector. Soon responsibility for storage and distribution was decentralized, but supplier contracts were still awarded nationally by COMED.

In Northern Transvaal Province, problems with unreliable public-sector distribution and frequent drug shortages led several regions to experiment with contracting different aspects of drug management out to private companies, eventually resulting in a prime vendor system for the entire province. COMED continues to conduct competitive tenders that establish the price and supplier for each product, but the Province Department of Pharmaceutical Services conducts its own competitive tender and awards a management contract for drug distribution. The contract combines four related services: ordering, storage, delivery to health units, and operating of the management information system. Early experience indicates that this approach has resulted in more reliable, less costly distribution and fewer shortages at health facilities (Möller et al. 1994).

Thailand: Pooled Procurement for Government Hospitals. For government hospitals in Thailand, decentralization of health services has led to substantial price increases as individual hospitals are faced with buying small quantities of drugs on the local market. In response to this problem, government hospitals in some areas have begun forming group purchasing cooperatives to agree on a standard list of items from the national essential drugs list and conduct tenders to establish the supplier and prices for each item. Individual hospitals then purchase directly from the contracted supplier. Only suppliers certified by the national drug regulatory authority are considered. Individual hospitals are responsible for determining the quantities they require, paying suppliers, managing their drug stocks, and monitoring drug use. This approach has allowed hospitals to get the price and quality assurance benefits of central supply while maintaining the benefit of decentralization through local control of quantification, supply management, and financial management.

United States: Group Purchasing through the Prime Vendor System. Over 75 percent of the US pharmaceutical market is served through the prime vendor system, in which a purchasing group has established separate procurement contracts with suppliers and with a prime vendor. The purchasing group may be a large managed-care insurance program, a branch of the US Public Health Service, or a group of local health facilities. The prime vendor orders contract drugs, maintains sufficient stocks to provide a service level of at least 90 percent, and delivers drugs to the individual health units. The health units that are part of the purchasing group order from the prime vendor and pay the prime vendor directly.

The Texas Association of Community Health Centers (TACHC) is one successful group purchasing program. In response to rising drug costs and declining government funds, TACHC was formed in 1986 by a group of twenty-four members (clinics and networks of clinics) serving primarily low-income patients. By 1994, there were thirty-five members in four states. Like all US procurement groups, TACHC uses estimated quantities, with no guaranteed purchases; group members order as needed at the contract price. The TACHC purchasing group negotiates one set of contracts with pharmaceutical companies for drug prices, and another contract with a prime vendor for wholesale warehousing and distribution. In 1986, TACHC paid a 5 percent prime vendor fee; in 1994, the fee was 1.75 percent over the pharmaceutical company contract price, including all shipping costs. With these low prime vendor fees, it makes little sense for TACHC to operate its own warehousing and distribution system (Rankin 1995).

Zimbabwe: Different Systems for Different Drugs. In the Zimbabwe Essential Drugs Action Programme (ZEDAP), different systems are used for different categories of drugs. High-usage drugs on the essential drugs list are procured, stocked, and distributed in bulk through the CMS. For high-cost, slow-moving specialist items, direct delivery contracts are used. In the past, such items were bought and stocked centrally, but demand was highly variable, resulting in frequent costly expirations. For most specialist items, an annual tender is conducted to fix the price for the year. Drugs are then ordered as needed by the roughly two dozen national hospitals and NGO hospitals that require these drugs. Orders are delivered directly to the hospitals. For government hospitals, payment is made centrally under proper authorization. Finally, for cancer agents and some other highly specialized drugs, no contract exists. Instead, drugs are purchased by the ministry's pharmaceutical division by individual order, with permission from the secretary of health.

Country Study 6.4 Direct Delivery in Indonesia

With a population of nearly 190 million people spread over 3,000 islands spanning a distance greater than the width of the United States, Indonesia presents a particular challenge for public-sector drug logistics. For over a decade, most essential drugs for primary health care have been supplied through a system in which drugs are delivered directly to nearly 300 district drug depots (GFKs).

Supply Sources. The essential drugs list is divided into categories that determine the source of supply: list A (forty-two drugs from Indo-Farma), list B1 (thirty-four drugs from Kimia Farma), list B2 (fifty-seven drugs from Pharpros), and list C (seven drugs from private manufacturers). Indo-Farma, Kimia Farma, and Pharpros are public-sector manufacturers. Other drugs on the national essential drugs list are procured from private manufacturers through competitive regional tenders.

Financing. Financing is provided by a combination of central government funds, the health insurance scheme for civil servants, provincial and district budgets, and specialized national programs (see Country Study 40.1). The national budget and insurance funds, which together account for 80 percent of the drug budget, use the same basic supply sources.

Quantification of Drug Requirements. Annual estimates of drug requirements are submitted through provincial offices by each district. Districts are expected to base their estimates on consumption records. Since drug prices and drug budgets for the major funding sources are known, districts can make informed choices to obtain the greatest therapeutic benefit within the available budget.

Distribution. Nearly all essential drugs are delivered directly to the country's 296 GFKs, from which drugs are distributed to government hospitals, health centers (6,954 in 1995), and auxiliary health centers (18,000 in 1995). GFKs are managed by pharmacists and assistant pharmacists according to a GFK management manual.

Drugs on lists A, B1, and B2 are distributed to GFKs from depots managed by Kimia Farma. Drugs on list C and other essential drugs are delivered directly to GFKs from private wholesalers' warehouses. There is no national CMS, and only a small number of drugs for diarrheal diseases, nutrition, and a few other specialized programs are distributed through provincial depots.

Coordination Complexities. District-level quantification and direct delivery to the GFKs are essential for supplying such a vast country. With multiple funding and supply sources, however, the government is continually working to improve record keeping, needs estimation, information flow, distribution schedules, and coordination.

Sources: Andajaningsih 1995; WHO/DAP 1989.

As with revolving drug funds operated by the government (see Chapter 44), the greatest concern with fully private supply is equity of access for the poor, children, patients with communicable diseases, and other target groups.

Comparison of Supply Systems

The five supply systems are compared in Figure 6.2. The systems vary with respect to the role of the state and the degree of private-sector involvement. The CMS approach demands the most of the central government in terms of human and physical resources, because it operates virtually the entire distribution system.

With an autonomous supply agency, direct delivery system, or prime vendor system, the role of the government changes from direct operations to a combination of direct operations and contract coordination and monitoring. These systems do not require a large central government distribution infrastructure, but they do require a drug procurement office (DPO) or its equivalent to manage contracts and monitor performance effectively.

A CMS or autonomous supply agency approach can be used when the local private sector is not well developed. However, the efficiency of a direct delivery or prime vendor system depends on a well-developed private sector.

Drug supply systems need to achieve two main objectives: (1) high service level, as measured by low rates of shortages and stockouts, and (2) efficiency, as measured by having low total costs for a given level of service. Autonomous supply agencies, direct delivery contracts, and prime vendor systems offer different approaches to create the flexibility, competition, and clear performance targets that help achieve these objectives.

≡ 6.3 Decentralization and Drug Management

Selection, procurement, and distribution can be effectively managed in centralized, partially decentralized, or fully decentralized systems. Of the four main functions in the drug management cycle, only local distribution and drug use are, by their nature, decentralized. Most other functions could be performed at the national, provincial, district, or local level.

Much attention has been given to decentralization. But what is meant by decentralization? The term is used to describe at least three different approaches to transferring power from central authorities: delegation, devolution, and privatization.

Delegation describes the assignment of responsibility for specific tasks to lower-level units within the health system, with overall control remaining at the central level. In Indonesia, quantification is delegated to the districts, although compiling drug orders and determining final order quantities remain central functions (see Country Study 6.4).

Devolution refers to the transfer of power (responsibility, authority, and accountability) to lower-level units, which

TWO FACES OF THE PRIVATE SECTOR

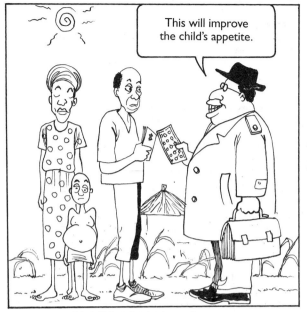

PROFIT BEFORE PEOPLE

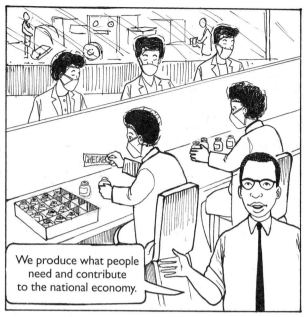

A REASONABLE RETURN FOR
RESPONSIBLE INVESTMENT

are then outside the direct control of the central level. In Thailand, decentralization of procurement to local hospitals meant that hospitals could establish their own procurement arrangements, free from central interference (see Country Study 6.3).

Privatization is properly defined as the transfer of ownership from the public to the private sector. But the term is also applied, less precisely, to contracting government services to the private sector (as with direct delivery contracts) or introducing private-sector features into the public sector (as with government-owned but semi-autonomous supply agencies).

Decentralization in any of these forms is intended to improve the responsiveness, quality, and efficiency of health services. Decentralization aims to achieve these benefits through greater local involvement, more direct public accountability, increased flexibility to adjust to local circumstances, more rapid and more accurate communication, and quicker adaptation to changing conditions. Improvements are far from certain, however. Problems that have occurred with attempts to decentralize drug management functions include

lack of capacity: Decentralization of drug management responsibility may be implemented without ensuring that there are sufficient local staff and management capacity to sustain services.

lack of financial resources: Responsibility is sometimes decentralized without providing an adequate budget or

financing system at the levels where responsibility is placed. In this case, decentralization simply becomes abandonment of responsibility.

increased corruption: Because of the money involved, interference for personal gain is common in drug supply systems. Although decentralization is meant to improve accountability, it sometimes makes it easier for local officials or other special interests to profit.

increased cost: Decentralization of procurement usually means smaller order quantities. It can result in higher prices for essential drugs, although this problem can be overcome with central contracts coupled with decentralized ordering.

decreased drug quality: Selecting reliable suppliers and monitoring drug quality are difficult at the local level if there is no unified national system.

For managing drug supply, it is useful to think in terms of a task-specific approach to decentralization. Tasks better performed centrally include those that require specialized skills, involve economies of scale, or depend on extensive or rapidly changing technical information. Examples of such tasks include development of essential drugs lists, preparation of standard treatments, management of competitive tenders, selection and monitoring of suppliers, quality assurance, and development of training programs in rational drug use.

Tasks that can be decentralized include those that do not require uncommon technical skills and those for which local information is required. Decentralization is appropriate when local circumstances vary significantly throughout the country and local interests favor improved performance. Examples of such tasks include adaptation of drug lists or standard treatments to local needs, quantification of drug requirements, coordination of local distribution, training in rational drug use, and monitoring of drug use at health facilities.

Thailand's approach to pooled procurement by government hospitals provides an example of a task-specific approach. Procurement is based on the national essential drugs list, and suppliers are selected from those that the national drug control authority has certified as following good manufacturing practices. Tendering is centralized at the level of the hospital purchasing group in order to obtain lower bulk prices. Quantification of drug requirements, payment for drugs, receipt and storage, and supervision of drug use are all decentralized to the level of the individual hospital.

≡ 6.4 Meeting Health Needs through Private Channels

Private pharmacies and other private drug outlets exist in virtually every country in the world. The percentage of total pharmaceutical expenditures that pass through the private sector varies from under 10 percent in some small, relatively isolated countries to over 90 percent in countries with a well-developed private sector and limited public-sector drug supply. By retail value, the majority of pharmaceuticals in many developing countries flow through the private sector.

Purchasing of drugs is a leading health expenditure in household surveys from developing countries. Doctors, other clinicians in private practice, and practitioners in the informal health sector commonly dispense pharmaceuticals, often deriving more income from drugs than from consulting fees.

Changes in national policy, declining government financial resources, or other trends may lead to an increasing role for the private sector. Governments' inability to provide regular drug supplies may push more patients to the private sector.

From a public health perspective, the objectives for government involvement with the private pharmaceutical sector are to ensure

- drug quality, safety, and efficacy
- drug availability (geographic access)
- drug affordability (economic access)
- rational drug use

Measures that may help achieve these objectives are outlined in Figure 6.4 and described briefly below.

Figure 6.4 Measures to Meet Health Needs through the Private Pharmaceutical Sector

Drug Quality, Safety, and Efficacy
- licensing and inspection of distribution premises and professionals
- licensing and inspection of manufacturers
- drug registration
- postmarketing surveillance

Availability (Geographic Access)
- licensing of importers, wholesalers, retailers
- incentives for wholesalers, retailers
- training of pharmacy aides and other drug sellers
- dispensing clinicians
- community drug schemes

Affordability (Economic Access)
- insurance coverage
- price information
- price competition through generic substitution
- price regulation: producer and distributor prices
- price regulation: retail margins

Rational Drug Use
- regulation of drug information and promotion
- basic undergraduate and continuing education of health professionals
- licensing of prescribers and dispensers
- public and patient education

Drug availability and affordability are of particular concern when government health services do not exist or are not able to provide drugs for poor, medically needy, geographically isolated, or otherwise underserved populations. In countries where a large proportion of the population is poor and government health services lack sufficient resources, ensuring universal access to drugs is particularly challenging.

The following discussion provides an overview of options, not a checklist of recommended actions. Government supervision of the private pharmaceutical market involves complex and often contentious issues. Public health objectives may conflict with commercial interests. Ideological or political considerations not directly related to either public health or commercial perspectives may further cloud discussions. Governments must carefully explore and understand these options in context.

Drug Quality, Safety, and Efficacy
Ensuring drug quality, safety, and efficacy is a fundamental responsibility of the government. Major tasks involved in drug regulation include licensing and inspection of distribution premises and professionals, licensing and inspection of manufacturers, drug registration, and post-marketing surveillance. Postmarketing surveillance includes monitoring and testing of drug quality and reporting of adverse drug reactions.

Effective drug regulation requires up-to-date drug legislation and regulations; a drug regulatory authority that is adequately staffed, financed, and equipped; and national commitment to implementing the measures necessary to ensure quality, safety, and efficacy. Specific aspects of drug legislation and regulation are discussed in Chapter 7.

Availability

A basic range of essential drugs should be available throughout the country. Availability can be improved through licensing requirements and incentives aimed at broadening the distribution network, training of pharmacy aides and other drug sellers, reliance on dispensing clinicians, and community drug schemes.

Importer, Wholesaler, and Retailer Licensing and Incentives. Availability of essential drugs is frequently a problem in distant and sparsely populated rural areas. Licensing of wholesalers may be used to increase drug availability by requiring distribution to drug outlets in all geographic areas and by requiring that each wholesaler provide the full range of a specified list of essential drugs. To encourage new services in relatively underserved areas, guidelines may be established for the minimum distance between drug outlets, or limits may be placed on the number of drug outlets per population in a given town or district.

Although such provisions would seem to promote equity, they may conflict with producer-wholesaler arrangements and face other practical difficulties, depending on the structure of the local market. Service and price competition may be reduced if the number of registered wholesalers and retailers is limited.

An alternative to licensure restrictions is financial incentives to expand services to remote and underserved areas. Possibilities include rural-urban pharmacy cross-subsidy systems, higher retailer margins or reimbursement rates, or tax reductions for providing services in remote areas.

Training of Pharmacy Aides and Other Drug Sellers. In many countries, a large share of drugs—even prescription drugs—is sold by untrained people. Economic factors contribute to the problem, but many countries also lack trained pharmacists. Recognizing this reality, a number of countries have established training programs to promote safe dispensing by pharmacy aides.

It is often assumed that profit-making and public health concerns are incompatible. Yet for many common illnesses, there are pharmaceutical products that are safe, effective, and profitable to dispense. Controlled field studies have demonstrated that drug sellers can be trained with special interactive methods to reduce their use of antibiotics and antidiarrheals and increase their dispensing of oral rehydration salts for simple diarrhea.

Dispensing by Clinicians. In many parts of the world, doctors, nurses, and other clinicians in private practice both prescribe and dispense drugs to their patients. Where drugs are hard to obtain or are distributed by untrained drug sellers, dispensing clinicians provide an important service. But clinicians often generate more income from drugs than from consultation fees. This creates an obvious and well-documented incentive to overprescribe.

It has been suggested that dispensing by clinicians be limited to rural and other areas with limited access to pharmacies, and that clinicians dispense drugs at cost rather than for profit. A pragmatic approach might be to accept dispensing by clinicians as one approach to increasing access to drugs, but at the same time to promote prescribing practices that are both therapeutically sound (see Chapter 30) and financially rewarding.

Community Drug Schemes. Drugs may also be made available through community drug schemes that emphasize essential drugs, low prices, and rational drug use. Community drug schemes are often initiated in areas with limited geographic or economic access to drugs. The considerable experience that has accumulated with community drug schemes and other forms of revolving drug funds is mixed, with some examples that support the arguments of both proponents and opponents (see Chapters 37, 40, and 44).

Affordability

Cost can be a major barrier to adequate treatment, particularly in low-income countries and for the poorest members of society. Possible mechanisms to increase economic access to essential drugs include increased insurance coverage, price information, price competition through generic substitution, regulation of producer and wholesaler prices, and regulation of retail markups or profit margins.

Insurance Coverage. Health insurance in various forms covers a large portion of the population in many high-income and some middle-income countries. It covers only a small, though growing, portion of the population in low-income countries. Important elements of insurance include risk-sharing and prepayment. Insurance spreads the burden of payment for illness among all the members of the scheme whether they are ill or healthy, poor or nonpoor.

National social insurance schemes, private voluntary insurance, managed care, and community prepayment schemes can increase access to essential drugs. Insurance programs, particularly of the managed-care type, have an incentive to control costs and promote rational drug use.

At the same time, there are a number of threats that may undermine the use of insurance to increase equity, access, and efficiency (see Chapter 40).

Price Information. Policy-makers, health professionals, people in the distribution chain, and consumers need complete, accurate, up-to-date information on drug prices. When they have information about drug prices and generic drugs, consumers can exert pressure on both prescribers and dispensers to control prices. Methods for communicating price information include

- ► listing prices or relative price information in therapeutics manuals;
- ► printing retail prices on drug packages;
- ► regular publication of a pharmaceutical pricing guide or manual;
- ► publication of selected pharmaceutical prices in local newspapers or other media.

Price comparisons over time and among countries can be useful to monitor pharmaceutical price differentials and the effects of various drug policies. Such comparisons can be complex and confusing, however. A pharmaceutical price index, based on the same principles that consumer price indexes use to monitor inflation, is one approach to making such comparisons. WHO has described such a method for calculating the value of a "basket of drugs" (WHO 1994).

For comparison purposes, world market prices for several hundred essential drugs are published annually by Management Sciences for Health (MSH 1995). In addition, bulk prices for several dozen active pharmaceutical raw materials are published by the International Trade Centre in conjunction with WHO (ITC 1995).

Price Competition through Generic Substitution. Competitive bulk procurement by generic name is a central feature of most essential drugs programs in developing countries and of many large hospitals and health services in developed countries. In the private market, price competition may be encouraged through incentives for prescribing and dispensing by generic name.

Over 90 percent of drugs on most national essential drugs lists are available by generic name. In many countries, the majority of patents on brand-name drugs sold in the private sector have expired and the drugs can therefore be sold by generic name. A number of countries have adopted policies that encourage generic prescribing and dispensing, yet large generic drug markets have developed in a relatively small number of countries (see Country Study 6.5).

Since at least the early 1970s, various countries have initiated efforts to promote generic drugs in the private sector. Problems faced by these initiatives have included difficulty in ensuring drug quality, inadequate preparation of health professionals, failure to address financial incentives at the dispensing point, and the incorrect assumption that public demand already exists for cheap generic drugs.

Experiences to date suggest four main factors that influence the growth and stability of the generic drug market in a country: supportive legislation and regulation, quality assurance capacity, public and professional acceptance, and economic factors (see Figure 6.5).

Policies based only on clinicians' voluntary decisions to prescribe by generic name have met with limited success. But laws that mandate generic substitution from the outset often elicit strong resistance. Generic substitution laws sometimes evolve from permitting substitution (brand-name dispensing is assumed unless the prescriber, dispenser, or patient requests generic substitution), to encouraging substitution (dispensing of a low-cost generic substitute is assumed unless otherwise specified), to requiring substitution of a lower-cost generic equivalent, if available (see the example from the United States in Country Study 6.5). When generic prescribing and dispensing evolve through these stages over a period of several years, clinicians, pharmacy staff, and consumers have an opportunity to become comfortable with generic substitution. However, this process may be too long for countries under pressure to quickly make affordable drugs more widely available.

Generic substitution is most readily implemented when reimbursement is involved—if the government is paying for the drugs, it is possible to implement controls such as reference pricing (see below). However, even without a reimbursement program, economic incentives at the retail level can contribute to the success of a generic substitution program. Once a generic market begins to develop, generic producers, importers, and distributors become advocates for further development of generic drug use. Whereas price regulation tends to generate uniform opposition from private producers and distributors, generic drug use tends to develop advocates within specific segments of the pharmaceutical market. In any case, generic drugs should be subject to the same quality standards as those applied to drugs sold by brand name. Quality assurance must exist not only in fact but also in the perception of health professionals and the public.

Price Regulation: Producer Prices. Increasing generic drug use makes essential drugs more affordable. At the same time, many countries adopt systems of direct price regulation. It is useful to separate regulation of producer prices

---

Country Study 6.5 Promoting Generic Drugs

European Community. As of the mid-1990s, generic dispensing differed greatly among the countries of the European Community. In Denmark, generic substitution was possible with the doctor's agreement, and generic drugs represented about 60 percent of prescription volume and 30 percent of sales value. In the United Kingdom, Germany, and the Netherlands, generic substitution was strongly encouraged, and 20 to 40 percent of prescriptions were dispensed generically. Except for Germany, these countries had low to average per capita drug consumption compared with that of the entire European Community. Countries such as Belgium, France, and Italy tended to have relatively low generic drug use—often less than 2 percent of sales value. The wide variation in generic dispensing among these countries—which are generally able to ensure the quality of generic products—illustrates the impact that national policies and different local circumstances can have on generic drug use.

Indonesia. A 1989 ministerial decree made the prescribing and dispensing of generic drugs compulsory in public health facilities and encouraged the use of generic drugs in the private sector. The Ministry of Health initiated a campaign to promote generic drug use by health professionals and the community. Production of "logo generic drugs" was led by state-owned manufacturers, but private manufacturers entered the market with government encouragement. By the mid-1990s, thirty pharmaceutical companies (four state owned and twenty-six privately owned) were producing generic drugs, nearly 200 commonly used essential drugs were commercially available by generic name, 408 pharmacies were obligated to provide generic drugs, the market in monetary terms had tripled over a five-year period, and generic dispensing had risen to about 15 percent of prescriptions (Andajaningsih 1995).

Philippines. The Generics Act of 1988, passed unanimously in congress, was the first legislation enacted to operationalize the Philippine National Drug Policy (PNDP). The act provided for mandatory use of generic names on labels, advertising materials, and prescription slips; encouraged pharmacists to provide information to clients on generic drugs and their prices; provided incentives for manufacturers of generic products; and advocated the dissemination of public and professional information on the generics law and on the rational use of drugs.

A consultative process was facilitated by the establishment of the Task Force on Pharmaceuticals, which included health professionals, drug industry representatives, health NGOs, consumer groups, and academics. Implementation approaches were sequenced to promote early high-visibility successes and impact. For example, generic labeling was begun with products having single active ingredients; labeling rules overall were put in place before generic prescribing and dispensing were mandated. The political process leading to enactment of the generics law, though broad-based, required some compromises. Professional and industry lobbying resulted in doctors being allowed to place their choice of brand names in parentheses on prescriptions. No controls on prices were included in the final law. Implementation of some elements of the law was postponed to gain cooperation. Despite these efforts, acceptance of generic prescribing and dispensing has been slow. This emphasizes the need for a persistent, long-term approach to promoting generic drug use.

United States. In the United States, generic dispensing was greatly encouraged by the 1984 Drug Price Competition and Patent Term Restoration Act (Waxman-Hatch Act), which facilitated registration of generic drugs. But laws governing generic substitution at the time of dispensing are made at the state level. A few states began with laws that permitted but did not encourage substitution. During the 1980s, states began to enact laws that more strongly encouraged generic dispensing, particularly for patients whose prescriptions were financed in whole or in part with public funds. As a result of these laws and the reimbursement limitations of government programs such as Medicaid and private insurance organizations, generic dispensing in the United States rose from about 18 percent of new prescriptions in 1984 to nearly 40 percent in 1994.

Source: WHO 1996.

---

from regulation of distribution margins. Although there a number of variations, controls on producer prices fall into three categories (Mossialos et al. 1994; Ballance et al. 1992):

1. *Cost-plus pricing:* Prices are negotiated between the manufacturer and the national authority, based on raw materials costs, production costs, marketing costs, other producer costs, and a reasonable allowance for profit.

2. *Reference pricing:* Reference pricing—also known as yardstick, benchmark, comparative, or leader pricing—sets or limits the price for an individual drug by comparison with the price of other drugs. *Internal* reference pricing is based on comparison with drugs already on the national market that have similar therapeutic effects. *External* reference pricing considers the price of the identical or comparable drugs marketed in other countries.

3. *Profit-based pricing:* Control of profits or return on capital investment is considered on a company-by-company basis, with target profit levels set in part on an assessment of the company's risk. Within overall profit limits, companies are free to set the prices of individual products.

Cost-plus pricing depends on being able to obtain accurate information on actual production, marketing, and other costs. Reported costs can be manipulated through various accounting practices. Reference pricing is more transparent and requires virtually no information from companies (or their accounting systems). Discussions center on the question of generic and therapeutic

Figure 6.5
Generic Drug Use: Some Enabling Factors

Supportive Legislation and Regulation
- ► abbreviated registration procedures (focus on quality)
- ► product development and authorization during patent period
- ► provisions that permit, encourage, or require generic prescription and substitution
- ► development of substitution, nonsubstitution lists
- ► requirement that labels and drug information contain generic names

Quality Assurance Capacity
- ► procedures to demonstrate bioequivalence
- ► national quality assurance capability
- ► national drug manufacturer and drug outlet inspection capability

Professional and Public Acceptance
- ► phased implementation, beginning with permission to substitute
- ► required use of generic names in all education and training of health professionals
- ► brand-generic and generic-brand name indexes available to health professionals
- ► required use of generic names in clinical manuals, drug bulletins, other publications
- ► consumer awareness

Economic Factors
- ► public and professional price information
- ► reference pricing for reimbursement programs
- ► retail price controls that favor generic dispensing
- ► support by social and private health insurance organizations
- ► incentives for generic drug industry
- ► tradeoffs with industry (reduced price regulation, increased patent protection)

substitutability. Profit-based pricing depends on having access to companies' financial information.

Pharmaceutical price regulation is common in both developed and developing countries, although there is little agreement on its overall impact (Redwood 1993; Zerda Sarmiento 1995). Proponents of price regulation believe that it lowers individual drug prices, lowers total drug expenditures, improves price information for insurers and consumers, and is necessary because market forces alone cannot ensure competition. Opponents believe that price regulation is cumbersome, encourages manipulation of accounting practices, creates scarcities (real or artificial), has no impact on patient or overall health expenditures (because it encourages the use of drugs and the use of more expensive drugs), reduces innovation and competition, and is unnecessary for most therapeutic needs if essential drugs are sold by generic name.

When price regulation has been effectively enforced, it has been shown to control both individual drug prices and increases in drug prices. Price control is most effective when the agency controlling prices is also paying for the drugs consumed by patients—reimbursing either the dispenser or the patient. However, the effect of price regulation on overall drug expenditures—either at the individual level or at the national level—and on therapeutic outcome is less certain (Redwood 1993). The effect of lowering individual drug prices may be offset by prescribing and dispensing greater quantities of drugs or a different (and more costly) selection of drugs. Poorly conceived price regulation systems may have unintended consequences—and sometimes the opposite of those intended. It is important to evaluate the economic reasoning behind price regulation policies and to anticipate the economic responses of producers, distributors, and consumers.

Price Regulation: Distribution Markups. Although considerable attention is paid to controlling producer prices, over half of the final selling price of a drug may reflect distribution margins—markups charged by importers, wholesale distributors, and retail outlets. The structure of distribution markups is critical, because it strongly influences dispensing incentives and advice at the point of purchase.

There are at least five methods used to regulate distribution margins for pharmaceuticals:

1. *Cost plus fixed percentage:* The most common approach is for wholesalers and retailers to add a fixed percentage to the price they pay.
2. *Cost plus declining percentage:* Some countries have adopted markups based on a declining percentage—the more costly the drug, the lower the markup.
3. *Cost plus fixed dispensing fee:* To reduce the incentive to dispense higher-cost drugs, some countries have adopted a system of fixed professional dispensing fees. For example, a pharmacist would charge $1 per prescription plus the wholesale cost of the drug.
4. *Cost plus differential dispensing fee:* To encourage generic dispensing, public and private insurance scheme may reimburse pharmacies based on drug costs plus a differential professional dispensing fee—for example, $2 for a generic prescription and $1 for a brand-name prescription.
5. *Maximum allowable price:* The maximum sale price or reimbursement level is fixed by a government price control agency. Price control can take the form of reference pricing for identical generic products or therapeutic categories, or the establishment of a source for each individual product on the market. Such methods are cumbersome, and governments often struggle to update prices and enforce the policies and regulations.

Fixed dispensing fees create a double incentive for dispensing lower-cost drugs. First, the pharmacist is likely to

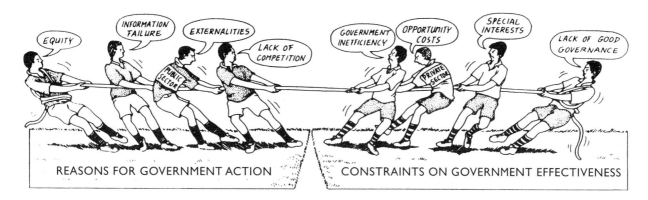

REASONS FOR GOVERNMENT ACTION | CONSTRAINTS ON GOVERNMENT EFFECTIVENESS

sell more when dispensing drugs whose final price to the customer is lower. Second, the stock-keeping costs of high-priced brand-name drugs are considerable. Selling more lower-cost drugs reduces the overall cost of maintaining drug stocks.

Distribution markups include two components: the markup for the wholesaler and the markup for the retailer. The final price paid by the customer represents the sum of the producer's price ("cost" in the above list), the wholesale markup and the retail markup. Different methods exist for combining producer price regulation and regulation of distribution markups. It is beyond the scope of this manual to describe and illustrate these methods. It should be recognized, however, that pricing structures establish incentives and disincentives that have a major impact on drug consumption patterns. They may also have unexpected effects on other aspects of the system. In some countries, fixed prices that are slowly updated produce an incentive to register more new products—many of which are only slightly different from older products—in order to negotiate higher prices. The *World Development Report* of 1993 reported more than 50,000 products officially registered in Brazil, due primarily to its pricing policy.

Rational Drug Use

Although greater competition and economic incentives may lead to managerial efficiency in the private sector, they often lead to therapeutic inefficiency. Profit motives may lead to overtreatment of mild illness, inadequate treatment of serious illness, misuse of anti-infective drugs, and overuse of injections. Consumers often buy subtherapeutic doses of drugs such as antibiotics and fail to adhere to correct advice for taking the drugs roughly half the time.

Promoting rational drug use in the private sector involves regulation of drug information and promotion (see Chapters 7 and 30), basic undergraduate and contin-

uing education of health professionals (see Chapters 31 and 32), licensing of prescribers and dispensers (Chapter 7), and public and patient education (Chapter 33).

≡ 6.5 Private Nonprofit Essential Drug Services

Nonprofit health care providers, including mission and charitable health services and other NGOs, play an important role in the financing and provision of health services in many countries. The share of health services and financing provided through the private nonprofit health sector varies considerably among countries, but in low-income countries it can range up to 50 percent of curative services (Bennett and Ngalande-Bande 1994; Gilson et al. 1994). NGOs can play an important role in promoting the concept of essential drugs and in supplying essential drugs.

Incentives for NGOs

To the extent that NGOs target their services to rural populations, mothers and children, the urban poor, and other underserved groups, it is in the interest of the government to encourage the growth and development of such organizations. Government incentives and subsidies for NGOs may include annual lump-sum grants, temporary assignment of ministry health personnel, payment of NGO staff, permission to purchase drugs from government stores, exemption from import duties (sometimes limited to drugs on the national essential drugs list), and payment of retirement benefits (WHO 1994). Providing access to government drug stores and exemption from import duties are particularly important for encouraging NGOs to provide essential drugs for their patients. Ethiopia, Ghana, Malawi, Tanzania, Uganda, Zambia, and Zimbabwe are among the countries that have allowed specific NGOs to purchase drugs from government medical stores—in some cases, at subsidized prices (WHO 1994).

Country Study 6.6 MEDS: An NGO Essential Drugs Service in East Africa

The Mission for Essential Drugs and Supplies (MEDS) program was established in 1986 by two Kenyan religious organizations, the Catholic Secretariat and the Christian Health Association, to supply good-quality essential drugs at a reasonable cost to more than 500 church-managed health units throughout Kenya. These units constitute roughly 36 percent of the country's rural health services.

MEDS supplies drugs for over 300 hospitals, health centers, and dispensaries. It also sells to several international NGOs for their local operations. The MEDS program has the approval of the country's Ministry of Health (MOH) but is autonomous from both its church parents and the government. It uses a revolving fund, financed by governmental and nongovernmental organizations in three European countries, by its Kenyan sponsor organizations, and by its clients' drug purchases. It has received consulting advice from WHO/DAP.

One of MEDS's methods for keeping drug prices down while keeping supply constant has been bulk buying from local producers; about 70 percent of the drug items are of local origin, and still more would be purchased locally if local prices were competitive for drugs of comparable quality. Thirty percent of drugs have been imported from Zimbabwe and Europe (requiring foreign currency). The costs of imported drugs have been increased by the Kenyan value-added tax and a levy of 1.5 percent, even on donated drugs.

In early 1993, a serious situation emerged with the sudden free float of the Kenyan shilling, which resulted in immediate price rises of up to 50 percent. MEDS tried to keep its own price rises to 10 percent the following month, but with considerable difficulty. One measure taken was implementation of thirty-day payment terms from the units being supplied, as these were the terms imposed on MEDS by importers and wholesalers.

Bulk purchasing has involved maintaining sizable storage and distribution facilities, as well as quality control operations and sales to at least four international NGOs for their local operations. A management staff of fifteen administrators has been assisted by fifteen warehouse personnel. Hospitals and health centers are charged a fixed price for the costs of transport, paying on ninety-day terms. Some hospitals failed to pay for the drugs and transportation costs, and new orders were refused until accounts were paid.

MEDS has provided training for program staff and health facility personnel about the rational use of essential drugs. This training is important because the program's success depends on the proper and efficient use of available drug resources. Training, initially supported by MOH and foreign funding (both later withdrawn), uses up a large percentage of MEDS's resources, and many local training needs remain unmet. In 1993, the staff training team comprised nine people, three of them medical professionals; 227 people were trained in 1993. A 1993 evaluation showed that drug consumption by the units declined after training, and there was a switch to ordering from the essential drugs list.

Sources: MEDS 1990, 1993.

Nonprofit Essential Drug Supply Services

Beginning in the late 1970s, coincident with the introduction of the essential drugs concept by WHO, mission or other nonprofit health associations in some countries began to create their own agencies to procure and distribute essential drugs. These NGOs generally develop their own essential drugs list, often based on the WHO model. NGOs obtain drugs from the national parastatal (where one exists), local manufacturers, international nonprofit suppliers, or other foreign suppliers. Financing usually comes from a combination of external donations, local donations, and drug fees.

Ghana, India, Kenya, Nepal, and Nigeria are among the countries in which NGOs operate essential drug supply services. Country Study 6.6 describes the origin and operation of Kenya's Mission for Essential Drugs.

Despite some financial and organizational difficulties, many NGO essential drug services have been very successful. Sudden currency devaluations have temporarily disrupted supply in some countries, and product quality control has been problematic for such organizations.

For NGOs that lack the capital or organizational capacity required to establish their own central store, the direct delivery or prime vendor system offers a means to obtain more favorable prices on a limited range of locally procured essential drugs.

≡ 6.6 Public Roles in Supplying Essential Drugs

Clarifying public-sector roles in essential drugs programs should be a central concern in the development and review of national drug policies. Ultimately, the roles a government assumes in providing and promoting essential drugs depend on the circumstances of the individual country. Important considerations in developing a strategy for public-private collaboration in the pharmaceutical sector are

Analysis of the national development environment: Within the context of economic, development, and industrial policy, what is the overall government approach to the roles of the public and private sectors? What have been the experiences in other sectors with the mix between private and public provision and financing of services?

Pharmaceutical sector analysis: What is the current status of the public pharmaceutical sector with respect to financing, human resources, physical infrastructure, management systems, and overall performance? What is the current status of the private sector with respect to these elements?

≡ Assessment Guide

National Drug Financing and Distribution
- ► Which drug financing sources are used (government budgets, private out-of-pocket purchases, insurance [compulsory, voluntary], other sources)?
- ► What is the percentage breakdown among public, private, NGO, and donor health spending?
- ► What is the structure of the drug distribution system (state wholesale monopoly, private wholesale distributors, NGO drug supply agency, centralized distribution for government facilities, other distributors)?

Drug Supply for Government Health Services
- ► What system is currently used (central medical stores, autonomous supply agency, direct delivery, prime vendor, or fully private supply)?
- ► Which alternative supply systems were considered?
- ► How well is the current system performing (see note)?

Autonomous Drug Supply Agency (if applicable)
- ► Does it have an independent and effective management board?
- ► What are the qualifications of the senior managers?
- ► What measures to ensure efficiency and monitor performance are in place?
- ► Are there adequate financing and financial controls?
- ► How is the system performing in terms of cost and delivery (see note)?

Direct Delivery and Prime Vendor Contracts (if applicable)
- ► Are contracts effectively monitored?
- ► Is there sufficient competition to ensure low prices and good service?
- ► Are there adequate financing and financial controls?
- ► How is the system performing in terms of cost and delivery (see note)?

Performance Indicators for Drug Supply
- ► Are indicator drugs currently available at health facilities?
- ► What is the frequency of stockouts for indicator drugs at health facilities?
- ► What is the average duration of stockouts for indicator drugs at health facilities?
- ► What is the average time between order and delivery for indicator drugs for regular orders?
- ► What percentage of supplier drug prices are the average distribution costs (administration, storage, transport)?

Measures Affecting Private Supply Channels
- ► What licensing provisions and incentives to increase geographic access through private wholesalers and retailers are in place?
- ► What kind of training and certification of pharmacy aides and other drug sellers is there?
- ► What types of policies, legislation, and regulations on clinician dispensing are there?
- ► What price information is available to health professionals and the public?
- ► What measures are there to encourage generic substitution?
- ► What percentage of prescriptions is filled with low-cost generic equivalents?
- ► Is there a system for regulating producer prices?
- ► What are the wholesale and retail margins based on (percentage, declining percentage, dispensing fee, differential dispensing fee)?

Note: Supply system performance should be measured at least annually. Most indicators can be measured at regional and other supply depots as well as at health facilities. Whenever possible, annual figures should be compared for the most recent year and two preceding years (three years total). See Chapter 36 for a discussion of indicator drugs. See assessment guides for Chapters 13 and 21 for additional procurement and distribution indicators, respectively.

Comparative advantages of public and private pharmaceutical sectors: Given the current level of development and performance in the public and private sectors, what are the advantages of promoting one over the other? Are there likely to be clear-cut benefits in changing the status quo?

Costs versus benefits of expanded private-sector involvement: Any change will involve costs and benefits. Do the potential economic and health care benefits of expanded private-sector involvement outweigh the likely costs of such expansion?

Phasing in of changes in the pharmaceutical sector: Even if good information and sound judgment lead to the conclusion that the public role in the pharmaceutical sector should change, it should not be assumed that such a shift can occur immediately and in one step. Phasing in of changes may lead to a smoother transition.

Monitoring of changes: Finally, it is essential that the objectives of government action be clearly specified and that indicators be identified and monitored to determine whether the objectives are being met. Such monitoring is especially important if changes are being made in phases and if there is an opportunity to hasten, delay, or modify implementation based on experience.

Each country must assess its own situation to determine which strategies seem best suited to the circumstances. The concepts presented here and the experiences of other countries should provide a framework for identifying options and making choices, keeping the key public health objectives in mind: increasing the availability and affordability of essential drugs, promoting rational use of drugs, and ensuring acceptable drug quality. ■

≡ References and Further Readings

★ = *Key readings.*

Andajaningsih. 1995. *Country report: Indonesia.* Presented at International Conference on National Medicinal Drug Policies, Sydney, October 8–11.

★ Ballance, R., J. Pogány, and H. Forstner. 1992. *The world's pharmaceutical industries: An international perspective on innovation, competition and policy.* Prepared for United Nations Industrial Development Organization (UNIDO). Aldershot, England: Edward Elgar Publishing Limited.

★ Bennett, S., G. Dakpallah, P. Garner, L. Gilson, S. Nittayaramphong, B. Zurita, and A. Zwi. 1994. Carrot and stick: State mechanisms to influence private provider behaviour. *Health Policy and Planning* 9(1):1–13.

Bennett, S., and E. Ngalande-Bande. 1994. *Public and private roles in health: A review and analysis of experience in sub-Saharan Africa.* Geneva: WHO, Division of Strengthening of Health Services.

★ Gilson, L., P. Dave Sen, S. Mohammed, and P. Mujinja. 1994. The potential of health sector non-governmental organizations: Policy options. *Health Policy and Planning* 9(1):14–24.

★ Helfenbein, S., R.-L. Kolehmainen-Aitken, and W. Newbrander. 1995. Decentralizing health and family planning services. *Family Planning Manager* 4(2):1–26.

Hessou, C. P., and M. P. Fargier. 1994. Benin central purchasing office for essential drugs: A new experiment. *Essential Drugs Monitor* 18:8–9.

ITC (International Trade Centre). 1995. *Pharmaceutical raw materials/essential drugs report. Market news service.* UNCTAD/GATT. Geneva: ITC.

★ McPake, B., and E. Ngalande-Bande. 1994. Contracting out health services in developing countries. *Health Policy and Planning* 9(1):25–30.

MEDS (Mission for Essential Drugs and Supplies). 1990. *Report of the MEDS operations and proposal for 36 months extension of funding.* Nairobi, Kenya: MEDS.

MEDS (Mission for Essential Drugs and Supplies). 1993. *Report of an annual conference.* Nairobi, Kenya: MEDS.

Mills A., J. P. Vaughan, D. L. Smith, and I. Tabibzadeh. 1990. *Health system decentralization.* Geneva: World Health Organization.

Möller, H., B. Pharasi, and R. S. Summers. 1994. *Evaluation of pharmaceutical services in the Northern Transvaal Province.* School of Pharmacy, MEDICOS Pharmacy Project and Center for Health Policy, University of the Witwatersrand, South Africa, Medical University of Southern Africa.

Mossialos, E., C. Ranos, and B. Abel-Smith, eds. 1994. *Cost containment, pricing and financing of pharmaceuticals in the European Community: The policy-makers' view.* Vol. 1. Athens: LSE Health and Pharmetrica S. A.

MSH (Management Sciences for Health). 1995. *International drug price indicator guide* (updated annually). Washington, D.C.: MSH.

Muschell, J. 1995. *Privatization in health.* Technical briefing note WHO/TFHE/TBN/95.1. Geneva: WHO Task Force on Health Economics.

★ Rankin, J. 1995. *Engaging the private sector in the public pharmaceutical system.* Presented at International Conference on National Medicinal Drug Policies, Sydney, October 8–11.

Redwood, H. 1993. *Price regulation and pharmaceutical research: The limits of co-existence.* Felixstow, Suffolk, UK: Oldwicks Press Limited.

WHO (World Health Organization). 1994. *Public/private collaboration for health: National health systems and policies.* WHO/SHS/NDP/94.2. Geneva: WHO.

WHO/DAP (World Health Organization/Action Programme on Essential Drugs). 1989. *Review of the drug programme in Indonesia: Report of a WHO mission, October 16–November 3, 1989.* DAP/90.11. Geneva: WHO/DAP.

WHO/DAP (World Health Organization/Action Programme on Essential Drugs). 1994. *Indicators for monitoring national drug policies.* WHO/DAP/94.12. Geneva: WHO/DAP.

Zerda Sarmiento, A. 1995. *Alternative drug pricing policies in the Americas: Health economics and drugs.* WHO/DAP/95.6. Geneva: World Health Organization.

Part I Introduction	**Part II** **Policy and Legal Framework**	Part III Drug Management Cycle	Part IV Management Support Systems

5 National Drug Policies
6 Drug Supply Strategies
7 Pharmaceutical Legislation and Regulation
8 Legal Aspects of Drug Management
9 Pharmaceutical Production Policy

Chapter 7
Pharmaceutical Legislation and Regulation

≡ **Summary**

Realistic and effective laws and regulations are needed for the pharmaceutical sector because

- ▶ *pharmaceuticals concern the whole population;*
- ▶ *many parties are involved—patients, health providers, manufacturers, and salespeople;*
- ▶ *there are serious consequences from the lack or misuse of drugs;*
- ▶ *informal controls are insufficient.*

Countries may choose to develop new legislation or to revise existing laws. When starting afresh, it is useful to prepare a general law. Models exist, and expert assistance is readily available. Once the law is passed, regulations made under it can bring its various provisions into operation, one by one, as the necessary resources and experience are acquired.

In drafting or revising legislation, a country should

- ▶ *inventory the laws and regulations already in force;*
- ▶ *determine what type of legislative instrument is required;*
- ▶ *involve both legal and health experts;*
- ▶ *keep all interested parties informed.*

National drug legislation generally includes provisions relating to the availability, marketing, prescribing, labeling, dispensing, and sometimes pricing of pharmaceutical products, as well as the licensing, inspection, and control of personnel and facilities. A regulatory authority is usually established for administrative control. Drug registration is often a major element in legislation to ensure that individual drugs meet the criteria of efficacy, safety, and quality.

Countries that need to introduce comprehensive legislation can seek guidance from the experiences of others and from World Health Organization (WHO) guidelines (1995).

≡ 7.1 The Role of Pharmaceutical Legislation and Regulation

Clearly, society needs to operate according to some set of generally understood rules. These rules, whether they relate to medicines, education, farming, or crime, are only partly created by written law. Many unwritten conventions for individual and institutional behavior are generally accepted simply because they serve the interests of society.

Why Laws and Regulations Are Necessary

The approach to pharmaceutical law and regulation can be best understood by first considering why laws are necessary in society, and what forms they take.

On some matters, people may want to agree voluntarily but explicitly—verbally or in writing—on what they propose to do together. Rules such as these may be written down in letters, contracts, or codes. The rules of a sports club are in that category: they are simply agreed upon among the members; the government has nothing to do with them.

Governments generally become involved and make laws and regulations in the following situations:

- ▶ When a matter involves a large number of people, perhaps the entire population;
- ▶ When a matter is complex and involves many parties, requiring detailed rules for their interaction and functioning;
- ▶ When failure to follow basic rules has serious and widespread consequences;
- ▶ When existing informal rules are insufficient or are not respected.

Although written laws are sometimes thought to be all-powerful, that is not always the case. Occasionally, a law remains ineffective because there is insufficient political will or too weak an infrastructure to enforce it, or because the law does not really meet the needs of society. A law that is designed to take into account as many interests as possible, and that does not demand more resources than society can reasonably muster, has a good chance of achieving its purpose.

The Difference between Laws and Regulations

Laws today are usually written in fairly general terms to meet present and possibly future needs. Laws usually have language that enables the government to issue regulations based on the law. Regulations can be passed more rapidly and simply than laws, sometimes requiring, for example, only the approval of a single minister on the advice of experts. They can also be altered more easily. Once approved, a regulation has the same power as the law itself.

Pharmaceutical Laws and Regulations

Pharmaceuticals involve many parties, including patients, doctors, other health workers, salespeople, and manufacturers. Thus, it is easy to see why laws and regulations are needed. The field also involves important risks: people can die from a lack of medicines, but also from drugs that are impure, wrongly prescribed, or used to excess. Although this point is widely accepted, there are those who argue that medicines—like many other commodities—should be subject only to the control of the ultimate user. But drugs are indeed different, as discussed in Chapter 1.

Additionally, informal controls are insufficient: charlatanism or quackery (that is, the deliberate sale of remedies known to be worthless) is centuries old, and firm action may be needed to put a stop to it. The United Kingdom, for example, reported twenty to thirty incidents of counterfeit medicines in 1994.

The approach to pharmaceutical regulation should not be purely repressive: rules creating a positive situation tend to be more effective than those that merely prevent harm from being done. Finally, a law will work only to the extent that it meets society's needs. A country should not rush into legislation on medicines before the situation is clear.

Evolution of Policy and Law

There may be a long preparatory period before the sort of consensus develops that can form the basis for a law. It is sometimes preferable to work for a while with informal agreements among parties so that generally accepted rules of behavior can develop in practice; the law then serves to confirm and formalize them.

Whether or not there is a national drug policy, countries need effective, enforceable legislation and regulation. This may take the form of a single national drug law that deals with all the issues or a series of complementary laws, each introduced when the time is right. In some countries, certain aspects of the drug sector are governed by national laws, and other aspects, such as pharmacy and medical practice, are governed by state laws. This chapter focuses on a single, comprehensive drug law at the national level. Most of the issues discussed are also applicable in situations where legal responsibility is divided between national and state governments.

A law on medicines must, first and foremost, clearly define what all the parties—manufacturers, doctors, pharmacists—are required to do, so that no serious misunderstanding is possible. Drug registration laws and regulations, for example, make clear what a manufacturer needs to do to obtain a license to sell a drug. They define how a registration body should assess the proposal to reach a fair decision reflecting society's needs.

A good law also creates administrative bodies to put rules into practice—for example, a national drug authority with broad competence, or separate organs to deal with the practice of pharmacy, inspection of factories, and advertising of medicines.

It can be tempting to try to achieve too much, too

Country Study 7.1 The Slow Road to Policy and Law

Anyone who would like to develop drug policy and law overnight can learn some sobering lessons from the history of England:

1540 Pharmacists are found to be selling substandard drugs. The College of Physicians is therefore empowered to search pharmacies for drugs that are "defective" or "corrupted." This is one of the earliest examples of a government becoming concerned about drug quality.

1665 The writer Daniel Defoe writes during an epidemic of the plague how "the Corners of Streets were plastered over with . . . Papers of Ignorant Fellows, Quacking and tampering with Physick, and inviting the People to come to them for remedies." A law on drug advertising was still 320 years away.

1799 A writer in a medical journal proposes a "public board, for the examination, analyzation and approbation of every medicine . . . before it should be vended in any manner whatsoever." Not until 1928 did Norway become the first country in Europe to establish drug registration.

1850 A British physician reports on numerous deaths from the use of mercury as a medicine. Mercury-based drugs were still in use 100 years later.

1902 The British Medical Association exposes more than 200 "secret remedies," few of which have any effect.

1922 The official Salvarsan Commission studies and reports on the serious side effects of a new arsenic-containing drug used to treat venereal disease. Yet drugs of this type remained on sale without proper warnings for another generation.

Britain's current Medicines Act dates only from 1968. No other country in Europe did much better. Broadly speaking, European countries began to legislate on the quality of medicines only from about 1870, on their safety from 1930 to 1960, and on their efficacy only after 1970. Almost every step on the road was met with opposition from those who believed that their interests (particularly their incomes) were being threatened. Almost every legislative step was taken only after disasters with drugs had claimed many lives and had led to a public outcry.

---

quickly. It took more than a hundred years (some would say much longer) for drug policy and law to evolve in the industrialized world, as illustrated in Country Study 7.1. Sensible questions to ask are:

► What are the most important goals to achieve within five, ten, and fifteen years?
► What means are available to achieve them?
► In which order can they best be tackled?
► What help is available?

The answers to these questions provide a good starting point in developing both policies and the laws needed to support them.

Country Study 7.2 Legislative Complexities in Implementing a National Drug Policy

Following a series of five policy formulation workshops, the government of Kenya adopted the Kenya National Drug Policy in 1994. The process involved over fifty individuals from government ministries, universities, professional societies, and the private sector.

Specific components of the policy included public-sector drug supply, drug supply by the private sector and NGOs, veterinary drug supply, regulatory control, rational drug use, quality assurance, drug abuse, importation and exportation of drugs, local production, and personnel training and development.

Immediately following the final policy development workshop, senior officials and advisers met to prepare an implementation plan for the policy. It was recognized that some policy elements would require legislative changes, others would require regulatory adjustments, and still others would require changes in day-to-day operations of the Ministry of Health. No fewer than seven acts of parliament were involved, including:

Chapter 242	Public Health Act
Chapter 244	Pharmacy and Poisons Act
Chapter 245	Dangerous Drugs Act
Chapter 253	Medical Practitioners and Dentists Act
Chapter 254	Food, Drugs and Chemical Substances Act
Chapter 364	Animal Diseases Act
Chapter 504	Price Control Act

Laws and regulations are intended to complement each other. It is often most appropriate to begin with passage of a broad law, dealing with what may be achieved within the next decade. The various provisions of the law are then brought into operation through regulation, step by step, addressing the most important things first. For instance, it may be urgently necessary to set up a new drug distribution system, but drug registration can wait for several years while essential drugs are procured through reputable channels where they are controlled for quality. Similarly, laws regarding factories need to be brought into effect only when a number of factories are actually established.

Drafting and Revising Drug Legislation and Regulations

Before drafting any new law, it is important to inventory the laws and regulations already in force. Even if there is no general drug law, there are likely to be pieces of legislation that touch on the field—for example, laws on narcotics and the licensing and responsibilities of pharmacists. There may be a general drug law that is out-of-date and should be replaced rather than merely amended. It is essential to determine to what extent existing laws and regulations contribute to attaining the national policy objectives.

Because concepts of drug policy are modern, legislation more than twenty years old may not be relevant to them; it may be simpler to start over. Country Study 7.2 illustrates, however, the number of currently existing laws that may be affected by a comprehensive national drug policy.

The second step is to have drafters and experts meet to decide what type of legislative instrument is required. The most straightforward model is likely to be a comprehensive law that deals in outline with all the relevant issues, each main section taking up a particular matter. Sections can then be brought into operation one at a time, through the passage of regulations.

In countries with a long history of regulation, laws on pharmacists and the registration of medicines and regulations on prices and costs are likely to be separate, because they came into being at different times. In starting afresh, however, and particularly if the laws on these matters are outdated or incomplete, it may be easier to pull together all relevant elements in a single law. Three approaches for revising existing law or starting afresh are illustrated in Country Study 7.3.

Ideally, the task of writing the law should be entrusted to a group of legal and health experts who are familiar with all the issues, but few countries can assemble such a group. Rather than solving the problem by copying laws from abroad, countries can obtain assistance from international and bilateral agencies to draft new drug legislation that meets the country's own needs.

An excellent bibliography that describes good and bad experiences is available to support this work (WHO/DAP 1994). National and regional meetings of drug regulatory authorities also provide opportunities for learning how to approach the problem and identifying expert colleagues who can be called on for advice.

At all stages, it is important to discuss early drafts of the law with all interested parties, including the health professions, trade and industry groups, other concerned government departments (such as those handling commerce and education), and consumer groups. The greater the consensus, the greater the chance that a law will be passed and will work in practice.

≡ 7.2 Basic Elements of National Drug Legislation

A well-defined set of elements, with slight modifications, constitutes the initial requirements for a strong and comprehensive national drug law. These elements, though basic, are sufficiently wide and varied in their scope to meet most of the objectives of any modest national drug policy. A model for national drug legislation, showing the various key elements, is presented in Figure 7.1. This model is intended to support the efforts of small national drug regulatory authorities in countries where only one or two professionals are available to deal with pharmaceuticals and related products.

≡ 7.3 Key Provisions of National Drug Legislation

Pharmaceutical products are universally recognized as being different from ordinary items of commerce (such as an article of clothing or a household appliance) and as requiring handling by specially trained health professionals. Medicines are subject to numerous controls at all levels, and legal authority is granted to regulate their availability, marketing, prescribing, labeling, dispensing, and occasionally related activities such as pricing.

An effective national drug law is a primary means of ensuring that drug policy goals are achieved while the unique character of pharmaceutical products, personnel, and facilities is preserved. The law may specify what products can legally be imported (for example, those included on the national drug list and possessing a WHO-type certificate of quality) and who is legally qualified to prescribe and dispense them—thus promoting certain national drug policies.

Likewise, through its control of the manufacture, storage, distribution, and sale of pharmaceutical products, a government is better able to ensure compliance with a national policy of having essential medicines of sufficient quality, safety, and efficacy universally accessible for their intended purposes. The processes of licensing and registration can grant authorization only to those personnel, products, and facilities that conform with the national drug law. For example, counterfeit or dangerous drugs can be taken off the market, and sanctions can be taken against those responsible for introducing them illegally.

The promulgation of regulations, the collection of licensing and registration fees, and the enforcement of the national law and its regulations are legally delegated to an agency—usually called the drug regulatory authority—headed by a commissioner or director who is responsible to a cabinet-level person, such as the minister of health. For example, in the United States, the basic national drug law is called the Federal Food, Drug, and Cosmetic Act, which is enforced by the Food and Drug Administration (FDA). For controlled substances, additional restrictions are imposed by the Drug Enforcement Administration (DEA). Wholesale distributors, pharmacy practice, and medical practice are regulated by individual states.

Country Study 7.3 Three Approaches to Changing Pharmaceutical Legislation

India: Revising and Updating Existing Legislation. India introduced legislation in 1982 (Act No. 68) amending the Drugs and Cosmetics Act of 1940. The latter act had been amended from time to time, but there had been a ten-year interval since the last change. The original act provided for the establishment of a Drugs Technical Advisory Board, a Central Drugs Laboratory, and a Drugs Consultative Committee. It prohibited the importation, sale, or manufacture of any misbranded or adulterated drug or of any drug that was not of the standard quality; imports were permissible only under license. The act was also written to allow for additional rules and regulations to be made, and the Drug and Cosmetics Rules were enacted in 1945.

Since the basic framework was already in place, the Drugs and Cosmetics (Amendment) Act of 1982 simply broadened the scope of the original act and strengthened the government's power to prohibit the import, manufacture, sale, or distribution of drugs in accordance with the public interest. More severe penalties for noncompliance were adopted, and fees for the inspection of premises were modified. Since the original act was kept intact, the case law related to its provisions continued to have the same binding force.

Sri Lanka: Replacement of Existing Legislation by Entirely New Legislation. Prior to the enactment of the Cosmetics, Devices, and Drugs Act No. 27 of 1980, the Sri Lankan law on drugs was embodied mainly in the Food and Drugs Act, a statute modeled on British legislation. Although Sri Lanka was independent in 1950 when the Food and Drugs Act was enacted, the British legal system, which had been applied for nearly 150 years, continued to have a pervasive influence on the lawmaking and judicial processes. Besides the Food and Drugs Act, numerous other laws contained provisions that were relevant to drugs.

The Cosmetics, Devices, and Drugs Act of 1980 repealed the Food and Drugs Act. It established a Cosmetics, Devices, and Drugs Authority and a Technical Advisory Committee. It provided for a system of licenses for the manufacture, importation, sale, and distribution of drugs. Also, for the first time, it provided for a system of drug registration. It established standards in relation to various pharmacopeias and required that labeling and advertising be confined to drugs that conformed to these standards. Because these changes were so far-reaching, building them into the original Food and Drugs Act would have complicated the structure of that act. In these circumstances, a new piece of legislation was warranted.

Gambia: Enactment of Comprehensive Legislation Where None Existed Previously. A team of outside experts reviewed an existing noncomprehensive drug law that had been in operation for nearly ninety years and recommended a thorough revision and updating. This was accomplished by the enactment of the Medicines Act No. 2 of 1984. Because they were starting from scratch, they could profit from the experiences of many other countries in drafting legislation tailored to the particular needs of their country.

Source: Adapted from Jayasuriya 1985.

Figure 7.1 Elements of a Comprehensive Drug Law

A. General Provisions
1. Title*
2. Purposes*
3. Territorial extent
4. Application of other laws
5. Definitions*

B. Control of Availability and Marketing
1. Drug registration*
2. National essential drugs list/national formulary
3. Scheduling, prescription, and dispensing authority*
4. Labeling*
5. Generic labeling, manufacturing, and substitution
6. Information and advertising
7. Public education
8. Imposition of fees
9. Price control
10. Special products (herbal medicines, orphan drugs)

C. Control of Supply Mechanisms
1. Importation of drugs*
2. Exportation of drugs*
3. Controls, incentives, disincentives for local manufacture
4. Control of distribution, supply, storage, and sale*

D. Drug Control Administration
1. Organization and function*
2. Appeals against decisions of the drug control authority*

E. Powers of Enforcement
1. Prohibition of specified activities*
2. Penalties for each offense based on magnitude and occurrence*
3. Legal procedures for offenses*

F. Powers to Make Rules and Regulations

G. Repeals and Transitional Provisions
1. Repeal of sections of existing laws in conflict with the act
2. Transitional period to implementation

H. Exemptions from Provisions of the Law

*Elements for which model legislation has been developed by WHO.
Source: Adapted from Jayasuriya 1985; WHO 1994.

Uganda, like many other countries, chose to enact a specific national drug policy and authority statute in 1993, complemented by a separate act on the national medical stores, to deal with one of its major challenges. Both laws are excellent models of what a country can achieve as a follow-up to well-defined policies.

Defining the Roles of Various Parties
Because so many parties are involved with medicines, the laws need to clearly state the roles, responsibilities, and rights of each, ranging from practitioners, auxiliaries, nurses, and pharmacists to importers, manufacturers, and distributors. The legislation should establish the qualifications required for those handling drugs, or it must state who has the authority to set these standards (for example, a minister, by passing appropriate regulations).

Licensing, Inspection, and Quality Control
The law should create mechanisms to ensure that all responsible parties are licensed and inspected so that the community can rely on them. Doctors and nurses may be covered by other laws, but the drug law needs to ensure that the people who import, distribute, and sell medicines are approved (when properly qualified), registered, and inspected.

Drugs themselves require a special form of inspection. An inspector visiting a pharmacy or warehouse may have reason to suspect that drugs are not of sufficient quality or in good condition: they may be damp, dirty, or disintegrating. More often, samples need to be obtained for checking in the quality control laboratory, an essential part of the inspection system.

Some countries have their own quality control laboratories, either specifically for drugs or shared with other commodities (such as foods). A number of countries use regional laboratories, such as the ones serving East Africa or the Caribbean. Whatever the structure, the drug law needs to ensure that a quality control laboratory exists and has the capacity and equipment to do the job. The law should also provide the basis for a postmarketing surveillance system to report problems with adverse reactions and product quality.

Advertising and Promotion
Although many countries have rules to ensure that advertising is not misleading, these rules are generally not sufficient to cover medicines. With consumer products, a certain degree of exaggeration is often tolerated as the normal practice of the marketplace. But for medicines—with their capacity to kill or cure, and with claims that people cannot easily verify themselves—it is important that advertising (to health professionals and to users) be objective and reliable; if it is not, the risks may be great.

For these reasons, most drug laws now include a clause empowering regulations on drug advertising. In many countries, drugs intended to be prescribed by health professionals must not be advertised to the general public. All advertising must be consistent with the information verified when the drug was registered or approved for marketing, with modifications required by the regulatory authority on the basis of postmarketing experience.

Useful guides to the principles that should underlie honest drug promotion have been issued by WHO and separately by manufacturers (WHO 1988).

Sanctions
Because constant vigilance is needed if the public is to be protected, a drug law needs to have teeth. There is no use

concluding that drug quality is poor, a warehouse is rat-infested or damp upon inspection, or an advertisement is untruthful unless something can be done about it. The drug regulatory agency must use its authority to impose penalties when necessary: sanctions may be penal (fines or imprisonment) or simply corrective (banning the drug, closing down the warehouse). Sometimes a party has contravened the law so seriously that the appropriate sanction is determined to be loss of license to prescribe, import, or distribute. On occasion, all three sorts of penalties may be needed.

≡ 7.4 Drug Registration, Licensing, and Marketing Authorization

The licensing and inspection of manufacturers and importers, although important, do not provide assurance about the products. Many countries have evolved systems of drug registration to ensure that individual products approved for sale meet the following criteria:

Efficacy: The drug should be effective for the indications claimed. (Note that no drug is ever 100 percent effective. In practice, efficacy means that in the majority of cases there is a clinically significant and useful effect.)

Safety: The drug should not present risks that are disproportionate to its benefits. (Note that some patients may react disastrously even to the safest drugs; in practice, this has to be expected and does not alter the fact that in the great majority of cases side effects are minor or absent.)

Quality: The drug should be well made, as specified in the official pharmacopeia chosen as a standard.

Truth: All the information needed to use the drug properly (indications, doses, precautions, undesirable side effects) should be provided as part of the packaging.

Drug registration, also referred to as licensing or marketing authorization, is often a major element in national drug law. In its fully developed form, however, it is costly and labor-intensive. Establishing a drug registration system is generally not justified until a country has a significant volume of private-sector drug sales. The primary concern of many developing countries is ensuring a reliable flow of essential generic drugs from reputable suppliers into the public health system. Since these drugs have properties that have been recognized and documented for a long time, they do not need to be individually registered, assuming that sound procurement policies ensure that they come from reliable sources. Rather, they need only be subject to an abbreviated application procedure.

As a country's development proceeds, however, more resources become available, and priorities may change.

Figure 7.2 Stages in the Evolution of a Drug Registration System

Stage 1 Notification Procedure. Standard information is obtained on all pharmaceutical products offered for sale in the country and entered into a register. No judgment is made regarding the appropriateness of the drugs for sale in the country.

Stage 2 Basic Authorization Procedure. Drugs listed in the register are provisionally authorized to remain on sale. All new drugs that are to be sold require a license, which is issued after assessment for efficacy, safety, quality, and truth and completeness of packaging information.

Stage 3 Full Registration or Licensing Procedure. Full evaluation of individual products is conducted by examining detailed data from the manufacturer (and from the literature) to assess their quality, safety, and efficacy.

Stage 4 Re-evaluation of Older Drugs. All older drugs on the market are systematically reassessed.

The private sector may become more active, and multinational firms may begin actively promoting their new products to prescribers and even to the public. It is at this point that the need for a drug registration system arises.

A drug registration system can best be developed in stages, as shown in Figure 7.2.

In Stage 1, the information requested may be simply the product name and the name of the manufacturer. Later, this can be expanded to include nonproprietary names for active substances, composition (including inactive ingredients), pharmacological action, therapeutic classification, and claims made in the package insert. Having a complete register of what is on sale means that when information arrives from other countries or from WHO about problems with a particular drug (for example, toxicity, contamination, evidence of inactivity), authorities will be able to ascertain whether the drug is on sale in their country and take appropriate action.

Stage 2 requires assessment for new drugs. Because this is a costly and time-consuming procedure, countries can rely on policies established in other countries. Is the drug approved for sale in its home country, in a country of the European Community, or in the United States or Canada? If so, what claims have been made for it? Does it carry a WHO-type certificate indicating that it is manufactured under satisfactory conditions? The firm wishing to import the drug must provide documented answers to these questions. Drug authorities may consult other countries directly before deciding to accept or reject a product. WHO and other bodies hold international and regional meetings of regulatory authorities from different countries, which helps

Country Study 7.4 Harmonized Regulations in Latin America

Drug registration is a major element of pharmaceutical legislation throughout Latin America. There are formal requirements for the registration of all drug products, whether old or new to the market, in all countries of the region.

The pharmaceutical market in virtually all countries is characterized by the availability of a great number of products, many of them constituted of irrational or unacceptable combinations of active ingredients, and potentially interchangeable multisource products, but without any real evidence of bioequivalence. A few countries employ a set of pharmacological standards for the registration of known drugs and their combinations. Most countries require a free sales certificate for imported drugs, and a few have now altered their regulatory procedures to require the use of the WHO certificate of a pharmaceutical product.

The technical standards and procedures for drug registration have been established independently in different countries and vary widely. In many countries, they have been largely ineffective due to cumbersome procedures involving considerable delays and chronic shortages of technical resources.

Drug registration and approval requirements have been considered barriers to a global market and the free exchange of goods across national boundaries, prompting some to argue for deregulation measures, including automatic registration of a number of drugs, the establishment of "provisional registrations," and time limits for the processing of applications. The establishment of provisional registration in one country led to an immediate increase in the number of registered products from 4,500 to 12,000, with few products subsequently deregistered; the practice was abolished. These concerns have put enormous pressure on regulatory authorities to review, simplify, and harmonize their technical and administrative procedures.

In view of these pressures, as well as commonalities in language, culture, and the drug market throughout much of the region, a number of harmonization activities have taken place in recent years in Latin America.

▶ The Health, Labor, and Social Security Committee of the Latin American Parliament approved a declaration in 1992 outlining proposals for a common health policy and legislative agenda. In 1994, the committee reviewed drug policies throughout the region and proposed legislation concerning generic prescription and dispensing and recommended the use of therapeutic formularies.

▶ Efforts to standardize pharmacopeial requirements between the United States Pharmacopeia and the Mexican Pharmacopeia were begun in 1995.

▶ In 1993, negotiations were undertaken in Central American and Andean countries toward mutual recognition of registration systems, pharmacological standards, and drug formularies and harmonization of inspection systems.

▶ Argentina, Brazil, Paraguay, and Uruguay signed the Asunción Treaty, which established the Common Market of the Southern Countries (MercoSur) as of January 1, 1995.

Harmonized technical standards and common regulatory actions within MercoSur were established with the participation of regulatory authorities and industrial representatives. Specific technical groups were placed in charge of negotiating harmonized regulations and standards for drug substances, drug products, medical devices, and home products. Proposals adopted by the Council of Ministers of MercoSur become official regulations of the common market, although each country still includes them in its national regulatory scheme.

Harmonized regulations include good manufacturing practices for finished pharmaceutical products, parenteral products, medical devices, and active ingredients and the establishment of common guidelines for inspections. Although there is a consensus regarding requirements and procedures for the future registration of new drugs, no agreement has been reached for mutual recognition of products already on the market.

---

create trust across borders and facilitates informal work sharing. Approval of locally manufactured drugs requires inspection of the manufacturing premises and staff.

The task of full registration described in Stage 3 should never be taken up lightly—even a large regulatory agency can be overwhelmed by the vast amount of material that needs to be examined. Some groups of countries handle assessment jointly; others look at where else in the world the drug is licensed, and under what conditions. Country Study 7.4 describes the efforts of a number of Latin American countries to establish common standards and procedures for drug registration. Countries that have the resources to handle registration and licensing independently can often obtain technical advice and practical help from WHO and support from other countries with well-developed regulatory agencies.

Stage 4, the re-evaluation of older drugs on the market,

is the final stage in the development of a regulatory system and is very ambitious. Few industrialized countries have yet managed to complete it.

≡ 7.5 Establishing Effective Administrative Control

Countries can draw guidance from the experiences of others, but problems have arisen when overly complex provisions were adopted. Legislation and administrative practices must be attuned to available resources, and every opportunity must be taken to understand and use the information provided by regulatory authorities in other countries (WHO 1990a).

Required Resources

Figure 7.3 details the resources required to achieve effective administrative control; at a minimum, this includes a

Figure 7.3 Resources Required for Effective Administrative Control

Resources Required	Specific Function or Purpose
Personnel	Regulatory activities (licensing, registration, and so forth) Monitoring, inspection, and surveillance Enforcement
Physical and Infrastructure	Office space for regulatory and enforcement personnel Computers, software, and office equipment Quality control laboratories Vehicles for distribution, inspection, and enforcement activities
Technical	Preservice and in-service training Establishment of drug manufacturing processes, packaging, and so forth Collation of data Dissemination of information
Financial	Capital and recurrent expenditures Technical programs Payments for patents and royalties Payments for consultants Publications (forms, licenses, pharmacopeia)

Source: Adapted from Jayasuriya 1985.

drug regulatory authority with staff, a team of inspectors to visit warehouses and retailers, and a quality control laboratory.

Personnel are the key resource for making effective drug regulation possible. Because of the technical nature of their work, it is often prescribed by law that the inspectors be pharmacists. Others can be trained to undertake licensing, registration, and enforcement duties. Depending on the size of the country and the degree of pharmaceutical development, the entire staff may consist of only a few individuals. Computer software now greatly simplifies many of the administrative tasks of the regulatory agency, as illustrated in Country Study 7.5. Registration software that runs on IBM-compatible microcomputers is now available from the WHO Division of Drug Management and Policy.

Financing for Drug Administration

The law must provide a realistic mechanism for funding regulatory functions. Funds may be provided from general tax income and, increasingly, from charges levied on the manufacturers, importers, and distributors to cover the bulk of the costs of the drug control system. The level of charges may be set from year to year, but the nature of the charges can be defined in the law. Importers, for example, can be required to pay a fee when they submit a new drug application to the regulatory authority for con-

Country Study 7.5 Computerization of Drug Registration in the Philippines

In 1993 and 1994, the Bureau of Food and Drugs (BFAD) in the Philippines undertook a project to computerize drug registration. Different offices involved in the registration process were connected by terminal to a common database running under a UNIX multiuser operating system. Separate terminals were set up for entering initial product information, for product evaluation functions, for the laboratory, and for the office of the director, where final decisions are made. Another terminal was made available for clients to inquire about the status of their applications.

Reports can be generated using a report generator in the software system. These are not preformatted reports that can be generated at the "click of a button" but are customized for responding to questions or requests for information. Use of the report generator has required training.

Development of this new computerized system required streamlining of the registration system itself through a process of ongoing feedback and revision. After installation, the old and new systems were run in parallel until the new system was shown to be reliable. Staff within BFAD participated in both development and installation to ensure sustainability and maintenance of the system. Although there was some initial resistance to the new system, it has speeded up the registration process and is now well accepted by BFAD staff.

Source: Brudon-Jakobowicz 1994.

sideration, a supplementary fee when the license is issued, and an annual fee for as long as the drug remains on sale. Manufacturers might be required to relicense their products periodically (for example, every three or five years).

Guiding Principles for Small National Drug Regulatory Authorities

Drug regulation is not the only component of drug policy, and sometimes it is not even the most pressing one. Nonetheless, the existence of a national drug regulatory authority to ensure drug quality, safety, and efficacy is the best guarantee that the public is getting the medicines it deserves.

When a country is ready to introduce drug regulation, a recent work by WHO (1990a) provides useful guidance for authorities with limited human, financial, scientific, and technological resources. To be effective, a small drug regulatory authority needs to operate within the context of whatever national drug law and policy have already been defined and must be able to relate to other interested bodies, including organizations responsible for drug procurement in the public sector and the national formulary committee.

The responsibilities of the regulatory authority are to ensure that products conform to acceptable standards of quality, safety, and efficacy and that all premises and practices employed to manufacture, store, and distribute drugs ensure their continued conformity to these standards until they are delivered to the end-user. The authority manages a national reporting system on adverse reactions and drug quality problems. It also approves the packaging text and directions folder that accompany a drug to ensure that they are truthful, complete, and balanced.

These objectives can be accomplished effectively only if a mandatory system of licensing products, manufacturers, importing agents, and distributors is in place. A small authority has limited capacity to undertake these tasks. For imported drug substances, a small authority is dependent on information generated in the exporting country. This information is most effectively obtained through the WHO certification scheme on the quality of pharmaceutical products moving in international commerce (WHO 1990b and WHO/DAP 1995). As discussed in Chapter 18, this scheme must be supplemented by direct contacts with international agencies and other regulatory agencies to obtain necessary information.

In summary, the regulatory authority should be vested with legal powers to

▶ issue, alter, and revoke licenses for pharmaceutical products on grounds of quality, safety, and efficacy;

▶ ensure the safe and effective use of each product by controlling, through the terms of the license, the content of all labeling (including package inserts, associated prescribing information, and advertising) and the channels through which the product may legitimately be supplied;

▶ inspect and license all manufacturing premises, importing agents, wholesalers, distributors, hospital dispensaries, independent pharmacies, and other retail outlets to ensure that they comply with prevailing regulations and guidelines.

To implement these responsibilities, the authority must have the power to order that certain things be done and to prosecute those who contravene the law. To retain public confidence and respect, the authority must be seen as operating in an independent, authoritative, and impartial manner. It should be concerned exclusively with the deter-mination of standards and the implementation of controls. Although it needs to work closely with the body responsible for public drug procurement, it should not be responsible for procurement and should remain independent in its operations and decisions.

≡ 7.6 Evaluating the Effectiveness of Drug Legislation

Evaluating the effectiveness of drug legislation and accompanying regulations is not always easy. The process of evaluation depends on the types of performance indicators and criteria used and on the availability of adequate data. The questions in the Assessment Guide provide a helpful framework.

The most important factor in the effectiveness of drug laws and regulations is the extent to which the legislative framework is in tune with national policy and the existing situation in the pharmaceutical sector. Changes in policy need to be reflected in the legislation and in its implementation.

Measuring the effectiveness of a law on pharmaceuticals is easier for certain elements than for others. For instance, the registration process can be evaluated in relation to quantitative targets and time schedules to see whether the agency is on schedule.

The degree of noncompliance with a law or regulation may suggest not only the need to take action against those responsible but also the desirability of identifying the causes of noncompliance: it may be related to technical defects in the law or in its wording, or to operational problems of implementation that can be resolved. Drug enforcement personnel should periodically report on their perception of how the law functions and the types of problems encountered, to facilitate any necessary revisions. Many legislative and regulatory provisions can be improved and updated when the legislation is sufficiently flexible to allow for modifications by the regulatory agency.

Responsibility for evaluating the effectiveness of a drug law often falls on the regulatory authority established by law for policy-making, implementation, or both. Periodic self-evaluation to identify weaknesses in policy-making and implementation activities is important. The body must devise its own systems to judge whether it receives sufficient feedback and whether its operational effectiveness can be improved. ■

≡ Assessment Guide

Policy, Legislation, and Regulation

▶ Is there a national drug policy approved by the government? When was it last updated?

▶ Is there a comprehensive drug law? Is it a new law or a revision of an existing law? When was it last updated?

▶ Is the legislation flexible in allowing for the passage and revision of regulations in response to new scientific information and market changes?

▶ Is there a drug regulatory authority responsible for the promulgation of regulations and for enforcement?

Drug Selection and Registration

▶ Is there a system for drug registration? Is this a notification procedure? A basic authorization procedure? A full registration procedure? Is periodic renewal required?

▶ Is drug registration based on an assessment of a drug's efficacy, safety, quality, and truth of packaging information? Are pharmacological or therapeutic standards used?

▶ Are there different registration procedures for essential drugs, generic products, multisource drugs, or imported products from selected countries?

▶ Is the WHO certification scheme on the quality of pharmaceutical products moving in international commerce used systematically for the registration of imported drugs?

▶ Is there a system for the collection of data regarding the efficacy and safety (adverse effects) of marketed drugs?

Licensing, Inspection, and Control

▶ Do mechanisms exist for the licensing, inspection, and control of pharmaceutical personnel and for manufacturing, distribution, and dispensing facilities?

▶ Do inspectors use a checklist for inspecting different types of pharmaceutical establishments?

▶ How many inspections were made during each of the last three years for the different types of pharmaceutical establishments?

▶ Is there an audit system to evaluate the inspection system?

Advertising and Promotion

▶ Is there any specific regulation regarding therapeutic claims in drug labeling and promotion?

▶ Is there any legal provision for the compulsory use of generic names in drug labeling and promotion?

▶ Are there controls on drug promotion, and are these consistent with the WHO ethical criteria for medicinal drug promotion?

Compliance and Enforcement

▶ What measures exist for enforcement of pharmaceutical laws and regulations? Are they enforceable administratively or through court actions? Are statistics available about compliance and enforcement?

▶ During the last three years, how many drug products were eliminated from the register? How many batches of drug products were recalled from the market?

▶ Is there a system for reporting drug product problems? What types of and how many complaints were registered in the past three years, and what corrective measures were taken?

▶ How many violations have occurred with regard to drug advertising and promotion in the past three years? What corrective measures were taken?

▶ Are there any statistics about the reaction of the industry and consumers to regulatory actions?

≡ References and Further Readings

★ = *Key readings.*

Brudon-Jakobowicz, P. 1994. *The Philippines national drug policy: Review of the WHO/DAP supported components.* Geneva: WHO.

Dukes, M. N .G. 1985. *The effects of drug regulation.* Norwell, Mass.: Kluwer Academic Publishers.

Dunne, J. F. 1993. Global harmonization of regulatory requirements: World Health Organization, 1993. In *Sixth international conference on drug regulatory authorities: Report of the conference proceedings.* WHO/DMP/ICDRA/93.1. Geneva: World Health Organization.

Goldberg, A. 1986. Development of drug regulating authorities. *British Journal of Clinical Pharmacology* 22:67S–70S.

★ IFPMA (International Federation of Pharmaceutical Manufacturers Association). 1994. *The IFPMA compendium on regulation of pharmaceuticals for human use.* Geneva: IFPMA.

★ Jayasuriya, D. C. 1985. *Regulation of pharmaceuticals in developing countries.* Geneva: World Health Organization.

Vernengo, M. J. 1995. *El control oficial de los medicamentos:*

Situación, problemas, y propuestas. Washington, D.C.: Pan American Health Organization.

WHO (World Health Organization). 1988. *Ethical criteria for medicinal drug promotion.* Geneva: WHO.

★ WHO (World Health Organization). 1990a. Guiding principles for small national drug regulatory authorities. In *WHO expert committee on specifications for pharmaceutical products.* Technical report series, no. 790. Geneva: WHO.

WHO (World Health Organization). 1990b. WHO certification scheme on the quality of pharmaceutical products moving in international commerce. In *WHO expert committee on specifications for pharmaceutical products.* Technical report series, no. 790. Geneva: WHO.

WHO (World Health Organization). 1993. Drug regulation and developing countries. *WHO Drug Information* 7:1–3.

WHO (World Health Organization). 1994. *A legislative scheme for regulating medicinal products for adaptation by small national drug regulatory authorities with limited manpower and other resources.* WHO PHARM/93.244, January 1994, Annex 3. Geneva: WHO.

★ WHO (World Health Organization). 1995. *Guidelines for developing national drug policies.* Geneva: WHO.

WHO/DAP (World Health Organization/Action Programme on Essential Drugs). 1993. *Pharmaceutical authorization policies.* Prepared by the Andean subregion. WHO/DAP/93.2. Geneva: WHO/DAP.

WHO/DAP (World Health Organization/Action Programme on Essential Drugs). 1994. *Selected annotated bibliography on essential drugs.* WHO/DAP/94.5. Geneva: WHO/DAP.

WHO/DAP (World Health Organization/Action Programme on Essential Drugs). 1995. *Use of the WHO certification scheme on the quality of pharmaceutical products moving in international commerce.* WHO/DAP/94.21. Geneva: WHO/DAP.

World Bank. 1994. *Pharmaceutical policies: Rationale and design.* WB/HROWP 35. Washington, D.C.: World Bank.

| Part I | Part II | Part III | Part IV |
| Introduction | Policy and Legal Framework | Drug Management Cycle | Management Support Systems |

5   National Drug Policies
6   Drug Supply Strategies
7   Pharmaceutical Legislation and Regulation
8   **Legal Aspects of Drug Management**
9   Pharmaceutical Production Policy

Chapter 8
Legal Aspects of Drug Management

≡ Summary

Laws related to the field of pharmaceuticals rely on the basic principles embodied in any system of law. Three areas of law are relevant to drug management: commercial law, tort law, and criminal law.

Commercial law has to do with fair business practices and includes

- *contracts: binding agreements between two parties to ensure that each respects the agreement (for example, a procurement contract between a purchasing agency and a supplier);*
- *patents: rights granted to an inventor to protect that individual's right to profit from the invention (for example, a right granted to the developer of a drug product to distribute the product without competition for a specified period);*
- *trademarks: trade names and packaging intended to distinguish a specific product from other similar ones.*

Tort law is often referred to as the "law of improper behavior." Even in the absence of a formal contract, an individual may claim that another's behavior was improper, for example, that

an importer used misleading advertising about a drug. Because ideas of proper behavior vary, tort law may be difficult to enforce internationally.

Criminal law applies when the laws and rules of society are drastically broken, for example, when unapproved drugs are marketed or drugs are stolen from a warehouse.

As a country develops and its economy becomes more stable, it is likely to introduce labor laws pertaining to employment. These laws may cover such matters as

- *written contracts of service*
- *wrongful dismissal*
- *equal opportunity*
- *employment of the young*
- *working conditions*

Because the laws of different countries vary, international contracts should specify which system of law will govern disputes. The likelihood of such disputes can be reduced by dealing with firms of good reputation, even if there is a higher initial cost, and consulting with a reliable and experienced law office for advice.

≡ There are numerous systems of law in the world: Napoleonic civil law in the countries that have developed in the French tradition, Anglo-Saxon common law in countries with historical links to Britain, Muslim Sharia, and numerous others. Systems can look very different but still embody many of the same principles, simply because they handle the same sorts of situations. Every system of law, for example, provides penalties for stealing, procedures for drawing up agreements, and rules for inheriting property. The mechanics may be different, however, and so may the penalties for breaking the rules.

Differences in what society regards as just and proper behavior are reflected in the law. There are also differences in the extent to which nations have found it necessary to formulate written rules at all on certain matters. In every community there is an understanding of what constitutes honest behavior. It does not always need to be spelled out in laws and regulations.

The field of pharmaceuticals relies on the basic principles embodied in any system of law. Although many countries have passed laws and other rules relating specifically to drugs (discussed in Chapter 7), a great many more general laws also apply. Since pharmaceuticals are bought and sold, they fall under the laws that apply to

other commercial goods. Because money is involved, and because drugs can injure people, conflicts can arise that need to be settled by civil law. And finally, when things go drastically wrong, criminal law may need to be applied. Anyone working with drugs needs some understanding of these general laws.

Three areas of law are considered here: commercial law, tort law (governing improper acts), and criminal law. The first two are part of what is generally known as civil, or noncriminal, law.

≡ 8.1 Commercial Law

Commercial law is a loose term for all those rules related to how business ought to be fairly conducted. It includes, for example, the law of contracts, the law of patents, and the law of trademarks.

Contract Law

A contract is a binding agreement between two parties that may be individuals, companies, or even states. The purpose of the law of contracts is to set the rules that apply to these agreements—in particular, how they should be concluded and carried out to ensure that the parties make a clear bargain and that each side keeps the agreement. The term *contract* does not mean that it applies only when there is a written, signed agreement between two parties; it applies equally if one orders goods from a catalog by mail or by telephone, or even if one goes into a shop and buys goods. The purchaser must always be critical ("let the buyer beware"); reading the small print is the buyer's responsibility.

Clearly, one of the greatest risks in drug procurement contracts is to be supplied with drugs of inferior quality. The buyer may find it advisable to include a specific clause in a purchase order or contract to protect against this risk—for example, claiming the right to check samples in advance and to reject individual batches that do not meet the agreed-upon standards. See Chapter 17 for further discussion of procurement contracts.

The following general provisions of contract law help protect against common problems regarding payment for goods, nature of goods, sellers' claims, and suitability of goods.

When Goods Are Supplied at the Price and Time Agreed upon, They Must Be Paid For. If the buyer does not pay for them, the seller can go to court to claim the money due. It makes no difference whether the goods are medicines, shoes, or bananas.

Goods Must Be What They Are Stated to Be, and Not Substantially Different. If a supplier agrees to provide 10,000 tablets of penicillin to the central medical stores (CMS) and sends 10,000 tablets of ampicillin instead, the CMS can demand back any money that has already been paid. If payment has not been made, the CMS can refuse to pay and return the goods (or require the seller to collect them) at the seller's expense.

Claims Made to the Buyer Must Be True. If a consignment of tetracycline is sold to Kenya with the claim that a higher than usual price is justified because the packaging is waterproof, and the shipment is ruined because it was exposed to dampness, the supplier must at least replace it or return the money. In some cases, a court may hold the supplier liable for much more—for example, for paying the much higher costs incurred in replacing the ruined batch with emergency supplies.

Goods Must Be Broadly Suited to Their Obvious and Intended Purpose. For example, a bicycle lamp must work when one puts in a battery and presses the button. It can be difficult to apply some forms of commercial law to medicines, because they are unusual products; no medicine is likely to be effective in all cases. A remedy for indigestion cannot be guaranteed to cure every case, but if it has been shown that, as a rule, it relieves digestive problems, it will normally be regarded as effective. A patient

who is disappointed with the results of treatment cannot claim reimbursement. In contrast, a batch of antacid tablets that are so tough that they pass right through the digestive system and never dissolve is clearly not suitable for any medical purpose. In this case, a purchaser is entitled to a refund.

Of course, contracts apply not only to the buying of goods but also to the provision of services—for example, those provided by a doctor or pharmacist to a patient. There is not likely to be a written contract (except perhaps when the patient enters a hospital for an operation), but there is clearly an implied agreement to treat and be treated. One of the unwritten rules in that agreement is that a professional must act with due care and skill.

In a classic case in the United States, a doctor wrote a prescription for an oral contraceptive. The pharmacist misread it and issued a tranquilizer to the woman; she became pregnant, and the pharmacist was ordered to pay the ensuing costs. This is an extreme case, but where drugs are concerned, doctors and pharmacists have often been found liable for choosing the wrong drug, prescribing or dispensing an overdose, not instructing the patient in the proper use of a drug, or writing an illegible prescription that is misread.

Patent Law

A patent is an exclusive right granted by a government to exploit an invention. Patent law, although it differs in detail from one country to another, is intended to protect the inventor from others who would like to profit from the invention. Because of agreements between countries, patents are often enforceable internationally.

There has been much controversy about drug patents. The "inventors" or developers of most of the drug substances used in medicine today have been large drug companies or institutes working closely with such companies. They claim that the long-term protection of their products via patents enables them to charge the prices needed to recover their research and development costs. Because patents generally relate to the process by which the drugs are made, and the methods are often described so broadly that they protect every possible way of making the substance, patents can completely shield a company from competition for the period of the patent—seventeen years in many countries, and in some cases (in the European Community, for example) up to twenty-five years. To illustrate: Company A, a patent-holding company, would likely succeed in a legal action and would be able to recover damages if Company B attempted to manufacture and distribute Company A's product. Company A would

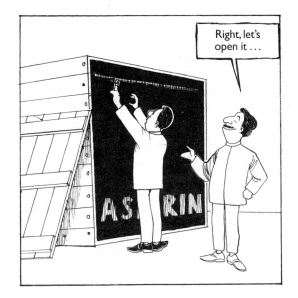

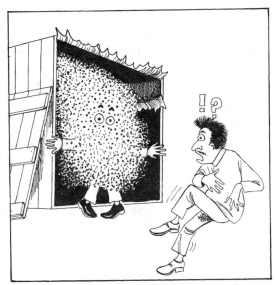

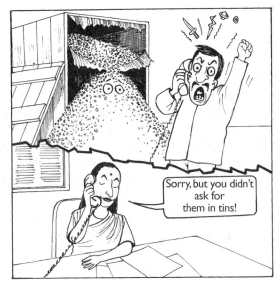

KNOW YOUR CONTRACT LAW

also have a good chance of winning an action for damages against any wholesaler in a third country that was distributing the product made by Company B.

Consumer groups and some national governments have claimed that patent protection is abused and that drug prices are sometimes so high as to deprive patients of needed treatments. In response, some countries, such as Canada, have enacted legislation to authorize the breaking of patents—for example, by obliging the originator to license others at a reasonable fee—if it is felt that the patents are being misused.

Many commonly used drugs are no longer under patent, having been developed and introduced more than twenty-five years ago. By the end of 1994, 95 percent of the 200 drugs most widely used in the United States were out of patent, including almost every drug likely to be included on an essential drugs list. In consequence, developing countries find that almost all the drugs required to fill their basic needs are now being made by multiple companies in competition with one another and can be obtained at much lower prices than previously.

Given this reality, the inclusion of many patented drugs on a country's essential drugs list could raise questions about the process by which the list was drawn up. Although the appearance of an important new drug providing a genuine breakthrough in treatment is always possible, many new drugs or new dosage forms claiming particular advantages may not offer any real benefit. In these cases, a careful medical assessment is needed to determine whether inclusion of the new patented drug at its higher price is justified.

Although almost everyone agrees that an inventor should be financially rewarded for pharmaceutical discoveries, the amount of the reward is a separate question, particularly when human lives are at stake and limited budgets are available to purchase lifesaving drugs. If patent protection is being claimed by a manufacturer, the following issues should be kept in mind:

► Is the product patented in the purchasing country? In the seller's country?
► Does the patent apply to the substance or to the production method? Often a substance patent has run out but the production method patent is still valid. In this case, there may be another production method for the substance.
► Patents are sometimes claimed unlawfully: a company claiming patent protection may not be the inventor, or it may have contracted out production rights to other companies for certain areas or even worldwide.

► A company claiming patent protection should indemnify the purchasing country against any risks or costs associated with claims of patent infringement made by other companies; conflicts should be between competing companies.

Because the language of patents can be complex, including numbers and formulations, it may be difficult for a layperson to read and understand them. Legal assistance may be needed.

One final point: some drugs are out of patent in one country but still protected in another. When finalizing a national list of essential drugs and before placing orders for them, it is wise to have the list checked for patents by an expert. This can be done, for example, through the World Health Organization (WHO). Contracts to procure a drug should include a clause making the supplier responsible for ascertaining that the product can be provided without contravening patents and absolving the buyer of liability if a patent holder should challenge the contract and seek damages. Although patent law differs from country to country, buyers should ensure that their own law will be respected first.

Trademark Law

A trademark is a product's trade name and a description of its package, which a producer is likely to register in countries where the product is being distributed. Since the trademark is the means by which a product is recognized, it is important that other companies be prevented from marketing products that could easily be confused with the original. Companies that copy trademarks may be selling pirated or counterfeit products.

If Company A has an officially registered trademark for a successful product (for example, a headache remedy based on aspirin with the name "Hedly" and a green and yellow package with the symbol of a lion in a triangle), and Company B begins to sell another remedy (based on paracetamol) with a similar name ("Hedlo") and similar packaging, Company A would likely succeed in suing Company B in all countries with strong trademark laws where B's product was marketed. Company B might argue that its product is different, but the courts would probably determine that the intent was to mislead and confuse the buyer and pull trade away from Company A.

Distributors occasionally create deliberate confusion by claiming that a product has patent protection when all that is protected is the trademark. Care must be taken to distinguish the two.

≡ 8.2 Tort Law

A tort is often defined as a private or civil wrong done by one party to another. The law of torts (in some countries known as the law of improper behavior) concerns rules that people are normally supposed to obey in their relationships with one another, even when they do not have a formal contract. These are generally considered to be matters of common decency. The law becomes involved to protect those who have suffered because someone else has not respected the rules.

Someone who suffers as a result of improper behavior may be able to seek damages or compensation in court from whoever was in the wrong. For example, if an importer advertises that a medicine can be used safely by young children when it is commonly known to be too strong for them, the importer could be liable for damages if children become ill, even though there is no contract. If a forklift truck entering the CMS drops medical equipment in the street and injures a passerby, the CMS may be liable for costs resulting from injury, treatment, and loss of working capacity.

A word of warning: because ideas of decency and proper behavior vary from one society to another, so does the law of torts. It may be difficult to enforce a claim internationally under this type of law.

≡ 8.3 Criminal Law

Criminal law is society's last resort when certain basic rules of behavior are so drastically broken that punishment by the state is called for in the form of a fine or a period of imprisonment. In criminal cases involving medicines, drug authorities may push for more severe penalties than the law would otherwise provide, and the courts are often inclined to impose heavier penalties because the crimes can have such serious consequences. In cases in which legal sanctions might include withdrawal of a license, for example, a drug authority might be permitted to prosecute an offender before a criminal court. Some examples follow.

► A firm imports and sells an unregistered drug in a country where all new drugs must be assessed and approved on grounds of efficacy and safety by a registration authority before they can be sold. The risks to the population are clear, and the firm is fined. The pharmaceutical law explicitly states that this is a criminal offense and prescribes the possible penalties.

► Thieves break into the CMS at night and steal a large quantity of tetracycline. The crime falls under the general criminal law and is punished just as if the thieves had stolen automobile tires from a garage.

► A drug company claims unjustifiably that its anti-inflammatory drug has less serious effects on the stomach than other drugs of the same type. In this British case, the medical director of the company was criminally prosecuted and received a heavy fine at the instigation of the Department of Health for contravening the section of the Medicines Act relating to truth in advertising and promotion.

≡ 8.4 Labor Law

Employment laws are generally made with private business in mind, although they are often stricter in the public sector and with autonomous state corporations (that is, companies set up and owned by the state but having a large degree of independence, such as a drug corporation might have). A company is not, as a rule, entirely free to employ and dismiss whomever, whenever, and on whatever grounds it likes. The further a country has developed and the more stable its economy has become, the more likely it is that basic rules have been introduced in the national law covering such matters as contracts, dismissal, equal opportunity, employment of the young, and working conditions.

Written Contracts of Service. Even for the simplest jobs, a written agreement may be needed and may be of benefit. It can indicate, for example, the conditions under which someone is employed, the jobs to be done, the way in which the work will be assessed, and the circumstances in which the employee may be dismissed.

Wrongful Dismissal. Some developing countries have introduced laws protecting employees against dismissal without sound reasons (for example, because of illness or pregnancy) or without sufficient notice.

Equal Opportunity. Rules are likely to indicate that in hiring employees there must be no discrimination (such as against women or against people of a particular race or belief).

Employment of the Young. Employment of children is generally forbidden; some laws provide for young people to be employed part-time while at school.

Working Conditions. There are likely to be limits on working hours, provisions to prevent work under grossly unhealthy conditions, and some provision for annual leave. These conditions, and the extent to which they are actually enforced by inspectors and courts, vary a great deal from country to country; a business law office should be consulted to provide basic advice on employment of staff, and preferably some model contracts.

It is impossible to generalize about government service, but the employment rules may be substantially different from those in private business. Although the salaries and wages paid are often much lower than in the private sector, this may be compensated for in various ways, such as with guarantees of employment or provision of housing. These differences can cause complications if government bodies are "privatized," as may happen with a drug procurement and warehousing operation.

≡ 8.5 Laws Governing International Agreements

Almost all laws are written with the lawmaker's own country and people in mind. With people and goods moving increasingly from one country to another, questions about which system of law applies often arise. If, for example, the CMS of Tanzania signs a contract to buy drugs from France, will the agreement fall under Tanzanian law or French law? The matter becomes particularly important if a disagreement arises. For example, suppose some of the goods arrive damaged. When the contract was written, no specification of legal jurisdiction was included. Which court should adjudicate the matter? In regard to contracts, there is a system known as *private international law* (or sometimes *conflict of laws*) that helps resolve the issue. The principles differ somewhat from country to country, but one piece of advice is generally valid: when drawing up an international contract (such as to buy goods or to employ a foreign citizen), a statement should be included as to which system of law will govern disputes.

The legal system in the country of one of the parties signing the agreement is usually chosen, or perhaps the country where the goods currently are or where payment is to be made. It is advisable to choose the system that seems most relevant to the situation and to the risks. If, for example, goods are being bought abroad and the concern is that the supplier may not deliver, involvement of the courts in the supplier's country may be the best way of ensuring delivery. Goods transported in boats or trains belonging to a third country, often Liberia or Panama, are not necessarily well protected, and the law of that country may not safeguard the goods. This does not alter the fact that the seller should be responsible for ensuring that they arrive. There is no guarantee that the courts of the country selected will agree to adjudicate any case that arises, but if the choice has been a commonsense one, it will probably be respected.

An alternative is to indicate some other body to settle disputes. In commercial contracts with some countries, the chamber of commerce may be asked to act as arbitrator. Arbitration is often a much better way of settling disputes than court proceedings, which may be costly and

---

≡ Assessment Guide

Commercial Law: Contracts, Patents, and Trademarks

► Do purchase orders or other contracts for the procurement of drugs include clauses enabling the checking of samples or other measures to ensure that purchased drugs are of a certain quality?

► How are patent issues handled in drug procurement contracts?

► Do contracts for the purchase of drugs from another country specify which system of law will cover disputes?

► How many drugs on the drug list are under patent? Are substitutes available that are not under patent and thus cost less?

► Which products on the drug list have officially registered trademarks?

► Is legal guidance sought on matters pertaining to pharmaceuticals from a reputable and experienced government lawyer or law office?

Criminal Law

► Do pharmaceutical laws exist that ensure that the public is protected from undue risks? Are these laws enforced?

Labor Law

► Do labor laws exist to cover such matters as written contracts of service, wrongful dismissal, equal opportunity, employment of the young, and working conditions?

---

take many years. It is important to find a suitable arbitrator who is fair, sufficiently expert in the field concerned, and trusted by both parties.

One word of warning: international disputes are often not effectively settled by the courts, or even by arbitration. An unscrupulous foreign seller of a dangerous or defective product may be able to escape liability because of the time and expense involved in bringing an international action. The supplier can change its name, address, domicile, and legal or corporate form and be out of reach of the courts. And the law may be unclear. Even between industrialized countries with a long history of personal-injury litigation, it remains difficult to claim compensation for drug injury from a foreign manufacturer of a bad product. Dealing with a firm of good reputation may be worth paying a higher price.

Obtain the advice of a reliable law office when entering into large contracts. Make sure that the other party to a contract is a well-established firm and not a company that may be here today and gone tomorrow.

≡ 8.6 A Word on Working with Lawyers

Lawyers are sometimes looked upon as people to be consulted primarily when something has gone wrong. It is much more sensible to bring a lawyer in earlier, to make sure that things have the least possible chance of going wrong. A good lawyer can give advice on many of the formal documents required in drug management, ranging from agreements of employment to the operations manual of the CMS. Legal language is sometimes complex, but its aim is to avoid ambiguity and vagueness and thereby lessen the chance of misunderstanding.

The legal profession, like the medical profession, has a large number of specialties; the lawyer in the ministry of justice who has helped draft the law on pharmaceuticals is almost certainly not the right person to give advice on procurement contracts or personnel disputes. A good link to a first-rate law office specializing in the various forms of business law is likely to be a sensible move. ■

≡ References and Further Readings

Downs, D. E., ed. 1992. *Understanding the freight business: A quick-reference manual for all those engaged in the operational aspects of forwarding cargo from producer to consumer*, 4th ed. Egham, Surrey, England: Micor Freight UK.

Spilker, B. 1994. Legal activities and issues. In *Multinational pharmaceutical companies: Principles and practices*. New York: Raven Press.

Part I Introduction	**Part II** **Policy and Legal Framework**	Part III Drug Management Cycle	Part IV Management Support Systems

5 National Drug Policies
6 Drug Supply Strategies
7 Pharmaceutical Legislation and Regulation
8 Legal Aspects of Drug Management
9 Pharmaceutical Production Policy

Chapter 9
Pharmaceutical Production Policy

≡ Summary

Policy-makers must be concerned about pharmaceutical production for the same reasons that underlie other policy and legal decisions: drugs can be dangerous as well as lifesaving. Health professionals and patients have no ready way of making judgments about drugs without public surveillance as a guide.

Problems of lack of access, high prices, and poor drug quality in many markets have prompted public and political interest in finding reasonable alternatives to dependence on outside suppliers. These alternatives have often been formulated in terms of local production to promote self-sufficiency, achieve independence from powerful international suppliers, develop local industrial capacity, and create jobs. Basically, the reasoning has been: if we develop our own production capacity, we'll be free from dependence on unreliable outsiders. To ensure that major public needs are met, the public sector has often become involved in local production.

Experience over the last two decades has demonstrated that this perspective is sometimes flawed. Ample evidence indicates that production by public agencies is often not the wisest course. Many failed attempts at such production, together with rapidly expanding markets and communication systems, have reduced earlier pressures for direct public-sector involvement in manufacturing. The principal policy question is often not make or buy but rather what to buy and where to buy it.

Three important findings of the last twenty years guide this chapter:

1. Drugs are potentially lifesaving and life-threatening.

Drug production requires precise standards, quality control, a skilled labor base, capital, and management. Modern drug production often uses raw materials that are most economical in the international market. This means that high-quality, low-cost drugs are not likely to be produced from the raw-materials stage in countries that do not have the required market size and resources in terms of skilled people, technology, and quality control.

2. Where private manufacturing initiatives have proved successful, pharmaceutical manufacture has remained a highly profitable industry. As Country Study 9.1 illustrates, in a market that is large enough, local manufacturers can carve out a role even when they are starting way behind the international producers. Section 9.1 describes the range of production options, from primary manufacture of raw materials to the packaging of finished products, that policy-makers must consider.

3. Since consumers are unable to judge medicines safely on their own, policy-makers must be concerned about regulating production quality, whether drugs come from international or domestic sources. Whether policy-makers take an active or a passive role, they must recognize that the regulations and incentives existing in a country always affect drug production. The most constructive stance may be to shape policies and working regulations that promote the goal of reliable access to effective, safe, and inexpensive medicines rather than focusing on where the production takes place.

≡ 9.1 Levels and Types of Local Production

Today, most countries are part of the global pharmaceutical market, and few try to be entirely self-sufficient. Raw materials, which form the backbone of the industry, are produced and traded as commodities worldwide. Almost all countries, even the large ones, actively acquire at least some raw materials, machinery, and packaging goods abroad—at the most economical prices and at different stages of production—and then complete the process efficiently at home. It is a matter of competitive advantage, not imaginary independence in an increasingly interdependent world economy.

Three different levels of production are recognized: primary, secondary, and tertiary.

Primary Production

Primary production is the manufacture of raw materials, such as the active ingredients and ancillary substances used in pharmaceutical formulations, or intermediary products and packaging materials. Some countries may not have all the infrastructure needed—a pool of skilled workers, industrial technology, the research and development base, quality control experience, capital, reliable utilities—as well as the potential market size to make primary production an initial goal. Rather, since the basic commodities are most efficiently produced in large volumes—much greater than the markets could absorb in many countries—they tend to be traded and bought internationally like steel, some foodstuffs, and other chemicals.

Secondary Production

Secondary production is the large-scale processing of finished dosage forms from raw materials or intermediate products, often from both local and imported sources. Production of sterile preparations (such as small injections, antibiotics, and intravenous fluids) and nonsterile

Country Study 9.1   The Growth of Kenya's Pharmaceutical Market

Over the last twenty years, Kenya's pharmaceutical market has increased eightfold, from a base that consisted of virtually all imported medicines. The essential drugs concept was adopted in 1981 with external donor support, and the market has moved from a completely import-dominated market to the point where more than twenty local producers hold a 25 percent market share. This growth in local capacity occurred in the face of many constraints: foreign exchange controls and taxes on raw materials, machinery, and packaging imports (when finished drugs were admitted duty free); slow and cumbersome payment procedures for local purchases, resulting in local suppliers using their own capital or borrowing at market interest rates of 30 percent; and external-source requirements attached by donors.

Despite these constraints, local production grew with the development of the economy, indicating that local knowledge and access count. Pharmaceuticals remained a profitable product line for local manufacturing despite substantial international competition.

preparations (oral solids, liquids, and topical preparations) can be carried out with either locally produced or imported packing materials. This stage of production uses modern, high-speed, precision equipment to turn out pills, capsules, and liquids in huge quantities, often at very low unit costs, which small facilities cannot compete with.

Tertiary Production

Tertiary production includes packaging and labeling finished products from primary and secondary sources into bulk packs, smaller dispensing packets, bottles, or course-of-therapy units for individual use. The initial quality of the pharmaceutical product established in the earlier phases of production must be maintained in the tertiary and final step. This type of production is often developed first in many countries as a profitable and productive contribution that also builds industrial skill and experience.

≡ **9.2   Status of Local Production**

As of 1992, worldwide pharmaceutical production capacity was distributed as follows:

- Ten countries had a sophisticated pharmaceutical industry and a significant research base (eight Western European countries, plus Japan and the United States).
- Seventeen countries had innovative capabilities: a sound production capacity and at least one new molecular entity marketed between 1961 and 1990 (several other European countries, Argentina, Australia, Canada, China, India, Israel, Mexico, Republic of Korea, and the former Soviet Union).

- Fourteen countries produced both therapeutic ingredients and finished products (a mixture of European and higher-income Latin American and Asian countries).
- Eighty-nine countries from virtually every continent produced only finished products from imported ingredients.
- Fifty-eight countries and areas had no pharmaceutical industry (primarily low-income African countries and islands with small populations).

Moving from one category to the next requires substantial technical and financial resources.

≡ **9.3   Policy Issues That Affect Local Production Decisions**

In general, the policy-maker's concerns should focus on the effects that a policy will have on someone else's decisions about production. In short, the policy-maker's best contribution may be to establish a fair and consistent operating environment for those who must assess the risk of producing medicines, and then let the market work. This boils down to creating a base of effective national drug legislation and enforceable regulations by which to stimulate and modulate the market.

The greatest challenge for policy-makers is often not creation of a comprehensive policy but rather creation of policy elements that are constructive next steps and that build on existing reality and local institutional capacities. Many countries are limited in their capacity to monitor, supervise, and regulate. Policies need to take into account a country's capacity to implement and enforce them.

Figure 9.1 lists many of the factors and policy issues that have an impact on production decisions. Each issue contains elements that may favor, hinder, or leave the production decision unaffected. In general, policy-makers should concentrate on promoting guidelines that support the essential drugs concept: improving the prospects of access to low-cost, high-quality, effective medicines. Producers can make their own decisions about what and how much to make, and essential drugs program managers can concentrate on choosing to buy from the best sources, domestic and international.

Market Factors

Population size and distribution combine with per capita income to determine how many potential clients will be able to buy medicines. Although aspirations for health are high, difficult economic times can create falling real personal incomes and low government capacity to provide health services; both limit actual market size in

Figure 9.1 Factors Influencing Local Production Decisions

Market Factors
- ► population size, geographic distribution, and income levels
- ► existing local production capacity (competition)
- ► barriers to imported products (degree of protection)
- ► size, reliability, and preference of public-sector market

Regulatory and Legal Provisions
- ► ease of registration, registration preference
- ► product and process patent protection
- ► good manufacturing practices and enforcement of standards
- ► generic labeling, prescribing, and dispensing laws and practices

Investment and Industrial Development Environment
- ► tax or other investment incentives
- ► industrial development funds (access to start-up capital)
- ► ownership requirements (limits on foreign ownerships, requirements of local ownership)
- ► repatriation of profits (foreign investors)

Physical and Human Infrastructure
- ► cost and reliability of water, power, and other resources
- ► availability of technical specialists
- ► availability of skilled production staff

Economic Incentives and Disincentives
- ► price controls
- ► access to foreign exchange
- ► export incentives

Duties and Import Controls
- ► active pharmaceutical ingredients (versus finished products)
- ► inactive pharmaceutical ingredients and other raw materials
- ► packaging materials
- ► specialized pharmaceutical equipment
- ► nonspecialized equipment

---

many countries. Local competitors or importers also need to be taken into account, along with the possibility of a preference in the public-sector market for local production. Projects supported by the international banks often include a local production preference of 10 to 15 percent in competitive bidding to encourage domestic industry. Barriers to importation may assist local producers initially, but they may increase local prices paid by consumers (and public health organizations) and foster a misinterpretation of international competitive potential that may not be realized.

Regulatory and Legal Provisions

As discussed in Chapter 8, drug registration requirements are rules to limit dangerous, unproven, or useless items and to promote the availability of effective, essential drugs. However, a cumbersome or corrupt registration process can limit a producer's incentives to offer a product. From the producer's viewpoint, the important issues related to registration are the speed, fairness, and expense of the process. If the process is arduous, individual products need to have a substantial market potential to merit the investment in registration.

Countries vary in their use and recognition of patent laws, which can cover both the individual products (that is, the chemical formulations) and the industrial processes by which the products are produced. The trend is toward more consistency among countries, and potential producers must expect to encounter patent protections and licensing by patent holders. Most local production decisions stem from a summary appraisal of the market that combines nonpatent or generic drugs and those to be manufactured on license by current patent holders. As patents expire, the drugs become candidates for direct local registration and production.

Production standards, often known as good manufacturing practices (GMPs), are quality requirements that have been adopted as guidelines by the industry and the World Health Organization (WHO). More exacting standards are required by some countries to further ensure quality, and any hope for an export market increasingly requires compliance with GMPs. Given the international nature of pharmaceutical trade and production, the rationale for local production at some lower standard is shrinking; such products will be exposed in the world market, as evidenced by the recent trend toward increased plant inspections of international suppliers by regulatory agencies. Currently, developing countries vary greatly in their capacity to monitor GMPs. In 1995, for example, 35 percent of foreign plant inspections by the US Food and Drug Administration (FDA) found serious manufacturing deficiencies, compared with 1 percent in US plants, prompting an increase in planned plant inspections for the future (*New York Times*, October 29, 1995).

Investment and Industrial Development Issues

Tax treatment and local development incentives can affect the cost of production start-ups through direct subsidies, assisted capitalization schemes, training support, or tax abatement. Given the huge and complex investment necessary for an effective research-based pharmaceutical industry, incentives for research and development by local government may or may not be useful instruments in affecting local production decisions.

Partnering with international companies is often the most common form of local production support, with joint ventures and majority or minority ownership shares depending on the strength of the local economy and political and market potential. The potential for profit repatriation by the external partners is critical.

Physical and Human Infrastructure

The reliability of water, power, and environmental controls and the availability of skilled technical and production staff are central to the production decision. In the short term, human resources can be supplemented from external sources, but production decisions are long-term investments that require sustainable, local staffing.

Economic Incentives and Disincentives

Pharmaceutical production involves a worldwide marketplace, and the raw materials that constitute about half of production costs are traded widely as competitive commodities. Reliable, rapid access to foreign exchange is essential. The pharmaceutical industry is commonly one of the most price-controlled industries, which can help as well as distort a production decision; price controls, by definition, distort the marketplace. High prices may produce short-term profits but disguise inefficiencies; low prices can discourage producers from competing. Disincentives can cause prescribers and dispensers to use too much or too little of a medication or cause distributors to distort their pricing and accounting practices. International firms may create internal (transfer) prices among partner companies as devices to hide profits and justify higher prices. Price controls in the form of allowable markups at steps in the distribution process or dispensing fees set by the provider may be applied differentially to brand-name and generic products or to essential drugs, creating incentives that the potential producer must evaluate.

Legislated incentives (tax protection or start-up subsidies) to promote exports can be illusory and are unlikely to be a major factor for most developing-country production. Only 5 percent of developing-country pharmaceuticals are exported on average; they offer little competitive advantage, because production must begin with imported raw materials.

Duties and Import Controls

Differential taxation of pharmaceutical materials, both imported and local, can significantly affect the production decision. If the public policy goal is to create a level playing field for producer decisions on what and where to produce, there should be no difference in the tax treatment of raw materials, both active and inactive ingredients, and finished products. If packaging materials and production equipment are heavily taxed, it will deter local industrial development.

Country Study 9.2 Local Public-Sector Production Problems

► One Latin American ministry created an "in-house" pharmaceutical factory to produce essential drugs for its own system. There was little connection with the ministry market, however, and the product line drifted into over-the-counter preparations and beauty aids, largely missing its original purpose.

► In another semi-autonomous government laboratory, production of essential drugs is usually two to three years behind schedule, throwing ministry purchasing into turmoil and resulting in higher prices because of emergency purchases.

► A parastatal company in East Africa faced multiple problems in producing drugs at competitive prices. Inadequate capitalization and inadequate foreign exchange allocation left the firm unable to purchase enough raw materials to operate at the break-even level of 60 percent capacity. For the drugs that were produced, containers of inadequate quality—metal tins without aluminum coating—were all the local suppliers had, and these had to be lined with polyethylene bags, adding to production costs. Plastic containers were tried, but the lids fit poorly, as a proper mold could not be obtained locally at reasonable cost. The cardboard used for boxes to pack intravenous fluids collapsed when stacked, and the containers broke when transported over rough roads. When the government attempted to purchase drugs on tender from the company, it could not meet the competitive prices on the market, and as a result of a structural adjustment program, the company has been put up for sale.

► For political reasons, a Latin American government was obligated to purchase a nonfunctional private facility as a means of expanding its production capacity. Originally constructed to produce small quantities of a large number of sterile injectable products, it had never functioned because of an inadequate water supply, which rendered it useless as a production facility. In addition, the plant lacked the production capacity, types of equipment, and storage capacity to produce the priority items required by the ministry.

≡ 9.4 Assessing the Feasibility of Local Production

Studies that document the failures of public-sector production abound (see Country Study 9.2). More promising results have been achieved following vigorous policy stimulation of local private production, as in Bangladesh (Country Study 9.3), and even in cases of policy neglect, such as Kenya (see Country Study 9.1).

Despite the case made here that actual production decisions should be left to private-sector and market forces, policy-makers must sometimes respond to pressures to become more involved in decisions about pharmaceutical production. A feasibility study is required, which may serve either as a warning to avoid a hasty decision to

Country Study 9.3 Promoting Local Production of Essential Drugs in Bangladesh

The government of Bangladesh enacted major drug policy reform in 1982. Prompted by financial and health concerns and fueled by the nationalistic fervor of a new government, the National Drug Policy (NDP) set out to promote domestic production of pharmaceuticals and, specifically, the production of essential drugs.

Prior to 1982, essential drugs were largely unavailable to large segments of the population, although there were 3,500 brands of pharmaceuticals on the market. Imports of raw materials (US$30 million) and finished products (US$12–15 million) strained both the health budget and the limited foreign exchange reserves. The local production that was already taking place was dominated by eight multinational firms that produced 75 percent of the total value of production.

In its policy announcement, the new government's Expert Committee on Drugs stated that "wastage of foreign exchange through the production and/or importation of unnecessary drugs or drugs of marginal value have to be stopped." The NDP created a restricted national formulary of 250 essential drugs, later increased to 302, and banned 1,666 products that were useless, ineffective, or harmful. Measures were included to promote local manufacture of the formulary drugs and to restrict the activities of foreign firms, preventing them, for example, from importing a drug if the same or a similar product was produced locally.

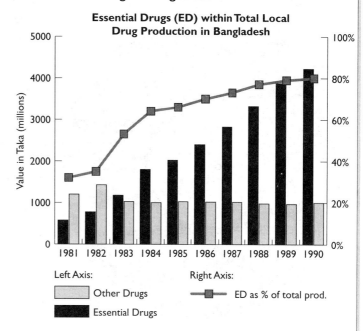

Essential Drugs (ED) within Total Local Drug Production in Bangladesh

Left Axis:
- ☐ Other Drugs
- ■ Essential Drugs

Right Axis:
- ■— ED as % of total prod.

Source: Drug Administration, government of Bangladesh. Reprinted from Michael R. Reich, "Bangladesh pharmaceutical policy and politics," *Health Policy and Planning* 9(2): 135, by permission of Oxford University Press.

Note: There were forty-five essential drugs until 1987; then there were seventy-three.

Strong resistance was forthcoming from the domestic and international pharmaceutical industry, which feared the restrictions imposed by the national formulary; from the Bangladesh Medical Association, which felt that it was not sufficiently consulted; and from foreign governments, which asserted that the policy would discourage private investment.

In the decade following enactment of the policy, however, results were dramatic, leading the Bangladesh pharmaceutical industry association to change its initial position to one of support. The value of local production increased by more than 217 percent in local currency terms. Nationally owned companies, which had produced 35 percent of all drugs (by value) in 1981, were producing over 60 percent in 1990. By 1991, the top three firms in pharmaceutical sales were Bangladeshi owned. As shown in the accompanying figure, essential drugs rose from 30 percent of all local production (by value) in 1981 (for forty-five items) to nearly 80 percent in 1990 (for seventy-three items).

Further, through price controls on imported raw materials and increased competition among manufacturers, the NDP reduced the cost of essential drugs to the government and to consumers. One study estimated that if dependence on imported drugs had continued, and if local manufacturers had continued to produce useless and ineffective products, more than US$620 million would have been wasted.

Opponents of the policy continue to argue that the NDP has driven away foreign investment, hampered the growth and development of the pharmaceutical industry by excessive regulation, and deprived patients of access to the latest lifesaving drugs. They have also raised issues about poor product quality under the NDP, criticizing the adequacy of quality control facilities within manufacturing firms and the government's inspection and enforcement mechanisms.

The government and other supporters of the policy recognize that although many of these criticisms are unsubstantiated, there is room for improvement, particularly in implementing some aspects of the policy. Recognizing too the continuing challenge of maintaining a balance between commercial and health interests, the government has invited representatives from the medical establishment and drug industry to participate in efforts to review regulatory and quality control mechanisms that will contribute to more effective implementation of the NDP.

Sources: Reich 1994; Chetley 1993.

consider manufacture or, if the decision is made to do so, to establish an appropriate framework, timetable, and resource plan for analysis. Figures 9.2 and 9.3 illustrate the project investment cycle and the complexity of the analysis process *only* for the feasibility stage. The issues to be considered in a careful investigation include marketing analysis, raw materials and supplies, location, engineering and technology, organization and overhead costs, human resources, implementation planning and budgeting, financial analysis, and investment appraisal.

Figure 9.2 Preinvestment, Investment, and Operating Phases of the Project Cycle

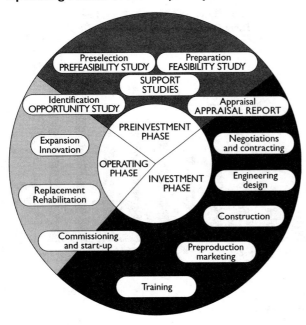

When a project feasibility analysis is carried out in the public sector, many different government agencies (ministries of treasury, industry, and commerce, as well as the ministry of health) must be involved to appraise the forces and issues that will determine the outcome of the analysis. The complexity of these negotiations means substantial time commitments from senior analysts and policy-makers. Although experience suggests that governments and public programs are usually unlikely to be successful producers of pharmaceuticals, Sri Lanka, Indonesia, and Nepal have demonstrated that some can be. Nevertheless, the vast majority of all worldwide production is done by private companies that have learned from experience how to manage the process efficiently. ∎

Figure 9.3 Information Flow for an Industrial Feasibility Study

Revenues and Marketing Costs	Operating Costs	Investment Costs	Financial Analysis
Sales program and revenue	Production program	Land, site	Fixed investment
Marketing costs	Raw materials and factory supplies	Civil engineering	Preproduction expenditures
Marketing personnel	Production personnel	Environmental protection costs	Net working capital
Wages, salaries	Wages, salaries	Technology	Total investment
	Land, site, related annual costs	Machinery, equipment	Source of finance
	Technology costs	Cash flow (working capital)	Balance sheet
	Factory overheads		Net income statement
	Administrative overhead costs		Net present value, internal rate of return
	Total costs of products sold		

Source: Adapted from Behrens and Hawranek 1991.

≡ Assessment Guide

Market Factors
- ► What are the size, distribution, and income of the population?

Regulatory Environment
- ► What is the status of laws on drug registration and patent protection?
- ► What is the status of laws on manufacturing, labeling, and prescribing standards?

Investment Environment
- ► What tax incentives and ownership requirements exist?

- ► Are there restrictions on profit repatriation?

Physical and Human Resources
- ► Are water and power available?
- ► Are technical and production staff available?

Economic Incentives
- ► Are there export incentives or price controls?
- ► Is there easy access to foreign exchange?

Duties and Import Controls
- ► Are there import duties on pharmaceutical ingredients, packaging materials, and equipment?

≡ References and Further Readings

★ = *Key readings.*

★ Ballance, R., J. Pogány, and H. Forstner. 1992. *The world's pharmaceutical industries: An international perspective on innovation, competition, and policy.* Brookfield, Vt.: Ashgate Publishers.

Behrens, W., and Hawranek, P. M. 1991. *Manual for the preparation of industrial feasibility studies* (revised and expanded edition). Vienna: United Nations Industrial Development Organization (UNIDO).

Chetley, A. 1985. Drug production with a social conscience: The experience of GPL. *Development Dialogue* 2:94–107.

Chetley, A. 1993. The future of the Bangladesh national drug policy. *Essential Drugs Monitor* 15:10–11.

Dukes, M. N. G. 1985. Towards a healthy pharmaceutical industry by the year 2000. *Development Dialogue* 2:108–20.

Hanushek, E. A., and W. S. Comanor. 1986. The political economy of the pharmaceutical industry. *Journal of Economic Literature* 24:1178–1217.

MSH (Management Sciences for Health). 1995. *International drug price indicator guide* (updated annually). Boston: MSH.

Reich, M. R. 1994. Bangladesh pharmaceutical policy and politics. *Health Policy and Planning* 9:130–43.

Spilker, B. 1994. *Multinational pharmaceutical companies: Principles and practices,* 2d ed. New York: Raven Press.

Spivey, R. N., A. I. Wertheimer, and T. D. Rucker, eds. 1992. *International pharmaceutical services: The drug industry in twenty-three major countries of the world.* New York: Pharmaceutical Products Press.

WHO/CDD (World Health Organization/Control of Diarrhoeal Diseases Programme). 1985. *Oral rehydration salts: Planning, establishment, and operation of production facilities.* WHO/CDD/SER/85.8. Geneva: WHO/CDD.

Part III
Drug Management Cycle

Part I	Part II	**Part III**	Part IV
Introduction	Policy and Legal Framework	**Drug Management Cycle**	Management Support Systems
		A Selection	
		B Procurement	
		C Distribution	
		D Use	

Section A
Selection

Part I	Part II	Part III	Part IV
Introduction	Policy and Legal Framework	**Drug Management Cycle**	Management Support Systems

A Selection ▶	**10 Managing Drug Selection**
B Procurement	11 Treatment Guidelines and Formulary Manuals
C Distribution	
D Use	12 Essential Medical Supplies and Equipment

Chapter 10
Managing Drug Selection

≡ Summary

The rationale for selecting a limited number of essential drugs is that it may lead to better supply, more rational use, and lower costs. Essential drugs are those that are deemed to satisfy the health care needs of the majority of the population and that should be available in the appropriate dosage forms and strengths at all times. Because it has a considerable impact on the quality of care and the cost of treatment, the selection of drugs is one of the most cost-effective areas for intervention.

A list of essential drugs may be selected for use in one or more health facilities or for the public sector as a whole. In the latter case, the list usually indicates the level of the health care system where each drug may be used. It can also be considered a supply list. A formulary manual contains summary information on a selected number of drugs, usually based on an essential drugs list. Treatment guidelines are systematically developed statements that assist prescribers in deciding on appropriate treatments for specific clinical problems. Whereas a formulary is drug centered, treatment guidelines are disease centered, presenting treatment alternatives and recommending a treatment of first choice.

The process of selecting essential drugs begins with defining a list of common diseases for each level of health care. The treatment of first choice for each health problem is the basis for the list of essential drugs, the national formulary, and the treatment guidelines. The supply system should supply the drugs that have been selected.

Essential drugs should be selected on the basis of (1) relevance to the pattern of prevalent diseases, (2) proven efficacy and safety, (3) adequate scientific data and evidence of performance in a variety of settings, (4) adequate quality, (5) favorable cost-benefit ratio, (6) desirable pharmacokinetic properties and possibilities for local manufacture, and (7) availability as single compounds. The drugs should be identified by the international nonproprietary name (INN) or generic name.

General acceptance of an essential drugs list can be promoted by wide consultation with senior specialists and experts, including professional organizations and academic institutions. An open and transparent system of regular updates is an absolute prerequisite for maintaining the authority and acceptance of an essential drugs list or formulary list. The essential drugs concept can be applied in any country, in the public and private sectors, and in rural areas as well as referral hospitals.

≡ 10.1 Introduction

Pharmaceuticals may constitute up to 40 percent of the health care budget in developing countries, yet large portions of the population frequently lack access to even the most essential drugs. The limited funds available are frequently spent on ineffective, unnecessary, or even dangerous drugs.

As many as 70 percent of the pharmaceuticals on the world market today are duplicative or nonessential. Many are minor variations of a prototype drug and offer no therapeutic advantage over other drugs that are already available. Other drugs show high toxicity relative to their therapeutic benefit. In some cases, drugs are newly released with insufficient information on efficacy or toxicity. Finally, many new products are for therapeutic indications not relevant to the basic needs of the population. They are nearly always more expensive than existing drugs.

With so many different drugs available, it has become impossible for prescribers to be up-to-date and to compare alternatives. The variety of available products may also contribute to inconsistent prescribing within the same health care system or health facility. With regard to procurement, purchasing power is significantly lessened by the large number of duplicate and nonessential drug products.

In short, pharmaceuticals can provide great benefits, but their cost is substantial. The selection of drugs has a considerable impact on the quality of care and the cost of treatment, and it is therefore one of the areas where intervention is most cost-effective.

≡ 10.2 Practical Implications of the Essential Drugs Concept

The World Health Organization (WHO) has defined essential drugs as those that satisfy the needs of the majority of the population and therefore should be available at all times. The rationale for the selection and use of a limited number of essential drugs is that it leads to an improved supply of drugs, more rational prescribing, and lower costs. This is a global concept that can be applied in any country, in the private and public sectors, in referral hospitals as well as primary health care units, and in both urban and rural areas. For example, limited lists are increasingly being developed by consensus, introduced, and enforced as health service, hospital, or local outpatient formularies in North America and the European Community.

Under optimal circumstances, the registration of drugs for the private and public sectors should be based on an evaluation of efficacy, safety, and quality. In some countries, cost and need are also criteria for drug registration. In such cases, the selection of essential drugs takes place during drug evaluation, approval, and registration and is therefore applicable to the public as well as the private sector.

More commonly, the selection and use of essential drugs are limited to public-sector health facilities. For each level of health care in the public sector, a limited list of essential drugs is prepared as the basis for the supply of drugs, for prescribing in the public sector, and for the training of health workers. This is especially relevant for medical and paramedical training institutions and teaching hospitals, as they have an important influence on the prescribers of the future.

Although there are many different settings in which a list of essential drugs can be used, the criteria for selection are basically the same. Box 10.1 summarizes the criteria recommended by WHO (1995).

There are many reasons to support the use of a limited essential drugs list. First, it is only fair that basic health services be accessible to everyone before more expensive services are made available to a small, usually urban proportion of the population.

Second, because the availability of drugs in the public sector is erratic in many countries, a regular supply of most drugs on the essential drugs list would result in a real health improvement.

Third, when the limited list of essential drugs represents prescribers' consensus on drug treatments of first choice, its use may improve the quality of care by ensuring that patients receive the treatment of choice as well as similar treatments from different providers. It also allows prescribers to become more familiar with a smaller number of drugs. This contributes to improved recognition of actual benefits and limitations of specific drug therapy, as well as to the detection and prevention of adverse drug reactions.

Fourth, improved effectiveness and efficiency in patient treatment lead to lower health care costs. Therefore, it is not true that the selection of essential drugs is necessary only because of a lack of funds in developing countries or that it compromises the quality of care. The essential drugs concept is increasingly being accepted as a *universal* tool to promote both quality of care and cost control.

Fifth, for public-sector supply programs, there are advantages to concentrating procurement and logistics efforts on a limited number of drugs, including reduction in the number of different products that must be stocked, distributed, and monitored. Essential drugs are usually

Box 10.1 WHO Criteria for Selection of Essential Drugs

Essential drugs are those that satisfy the health care needs of the majority of the population; they should therefore be available at all times in adequate amounts and in the appropriate dosage forms.

The choice of such drugs depends on many factors, such as the pattern of prevalent diseases; the treatment facilities; the training and experience of the available personnel; the financial resources; and genetic, demographic, and environmental factors.

Only drugs for which sound and adequate data on efficacy and safety are available from clinical studies, and for which evidence of performance in general use in a variety of medical settings has been obtained, should be selected.

Each selected drug must be available in a form in which adequate quality, including bioavailability, can be ensured; its stability under the anticipated conditions of storage and use must be established.

When two or more drugs appear to be similar in the above respects, the choice between them should be made on the basis of a careful evaluation of their relative efficacy, safety, quality, price, and availability.

In cost comparisons between drugs, the cost of the total treatment, not only the unit cost of the drug, must be considered. The cost-benefit ratio is a major consideration in the choice of some drugs for the list. In some cases, the choice may also be influenced by other factors, such as pharmacokinetic properties, or by local considerations, such as the availability of facilities for manufacture or storage.

Most essential drugs should be formulated as single compounds. Fixed-ratio combination products are acceptable only when the dosage of each ingredient meets the requirements of a defined population group and when the combination has a proven advantage over single compounds administered separately in terms of therapeutic effect, safety, or patient adherence to treatment.

Source: WHO 1995.

available from multiple suppliers. With increased competition, more favorable prices can be negotiated. In addition, by limiting the number of different drugs used to treat a particular clinical problem, larger quantities of the selected drug will be needed, with potential opportunities to achieve economies of scale. It is also easier to ensure the quality of a small number of drug products.

Finally, the selection of a limited number of essential drugs facilitates efforts to provide drug information and education, both of which further rational prescribing and use. Objective drug information and training materials are so scarce in most developing countries that their provision is considered very beneficial by physicians and other health care workers. Thus, although the number of pharmaceutical products for public health use could be limited by an essential drugs list, the practical availability of drugs and corresponding drug information and training materials may be increased. Patient education and efforts to promote proper use of drugs by patients can also be enhanced by focusing on these drugs.

The potential advantages of using a limited list of essential drugs are summarized in Figure 10.1. These advantages do not, however, follow automatically. The essential drugs list is only a starting point, not an end in itself. For countries to realize its advantages, the selection of essential drugs must be followed by other actions outlined in this manual, including preparation of standard treatment manuals, improvements in procurement and distribution, and efforts to promote rational drug use.

≡ 10.3 Selection Criteria

For a national essential drugs list to be credible and accepted, explicit criteria must be defined and published. The final selection criteria should be based on thorough discussions and acceptance by influential prescribers. The following WHO criteria for the selection of essential drugs are frequently adopted and modified to fit local requirements:

- ► relevance to the pattern of prevalent diseases;
- ► proven efficacy and safety;
- ► evidence of performance in a variety of settings;
- ► adequate quality, including bioavailability and stability;
- ► favorable cost-benefit ratio in terms of the total treatment cost;
- ► preference for drugs that are well known, with good pharmacokinetic properties and possibilities for local manufacture;
- ► single compounds.

These criteria, which were arrived at after prolonged deliberation, are described in greater detail in Box 10.1.

The choice of drugs depends on the staff's capacity to use them effectively. Consequently, it is important to know the extent of staff training and the availability of support facilities for each level of the health care system before deciding where individual drugs will be made available. For example, cancer drugs are expensive, have serious side effects, and require frequent laboratory monitoring. Therefore, such drugs might be limited to a few designated cancer treatment centers, as occurs in Zimbabwe.

Safety and efficacy appear to be obvious criteria, but controversies may arise, as in the case of metamizole (dipyrone). Because of unacceptable toxicity, this drug for the symptomatic treatment of pain and fever has been

Figure 10.1 Advantages of a Limited List of Essential Drugs

Supply
- ► Easier procurement, storage, and distribution
- ► Lower stocks
- ► Better quality assurance
- ► Easier dispensing

Prescribing
- ► Training more focused and therefore easier
- ► More experience with fewer drugs
- ► No irrational treatment alternatives available
- ► Focused drug information
- ► Better recognition of adverse drug reactions

Cost
- ► Lower prices, more competition

Patient Use
- ► Focused education efforts
- ► Reduced confusion and increased adherence to treatment
- ► Improved drug availability

withdrawn from various countries, but others (mostly developing countries) continue to allow metamizole to be marketed.

In choosing among drugs of similar safety and efficacy, the total cost of treatment should be considered. Care must be taken, however, in making the comparison. For example, ampicillin may be cheaper than amoxicillin in a tablet-to-tablet comparison but more expensive in a course-of-therapy comparison, since ampicillin must be taken more often. Because drug costs vary from country to country, cost comparisons should be country specific.

Decision-making becomes more complicated when more expensive drugs are also more effective, as in the case of certain antibacterial, antitubercular, or antimalarial drugs for resistant organisms. In such cases, the cost of cure may actually be less for drugs that are more expensive based on a tablet-to-tablet (dose-to-dose) comparison. Chapters 3 and 11 discuss how cost-effectiveness analysis can guide such decisions.

Thus, although all the criteria appear reasonable and almost self-evident, considerable room exists for discussion about the relative merits of individual drugs. Before such a discussion occurs, members of the selection committee should review, discuss, and come to a common understanding of the selection criteria and the quality of the evidence to support the choices.

≡ 10.4 Use of International Nonproprietary (Generic) Names

Each drug on the market has a chemical name (for example, 6-{D(-)-,α-amino-α-phenylacetamido}-penicillinic acid) and an international nonproprietary name (INN) or

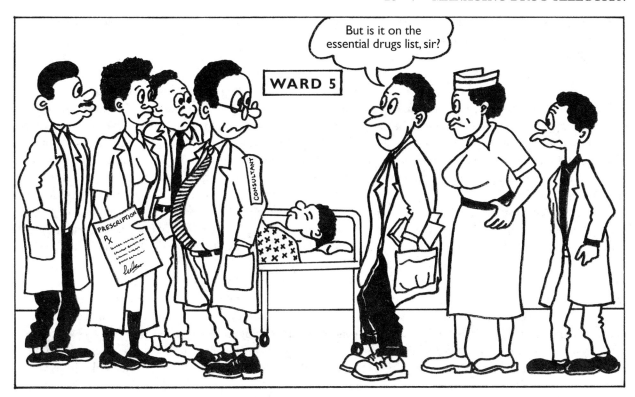

generic name (ampicillin). The INN is the drug's official name, regardless of who manufactures or markets it. A proprietary, commercial, trade, or brand name is chosen by the manufacturer to facilitate recognition and association of the product with a particular firm for marketing purposes.

For most common drugs there are several branded products that all contain the same active ingredient and therefore share the same INN. For example, the *Monthly Index of Medical Specialties* (MIMS) Middle East lists over twenty different brand names of oral ampicillin. In Pakistan there are over 100 preparations containing paracetamol, most of them with different brand names.

INNs are assigned through WHO following a well-established procedure. Official INN listings are in Latin, English, French, Spanish, and Russian. National nonproprietary names sometimes differ from INNs. For example, in the United States, acetaminophen is used instead of paracetamol; in the United Kingdom, frusemide is used for furosemide. Public health programs should therefore specify that the INN be used as the generic name for a drug, except when the official national nonproprietary name differs from the INN.

The use of generic names for drug purchasing as well as prescribing carries considerations of clarity, quality, and price. Proponents of generic drug purchasing and prescribing point out that

▸ generic names are more informative than brand names and facilitate purchasing of products from multiple suppliers, whether as brand-name or as generic products;
▸ generic drug products are often cheaper than products sold by brand name;
▸ generic prescribing also facilitates product substitution, whenever appropriate.

Opponents argue that the quality of generic drugs is inferior to that of brand-name products.

With regard to clarity, the generic name helps identify the class of drug. The common stem of the INN usually indicates a "family" of drugs. For example, the names of all benzodiazepines end with *-zepam* (diazepam, temazepam, nitrazepam), and beta-blockers share the stem *-olol* (propranolol, atenolol, metoprolol). In addition, it is obviously much easier for students and prescribers to learn one generic name rather than a host of different brand names. However, to many students it may seem easier initially to memorize a brand name, as these are usually designed to sound attractive. The confusion comes later, when the students are confronted with many different names for the same drug.

With regard to price, the patents on many common drugs have expired, allowing other manufacturers to produce and market equivalent products by the drugs' generic names. These generic drug products are usually sold at a lower price than the branded equivalents. Therefore, the use of the generic name introduces elements of price competition. The wholesale price difference between the original branded product and its generic equivalents may be considerable. However, as the actual manufacturing costs are comparable, suppliers of brand-name drug products can frequently match generic product suppliers in international tenders; they may even undercut generic prices if they are specifically aiming to increase or maintain a market share.

This element of price competition is also valid at the retail level. If a prescription is written using the generic name of the drug, the pharmacist may dispense an equivalent product with a price that is more attractive to the consumer but that also meets quality standards. In general, all products registered for sale in a country (whether as brand-name or generic products) should comply with established quality standards. One further step is the concept of *generic substitution* that is accepted in an increasing number of countries: even if the prescription is made under a brand name, the pharmacist may substitute a generic equivalent unless the prescriber specifically indicates that this should not be done, by writing "do not substitute" on the prescription. This measure may lead to large savings in drug costs (see Chapter 6).

Quality control and naming of drugs are completely separate issues. Generic drugs from reliable suppliers are as safe, effective, and high in quality as drugs with well-known brand names. At the same time, brand-name drugs from a manufacturer with inadequate procedures for quality control can be of poor quality, despite the brand name. Also, although any drug can be counterfeited, there are more incentives for counterfeiting brand-name drugs. In countries with strong drug regulatory systems, drug products sold by generic name have the same low rate of recall as brand-name products. Some pharmaceutical companies also sell their branded products under the generic name, for a much lower price.

Bioequivalence is often misused as an argument against the use of generic equivalents. For many drugs, the variation in bioavailability among individual patients is much larger than the variation among products of different manufacturers. In fact, bioavailability is clinically relevant for only a relatively small number of drugs. WHO published the following short list of drugs (from the *Model List of Essential Drugs*) that are widely considered to pose bioavailability problems: furosemide, griseofulvin, chloroquine, digoxin, ampicillin, levodopa, erythromycin, metronidazole, isoniazid, phenytoin, phenoxymethylpenicillin, mebendazole,

tetracycline, and tolbutamide (WHO 1990). (Drug quality and bioequivalence are discussed in Chapter 18.)

≡ 10.5 Essential Drugs Lists in Context

An essential drugs list names the drugs considered optimal treatment choices to satisfy the health care needs of a given population. In its simplest form, it is used for one health facility (for example, a hospital) or for a group of health facilities to indicate which drugs should be procured and prescribed. In most developing countries, the ministry of health has developed a *national essential drugs list* for the public sector. Some national essential drugs lists indicate, for each level of care, the drugs that should be procured, distributed, and used. This is called a *leveled essential drugs list*. In fact, it is a combination of separate lists for dispensaries, health centers, district hospitals, and referral hospitals, with the number of drugs increasing with the level of care. The criteria for inclusion usually focus on efficacy, safety, need, and cost (see Box 10.1). Drugs are identified by the INN or generic name, without specifying the manufacturer. For practical purposes, the lists can be considered *supply lists*, defining the range of drugs for the different levels of care and indicating dosage form and, sometimes, pack size and other specifications. A sample page of a list, organized by levels of use, is reproduced in Figure 10.2. The number of drug products on a variety of national essential drugs lists is given in Figure 10.3.

Lists of Registered Drugs

Adoption of a national list of essential drugs, usually limited to the public sector, does not necessarily mean that no other drugs are available in the private sector. In many countries, the marketing of pharmaceutical products requires prior evaluation, approval, and licensing by the national drug regulatory authority. The criteria for approval and licensing include efficacy, safety, and quality, but some countries also consider cost and need. Drug registration is discussed in greater detail in Chapter 7. The list of registered drugs includes all drug products that have been licensed.

The number of drug products that are licensed may be many times greater than the number of drug products on the essential drugs list for two reasons. First, equivalent drug products produced by different manufacturers are registered separately (the product is registered, not the active substance). Second, there are drugs that may not be considered essential for use in the public sector, yet their efficacy, safety, and quality are such that they can be available in the private market. For example, in the United

Figure 10.2 Example of Level-of-Use Categories, Kenya Essential Drugs List, 1993

Therapeutic Class and Item Description	Unit of Pack	Level of Care						
		KNH	PGH	DH	SDH	HC	DISP	CHW
6. Anti-infective drugs								
6.2.a. Antibacterials—oral liquids								
Amoxicillin suspension 125 mg/5 mL	Bottle	■	■	■	■	■		
Amoxicillin + clavulanic acid 156 mg/5 mL	100 mL bottle	■	■	■				
Clindamycin oral suspension 75 mg/5 mL	10 mL bottle	■	■	■				
Cloxacillin syrup 125 mg/5 mL	100 mL bottle	■	■	■				
Cotrimoxazole suspension 200:40/5 mL	50 mL bottle	■	■	■	■	■	■	
Erythromycin ethyl succinate syrup 200 mg base/5 mL USP	100 mL bottle	■	■	■				
Metronidazole suspension 200 mg/5 mL	Bottle	■	■	■	■			
Nystatin oral suspension 100,000 units/mL	24 mL bottle	■	■	■	■	■		
Penicillin V syrup 125 mg/5 mL	100 mL bottle	■	■	■	■	■	■	
6.2.b. Antibacterials—oral tablets/capsules								
Amoxicillin caps 250 mg	1,000	■	■	■	■	■		
Amoxicillin 250 mg + clavulanic acid 125 mg tabs	1,000	■	■	■				
Chloramphenicol caps 250 mg	1,000	■	■	■				
Clindamycin HCl caps 150 mg	1,000	■	■	■				
Cotrimoxazole tabs 400:80	1,000	■	■	■	■	■	■	
Doxycycline HCl tabs 100 mg	1,000	■	■	■	■	■	■	
Erythromycin stearate tabs film coated 250 mg	1,000	■	■	■	■			
Nitrofurantoin sodium tabs 100 mg	1,000	■	■	■	■			
Penicillin V tabs 250 mg	1,000	■	■	■	■	■	■	
Tetracycline HCl caps 250 mg	1,000	■	■	■	■	■	■	

Source: Reprinted with permission of Ministry of Health, Government of Kenya.

Notes: KNH = Kenyatta National Hospital; PGH = provincial general hospital; DH = district hospital; SDH = subdistrict hospital; HC = health center; DISP = dispensary; CHW = community health worker.

Kingdom, the list of drugs available free of charge through the National Health Service contains several laxatives; if a particular patient wants another brand, it is available for sale but without reimbursement. Figure 10.4 illustrates the relationship between the list of essential drugs and the list of registered drugs.

Formulary Manuals

The term *formulary* can be confusing. It is useful to distinguish between the formulary list as a selection tool, the formulary manual as a source of drug information, and the formulary system as a drug management process.

A *formulary list* is a list of drug products approved for use in a specific health care setting. It may be a national formulary list, a provincial list, a hospital list, or a list reimbursed by a health insurance program. In most developing countries, *formulary list* is synonymous with *essential drugs list.*

A *formulary manual* contains summary drug information. It is not a full textbook, nor does it usually cover all drugs on the market. Instead, it is a handy reference that contains selected information that is relevant to the prescriber, dispenser, nurse, or other health worker. It commonly includes the generic name of a drug, indications for use, dosage schedules, contraindications, side effects, and important information that should be given to the patient. A formulary is drug centered, as it is based on monographs for individual drugs or therapeutic groups. Formularies may or may not contain evaluative statements or comparisons of drugs. Some formularies also include comparative price information, which can help guide prescribing decisions.

A national formulary manual is based on the national list of essential drugs. The *Malawi National Formulary* is an example of such a manual. The *British National Formulary* includes most of the drugs registered for use in the United Kingdom; even though drug selection is not as limited there as it is in developing countries, there are general evaluative statements at the beginning of each section, and the formulary indicates the drugs whose costs are not

Figure 10.3 Number of Drug Products on Selected National Essential Drugs Lists

Country	National Hospital[a]	Provincial Hospital[b]	District Hospital[c]	Health Center[d]
Bangladesh	—	280	150	45
Bhutan	312	251	202	91
Cambodia	190	110	71	—
Ecuador	—	410	370	131
Guinea	341	170	102	69
Kenya	256	255	223	75
Malaysia	1,048	578	578	136
Zimbabwe	592	414	337	83

[a] Tertiary care and specialized units.
[b] General and specialist care.
[c] General medical care.
[d] Paramedical care; in many developing countries, one or more lower levels are distinguished, such as dispensary (25–40 drugs) and community health worker (12–18 drugs).

reimbursed through the National Health Service. The development of a formulary manual is discussed in Chapter 11.

Finally, the term *formulary system* is used in some settings to encompass the whole system for developing, updating, and promoting the formulary (essential drugs) list. A fully developed formulary system usually includes, in addition to the formulary list and formulary manual, regular newsletters or bulletins, guidelines for the use of nonformulary drugs, and methods for evaluating the need for changes in the formulary list or manual. The formulary system in the hospital setting is discussed in Chapter 38.

Treatment Guidelines

Treatment guidelines (standard treatment guidelines, treatment protocols) are systematically developed statements that assist prescribers in deciding on appropriate treatments for specific clinical problems. These guidelines usually reflect the consensus on the optimal treatment options within a health facility or health system. The information is disease centered, emphasizing the common diseases and complaints and the various treatment alternatives. Information on drugs is usually limited to strength, dosage, and duration. Most guidelines indicate a treatment of first choice. Some include diagnostic criteria for starting the treatment or for choosing among treatment alternatives. The development of treatment guidelines is discussed in Chapter 11.

The key difference between a formulary manual and a treatment guideline is that the former is drug centered, concentrating on drug information and usually not providing comparisons among different drugs, whereas the latter is disease centered, listing treatment alternatives and indicating a treatment of choice.

Figure 10.4 The Essential Drugs Target

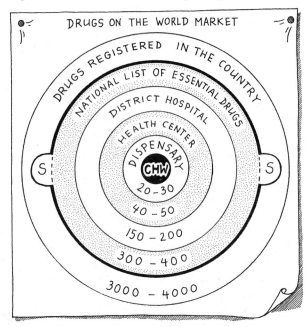

Notes: S = specialist drugs available selectively to special hospitals and departments in the public sector; CHW = community health worker, who typically has an essential drugs list of 12 to 18 items.

≡ **10.6 Approaches to Developing Essential Drugs Lists, Formularies, and Treatment Guidelines**

Essential drugs lists, formularies, and treatment guidelines are interdependent and should be developed in a systematic way. The most logical approach is based on the needs of patients and on the job descriptions of health workers. The first step is to prepare a list of common health problems. A first-choice treatment for each health problem on the list may be limited to one or more drugs or to various forms of nondrug treatment. This choice of treatment can be the basis for two important documents: the *list of essential drugs* for that level of care, which is a direct result of the selection; and a set of *treatment guidelines* for that level of care, which requires additional clinical information (diagnostic signs and symptoms and treatment algorithms).

This approach works best for the primary health care level. The number of diseases and complaints may be too long or too complex to be practical for a hospital, although the approach could be applied at the departmental level.

In practice, some sort of drug list is already available in most settings and can serve as a starting point. This list is critically reviewed by therapeutic group, and as in the WHO *Model List of Essential Drugs*, first-choice drugs and alternative or complementary drugs may be indicated.

The lists of essential drugs for each level of care should

Figure 10.5 Common Health Problems Guide Selection, Training, Supply, and Drug Use

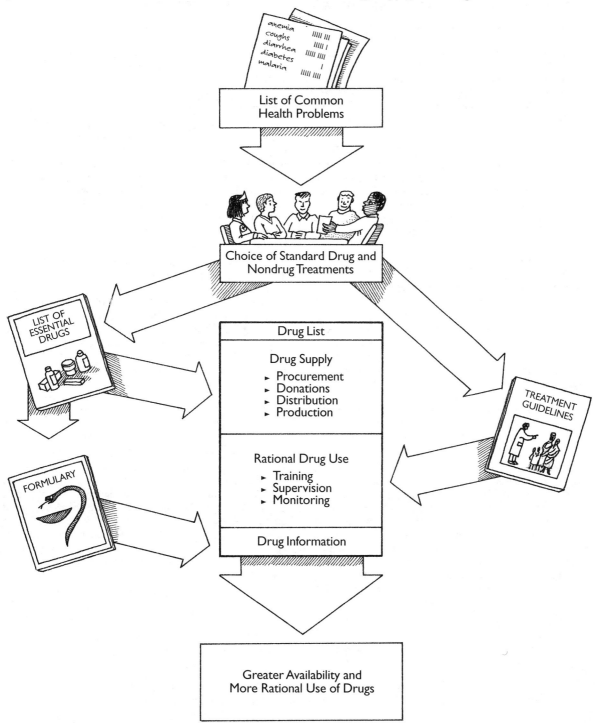

be combined into one *national list of essential drugs* (see Figure 10.5). This list is the basis for developing the *national formulary*. This approach ensures that the supply of drugs, which is based on the national list of essential drugs, is consistent with the treatment guidelines in public-sector facilities and training institutions and that summary drug information is available for all drugs supplied in the public sector.

Using another approach, the *list of registered drugs* can be critically reviewed to select a much shorter *national list of*

Country Study 10.1 Approaches to Updating Essential Drugs and Formulary Lists

Bhutan. A participatory approach was used to update the national essential drugs list (NEDL). A form was developed, and health workers at all levels were invited to propose additions and deletions to the national list. Suggestions were also requested for the level of use for each drug. The proposals were compiled by the essential drugs program coordinator for the National Selection Committee, which made the final decision. The current NEDL consists of 312 drugs and indicates their level of use.

Eastern Caribbean Drug Service (ECDS). The ECDS is a group purchasing service for seven small Caribbean countries. Procurement is limited primarily to the ECDS Regional Core Formulary. Drugs are selected by the ECDS Technical Advisory Subcommittee (TAC), which consists of one member appointed by each participating country (generally the chief medical officer or a comparable ministry appointee) and the central stores managers from each country. The ECDS managing director and assistant managing director are nonvoting members of the TAC. The formulary list is subject to continual review. Changes are based on the evaluation and approval of written requests (see Figure 10.6).

United States Public Health Service (USPHS). Most drugs for the Oklahoma area of the USPHS are procured centrally, based on a formulary list. Each hospital in the area has a pharmacy and therapeutics committee that reviews drug needs and drug utilization for the hospital and its health centers. The formulary list is revised each year. Hospitals submit suggested additions and deletions to the area pharmacist, who compiles the suggestions. In a representative fashion, the chairpersons from each hospital pharmacy and therapeutics committee then meet at area headquarters to review and decide on the proposed revisions.

World Health Organization. Since publication of the first *Model List of Essential Drugs* in 1977, the list has been updated every two to four years, with revisions appearing in 1979, 1983, 1985, 1988, 1990, 1992, and 1995. The list is updated by an expert advisory committee that consists primarily of clinical pharmacologists and physicians. A major change that occurred with the 1985 list was the introduction of complementary drugs, which allowed substitution of therapeutic equivalents. Over the first fifteen years, the number of drugs on the list increased slightly, but most changes involved

replacement of one preparation with a more therapeutically appropriate or cost-effective preparation. For example, amoxicillin replaced ampicillin, and doxycycline replaced tetracycline. Nevertheless, the list contains fewer than 300 active ingredients.

Zimbabwe. The first Essential Drug List for Zimbabwe (EDLIZ) was produced in 1985. The list contained 581 formulations, 224 of which were allowed at the clinic level. As of 1994, the list had been revised three times and included 409 drugs and vaccines in 592 formulations. The number of formulations available at the clinic level had been decreased to 83, with an additional 259 for district hospitals (general practitioners), 77 more for provincial hospitals (with some specialists), and another 154 for specialists' use only. Twenty-four drugs are featured in a supplementary list and can be imported without prior permission from the Ministry of Health for rare life-threatening conditions.

Revisions are carried out by the National Drug and Therapeutics Policy Advisory Committee (NDTPAC), which meets regularly. Its members include a professor from the Department of Pharmacy, University of Zimbabwe (UZ); a general practitioner; the clinical pharmacist, Department of Pharmacy, UZ; a professor from the Department of Medicine, UZ; a professor from the national teaching hospital; the professor of clinical pharmacology, UZ; and the president of the national pharmacy association (private sector). The secretariat for the NDTPAC includes the director of pharmacy services, Ministry of Health and Child Welfare; the registrar, Drugs Control Council; the controller, Government Medical Stores; and the project coordinator, Zimbabwe Essential Drugs Programme.

The revision process is continual and takes about two years. It is actually restarted as soon as a new list is issued. In this way, the merits of all new developments can be discussed and evaluated as soon as they arise. The committee has called on a panel of forty specialists for their views and contributions, and another eighty persons have been asked for comments and opinions. All medical disciplines, as well as pharmacists, buyers, and health economists, are represented, to arrive at the most economical choice with the widest possible coverage for medical conditions prevalent in Zimbabwe.

---

essential drugs. Based on this list, drugs and therapeutics committees in individual health facilities can choose a treatment of first choice for that facility or district. Drug selection at the facility level is especially valuable when the national list of essential drugs is too long for individual facilities. It further ensures maximal involvement, acceptance, and compliance by the prescribers concerned.

For most countries, drug selection by committee is the preferred approach. It minimizes the opportunity for private interests to influence the decision-making process. Furthermore, the judicious selection of committee members with relevant backgrounds and previous experience

can facilitate the rational selection of drugs (see Country Studies 10.1 and 10.2).

The selection of essential drugs for the public sector can be done at the national level by an officially appointed committee or by regional or local officials. An advantage of national-level selection is the potential for improved efficiency and economy of central procurement; regional or local staff should be included in the committee. In large countries, regional selection and procurement may be more appropriate.

The greatest efficiency is possible when drug selection is coordinated with other activities in the supply process.

This can be achieved, in part, by including representatives from the ministry of health, the purchasing department, and regional and local health facilities, including medical and paramedical prescribers. Technical experts should include one or more clinical pharmacologists, an internist, an infectious disease specialist, a pediatrician, a surgeon, one or more hospital and district pharmacists, a hospital director, and other specialists as needed. Representatives of disease control programs (such as malaria, tuberculosis, and AIDS programs) can be co-opted to attend certain meetings. Committee members should serve for several years with staggered terms, so that the committee retains some experienced members each year. Committee members should be known for their integrity, honesty, and dedication; ideally, they should not have relationships with any drug manufacturer or distributor, nor be closely related to any person who does.

The most practical approach to drawing up a list for the first time is to have it prepared by one or two experts, preferably based on the WHO *Model List of Essential Drugs* and using the WHO criteria for selection (see Box 10.1). The full committee can then review the draft and finalize the list. After publication of the first national list, the committee should meet at least every two years to update it. Its decisions should again follow the established criteria. The use of a revision form may facilitate rational additions and deletions (Figure 10.6). It provides a mechanism for prescribers to participate constructively in the selection process, and since the form requires a certain amount of effort on the part of the petitioner, it may reduce requests for items that are not really needed.

The same basic principles apply at the hospital level. The selection of drugs should be made on the basis of the national list of essential drugs, using similar criteria. The list should be made by a hospital drugs and therapeutics committee, ideally convened by a clinical pharmacologist, with senior clinicians and the hospital pharmacist as members. This committee could also advise on prescribing policies and should, from time to time, review the prescribing patterns in the facility through simple prescription surveys (see Chapter 29). Such committees are now mandatory in several countries. In countries where there are limited numbers of qualified staff, the first priority is to establish such committees in the teaching hospitals to serve as models for the rest of the country and for future generations of prescribers.

Lists of essential drugs and treatment guidelines should also be drawn up for the lower levels of health care, such as health centers and dispensaries. Paramedical workers and teaching staff such as nurse tutors should be involved in the process. This is usually done at the national level.

Country Study 10.2 Updating the National Essential Drugs List of Kenya

Kenya was one of the first African countries to recognize the importance of the essential drugs concept and developed its own essential drugs list in 1981, based on the WHO model. In 1992 the Ministry of Health decided to intensify its efforts to rationalize the pharmaceutical sector. These efforts included updating the essential drugs list, rigorously implementing the list as the basis for drug management in the public sector, and developing clinical treatment guidelines.

It was decided early on that the review of the essential drugs list and the development of clinical guidelines should be done in tandem. Draft treatment guidelines for the most common diseases and complaints had been prepared by the Ministry of Health, in consultation with university teachers and specialists in provincial hospitals, and distributed widely for comments. Review of the essential drugs list was begun by comparing the drugs from the 1981 national list with those mentioned in the draft treatment guidelines, alongside the 1992 WHO *Model List of Essential Drugs*.

It was decided to hold two national workshops simultaneously in the same location, one for refining the treatment guidelines and the other for revising the list. This facilitated interaction between the two groups and ensured that the new essential drugs list was in keeping with national clinical practice.

The participants in the drug list workshop were mainly government pharmacists from different departments, joined by a professor of clinical pharmacology and a clinical pharmacist from the University of Nairobi, a senior nursing officer, and the head of the Kenya Essential Drugs Programme. The group based its deliberations on the WHO criteria for the selection of essential drugs (see Box 10.1) and consulted frequently with the clinical guidelines group. Emphasis was placed on drugs required to meet the health care needs of the *majority* of the population.

The two workshops concluded with a final joint session, in which a revised list conforming to WHO criteria was approved. This list included 195 drugs in 256 dosage forms and strengths (fewer than the 1981 version) and was divided into seven levels of care. The process that was followed resulted in a common base of understanding and commitment toward both the essential drugs list and the treatment guidelines.

The revised essential drugs list was printed in a twenty-eight-page booklet, which included background information, selection criteria, and listings by therapeutic category and level of care (see Figure 10.2), as well as an alphabetical listing with store codes and packing units. This booklet has been distributed to all public-sector hospitals, missions, professional associations, and local manufacturers.

The national drug policy adopted in September 1993 stated that the essential drugs list would be used for (1) public education and information; (2) public-sector procurement, prescribing, and dispensing; (3) paramedical and medical graduate education; (4) in-service training programs for health professionals; (5) preferential import duties and value-added taxes on drugs; (6) selective support for the local pharmaceutical industry; (7) pricing policies; and (8) controlling drug donations.

Figure 10.6 Sample Form for Proposing Revisions in Essential Drugs Lists

ADDITION/DELETION/SPECIAL AUTHORIZATION FORM

√ Formulary Addition ___ Deletion
___ Request for Special Authorization

Section A To be completed by doctor	Ciprofloxacin Name(s) of medication (generic and brand) Name of manufacturer Desired dosage: √ Tablet ___ Capsule ___ Injection ___ Other (specify): _____ Estimated usage: √ Routine ___ Emergency ___ Clinical Evaluation Is similar-acting medication stocked now in pharmacy? ___ Yes √ No If yes, please explain advantages of this medication: Ndowa N. Guc-Havave Name of requesting medical/dental officer Clinic/hospital Ndowa January 16, 1998 Signature Date **Forward completed form to attention of:** **Chairman, National Formulary Committee**
Section B To be completed by medical supplies officer	**Central Medical Stores Report** Cost of requested medication: 32-65 (250 mg Tab) Cost of similar-acting item stocked: N/A Remarks (advantages, disadvantages): Ciprofloxacin has been added to the WHO Model List of Essential Drugs (1995, Tech. Rep. Series 850) Gerritt Dawee February 12, 1998 Medical Supplies Officer Date
Section C To be completed by formulary committee	**Formulary Committee Report** Determination: ___ Rejected √ Approved: S (Specialist Use) Level of Use Reasons: LEAST COSTLY ORAL MEDICATION PROVIDING 95% CURE RATE IN THESE SEXUALLY TRANSMITTED INFECTIONS (NB—RESTRICTED TO THESE INDICATIONS ONLY). Vanyaganya. F. March 14, 1998 Formulary Committee (Chairman) Date

---

(Formulary Addition/Deletion & Special Authorization / Page 2)
Pertinent Pharmacological Data on Medication

Therapeutic Action and Indications for Use:

As a third-line treatment of chancroid and/or gonorrhea
Note: (A) First-line drugs are now marginally efficacious. (1)
(B) Prolonged courses of erythromycin (second-line treatment of chancroid-haemophilis ducreyi) do not heal ulcers.

Side Effects, Toxicity, and Precautions:

Side effects:
CNS stimulation; hypersensitivity reactions; interstitial nephritis; photosensitivity; dizziness or lightheadedness; headache; nervousness; insomnia; gastrointestinal disturbances.
Relative contraindications:
Hypersensitivity; renal function impairment.
Caution: There is limited experience of the effect of concurrent HIV infection on adverse effects profiles.
(2)

Dosages (Maximum and Minimum):

500 mg as a single dose in adults.

References:

(1) Ndowa et al., "Efficacy of STD Treatment Regimens in a Genito-Urinary Clinic in Havave." Centr. Afr. J. Med. 3, 1995, pp. 36-40.
(2) USP-DI 1994 and manufacturer's product data sheet.

Source: Organization of Eastern Caribbean States/Eastern Caribbean Drug Service 1994.

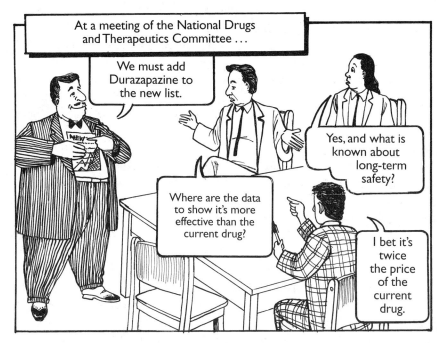

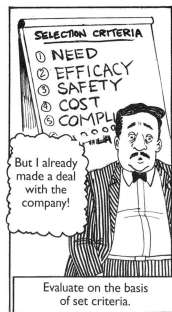

Evaluate on the basis
of set criteria.

≡ 10.7 Therapeutic Classification Systems

Essential drugs lists and national formularies are best organized according to therapeutic category. In addition, analyses of drug requirements, drug consumption, or drug prices are often facilitated by listing drugs according to their therapeutic class. There are countless therapeutic classification systems in use throughout the world. Some, such as the British national formulary system, are organized by target organ or disease condition (for example, eye, infections). Others, such as the American Hospital Formulary Service system, are organized by pharmacologic-therapeutic action. The Nordic ATC system combines *a*natomic, *t*herapeutic, and *c*hemical criteria to classify drugs.

Existing therapeutic classification systems also differ in their complexity; some systems may have five or six levels of subdivision. The level of complexity should be appropriate to the intended use of the system. In general, public drug supply programs should strive for a noncomplex therapeutic classification system that is readily understood by midlevel medical workers and trained supply clerks as well as by pharmacists and physicians.

Increasingly, essential drugs programs are adopting the classification scheme employed in the WHO *Model List of Essential Drugs*. This relatively straightforward system has been adopted by the United Nations Children's Fund (UNICEF) and by most international nonprofit suppliers of essential drugs. Therefore, price comparisons and ordering are easier if this system is adopted by national or local programs.

≡ 10.8 Sources of Information

In most developing countries, the sources of current information available for drug selection decisions are limited. (Chapter 30 discusses sources of drug information and how to assess them.)

Many academicians prefer to base the selection of essential drugs on information from original research articles, which requires compiling articles from journals for comprehensive review. The randomized controlled trial is becoming the "gold standard" both to establish drug efficacy and to determine the comparative efficacy of different drugs for the same clinical problem. Results from such studies are not easily obtainable, unfortunately, so selection decisions must usually be made on the basis of the best available evidence.

Many respected reference texts and periodicals, such as drug bulletins, critically assess and synthesize the best available evidence. Of the many valuable resources that could be consulted, *Martindale: The Extra Pharmacopoeia* is particularly useful, as it contains summaries on over 5,000 drugs and information on the composition of 46,000 medicinal preparations. The American Medical Association *Drug Evaluations Annual* and the *British National Formulary* contain comparative evaluations of individual drugs or of therapeutic groups. Independent drug bulletins, such as the *Medical Letter on Drugs and Therapeutics* and the *Drug and Therapeutics Bulletin*, regularly prepare comparative reviews of drugs and therapeutics.

The WHO *Model List of Essential Drugs* is a useful reference, derived from the consensus of recognized international experts and updated every two to four years. The drugs that appear on this list are widely acknowledged to be safe, efficacious, cost effective, and of acceptable quality. Consulting essential drugs lists from other countries may also be useful. WHO provides a listing of other essential drugs lists, formularies, and treatment guidelines that may be useful for drug selection (WHO/DAP 1994).

Sufficient information on efficacy, safety, and dosages, particularly for risk groups such as children, pregnant women, and the elderly, is often difficult to obtain for newly released drugs. Since the relative merits of newly marketed drugs are not known until experience with the drug has accumulated or appropriate comparative trials with other drugs are undertaken, it is advisable to delay the inclusion of such new drugs until sufficient information is available from reliable independent sources.

≡ 10.9 Implementing and Updating Essential Drugs Lists

The development and use of lists of essential drugs have enormous implications for drug procurement, local production, supply, training, prescribing, and supervision. However, many essential drugs lists, treatment guidelines, and formulary manuals have been developed, printed, and forgotten. There are many reason for such failures.

Reasons for Failure

Probably the most common reason for failure is not involving as wide a group of national experts and politicians as possible. Lists and guidelines that have been developed by individuals, departments, or institutions operating in isolation, or that are not updated regularly, are bound to fail. They lack credibility, and other interested parties will not accept the result. Another common mistake is a lack of both a purpose and a drug policy framework. Such weaknesses provide an opportunity for pressure groups to defeat the endeavor. Also, if the whole selection process lacks openness, or if no procedure for suggestions and additions exists, the result is likely to fail. Lastly, failure can result if the selection is perceived as unrealistic (for example, when sophisticated drugs are listed for lower health care levels when resources are scarce).

Gaining Acceptance of Essential Drugs Lists

The development and use of a national list of essential drugs are cornerstones of a national drug policy. The formulation and acceptance of such a policy are, in most cases, based on the concept of essential drugs and lead to the development of a list. An essential drugs list can be developed without a drug policy, but agreement on the purpose and use of the list is imperative.

In developing a national list of essential drugs, it is important to obtain the support of professional organizations, such as the national medical and pharmaceutical associations. They should be consulted from the start and should be informed about the reasons for developing a list and the selection criteria. The same applies to senior clinicians and teachers from medical and pharmacy schools, who are often leading national figures involved in the process of drug registration. Arguments in favor of the essential drugs concept and the advantages of a limited list of drugs (see Figure 10.1) should be discussed with these individuals. The acceptance of the list by senior specialists and other health care workers can be further enhanced by their involvement in the development of the list, treatment guidelines, and formulary manual (see Chapter 11) and by generous acknowledgment of their contributions (see the example of Zimbabwe in Country Study 11.1). The obvious advantages of a consistent set of training and information materials and a corresponding system of drug supply offset most professional resistance.

When the list is completed and printed, it is important to give it national prominence and credibility through a launching campaign. This should involve the highest possible government officials, such as the minister of health or the president, and intensive press coverage. A national conference can emphasize topics such as the advantages of the list, the national consensus in defining the health needs of the population at large, and the cost-effective use of limited resources.

Authority of Essential Drugs Lists

It is important to specify the purpose of the list at an early stage. Will procurement and distribution of drugs in the public sector be limited to the list? Is a change in legislation or regulation needed for this, or a decree? Will exceptions be allowed? If so, on what grounds and by which authority?

There will also be pressure to provide drugs not on the essential drugs list. Exceptions to the official list must be controlled through *administrative* or *budgetary* methods. Health services often require a written request for special authorization of nonlisted drugs (for example, the form in Figure 10.6) and have procedures for evaluating and approving such requests. There may also be a budgetary maximum for such exceptions—a maximum of 5 to 10 percent of the drug budget, for example. Such a budget for nonlisted drugs is usually effective in ensuring acceptance of the list by district authorities and clinical specialists;

≡ Assessment Guide

Management Structure of the National
Essential Drugs List (NEDL)
- ► Has an NEDL been officially adopted and distributed countrywide?
- ► Is there an official drug committee whose duties include updating the NEDL?
- ► Has the NEDL been updated and distributed countrywide in the past five years?
- ► Is there a national drug policy statement to promote and define the use of the NEDL?

Outcome of the Selection Process
- ► What are the total number of drugs on the NEDL list (in dosage forms and strengths) and the number of drugs per level of health care?

Use of the NEDL (Public Sector)
- ► Is procurement in the public sector limited to drugs on the NEDL?
- ► What is the value of drugs from the NEDL out of the total value of drugs procured?

- ► What percentage of health facilities has a copy of the NEDL available?
- ► What is the number of drugs from the NEDL out of the total number of drugs prescribed?
- ► Do drug donations comply with the NEDL?
- ► Is the concept of essential drugs part of the curriculum in the basic training of health personnel?

Use of the NEDL (Private Sector)
- ► Is the NEDL used to promote national pharmaceutical production?
- ► Is there at least one major incentive for selling essential drugs at low cost?
- ► Are essential drugs sold under INNs in private drug outlets?
- ► Out of the fifty best-selling drugs in the private sector, how many are on the NEDL?

without such a safety valve, many lists are perceived as too rigid and are likely to be undermined. In addition, if certain nonformulary drugs are commonly ordered, they can be considered for inclusion when the list is revised.

Finally, an open and transparent system of regular updates is an absolute prerequisite to maintain the authority and acceptance of an essential drugs or formulary list. ∎

≡ Glossary

Bioavailability: The rate and extent of availability of an active ingredient from a dosage form as measured by the concentration/time curve in the systemic circulation or its excretion in the urine.

Branded generics: Generic pharmaceutical products marketed under brand names.

Drug: Any substance in a pharmaceutical product that is used to modify or explore physiological systems or pathological states for the benefit of the recipient.

Drug product: A unique combination of drug(s), strength, and dosage form (for example, ampicillin 500 mg capsule).

Efficacy: The ability of a drug to produce the purported effect, as determined by scientific methods.

Formulary list: A list of drugs approved for use in a specific health care setting.

Formulary manual: A manual containing clinically oriented summary pharmacological information about a selected number of drugs. The manual may also include administrative and regulatory information pertaining to drug prescribing and dispensing.

Formulary system: The principles, criteria, procedures, and resources for developing, updating, and promoting the formulary (essential drugs) list.

Generic name: The approved or nonproprietary name of a drug. It is generally the international nonproprietary name given by WHO.

Generic pharmaceutical products: Products marketed by any producer under nonproprietary or approved names.

Multisource pharmaceutical products: Pharmaceutically equivalent products, available from different manufacturers, that may or may not be therapeutically equivalent.

Pharmaceutical equivalents: Products that contain the same amount of the same active substance(s) in the same dosage form, meet the same or comparable standards, and are intended to be administered by the same route.

Pharmaceutical product: A dosage form containing one or more drugs along with other substances included during the manufacturing process.

Therapeutic equivalents: Pharmaceutically equivalent products whose effects with respect to both safety and efficacy are essentially the same, when administered in the same molar dose, as can be derived from appropriate studies (bioequivalence, pharmacodynamic, clinical, or in vitro studies).

≡ References and Further Readings

★ = *Key readings.*

MSH (Management Sciences for Health). 1992. Selection and formulary management (trainer's and participant's guides). In *Managing drug supply training series.* Part 1: *Policy issues in managing drug supply.* Boston: MSH.

OECS/ECDS (Organization of Eastern Caribbean States/Eastern Caribbean Drug Service). 1994. *Regional drug formulary and therapeutics manual.* 4th ed. Castries, St. Lucia: OECS/ECDS.

WHO (World Health Organization). 1990. *Expert committee on specifications for pharmaceutical preparations.* 31st report. Technical report series no. 790. Geneva: WHO.

★ WHO (World Health Organization). 1995. *The use of essential drugs.* Technical report series no. 850. Geneva: WHO.
   Contains the WHO *Model List of Essential Drugs,* which is reviewed every two years, as well as background information on the essential drugs concept and criteria for the selection of drugs.

WHO/DAP (World Health Organization/Action Programme on Essential Drugs). 1994. *National, regional, and international essential drugs lists, formularies, and treatment guides.* WHO/DAP/94.2. Geneva: WHO/DAP.
   A regularly updated list of published essential drugs lists, formularies, and treatment guidelines.

WHO/PAHO (World Health Organization/Pan American Health Organization). 1984. *Development and implementation of drug formularies.* Scientific publication no. 474. Washington, D.C.: WHO/PAHO.

| Part I | Part II | Part III | Part IV |
| Introduction | Policy and Legal Framework | **Drug Management Cycle** | Management Support Systems |

A Selection ▶	10 Managing Drug Selection
B Procurement	**11 Treatment Guidelines and Formulary Manuals**
C Distribution	
D Use	12 Essential Medical Supplies and Equipment

Chapter 11
Treatment Guidelines and Formulary Manuals

≡ Summary

Treatment guidelines are disease oriented and reflect a consensus on the treatments of first choice for a range of medical conditions. A formulary manual is drug oriented and contains summary drug information on a selected number of drugs, sometimes combined with practical prescribing and dispensing information. They can both be developed for different levels of health care.

The development process of these publications (the formulary process) is a continual effort, not limited to the one-time production of a set of treatment guidelines or a formulary manual. The process includes gaining acceptance of the concept, preparing a text on the basis of wide consultation and consensus building, implementing an introductory campaign and training activities, and undertaking regular reviews and updates.

Treatment guidelines can be made for one institution, such as a hospital; for one level of care, such as all health centers; or for a region or nation. Treatment guidelines are a powerful tool to promote rational prescribing, provided they are based on extensive involvement of the end-users. Their development is a good opportunity to integrate the technical advice of different disease programs into an overall training program. Treatment guidelines should be used as the basis for undergraduate medical and paramedical training, for in-service training, for supervision, and for medical audit. The range of drugs included should be limited to drugs on the national list of essential drugs.

A national formulary should be developed by a formulary subcommittee within the national drug committee. Both committees should ensure the full participation of prominent specialists and health opinion leaders in the process. One or two editors should be commissioned to draft and edit the formulary. A hospital formulary can be drawn up through a similar procedure.

To maintain the credibility of the information, a system for regular updates and for incorporation of accepted amendments into the next edition is essential for both formularies and treatment guidelines.

This chapter builds on concepts introduced in Chapter 10, which should be read first.

≡ 11.1 Need for Local Reference Manuals

Once a national essential drugs list has been agreed upon and adopted, the next step is the development of standard treatment guidelines and a formulary manual.

The procedures to develop an essential drugs list, a set of treatment guidelines, or a formulary manual are similar; together they could be called the formulary process. General information on the selection of drugs and the development and maintenance of a list of essential drugs is given in Chapter 10. In this chapter, the specific aspects of the formulary process are outlined in relation to developing treatment guidelines or a formulary manual.

Treatment Guidelines

The terms *standard treatment guidelines, treatment protocols,* and *prescribing policies* are all used to indicate systematically developed statements to help practitioners or prescribers make decisions about appropriate treatments for specific clinical conditions. Treatment guidelines exist for different levels of health care, ranging from general prescribing guidelines for paramedical workers in rural areas to detailed protocols for tertiary health care centers in wealthy urban areas.

Standard guidelines benefit health officials, supply management staff, health care providers, and patients (Figure 11.1). Together with a national list of essential drugs, treatment guidelines are powerful tools to promote the rational use of drugs. They offer an opportunity to ensure that the training of health workers is based on a logical approach to treatment and on a consensus about the selection of essential drugs. The technical advice of different vertical disease-oriented programs (malaria, diarrheal diseases, schistosomiasis, tuberculosis, sexually transmitted diseases [STDs], AIDS, and many others) can be integrated into one set of national treatment guidelines. These comprehensive guidelines are a logical starting point for integrated training and an excellent basis for drug supply in the public sector. Treatment guidelines should be used for in-service training, supervision, and medical audit. They can also assist in the standardization (and rationalization) of prescribing patterns in countries with large numbers of foreign-trained medical graduates.

In developing standard treatment guidelines, the starting point is a list of common diseases and complaints. On the basis of this list of health problems, a treatment of choice is defined for each diagnosis or problem. The treatment guideline should include only drugs on the national list of essential drugs. In fact, the treatment choice should underlie the list of essential drugs (see Chapter 10). This ensures that the supply system, based

Figure 11.1 Potential Benefits of Standard Treatment Guidelines

For Health Officials
- Identification of cost-effective treatments for common health problems;
- Basis to assess and compare quality of care;
- Vehicle for integrating special programs (control of diarrheal disease, acute respiratory infection, tuberculosis, malaria, and so on) at the point of the primary health care provider.

For Supply Management Staff
- Identification of which drugs should be available for the most commonly treated problems;
- Facilitation of prepackaging of course-of-therapy quantities of commonly prescribed items;
- Drug demand more predictable, so forecasting more reliable.

For Health Care Providers
- Expert consensus on most effective, economical treatment for a specific setting;
- Opportunity for providers to concentrate on correct diagnosis;
- Quality-of-care standard;
- Basis for monitoring and supervision.

For Patients
- Encouragement of adherence to treatment through consistency among prescribers;
- Most cost-effective treatments are provided;
- Improvement in availability of drugs;
- Better treatment.

on the list of essential drugs, supports the treatment guidelines.

Unlike the drug information in a national formulary manual, which tends to be noncontroversial, treatment guidelines may generate considerable differences of opinion among prescribers. Reaching consensus is much more difficult, and the developmental process takes much more time. Wide consultation is a key condition for acceptance and impact.

Formulary Manual

A formulary manual contains summary drug information on a selected number of drugs. It is drug centered, and the information is usually organized in therapeutic groups. In most developing countries, the national formulary is limited to drugs on the national list of essential drugs. A *therapeutic formulary* includes detailed and comprehensive therapeutic information on each of the drugs listed and may also include guidelines on rational prescribing and dispensing. The distinction between a formulary and treatment guidelines then becomes less clear, as is the case with the *British National Formulary* (BNF).

Although there are several reference texts available that include comprehensive drug information, these may not be appropriate for all settings. A national formulary

concentrates on drugs relevant to a particular country. For example, it would exclude information on drugs that are not available in the country, or that are overly expensive. It would also put less emphasis on uncommon, irrelevant, or minor side effects. But it should include information that may be missing in other texts on nationally important drugs, such as those used for tropical conditions or for locally common diseases that may be rare in other countries. It would also include information on specific treatment considerations (for example, G6PD deficiency, sickle cell anemia, HIV infection). Recommended dosage schedules can be adapted to national requirements, special storage guidelines may be added, and specific national problems (overuse of injections, polypharmacy) can be addressed.

≡ 11.2 Treatment Guidelines

The process of developing treatment guidelines is similar to that of developing an essential drugs list or formulary manual (see Country Study 11.1), and only those aspects specific to treatment guidelines are discussed here.

Establishment of an Editorial Committee

For national treatment guidelines, the editorial committee can be a subcommittee of the national drugs and therapeutics committee and is likely to be different from the national formulary committee. The committee should include one or two senior editors who have final responsibility for the guidelines, one or two interested clinical specialists, and several end-users (general practitioners, medical assistants, nurses). It is not necessary to have all medical specialties represented on the committee, as they can be co-opted to prepare or review the relevant chapters.

Before starting the work, and especially before inviting other experts to write chapters or sections, the editorial committee has to make several important decisions on target groups, choice of authors, and editing and reviewing of the manuscript.

Targeting Different Levels. The length and format of the publication depend on the target group and the level of detail. A key question is: should all information for all levels of health workers be presented in one publication, or should different publications be issued for different levels of care? One publication for all levels can serve as a complete reference for all recommended treatments. It also allows practitioners at the lower levels to read about treatments that are recommended at the higher levels, which may be an advantage in emergency cases and is, at the least, educational. In addition, the production process is easier, and the publishing costs are reduced.

Country Study 11.1 Production and Use of Treatment Guidelines

Australia. Started as a hospital-based initiative, the *Antibiotic Guidelines* were first issued in Victoria in the late 1970s. They were used as a teaching document for medical students and interns and, more importantly, as an audit standard against which prescribing patterns in the wards could be compared. More and more hospitals became involved, and subsequent editions of the booklet were increasingly used in other regions of the country. New editions were introduced with marketing campaigns that were very professional and inventive, using posters, advertisements, drug use studies, and face-to-face education. These campaigns, together with the widening range of professionals involved in subsequent editions, greatly improved the acceptance of the guidelines.

Since 1992, the regular production, promotion, and evaluation of a comprehensive set of therapeutic guidelines are recognized by the government as essential components of the Australian national drug policy. The series, which is produced by the Victorian Medical Postgraduate Foundation Therapeutic Committee, now includes guidelines on analgesic, antibiotic, cardiovascular, gastrointestinal, psychotropic, and respiratory drugs. The authorship of the various booklets has progressively widened to better represent general practice needs and to involve all states and territories of Australia. A network of general practitioners has been recruited to provide feedback. Each booklet is updated every two years.

Nicaragua. A series of therapeutic guidelines existed in Nicaragua, and although they were technically sound, their presentation was unattractive and the language was more appropriate for doctors than for paramedical workers. In addition, the material was contained in several booklets, and many health facilities did not have a complete set.

Development of the new guidelines for rural health workers included a three-day workshop attended by health workers who were stationed alone in ten "sentinel" health posts, with nurses, physicians, and pharmacists from the surrounding areas. The group identified the most common diseases treated in the health posts and drew up a corresponding list of essential drugs. The resulting draft booklet was widely field-tested. It was then decided to revise and expand the handbook to the national level with a bottom-up approach, again calling on the experience of end-users. The draft was also reviewed by a multidisciplinary group of specialists at the regional, provincial, and university levels. The product was an extensive, illustrated,

440-page learning and action guide for local health workers, *Buscando remedio* (Seeking a Remedy), published by the Autonomous University of Nicaragua and Medicus Mundi, France.

Sudan. In Sudan, the national treatment guidelines were written by one national expert (physician) and one expatriate pharmacist. There were several rounds of consultation with local experts. The general approach was to give relevant prescribing information on all drugs on the national list of essential drugs. The manual, consisting of about 300 pages, was first printed by the national essential drugs program. Later it was officially issued by the national medical association as the *Sudan National Formulary* and given to each medical student and doctor. A separate, shorter version was later prepared for paramedical workers. This covered only the diseases and essential drugs relevant to that level; it was issued in Arabic. Both guidelines are now widely used in basic and in-service training.

Zimbabwe. In Zimbabwe, a set of treatment guidelines ("modules") was developed for paramedical workers. Each module was written by an author who was close to the target audience, such as a paramedical tutor. Each draft module was reviewed by a group of about ten health workers, which included one medical doctor and several tutors. The majority were representatives of the target audience (nurses, medical assistants).

During the first three days of a five-day workshop, the draft was discussed in detail, and the text was revised on a portable computer and printed. On the fourth day, the participants all went into the field to use the new draft in a real-life training session. On the fifth day, their field experiences were used to adapt the draft. The final draft text, with illustrations and layout of each module, was prepared by the two series editors using simple desktop publishing software.

This draft was then sent out for comments to 300 opinion leaders and reviewers and revised again. The names of the primary author, primary reviewers, and series editors were printed on the cover of each module. Since each of the fifteen modules was written and reviewed by different groups of ten to twenty health workers, several hundred people were involved in the process. This is one of the reasons that the series was so well accepted and has been in use for many years.

In contrast, separate guidelines for different levels of health care can recommend treatments focused on drugs supplied to that level, so that no unavailable drugs are recommended. The language, illustrations, and presentation can be adapted to the end-users (paramedical prescribers, for example). Training is easier, and the manual is smaller and easier to use, making translation more feasible.

Several developing countries with large proportions of paramedical prescribers have produced separate national treatment guidelines for general practitioners and for paramedical prescribers (such as clinical officers, medical assistants, and nurses). The former are pocket-size books with

treatment guidelines in a condensed format; the latter use simpler language, are extensively illustrated, and recommend only drugs that are available at rural health facilities. One set of guidelines is usually sufficient in countries where primary health care is delivered mainly by physicians.

Choice of Authors. The choice of authors is another important decision. The most practical approach is to invite a number of authors to draft first texts of separate chapters. The authors should be recruited from the level of prescribers for which the guidelines are intended. For example, it may not be practical to invite a university specialist to write treatment guidelines for dispensing nurses;

Figure 11.2 Sample Annotated Page from Malawi Standard Treatment Guidelines (MSTG)

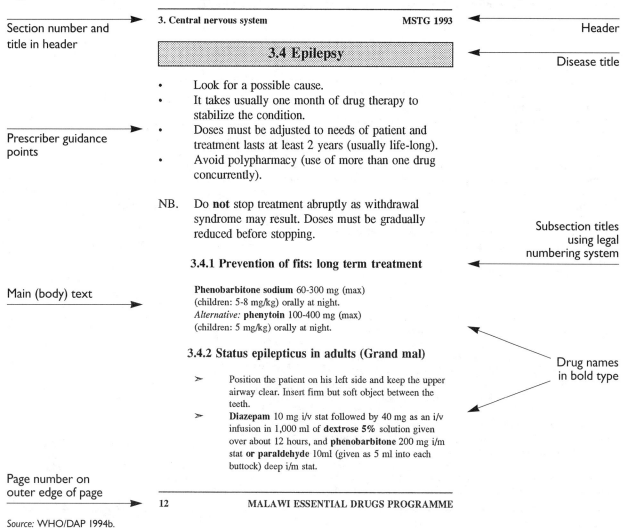

Section number and title in header

3. Central nervous system   MSTG 1993

Header

3.4 Epilepsy

Disease title

- Look for a possible cause.
- It takes usually one month of drug therapy to stabilize the condition.

Prescriber guidance points

- Doses must be adjusted to needs of patient and treatment lasts at least 2 years (usually life-long).
- Avoid polypharmacy (use of more than one drug concurrently).

NB. Do **not** stop treatment abruptly as withdrawal syndrome may result. Doses must be gradually reduced before stopping.

Subsection titles using legal numbering system

3.4.1 Prevention of fits: long term treatment

Main (body) text

Phenobarbitone sodium 60-300 mg (max)
(children: 5-8 mg/kg) orally at night.
Alternative: **phenytoin** 100-400 mg (max)
(children: 5 mg/kg) orally at night.

3.4.2 Status epilepticus in adults (Grand mal)

➤ Position the patient on his left side and keep the upper airway clear. Insert firm but soft object between the teeth.

➤ **Diazepam** 10 mg i/v stat followed by 40 mg as an i/v infusion in 1,000 ml of **dextrose 5%** solution given over about 12 hours, and **phenobarbitone** 200 mg i/m stat **or paraldehyde** 10ml (given as 5 ml into each buttock) deep i/m stat.

Drug names in bold type

Page number on outer edge of page

12   MALAWI ESSENTIAL DRUGS PROGRAMME

Source: WHO/DAP 1994b.

a nurse-tutor would be better equipped for that task, although the author can consult relevant specialists and have them review the draft. Several production issues—for example, the specifications for text and presentation (see Section 11.4)—should be addressed early in the process (Figure 11.2).

Reviewing and Editing the Draft. The editors of the guidelines should unify the draft chapters into one consistent document before sending the draft text out for review by a large number of experts. As mentioned above, it is usually more difficult to reach consensus on a treatment of first choice than on the factual drug information that is included in a national formulary. In addition, there is bound to be more opposition after the guidelines have been published. Several rounds of consultation, involving an increasing number of experts and professional associations, can do a great deal to resolve objections.

Information in Treatment Guidelines

Treatment guidelines are disease oriented (in contrast to formularies, which are drug oriented). This means that the treatment of choice is presented for each common health problem, together with basic information needed by the prescriber. Any appropriate nondrug treatments should always be included. Alternative treatments may be listed, with an indication of when they should be used. Comparisons of the costs of different treatments may also be included in the analysis, with the "best" treatment dependent on circumstances (such as drug resistance) or selection criteria (Box 11.1).

Treatment guidelines necessarily repeat some information that is also presented in the national formulary. It is not necessary, however, to include all drug information—only that which is needed to make rational treatment decisions.

Box 11.1 Cost-Effectiveness Analysis for Choosing Standard Treatments

Even when funds are limited, the *cheapest* treatment for a specific health problem may not be the *best* treatment. A cost-effectiveness analysis (CEA, see Chapter 3) may help organize cost and effectiveness information to guide decisions about first- and second-line treatments. This is particularly true when higher-cost treatments are also more effective, such as for certain antibacterial, antitubercular, or antimalarial drugs for which drug resistance is high. A CEA can also be useful to establish standard guidelines for chronic diseases such as hypertension and for antibiotic prophylaxis for surgery.

The accompanying table provides an example of a CEA that compares standard and short-course chemotherapy for tuberculosis. In this study, standard therapy consisted of twelve months of treatment involving isoniazid, streptomycin, and thiacetazone. Short-course therapy lasted only six months and also involved more costly rifampicin and pyrazinamide. Both approaches involved hospitalization during initial treatment. Costs included not only drugs but also all program costs, including health staff, program administration, laboratory reagents, hospitalization costs, and vehicle costs.

Short-course chemotherapy was clearly more effective: 85 percent cure rate versus 60 percent for standard chemotherapy, and one-third as many cases requiring retreatment. Unfortunately, short-course chemotherapy was also three times as expensive per case treated as standard chemotherapy: US$155 versus $54. When the average cost per *case cured* is considered, however, short-term chemotherapy is actually cheaper: $232 per case cured versus $301 for standard chemotherapy. In this example, cost effectiveness can also be expressed in terms of cost per death averted (considering deaths of the immediate patient and deaths avoided because of reduced transmission) or cost per year of life saved (considering remaining life expectancy of those whose lives were saved). By each cost-effectiveness measure, the additional cost of short-term chemotherapy is more than offset by its higher initial cure rate and lower retreatment rate. Thus, although short-course chemotherapy is much more costly per treatment, it is actually a better choice than standard chemotherapy in both human terms (more lives saved) and economic terms (more cost effective).

A CEA may be carried out using only information on cure rates and drug costs. However, a truer picture usually emerges if broader measures of effectiveness are used (morbidity, including disability, as well as mortality) and if all costs are included. For example, in an area of moderate resistance, a more effective second-line antimalarial may not be more cost effective when only drug costs are considered, but it may prove more cost effective when additional costs are considered, such as hospitalization of patients who fail to respond to first-line treatment.

Cost Effectiveness of Different Treatments

	Standard Chemo-therapy	Short-Course Chemo-therapy	Short-Course as Percentage of Standard Chemotherapy
Effectiveness:			
Cure rate (percent)	60	85	142%
Cases requiring retreatment (number)	30	10	33%
Average cost (US$) per:			
Case treated	54	155	287%
Case cured	301	232	77%
Death averted	76	57	75%
Year of life saved	3.4	2.6	76%

Source: Murray et al. 1993.

Diagnostic Criteria. Diagnostic criteria are especially important when a disease may present in different stages of severity (for example, dehydration). They need to indicate when treatment is needed and when it is not, such as in the treatment of fever or cough. Required investigations may be included.

Treatment of First Choice. The section on the first-choice treatment (drug or nondrug) contains the most information for the prescriber. It should include the choice of drug, its usual dosage schedule, and, when needed, adapted dosage schedules for children, for patients with concurrent liver or renal diseases, for pregnant patients, for the elderly, and for other high-risk groups.

Cost of Treatment. Information on the cost of treatment is useful if alternatives are proposed. However, it means that the guidelines have to be updated regularly. The information can also be presented as price ranges, such as "cheap," "moderate," and "expensive," or as price ranges identified as "A," "B," and "C." These categories are unlikely to change substantially.

Important Contraindications and Side Effects. The section on contraindications and side effects should list both relative and absolute contraindications; groups at special risk (the elderly, patients who are pregnant, breastfeeding, or have liver or renal disease) must be highlighted. Side effects should be broken down into reactions that are self-limiting and those that may require a change in therapy.

Important Drug Information, Warnings, and Precautions. This highlights the information that the patient should be given by both the prescriber and the dispenser.

Referral Criteria. These criteria describe when to refer the patient to a higher level of care. For example, *if the patient's condition does not improve within four hours, refer the patient to a hospital.*

Index. Although treatment guidelines are usually disease centered, many prescribers also use them to check on specific drugs or dosage schedules. For this reason, an index with both drug names and health problems makes the manual more useful.

Use of Treatment Guidelines

Treatment guidelines should be used for basic training of health workers, in-service training, supervision, reference, and medical audit. They are potentially valuable in promoting the rational use of drugs, as many prescribers recognize them as useful references. Because they are related to the list of essential drugs, they should also serve as the basis for the supply of essential drugs.

It was originally hoped that the availability of guidelines would change irrational prescribing patterns. However, it has become apparent that sending treatment guidelines to all prescribers is not enough to bring about an improvement in prescribing practices. To be effective, they must be properly introduced to the prescribers, and their use should be monitored.

All relevant health workers should have their own copies of the guidelines, and training courses should be organized to introduce the guidelines and teach health workers how to use them. In Zimbabwe a separate (short) training module was prepared and used to teach health workers how to use the new edition of the national treatment guidelines. This module included some of the new tables and one or two exercises on how to use the index of the new edition.

Treatment guidelines for paramedical prescribers are usually well received and are common in developing countries; this is also true of national treatment guidelines for general doctors. National guidelines for tertiary care are rare, but general care guidelines are often used in tertiary institutions. In Zimbabwe, treatment guidelines for oncology have been developed. In developed countries, treatment protocols are usually drawn up for specific diseases (hypertension, diabetes, certain types of cancer) or for single hospital departments (prescribing policies in the pediatric department of a teaching hospital, for example).

Treatment guidelines have the strongest long-term impact if they are frequently updated, widely distributed, integrated in the basic curriculum of medical and paramedical teaching institutions, and used for audit (see Country Study 11.2). This is especially true when the turnover and transfer of field staff is so frequent that the effect of in-service training is quickly diluted.

≡ 11.3 Formulary Manuals

As noted in Chapter 10, the term *formulary* can be applied to a simple formulary list, the formulary manual (the

---

Country Study 11.2 Two Decades of Standard Treatment Manuals in Papua New Guinea

In November 1973, a national workshop of senior medical specialists, senior nurses, and senior administrators passed a resolution calling for each of the four major disciplines (adult medicine, pediatrics, surgery, and obstetrics-gynecology) to prepare within twelve months a handbook of standard treatments for no more than fifteen of the most common conditions in each discipline. The first to be produced was the pediatrics manual, which came off the press in December 1974. Adult medicine and obstetrics-gynecology pocket manuals have since been produced. The pediatrics manual has been revised at least three times. Health workers in both the government and the private sector have been provided with copies of the manuals. The manuals have been used by medical and nursing students. Most importantly, drug supply has been matched to the recommended treatment.

Key features of the standard treatment manuals, as they have been implemented in Papua New Guinea, include

simplicity: The number of health problems is limited in each of the main manuals. For each health problem, a few key clinical diagnostic criteria are listed. Finally, drug and dosage information is clear and concise.

credibility: The treatments were initially developed by the most respected clinicians in the country. Revisions based on actual experience have added to the credibility of the manuals.

use of the same standards for all levels: Doctors and other health care providers use the same standard treatments. The referral criteria differ, but the first-choice treatment for a patient depends on the patient's diagnosis and condition—not on the prescriber.

provision of standards for drug supply: The standard treatments are coordinated with the supply of drugs. If changed circumstances require a new drug for the standard treatment, the supply system responds.

introduction in preservice training: Standard treatment manuals are distributed during preservice training, and their use becomes habitual.

regular updating: As bacterial resistance patterns change or other factors alter therapeutic preferences, the standards are revised to reflect current recommendations.

durability and convenience: The standard treatments are published as small, durable pocket manuals, which are convenient to carry and use.

An assessment found that the treatment manuals were widely available and widely used. Analysis of prescription records has shown considerable adherence to the standard treatments.

Source: WHO/DAP 1987 and contributors.

---

subject of this discussion), or a fully developed formulary system. A formulary system develops from the essential drugs or formulary list and the formulary manual. It includes drug information and other services that support good drug management and the rational use of drugs. As with treatment guidelines, the production of a formulary manual is one step in an ongoing process.

Figure 11.3 Information in a Formulary Manual

Introductory Information

► Acknowledgments (individuals and agencies who contributed, explanation of how drug information is presented in manual);
► List of abbreviations;
► Introduction (development of manual, intended uses).

Basic Information for Each Drug

► Generic name;
► Dosage form(s) and strength(s);
► Main indications (diseases and conditions for which a drug is given);
► Pharmacology (may include pharmacokinetic data);
► Contraindications (reasons not to give the drug);
► Precautions (such as pregnancy, breastfeeding, certain health conditions);
► Side effects (major and minor, with estimated frequency);
► Dosage schedule (dosage form, frequency, duration, pediatric dosage, dosage adjustments for the elderly and for renal or liver disease);
► Instructions and warnings;
► Drug interactions (most common or severe).

Supplementary Information on Each Drug

► Price;
► Level-of-use code;
► Regulatory category (prescription only, over-the-counter, controlled narcotic drugs);
► Storage guidelines;
► Patient counseling information;
► Labeling information;
► Brand names and synonyms;
► National essential drugs list reference number;
► Stores catalog number.

Prescribing and Dispensing Guidelines

► Rational prescribing;
► Principles of prescription writing;
► Use of placebos;
► Special requirements for inpatient prescriptions;
► Guidelines on quantities to be supplied;
► Special requirements for controlled drug prescriptions;
► Prevention and reporting of adverse drug reactions;
► Dispensing guidelines (correct dispensing practices, patient counseling);
► List of cautionary and advisory labels;
► Table of drug interactions (highlighting most common and most severe).

General Drug Use Advice (Optional)

► Use of intravenous (IV) additives (general guidance, table with recommended quantities);
► Prescribing in special situations (pregnancy, breastfeeding, renal or liver disease, the elderly, children, terminal care);
► Poisoning (general information, antidotes for common poisons, telephone for poison center if one exists);
► Treatment of snakebites, insect stings.

Other Components

► Metric units;
► Adverse drug reaction reporting form;
► Formulary revision form;
► Indexes (by generic name, brand name, therapeutic category).

Information in a Formulary Manual

The information is usually presented in the form of drug information sheets or drug monographs. Such sheets can also be used as the basis for developing drug package inserts for locally manufactured drugs for prescribers or patients.

In most developing countries, the drugs included in the national formulary are limited to those on the national list of essential drugs. However, a formulary manual may also include some information on commonly used drugs whose use is *not* recommended, stating exactly why these drugs are not recommended and discouraging their use.

Figure 11.3 outlines information that may be included in a formulary manual. Acknowledgments should list all persons or agencies that contributed to the formulary; this enhances its authority and credibility. The introduction should briefly describe the development process and the manual's intended use.

Basic information for each drug should be easy to read and complete but concise. The format and wording should be carefully chosen so that the information can be easily understood.

If cost information is included, the formulary must be updated regularly. Price information can be presented as treatment cost per day or as cost per course of treatment. This information can be presented in tables or bar charts. Information that prescribers or dispensers should give to patients to ensure that the drug is used correctly should be specific. Cautionary and advisory labels can be mentioned as a letter code (for example, A: do not use alcohol).

A section on prescribing and dispensing guidelines helps promote rational drug use. General points to consider before writing a prescription include the use of generic names, the importance of nondrug treatment and simple advice, suggestions for dealing with patients' demands for injections and other expensive dosage forms, and the limited usefulness of combination drugs. Principles of prescription writing include writing legibly in ink, stating the weight or age of children, writing the full generic name of the drug, not using unofficial abbreviations, and always stating the full dose regimen.

Dispensing guidelines may include correct dispensing practices and types of patient counseling information to be given (see Chapters 32 and 33). A list of cautionary and advisory labels can be included. Each of these can be numbered and cross-referenced in the drug sheets.

A comprehensive index of all drug groups and drug names (including brand names in italics, where appropriate) should be given at the end of the publication. A good index greatly enhances the usefulness of the formulary and the accessibility of its information.

The first edition of the formulary will generate many comments. It is worthwhile to invite and structure such comments by including a *formulary revision form*, containing a request for supporting references.

Developing a Formulary Manual

The production and maintenance of a formulary manual are major tasks requiring discussion and planning. A clear and systematic process for its development, printing, and distribution should be agreed upon, with sufficient time, personnel, and resources allocated.

Many aspects of the formulary process have already been described for essential drugs lists and for treatment guidelines (Chapter 10). The process for developing a formulary manual or national formulary is not very different, and only some specific aspects are discussed here.

Establish a National Formulary Committee. The formulary committee could be the national drug committee itself or a smaller subcommittee of it. Ideally, the formulary committee should include a clinical pharmacist or pharmacologist, a physician, and additional prominent medical specialists, as required, to prepare or review sections related to their areas of expertise for accuracy and completeness.

Secure Agreement on the Content, Structure, and Format of the Formulary. The formulary committee should propose the content, structure, general arrangement of the information, and layout for approval by the national drug committee. The committee should use models such as the BNF to save time and effort. Specific issues to be addressed regarding the nature, content, and format of the formulary are summarized in the next section.

Appoint an Editor. One person (or a maximum of two co-editors) should be appointed to draft the text of the formulary. The editor should have an understanding of the pharmaceutical, pharmacological, and clinical aspects of the information required and of the level of language appropriate for the target audience.

Review the Draft. Once the first draft has been produced, it should be presented to the formulary committee for review. The committee should call upon other experts to resolve issues in dispute or to assist in the review of specialized drugs or topics. The accepted amendments are then incorporated into the text. This second draft should be widely circulated among the members of the national drug committee and any other invited reviewers for further comment.

A special national meeting involving committee members and guest participants, including future users of the formulary, is then called to discuss any outstanding issues and give final approval to the form and content of the document. It is important for the credibility and acceptability of the formulary that all relevant opinions be considered and that key health policy-makers be included in the process, even when their expected contributions may be minimal. In this way, all participants will consider the formulary as partly their own creation and thus be more committed to ensuring its acceptance and widespread use.

Revise and Produce New Editions. As therapeutic practices change and amendments are made to the national list of essential drugs, these must be reflected in the formulary, along with proposed revisions submitted by users. Once a sufficient number of revisions has been received and accepted, it is necessary to repeat the development process to produce a new edition. It is important that new editions be produced regularly to maintain the usefulness and credibility of the formulary.

Between editions, new information can be disseminated through circulars or drug bulletins. Prior to the production of a second edition, readers' opinions on the general usefulness, design, and layout of the manual can be sought through a survey.

Practical Issues in Formulary Development

In developing a formulary, consideration needs to be given to such issues as sequencing, presentation of the information, which information to include, size of the publication, inclusion of brand-name drugs, and pricing choices (see Country Study 11.3).

Sequence of Drug Monographs. Structuring the drug information by therapeutic class is better than following alphabetical order. It places each drug in its therapeutic context and helps minimize duplication of drugs. It is recommended that the therapeutic classification of the national list of essential drugs (Chapter 10) be used. A short overview of the recommended drugs in the therapeutic group could be included as an introduction to the chapter (as is done in the BNF).

Presentation of Drug Information. Information on drugs can be presented in text or tables. Tables are useful if the information is brief and for comparisons among drugs. When information is more extensive, however, text is more appropriate.

Information on Drugs Not on the National List of Essential Drugs. Should information be included on drugs that are not recommended but are being used in some settings or that complement drugs on the list? Alternatively, information on these drugs can be provided through a drug information circular or drug bulletin, as well as through training of prescribers. Including private-sector drugs that are not on the national list of essential drugs duced in portable form. And including information that is not relevant to the public sector may induce an unwanted demand for items that are not on the national list of essential drugs.

Size of the Publication. A formulary can be pocket-size for day-to-day use or a larger desktop reference for occasional use. The size is determined primarily by its intended use. If the focus is on individual drugs, the formulary is probably most useful as a desktop reference. If it is more comparative and evaluative, with information on indications, dosages, and cost, including drugs of first choice, it should probably be pocket-size. A loose-leaf edition is not recommended, because pages tend to disappear and updates are not always properly inserted.

Inclusion of Brand-Name Drugs. Although the drug monographs should always appear under the generic name of the drug, it may be useful to list common brand names. If these names are included, they should appear in italics, both in the main text and in the index, so that they are easily identifiable. This enables prescribers who are not yet familiar with generic names to locate the required monograph easily. Cross-references are helpful.

Provision of National Formularies Free of Charge. The production of a formulary is time-consuming and costly, and it may be necessary to recover some of these costs. It may be possible to provide the formulary free to public-sector health workers and students and to charge the full price to the private sector. Ideally, it should be distributed without charge to everyone in the target audience.

Hospital Formularies

In many countries, especially those with highly developed health systems, hospitals develop their own formulary manuals. The advantage is that the formulary can be tailored to fit the particular requirements of the hospital and to reflect departmental consensus on first-choice treatments from the national list of essential drugs.

The process is similar to that discussed above. A hospital formulary committee is given responsibility for producing and subsequently revising the formulary. Additional information presented in hospital formularies may include details of recommended hospital procedures, hospital antibiotic policy, and guidelines for laboratory investigations and patient management. Hospital formularies usually reflect consensus on the treatment of first choice and thus are not always distinct from treatment guidelines.

≡ 11.4 Production Issues

Production issues for treatment guidelines and formulary manuals are similar. In addition to the information in

makes the formulary more comprehensive and interesting to a wider audience. However, inclusion of these drugs means that many more monographs have to be prepared, making the publication much larger and not easily pro-

Figure 11.4 Sample Pages from *Malawi National Formulary*, Second Edition, 1991

12.5 CARDIAC GLYCOSIDES

DIGOXIN (TABLETS)

Presentation: Tablet, 250 micrograms or paediatric tablet, 62.5 micrograms
MSDL: 12.5.(i).(a) or (b)

Indications: Heart failure, supraventricular arrhythmias, especially atrial fibrillation

Contraindications: Bradycardia, supraventricular arrhythmias caused by Wolff-Parkinson-White syndrome

Dose/Administration: (Adult) (1) Rapid oral digitalisation: 1-1.5 mg in divided doses over 24 hours followed by 125-250 micrograms once daily
(2) Slow oral digitalisation: 125-250 micrograms twice daily for 1 week, then reduce accordingly
(3) Maintenance (all routes): 250-700 micrograms daily as required, best given in divided doses except in an emergency.

NB. It is recommended that digoxin therapy in elderly patients be carried out gradually with smaller doses

(Child) (1) under 1 month and over 1 year:
- loading dose: 5 micrograms/kg/dose every 8 hours for 3 doses
- maintenance dose: 5 micrograms/kg/dose twice daily
 (2) between 1 month and 1 year:
- loading dose: 10 micrograms/kg/dose every 8 hours for 3 doses
- maintenance dose: 10 micrograms/kg/dose twice daily

Adverse reactions: Nausea, vomiting, anorexia, confusion, arrhythmias, heart block

Precautions: Give lower doses in renal failure and the elderly; recent infarction hypothyroidism; avoid hypokalaemia

Page 138   MNF 1991

---

12. CARDIOVASCULAR AGENTS

Drug interactions: See Appendix 1

Notes: The paediatric tablets should be used in preference to the elixir, 12.5.(i).(c), for children able to swallow solids

CMS code: A0146 (250 micrograms) A0145 (62.5 micrograms)

Distribution code: D   **Price code:** B (250 mcg) C (62.5 mcg)

DIGOXIN (ELIXIR)

Presentation: Elixir, 50 micrograms/ml **MSDL:** 12.5.(i).(c)

Indications, etc: As for tablet, 12.5.(i).(a)

Notes: (1) The elixir should not be diluted
(2) Use of the elixir should be reserved for very small babies not able to be given paediatric digoxin tablets, 12.5.(i).(b)
(3) Doses should be precisely measured using the pipette provided with the preparation

CMS code: E0264   **Distribution code:** D   **Price code:** D

MNF 1991   Page 139

Section 11.3, the following practical advice is useful for producing local reference manuals. The Malawi Essential Drugs Programme documented its experience in a World Health Organization (WHO) document that includes useful tips and descriptions of how problems were solved (WHO/DAP 1994b).

Manuscript Production and Layout

It is important to define a standard style for chapters, tables, and monographs before requesting outside experts to write sections of a publication (treatment guidelines or formulary manual). If this is not done, large differences in approach, level of detail, and style (for example, for headings, abbreviations, and use of bullets) can be expected. It is cumbersome, time-consuming, and expensive to correct these differences at a later stage. It is a good idea to include one or two examples and a few sample pages along with instructions to the writers.

If the manual will be produced using an in-house computer and word-processing program, staff should be familiar with word-processing features that can assist in producing a well-organized, easy-to-use manual. These features include page formatting, headers and footers, functions for creating and editing tables, automatic generation of tables of contents and lists of key words (to assist the indexer), and functions for creating standard layouts.

Printing

Time and money can be wasted if the treatment guidelines or formulary manual is printed in the wrong format or to the wrong quality standard. Key aspects of printing include page size, paper quality, printing quality, cover design, quality of cover material, and binding. As noted earlier, the most widely used standard treatment and formulary manuals are pocket-size.

Since printing is a specialized field, it is worth talking with a few printers to learn which options are available locally. What are the different qualities of paper and cover material? How long will they last? What are the different methods of printing, and how easy is it to read manuals and books printed by each method? Small print can be read much more easily when produced on a high-quality printing press. What binding options exist—hardcover binding, spiral binding, gluing, stapling, or loose-leaf binding? How durable and how costly is each option? Since seemingly small decisions can have a significant effect on printing costs and quality, printers should also be asked about cost-saving measures.

The cover is the most visible part of the manual. Careful thought should be given to its content and to the selection of a professional artist or designer.

To avoid unpleasant surprises, all these features should be specified precisely in the agreement with the printer, just as drug quality is specified in procurement contracts. Specifications should include the size, type, and weight (thickness) of paper to be used; the type and thickness of cover material; and the type of binding.

Price quotations from several reputable, reliable printers should be obtained, based on the specifications. A tender may be necessary or required by policy or regulation. In choosing a printer, one should also consider the quality of earlier books produced by the printer. Once the printer has been chosen, a contract is drawn up, including the exact specifications for the publication.

In view of the importance of the information as a reference, the page proofs should be checked very carefully. A typographical error in a dosage, for example, could be fatal.

In estimating the number of copies required, consideration should be given to a potential increase in the target audience in the time between editions. The number of copies required is commonly underestimated. Since it is usually relatively cheap to increase the number of copies, including an extra margin of at least 10 to 20 percent is recommended.

Distribution

A clear, systematic, and realistic distribution plan should be drawn up before the manual is sent to the printer. Apart from distribution through government mail, alternative strategies are distribution through workshops, professional associations, or sales or adding the manuals to regular drug supplies. Whatever method is chosen, the introduction and distribution costs should be included in the budget. A procedure should be set up to monitor distribution and to handle requests for additional copies.

≡ 11.5 Implementing Treatment Guidelines and Formulary Manuals

Once the treatment guidelines manual or formulary manual has been printed and distributed, work is still required to ensure its acceptance and widespread use. The quality of the materials contributes to their acceptance. However, acceptance can be improved by ensuring that drug availability matches the guidelines, by using the materials for teaching and examination at all levels of training, and by using the manual to set standards for drug utilization review. Finally, treatment guidelines and formulary manuals need to be publicized (see below).

Common Failures

The most common failure in the implementation of treatment guidelines and national formularies is a lack of credibility and acceptance, due to failure to involve a wide range of national experts and established training institutions in the production. A common mistake with treatment guidelines is the selection of drugs that are too sophisticated, too expensive, or not generally available at the relevant level of health care. In tertiary care, treatment guidelines based on essential drugs are sometimes regarded as second-class medicine or as an infringement on clinical freedom.

Gaining Acceptance for Treatment Guidelines and Formulary Manuals

As with essential drugs lists, acceptance should be sought from the start of the development process. The more involved people are, the more likely they are to accept, use, and defend the outcome. The drafting committee should therefore be generous with its acknowledgments, since experts whose names are printed inside will have a strong sense of ownership with regard to the manual (see Country Study 11.1, Zimbabwe example). It is also important to involve health workers of different levels, including rural health care and training institutions, in both the development and the review process. A broad range of opinions on the proposed content and format of a first edition and subsequent revisions should be solicited.

After the materials are printed, a careful introduction campaign is needed to promote their general acceptance and use. This may include the official launching of the publication by a high official, press reviews, introductory workshops in key educational institutions, articles in drug information circulars and drug bulletins, or a competition for the design of the cover or formulary logo. The cost of such a campaign should be included in the planning.

If possible, free copies should be made available to all health workers and all types of students (nursing, pharmacy, paramedical, and medical). In many countries, these people have such difficulty obtaining good training and reference materials that they are likely to use their manuals extensively. This means that students will be using the right drug and therapeutic information from the start of their studies. This effect is further enhanced if the material is officially adopted by the training institutions.

≡ Assessment Guide

Management Structure
- ▸ Is there a national committee responsible for managing the formulary process?
- ▸ Are there drugs and therapeutics committees in major hospitals?

Outcome of the Formulary Process
- ▸ Is there a national therapeutic guide with standardized treatments?
- ▸ Is there a national formulary manual with basic drug information?
- ▸ Are the treatment guidelines and formulary manual consistent with the national list of essential drugs?
- ▸ Do the treatment guidelines cover common problems such as acute respiratory tract infections, diarrheal diseases, sexually transmitted diseases, tuberculosis, leprosy, hypertension, diabetes, and epilepsy?

Use of Treatment Guidelines and Formulary Manual
- ▸ Is there a national drug policy statement to encourage the use of the treatment guidelines and formulary manual?
- ▸ Are the treatment guidelines and formulary manual used for basic and in-service training of health personnel?
- ▸ What percentage of public-sector health facilities has a copy of the treatment guidelines and/or formulary manual?
- ▸ What percentage of prescriptions in public-sector health facilities complies with the treatment guidelines?

The cost of providing copies to students as well as health workers should be included in the budget.

Authority of Materials

As with the list of essential drugs (Chapter 10), the credibility and acceptability of the treatment guidelines and formulary manual can be maintained only if a transparent process for reviewing and updating them is in place. Especially for treatment guidelines, a second edition will be needed soon after the first. Mistakes will undoubtedly have occurred that need correction, and comments and proposals for change are bound to be received from people who may not have taken the trouble to comment on the first draft. ∎

≡ References and Further Readings

★ = *Key readings.*

Herxheimer, A. 1987. Basic information that prescribers are not getting about drugs. *Lancet* 1:31–32.

★ Laing, R. O., and R. Ruredzo. 1989. The essential drugs program in Zimbabwe: New approaches to training. *Health Policy and Planning* 4:229–34.

MSH (Management Sciences for Health). 1992. Selection and formulary management (trainer's and participant's guides). In *Managing drug supply training series.* Part 1: *Policy issues in managing drug supply.* Boston: MSH.

MSH (Management Sciences for Health). 1995. Standard treatments (trainer's and participant's guides). In *Promoting rational drug use.* Boston: MSH.

Murray, C., K. Styblo, and A. Rouillon. 1993. Tuberculosis. In *Disease control priorities in developing countries,* ed. D. Jamison, W. Mosley, A. Measham, and J. Bobadilla. New York: Oxford University Press.

WHO/DAP (World Health Organization/Action Programme on Essential Drugs). 1987. *Assessment of the pharmaceutical supply system of Papua New Guinea.* WHO/DAP/87.7. Geneva: WHO/DAP.

WHO/DAP (World Health Organization/Action Programme on Essential Drugs). 1994a. *National, regional, and international essential drugs lists, formularies, and treatment guides.* WHO/DAP/94.2. Geneva: WHO/DAP.

★ WHO/DAP (World Health Organization/Action Programme on Essential Drugs). 1994b. *Producing national drug and therapeutic information: The Malawi approach to developing standard treatment guidelines.* WHO/DAP/94.14. Geneva: WHO/DAP.

★ WHO/PAHO (World Health Organization/Pan American Health Organization). 1984. *Development and implementation of drug formularies.* Scientific publication no. 474. Washington, D.C.: WHO/PAHO.

Formularies and Treatment Guidelines

★ British Medical Association and the Royal Pharmaceutical Society of Great Britain. Updated every six months. *British national formulary.* London.

Malawi Ministry of Health. 1993. *Malawi standard treatment guidelines.* Lilongwe.

★ Médecins sans Frontières. 1988. *Clinical guidelines: Diagnostic and treatment manual.* Paris: Hatier.

★ Ministry of Health and Child Welfare. 1994. *EDLIZ (essential drugs list for Zimbabwe).* Harare, Zimbabwe.

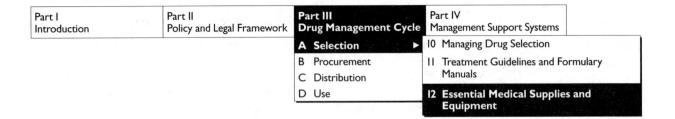

Part I	Part II	**Part III**	Part IV
Introduction	Policy and Legal Framework	**Drug Management Cycle**	Management Support Systems

A Selection ▶	10 Managing Drug Selection
B Procurement	11 Treatment Guidelines and Formulary Manuals
C Distribution	
D Use	**12 Essential Medical Supplies and Equipment**

Chapter 12
Essential Medical Supplies and Equipment

≡ Summary

In many aspects of selection and management, medical supplies and equipment are similar to drugs and are just as essential in providing effective and efficient medical services. Even though supplies and equipment may consume up to 40 percent of the amount spent on drugs, they are rarely given as much attention as essential drugs.

Three main issues associated with supplies and equipment are lack of policies, lack of standardization, and lack of quality assurance. A national list of medical supplies and equipment should be developed, which is based on expected types of tests, treatments, and interventions at different levels of health care. Lists of supplies and equipment tend to become long, and the items should be standardized as much as possible. Such a national list is useful to

 ► *define priority items and help ensure that the most essential items are available where needed;*

 ► *promote cost-effective use of scarce financial resources;*
 ► *reduce the number of items through standardization;*
 ► *serve as the basis for training staff and technicians.*

The four main criteria in the selection of equipment are (1) local possibilities for servicing and spare parts, (2) local availability of essential supplies (such as chemicals and filters), (3) a well-established brand of simple and sturdy design, and (4) local possibilities for training staff in its use and maintenance.

Before procuring medical supplies and equipment, the minimum specifications should be defined in close collaboration with technical staff. These specifications are needed for the procurement department and for claims in case of faulty products.

≡ In terms of selection and management, medical supplies and equipment are rarely given as much attention as drugs. For some reason they are regarded as less important, yet they are as essential to patient care as drugs. Their cost is considerable as well. In most developing countries, the cost for medical supplies can be as much as 30 to 40 percent of the amount spent on drugs, with a few expensive items usually responsible for a large percentage of the total cost.

Medical supplies and equipment include a large, heterogeneous group of items. *Supplies* comprise mainly disposable items (such as cotton, dressings, disposable syringes) or items with relatively short life spans (such as reusable syringes or catheters). The term *equipment* encompasses both capital equipment and recurrent equipment, the former being long-lasting, durable goods such as autoclaves, and the latter including goods with shorter life spans such as thermometers or sphygmomanometers. The distinction between supplies and equipment is not always clear. For example, thermometers are pieces of equipment, but they are purchased so frequently that they are sometimes referred to as supplies.

It is a challenge to find good data on the consumption and cost of medical supplies, and especially of individual items. The number of different items and brands is much larger than the average number of essential drugs, and the specifications are much less standardized. Another problem springs from the records used to compile data. Are different sizes of X-ray films, or all sizes of syringes, regarded as one item? In some countries, drugs and other medical supplies come under different management structures or different budgets, which makes intercountry comparisons difficult.

This chapter concentrates on practical aspects in the selection of medical supplies, with emphasis placed on those aspects that differ from the selection of drugs as described in Chapters 10 and 11. In addition, some aspects of procurement, storage, and distribution that are particular to medical supplies are presented.

≡ 12.1 National Equipment and Medical
       Supplies Policy

Three main problems associated with medical supplies and equipment are lack of policies, lack of standardization, and lack of quality assurance.

The absence of an effective equipment policy and lack of standardization of supplies can lead to wasteful and expensive overpurchasing and overstocking. In most supply organizations, the number of different items of medical supplies and equipment is about three to five times greater than the number of essential drugs. The government supply system in Cyprus carries about 2,500 items; the government medical stores catalog in Zimbabwe, which has already been standardized and is very selective, includes about 1,200 (see Country Study 12.1). Although medical supply items are not generally subject to expiry (with the notable exception of many sterilized items), there are many examples of accumulating stocks of instruments and spare parts that have been ordered but are no longer required or are not compatible with newer types of equipment.

Country Study 12.1 Revising the Medical Stores Catalog in Zimbabwe

In Zimbabwe, the medical stores catalog is a leveled list of essential equipment, instruments, and supplies. It contains the stock number, description, price, level of use, and VEN (vital, essential, nonessential) category for each item on the list. The list is considered a national list, and it is revised every two years.

The list is divided into three levels, according to the knowledge and expertise required to use the items properly. C-level items are the most generally accessible items, meant for clinics where no doctor is available as well as any higher-level institution. B-level items are meant for (mainly district) hospitals, institutions that employ a doctor or clinical officer, and any higher-level medical institutions. A-level items are meant for use in provincial and general hospitals. These hospitals employ a number of specialists and function as referral hospitals for the district-level facilities. S-level items are meant for use only by specialists in the provincial general hospitals and national referral and teaching hospitals. This means that surgical items marked "S" can be requested only when the requesting institution has a surgical specialist attached to it.

Many participants contribute to the revision process, and comments are invited from government and private health workers at all levels of care, including the manufacturing industry and importers. During a national workshop, groups of items are reviewed by working groups. Proposals for changes are discussed and finalized in plenary sessions.

Most participants consider the process a positive one with numerous advantages. The discussions produce many valuable and sometimes unexpected comments by the end-users. An additional benefit of the national workshop is that there is less need for time-consuming visits by sales representatives to the procurement department of the government medical stores. Instead, representatives are invited to attend the review meeting and can propose new products or alternatives to items already on the list. This procedure works well, as few products are so revolutionary that they need to be procured immediately and cannot wait until the next review of the list.

The general impression has been that experienced hospital matrons and theater nurses have a better understanding of what is needed than most doctors and surgeons, and that good sales representatives know more about their products than their directors and sales managers.

A sound national equipment policy with a list of essential medical supplies can be effective in simplifying supply issues, reducing costs, and promoting efficient provision of health care. The policy specifies what medical equipment and supplies should be used in which types of medical tests, interventions, and operations. Since different medical procedures are carried out at different levels of health care, the policy defines the sets of supplies and equipment that will be needed at each of these levels. A good example of an equipment and supplies policy can be found in Country Study 12.2.

Drawing Up the List

From this policy, lists of essential equipment and supplies can be drawn up according to level of care. These lists are useful to

- define priority items and help ensure that the most essential items are available where needed;
- promote careful use of scarce financial resources;
- promote standardization, which simplifies supply management and reduces stock costs;
- provide the basis for training of staff and maintenance technicians.

Like drugs, equipment and medical supplies should be selected on the basis of need. For example, selection can be based on the instruments and supplies that are needed for an intravenous infusion, an uncomplicated delivery, or a suture.

A national committee for medical supplies and equipment should then combine the lists for each level of care into one national list of essential medical supplies and equipment. Like the list of essential drugs, this list should be the basis for standardized procurement and distribution of supplies and equipment, as well as for training.

Managing the Medical Supplies and Equipment List

The list of essential equipment and supplies should contain a complete and clear description of each item, including stock number, type, standard pack size, and the most recent unit price. VEN categories (see Chapter 41) are also useful to identify those items that should never be allowed to run out of stock. For long lists, it is probably better to group the items by category (disposables, small equipment, chemicals, bandages, dressings) and use the stock or catalog number to identify the category. Shorter lists, such as those for lower levels of health care, can be organized alphabetically. These can also be used as standard order lists.

Without effective limits, a list of medical supplies tends to be long. It is therefore important that the items be standardized as much as possible, in order to minimize costs and prevent confusion. A model list of the most common items is given in Annex 12.1. This list is based on information supplied by a number of essential drugs programs and international suppliers. It may seem short, but if all these items are always available, most basic needs can be met.

There is usually pressure to include more items on the list. Doctors who were trained overseas may want to bring their treatment habits with them, or even impose them on other health workers. It is not easy to resist such pressure,

Country Study 12.2 Uganda's Medical Equipment Policy

In 1991, most medical equipment in Uganda was dilapidated, difficult to maintain, and procured from many different suppliers, with donated equipment originating from a number of different countries. In the face of this chaos, the government decided to formulate a medical equipment policy.

A national committee composed of experts in medicine, surgery, and pathology; medical engineers; and administrators was chaired by the chief surgeon. As it developed the policy, the committee was guided by the following criteria: standardization; technical suitability; general maintenance; and cost, which took into account investment costs, maintenance costs, running costs, and depreciation.

The committee formulated a policy to guide the procurement and supply of equipment and spares to different levels of health care. The result of their deliberations was a document that spelled out clear specifications for most items. The policy is now used to guide the procurement department of the government medical stores and is also used as a donor guideline.

Figure 12.1 Sample Product Specifications

Minimum Quality Requirements for Hydrophilic Absorbent Gauze

Raw material: 100 percent cotton, bleached and scoured
Minimum number of warp and weft threads per inch: 19 x 15
Total of warp and weft threads per cm: 13
Net weight per square meter: 17 g
Net weight per roll: 1,392 g
Products comply with BP88
Packing details: Per piece in white polyethylene bag; 20 pieces in export carton

Source: IDA Newsletter no. 7 (November 1993).

Note: Not only price but also standard pack size and quality need to be considered when placing an order. For example, in this case, a lower number of threads per square centimeter can result in a weight difference (and loss of absorption capacity) of up to 40 percent among products of various suppliers.

but a standardized list, drawn up by committee and with procedures for regular updates, is probably the best solution. An argument often heard in favor of a wide selection is that wastage is reduced by having many different sizes of certain items. In general, however, it is less expensive to standardize on one or two common sizes of selected items than to pay the extra costs of handling, distributing, and storing many different sizes. When standardization is not in place, wastage due to expiry is also likely to be higher. Examples of items for which standardization is often possible are dressings, endotracheal tubes, needles, scissors, sutures, and syringes.

Another argument in favor of expanding the list, and one that has to be taken into consideration, is that facilities have different types of equipment that require special parts and supplies. Although this may be true when many different brands of equipment are on hand, the long-term answer is to standardize the capital equipment instead of continuing to stock many different types of spares.

Minimum Specifications

In addition to a catalog or list of essential items, a separate set of technical specifications for the items must be developed. These specifications must be prepared by technically qualified personnel and must be as accurate and precise as possible. They are essential to the procurement department or tender board to ensure the quality of the items. They are also needed for any claim if poor-quality goods have been received. An example of product specifications is given in Figure 12.1.

≡ **12.2 Selecting Medical Supplies**

Many supply items, such as syringes, needles, and gloves, are available as either disposable or reusable items. The national policy on the use of disposable or reusable items may differ from one country to another. Important factors to consider in making a choice are listed in Figure 12.2. If reusable products are chosen, it is essential to buy products that can be autoclaved.

Disposable and Reusable Items

In countries with limited funds for medical supplies, the main problem with using disposable syringes and needles is that they are expensive and sometimes out of stock; because of this, they are often resterilized and used again. Two problems arise: first, these disposables are not meant to be sterilized (resulting in air leakage and inadequate dosing); second, the method of sterilizing is often inadequate. It is common to see a few "disposable" needles and syringes floating in a pan of water, with or without a lid, which may or may not have been boiling for some time. Boiling only disinfects and does *not* sterilize! The same applies for soaking the disposables in a disinfectant solution. Where stockouts are a problem, every health facility should probably keep a few reusable syringes and needles in reserve. This implies that a national policy for using *only* disposable or *only* reusable materials is not always practical.

The United Nations Children's Fund (UNICEF) and the World Health Organization (WHO) have, in recent years, tried to solve the problem of the reuse of disposables by creating "autodestructing" disposable syringes and needles, which are made in such a way that they can be used only once. Although originally more expensive than ordinary

Figure 12.2 Advantages and Disadvantages of Disposable Items

Disposables	Reusables
Advantages	Advantages
▸ No sterilizer and running costs ▸ No labor cost ▸ Safer; less risk of disease transmission (if not reused)	▸ Cheaper to purchase ▸ Need less storage space ▸ Less waste
Disadvantages	Disadvantages
▸ Usually more expensive ▸ Bulky ▸ Wastage problem ▸ Unsafe if reused (cannot be sterilized)	▸ Need sterilizing equipment, running costs, and continuous supply of bags, autoclave control tape, and glove powder ▸ Time-consuming to sterilize ▸ Less safe; risk of transmitting disease if not cleaned and sterilized properly

disposables, they are now produced in such large numbers that the price difference has nearly disappeared. The carton in which they are supplied serves as a safe disposal box, with an inner lining that can easily be burned. The plastic melts all needles and syringes into one block, which can be safely disposed of.

When buying disposable components for special equipment, it is important to make sure that what is purchased will actually fit. Some equipment uses standard disposables; other equipment requires product-specific supplies. This is an example of the risk of not considering recurrent costs when buying equipment.

It is necessary to be very careful when preparing the specifications for items that are to be used together. Will the catheter or the syringe fit on the needle (fittings Luer/Luer) or is an adapter required (fittings Luer/Record)? Record was the old standard for fittings, and some sundries with this fitting can still be found. All new supplies should have Luer fittings.

Needles and Syringes

Injections are overused in many countries. In view of their cost and the risk of transmission of disease, this practice should be discouraged as much as possible. Nevertheless, every health facility should keep on hand enough syringes and needles to provide sterile items for each injection.

In primary health care, injection equipment is needed for immunization and for drug treatment. For immunization, a 2 mL syringe with a subcutaneous needle (23 G × 1 inch, 0.6 × 25 mm) is used. For intramuscular injection of drugs in suspension or oil, a 5 mL syringe with a thick needle is needed (19 G × $1^1/2$ inches, 1.1 × 40 mm).

Ideally, a finer needle should be used for other intramuscular and intravenous injections, but it is not essential.

In most hospitals or districts, the range of different syringes and needles can be simplified. It is not necessary to have all possible sizes available.

Sutures

At the primary care level, two kinds of sutures are usually sufficient: a resorbable chromic catgut suture with needle for deliveries, and a nonresorbable monofilament or braided suture with needle for wound suturing and minor surgery.

In district and specialist hospitals, some additional types of sutures are needed, but not the wide range that is usually found in stock, at considerable cost. There are round and cutting needles of different sizes, with catgut, nylon, silk, or Dexon threads in five to ten different thicknesses; the number of varieties is nearly unlimited. Discuss with senior staff (surgeon, senior nursing officer) the minimum range that should be available. A sample list is included in Annex 12.1.

Gloves

Gloves are necessary for staff in dressing and delivery rooms, operating rooms, and laboratories where blood samples are handled. Gloves are used to protect personnel from infection by microorganisms from a patient's body fluids. In surgery, they are also used to protect the patient against infection with microorganisms from the surgeon's hands. The risk of HIV transmission has increased awareness and underscored the importance of using good-quality products with a low risk of pinholes and cuts.

There are many different types of gloves: thick rubber gloves used by cleaners and mortuary workers; thin, plastic, nonsterile disposable gloves to handle infected materials (dressings); plastic or rubber nonsterile but reusable plastic gloves; sterile disposable surgeon's gloves; and reusable rubber surgeon's gloves, which can be sterilized several times. It is important to match the correct gloves to the task.

Common errors are cleaners using rubber surgeon's gloves, and surgeons wearing resterilized disposable gloves (often patched with small pieces of rubber to repair the holes). Latex rubber gloves are preferred over plastic for procedures in which contact with a patient's body fluids is likely. Even wearing two or three layers of gloves does not reduce the risk of needle-stick injury.

≡ 12.3 Selecting Instruments and Equipment

Over the years, a tremendous amount of surgical, laboratory, anesthesia, and other special instruments and

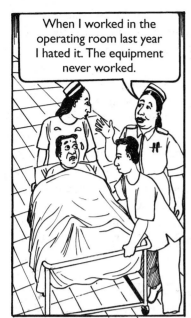
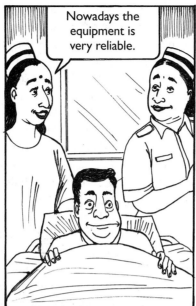
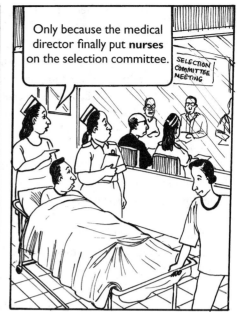

INVOLVEMENT OF NURSES IN EQUIPMENT SELECTION

equipment, as well as spare parts, can build up. Such an accumulation is enough to defeat all but the best inventory and stock control systems. This problem cannot be solved easily, and only a few general remarks are made here.

The world is still not united in several important areas, such as electrical and metric systems. Around the world, there are at least four different types of electrical plugs; two voltage systems, with 110 or 220 volts and 50 or 60 cycles per second; three different weight and volume measurement systems; and instructions in dozens of different languages. In addition, for equipment such as gauges on gas containers, different companies may use different internal standards. This creates immense problems for countries that have not managed to standardize their equipment or that receive equipment from a number of different donors.

The obvious strategy for tackling this problem is to standardize equipment and instruments as much as possible. When the standard types and brands have been chosen, a list of standard equipment with specifications should be prepared to serve as a guideline for the procurement department. These standards should also be communicated to the main donor agencies and should be used as much as possible for donated equipment. It may be necessary to refuse certain donations.

For surgical instruments, stainless steel is generally more expensive but lasts longer and can be sterilized. Polypropylene is cheaper but less durable and does not always survive the autoclave. The material should be verified in advance and specified when ordering the equip-

ment. It is not advisable to buy low-quality stainless-steel products, since they may rust or screws may come loose. Procurement from reputable suppliers is recommended even if the prices are higher.

Expertise is required in the purchase and maintenance of medical equipment. Consulting experts at an early stage of the procurement process may prevent later problems (Bloom and Temple-Bird 1994).

≡ 12.4 Donated Supplies and Equipment

When donors are involved in providing medical supplies and equipment, problems related to the lack of standardization and to maintenance may arise. First, many donors prefer to assist only in the buying of equipment, leaving the recipient to solve the problem of paying for installation, maintenance, and recurrent costs. Second, many donors are more sensitive to the demand for orders from their national manufacturers than they are to the recipient's technical requirements. Thus, a look around the storerooms in many countries reveals equipment that has never been used or has broken down and cannot be repaired, due to a lack of spare parts and local service facilities or a lack of instructions in the local language. Third, a donor's policy may differ from the national policy, for example, in relation to the use of disposable syringes. In general, much of the lack of standardization of equipment in developing countries is caused by donated equipment.

Most of the principles of drug donations, as presented in Chapter 20, apply equally to medical supplies and equipment. Nevertheless, there are a few specific issues regarding donations of equipment that should be kept in mind. The most important is the provision for maintenance and spares. As mentioned above, this should be the first criterion used in choosing equipment for procurement; it should also be the first argument for acceptance of a proposed donation.

At present, the best guidelines for equipment donations are the *Equipment Donations Guidelines* of the Christian Medical Commission of the World Council of Churches. The main points, as summarized below, include responsibilities for both donors and recipients.

Responsibilities of Recipients
- ▶ Standardize equipment as much as possible.
- ▶ Involve technical departments in formulating a request for support.
- ▶ Clearly specify the items to accompany the equipment.
- ▶ Make a checklist of these three points for submission to the donor.

Responsibilities of Donors
- ▶ Communicate with the recipient before donating equipment.
- ▶ Supply fully operational equipment.
- ▶ Supply all technical documents.
- ▶ Supply the requirements of consumables and spare parts for two years.
- ▶ Ensure proper packaging and shipping.
- ▶ Offer technical assistance in the training of end-users and maintenance staff.
- ▶ Understand and respect important laws and regulations in the recipient country (for example, with regard to payment of customs duties).

≡ 12.5 Management of Medical Supplies

In principle, managing medical supplies and equipment is similar to managing drug supply. Chapters in the procurement and distribution sections of this book discuss the general management aspects of procurement, storage, and distribution in detail. The subsections that follow are limited to a few aspects specific to the management of medical supplies and equipment.

Procurement

Procurement of medical supplies is not substantially different from drug procurement. There are a limited number of items that are responsible for a large proportion of the budget, and these can be identified by ABC analysis

(see Chapter 41). It is obvious that these A items should be procured through tender. As with drugs, the tender should be restricted to prequalified suppliers to ensure quality.

The quality specifications of drugs can usually be summarized by referring to existing pharmacopeias, such as the *British Pharmacopoeia*. Unfortunately, such standardization rarely exists for supplies and equipment, making it important to prepare detailed specifications for each item (see Figure 12.1). Without these, it is difficult to issue the tender, evaluate bids, and claim any damages in case of faulty products.

For several items, local procurement may be much more attractive than importation. Typical examples are cotton and dressing materials. Both of these items are easy to manufacture and bulky to transport. In addition, they take up enough storage space to make frequent deliveries cost effective; such deliveries can be provided more easily and at less expense by local producers.

In addition to the few items that are needed in large quantities, there are numerous other items of which only small quantities are necessary. Many of these have to be imported, but neither their cost nor their volume makes it worthwhile to put them through the tender process. It is usually much more cost effective to buy these items through international nonprofit suppliers such as Equipment for Charitable Hospitals Overseas (ECHO; see Box 12.1), UNIPAC, or the International Dispensary Association (IDA).

There will always be requests for the procurement of items that are not on the national list of essential supplies. For such items, for new items that have not yet been included on the list, or for new items with an expected low turnover, the following questions should be asked before an order is placed:

- ▶ Is the item really necessary? Can and will it be used in the place for which it is being ordered?
- ▶ Is there a local alternative?
- ▶ Can spare parts or means of maintenance be consistently obtained?

Storage

Although most medical and surgical supplies are quite durable, some contain specific expiration dates, and others are subject to spoilage if left unused for too long. Other items are sensitive to heat and humidity. Many sterile products, even if properly packed by the manufacturer, remain sterile only if stored correctly. Many have an expiry date and may lose sterility under tropical conditions.

Insufficient attention is frequently paid to the storage requirements of medical supplies. In some places, storage conditions are poor, with leaking roofs, dust, extreme heat, and rodents. Under such circumstances, the financial waste due to damaged supplies is considerable, and investing to upgrade the stores, particularly at the central and regional levels, is likely to be cost effective.

In selecting supplies and in defining the specifications for them, one should consider the anticipated storage conditions. Guidelines for storage should be prepared and described in the list of essential supplies.

Distribution

Preprinted standard requisition lists of medical supplies, organized by level of health facility, are useful tools to simplify the distribution of supplies and promote the rational use of limited resources. Such lists indicate to the end-user the range of items that are available within the system, with their specifications, pack sizes, and stock numbers. The lists can also include the current unit price. In addition, such lists facilitate checking procedures for ensuring that only approved items are ordered and supplied.

The lists should specify the maximum amounts of all critical items to be kept in the health facility or hospital ward. The amount ordered would then be the difference between the stock on hand and this maximum quantity. For health facilities with four shipments per year, the maximum amount could reflect three months' use; for hospital wards or departments, a two-week supply is probably reasonable.

Many medical supplies (gloves, catheters, and sutures) come in various sizes and materials. One of the most difficult aspects of stock management of medical supplies is to ensure that the specifications for the items (size, material, pack size) are all correct.

It remains a challenge to put together a requisition form that is clear to everybody: should it list single units or packages (for example, one syringe or a box of 100, one bandage or a pack of twelve)? How should the list be organized—strictly alphabetically or by class? Should an alphabetical list mention *Bandage, crepe,* or *Crepe bandage*? If the list is by class, should all plastics be listed together or classed as disposables, nondisposables, or something else?

The best solution for the central store and highest-level health facilities is a full list of items organized in groups and using the common pack size of items as the counting unit. For the lower levels of health care or for individual hospital wards, a short alphabetical list and standard order form can be used, with single items as the counting unit. Whatever the system, it is important to be logical and test the form with some end-users.

Box 12.1 ECHO: Nonprofit Equipment Supplier

ECHO was established in London in 1966 to assist rural health care workers in developing countries to obtain essential medical supplies and equipment. At first, medical and surgical materials were obtained free ("surplus to requirements") from British hospitals. They were cleaned, repaired, and then sent to rural mission hospitals in developing countries.

As ECHO's nonprofit and needs-based approach succeeded around the world, the organization grew rapidly, always focusing on the practical requirements of developing-country health care workers. Robust new medical equipment of appropriate technology was designed and manufactured in the United Kingdom for ECHO. Items such as mobile spotlights, microscopes, and obstetric beds were manufactured for ECHO and supplied by it to many developing countries. A full range of essential medical supplies and equipment was developed—a range so broad that ECHO was called upon to re-equip hospitals and medical stores and to supply relief and emergency aid programs. Nine years after its founding, ECHO began to supply generic pharmaceuticals, and the demand for these also grew rapidly.

ECHO's purpose continues to be to offer a comprehensive medical supply service for the relief of illness abroad, regardless of race, caste, or creed. ECHO can make its low-cost medical supplies and drugs available to mission, charity, and government hospitals as well as to rural health care units in developing countries worldwide.

With rapid growth has come an awareness of ECHO's responsibility to maintain focus and to channel its growth to achieve the most effective continuing support of health care workers. A technical department has been set up to repair and recondition used equipment such as infant incubators, cardiac monitors, and anesthesia machines. These machines are then supplied at a fraction of the cost of equivalent new items. ECHO supports the equipment by sending out spare parts and by supplying manuals and technical information.

A logical extension of such technical support has been to develop training of hospital engineers in field situations. ECHO has supported the establishment of two technical training workshops in East Africa, one in Uganda and one in Tanzania. At these workshops, groups of national hospital engineers from rural units are trained in the preventive maintenance and repair of a wide range of hospital equipment.

A key focus of ECHO's growth is to respond to new developments and problems in health care worldwide. In response to the HIV and AIDS crisis, ECHO supplies low-cost, simple HIV testing kits, as well as a wide range of supporting materials.

ECHO has prepared model lists of essential medical supplies for first-level (simple health clinic) and second-level (district hospital) health care facilities in developing countries (see "References and Further Readings").

Consumption Monitoring

Cost awareness among end-users can be created by having the nursing officer in charge keep a stock register for selected supplies at the health facility or hospital ward. Each facility should develop its own list, but in general, the list should include syringes and needles, absorbent gauze, cotton, adhesive tape, disinfectants, and soap. Unit prices should be included on the requisition form.

Regular monitoring of the consumption of medical supplies and equipment is useful to plan for future requirements, allocate supplies, and identify wards and facilities that have higher-than-expected consumption of particular items. Such a simple system can be an important deterrent to the misuse of supplies.

Consumption monitoring is not necessary for all items. Initially, it can be limited to those items that are most attractive, most prone to misuse, or most valuable. Monitoring reports can be produced quarterly. Each ward or unit should be listed separately.

Over time, usage indicators can be developed along the lines of those that already exist for drugs. An example of a usage indicator would be: *number of rolls of cotton per month per 100 medical admissions*. Such an indicator becomes a useful tool for comparing consumption among medical wards and for planning future requirements.

≡ 12.6 Supplies for Other Services

There are other medical services that need a certain number of instruments, basic equipment, reagents, chemicals, and spare parts. Some of these services are briefly discussed below. A few practical lists of basic requirements appear in References and Further Readings.

Laboratory Services

The extent of laboratory services may vary considerably from one country to another, and this situation has implications for the supply system. In most developing countries, laboratory services exist at the district hospital, and sometimes in facilities at lower levels, for collecting specimens and performing simple analyses. The selection of laboratory equipment, instruments, and supplies should be needs driven and based on the range of tests required at each level. Examples of such lists are available (Hogerzeil and Hofs 1986; IDA annual updates; WHO 1987). Many laboratory supplies are used in machines, such as chambers for the hemoglobin test and test tubes

for the centrifuge. It is particularly important to ensure that reagents and machines are compatible and that maintenance services can be provided locally. Reagents may be produced locally by the central laboratory or the hospital pharmacy.

Dental Services

The extent of dental services is often limited in developing countries, due to a lack of dentists and dental technicians. Comprehensive services are available only in dental clinics in the major towns or at the regional hospitals. The care provided at lower levels usually consists of diagnosis, tooth extraction, and temporary fillings. The equipment and supplies needed for each level of health care should be listed on the basis of the available services. Halestrap (1987) has provided a model list of supplies for dental first aid.

Family Planning Services

Family planning services in many developing countries are largely donor supported. The donor provides contraceptive supplies and trains local health workers. Unfortunately, in many cases, the donor also decides which methods and brands are to be used. Procurement and distribution of supplies are often carried out separately from the regular governmental system.

Immunization Services

Immunization services are also largely donor supported in some countries. UNICEF is the main donor of both equipment and services. The extent of cooperation between UNICEF and the ministry of health may vary, and, as with family planning, the involvement of national staff on the managerial level may be limited. Lists of essential supplies are available (WHO 1984).

There is no reason that supplies and equipment for laboratory, dental, family planning, and immunization services should not be part of medical supplies in general. However, the responsibility for such supplies may lie with different departments in the ministry of health. To ensure optimal management and a rational supply process, these units should play a consultative role in selecting items and estimating national needs, in the same way that nurses and doctors are involved in the selection of drugs and general medical supplies. This is also the most rational use of human resources, ensuring experienced management and releasing busy professionals for more urgent tasks. ■

≡ Assessment Guide

Management Structure
- ► Has a national list of essential medical supplies and equipment (NLEMSE) been officially adopted and distributed countrywide?
- ► Is there an official committee whose duties include updating the NLEMSE?
- ► Has the NLEMSE been updated and distributed countrywide in the past five years?

Outcome of the Selection Process
- ► How many items does the NLEMSE contain? How are the items classified?
- ► Is the NLEMSE divided into levels of health care? How many items are there for each level?

Use of the NLEMSE
- ► Is there a national drug policy statement to encourage the use of the NLEMSE?
- ► Is procurement in the public sector limited to items on the NLEMSE?
- ► What is the ratio of value of items from the NLEMSE procured in the public sector to the total value of medical supplies and equipment procured in the same sector?
- ► Do drug donations comply with the NLEMSE?
- ► Is the NLEMSE used for the training of health workers and maintenance personnel?

≡ References and Further Readings

★ = *Key readings.*

General
★ Bloom, G., and C. Temple-Bird. 1994. Medical equipment management. In *Health and disease in developing countries*, ed. K. S. Lankinen, S. Bergstrom, P. H. Makela, and M. Peltomaa. London: Macmillan.
★ Christian Medical Commission–Churches' Action for Health. 1993. *Equipment donations guidelines*. Geneva: Christian Medical Commission–Churches' Action for Health.
Equipment for Charitable Hospitals Overseas (ECHO). 1995. *Selecting medical supplies for basic health care*. Surrey, England: ECHO.
IDA (International Dispensary Association). *Price indicator*. Updated semiannually. Amsterdam: IDA.
UNICEF (United Nations Children's Fund). *Supply catalogue*. Copenhagen: UNICEF.
WHO/DAP (World Health Organization/Action Programme on Essential Drugs). 1990. *The new emergency health kit*. WHO/DAP/90.1. Geneva: WHO/DAP.

Surgery and Obstetrics
Cook, J., B. Sankaran, and A. E. O. Wasunna, eds. 1991. *Surgery at the district hospital: Obstetrics, gynaecology, orthopaedics, and traumatology*. Geneva: World Health Organization.

Dobson, M. B. 1988. *Anaesthesia at the district hospital*. Geneva: World Health Organization.
WHO (World Health Organization). 1991. *Essential elements of obstetric care at first referral level*. Geneva: WHO.

Laboratory and Vaccines
Hogerzeil, H. V., and M. Hofs. 1986. Essential reagents for rural medical laboratories in Ghana. *Tropical Doctor* 16:58–60.
IDA (International Dispensary Association). 1995. *Medical laboratories: Methods and materials*. Amsterdam: IDA.
WHO (World Health Organization). 1984. *Immunization in practice. A guide for health workers who give vaccines*. WHO/EPI/PHW/84.4. Geneva: WHO.
WHO (World Health Organization). 1987. *Laboratory services at the primary health care level*. WHO/LAB/87.2. Geneva: WHO.
WHO (World Health Organization). 1991. *Essential elements of obstetric care at first referral level*. Geneva: WHO.

Dental
Halestrap, D. J. 1987. *Simple dental care for rural hospitals (without a dentist)*. London: Teaching Aids at Low Cost.

Annex 12.1 Model List of Essential Medical Supplies

The following list was developed on the basis of answers to a survey questionnaire by about thirty supply agencies and managers of essential drugs programs in both developed and developing countries. More comprehensive lists are available from ECHO and IDA. The list can be used as a starting point and adapted to meet national or local needs. It indicates a basic range of essential supplies that would be needed at either a district hospital or a health center staffed by paramedical staff, catering to the usual range of interventions at that level of care (rehydration, intravenous infusion, wound disinfection and suturing, dressing, incision of abscess, and normal delivery).

Essential Medical Supply	Health Center	Hospital
Dressings		
Gauze, plain, 90 m x 0.9 m	■	■
Cotton, absorbent, 400 gms BP	■	■
Bandages, loose woven, 7.5 cm x 4.45 m BP	■	■
Adhesive, plaster, 2.5 cm x 4.5 m	■	■
Strapping, plaster, 10 m x 4.5 m BP	■	■
Plaster of Paris bandages, 20 cm x 2.75 m BP		■
Plaster of Paris bandages, 10 cm x 2.75 m BP		■
Towels, maternity	■	
Dressing, sterile paraffin medicated, 10 x 10 cm		■
Dressing, sterile paraffin medicated, 20 x 15 cm		■
Clinical thermometers (Centigrade)	■	■
Crepe or elastic bandages, 7.5 cm	■	■
Crepe or elastic bandages, 15 cm	■	
Syringes, Needles, Surgical Blades		
Syringes, tuberculin w/26 G needle	■	■
Syringes, insulin w/26 G needle 100 IU/mL		■
Syringes, disposable, 2 cc	■	■
Syringes, disposable, 5 cc	■	■
Syringes, disposable, 10 cc	■	■
Needles, disposable, 2.5 cm, 23 G	■	■
Needles, disposable, 3.75 cm, 19 G	■	■
Needles, scalp vein 21 G	■	■
Needles, scalp vein 25 G	■	■
IV cannulae, 18 G	■	■
IV cannulae, 22 G		■
Surgical blades size 24		■
Surgical blades size 22	■	■
Surgical blades size 15		■
Surgical blades size 11		■
Blades for safety razor	■	■
IV giving set	■	■
IV blood giving set		■
IV blood taking set		■
Sutures and Surgical Needles		
Catgut, chromic, no. 2/0 on 1/2 C, 30 mm RB needle	■	■
Catgut, chromic, no. 0, 1.5 m		■
Catgut, chromic, no. 1, 1.5 m		■
Catgut, chromic, no. 2, 1.5 m		■
Catgut, chromic, no. 3/0 on 1/2 C, 25 mm RB needle		■
Catgut, chromic, no. 5/0, revs. cutt. needle, dbl. end		■
Catgut, chromic, no. 0, on 1/2 C, 40 mm RB needle		■
Catgut, plain, no. 2/0, 1.5 m		■
Nylon suture, no. 2/0 on curved cutting 40 mm needle		■
Nylon suture, no. 0, without needle		■

Essential Medical Supply	Health Center	Hospital
Silk suture, braided, no. 2/0, 1.5 m		■
Silk suture, braided, no. 1, 1.5 m	■	■
Silk suture, braided, no. 3/0, on 1/2 C 25 mm needle		■
Silk suture, braided, no. 6/0, on 1/2 cutting needle		■
1/2 circle cutting needle no. 2	■	■
1/2 circle RB size 3		■
1/2 circle RB size 4		■
1/2 circle RB size 7		■
1/2 triangular pointed cutting size 3		■
1/2 circle triangular pointed cutting size 9		■
1/2 circle tapered cutting size 10		■
Gloves		
Glove, industrial size 7		■
Glove, surgeon's size 6.5	■	■
Glove, surgeon's size 7		■
Glove, surgeon's size 8	■	■
Glove, postmortem size 8		■
Glove, powder	■	■
Plastic exam. gloves, small		■
Plastic exam. gloves, medium	■	■
Plastic exam. gloves, large		■
Catheters		
Catheters, Nelaton-6 FG		■
Catheters, Nelaton-14 FG		■
Catheters, Foley, 30 mL-14 FG	■	■
Catheters, Foley, 30 mL-18 FG		■
Bags, urine, with outlet, sterile, 2000 mL	■	■
Bags, colostomy, 10 cm x 5 cm		■
Cord clamps or cord ties	■	■
Corrugated rubber drain, in sheets, 12 cm x 25 cm		■
Tubes—Nasogastric, Feeding, etc.		
Tubes, feeding, infant, size 4 FG	■	■
Tubes, feeding, infant, size 8 FG	■	■
Tubes, gastroduodenal, Levin's 10 FG		■
Tubes, gastroduodenal, Levin's 14 FG		■
Spatula, wood (applicator), 1.3 cm x 13 cm	■	■
Lubricant jelly (for tubes)	■	■
Endotracheal cuffed tubes, 5 m		■
Endotracheal cuffed tubes, 7 m		■
Endotracheal cuffed tubes, 9 m		■
Endotracheal tube, 3 mm		■
Other		
Autoclaving tape 1/2"	■	■
Plastic dispensing bag		■

BP = British Pharmacopoeia; G = gauge; C = circular; RB = round-bodied; FG = Foley gauge.

Section B
Procurement

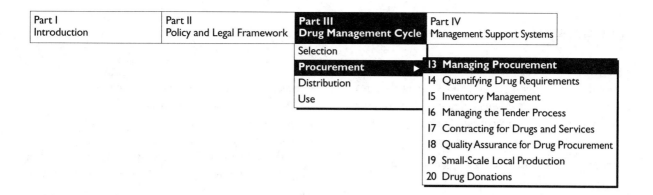

Part I Introduction	Part II Policy and Legal Framework	**Part III** **Drug Management Cycle**	Part IV Management Support Systems
		Selection	
		Procurement ▶	**13 Managing Procurement**
		Distribution	14 Quantifying Drug Requirements
		Use	15 Inventory Management
			16 Managing the Tender Process
			17 Contracting for Drugs and Services
			18 Quality Assurance for Drug Procurement
			19 Small-Scale Local Production
			20 Drug Donations

Chapter 13
Managing Procurement

164 PROCUREMENT

≡Summary

An effective procurement process ensures the availability of the right drugs in the right quantities, at reasonable prices, and at recognized standards of quality. Drugs may be acquired through purchase, donation, or manufacture.

The procurement cycle involves the following steps:
► review drug selections
► determine quantities needed
► reconcile needs and funds
► choose procurement method
► locate and select suppliers
► specify contract terms
► monitor order status
► receive and check drugs
► make payment
► distribute drugs
► collect consumption information.

The major procurement methods are open tender, restricted tender, competitive negotiation, and direct procurement, which vary with respect to their effect on price, delivery times, and workload of the procurement office.

Key principles of good pharmaceutical procurement include:
► procurement by generic name;
► limitation of procurement to the essential drugs list;
► procurement in bulk;
► formal supplier qualification and monitoring;
► competitive procurement;
► sole-source commitment;
► order quantities based on reliable estimate of actual need;

► reliable payment and good financial management;
► transparency and written procedures;
► separation of key functions;
► product quality assurance program;
► annual audit with published results;
► regular reporting of procurement performance indicators.

Alternative systems for supplying drugs to public health systems include the central stores system, autonomous supply agency system, direct delivery system, prime vendor system, and private pharmacy system. All involve pharmaceutical procurement.

Procurement may proceed under different models—annual purchasing, scheduled purchasing, or perpetual purchasing. Different combinations of these models may be used at different levels of the system or for different drugs. Whichever combination of supply systems and purchasing models is used, most public-sector drug procurement involves group purchasing, whereby one procurement office, whether public or private, negotiates contracts for members of a group with similar needs and interests.

Effective procurement is a collaborative process between the procurement office, with requirements for trained staff and appropriate management systems, and technical and policy committees, which make final decisions as to which drugs to buy, in what quantities, and from which suppliers.

Key considerations for financial sustainability include access to funds for drug purchase and support of the procurement office, access to foreign exchange for international procurement, and reliable payment mechanisms.

≡The pharmaceutical procurement system is a major determinant of drug availability and total health costs. In most developing countries, drug purchases represent the single largest health expenditure after personnel costs. Drugs also consume the major share of health-related foreign exchange.

An effective procurement process should

► procure the right drugs in the right quantities;
► obtain the lowest possible purchase price;
► ensure that all drugs procured meet recognized standards of quality;
► arrange timely delivery to avoid shortages and stockouts;
► ensure supplier reliability with respect to service and quality;
► set the purchasing schedule, formulas for order quantities, and safety stock levels to achieve the lowest total cost at each level of the system;
► achieve these objectives in the most efficient manner possible.

Given the impact of procurement activities on the operation and effectiveness of health services, it is essential that these activities be performed by trained staff using sound procedures, working in adequate offices with good communications, and with access to reliable inventory and consumption information. Good procurement management demands medical, pharmaceutical, managerial, economic, and often political expertise.

When a health system sets up a pharmaceutical procurement program, it is, in effect, developing a group purchasing program for health regions, districts, and individual health facilities. The purchases of group members may be financed centrally through government allocations or donor contributions, in a decentralized way through drugs fees, or through some combination of financing alternatives. Procurement may be managed through any of several organizational arrangements described in Chapter 6 and discussed later in this chapter.

Over the last twenty years, formal group purchasing programs have become common, and the factors that make them successful are known. Some countries have established successful public-sector procurement programs sharing many similar features. In other countries, procurement continues to be less successful, in spite of extensive reform efforts and substantial financial assistance from aid agencies.

Although the procurement chapters in this manual are written primarily with public-sector group purchasing programs in mind, the principles and procedures can be applied to either public or private procurement at any level from a rural aid post to a national health program. The details of procurement at the various levels may be slightly different, but the basic steps are the same.

≡13.1 The Procurement Cycle

The procurement cycle includes most of the decisions and actions that determine the specific drug quantities obtained, prices paid, and quality of drugs received.

Procurement is defined here as the process of acquiring supplies from private or public suppliers or through purchases from manufacturers, distributors, or agencies such as the United Nations Children's Fund (UNICEF), the World Health Organization (WHO), or bilateral aid programs. These sources may be used individually or in combination to meet the entire range of drug needs.

Steps in the procurement cycle are illustrated in Figure 13.1 and discussed in Chapters 14–20 and 40–44.

≡13.2 Factors Influencing Drug Prices and Total Costs

Given the limited budgets of virtually all health programs, drug procurement costs must be a concern of all policymakers, senior officials, essential drugs program managers, and procurement staff. Drug procurement costs include several different components; some costs are obvious and some are not.

Unit Prices

What determines the tender price of a container of 1,000 amoxicillin tablets or ten ampoules of adrenalin? There are many considerations involved in drug pricing by manufacturers and distributors, and many factors that cause prices to vary from country to country. A fundamental principle is that increasing competition among suppliers usually decreases drug prices.

Several factors influence competition and pricing in any pharmaceutical market. One main issue is how many different drug products, and different generic versions of the same product, are on the market. This can be influenced by government policies on registration, licensing for manufacturing and distribution, authority to prescribe and dispense, generic substitution, and price control. In some markets, suppliers may offer discount pricing to the public sector that is not necessarily related to purchase volume to establish or maintain market share. As discussed in Section 13.3, the type of procurement method used greatly influences how much competition there is among potential suppliers. The strategies and issues discussed in Section 13.4 also directly or indirectly influence the degree of competition and the degree of discount pricing available to the health system.

Purchasing Models and the Total Variable Cost of Purchasing

Drug acquisition prices are only one part of the total cost of drug purchasing; the other important components are the costs associated with holding inventory, the costs of operating the purchasing system, and the extra costs incurred when stockouts occur (shortage costs).

Although procurement offices typically concern themselves mainly with drug acquisition costs, the other cost components may increase the total purchasing cost by 50 percent or more of the acquisition costs. For each country's situation, total purchasing costs can be minimized by choosing the optimal purchasing model, as defined by

- ▸ the interval between orders—options include annual (one order per year), scheduled (periodic orders, for example, every three months), and perpetual (orders are placed whenever stock falls to a specified level);
- ▸ the safety stock targets, which vary according to supplier lead times, patterns of consumption, and service level objectives;
- ▸ the formula used for calculating the order quantity, which may be a fixed or variable quantity.

The choice of purchasing models is discussed in Chapter 15; these are not always simple decisions. The purchasing model may differ from one level of the supply system to another, or from one type or class of drug products to another. For example, consider a supply system with a central medical stores (CMS) and several regional warehouses that serve hospitals and major health centers (which then distribute to primary care facilities). The CMS might purchase most

Figure 13.1 Procurement Cycle

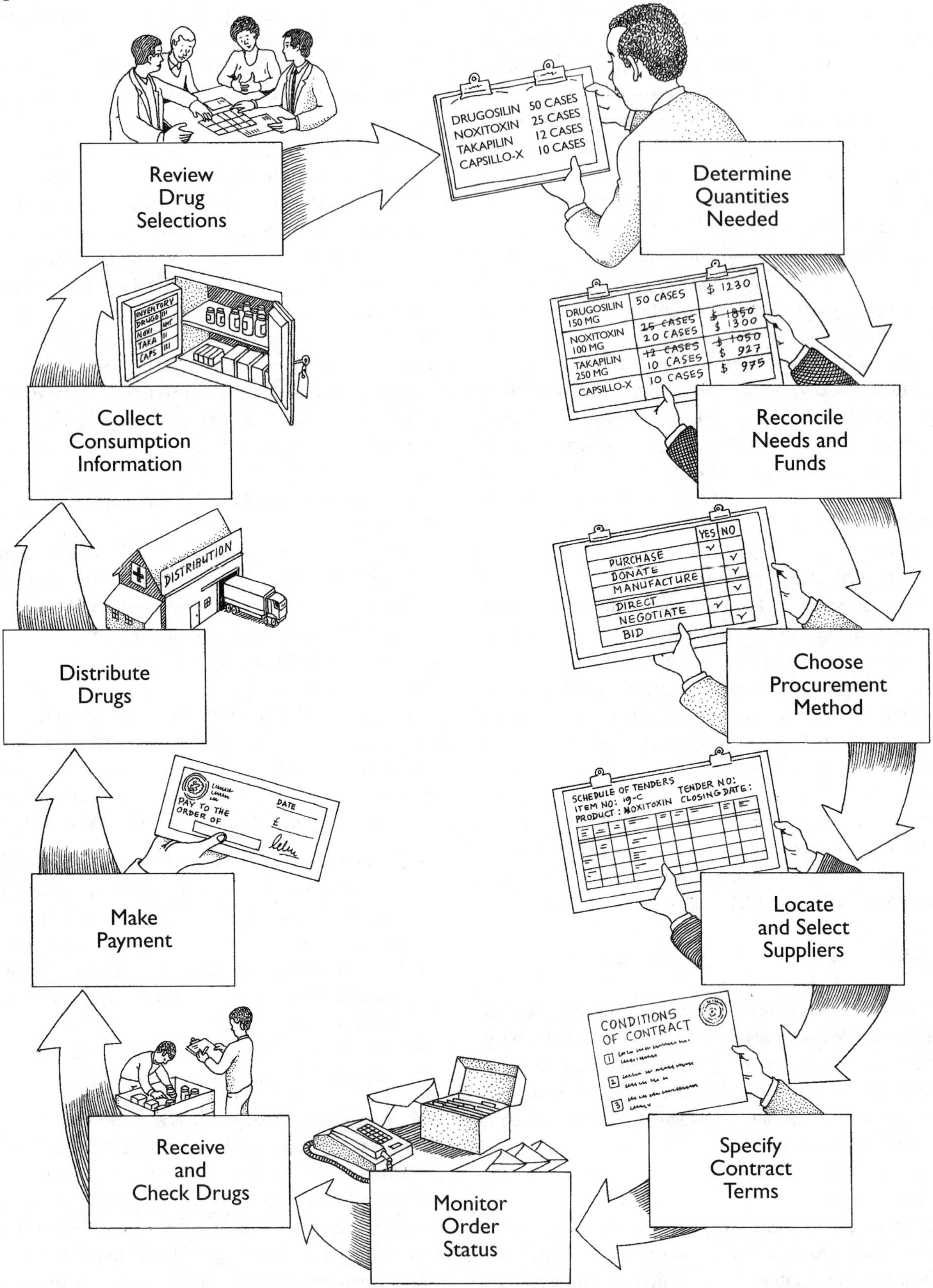

Figure 13.2 Impact of Hidden Cost on Total Cost

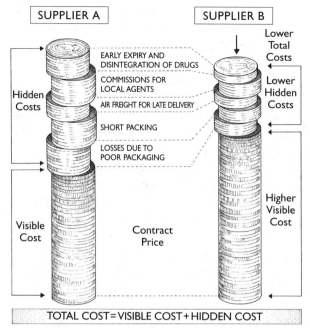

items through annual tender; however, in most countries, lower total costs can be achieved by purchasing at least some items more frequently. The regional stores might order from the CMS on a quarterly basis for most items. The health centers and hospitals might order most items monthly, with a weekly supplemental order, and so forth.

The purchasing model influences the types of procurement methods and purchasing contracts that can be used (see Section 13.3). However, this works both ways; individual country circumstances or laws may dictate one sort of procurement method or contract, which then limits the options for choosing the purchasing model. For example, if only fixed-quantity tenders are allowable under local laws, it will be difficult to implement a perpetual purchasing model. If all drugs are imported and average lead times are six to nine months, it will be difficult to avoid an annual purchasing system for most items.

The systems and formulas used to estimate needs and define order quantities vary with the purchasing model and with the availability of information on past consumption. The procedures for estimating needs for annual purchasing are discussed in Chapter 14; with scheduled or perpetual purchasing, order quantity can usually be determined by one of the formulas from Chapter 15. However, in some situations it may be necessary to use a procedure such as morbidity-based forecasting (see Chapter 14) to estimate needs for semiannual procurement.

The ultimate goal should be a combination of purchasing

models and distribution procedures that produces the lowest total costs to the supply system while providing the desired level of service to health facilities (and patients).

Chapter 41 presents total variable cost (TVC) analysis as a method for compiling and analyzing the total variable costs of inventory management: drug acquisition, inventory holding, purchasing operations, and shortage costs. These cost components have both stable and variable subcomponents, since some costs increase as the volume of activity increases, and some are stable through a wide range of activity levels (such as salaries of permanent staff). The TVC analysis examines stable and variable costs for potential savings and helps managers evaluate potential changes in procurement and distribution policy and procedure in terms of the likely impact on total variable costs.

Visible and Hidden Costs

As discussed above, the total variable cost has four components—drug acquisition prices, inventory holding costs, purchasing operations costs, and shortage costs. Some of these costs are easily visible to managers—the total expenditures for drug acquisition, or the salaries of procurement staff. However, the costs associated with shortages and poor supplier performance are not so obvious; hidden costs associated with poor performance by the supplier (or the procurement office) include

- ▸ increased acquisition costs due to emergency procurement, such as when a vital drug is ordered too late or the supplier fails to deliver on time;
- ▸ replacement costs when goods are lost or must be discarded because of poor packaging, improper shipping conditions, rapid spoilage, or short shelf life;
- ▸ replacement costs for short shipments, diluted liquid medications, wrong dosage forms, and so on;
- ▸ storage, port charges, and administrative expenses due to inefficient clearing procedures or lack of funds or proper documentation;
- ▸ health and economic costs of stockouts resulting from delay or default on delivery.

The potential impact of hidden costs on the total cost is illustrated in Figure 13.2. In this example, Supplier A has quoted a lower price, but additional expenses resulting from poor performance ultimately raise the total cost above that quoted by Supplier B. In a competitive tender, a large number of suppliers with varying technical and commercial backgrounds may tender, and their quoted prices will vary considerably. A system to investigate and monitor supplier performance is essential to minimize the impact of hidden costs.

≡13.3 Overview of Procurement Methods

There are numerous mechanisms by which governments, nongovernmental organizations (NGOs), and other organizations procure drugs. Virtually all pharmaceutical procurement methods, at any level of the health system, fall into one of four basic categories: open tender, restricted tender, competitive negotiation, and direct procurement. Each of these methods can be used with any of the standard purchasing models—annual, scheduled, or perpetual review—given the right sort of procurement contract.

Open tender: Open tendering is a formal procedure by which quotations are invited from any manufacturer or manufacturer's representative on a local or worldwide basis, subject to the terms and conditions specified in the tender invitation. International competitive bidding (ICB), as specified in World Bank (1993a) guidelines, is a tender open to all interested international manufacturers from World Bank member countries.

Restricted tender: In a restricted tender—also termed a closed bid or selective tender—interested suppliers must be approved in advance, often through a formal prequalification process that considers adherence to good manufacturing practices (GMPs), past supply performance, financial viability, and related factors. The prequalification process is often open to any supplier that wishes to apply.

Competitive negotiation: In competitive negotiation, the buyer approaches a limited number of selected suppliers (typically at least three) for price quotations. Buyers may also bargain with these suppliers to achieve specific price or service arrangements. Competitive negotiation is also called negotiated procurement or international or local shopping.

Direct procurement: The simplest, but usually most expensive, method of procurement is direct purchase from a single supplier, either at the quoted price or at a negotiated price. For single-source drugs (generally those under patent with no licensing agreements that allow other firms to manufacture the drug), the buyer has two choices—direct procurement or selection of an alternative drug.

In the initial stages of developing a new pharmaceutical procurement system, it may be best to start with a relatively simple purchasing method—some combination of negotiation with known suppliers, negotiating with international procurement agencies, and local tendering. This will bring supplies into the system quickly while a more elaborate tendering system is being developed. Some of the well-known international procurement agencies are listed in the annual *International Drug Price Indicator Guide* (MSH 1995).

International open tenders usually attract the most competitive offers and potentially the lowest prices. Although international tenders are sometimes limited to primary manufacturers, they should include reputable international procurement agencies to ensure that at least one reliable bid is received for most tendered products.

Virtually all professionally managed pharmaceutical procurement organizations—including private companies, international procurement agencies, and successful government drug procurement units—purchase most large-volume items by restricted tender or by competitive negotiation from a limited list of reliable suppliers.

Some procurement offices use a combination of methods: open or restricted tender for large-volume items, and competitive negotiation or direct procurement for lower-volume or emergency supplies (see Country Study 13.1).

An experienced pharmaceutical buyer may be able to purchase effectively using only competitive negotiations with known reliable suppliers. However, this requires excellent access to market intelligence and reliable, flexible access to funds for procurement. In most circumstances, procurement for the public sector is best done through formal competitive methods.

In many countries, laws and government regulations dictate the procurement method to be used, often based on the value of the goods being purchased. Chapter 16 focuses on the tender process and compares procurement methods (see Figure 16.1).

≡13.4 Good Pharmaceutical Procurement Practices

Pharmaceutical procurement practices vary widely from country to country. However, nearly two decades of experience with essential drugs programs and many more years of experience with large government-run pharmaceutical supply services in a number of countries (see Chapter 2) have suggested a number of key principles, which are summarized in Figure 13.3.

Procurement by Generic Name (International Nonproprietary Name)

Procurement by generic name—formally known as the international nonproprietary name (INN)—has become the standard for purchasing drugs that are available from multiple companies. Brand-name suppliers may compete, but their bids should be by generic name; they may offer lower prices for certain drugs than generic competitors, because they wish to keep their public-sector market share. It is reasonable to require that all drugs supplied to the health system be labeled with the INN featured

---

Country Study 13.1 Procurement through Combined Methods in Benin

The Benin Central Purchasing Office was established in 1991 as a single national supply and sales structure for essential drugs and medical supplies intended for public-sector health facilities and the private nonprofit sector. Following proce- dures defined by its Management Committee, the Central Purchasing Office makes purchases through selective tender, negotiated purchase, or direct purchase, as shown in the following table.

Method	Total Value	Purchasing Authority	Procedure
Restricted tender	over US$500,000	Tender Committee (composed of Central Office management, a representative from the Health Services Development Project, the two Technical Committee members, and a Ministry of Health representative)	One annual tender for drugs and another for medical supplies; Central Office undertakes prequalification of suppliers every two years and maintains supplier file (currently about thirty suppliers, 80 percent based in Europe); Central Office compiles list of specifications and file of invitations to tender; Tender Committee distributes invitations to tender to prequalified suppliers and analyzes and adjudicates tenders received
Competitive negotiation	US$70,000–$500,000	Technical Committee (consisting of two members, one representing development partners and one representing national institutions)	Central Office management analyzes supplier bids and submits results to Technical Committee for approval
Direct procurement	Up to US$70,000 (or above in cases of emergency)	Central Purchasing Office management	Direct negotiation with supplier; price compared with established international reference or determined on basis of three pro forma invoices

Source: Hessou and Fargier 1994.

---

prominently, in addition to any brand name that may be on the label.

Procurement Limited to Essential Drugs List or Formulary List

Virtually no health program can afford to purchase all drugs available on the market. A limited drug list or formulary, defining which drugs will be purchased, is one of the most effective ways to control procurement costs. It simplifies other supply management activities and reduces inventory holding costs as well (see Chapter 15).

The first step is to avoid generic duplication; after this, there are two main options for reducing the procurement list. The first combines the standard formulary process discussed in Chapter 10 with therapeutic category analysis as explained in Chapter 41. For example, a program regularly purchasing cimetidine, famotidine, and ranitidine (all therapeutically similar antiulcer drugs) might save substantial sums by restricting the formulary to one of these drugs and combining the estimated purchase volume into a single, much larger quantity of the drug selected.

The second approach also includes formulary selection and therapeutic category analysis and then takes them one step further through competitive tender within a selected therapeutic subcategory (as discussed in Chapter 41). The drug selection committee determines which subcategories are appropriate for category-based tendering and which drugs in those subcategories are acceptable equivalents. Then the tender request specifies only the therapeutic category rather than individual drug products. This strategy has been used for several years in some purchasing groups in the United States and in the eastern Caribbean and is similar to strategies used in Europe for establishing reimbursement prices.

Any change from one therapeutically similar product to another should be carefully considered, particularly for drugs used in chronic treatment; patients using these drugs need to be monitored during the changeover.

Efforts to limit the drug list by reducing therapeutic duplications will meet resistance both from drug suppliers whose products are removed from the procurement list and from some doctors (and some patients) who prefer a wider range of choices. Suppliers may issue dire public warnings of adverse impact on public health and patient care if their drugs are not purchased. The health system needs to be prepared to counter these claims with carefully designed information dissemination programs.

Resistance from doctors can often be overcome by

Figure 13.3 Good Pharmaceutical Procurement Practices

Procurement by Generic Name
► Use generic names (international nonproprietary names) for fair competition.
► Specify quality standards, not specific brands, for drugs with bioavailability problems.

Procurement Limited to Essential Drugs List or Formulary List
► Select safe, effective, cost-effective drugs.
► Use formal approval procedures for procurement of non-listed drugs.

Procurement in Bulk
► Concentrate purchases on limited list to increase quantities, reduce price.
► Specify divided deliveries.

Formal Supplier Qualification and Monitoring
► Use formal supplier qualification based on drug quality, service reliability, and financial viability.
► Approve suppliers before tendering (prequalification) or after (postqualification).
► Use a formal monitoring system to ensure continued supplier qualification.

Competitive Procurement
► Use competitive bidding on all but very small or emergency purchases to obtain the best prices.
► In restrictive tenders, only prequalified suppliers compete.
► In open tenders, suppliers must be evaluated after submission of bids.

Sole-Source Commitment
► All contracted drugs are procured from winning supplier.
► Enter into no separate deals with noncontracted suppliers.

Order Quantities Based on Reliable Estimate of Actual Need
► Develop reliable consumption records and morbidity data.
► Systematically adjust for past surpluses, shortages, stockouts.
► Adjust for expected program growth and changing disease patterns.

Reliable Payment and Good Financial Management
► Develop mechanisms for prompt, reliable payment.
► Prompt payment may bring down drug prices as much as bulk discounts.
► Financial mechanisms that establish separate drug accounts (for example, revolving drug funds) may allow the procurement cycle to operate on a separate schedule from the treasury cycle.

Transparency and Written Procedures
► Develop and follow written procedures for all procurement actions.
► To the maximum extent possible, make information on the tender process and results public.

Separation of Key Functions
► Separate key functions that require different expertise.
► Functions that involve different committees, units, or individuals may include selection, quantification, approval of suppliers, and award of contracts.

Product Quality Assurance Program
► Establish and maintain a formal system for product quality assurance.
► Include quality assurance product certification, inspection of shipments, targeted laboratory testing, and reporting of suspect products.

Annual Audit with Published Results
► Conduct an annual audit to assess compliance with procurement procedures, promptness of payment, and related factors.
► Present results to the appropriate public supervising body.

Regular Reporting on Procurement Performance
► Report key procurement performance indicators against targets at least annually.
► Use key indicators such as ratio of prices to world market prices, supplier lead times, percent of purchases made through competitive tendering, and planned versus actual purchases.

---

documenting the cost savings possible with the restricted procurement list and pointing out the benefits of year-round access to the limited list rather than sporadic access to a larger list of drugs.

Procurement in Bulk

Larger procurement volume makes favorable prices and contract terms more likely. Pooling of procurement volume from many facilities or from several states or countries, restriction of the drug list, and elimination of duplication within therapeutic categories lead to higher volumes for single items. In addition, the commitment to award a single contract for the entire volume of each item raises suppliers' interest in bidding and provides an incentive for them to offer competitive prices.

A contract award to a single supplier does not mean that the entire volume must be shipped at once. Many procurement services specify, as part of contract terms, divided deliveries over the period of the contract, sometimes to multiple delivery points. As discussed in Chapter 16, many supply systems use estimated-quantity tenders, with orders placed throughout the contract period as needed, using either a scheduled or perpetual purchasing model (see Chapter 15). These strategies allow optimal use of available storage and transport capacity, reduce inventory holding costs, and ease cash flow constraints.

Formal Supplier Qualification and Monitoring

All suppliers should be pre- or postqualified through a process that considers product quality, service reliability (and delivery time), and financial viability. The process for evaluating new suppliers can include formal registration, reference checks with past clients and international agencies, test purchases in small quantities, and informal local information-gathering (see Chapter 16). By first eliminating substandard suppliers from the tender process, prequalification ensures that the lowest tenderer is qualified and thus expedites adjudication. With postqualification, the supplier evaluation is done after bids have been received. Countries that do not have functional quality assurance testing laboratories must implement vigorous efforts to check references of new suppliers and should buy only from suppliers that are known to provide quality products.

Successful procurement agencies ensure continued good performance by suppliers through a formal monitoring system that tracks lead time, compliance with contract pricing terms, partial shipments, remaining shelf life, compliance with packaging and labeling instructions, and compliance with other contract terms. A file for each supplier should have copies of registration papers, references, special correspondence, complaints, and other anecdotal information. The information system should track the number and value of tender contracts awarded chronologically and the value of total purchases from the supplier by year.

Procurement programs using restricted tenders should make special efforts to seek out potential new suppliers to maintain competitive pressure on established suppliers.

Competitive Procurement

As discussed in Section 13.3, there are four main methods for purchasing drugs—restricted and open tenders, competitive negotiations, and direct purchase from a single-source supplier. Since inducing supplier competition is key to obtaining favorable pricing, public-sector programs should use some sort of competitive bidding program for all but very small or emergency purchases, if there are multiple suppliers for the needed items.

Sole-Source Commitment

Except when each health facility purchases drugs independently, all public pharmaceutical procurement systems are group purchasing programs. Effective purchase volume is maintained only if group members purchase all contracted drugs from the suppliers that hold the group contracts. Country Study 13.2 describes effective group purchasing by the Eastern Caribbean Drug Service.

If group members are free to make separate deals with other suppliers at will, the suppliers that participate in tenders will have little incentive to offer the best possible discounts to the group. The lack of "sole-source commitment" is one reason the CARICOM (Caribbean Community) purchasing program for the public sector was unsuccessful in the early 1980s.

The sole-source commitment must be monitored and enforced. Local or regional suppliers may offer low prices on a short-term basis in an attempt to break the purchasing cartel, but group members must resist these offers; otherwise, the group will fail and prices will rise to previous high levels.

Order Quantities Based on Reliable Estimate of Actual Need

Accurate estimates of drug requirements are needed to avoid stockouts of some drugs and overstocks of others. In addition, suppliers are most apt to compete for an estimated-quantity supply contract if they believe that the quantities specified are reasonably accurate.

The most accurate way to quantify pharmaceutical needs is to start with accurate past consumption data from all units being supplied. These data should be tempered by known or expected changes in morbidity patterns, seasonal factors, service levels, prescribing patterns, and patient attendance. Unfortunately, in many countries, consumption data are incomplete or do not reflect real need because the supply pipeline has never been full. In such cases, the morbidity-based and adjusted consumption techniques discussed in Chapter 14 may be needed for procurement quantifications.

Expert technical assistance in quantification may be useful in initial phases of the procurement program, with local officials participating to gain an understanding of the methodology.

When funds are not available to purchase all the drugs listed in estimates, it is necessary to reduce the list according to health system resources. The following three tools, discussed in more detail in Chapter 41, can help with prioritization:

VEN (vital, essential, nonessential) analysis classifies drugs in two or three categories, according to how critical the drug is for treating commonly encountered diseases. Priority is given to vital drugs.

Therapeutic category analysis applies cost-effectiveness, cost-benefit, and/or cost-minimization methods to help select the best drugs for treating common diseases.

ABC analysis assembles data from recent or projected procurements to determine where money is actually being spent, allowing managers to focus first on high-cost items when considering ways to reduce procurement costs.

Reliable Payment and Good Financial Management

Prompt, reliable payment can have as great an influence on bringing down drug prices as bulk discounts (see Country Study 13.2). Financial mechanisms such as decentralized drug purchasing accounts may allow the

Country Study 13.2 Pooled Procurement through the Eastern Caribbean Drug Service

The Eastern Caribbean Drug Service (ECDS) was established in 1986, with U.S. Agency for International Development (USAID) support, to manage the procurement process on behalf of member countries of the Organization of Eastern Caribbean States (OECS).

Prior to ECDS, the drug supply systems of OECS member countries were beset with problems: disorganized procurement and management functions and poorly trained staff contributed to chronic drug shortages in health facilities. Due to fiscal constraints, countries were slow to make payments to suppliers and incurred large surcharges. The drug prices paid by OECS states ranged 30 percent or more above those paid by other countries of the Caribbean, such as Barbados.

Design of the ECDS procurement program incorporated a number of key features:

Selective list: Procurement under ECDS is based on the *Eastern Caribbean Regional Drug Formulary*, compiled from individual country drug lists. Country-level purchasing officers may purchase nontender items independently.

Pooled quantities: Each year, participating countries project their expected purchases of formulary items and forward these estimates to ECDS, where ECDS management and technical staff review them. The individual projections are then aggregated into a single tender list.

Competitive bidding: Suppliers are prequalified for the ECDS restricted tenders. Prequalification is based on submission of a vendor registration form and reference checks with international agencies and procurement agencies that are listed as references. A single contract award is made for each tendered product to a primary and a secondary supplier. Unless quality or performance issues are a concern, the lowest tender price receives the primary award. There are no split tenders.

Supplier monitoring and quality assurance: The performance of all contract suppliers (lead times, partial shipments, quality problems) is monitored and reviewed annually to determine which suppliers should continue as registered participants. ECDS solicits verbal and written reports from member countries concerning potential product problems and follows up with testing at the Caribbean Regional Drug Testing Laboratory.

Variable purchase quantities by group members: ECDS estimates of purchase volume are not binding on individual countries or on ECDS, and there is no fixed procurement quantity or delivery schedule. All OECS member states are charged the same contract price, regardless of volume, for the duration of the contract period. All tender prices are CIF (cost, insurance, and freight) direct to the member country.

Sole-source commitment: Member countries are required to purchase items listed in ECDS contracts solely through the ECDS system, from contracted suppliers. ECDS monitors this annually, and there have been few violations.

Reliable payment mechanism: Payments to suppliers are managed by the Eastern Caribbean Central Bank (ECCB), where each participating country maintains a special revolving drug account. According to policy, ECDS will not forward a new order by a country to the contract supplier unless sufficient funds are on deposit in the ECCB account to pay for all outstanding orders. This system has encouraged suppliers to participate in the system without demanding prepayment, cash on delivery, or letters of credit on delivery.

Fifteen percent fee to group members: With each order, an administrative fee of 15 percent of the payment amount is made by ECCB to the ECDS account. This fee covers all ECDS operating expenses; no additional budget allocations have been required. ECDS became financially self-supporting in 1990.

The results of the ECDS procurement program have been extremely positive. Participating countries benefited from an average 44 percent reduction in acquisition price for tender products in the first ECDS tender cycle (1987–88). The figure below illustrates the price reductions experienced by individual countries, based on a market basket of the top twenty-five products in each country. Prices have continued to be well below those paid by the private sector, and below the prices paid by larger public-sector systems such as that of Barbados.

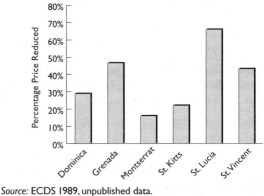

Average Price Reductions through Group Purchasing

Source: ECDS 1989, unpublished data.

---

procurement cycle to operate independently from the treasury cycle. Revolving drug funds can help achieve this separation by establishing their own bank accounts and their own working capital.

Efficient financial management systems are especially important if funds are limited and procurement priorities must be set. Being able to order drugs when needed and to pay for them on time has a positive effect on reducing both prices and stockouts.

Transparency and Written Procedures

The appearance and reality of fairness are essential to attract the best suppliers and the best prices. This can be achieved by maintaining transparent tender procedures: formal written procedures should be followed throughout the tender, and formal, explicit criteria should be used to make procurement decisions. Broad-based committees should have the sole authority to make contract awards. Information on the tender process and results should be public, to the extent permitted by law. At a minimum, both bidders and health units should have access to information on the suppliers and the prices for all winning contracts.

When the pharmaceutical tender process is secretive, it tends to be perceived as corrupt or unfair. There may be charges of cronyism. Whether true or not, such charges are damaging in that suppliers, health care providers, and patients lose confidence in the system. Unsuccessful suppliers may feel that they have no chance to win and consequently withdraw from future tenders (or submit only token bids). As the pool of potential suppliers decreases to a small set, price competition decreases and procurement prices will be much higher than necessary. Country Study 13.3 documents problems that can occur when the tender process is not transparent.

Separation of Key Functions

There are several key procurement functions, which typically require different expertise. In general, these functions should be handled by separate individuals, units, committees, or subcommittees. Such functions include

- selection of drugs;
- quantification of drug requirements;
- preparation of product specifications;
- approval of suppliers (prequalification or postqualification);
- adjudication and award of tender.

Without separation of functions, the procurement process is much more susceptible to influence by special interests. Suppliers or procurement personnel may be able to bias drug selection, manipulate orders to increase the quantities of certain drugs, prejudice supplier qualification decisions, manipulate the final award of tender, and slant product specifications to limit competition (by selecting less common dosage forms, for example).

Separation of key functions contributes to professionalism and accountability. Section 13.5 describes ways in which a procurement system can be organized to separate these functions.

Product Quality Assurance Program

An effective procurement program must ensure that the drugs purchased and distributed are of high quality, according to international standards. Chapter 18 discusses four components of an effective quality assurance system:

- selecting reliable suppliers of quality drugs;
- using existing mechanisms such as the WHO certification scheme (WHO 1995a);
- reporting product problems and performing post-marketing surveillance;

Country Study 13.3 Problems with Lack of Transparency in Tenders

In one Latin American country, the procurement office conducts two major tenders each year and separate procurements for items that either were not included on the tenders or were on the tenders but for which contracts were not awarded.

A survey of private-sector pharmaceutical companies in the mid-1990s found complaints that the process for evaluating tender offers and awarding contracts was not transparent. The procurement office did not release competing prices or winning bid prices, so companies had no way of knowing whether their offers were competitive or whether they were rejected for reasons not related to price.

The procurement office relied totally on postqualification, with criteria not clearly defined in writing, and contract awards were based on the subjective judgments of the purchasing committee. The survey found that competing companies had no confidence that their offers were fairly evaluated.

The procurement office did not always award contracts for all items on the tender, even though offers were received; criteria for determining the acceptability of offers were undefined, again lending an air of subjectivity to the process.

Quantities purchased did not correspond with annual estimates of need, and there were no defined procedures for procurement priorities and quantities of items on tenders.

Tender procedures were heavily centralized, with procurement office management determining which drugs to purchase and which suppliers would receive contracts, leading to questions about the transparency of the tender process. Although two Ministry of Health (MOH) representatives were on the purchasing committee, the procurement office had three members, and no representatives of health facilities were involved in the decisions.

One private-sector company reported that a contract that had been awarded was unilaterally canceled by the procurement office, and a separate contract for the same item was awarded to another company. The original company had already manufactured the quantity ordered, to MOH specifications for generic drugs.

Some companies stopped participating in the tender process, believing that they had no chance to win a contract. Only twenty-seven of more than one hundred local manufacturers participated in the first 1994 tender. On average, only two offers were received for each product, with a high of six for multivitamins. For forty-three of the seventy-eight products requested, only one offer was received. In the second 1994 tender, twenty-eight out of forty-eight products had multiple offers; the lowest price was not accepted in three cases (11 percent). Contracts for twenty products were not awarded, although offers had been received.

- performing targeted quality assurance testing.

When introducing drug procurement by generic name and new suppliers whose products are not familiar in the country, the procurement program must be particularly alert to product quality issues.

Some products vary substantially in formulation and bioavailability from supplier to supplier. When this difference is therapeutically significant, purchasers should be cautious about making changes in supplier from year to year, and particularly in accepting unknown suppliers. The Eastern Caribbean Drug Service (see Country Study 13.2) has identified a total of thirteen drug products that are deemed "critical"; they are tendered under generic name, but a new supplier's products must demonstrate pharmaceutical equivalence through testing before a change is made.

Even when new products are completely equivalent in content and effect, changes in dosage form can be problematic, requiring patient and provider re-education. For drugs used primarily in chronic therapy, there should be a significant cost benefit before changes are made.

Annual Audit with Published Results

At least once a year, the procurement unit should undergo an audit, which is a formal examination and verification of accounting books and records by accountants who specialize in audit procedures. *Internal audits* are conducted by auditors from within the government or organization. *External audits* are conducted by auditors from outside and are generally considered more credible, even if the process and findings are the same.

The annual external or statutory audit, conducted by a registered or licensed auditor, should include tests to ensure that the assets of the organization are safeguarded and accounted for; that the systems of internal controls and procedures are adequate to account for all the income and expenditures of the organization; and that the organization is complying with its constitution, rules and regulations, and management. This includes compliance with procurement procedures, promptness of payment, and inventory control.

The auditor should issue a statutory audit report in accordance with legal regulations of the jurisdiction and, in addition, should issue a detailed letter of comment to the management of the organization and to the appropriate public supervisory body.

Regular Reporting on Procurement Performance

The recent introduction of standard *indicators* for monitoring performance and program implementation (see Chapters 4 and 36) has been a significant advance in drug management. Standard indicators allow comparison of actual performance with targets, over time and among countries. Some indicators use a standard list of ten to twenty *indicator drugs* (also called tracer drugs or market basket of drugs; see Chapter 36).

The procurement office should be required to report on key procurement performance indicators at least annually. The assessment guide at the end of this chapter suggests some procurement indicators. Indicators such as average supplier lead time and percentage of key drugs in stock should be used to assess performance on a continuing basis. These indicators can be adapted by mission drug services, other nongovernmental organizations (NGOs), and even private health institutions seeking to control their drug costs. Figure 13.4 provides actual indicator data from several countries.

≡13.5 Organization and Management of the Procurement System

One important policy issue facing senior managers is how the procurement program will be structured and how responsibilities will be divided. Chapter 6 describes five different systems currently being used by governments to supply drugs to their health services:

Central stores system: Conventional central medical stores (CMS) approach, in which drugs are procured and distributed by a centralized government unit.

Autonomous supply agency system: Bulk procurement, storage, and distribution managed by an autonomous or semi-autonomous supply agency, *not* directly managed by the government.

Direct delivery system: A "non-CMS" approach, in which tenders establish prices and suppliers for each essential drug, which is delivered directly by suppliers to individual districts and major facilities.

Prime vendor system: Contracts for drug pricing negotiated with suppliers, and a separate contract negotiated with a single prime vendor to warehouse and distribute drugs for districts and major health facilities.

Fully private supply: Public-sector patients obtain pharmaceutical services from private pharmacies. Government may or may not reimburse the cost of those services, less any copayments. Reimbursement may go directly to the pharmacy based on claims submitted or to the patient (meaning that the patient pays the pharmacy and submits a reimbursement claim).

The important point in most models is the concept of group purchasing (also known as pooled procurement), whereby one procurement office, whether publicly or privately managed, negotiates drug supply contracts for members of a group with similar needs and interests (see Country Study 13.2). Group purchasing offers several potential advantages:

▶ Economies of scale reduce the cost of managing procurement.

▶ It is usually easier to sustain an effective program with only one procurement unit to staff and manage.

▶ A single procurement list for a large group of facilities increases effective volume and promotes reduced prices.

▶ Systems of finance and payment may be more readily managed to encourage suppliers to compete for contracts and to perform appropriately.

There are also potential drawbacks to a centralized procurement program:

▶ If it does not function well, all group members suffer: although the prices may be theoretically better than with individual facility procurement, the system may not provide the medicines needed in time to provide continuous care to patients.

▶ Without significant input from the participating facilities, it is likely that the centralized services will not meet users' needs very well.

▶ If there is substantial corruption in the central agency, the program will never function effectively.

Pharmaceutical purchasing and distribution systems have traditionally been heavily centralized in many countries, with little management input from lower levels. Many of these countries are now decentralizing procurement to the regional, state, or even local facility level, either by choice or because the central system has collapsed.

Decentralized management is not, however, a panacea. Potential problems include significantly higher prices, irrational procurement patterns based on the whims of prescribers or local procurement offices, irregular supply due to local inefficiencies, lack of access to funds, or poor management.

Worldwide experience suggests that group purchasing through one procurement office continues to offer clear advantages over totally decentralized procurement. However, group purchasing may be effectively combined with any of the supply system models mentioned above.

Supervision by Senior Management

Without political commitment to efficiency and active supervision by senior management, the procurement system will not function efficiently, regardless of how it is organized. The lack of modern financial management, accounting systems, and management and supervisory responsibility has doomed many pharmaceutical systems to chronic failure.

Figure 13.4 Comparison of Procurement Indicator Results for Nine Countries

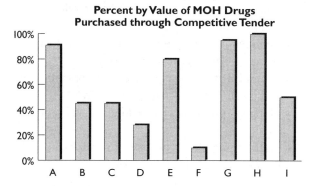

Percent by Value of MOH Drugs Purchased through Competitive Tender

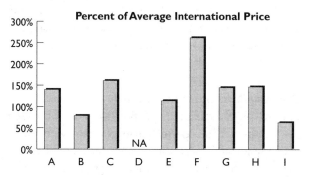

Percent of Average International Price

Key
A Mozambique 1993
B Ghana 1993
C Ecuador 1993
D Ecuador 1994
E El Salvador 1993
F Guatemala 1992
G Jamaica 1992
H OECS countries (Eastern Caribbean) 1993
I Nepal 1993

To manage the drug supply system, senior managers should demand and use regular reports from procurement and distribution agencies and from health facilities on expenditures, purchases, stock levels, order status, lead times, and budget status. If a system lacks the capacity to produce these reports in a timely manner, the tools to provide them should be top-priority components of new projects and programs. Senior managers should also maintain regular communications with facilities and staff; systems do not work very well if the senior managers have never visited any facilities outside the capital.

Many operations-level procurement managers have not had formal management training and may fail to appreciate the importance of setting such realistic and quantifiable procurement objectives as

▶ acquiring quality supplies at the best possible price;

▶ ensuring prompt and dependable delivery;

▶ following procedures that are transparent and not influenced by special interests;

► maintaining a procurement pattern that produces an even workload and constant supply to clients;

► achieving efficiency through use of appropriate systems and procedures;

► limiting total procurement operating costs to a given percentage of drug purchase costs;

► ensuring that revenue is adequate to support the office, and that finances are managed effectively;

► filling key positions with well-trained and motivated staff;

► maintaining effective working relationships with senior management and with clients.

It is the responsibility of senior management to make sure that these considerations are properly addressed and particularly to enforce transparency and fairness in the purchasing process.

Responsibilities in the Procurement Process

Effective procurement is a collaborative process between the procurement office, which manages many of the steps, and technical and policy committees, which should usually make the decisions about which drugs to buy, in what quantities, and from which suppliers. In a complex setting (such as a procurement program at the national level), the following division of responsibilities may be appropriate.

Procurement Office. The procurement office, which may be government operated or independent, collates information on drug needs, develops a proposed procurement list (based on clients' requirements), manages the tendering process and negotiates supply contracts (unless there is a separate tender board), and monitors performance of suppliers and clients.

Staff of the procurement office should not have the deciding voice in determining which products are purchased and which suppliers receive contracts; these decisions should be made by committees that include representatives from client facilities. This separation of powers helps ensure broad ownership of the system and avoid conflicts of interest. If the procurement office is independently operated, it is important that its operations be supervised by a board of directors that includes senior policy-makers of the health system.

Tender Board. In many countries, tendering and contract negotiation are done according to law by a government tender board, which either reports to the finance ministry or is independent of any ministry. In such situations, the procurement office prepares the list of requirements, and the tender board manages the tender process. The tender board also decides which suppliers get contracts in some cases; in others, the tender board makes rec-

ommendations to health officials. Whichever system is followed, it is essential that the health system provide technical input into the contract decision.

Drug Selection Committee. Often the same as the formulary committee or pharmacy and therapeutics committee, the drug selection committee should be composed of knowledgeable practitioners who evaluate competing drug products in various therapeutic categories to select those products that are most essential to the health system. A senior physician frequently serves as chair of the committee, and a pharmacist as organizing secretary. The committee reviews requests for additions to the procurement list, compares the cost effectiveness of drugs on the list, and recommends which drugs will be purchased and, when necessary, which drugs should be cut to accommodate budget constraints; it also determines which therapeutic categories, if any, are suitable for open tender by therapeutic class. The committee needs access to current, unbiased drug information and members who can synthesize such information for selection decisions.

Procurement/Tender Committee. A health system procurement committee should make final decisions on drug selection, procurement quantity, and supplier selection and approve the exact specifications for product description, packaging and labeling, and quality assurance standards. Such decisions should be based on recommendations from technical committees and subcommittees. The procurement committee reviews information on suppliers and determines which should participate in tenders (if a restricted tender is used) and which suppliers should receive contracts (unless such decisions are made by a separate tender board). The procurement committee should include senior officials from the highest level of government served by the procurement system, as well as officials from user facilities in the system. For example, a federal government program that serves teaching hospitals and regional health systems might include two or three representatives of the ministry of health, two or three representatives of regions, and one or two representatives of teaching hospitals.

In some countries, separate subcommittees are responsible for developing product specifications and for investigating suppliers' qualification for participation in tenders.

Procurement Office Staffing and Management Systems

The structure of the procurement office depends on the scope of the program, the availability of funds, and whether the office is managed as a government entity or as an independent agency.

Staffing Requirements. In general, the procurement office needs a director, an assistant director, and experienced technical staff, with at least one pharmacist capable of providing input for the development and refinement of procurement lists based on pharmacoeconomic principles.

Accounting and finance officers are necessary to manage the accounts and (in some systems) manage payment to suppliers. Automated offices need computer operators and at least one computer professional. Also needed are one or more clerical managers, one or more secretaries or clerks, a receptionist or telephone operator, maintenance staff, and, in some systems, a driver and security staff.

Staff in key procurement and distribution positions must be well trained and highly motivated, with the capability to manage the procurement process effectively. Unfortunately, in many countries, people are transferred just as they become competent in a position, and a new cycle of training and time lag between appointment and competence must begin.

Salaries for Procurement Staff. When procurement office salaries are too low to support an individual or a family, or much lower than for equivalent work in the private sector, corrupt practices and neglect of duties are much more likely to occur. These kinds of problems increase budgetary and/or donor funding requirements to replace the theft and waste that are inevitable in these circumstances. It is usually more cost effective to pay reasonable salaries in the first place and implement tough controls.

In some countries, restructuring the procurement office as an independent parastatal or privatized unit may be the only way in which adequate salaries can be paid to key staff.

Communications and Market Intelligence. To succeed in the international market, procurement programs need two sorts of key information: comparative price data and information about suppliers' capacity, reliability, and quality. Many procurement agencies work in an information vacuum, with no access to information on prices or on the performance record of international suppliers, and are essentially at the mercy of the suppliers.

Access to market intelligence depends on communications capacity. A fax and external telephone line are essential in modern procurement, even if all procurement is done through local suppliers. For international procurement, direct access to an overseas line is mandatory. Electronic communication (E-mail) is becoming more common throughout the world, and most procurement agencies of the future will need this capacity.

Comparative price information is currently available to countries through the *International Drug Price Indicator Guide* (MSH 1995). Options for obtaining and evaluating information about pharmaceutical suppliers are discussed in Section 16.4 of Chapter 16. A central repository of international information on worldwide supplier performance and tender pricing would be useful but has not proved feasible to date.

Tracking Performance of the Procurement System. A reliable management information system (MIS) is one of the most important elements in procurement. Lack of a functioning MIS or the inability to use it appropriately is a key cause of program failure.

The MIS must track all orders placed, the number and status of shipments and receipts, compliance with contract pricing, lead time of each order, payments made by the office or by group members, performance bond status, and the results of any investigations related to product quality.

It is important that the information system also track the performance of purchasing group members: number of orders placed, payments made, quantities actually purchased compared with estimates, purchases from all contract suppliers, and (if possible) drug purchases from noncontract suppliers. In all but the smallest procurement systems, the information system should be computerized.

Computerized procurement information systems depend on appropriate software (as discussed in Chapter 46). Key staff must be familiar with the software, and competent data entry personnel must be available.

Procurement Manuals. Achieving and sustaining an efficiently functioning procurement system are complex and demanding jobs. One key is the use of written policies and procedures that spell out how the procurement process should be managed and how the procurement system should operate. A comprehensive procedures manual can be time-consuming to develop but worthwhile if it is actively used to orient and manage staff. Good examples of procedures manuals are available that can be adapted to individual countries' requirements.

The *Eastern Caribbean Drug Service Procurement Manual* (MSH 1990) is a useful example for programs that base their tenders on prequalified suppliers and contracts that involve estimated quantities with periodic orders by purchasing group members. The *Nigeria Essential Drugs Project Drug Procurement Procedures and Documents Manual* (NEDP/MSH 1992) incorporates prequalification into World Bank international competitive bidding (ICB) procedures, with guaranteed quantity contracts and local supplier preference. Templates for bidding documents and procurement contracts are included in both these procurement manuals. UNICEF and the International Dispensary Association (IDA) have also developed standard procurement contracts and procedures. For purchasing through World Bank–financed loans, the World Bank's *Standard*

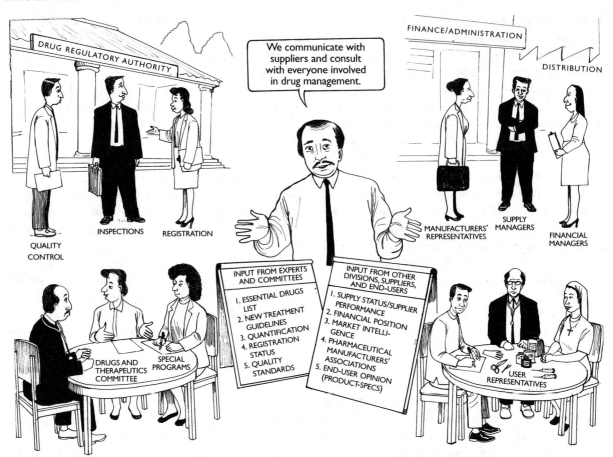

GOOD COMMUNICATION IS ESSENTIAL TO THE PROCUREMENT PROCESS

Bidding Documents for Procurement of Pharmaceuticals and Vaccines (World Bank 1993b) and *Procurement Technical Note 4.3.2* (World Bank 1993a) are essential references.

≡13.6 Financial Sustainability

Procurement programs cannot function effectively when funds are chronically inadequate. Traditionally, many countries have relied totally on the public budget to support drug procurement, with drugs provided free to both inpatients and outpatients. In some countries, pharmaceutical purchases have consumed 20 to 40 percent of the total public health budget. The reality is that few countries have sufficient budget capability to purchase enough drugs to cover the needs of all inpatients and outpatients, without supplementing the budget with some sort of cost recovery and/or donor support.

Sources of Funds for Pharmaceutical Procurement

Sources of funds for pharmaceuticals include government financing, user fees, health insurance, community co-financing, and donor financing. These options are described in Chapter 40 in terms of their efficiency, equity, sustainability, and feasibility.

The most important considerations for procurement are availability of funds, adequate access to foreign exchange, and regularity of access to funds. Government funds are sometimes released irregularly throughout the financial year, and regulations often specify that funds must be spent in the year for which they are allocated or be returned to the treasury. Together, these factors may make it difficult to operate proper procurement systems and to obtain the best prices.

Strategies such as decentralized financial management and revolving drug funds are increasingly being employed to separate drug procurement from the annual treasury cycle. This separation also usually requires some form of cost recovery, which is managed by the decentralized mechanism.

Uncoupling the procurement cycle from the treasury cycle has substantial management advantages. Inventory management improves when drugs can be ordered when needed rather than at an arbitrary point in the government fiscal year. When suppliers know that orders will be placed promptly after tendering and that payment will be made upon delivery, prices will be much more competitive.

Drug financing issues that affect the procurement system are discussed in Chapters 40–44. These issues include the actual revenue potential of user fee programs, equity aspects of user fees, management and accountability requirements for successful user fee programs, the role of health insurance and other social financing mechanisms, the role of donor financing, and related issues. For donor financing, grants and loans should be clearly distinguished: loans may be necessary to finance the start-up capital for a revolving drug fund or for a major emergency but are an undesirable mechanism for financing the recurrent costs of supplying drugs.

Access to Foreign Exchange

Pharmaceutical procurement almost always requires the largest outlay of foreign exchange in the health system. Shortage of foreign exchange continues to be a main constraint on international procurement in many countries and is often a primary rationale for seeking donor support for pharmaceutical purchases. In situations in which foreign exchange is constrained, it is important that procurement and pharmaceutical management systems be maximally efficient, that the best use be made of local supply sources, and that the best possible prices be obtained in international procurement. Sound documentation of actual needs and of efficient use of funds may help justify increases in foreign exchange allocation from the ministry of finance or central bank.

Reliable Payment Mechanism

Sustained low drug prices are possible only when a procurement program can guarantee prompt payment in full according to contract terms. Due to past payment problems, many countries are forced to pay in advance through irrevocable letters of credit for international purchases and, in some cases, for local purchases.

In the international market it is possible to develop a payment mechanism that does not require advance payment to suppliers. One example is the revolving drug fund described in Country Study 13.2; it should be emphasized that suppliers care only about payment performance, not the design of the payment scheme.

Revolving drug funds work only if there is the political will and financial capacity to replenish deposits in the fund each time purchases are made. The fund will soon vanish if this is not done. Examples are numerous: One cautionary tale comes from Central America, where a donor provided capital for revolving funds in several countries. Within a few years, all but one of the funds were totally decapitalized. One country continued with the program, but it experienced periodic problems with replenishing the account after purchases were made, resulting in delays in procurement and stockouts in health facilities.

Financial Support for the Procurement Office

Procurement services may be part of the warehouse and distribution operation or set up as a separate procurement office. In either case, salaries and operational costs of the procurement function must be covered. Options include

- support through the government budget;
- a periodic percentage payment to the office from group members, based on the invoice value of shipments;
- a percentage payment from group members at the beginning of the procurement cycle, based on the projected value of the total procurement, or at the end of the cycle, based on the actual value of total shipments;
- a regular payment from suppliers that ship to group members, based on a percentage of the invoiced value of the shipment (this method may be contrary to some countries' procurement integrity regulations);
- payment from group members in the form of a flat annual fee, based on total expenses divided by the total number of areas and independent institutions served.

The proper choice depends on the situation. There is some risk in tying a procurement office's reimbursement to the value of purchases by user facilities, as this may set up an incentive for the procurement office to increase, rather than decrease, prices and total purchases. Therefore, if this approach is used, checks and balances must be put in place, such as requiring that all major procurement decisions be made by user representatives. ■

180   PROCUREMENT

≡ Assessment Guide

Procurement Performance Indicators

► Percentage by value of ministry of health (MOH) drugs purchased through a central procurement system;

► Percentage of average international price paid for last regular procurement (indicator drugs);

► Percentage by value of MOH drug purchases that are on the essential drugs list or national drugs formulary;

► Percentage by value of MOH drugs purchased through competitive tender;

► Percentage by value of drugs purchased from local manufacturers;

► Average lead time for a sample of orders (calculated separately for all suppliers, local manufacturers, foreign suppliers);

► Average time for payment for a sample of orders (calculated separately for all suppliers, local manufacturers, foreign suppliers);

► Percentage of drugs (batches) subjected to quality control testing compared with target percentage to be tested;

► Percentage of drugs (batches) that failed quality control testing.

Procurement System Procedures

► What type of system is used to supply drugs to public facilities (CMS, autonomous agency, direct delivery, prime vendor, private pharmacies)?

► What type(s) of purchasing models are used at each level of the supply system (annual, scheduled, or perpetual)?

► How are order and tender quantities determined at each level of the system?

► How are suppliers selected for tender or negotiation—is there a formal qualification process?

► Is procurement done using generic names, brand names, or a mix?

► Are therapeutic equivalent drugs purchased through therapeutic subcategory tendering?

► How are lead times factored into ordering formulas and safety stock requirements?

► Are purchases limited to items on the formulary or essential drugs list?

► What constraints limit successful procurement in the public-sector drug supply system?

Procurement System Responsibilities

► Which agency or office is responsible for procurement of drugs and, if different, vaccines, contraceptives, diagnostics, and medical supplies?

► How are procurement responsibilities divided for drug selection, needs estimation, tender management, and contract awards?

► Are written procedures for tenders and contract awards in place and regularly followed? Is the tender process transparent?

► What type of procurement management information system is used, and what kinds of reports are produced?

► How does the purchasing office obtain information on comparative prices and new supplier performance?

► What kinds of computers and computer applications are used to manage procurement?

► Is information available to carry out ABC, VEN, or total variable cost analyses?

► What procedures are used for monitoring supplier performance and enforcing procurement contracts?

Procurement Finance

► What are the usual payment terms, payment lead times, and current debts owed to local and international suppliers?

► Is there a problem with foreign exchange status in the public sector? If so, what impact does this have on drug procurement?

► Are funds available as needed or is there a fixed schedule for release of funds (and what approvals are needed)?

► Do cost recovery and/or drug revolving funds contribute significantly to procurement financing?

► To what degree is procurement financed by donors or by loans from development banks?

≡Glossary

ABC value analysis: Method by which drugs are divided, according to their annual usage (unit cost times annual consumption), into Class A items (the 10 to 20 percent of items that account for 75 to 80 percent of the funds spent), Class B items (with intermediate usage rates), and Class C items (the vast majority of items with low individual usage, the total of which accounts for 5 to 10 percent of the funds spent). ABC analysis can be used to give priority to Class A items in procurement, inventory control, and port clearing.

Active ingredient: That portion of a drug that has therapeutic properties.

Annual purchasing: An inventory control system in which drug requirements are determined and orders are placed once each year.

Back order: An order for a product that is currently out of stock. Back orders are filled when a new supply of the product becomes available.

Basic unit: The smallest unit in which a drug can be conveniently dispensed or administered. It is used in quantification, reorder formulas, and comparison of prices of different-sized bottles or vials. Typical basic units are tablet or capsule, mL (for liquids), and gm (for ointments and creams).

Batch: The quantity of a drug produced in one production run.

Bid bond: A form of financial guarantee provided when a bid is submitted. The bond is forfeited if the successful bidder withdraws the offer or refuses to agree to the announced contract requirements.

Bulk purchasing: Procurement of drugs in large quantities in order to obtain lower unit prices. Generally done in a bid system in which all drugs are identified by their generic (INN) name.

Call for offers: A publicized invitation to bid. Used in tender or bid purchasing. Includes product specifications, required delivery date, closing date for submitting offers, and other requirements of participation.

Certificate of manufacture: A document accompanying a commercial invoice that is presented to the buyer's bank—usually one of the requirements of a letter of credit—certifying that the products have been manufactured, are ready for shipment, and are in safekeeping.

CIF (cost, insurance, freight): When a seller quotes CIF, the costs of goods, marine insurance, and transportation to the named destination point are included.

Competitive negotiation: A procurement method by which the buyer approaches a small number of selected potential sellers and bargains with them directly to achieve specific price or service arrangements.

Compound: To mix together the ingredients of a prescription or drug formula. Generally refers to a manual process performed for individual orders by a dispenser or pharmacist.

Consumption: The rate at which items are issued to clients or patients. This is also called demand (which is, in strict terms, the rate of requests or orders). Consumption is usually measured in terms of units consumed within a specific period.

Consumption-based estimate: Prediction of future drug requirements on the basis of historical information on drug consumption.

Direct procurement: The simplest but usually most expensive method of procurement, in which an item is purchased from a single supplier at its quoted price.

Disintegration: The breaking up of a tablet or capsule into granules or aggregates in an aqueous fluid.

Dissolution: The breaking down of fine particles into molecules or ions homogeneously dispersed in an aqueous fluid.

Estimated-quantity contract: A supply contract for a fixed period that stipulates an estimated total quantity, with the actual total quantity determined by orders placed as needed at the contract price during the contract period.

Excipient: An inert substance used to give a pharmaceutical preparation a suitable form or consistency.

Expiry date: The date appearing on a drug product and established by the manufacturer, beyond which the manufacturer will not guarantee the potency, purity, uniformity, or bioavailability of the product.

External packaging: The case, crate, carton, or other container in which individual packages are placed.

Financial guarantees: Deposits in the form of earnest money, bid bonds, performance bonds, or retention money required of suppliers to guarantee their participation once they have submitted bids or to ensure the complete fulfillment of contractual obligations by the supplier that wins the bid.

Freight: The fee charged for carrying goods. The word is also applied to the items to be carried, but the correct term for them is *cargo*.

GMPs (good manufacturing practices): Performance standards for pharmaceutical manufacturers established by WHO and many national governments; they include criteria for personnel, facilities, equipment, materials, manufacturing operations, labeling, packaging, quality control, and, in most cases, stability testing.

Group purchasing: Purchasing done by one procurement office on behalf of a group of facilities, health systems, or countries. Group members agree to purchase certain drugs exclusively through the group.

Hidden costs: Costs in addition to the contract price that are not paid to the supplier but are real costs to the supply system. These include costs associated with poor quality, late deliveries, defaults on deliveries, short packing, and other factors.

Identity: Presence of the correct active ingredient in a drug product.

Immediate container (package): The individual jar, bottle, box, blister pack, or other container in which a single group of items is packed.

International procurement services: Organizations such as UNICEF, WHO, IDA, ECHO, and other groups that supply drugs on a nonprofit basis.

Inventory: The sum of all items held in stock.

Inventory holding cost: Also known as *carrying cost*. The cost of holding one unit of an item in stock for a year. It may be expressed as a monetary amount or a percentage of purchase cost. This includes capital costs, costs associated with storage space, utilities, handling costs, losses due to waste and theft, and storehouse administrative costs. These costs may be 20 to 40 percent of the purchase price for a year.

Inventory value: The sum of the number of units of each item on hand or in storage in the system, times the current unit price of each item.

Issue unit: The quantity or size of each item counted as one inventory issue unit in the stock records. For example, in some supply systems, the unit for tetracycline capsules might be one bottle of 100 capsules, and in others it might be one capsule. This is not necessarily the same as the basic unit or comparison unit, although they may be the same (see Chapter 46 for a discussion of units).

Item: A unique product for inventory purposes. In drug supply, an important issue is whether generic equivalent items are treated as the same item or whether different brands of the same generic product are treated as different items. The item is sometimes called a stock-keeping unit (SKU), which is *not* the same as an *issue unit*.

Lead time: The time interval needed to complete the procurement cycle. It begins at the time the need for new stock is recognized and ends when that stock is received and available for issue.

Lead-time analysis: A systematic study of the components of lead time, aimed at discovering areas in which lead time can be reduced.

Line item: A product listed on an order or invoice. Each separate product on the document is one line item, no matter what quantity of the product is listed.

Make or buy: A management decision that involves the analysis of the cost and potential benefits of manufacturing a product rather than buying it on the open market.

Open tender: The formal procedure by which quotations for the supply of drugs under their generic names are invited from any local or international manufacturer or representative, subject to the terms and conditions specified in the tender invitation.

Opportunity cost of inventory: The cost of monies tied up in inventory. If average inventories increase, then capital invested in inventory increases proportionally. Since these funds invested in inventory could be used for other expenditures, they should be valued at current bank interest rates.

Order quantity: The amount of stock to be ordered (or that has already been ordered) via requisition or purchase order from a supplier or supply point.

Order status: The status of an order with respect to the specific tasks that must be performed for the order to be delivered to the buyer.

Payment terms: The conditions arranged between a buyer and a seller regarding the method of reimbursement. Letters of credit and commercial or deferred terms are the most common.

Performance bond: A form of financial guarantee that the supplier deposits when accepting the contract. This amount is forfeited if the supplier defaults on the contract.

Perpetual purchasing: A procurement model in which stock levels are reviewed continually, and orders are placed whenever stock levels fall below designated or calculated reorder points.

Pooled procurement: Another name for group purchasing.

Population-based estimate: Prediction of future drug requirements based on the demographic composition of the population, disease patterns, and norms for treatment.

Port clearing: The process of locating items in port, obtaining the proper import documentation, paying the necessary fees, and inspecting the drugs for damage during transit.

Potency: The extent to which a drug contains the specified amount of the active ingredient.

Procurement: The process of acquiring supplies, including those obtained by purchase, donation, and manufacture.

Procurement period: The period of time between an order to a supplier and the next scheduled order.

Product file: A card or ledger file that records the technical specifications and performance of suppliers for each product.

Purchasing costs: All costs involved in placing and monitoring an order, including communication costs, the cost of preparing an order or tender and of subsequent negotiations, the staff time involved in routine checking of inventory levels, costs of receiving goods, any related special fees, and administrative costs. In practice, the cost of each order is estimated by dividing the total annual direct and indirect costs of the purchasing department by the number of orders placed in the year.

Purity: The extent to which drugs are free from potentially harmful contaminants, significant quantities of other drugs, bacteria, or other microorganisms.

Quality assurance: The management activities required to ensure that the drug that reaches the patient is safe, effective, and acceptable to the patient.

Quality control: The testing of drug samples against specific standards of quality.

Quantification: Estimation of the quantities of specific drugs needed. Financial requirements for purchasing the quantities are also usually calculated.

Restricted tender: Procurement procedure in which participation in bidding is limited to suppliers that meet certain prerequisites or have previously registered as suppliers.

Retention money: See **Performance bond**.

Scheduled purchasing: Procurement model in which stock levels are reviewed periodically at set times during the year and orders are placed as necessary.

Secondary manufacture: The processing of medicinal substances, usually together with excipients, to produce a pharmaceutical dose form.

Shelf life: The length of time a material may be stored without affecting its usability, safety, purity, or potency.

Shortage cost: If emergency supplies are purchased to address a stockout, any increment in purchase price is a shortage cost. This cost is more difficult to quantify than holding cost but may still be significant. Loss of customers, decreased goodwill, and decreased sales are also real shortage costs if drug sales are involved.

Specifications: A precise description of an item to be procured, including any special requirements.

Stock: The items stored in the warehouse or facility (or health system). There are several types of stock:

Pipeline stock: Stock that is in transit at various stages of the purchasing and distribution cycles.

Quarantine stock: Stock that has been physically received in the storage facility but is held separately and not available for issue. There may be a need to confirm product quality or compliance with the contract, or the transfer to working stock might be delayed pending completion of necessary documents.

Safety stock: The buffer or minimum stock that is kept on hand to protect against stockouts. If there is no safety stock, stockouts will occur when deliveries are delayed or when there is an unexpected increase in demand. In theory, the safety stock is separate from the working stock, but in practice there is no separation of the two, and safety stock sometimes must be issued.

Seasonal stock: Stock that is acquired with the expectation that it will be needed to satisfy seasonal demand—for example, cough and cold medications in the winter. This stock is also part of the working stock once it is in the warehouse.

Vertical program stock: Stock that is not available on open request but is held for sole use by a vertical program, such as family planning or Expanded Programme on Immunization (EPI). This stock may also be separated into working stock and safety stock.

Working stock: Stock that is on hand in the warehouse or storeroom and is shipped to requesting operating units. Working stock fluctuates as orders are filled and new stock arrives.

Other stock: Stock that is not usually issued but may be needed for purposes such as shipping or repackaging. May include items such as shipping tape, boxes, and labels.

Supplier: Any individual or company that agrees to provide medications, regardless of whether that party is the manufacturer.

Supplier file: A record kept for each supplier indicating when orders were placed, when they were received, what kind of service the supplier provided, and the quality of the product provided.

Supplier reliability: The past performance of a supplier in terms of the drug and packaging quality, timeliness of delivery, and level of service provided.

Tendering: The procedure by which competing bids are entered for a particular contract.

Trade terms: A set of standard terms to describe the buyer's and seller's responsibilities in international trade—a list is found in Chapter 17.

VEN system: A system of setting priorities for purchasing drugs and keeping stock, in which drugs are divided according to their health impact into vital, essential, and nonessential categories.

Wholesaler: A dealer who purchases supplies from a manufacturer and resells them to the ultimate buyers.

≡ **References and Further Readings**

★ = *Key readings.*

Broun, D. 1994. *Procurement of pharmaceuticals in World Bank projects.* Washington, D.C.: World Bank.

★ FIP (Fédération Internationale Pharmaceutique). 1992. *FIP guidelines for drug procurement.* Amsterdam: FIP.

Hessou, C. P., and M. P. Fargier. 1994. Benin central purchasing office for essential drugs: A new experiment. *Essential Drugs Monitor* 18:8–9.

HID (Health Information Designs). 1988. *USAID handbook and field operations manual for pharmaceutical procurement in Latin America and the Caribbean.* Arlington, Va.: HID.

IDA (International Dispensary Association). 1994. *General purchase conditions of the International Dispensary Association: Nonprofit procurement of medicines and medical supplies.* Amsterdam: IDA.

MSH (Management Sciences for Health). 1990. *Eastern Caribbean Drug Services procurement manual.* Boston: MSH.

MSH (Management Sciences for Health). 1992a. *Managing drug supply training series.* Part 1. *Policy issues in managing drug supply.* Boston: MSH.

MSH (Management Sciences for Health). 1992b. *Managing drug supply training series.* Part 2. *Financing and financial management of drug supply.* Boston: MSH.

MSH (Management Sciences for Health). 1992c. *Managing drug supply training series.* Part 3. *Supply management.* Boston: MSH.

★ MSH (Management Sciences for Health). 1995. *International drug price indicator guide.* Boston: MSH.

NEDP/MSH (Nigeria Essential Drugs Project and Management Sciences for Health). 1992. *Drug procurement procedures and documents manual.* Boston: MSH.

UNIDO (United Nations Industrial Development Organization). 1987. *A study to assist in improving management skill for procurement of pharmaceutical chemicals, their intermediates, and drugs (pharmaceutical formulations).* Vienna: UNIDO.

WHO (World Health Organization). 1984. *Report of a WHO meeting on drug policies and management: Procurement and financing of essential drugs.* Geneva: WHO.

WHO (World Health Organization). 1995a. *The use of essential drugs.* Technical report series no. 850. Geneva: WHO.

WHO (World Health Organization). 1995b. *Use of the WHO certification scheme on the quality of pharmaceutical products moving in international commerce.* Geneva: WHO.

★ World Bank. 1993a. *Procurement technical note number 4.3.2: Procurement of pharmaceuticals and vaccines.* Washington, D.C.: World Bank.

★ World Bank. 1993b. *Standard bidding documents for procurement of pharmaceuticals and vaccines.* Washington, D.C.: World Bank.

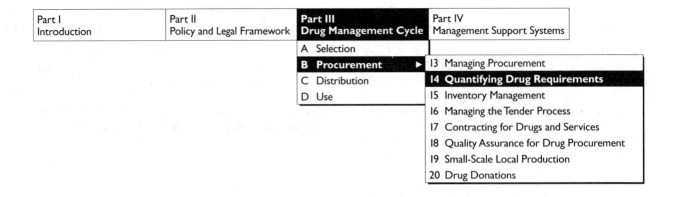

| Part I | Part II | **Part III** | Part IV |
| Introduction | Policy and Legal Framework | **Drug Management Cycle** | Management Support Systems |

A Selection
B Procurement ▶ 13 Managing Procurement
C Distribution **14 Quantifying Drug Requirements**
D Use 15 Inventory Management
16 Managing the Tender Process
17 Contracting for Drugs and Services
18 Quality Assurance for Drug Procurement
19 Small-Scale Local Production
20 Drug Donations

Chapter 14
Quantifying Drug Requirements

≡ Summary

The methods and strategies described in this chapter can be used as tools to

> ► *prepare and justify a drug budget;*
> ► *plan for new and expanding programs;*
> ► *optimize drug budgets based on priority health problems to be treated and the most cost-effective treatment approaches;*
> ► *calculate emergency needs for disaster relief and epidemics;*
> ► *resupply an existing supply network that has become depleted of products;*
> ► *compare current drug consumption with public health priorities and usage in other health systems.*

The quantification method selected must be chosen in light of the resources and information available.

The consumption method, which uses data on drug consumption, gives the most accurate prediction of future needs. Large, well-established drug supply systems rely primarily on the consumption method. To be reliable, the consumption data must come from a stable supply system with a relatively uninterrupted supply and a full supply pipeline. Consumption data may or may not reflect rational prescribing and use of drugs.

The morbidity method forecasts the theoretical quantity needed for the treatment of specific diseases. This method requires reliable data on morbidity and patient attendances (visits to health facilities) and uses standard treatment guidelines to project drug needs. This is the most complex and time-consuming method, and there can be major discrepancies between projections and subsequent utilization. Still, this method is often useful and may be the most convincing approach for justifying a budget request.

If there is no reliable information on past consumption or morbidity, it is possible to extrapolate utilization from other facilities, regions, or countries. The adjusted consumption method is flexible enough to apply to various situations and can be either population or service based. Service-level quantification of budget requirements can be applied when only budget requirements, and not specific drug quantities, are needed. It provides a clear, logical, one-page justification of drug financing requirements.

There are several critical issues common to all methods. The drug list is the central component and must be produced in a format suitable to the type of quantification. In a new supply system, or one in which shortages have been widespread, quantification estimates must be adjusted because the supply pipeline must be filled. The lead time has a major impact on quantities required for safety stocks. In virtually all supply systems, it is necessary to adjust for losses due to wastage and theft.

Quantification estimates can be cross-checked by combining different methods. No matter which method is used, there may be a gap between the initial estimates of drug needs and the allocated budget. The quantification process itself may help justify an increase in the budget, but often the quantification estimates have to be adjusted and reconciled to fit available funds. The choice between manual and computerized quantification may be dictated by circumstances, but the process is much easier with computer assistance. Quantification can be centralized, or it can be decentralized to staff of peripheral warehouses and health facilities. The personnel and time requirements depend on the quality and accessibility of source data and on the type and scope of quantification. A large-scale quantification often requires several months to carry out.

≡ 14.1 Methods of Quantification

Drug needs can be quantified by using one or a combination of four standard methods. Quantification involves estimating the quantities of specific drugs needed for a procurement. Most quantification exercises also estimate the financial requirements to purchase the drugs. The quantification methods described in this chapter are normally used to forecast needs for an annual or semiannual procurement. They are not usually used to calculate routine order quantities in an established supply system that uses scheduled purchasing (periodic orders) or perpetual purchasing (orders placed whenever need arises). In such situations, one of the reorder formulas presented in Chapter

15 is used to calculate the optimal order quantity and order interval for each item. The goal is to maintain the most cost-effective balance between service levels and inventory costs.

Major Options for Quantification

The four general methods discussed in this chapter are

1. consumption method
2. morbidity method
3. adjusted consumption method
4. service-level projection of budget requirements

The *consumption method* uses records of past consumption of individual drugs (adjusted for stockouts and projected changes in drug utilization) to project future need (see Section 14.4).

The *morbidity method* estimates the need for specific drugs based on the expected number of attendances, the incidence of common diseases, and standard treatment patterns for the diseases considered (see Section 14.5).

The *adjusted consumption method* uses data on disease incidence, drug consumption or utilization, and/or drug expenditures from a "standard" supply system and extrapolates the consumption or utilization rates to the target supply system, based on population coverage or service level to be provided (see Section 14.6).

Service-level projection of budget requirements uses the average drug procurement cost per attendance or bed-day in different types of health facilities in a standard system to project drug costs in similar types of facilities in the target system (see Section 14.7). This method does not estimate quantities of individual drugs.

Relative Predictive Accuracy of Quantification Methods

Quantification of drug requirements is inherently imprecise, due to the many variables involved. Useful results depend as much on art as on science.

The most precise method for forecasting drug usage is the consumption-based approach, provided the source data are complete, accurate, and properly adjusted for stockout periods and anticipated changes in demand and use. This method does not normally address the appropriateness of past consumption patterns, which may or may not correspond with public health priorities and needs. Thus, irrational drug use may be perpetuated by total reliance on the consumption method. If stockouts have been widespread for long periods, it may be impossible to apply this method accurately.

Morbidity-based quantification is the most complex and time-consuming. In many countries, it is very difficult to assemble valid morbidity data on more than fifty or so diseases; therefore, some needs will be overlooked in the quantification. Data on patient attendance are often incomplete and inaccurate, and it is difficult to predict what percentage of prescribers will actually follow the standard treatment regimens used for quantification. Despite these constraints, this method may still be the best alternative for planning a procurement or for estimating budget needs in a supply system or facility in which a limited range of health problems accounts for virtually all drug consumption, such as a small primary care system or a special-purpose hospital.

Adjusted consumption is the method generally used if neither the consumption-based nor the morbidity method is feasible. This method is most likely to yield accurate projections when used to extrapolate from one set of facilities to another set that serves the same type of population in the same type of geographic and climatic environment. If the method is applied by drawing standard data from another country (such as the Nordic utilization data), the results will be only a rough estimate of need. Even when target and standard facilities are closely matched, quantification estimates are suspect, because it is a big leap to assume that disease incidence, utilization patterns, and prescribing habits will be essentially the same in both settings. Still, this method may be the best alternative in the absence of suitable data for the consumption- or morbidity based method. It is also useful for cross-checking projections made with other methods.

Service-level projection of budget requirements produces a rough estimate of financial needs for drug procurement. The method relies on two assumptions: that the "standard" system (used for comparison) and the target system are comparable in terms of patient attendance and bed-days per type of facility, and that the patterns of drug use are roughly the same in both systems. Despite its limitations, this method can be useful in predicting drug costs in a new system or in a system in which no data are readily available. Figure 14.1 summarizes the applications and limitations of the four major quantification methods.

≡ 14.2 Applications of Large-Scale Quantification

Large-scale quantification is normally appropriate for

Forecasting for large-scale procurement: Formal quantification is mandatory before each annual or semiannual procurement. These estimates need to be accurate to avoid stockouts, emergency purchases, and overstocks and to maximize the impact of procurement funds. The consumption method is the first choice, cross-checked to assess the appropriateness of usage patterns. When consumption data are unreliable, it may be necessary to apply the morbidity and/or adjusted consumption methods for an initial quantification, switching to the consumption method once reliable data can be compiled (see Country Study 14.1).

Estimating budget requirements: In many countries, the annual pharmaceutical procurement budget is determined by adding a fixed percentage to last year's request or allocation to allow room for expected cuts by the ministry of finance. Both budget requests and cuts are frequently prepared without reliable estimates of actual

Figure 14.1 Comparison of Quantification Methods

Method	Uses	Essential Data	Limitations
Consumption	First choice for procurement forecasts, given reliable data Most reliable predictor of future consumption	Reliable inventory records Records of supplier lead time Projected drug costs	Must have accurate consumption data Can perpetuate irrational use
Morbidity	Estimating need in new programs or disaster assistance Comparing use with theoretical needs Developing and justifying budgets	Data on population and patient attendances Actual or projected incidence of health problems Standard treatments (ideal, actual) Projected drug costs	Morbidity data not available for all diseases Standard treatments may not really be used
Adjusted consumption	Procurement forecasting when other methods unreliable Comparing use with other supply systems	Comparison area or system with good per capita data on consumption, patient attendance, service levels, and morbidity Number of local health facilities by category Estimation of local user population broken down by age	Questionable comparability of patient populations, morbidity, and treatment practices
Service-level projection of budget requirements	Estimating budget needs	Utilization by service levels and facility type Average drug cost per attendance	Variable facility use, attendance, treatment patterns, supply system efficiency

needs. This cycle can be broken with rational, well-documented quantification.

Although consumption-based quantification is the best guide to probable expenditures, the morbidity-based method may be the most convincing documentation for a budget request. Adjusted consumption is useful for checking and justifying either consumption or morbidity methods.

For some budgeting purposes, quantification may not need to specify individual drug quantities but only estimated financial requirements. This can be done by projecting costs using the service-level method.

Forecasting for new programs: When drugs are needed for a new full-service health system or vertical program (such as family planning or control of diarrheal disease), large-scale quantification serves two purposes: to establish funding requirements for procurement and to develop the initial procurement list. In most situations, the consumption-based method is not feasible, and some combination of morbidity-based and adjusted consumption methods must be used for the initial quantification.

Forecasting for assistance projects: A donor organization may undertake ad hoc quantification studies to plan procurement needs in the context of a development project. When local consumption data are not sufficiently reliable for quantification, the morbidity or adjusted consumption methods are required, either singly or in combination.

Estimating drug requirements in emergency relief situations: In emergencies such as floods or earthquakes, the first step is to provide emergency kits quickly (Chapter 27). As local health problems become clear, a morbidity-based method can be used to project requirements in the short and medium term, until the regular supply system can resume services. Country Study 14.2 describes quantification for a cholera epidemic in a Latin American country.

Comparing actual drug consumption with theoretical need: In most functional supply systems, the regular procurement quantification is based on past consumption. However, it is useful to periodically compare consumption with theoretical need based on public health priorities. The morbidity-based method provides the most informative comparison, but simply comparing consumption data from different systems is worthwhile.

≡ **14.3 Critical Issues in Quantification**

Several issues must be addressed in any large-scale quantification:

► preparing an action plan for quantification;
► using centralized or decentralized quantification;
► using manual or computerized methods for quantification;
► estimating the time required;
► developing the drug list;
► filling the supply pipeline;

Country Study 14.1 Large-Scale Quantification in Zimbabwe

The Zimbabwe Essential Drugs Action Programme (ZEDAP) was established in 1986. In 1987, quantification was done to predict the real national drug requirements and the costs in foreign and local currency terms. The drug purchase was expected to cover all public health care facilities, and the sources of supply would likely be both local and foreign.

A WHO team consisting of a physician, a pharmacist, and an economist worked with Zimbabwean staff to produce the estimates, using a computer spreadsheet program to facilitate the calculations.

The vast majority of the estimates were made using the morbidity method, since standard treatment guidelines had already been developed and published. Data for health problem frequency (morbidity) were not available for all facilities but were extrapolated using standard facilities at four different levels to represent health problem frequency for (1) central hospital inpatients, (2) general and district hospital inpatients, (3) all hospital outpatients, and (4) rural health center patients. The common denominator used was patient cases for the hospitals and population coverage for the health centers. Standard treatment guidelines and health problem frequency were differentiated for patients under five years old and those aged five years or older.

Intravenous solutions and drugs for psychiatric patients were estimated using the consumption method.

The team estimated requirements and costs for 159 essential drugs. The estimated cost was combined with costs for other essential drugs not included in the quantification to prepare a budget proposal, which was approved by the Ministry of Finance.

Since this exercise, annual quantification exercises continue, with regional and provincial stores managers meeting for three days a year to prepare an annual procurement list. The consumption method is now the basis for calculations, although population figures, morbidity data, and prescribing practices are considered in the decisions.

► considering the impact of lead time;
► adjusting for losses due to wastage and theft and for program growth;
► cross-checking estimates produced by quantification;
► estimating total procurement cost;
► adjusting and reconciling final quantities.

Preparing an Action Plan for Quantification

Perhaps the most critical step in any large-scale quantification is preparing and then following a sound action plan through each step of the quantification. Essential points include:

► Name the official or office that will manage the process and define roles and responsibilities;

► Form a working group to coordinate activities of the offices, departments, and facilities involved;
► Define the objectives and coverage of the quantification;
► Examine the availability of data and choose the best quantification method in light of objectives and available data and resources (personnel, funding, computer capacity);
► Develop drug lists and data collection forms;
► Develop standard treatment guidelines (if applicable);
► Train staff in the applicable quantification method and in data collection and analysis;
► Develop a workplan and timeline for quantification, with realistic deadlines for each phase;
► Manage quantification according to plan (adjusting for inevitable delays and unexpected constraints);
► Adjust estimated quantities as needed;
► Evaluate the quantification process and plan improvements to resolve problems encountered.

The World Health Organization (WHO) manual *Estimating Drug Requirements* (WHO/DAP 1988) discusses how to develop a good action plan and manage the quantification process.

Using Centralized or Decentralized Quantification

Most supply systems have traditionally managed large-scale quantification at the central level. The increasing trend toward decentralizing this responsibility adds significantly to ownership of the results at health facilities and, if managed properly, can improve the accuracy of the results. However, a centralized approach is generally more efficient when the supply system is in equilibrium, with adequate supply to all levels.

A common approach to decentralizing quantification is to have each responsible office or facility compile its own estimates, based on a common list of approved drugs. The list can be sent directly to the procurement office, which compares the list with past consumption, clarifies any questions directly with the client, and compiles the master list for procurement. Reviews at the district and province levels before submission to the procurement office may increase the validity and ownership of estimates, at the cost of adding time to the process.

It is important to make sure that consumption is not double counted: that is, if all drugs come to facilities through a central warehouse, and a needs estimate is submitted by both the central warehouse and the client facilities that order from the warehouse, the total estimate for

Country Study 14.2 The Morbidity Method and a Cholera Epidemic in a Latin American Country

In 1991, a cholera epidemic in Latin America spread rapidly to most regions of one country within six months. A quantification was carried out to determine drug supply needs to treat cholera patients.

Target Coverage. All cholera patients requiring treatment through hospitals, clinics, and community health workers were to be covered.

Drug List. The drugs to be included were not clear, since average treatment practices were not known and standard treatment guidelines had not yet been developed. A team collected data from sample patient charts and focused surveys to determine current treatment practices.

Source of Supply. Products were to be purchased from both local and international suppliers. All cost estimates were converted to US dollars for purposes of consistency.

Data. Since demand had increased dramatically for drugs used to treat cholera, stockouts were common and consumption data were not reliable. Fairly accurate morbidity data were readily available, reported weekly via fax to the central level.

Resources for Quantification. A team of local and international specialists collected and analyzed data on disease incidence and current treatments and developed a computer spreadsheet for forecasting.

The morbidity method was used to calculate supply needs based on current epidemiological data, with two alternatives for treatment: current average treatment practices, and WHO treatment guidelines. The accompanying graph illustrates the projected annual supply costs for both calculations. Note the huge difference in total costs of the alternative treatment regimens. Total drug costs were more than two times higher with current treatment practices, with the excess almost exclusively due to overuse of lactated Ringer's IV solution when oral rehydration solution (ORS) could be safely substituted.

The results of calculations were presented to the national cholera committee, which agreed to a switch to WHO guidelines.

Policy-makers used the comparative cost information in educational activities to improve prescribing practices.

Annual Drug Costs

Note: Costs in millions of U.S. dollars.

each drug should be either the total of all facility estimates (plus central warehouse safety stock) *or* the central warehouse estimate, whichever is deemed more accurate.

Using Manual or Computerized Methods for Quantification

It is possible to conduct an accurate drug quantification without computerization. However, computers using spreadsheet or database software make the process much easier. The examples of quantification tables in this chapter were constructed with a standard spreadsheet program.

Computerized quantification has three major advantages: speed, accuracy, and flexibility. The process is much faster because the formulas can be programmed into the software, and once the data for basic assumptions are entered, the calculations are done automatically. The computer itself will not make errors in computation; if the data are entered correctly and the formulas are correct, the calculated answer will be correct. Finally, it is much easier to do "what-if" analysis by making changes to quantities of various items to see what happens to the total procurement costs. Tables constructed manually need to be retyped or rewritten, and all sums need to be recalculated each time a change is made. With a computer, the recalculation and reprinting are done at the touch of a key. Once a computerized drug list and quantification model have been developed, they can be reused repeatedly.

Estimating the Time Required for Quantification

Large-scale quantification is time-consuming, and a realistic time frame must be established for all the steps in the quantification plan. The time frame depends largely on how many levels of the supply system are involved and the type of data available. In multilevel systems in which data are incomplete, it will almost certainly require several months to produce a useful quantification.

Organizing the Drug List

The drug list is the central component of any quantification process. It is not possible to calculate quantities needed until it is known which products are needed. Specifications for each drug on the list should include

- ► drug description, generic name, or international non-proprietary name (INN);
- ► a local trade name, if any, in addition to the generic name;
- ► dosage form, such as tablet, suppository, ampoule for injection;
- ► strength—for example, 250 mg, 95 percent;
- ► basic unit, such as tablet, tube, mL, bottle;
- ► package size in basic units;
- ► projected purchase price per basic unit or per package.

In computerized quantification, data management is easiest when a separate field is provided for each of these specifications (see Chapter 46).

The drugs on the list need to be sorted according to the type of quantification and the type of facilities and personnel that will be recording data. The list must be provided in a form useful for retrieving information quickly and correctly. For example, if drugs are stored and records are arranged by dosage form (all tablets and capsules together, all injections together), the list should be organized by dosage form. If items are stored by therapeutic class, the list should be organized by therapeutic class, and so on. If the process involves decentralized data collection, the list should be distributed on data collection forms to each level and facility responsible for quantification at least three months before the estimates are needed for procurement.

For decentralized quantification, all facilities should submit estimates directly on the list (or a computerized facsimile). This allows the compilation of one master list in a reasonable time, comparison of estimated quantities among facilities, and verification and adjustment of estimates. Dosage forms and strengths should match those included in standard treatment guidelines and those available from likely sources of supply. If 500 mg tablets are quantified but suppliers offer only 300 mg tablets, it will be difficult to make a conversion.

Drug lists for quantification are often derived from past procurement or formulary or essential drugs lists. Procurement lists from previous purchases may contain specifications and the last prices paid, but they may not represent rational drug selection nor comply with the formulary or essential drugs list. Essential drugs lists or drug formulary lists that have been regularly updated should be the basis for the quantification list, since they reflect drugs needed for current morbidity patterns (see Chapters 10 and 11).

Filling the Supply Pipeline

The supply pipeline refers to stock levels within the supply system and the number of supply points at each level, as discussed in Chapter 21. The number of levels, the frequency of requisition and delivery, and the amount of safety stock at each level all influence the amount of drugs needed to fill the pipeline and, hence, the amount that must be procured when a program is started or expanded. Underestimation of stock in the pipeline is a common cause of program failure, particularly when a revolving drug fund has been planned (see Chapter 44, Box 44.1).

Considering the Impact of Lead Time

The procurement order quantity should be sufficient to last until the next procurement cycle is completed. The steps of the procurement process needed to place an order may take several months. In addition, once an order is placed, several more months are often required for the drugs to arrive in the country, clear customs, and reach the central warehouse. The waiting period from the time an order is prepared until it arrives in the country is the lead time (Chapter 15). When lead times are underestimated, the likely results are shortages and more expensive emergency purchases.

Adjusting for Losses and Program Growth

Inevitably, some drugs will be lost due to damage, spoilage, expiration, and theft. If such losses are not considered in quantification and procurement, stockouts are likely to result. To prevent shortages, a percentage can be added to allow for losses when quantifying requirements. Many systems need to allow at least 10 percent for losses.

Not all drugs are equally at risk for loss—for example, some are more attractive to thieves than others. The drugs that are most at risk may vary from country to country. If it is possible to identify them, it may be feasible to adjust the quantities for those items by a higher percentage rather than applying the same adjustment to all items. One strategy is to allow a loss percentage only for vital items, accepting the risk of stockouts for other items.

Clearly, it is in the best interests of the health system to make every effort to control loss and wastage. Options for controlling theft are discussed in Chapter 39; Chapter 41 offers tips for analyzing expiry dates in a large drug inventory; and Chapters 23 and 24 provide suggestions for managing stock to avoid wastage.

In a supply system in which patient utilization or the number of facilities is growing, it is reasonable to assume that drug consumption will increase. In such situations, estimated quantities can be increased by a percentage corresponding to the rate of growth.

Cross-Checking the Results of Quantification

Since there will be some imprecision in the estimates no matter how rigorously the appropriate quantification methods are followed, it is always useful to check the estimates with a different quantification method. The two sets of data can then be compared to see which appears to be more realistic, considering the reliability of source data used for the two estimates. Figure 14.2 illustrates how three different forecasting methods produced different estimates for the same supply system in a Latin American country.

Cross-checking is a fundamental step to reconcile procurement quantities with available funds. It is also useful to cross-check consumption with theoretical need to get an idea of the rationality of drug therapy in the system. For example, if the supply system usually bases purchases on past consumption, cross-checking for high-volume, high-cost drugs using another method may reveal targets for interventions to promote more rational drug use.

Estimating Total Procurement Costs

When estimating the cost of drugs on a quantified list, the critical issue is determining the next purchase prices. It is not adequate to use the last purchase prices, because in most cases, doing so results in an underestimate of the actual next purchase prices, leading to insufficient funds when it comes time to place orders.

There are two basic ways to estimate the next purchase price of a drug; both are usually needed to estimate the cost for the full list of drugs.

The first option is to obtain data on current drug prices in the market where the drugs will be purchased. As discussed in Chapter 16, sources for price data include local suppliers, international procurement agencies, and references such as the *International Drug Price Indicator Guide* (MSH 1995).

The other option for estimating next purchase price is to adjust the last purchase price for factors such as

▸ international inflation for products bought internationally;

Figure 14.2 Comparison of Quantification Results

Drug	Consumption Estimate	Morbidity Estimate	Adjusted Consumption Estimate
ORS 1 L pkg.	11,290,000	18,650,000	14,850,000
Chloroquine 300 mg tablet	1,230,000	2,233,000	2,005,000
Paracetamol 500 mg tablet	20,960,000	14,010,000	22,320,000

▸ devaluation of local currency for products purchased internationally (if relevant)—this percentage is added to the price for drugs purchased on the international market;

▸ local inflation for products purchased on the local market, adding the appropriate percentage based on the current local situation.

Once price estimates are obtained, it is necessary to add percentages for shipping and insurance for drugs obtained from international sources (usually 15 to 20 percent) and any known fees, such as those paid to a tender board or for local customs duties.

Adjusting and Reconciling Final Quantities

Difficult decisions must often be made to reduce the number of drugs and/or the quantities of drugs until the estimated quantities and costs correspond with the available budget. These reductions may require policy decisions regarding priority diseases, priority age groups, priority facilities for supply, selection of less expensive therapeutic alternatives, and changes to standard treatment guidelines. Chapter 41 discusses several approaches to making reductions rationally, using specific tools such as VEN (vital, essential, nonessential) categories, ABC analysis, and therapeutic category analysis. Another way to provide a foundation for reduction is to cross-check the quantification with another method to find out where the quantified estimate is much higher than necessary based on known morbidity and attendance data or much higher than that in a comparable health system.

It may be tempting to eliminate adjustments for expected losses as the first step in reducing quantities, but this is a false economy unless losses will in fact be eliminated. If the losses are likely to occur, they must be incorporated into the final quantification, or stockouts will almost certainly result. It may be possible to cut the overall percentage allowed for losses by targeting the allowance to those items most at risk and/or eliminating the adjustment for nonvital drugs, with the expectation that some stockouts will result for drugs that are not covered.

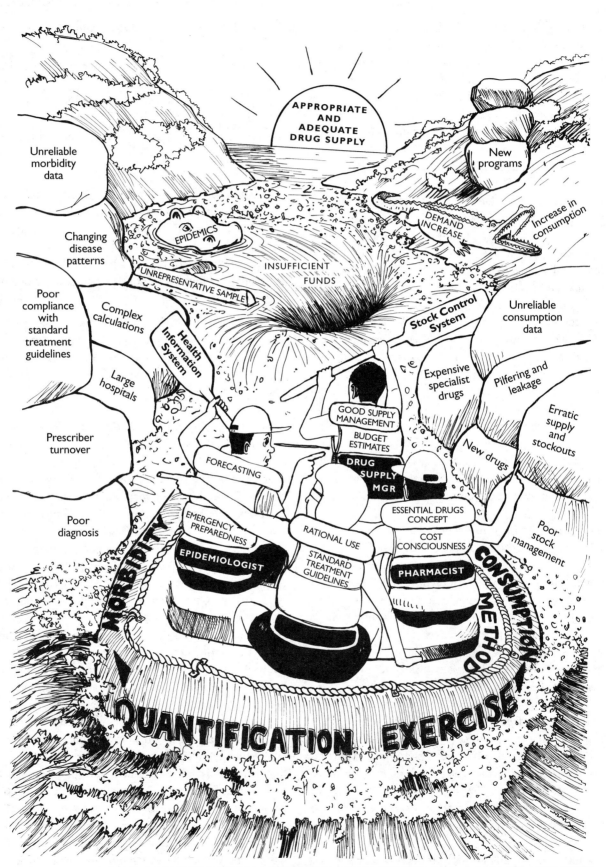

SUCCESSFUL DRUG QUANTIFICATION REQUIRES A TEAM EFFORT AND A MIX OF METHODS

≡ 14.4 Consumption Method

In the consumption method, a list is prepared of all drugs eligible for procurement, and the most accurate inventory records of past consumption are used to calculate the quantities needed for each drug.

Consumption during a recent period of six to twelve months is adjusted for stockouts to obtain the average monthly consumption. Then the average monthly consumption is multiplied by the number of months to be covered by procurement, and safety stock levels (in months) are also multiplied by the average monthly consumption. These two figures are added to get the gross needs during the period, with the stock on hand and any stock on order subtracted from the gross estimate, to derive the quantity to purchase. This quantification formula is the same as the consumption-based reorder formula described in Chapter 15.

The anticipated unit cost for each drug (not the last unit cost) is multiplied by the number of units to be purchased to obtain the expected purchase value for the entire quantity. All purchase values for individual drugs are added to obtain the total expected procurement cost. If this cost is greater than the budget, adjustments are made, as described in the previous section.

Example

Figure 14.3 shows a sample consumption-based quantification from an eastern Caribbean country in the early 1990s. This is not the complete quantification list, but it illustrates the estimates for nineteen drugs. Box 14.1 provides a summary of calculations used in consumption-based quantification.

Steps in the Quantification

Step 1. Prepare a List of Drugs to Be Quantified. The drug list should be prepared as described in Section 14.3, sorted into the order that will best facilitate data collection, and distributed to those officials and facilities that will enter consumption data.

Step 2. Determine the Period of Time to Be Reviewed for Consumption. If the procurement is to cover a twelve-month period, the consumption data for the past twelve months should be reviewed (if a full year's useful data are available). A twelve-month review may also be used for a procurement covering six months, but if there are significant seasonal variations, it may be better to use the same six-month period from the preceding year. A short review period such as three months is inadequate to plan a procurement to cover twelve months, unless the three months reviewed reflect a steady state of consumption for the entire year.

Step 3. Enter Consumption Data for Each Drug. For each drug on the list, enter

- ► the total quantity used during the review period, in basic units;
- ► the number of days in the review period that the drug was out of stock (if it is impossible to determine the number of days out of stock with accuracy, the estimated number of months out of stock during the period can be entered);
- ► the lead time for the last procurement (or the average from the last several procurements).

It is important to use the most accurate and current records available. The likely sources for consumption and lead-time data are

- ► stock records and distribution reports from a central distribution point;
- ► stock records and reports from regional or district warehouses;
- ► invoices from suppliers;
- ► dispensing records from health facilities.

If projected pricing data are available at this stage, it may save time to enter prices while entering consumption data (see step 10).

Step 4. Calculate the Average Monthly Consumption. The average monthly consumption is a key variable in the quantification formula and should be as accurate as possible. The simple approach is to divide total consumption by the number of months reviewed. If there were stockouts during that period, the average must be adjusted to include the consumption that would have occurred if stock had been available.

There are two ways to account for stockouts when computing average monthly consumption. The recommended method is illustrated in Box 14.1 as formula number one. Enter the total consumption and divide this by the number of months in the review period minus (the total number of days out of stock in the same period divided by 30.5 to convert to months). For example, consider the entry for ampicillin 250 mg capsules (the second item) in Figure 14.3. The total consumption for a six-month review period was 89,000 capsules. The drug was out of stock for thirty-four days in the six-month period. Therefore the average monthly consumption is:

$$C_A = 89,000 \div [6 - (34 \div 30.5)], \text{ or } 89,000 \div 4.8852 = 18,218$$

An alternative method, which is simpler but less precise, is shown as formula number two in Box 14.1. It uses the estimated number of months out of stock for adjusting

Figure 14.3 Consumption-Based Forecast for an Eastern Caribbean Country

Drug	Strength	BU	Pack Size	Total Consumption in Period (BU)	Days Out of Stock	Adjusted Average Monthly Consumption (BU)	Stock on Hand (BU)	Stock on Order (BU)	Safety Stock Level (BU)	Suggested Quantity to Order (BU)	Adjusted Order Quantity	Order Quantity (Packs)	Probable Pack Price (US$)	Value of Proposed Order (US$)
Ampicillin	500 mg	capsule	1,000	59,500	0	9,917	32,000	42,000	29,750	45,000	50,737	51	69.30	3,534.30
Ampicillin	250 mg	capsule	1,000	89,000	34	18,218	81,000	58,000	54,654	79,616	89,766	90	35.10	3,159.00
Ampicillin sodium injection	500 mg	ampoule	100	3,879	0	647	111	7,600	1,940	47	53	1	29.95	29.95
Ampicillin suspension 100 mL	125 mg/5 mL	bottle	1	4,128	0	688	1,513	3,000	2,064	3,743	4,220	4,220	0.75	3,165.00
Antihistamine decongestant elixir	250 mL	bottle	1	853	29	169	351	929	507	747	843	843	1.57	1,323.51
Antihistamine decongestant	(any)	tablet	500	50,000	0	8,333	0	62,500	25,000	37,500	42,281	85	12.00	1,020.00
Bacitracin antibiotic ointment	—	tube	1	2,414	31	484	3,400	100	1,453	2,313	2,608	2,608	0.54	1,408.32
Bendrofluazide	5 mg	tablet	500	141,500	30	28,208	142,000	50,000	84,623	146,490	165,168	330	1.90	627.00
Benzathine benzyl-penicillin injection	2.4 M.U.	ampoule	50	1,318	0	220	1,486	0	659	1,150	1,297	26	25.00	650.00
Cephradine injection	500 mg	ampoule	100	2,695	0	449	2,300	1,100	1,348	1,990	2,244	22	75.00	1,650.00
Chlorhexidine gluconate solution (Hibitan)	5%	liter	5	302	0	50	433	0	151	171	192	38	17.95	682.10
Chlorhexidine/cetrimide (Savlon)	5 liter	liter	5	438	0	73	418	250	219	209	235	47	14.70	690.90
Chlorpropamide	250 mg	tablet	1,000	162,000	0	27,000	169,000	0	81,000	155,000	174,763	175	8.99	1,573.25
Cimetidine (Tagamet) injection	200 mg	ampoule	10	1,090	0	182	2,580	0	545	0	0	0	8.36	0.00
Cimetidine	400 mg	tablet	1,000	24,000	0	4,000	23,500	25,000	12,000	0	0	0	42.00	0.00
Cloxacillin suspension 100 mL	125 mg/5 mL	bottle	1	882	0	147	1,446	0	441	318	359	359	1.00	359.00
Cotrimoxazole suspension 100 mL	200/40 mg/5 mL	bottle	1	1,152	0	192	374	1,930	576	0	0	0	0.75	0.00
Cotrimoxazole	400/80 mg	tablet	1,000	81,000	0	13,500	82,000	0	40,500	80,000	90,200	90	21.00	1,890.00
Dextrose in saline (IV) 1,000 mL	5%/0.9%	bottle	1	1,525	32	308	0	2,288	924	1,408	1,588	1,588	1.35	2,143.80

Total order cost: $23,906.13

Note: BU = basic unit.

Box 14.1 Consumption-Based Calculations

Formula Number	Objective of Formula	Calculations
1	Adjusted average monthly consumption (preferred)	$C_A = C_T \div [R_M - (D_{OS} \div 30.5)]$
2	Adjusted average monthly consumption (alternative)	$C_A = C_T \div (R_M - M_{OS})$
3	Basic safety stock requirements	$C_A \times LT$
4	Quantity to order	$Q_O = C_A \times (LT + PP) + SS - (S_I + S_O)$

C_A = Average monthly consumption, adjusted for stockouts
C_T = Total consumption during review period, in basic units
D_{OS} = Number of days an item was out of stock during the review period
LT = Average lead time (for projected supplier or worst case), in months
M_{OS} = Estimated number of months an item was out of stock during the review period
PP = Procurement period (number of months to be covered by order)
Q_O = Quantity to order in basic units, before adjustment for losses or program change
R_M = Review period in months (number of months of data reviewed for forecasting)
S_I = Stock now in inventory, in basic units
S_O = Stock now on order, in basic units
SS = Quantity needed for safety stock

---

consumption, omitting the step of converting days to months. Using the same drug from Figure 14.3, the drug was in stock for about five of the six months, leaving about one month out of stock. Therefore, the average monthly consumption is:

$$C_A = 89,000 \div (6 - 1) = 89,000 \div 5 = 17,800$$

Step 5. Calculate the Safety Stock Needed for Each Drug. Safety (buffer) stock is needed to prevent stockouts, although high levels of safety stock increase inventory holding costs and should be avoided (see Chapter 15). In some supply systems, the safety stock is set for each item at a fixed quantity or a fixed number of months' worth of consumption. However, the preferred method is to calculate the safety stock based on the average consumption and the expected lead time (see formula number three in Box 14.1). The average monthly consumption from step 4 is multiplied by the average lead time. This safety stock level should avoid stockouts, assuming that the item is reordered when only the safety stock remains, the supplier delivers within the projected lead time, and consumption is no greater than average. Using this formula, the safety stock for ampicillin 250 mg capsules in the example is 18,218 x 3 months = 54,654.

For vital items, it may be necessary to adjust the safety stock to cover variations in consumption or lead time. There are several options for adjusting safety stock levels (see Chapter 15). The simplest method multiplies the basic safety stock by an adjustment factor. For example, an adjustment factor of 1.5 would increase the safety stock of

ampicillin 250 mg capsules in Figure 14.3 to 81,981 capsules. If this sort of adjustment is done for all items, the cost of safety stock will increase substantially; therefore, adjustments should be made only when there is true uncertainty about the lead time or consumption.

Step 6. Calculate the Quantity of Each Drug Required in the Next Procurement Period. The suggested formula for calculating the quantity to order is shown as formula number four in Box 14.1. The calculation is done in three main steps. First, the average consumption is multiplied by the sum of the lead time and the procurement period, yielding the total needs before considering safety stock, stock on hand, or stock on order. The second step is to add the quantity needed for safety stock. Finally, the quantity of stock on hand and the stock on order are added together, and then subtracted from the previous total. Using the example of ampicillin 250 mg capsules from Figure 14.3, the quantity to order is:

$$Q_O = 18,218 \times (3 + 6) + 54,654 - (81,000 + 58,000) = 79,616$$

Since the ampicillin capsules are purchased in bottles of 1,000, this means that eighty bottles should be ordered.

Step 7. Adjust for Expected Changes in Consumption Pattern. Using the example of ampicillin 250 mg capsules from Figure 14.3, if it is expected that utilization will increase by 5 percent in the coming year, it would be reasonable to adjust the six-month forecast by 2.5 percent; this would raise the expected need by 1,990 capsules, bringing the total to 81,606 capsules (or eighty-two bottles of 1,000).

Some changes in consumption may be independent of trends in overall patient utilization. One example is predictable seasonal variation in the consumption of cough and cold remedies. A potential spike in an epidemic disease such as cholera is another example. If this is anticipated, it would be sensible to increase estimates for drugs such as ORS, parenteral solutions, and some antibiotics; this does not mean that the need for all drugs will increase by the same factor.

If it is known that a new formulary drug will replace an older drug by a substantial proportion, the estimate for the older drug should be reduced. If there are major efforts to alter prescribing patterns, it would be reasonable to anticipate at least some success by reducing the expected need for affected drugs by a small percentage. When there is a turnover in prescribing staff, the new prescribers may have different ways of treating common conditions that would substantially affect drug needs in some therapeutic categories. If such changes can be anticipated, it is wise to adjust the forecasts to avoid spending resources on drugs that will not be as popular as in the past.

Step 8. Adjust for Losses. To avoid stockouts, it is necessary to adjust quantification estimates to allow for losses, as discussed in Section 14.3. If the supply system from Figure 14.3 averaged 10 percent per year in losses, and this was applied to ampicillin 250 mg capsules, the allowance would add 8,160 capsules to the estimate from step 7, bringing the total purchase quantity to 89,766, or ninety bottles of 1,000 capsules.

Step 9. Compile Decentralized Quantifications (if Applicable). In a decentralized quantification, staff at each facility or storage point enter their own consumption quantities and stockout information, and the estimates of the individual facilities are totaled and compiled on the master quantification list.

Step 10. Estimate Costs for Each Drug and Total Costs. In order to estimate procurement costs, multiply the quantities estimated for each drug by the most accurate prediction of the expected next purchase price (not the last one), as discussed in section 14.3.

Once the expected price has been entered for each drug, multiply the price by the estimated quantity needed to obtain the total procurement value for each drug. Figure 14.3 uses the package price as the basis for making these projections, but in many cases it is preferable to use the basic unit price, because there is more flexibility in combining information from different sources to arrive at an average. The basic unit price is also preferable if it is unclear what package sizes will be ordered or if projections are based on average international prices from a

source such as the annual *International Drug Price Indicator Guide* (MSH 1995).

After the estimated procurement value has been calculated for each drug, the final step in the basic quantification process is to add up the estimated procurement values for all drugs to obtain the total expected cost for the procurement.

Step 11. Compare Total Costs with Budget and Make Adjustments. If the total expected procurement cost exceeds the available budget, there are really only two choices: either obtain more funds or reduce the number of drugs and/or the quantities ordered. Section 14.3 discusses rational ways to adjust the estimates.

≡ 14.5 Morbidity Method
The morbidity method uses data on patient utilization (attendances at health facilities) and morbidity (the frequency of common health problems) to project the need for drugs based on assumptions about how the problems will be treated. Readers who plan to undertake a morbidity-based quantification are strongly advised to obtain the WHO manual *Estimating Drug Requirements* (WHO/DAP 1988), which provides a more detailed discussion of the steps in this type of quantification.

The morbidity method requires a list of common health problems, an essential drugs list that includes therapy for the problems, and a set of standard treatments for quantification purposes (based on either average current practices or "ideal" treatment guidelines). For most health problems there are at least two alternative treatments, and a percentage must be assigned based on how frequently each regimen is used. Then, the expected incidence (number of treatment episodes) of each health problem must be estimated.

The quantification formula involves multiplying the quantity of each drug included in standard treatments for each health problem by the number of treatment episodes expected for the health problem. The expected total need for each drug is the sum of the estimates from all treatment regimens in which the drug is included. Then the estimates are adjusted to fill the supply pipeline, allowing for losses to theft and wastage. Finally, the expected cost is calculated based on the expected purchase price of each drug, and estimates are reconciled with available funds.

Given the limited data likely to be available on morbidity patterns and the difficulty in defining standard treatments that are meaningful for quantification, it is difficult to apply this method to more than fifty to one hundred health problems. This limits the method's utility for a complex health system with many types of health problems and several levels of health facilities. In general, the morbidity method is most useful when a relatively small number of different health problems are seen, such as in primary care and special-purpose facilities and programs.

Since a limited number of health problems are likely to be addressed in most morbidity-based quantification procedures, the resulting estimates for each drug must be adjusted to cover health problems not considered in the quantification, usually using some variant of adjusted consumption (see Section 14.6). Adjustments may also be required to fill the supply pipeline, to account for losses, and, in most cases, to reconcile the quantities needed with the funds available.

In a simple quantification for one health problem, such as cholera (see Country Study 14.2), or for a small group of health problems and drugs, the process can be done manually (although it is easier with a computer). A computer is virtually required to conduct a large-scale morbidity-based quantification covering a large number of health problems and drugs.

Figure 14.4 is a flow diagram that illustrates how the data inputs on population, percentage of coverage, health problems, standard treatments, and unit costs are used to calculate the quantities needed and projected procurement costs.

Example

Figure 14.5 is an example of morbidity-based quantification. This includes a health problem list using International Classification of Diseases (ICD) codes, sample standard treatment regimens for the same health problems, and morbidity estimates for a one-year period. All this information is combined to project drug requirements and to produce a procurement list.

Steps in the Quantification

Step 1. Specify the List of Problems. List the major specific health problems encountered (see Figure 14.5). If there is an existing information system that reports on diseases, those disease codes should be used; if there is no existing coding system, the ICD system should be used.

The health problem list should not be broken down into too much detail but should be defined according to the diagnostic capacity and health problems treated at each type of health facility. At the lowest level of the system, only a limited number of problems are recognized and treated; the range of problems diagnosed and treated normally increases at the health center, district hospital, and referral hospital levels.

Since treatments differ markedly for adult and pediatric

Figure 14.4 Morbidity Method

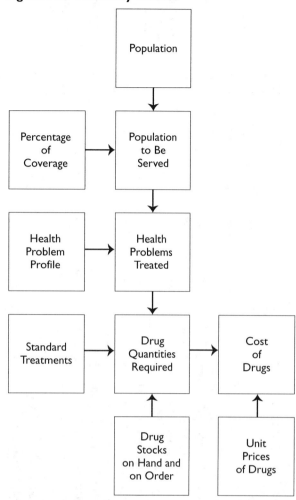

patients, it is important to include at least two categories (under five years and over five years) for most problems. Although it may be tempting to provide several categories (under five, five to twelve, thirteen to sixty-five, and over sixty-five), it is best to avoid overcomplicating the development of treatment guidelines (see below) and the process of compiling data on treatment episodes.

Step 2. Establish the List of Drugs to Be Quantified. The objective here is a list of essential drugs that covers the major health problems and forms the basis for standard treatment schedules. A current and appropriate national or health system formulary or essential drugs list should be used when available. If there is no official list, one needs to be developed (see Chapter 10); it may grow out of the process of developing standard treatments.

The drug list must be available in two formats—one organized in alphabetical order by generic name (INN) and one by therapeutic categories. The therapeutic category list is most useful in developing standard treatment

Figure 14.5 Drug Needs Based on Morbidity

Problem	Severity	Age Group	Episodes per 1,000 Contacts	Past Year Estimated Number of Episodes	Projected Number of Episodes	No. of Regimen	% Cases Treated with Regimen	Drug Product	Basic Unit	Basic Unit per Dose	Doses per Day	Number of Days	Basic Units per Episode	Total Basic Units Needed
Malaria	1	<5	364	1,136,921	1,193,767	1	100%	Chloroquine 150 mg base	Tablet	0.50	1	2	2.50	2,984,416
						2	80%	Paracetamol solution 120 mg/5 mL	mL	1.50	4	10	60.00	57,300,794
		>5	278	868,307	911,723	1	100%	Chloroquine 150 mg base	Tablet	2	2	2	10	9,117,228
						2	80%	Paracetamol 500 mg	Tablet	2	4	5	40.00	29,175,129
	2	<5	65	203,022	213,173	1	100%	Quinine injection 300 mg/mL	mL	0.50	3	1	1.50	319,759
						1	100%	Quinine 300 mg	Tablet	0.50	3	6	9.00	1,918,553
						2	100%	Paracetamol solution 120 mg/5 mL	mL	1.50	4	10	60.00	12,790,356
		>5	61	190,528	200,054	1	100%	Quinine injection 300 mg/mL	mL	2	3	1	6.00	1,200,326
						1	100%	Quinine 300 mg	Tablet	2	3	6	36.00	7,201,954
						2	100%	Paracetamol 500 mg	Tablet	2	4	10	80.00	16,004,343
Conjunctivitis	—	<5	53	165,541	173,818	1	100%	Tetracycline 1% eye ointment	5 g tube	1	3	7	1	173,818
		>5	38	118,690	124,624	1	100%	Tetracycline 1% eye ointment	5 g tube	1	3	7	1	124,624
Otitis media	—	<5	106	331,081	347,635	1	100%	Cotrimoxazole suspension	mL	5	2	10	100.00	34,763,531
						2	100%	Paracetamol solution 120 mg/5 mL	mL	1.50	4	10	60.00	20,858,119
						3	80%	Pseudoephedrine syrup	mL	2.50	4	5	50.00	13,905,412
		>5	29	90,579	95,108	1	100%	Cotrimoxazole 800/160 mg	Tablet	1	2	10	20.00	1,902,155
						2	100%	Paracetamol 500 mg	Tablet	2	4	5	40.00	3,804,311
						3	80%	Pseudoephedrine 60 mg	Tablet	1	4	5	20.00	1,521,724
Acute tonsillitis	—	<5	72	224,885	236,130	1	100%	Penicillin VK 125 mg/5 mL liquid	mL	5	4	5	100.00	23,612,964
						2	100%	Paracetamol solution 120 mg/5 mL	mL	1.50	4	10	60.00	14,167,779
		>5	33	103,072	108,226	1	100%	Procaine penicillin 3 MU injection	vial	1	1	1	1.00	108,226
						2	100%	Penicillin VK 250 mg	Tablet	1	4	5	20.00	2,164,522
						3	100%	Paracetamol 500 mg	Tablet	2	4	5	40.00	4,329,043
Gastritis, heartburn	—	<5	11	34,357	36,075	1	100%	Antacid suspension	mL	5	4	5	100.00	3,607,536
		>5	77	240,502	252,528	1	70%	Antacid suspension	mL	10	4	5	200.00	35,353,855
						2	30%	Cimetidine 300 mg	Tablet	1	4	5	20.00	1,515,165

Note: Based on 3,123,408 contacts in the past year; 5 percent expected rate of increase.

schedules, and the list organized by generic name is used for the procurement list.

Step 3. Establish Standard or Average Treatments. Standard or average treatment regimens are required for each health problem to forecast drug needs, as in Figure 14.5. This is the most complicated part of the method. There are two basic options for developing standard treatments: *average actual treatments* or *ideal standard treatments*. The components are the same, but there is an important difference between the approaches: *average* regimens are based on observed or reported practices and are more likely to predict what will actually happen, whereas *ideal* regimens define what should happen if prescribers follow the ideal guidelines. Country Study 14.2 illustrates how different the results can be between average current treatments and standard treatments.

Which should be used? Perhaps both, in a combination approach. For example, if one treatment regimen is viewed as ideal but another is commonly used, include both regimens in the guidelines for quantification and estimate the percentage of treatment episodes that will receive each of the two regimens.

In most quantification exercises, it *is* necessary to develop (or modify) the treatment guidelines (see Chapter 11). Ideal standard treatment guidelines should be developed by expert committees (with expert assistance, if needed). Unless there is reliable information on drug utilization and prescribing patterns, a special study may be needed to determine average actual treatment patterns; this can be combined with a study to determine morbidity patterns and incidence of health problems (see step 4).

Whichever option is used, the same information must be compiled:

- ▶ the percentage of treatment episodes in which the drug will be prescribed;
- ▶ the name of each drug and strength (see Section 14.3), with separate treatments listed for age level, as appropriate;
- ▶ the basic unit (see Section 14.3);
- ▶ the number of basic units in each average dose for the health problem in question;
- ▶ the average number of doses of each drug per day for the problem;
- ▶ the average number of days of treatment for each drug per episode.

These components are combined to project the quantity of each drug needed for each treatment episode (Q_E) in each standard treatment regimen. This projection is made by multiplying the basic units per dose (D_{CU}) by the num-

ber of doses per day (N_D). This result is multiplied by the length of treatment per episode, in days (L_D). The entire formula is:

$$Q_E = D_{CU} \times N_D \times L_D$$

In the example from Figure 14.5, three different drug products are prescribed for otitis media for both age groups; the drugs are the same, but the dose and dosage form differ. The quantity of cotrimoxazole suspension needed to treat otitis media in patients under five years old is calculated as:

$$Q_E = 5 \text{ mL} \times 2 \text{ doses/day} \times 10 \text{ days} = 100 \text{ mL}$$

This calculation is done for all drugs in all the standard treatment regimens.

If different treatment regimens (perhaps with multiple drugs) are used for the same disease according to its severity, separate standard regimens must be developed and assigned for each. This is illustrated by the malaria treatment guidelines in Figure 14.5.

For each regimen, the proportion of patients with each disease who will be treated with each different therapy is estimated. From Figure 14.5, in patients over five years old with gastritis, 70 percent are expected to be treated with antacid and 30 percent with cimetidine. In some situations, depending on treatment practices, it might be appropriate to allot 70 percent for antacid and 50 for cimetidine (because some patients will receive both drugs). Thus, the cumulative percentage may exceed 100 for a particular health problem.

If there are major differences in the way common problems are treated by different levels of prescribers, it may be useful to estimate how many (or what percentage of) treatment episodes of each disease will be managed by each category of prescriber, and then specify separate treatment regimens common for each prescriber category.

It is important that practitioners involved in developing standard treatment guidelines for quantification understand that the guidelines are only for quantification, and that a prescriber's freedom will not necessarily be curtailed as a result. In one West African country, a committee was formed to develop standard treatment guidelines for quantification, with the assistance of an outside expert. The committee met but decided that standard treatment guidelines would restrict doctors' freedom to choose a therapy and instead produced a simple therapeutics manual. When the external quantification team arrived in the country, there were no lists of common diseases with guidelines for quantification, and the process ultimately failed to produce a useful list for procurement.

Step 4. Collect Morbidity Data for Each Health Problem Treated. This step estimates the expected number of treatment episodes for each health problem from step 1. A treatment episode is "a patient contact for which a standard course of drug treatment is required" (WHO/DAP 1988, 6.1). Figure 14.5 shows one way to organize morbidity data for the health problems from step 1 and to estimate the number of treatment episodes.

Information from the regular health information system on morbidity patterns and treatment episodes can be used for quantification. In many cases, however, this information is not available, and a special study is needed in sentinel facilities, from which data can then (with caution) be extrapolated. The study can take two forms: a retrospective review of records in selected facilities (if those records are relatively accessible, complete, and accurate), or a prospective study in a sample of health facilities. The study must be completed prior to actually starting the quantification. There are some key issues in conducting these studies:

► Both the number of contacts and the number of treatment episodes must be obtained in the study of sample facilities.

► Only patient contacts that normally result in drug treatment should be counted, separate from those that do not (such as well-child programs).

► The sample data should specify the frequency of each health problem in terms of a common denominator, such as 1,000 inpatients or 1,000 outpatient visits (for example, number of acute diarrhea cases per 1,000 outpatient contacts).

► Separate frequencies must be developed for all age groups specified in the standard treatment guidelines. Figure 14.5 shows one format for doing this.

► It may be impossible to separate curative from non-curative contacts in a retrospective review of records. Even for curative contacts, not all patients who come to facilities with health problems receive drug therapy (although the vast majority do if there are drugs in stock). If this is thought to be important, the proportion of cases that will be treated with drugs can be estimated.

► If discrete types of prescribers (such as doctors versus paramedical staff) use different treatment regimens, the number of treatment episodes must be compiled separately for each prescriber type.

► The sample data should also specify the number of patient contacts per total population in the area served by the sample facilities. For example, if the total population in the sample area was 3.9 million,

and there were 3,123,408 patient contacts per year (as in Figure 14.5), on average there were 0.8 patient contacts per inhabitant. This average could be used to project the number of contacts in another area, as described in Section 14.6 on the adjusted consumption method.

Estimating Drug Requirements (WHO/DAP 1988) provides guidelines for surveying health facility records, doing a prospective study of morbidity, and constructing morbidity projections. Chapter 29 of this manual provides guidance for studying drug use in health facilities.

Step 5. Calculate the Number of Treatment Episodes for Each Health Problem. There are two options for calculating the number of treatment episodes. If the number of expected patient contacts (outpatient contacts, inpatient admissions, or both) can be estimated directly in the target facilities, the calculations are done in one step based on the number of contacts. If the information on contacts is not reliable, it must be estimated from the population in the area served and the frequency of contacts per inhabitant in the target population.

The estimated total number of patient contacts for the past year is divided by 1,000, so that the denominators of contacts and treatment frequency are the same. (The frequency of treatment episodes is usually expressed in treatment episodes per 1,000 contacts.) Next multiply the expected total number of contacts in thousands (N_C) by the expected frequency of the problem (F) to obtain the number of treatment episodes (E_T) based on last year's data. This must be done separately for each discrete age range used in the process. If there are multiple levels of treatment, the number of treatment episodes at each level must also be estimated.

In the Figure 14.5 example, there were 3,123,408 contacts, separated into two categories: under five years old and over five years old. Since the frequency of health problems is estimated per 1,000 contacts, the total number of contacts is divided by 1,000, yielding 3,123.4 groups of 1,000 contacts. Next, the number of treatment episodes must be adjusted for expected changes in patient utilization; in Figure 14.5, a 5 percent increase is expected. Therefore, the estimated number of treatment episodes for each age group and each health problem is multiplied by 1.05.

Step 6. Calculate the Quantity of Drugs Needed for Each Health Problem. For each health problem, the projected number of treatment episodes from step 5 (E_T) is multiplied by the quantity of basic units (Q_E) specified in the guidelines for each age group (and each level of disease severity from step 3). This result is then multiplied by the percentage of cases that are expected to be treated (P_T). The full formula is:

$$Q_T = E_T \times Q_E \times P_T$$

In Figure 14.5, 80 percent of patients under age five with malaria, severity level one, are expected to be treated with paracetamol solution. Therefore, the calculation is:

$$Q_T = 1,193,767 \times 60 \text{ mL} \times 0.8$$

This calculation yields a total of 57,300,816 mL needed for this treatment regimen.

Step 7. Combine the Estimates for Each Drug from the Various Health Problems into a Master Procurement List. This step combines the estimated quantities from different treatment regimens into one master list for procurement. For example, in Figure 14.5, paracetamol solution is included in four different treatment guidelines (malaria, severity one and severity two, otitis media, and tonsillitis). For the master procurement list, the four separate estimated quantities must be added to yield the total number of mL of paracetamol needed. Master list quantities usually then need to be adjusted to cover factors such as health problems not considered in the basic estimates, shortages in the supply pipeline, and losses due to theft and wastage.

Step 8. Adjust Quantities to Cover Other Health Problems. The reliability of morbidity-based quantification increases as the number of health problems addressed increases, but it is rarely feasible to get reliable data or estimates for all major health problems. In this situation, the morbidity-based quantification cannot predict total drug needs, and it is necessary to adjust for drug needs not addressed in the quantification. Otherwise, there will be stockouts.

Since reliable consumption data from the target system are not available for comparison (or that method would probably have been used for the quantification), the adjusted consumption method described in Section 14.6, or "expert opinion," may be used to estimate what percentage adjustment should be made to the morbidity-based estimates.

If data on drug utilization are available from another similar health system, it might be possible to extrapolate requirements for twenty or thirty commonly used drugs and determine the average percentage difference between the estimates produced by each method. For example, if the extrapolated method produces estimates that average 10 percent higher than those produced by the morbidity method, the quantities of all drugs could be increased by 10 percent.

An alternative is to survey local experts to determine what percentage of overall patient contacts have been cap-

tured in the list of health problems used for morbidity quantification. For example, if local experts agree that about 90 percent of the drug needs are covered in the standard treatments, estimated quantities could again be increased by 10 percent.

Step 9. Adjust for Filling the Pipeline and Current Stock Position. So far, the calculations assume that the supply pipeline (see Section 14.3) is relatively intact and that the procurement is only replacing drugs that are being consumed. If there have been major stockouts that need to be corrected, additional stock will be necessary to fill the pipeline.

If applicable, make adjustments for stock on hand, stock on order, and lead time as described in the consumption method (see Section 14.4, step 6) to finalize the preliminary estimates.

Step 10. Adjust Quantities for Expected Losses. This procedure is discussed in section 14.3. In most supply systems, losses are a reality, and unless they are considered in the quantification process, stockouts will be unavoidable.

Step 11. Estimate Costs for Each Drug and Total Costs. With adjustments made to cover needs for additional health problems, losses, and filling the pipeline (if necessary), the total estimated quantity can be divided by the purchase pack size to determine the number of packs to be ordered. For example, in Figure 14.5, 236,129,644 mL of penicillin UK solution are the estimated need. If this drug is produced in 100 mL bottles, 2,361,296 bottles should be ordered.

If the basic unit price is used as the basic estimate of cost, multiply it by the expected package size to determine the expected package price. If the available prices are based on package price, enter it directly.

To calculate the estimated procurement value, multiply the expected pack price by the estimated number of packages to be purchased. The prices used in the estimate should be the expected next purchase price, not the last purchase price (see Section 14.3).

Step 12. Compare Total Costs with Budget and Make Adjustments. Reduce the estimated quantities and/or the number of drugs to conform with budget realities, if necessary. The morbidity-based method lends itself to considering the relative therapeutic value of drugs on the list. In the example illustrated by Figure 14.5, it might be determined that since pseudoephedrine has not been proved to be useful in otitis media, the percentages allotted for this drug could be reduced. The important point is that when reductions are required, they should be made rationally, with the goal of maximizing the therapeutic benefit of expenditures.

≡ 14.6 Adjusted Consumption Method

Many supply systems face a severe information deficit, which limits accurate quantification. When neither consumption nor morbidity methods are feasible, the best option is extrapolating from consumption data from another region or health system. The adjusted consumption method uses known consumption data from one system, called the *standard*, to estimate the drug needs in a similar or expanded system, known as the *target*.

This method can be *population based*, defining drug use per 1,000 population, or *service based*, defining drug use per specified patient case, inpatient admission, or rural health center. A complete quantification may use a combination of the two methods, with different denominators for different products.

Example

Figure 14.6 illustrates the adjusted consumption method of extrapolating consumption of outpatient drugs from a standard health system to the target health system. The data in Figure 14.6 do not represent any particular country.

Steps in the Quantification

Step 1. Select the Standard System for Comparison and Extrapolation. The standard facilities should, if feasible, closely resemble the region or country for which the estimate is made in terms of geography and climate, patient population served, morbidity patterns, prescribing practices, and drug supply status. Representative standard facilities should be selected at each level of health care that has a different drug list, morbidity patterns, or prescribing practices. They should have an adequate and uninterrupted drug supply (but not greatly overstocked), fairly rational prescribing practices, and complete and accurate records of patient contacts and drug inventory movement. Of course, it may not be possible to find an ideal standard, but an effort should be made to select the best standard data available.

Step 2. Develop the Drug List. See section 14.3 for a discussion of issues.

Step 3. Establish the Time Period to Be Covered in Review. Determine the number of months' worth of data to be reviewed in the standard system.

Step 4. Review Records from the Standard System to Compile Contact or Population Data. Use available reports on patient contacts in the standard system; if reports are not already compiled with suitable data, a survey of standard facilities can be done to determine the number of patient contacts during the time period established. A similar survey might be carried out in the target system, but if

the target system has had a severe problem with stockouts, the attendance data may not reflect the number of contacts that can be expected once drugs are available.

Step 5. Establish the Denominator for Extrapolation. The denominator used to extrapolate consumption can be either population in the area served or number of patient contacts, depending on the data obtainable through step 4. Whichever one is used, the denominator is usually thousands of patient contacts or thousands of inhabitants in the region (as in Figure 14.6). In very large systems, it might be preferable to use tens of thousands or even millions of contacts or inhabitants.

Step 6. Determine the Consumption Rate in the Standard System. For each drug, produce an adjusted average monthly consumption (see Section 14.4). The average monthly consumption is multiplied by twelve to obtain the adjusted annual consumption. Then divide the adjusted annual consumption by the number of thousands of contacts or inhabitants to establish the consumption rate.

Step 7. Extrapolate the Standard System's Consumption Rate to the Target System. Multiply the standard consumption rate for each drug by the estimated number of thousands of contacts or inhabitants in the target system to yield the projected requirements in the target system.

Step 8. Adjust for Expected Losses. Because these are very rough estimates, and because it may be unclear what percentages of losses were experienced in the standard system, it may not be realistic to adjust for losses. However, if there are known losses, add a percentage allowance, at least for vital drugs (see Section 14.3).

Step 9. Estimate Costs for Each Drug and Total Costs and Make Adjustments. Multiply the projected quantities for each drug by the most accurate prediction of the next procurement cost and reconcile that with available funds, as discussed in section 14.3.

≡ 14.7 Service-Level Projection of Budget Requirements

This method is used to estimate financial requirements for drug procurement based on costs per patient treated at various levels of the same health system or, with great caution, based on data from other health systems. It does not forecast needs for specific drugs. It is more reliable to generalize from one region in a country to another region in the same country than it is to extrapolate to a different country.

Like the adjusted consumption method, this method produces rough estimates because there may be significant, but not always apparent, variations between the target health system and the system used as a source of standard data. Possible sources of error include prescribers in the

Figure 14.6 Adjusted Consumption

Drug	Strength	Basic Unit	Standard System Consumption: 50,000 Inhabitants, 32,500 Outpatient Contacts						Target System Extrapolation: 80,000 Inhabitants, Unknown Outpatient Contacts				
			Total Usage in 6-Month Period (BU)	Days Out of Stock	Adjusted Average Monthly Usage (BU)	Adjusted Annual Usage (BU)	Usage per 1,000 Inhabitants	Usage per 1,000 Outpatient Contacts	Projected Requirements in BUs Based on 80,000 Inhabitants	Pack Size	Order Quantity (Packs)	Probable Pack Price (US$)	Value of Proposed Order (US$)
Ampicillin	500 mg	Capsule	59,500	0	9,917	119,000	2,380	3,662	190,400	1,000	190	69.30	$13,194.72
Ampicillin	250 mg	Capsule	89,000	34	18,218	218,617	4,372	6,727	349,788	1,000	350	35.10	$12,277.56
Ampicillin suspension 100 mL	125 mg/5 mL	Bottle	4,128	0	688	8,256	165	254	13,210	1	13,210	0.75	$9,907.20
Antihistamine decongestant elixir 250 mL	—	Bottle	853	29	169	2,027	41	62	3,244	1	3,244	1.57	$5,092.48
Bacitracin antibiotic ointment	—	Tube	2,414	31	484	5,813	116	179	9,300	1	9,300	0.54	$5,022.14
Bendrofluazide	5 mg	Tablet	141,500	30	28,208	338,490	6,770	10,415	541,584	500	1,083	1.90	$2,058.02
Benzathine benzyl-penicillin injection	2.4 MU	Ampoule	1,318	0	220	2,636	53	81	4,218	50	84	25.00	$2,108.80
Chlorpropamide	250 mg	Tablet	162,000	0	27,000	324,000	6,480	9,969	518,400	1,000	518	8.99	$4,660.42
Cimetidine	400 mg	Tablet	24,000	0	4,000	48,000	960	1,477	76,800	1,000	77	42.00	$3,225.60
Cotrimoxazole	400/80 mg	Tablet	81,000	0	13,500	162,000	3,240	4,985	259,200	1,000	259	21.00	$5,443.20
Erythromycin	250 mg	Tablet	80,500	0	13,417	161,000	3,220	4,954	257,600	500	515	20.95	$10,793.44
Ferrous salt/folic acid	60/1 mg	Tablet	353,000	0	58,833	706,000	14,120	21,723	1,129,600	1,000	1,130	5.35	$6,043.36
Fluphenazine decanoate injection 10 mL	25 mg/mL	Vial	324	0	54	648	13	20	1,037	1	1,037	2.70	$2,799.36
Indomethacin	25 mg	Capsule	167,000	0	27,833	334,000	6,680	10,277	534,400	1,000	534	8.50	$4,542.40
Insulin Lente	100 IU/mL	Vial	4,504	0	751	9,008	180	277	14,413	1	14,413	3.91	$56,354.05
Methyldopa	500 mg	Tablet	191,000	32	38,579	462,954	9,259	14,245	740,726	500	1,481	30.00	$44,443.55
Nystatin skin cream 30 gm	100,000 IU	Tube	1,815	0	302	3,630	73	112	5,808	1	5,808	0.80	$4,646.40
Oral rehydration salts	—	Sachet	6,820	0	1,137	13,640	273	420	21,824	1	21,824	0.09	$1,964.16
Paracetamol elixir 150 mL	120 mg/5 mL	Bottle	2,934	0	489	5,868	117	181	9,389	1	9,389	0.94	$8,825.47
Paracetamol	500 mg	Tablet	319,000	0	53,167	638,000	12,760	19,631	1,020,800	1,000	1,021	6.95	$7,094.56
Penicillin VK suspension 100 mL	125 mg/5 mL	Bottle	1,447	0	241	2,894	58	89	4,630	1	4,630	0.75	$3,472.80
Salbutamol liquid 150 mL	2 mg/5 mL	Bottle	1,063	0	177	2,126	43	65	3,402	1	3,402	0.99	$3,367.58
Tetracycline HCl	250 mg	Capsule	62,000	0	10,333	124,000	2,480	3,815	198,400	1,000	198	12.00	$2,380.80
Vitamins, multiple	—	Tablet	259,000	0	43,167	518,000	10,360	15,938	828,800	1,000	829	3.20	$2,652.16
											Total Order Cost:		$222,370.22

Note: BU = basic unit.

Figure 14.7 Service-Based Budgeting of Essential Drug Requirements

Type of Facility and Patient (1)	Number of Facilities (2)	Average Annual Workload per Facility (3)	Average Cost per Attendance or Bed-Day (US$) (4)	Annual Drug Needs (US$) (5)
Provincial general hospitals	13			
Inpatients		176,000 bed-days	0.55	1,258,400
General outpatients[a]		195,000 attendances	0.55	1,394,250
Antenatal patients		19,500 attendances	0.15	38,025
District hospitals	42			
Inpatients		57,000 bed-days	0.50	1,197,000
General outpatients		85,000 attendances	0.50	1,785,000
Antenatal patients		11,000 attendances	0.15	69,300
Subdistrict hospitals	35			
Inpatients		21,500 bed-days	0.45	338,625
General outpatients		60,000 attendances	0.50	1,050,000
Antenatal patients		7,500 attendances	0.15	39,375
Rural health training centers	38			
Inpatients		20,000 bed-days	0.40	304,000
General outpatients		40,000 attendances	0.45	684,000
Antenatal patients		5,000 attendances	0.15	28,500
Health centers	315			
Inpatients		1,500 bed-days	0.20	94,500
General outpatients		32,000 attendances	0.40	4,032,000
Antenatal patients		4,000 attendances	0.15	189,000
Dispensaries	1,114			
General outpatients		18,000 attendances	0.30	6,015,600
Total				
Total				18,517,575
Per capita requirement				0.686
Subtotals				
Provincial general hospitals				2,690,675
District and subdistrict hospitals				4,479,300
Rural health training centers				1,016,500
Health centers and dispensaries				10,331,100
Total				18,517,575

Source: Adapted from Ministry of Health, Workload-Based Annual Budget for Pharmaceuticals and Non-Pharmaceuticals, Government of Kenya, 1992.
Note: The exchange rate used is 60 KSh to US$1. Population equals 27 million (estimate for 1993).
[a]This category includes (for all levels) adult and pediatric general outpatients, casualty, and specialty clinics.

target system using a different mix of drugs from those in the source system, variability in disease frequency and the number of patient attendances per facility, and differences in the effectiveness of procurement and financial management systems in the two systems.

The main requirement for this method is a fairly reliable estimate of average drug cost per patient attendance and average numbers of patient attendances at various levels of the standard health system. This information may not be readily available, but it can be compiled through a special study in one part of a health system where drug supplies are consistent and where treatment practices are considered to be representative. It is necessary to compile

▶ the average number of curative outpatient attendances, noncurative attendances, and inpatient bed-days for each type of facility in the source health system;

▶ the average cost per outpatient attendance, per non-

curative attendance, and per bed-day in each type of facility in the source health system.

Example

Figure 14.7 shows the method applied to estimate financial requirements for drug procurement, from Kenya.

Steps in the Quantification

Step 1. Establish the Categories of Facilities and Determine the Number in Each Category. List each type of facility to be considered in the first column. The number of facility categories used depends on the size and scope of the target health system. In Figure 14.7 there are six significant levels (see column 1). The number of facilities in each category is entered in the second column.

Step 2. Determine the Patient Contact Denominators for Each Type of Facility, and Compile or Estimate the Average Number of Patient Contacts of Each Type at Each Category

---

≡ Assessment Guide

Availability of Data
- ► Which records of drug usage are current and accurate at the medical stores and health facilities?
- ► What data and reports are maintained centrally (or at other levels of the health system) on outpatient attendances, inpatient bed-days, or other counts of patient contacts?
- ► For how many diseases is there reliable information on numbers of cases reported or treated annually?
- ► Are there official standard treatment guidelines for certain diseases? If so, how many diseases are covered, and how is compliance monitored?

Management of Quantification
- ► Is there a formal workplan and schedule for quantification?
- ► Is quantification done manually or by computer? If computers are used, which offices have computers, and what software program is used for quantification? Which levels of warehouses and facilities have computerized procurement and inventory records?
- ► Is quantification decentralized or managed centrally? Which offices and levels of the system are responsible for quantification?
- ► If quantification is decentralized, what training is or has been provided to responsible staff at peripheral facilities?

- ► Are preprinted quantification forms distributed to the facilities?

Quantification Methods
- ► What quantification methods are used to forecast drug and budget needs?
- ► Are actual procurement quantities and costs compared at the end of each year against the initial quantification estimates?
- ► Is the supply system pipeline functioning well, or have there been frequent or widespread drug shortages? If there have been shortages, do only certain drugs present problems, or do shortages exist for many different drugs?
- ► What information is used to predict procurement costs? If last year's prices are used, how are they adjusted?
- ► What standard formulas are used to calculate order quantities?
- ► Is there an essential drugs list or health system drug formulary that is used for quantification? Is procurement limited to drugs on the list?
- ► What techniques are used to adjust initial estimates to conform with budget realities?

---

of Facility. These data can be obtained from centrally available information or from a special-purpose survey to determine the average number of patient contacts for each category of facility. For each category, there may be several different types of patient contact that result in drug costs. Minimally, inpatient and outpatient costs and contacts should be separated.

In Figure 14.7 (column 3), in all but the lowest-level facility, contacts were separated into three types: inpatient, with bed-days as the common denominator; and general outpatient and antenatal visits, each with attendances as the denominator.

Step 3. Calculate the Average Cost per Contact. The average cost per attendance and or bed-day is derived by dividing the total drug purchases for the facility or facilities in the class by the total attendances or bed-days. In facilities

with both inpatients and outpatients, it is necessary to estimate the fraction of total procurement costs attributable to inpatients, outpatients, and noncurative visits. Column 4 in Figure 14.7 shows the average cost data.

Step 4. Calculate the Total Projected Drug Costs. Multiply the average number of patient contacts for each facility (column 3 in Figure 14.7) by the number of facilities (column 1). This result is then multiplied by the average drug cost for that type of patient in that type of facility (column 4), which estimates total financial requirements for each type of attendance in each type of facility (column 5). These totals are then summed to produce the total financial requirements. This is an estimate of the probable drug costs, on average, for each type of facility and for the system as a whole. The results are not necessarily applicable to any specific facility. ■

≡ References and Further Readings

★ = *Key readings.*

Hogerzeil, H. V. 1986. Estimating drug requirements: Standardized supply of essential drugs in Ghana. *Tropical Doctor* 16:155–59.

★ MSH (Management Sciences for Health). 1992. Planning drug requirements (trainer's and participant's guides). In *Managing drug supply training series.* Part 1. *Policy issues in managing drug supply.* Boston: MSH.

MSH (Management Sciences for Health). 1995. *International drug price indicator guide.* (Updated annually.) Boston: MSH.

Osore, H. 1989. Estimating drug requirements using morbidity data-based method: Cumulative country experience. *Tropical Doctor* 19:90–94.

Soeters, R., and W. Bannenberg. 1988. Computerized calculation of essential drug requirements. *Social Science and Medicine* 27:955–70.

WHO (World Health Organization). 1995. *The use of essential drugs.* Technical report series no. 850. Geneva: WHO.

WHO/CDD (World Health Organization/Control of Diarrhoeal Diseases program). 1991. Guidelines for cholera control. WHO/CDD/SER 80.4 REV 2. Geneva: WHO/CDD.

★ WHO/DAP (World Health Organization/Action Programme on Essential Drugs). 1988. *Estimating drug requirements: A practical manual.* Geneva: WHO/DAP.

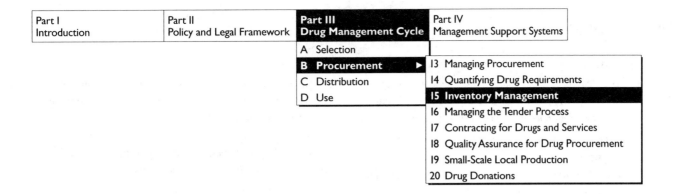

Part I Introduction	Part II Policy and Legal Framework	**Part III** **Drug Management Cycle**	Part IV Management Support Systems
		A Selection	
		B Procurement ▶	13 Managing Procurement
		C Distribution	14 Quantifying Drug Requirements
		D Use	**15 Inventory Management**
			16 Managing the Tender Process
			17 Contracting for Drugs and Services
			18 Quality Assurance for Drug Procurement
			19 Small-Scale Local Production
			20 Drug Donations

Chapter 15
Inventory Management

≡ Summary

This chapter discusses inventory management—the management of the routine ordering process. Seven basic issues must be considered for effective, efficient inventory management:

- *The supply system's purpose and the type of distribution system;*
- *Records and reports that will provide the foundation for inventory management;*
- *Selection of items to be stocked;*
- *The balance between service levels and stock levels;*
- *The policy on reordering frequency;*
- *The formula used to calculate reorder quantity;*
- *The control of costs associated with inventory management.*

The type of inventory management system needed depends first on the context—different systems are used for dependent demand systems (manufacturing) and independent demand systems (distribution of finished goods). Similarly, a different system may be needed in a push system as opposed to a pull system (see Chapter 21), although ordering has to be done in both push and pull systems. Clearly, most inventory management for drug supply concerns the distribution of finished goods.

Accurate and current stock records are essential to good inventory management. They are the source of information used to calculate needs, and inaccurate records produce inaccurate needs estimations (and problems with stockouts and expiry). Each inventory system should monitor performance with indicators and produce regular reports on inventory and order status, operating costs, and consumption patterns.

The primary reason for holding stock in a drug supply system is to ensure availability of essential items at all times. The selection of items to stock should be based on their value to public health and on the regularity and volume of consumption. VEN (vital, essential, nonessential) and ABC analyses are useful tools for defining which items on the formulary list must be held in stock.

Key issues in inventory management are service level and safety stocks. The service level is the measurement of service from a supplier or from a warehouse. The principal determinant of service level is safety stock—the higher the level of safety stock in the warehouse, the higher the service level. However, excessive safety stocks cause excessive inventory holding costs. The basic method for setting safety stock is multiplying the lead time by the average monthly consumption, but adjustments may be needed to cope with variations in consumption and lead-time patterns.

The ideal inventory model is the optimal stock movement pattern, in which inventory levels are minimized, consumption patterns are smooth, and suppliers always deliver on time, but this is rarely achieved in practice. The three common inventory models used in drug supply systems are defined by how often regular orders are placed with suppliers:

- *Annual purchasing (one regular order per year);*
- *Scheduled purchasing (periodic orders at set times during the year);*
- *Perpetual purchasing (orders are placed whenever stock becomes low).*

Average inventory levels (and holding costs) decrease with more frequent orders.

The basic formulas for calculating order quantity are relatively simple; two useful formulas are minimum-maximum and consumption based. Both incorporate several essential factors:

- *Average monthly consumption*
- *Supplier lead time*
- *Safety stock*
- *Stock on order*
- *Stock in inventory*
- *Stock back-ordered to lower levels*

The more complicated mathematical formulas, such as economic order quantity and exponential smoothing of demand, do not necessarily lead to better services than the simpler approaches and are not recommended for most drug supply systems. Whichever formulas are used, it is necessary to adjust purchase quantities to take into account factors such as seasonal demand, expected changes in utilization or prices, currency fluctuation, and availability of storage space.

Primary considerations in promoting efficiency are the costs of purchasing and of holding stock in inventory. A regular stock count and standard methods for valuing the inventory are needed to determine the base inventory value. Other relevant costs are the operating costs associated with procurement and with holding inventory. The objective of good inventory management is to maintain steady supply to operating units (and patients) while minimizing the costs of holding inventory and managing procurement. Compiling information on the total variable costs of inventory management (drug acquisition costs, inventory holding costs, purchasing operations costs, and shortage costs) allows managers to evaluate strategies for reducing costs.

≡ 15.1 Introduction

Inventory management is the heart of the drug supply system; in fact, the nonspecialist might say that inventory management *is* drug management. That would be simplistic, as the other chapters of this book demonstrate, but it is true that without a healthy inventory management system, the drug supply system as a whole will not be viable.

Inventory management for drug supply sounds easy—all that must be done is to order, receive, store, issue, and then reorder a limited list of items. In reality, the task is difficult, and in many countries, poor inventory management in the public drug supply system leads to waste of financial resources, shortages of essential drugs, and a decrease in the quality of patient care.

"Sick" inventory management systems generally feature subjective, ad hoc decisions about order frequency and quantity, inaccurate stock records, and a lack of systematic performance monitoring. These problems are directly related to ineffective management. In many cases there are no systematic procedures and rules to guide staff, a problem compounded by lack of understanding of the basic issues of proper inventory management on the part of managers.

Seven basic issues must be carefully considered when an inventory management system is being designed or revitalized:

1. Definition of the context in which the inventory management system must function;
2. Determination of the types of stock records and inventory reports needed;
3. Selection of items to be stocked;
4. Maintenance of a proper balance between service levels and stock levels;
5. Adoption of a model for reordering frequency;
6. Implementation of optimal reorder formulas;
7. Identification and control of variable inventory management costs.

To address these issues, managers must use mathematical formulas and models to set policies concerning stock levels, reordering frequency, and reorder quantity. Since inventory management is so important in all supply systems, public or private, a number of formulas have been developed over the years, some fairly simple and some involving complex calculations. In the great majority of drug supply situations, the simple models and formulas work as well as the complex models, so the simple ones are emphasized in this chapter.

≡ 15.2 The Context of an Inventory Management System

Before defining rules for inventory management, it is necessary to define the context in which an inventory management system operates. Two factors are relevant—independent versus dependent demand, and "push" versus "pull" logistics.

One factor that defines the context is whether the inventory system supports a supply system in which clients (health facilities) order finished products from a warehouse or other supply source, or whether the system supports primarily internal manufacturing; this determines whether the system is an independent demand system or a dependent demand system. The fundamental inventory management concepts and resulting procedures are quite different for the two systems.

Independent demand systems are applicable to the management of procurement and distribution of finished goods. The order intervals and quantities are derived from forecasts based on historical consumption by clients, tempered by knowledge of expected changes in consumption. Inventory levels are set to provide a defined level of service to clients, at an acceptable cost.

Dependent demand systems manage inventory requirements for raw materials and supplies based on what is needed for production in a manufacturing or repackaging operation. This is also known as a *materials requirement planning system*. Ordering intervals and quantities and inventory levels depend on projected production schedules. The just-in-time system is an example of inventory management in this context.

Because a typical drug supply system is involved mainly in the procurement and distribution of finished drug products, this chapter focuses on the independent demand system. However, in some drug supply situations (such as local manufacturing or repackaging), a dependent demand system would be more appropriate. Readers who need information on dependent demand systems should refer to "References and Further Readings" (Dear 1990; Waters 1992).

Another issue that defines the inventory management context is whether the logistics system is a pull system or a push system. In the *pull system*, operating units order drugs from a warehouse or supplier according to local determination of need. In the *push system*, a central authority orders drugs from suppliers and determines the quantities that will be shipped to the operating unit, based on the annual distribution plan and on information transmitted to the warehouse about need at the operating unit. The best-known example of a push system in drug supply is the ration kit system discussed in Chapter 27. Note that a push system has some features of a dependent demand system—a plan is set for distribution to operating units, and procurement is done to carry out that plan.

The inventory management methods discussed in this chapter can be applied in either a pull or a push system; the difference lies at which levels of the system ordering is done.

Before readers go further, it may be useful to review the procurement glossary at the end of Chapter 13, which contains commonly used terms that have a specific meaning in the discussion of inventory management.

≡ 15.3 Stock Records and Standard Reports

This section discusses the types of stock records and reports that form the foundation of effective inventory management.

Stock Records

Stock records are the core records in the inventory management system. They are the primary source of information used in the various reordering formulas discussed later in this chapter; they are also the source of data used to compile the reports discussed in this section. Stock records can be either manual or computerized. Commonly used manual stock records include

vertical file cards: File cards are stored vertically in alphabetical or numerical order in a card file or drawer.

"Kardex" system: File cards are stored in a visible-edge record tray system, with names and stock numbers on the lower edge, overlapped to provide an index.

bin cards: File cards are physically kept with the stock. This makes a visual check easy and serves as a reminder to keep records.

ledger system: Records are kept on ledger sheets in a bound or loose-leaf book.

Many supply systems maintain two stock records for each item, to improve accuracy and accountability. Typically, there is a bin card kept with the stock, combined with a ledger, Kardex, or computer system kept in the central office. The use of these record systems in a large warehouse is discussed in Chapter 23, and the maintenance of stock records in health facilities is treated in Chapter 24. Examples of manual and computerized stock records can be found in those chapters.

In most supply systems, computerization is desirable if the local situation can support automation. Computers are essential to manage an inventory of any size with perpetual purchasing. Moreover, a good software program, properly used, makes information retrieval and reporting much easier than a manual system (see Chapter 46). However, stock can still be controlled with manual records in most drug supply environments, if necessary.

The key point about stock records, whether manual or computerized, is that they must be current and accurate. It is impossible to manage the reordering process well if stock movement cannot be tracked.

Several factors contribute to inaccurate stock records; some are totally avoidable, but some are not:

► High-volume, repetitious entries lead to occasional entry errors just by the nature of the task.

► Drug names and descriptions are similar—there may be ten items that are different forms of the same drug, and an entry may be made for the wrong form.

► Duplicate entries for receipts or issues may be caused by duplicate paperwork provided separately to different clerks.

► Spoiled or junk stock may be destroyed but not written off the records.

► Theft produces inaccurate records, except when they are deliberately altered to conceal the theft.

► Physical stock counts may be rarely or never taken, or the records may not be reconciled after stock counts.

► Sloppy warehouse conditions may make it difficult to reconcile actual stock with recorded stock.

► Clerical and stock management staff may be poorly paid, poorly trained, and poorly motivated.

► There is often minimal supervision of warehouse staff or clerical staff, and limited effort by management to reconcile discrepancies.

Automation and newer technologies such as bar coding reduce some of the problems with inaccurate data entries, but this technology is still expensive to implement and does not solve all the problems. The best way to promote greater accuracy is better training and closer supervision, with spot checks of records and stock status by supervisors.

Physical Stock Counts. It is important to carry out stock counts, both for reordering purposes and for determining the inventory value. There are still some drug supply systems that never count stock and rely totally on inventory records, but most systems have a policy of conducting stock counts at least annually (although they may not really be carried out every year). The best approach to tracking the quantity actually in stock is *cyclic counting*.

In cyclic counting (sometimes known as continuous counting), inventory is divided into counting groups, and one group is counted each week (or each month), with reconciliation of discrepancies; another group is counted the next week (or next month), and so forth. It is generally accepted that a regular, cyclic stock-counting procedure is superior to an annual stock count. There are two main reasons for the change to cyclic counting:

1. With an annual stock count, a whole warehousing and distribution operation is shut down for a day or two to a week or more. This disrupts the supply system and causes frustration for warehouse and financial staff, who must rush to get the whole process completed as quickly as possible.
2. When discrepancies are found in an annual count, it is difficult to trace exactly where the problem arose during the year, so the records are simply corrected to reflect actual stock, and any losses are written off.

Cyclic counting, in contrast, can take place without interrupting normal operations. With more frequent counting, it may be possible to track down the source of discrepancies. Moreover, more frequent counting may make it harder for staff to pilfer stock.

One method of cyclic counting is to assign the counting frequency and timing by ABC category (defined in Section 15.4), counting A items three or four times a year, B items twice, and C items once; it may be worth adding to the A category any B or C items that are prone to disappear.

For best results, the staff who are counters in this process should not be the ones to reconcile discrepancies; a system of rotating different staff through both functions helps maintain the integrity of the process.

Activity Reports and Performance Monitoring

The most accurate stock records have little value if the information in them is not compiled in reports for use by the managers who make purchasing and stock management decisions. Two similar but separate types of reports are useful: periodic analyses and routine reports.

The inventory management system's health can be measured periodically using standard performance indicators. Box 15.1 lists performance indicators commonly used by commercial firms. The assessment guide at the end of the chapter cites indicators that have been tested in public supply systems.

Routine reports on purchasing and inventory management activities should be produced monthly to quarterly in a computerized system and at least annually in a manual system. The following lists illustrate the types of reports that are useful for improving inventory management.

Storage facilities should report on

Box 15.1 Performance Indicators Used by Commercial Firms

Inventory management performance indicators are used in commercial companies throughout the world to measure how effectively inventory is being managed; these indicators can and should be used in public drug supply systems when data are available.

Net sales to inventory: Also called *inventory turnover,* this is the total value of drugs distributed, minus write-offs, divided by the value of the inventory. The higher the ratio, the lower the average inventory level (and average holding cost). Most private companies would expect a turnover ratio of twelve or higher; in public drug supply systems, the ratio is dictated to some extent by the purchasing model, but a ratio of at least six is realistic in most cases.

Inventory shrinkage: The sum of beginning inventory value plus purchases, minus the sum of the cost of goods sold, plus ending inventory value. Ideally, this would be zero, but any value less than ten percent of inventory value is within expectations in most public drug supply systems.

Expense ratio: Total operating expenses divided by net sales (or value of drugs distributed). In one view, the lower this ratio, the more efficiently services are being managed.

Service level: The percentage of items ordered or requested that is filled from stock by the supplier or warehouse. From the public health viewpoint, the higher the service level, the better, as long as inventory costs do not rise to insupportable levels.

Average inventory holding cost: The average cost of holding inventory as a percentage of average inventory value. In a public drug supply system, 30 to 40 percent is a reasonable target.

Incremental ordering cost: The average incremental cost of placing each order. In a private company in an industrialized country, this might be $100 to $200 per order. It should be considerably lower in most public drug supply systems.

- ► stock position—stock on hand and on order, globally and by item, reported as absolute quantities and in terms of months' worth of consumption;
- ► beginning and ending inventory value, and the average inventory holding costs;
- ► changes in inventory value and any discrepancies noted during stock counts;
- ► consumption patterns for all stock items and an ABC analysis of consumption—with computer assistance, this can be done globally and for each operating unit;
- ► service level from suppliers to medical stores and from medical stores to health facilities;
- ► expiry status of drugs in inventory and estimate of how much stock is likely to expire before it can be used;
- ► quantity and value of obsolete stock waiting for disposal and stock destroyed or junked.

Purchasing and financial departments should report on

- budget status—expenditures versus targets, and amount remaining;
- purchases and expenditures, broken down by supplier and by operating unit;
- summaries of accounts payable to suppliers;
- status of outstanding orders;
- supplier performance;
- comparison of actual purchase price and projected cost;
- comparison of actual items purchased and original needs projections;
- operating costs attributable to stock management and to purchasing.

Accurate reporting is possible with either a manual or a computerized information system, but the information is much more readily compiled with computer assistance. Again, source data for the reports—stock records and purchasing records—must be maintained accurately and kept up-to-date. The key is that senior managers should demand these sorts of reports, use them in making policy decisions, and take corrective action when reports are not produced.

≡ 15.4 Selection of Items to Be Held in Stock
It is necessary to hold stock for several reasons:

To ensure availability: In the typical drug supply system, it is impossible to forecast demand with complete accuracy or to be certain about suppliers' performance. Inventory absorbs fluctuations in supply and demand and reduces the risk of stockouts.

To maintain confidence in the system: If there are regular stockouts, patients and staff lose confidence in the system, and patient utilization drops for both curative and preventive services.

To reduce the unit cost of drugs: Ordering drugs in bulk allows quantity discounts from suppliers and reduces shipping and port-clearing costs.

To avoid shortage costs: If emergency orders are needed to cope with stockouts, the unit cost is likely to be much higher than for a regular order. Also, when a drug sales program is operating, stockouts mean lost revenue, as clients go elsewhere for drugs.

To minimize ordering costs: Purchasing costs increase when items are ordered frequently. These costs include salaries and benefits for purchasing and accounting staff, office space costs, utilities, supplies, and other costs associated with tenders and regular orders.

To minimize transport costs: Drugs can be delivered less frequently, enabling transport resources to be used more economically.

To allow for fluctuations in demand: Changes in demand for specific drugs are often unpredictable, and an adequate inventory allows the system to cope with demand fluctuations.

It seems evident that drug supply systems need to hold a certain level of inventory; however, holding high stock levels has disadvantages (see Figure 15.1). Substantial capital can be tied up in inventory and thus be unavailable for other purposes. As inventories become larger, the costs for personnel, utilities, insurance, storage facilities, and other costs of holding stock increase. High inventory levels also increase the likelihood of losses due to spoilage, expiry, obsolescence, and theft. These adverse effects of high stock levels compel managers to focus on proper inventory management; otherwise, it would be simple to hold such large quantities of stock at all levels of the system that there would be no chance of shortages.

Most drug supply systems try to regularly stock all items that are on the formulary or essential drugs list (see Chapter 10). In many cases, items that are not on the approved list but are regularly requested by physicians are also routinely held in stock. Often no discrimination is made between vital and nonessential items, between high-cost and low-cost items, or between items that move quickly and those that are rarely used. This leads to an accumulation of slow-moving stock and excess capital tied up in inventory.

One way to decide which items should be stocked is to look at records of stock movement in and out of the storage facilities and identify the high-volume items that definitely need to be stocked, as well as items that have shown little or no movement in the past year. A good tool for reviewing stock movement is ABC analysis, which categorizes items by the volume and value of consumption during a specific period of time, usually one year. Class A items (10 to 20 percent of items, 75 to 80 percent of expenditures) are mostly high-volume, fast-moving drugs. Class B items are usually 10 to 20 percent of items and 15 to 20 percent of expenditures. Class C items often represent 60 to 80 percent of the items but only about 5 to 10 percent of expenditures; these are the low-volume, slow-moving items. Thus, Class C is a good place to look for items that might not be needed in stock at all times.

The VEN system is another system for categorizing stock as vital (V), essential (E), or nonessential (N). This system is sometimes modified to two categories—V and N. VEN analysis is often used to prioritize procurement when there are not enough funds to purchase all the items requested. The system can also help determine which items should be kept in stock and which can be ordered when needed. Clearly, V drugs would be more likely to be

Figure 15.1 Balancing Benefits and Costs in Inventory Management

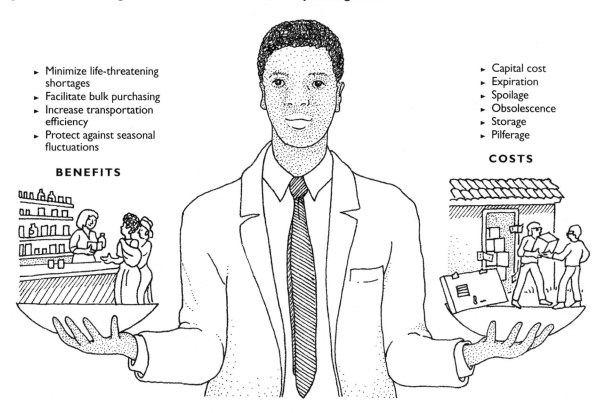

► Minimize life-threatening
  shortages
► Facilitate bulk purchasing
► Increase transportation
  efficiency
► Protect against seasonal
  fluctuations

BENEFITS

► Capital cost
► Expiration
► Spoilage
► Obsolescence
► Storage
► Pilferage

COSTS

regular stock items than N drugs. Both ABC and VEN analysis are discussed in detail in Chapter 41.

Not all drugs have to be stocked at each level of the system. One way of classifying stock versus nonstock items is according to the approved level of use. For example, a drug such as aspirin would be a stock item at all levels of the system, but a third-generation cephalosporin or a drug used in cancer chemotherapy might be a stock item only in tertiary care hospitals. Classifying drugs according to their eligibility for routine use at each level helps minimize stock levels and ensure that only qualified staff prescribe dangerous or expensive drugs.

Finally, the issue of local availability must be kept in mind. If a drug is vital to patient care (even if rarely used) but cannot be obtained quickly when it is needed, that drug will probably need to be kept as a stock item. When there are no local sources of supply and all drugs are imported, with long lead times, all drugs need to be held in stock somewhere in the system. In most countries, however, there are opportunities to purchase some drugs as needed from local sources, and it is worth considering which of those items need to be constantly held in stock.

Zimbabwe has started closely examining the stock status of formulary items. The Zimbabwe Essential Drugs Action Programme (ZEDAP) has separated the essential drugs list

(EDLIZ) into stock and nonstock items. As of 1994, ZEDAP decided that of the 592 drugs on the EDLIZ, 307 "less frequently used drugs" would not be stocked at medical stores and would be obtained through local private-sector sources when needed. ZEDAP produces a catalog of items on the essential drugs list that shows which items are routinely held in stock; the catalog is updated periodically throughout the year to illustrate central medical stores (CMS) stock status. This sort of catalog is recommended for all supply systems; it serves as a basic means of communicating which items are in stock and also provides the basic list for procurement consideration.

Whichever approaches are used to designate stock and nonstock items, some scheme for periodically re-evaluating the stock status is needed. If the system is computerized, the software can be programmed to automatically recategorize items at specified intervals based on recent patterns of stock movement.

≡ 15.5 Service Level and Safety Stock

Once the decision has been made about which items will be routinely held in stock and which will be ordered only when they are needed, the discussion turns to how much stock should be held at each level of the system. There are likely to be different points of view: stock controllers and

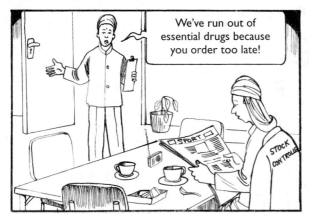

WHY DOES STOCK CONTROL WORK IN SOME SITUATIONS BUT NOT IN OTHERS?

clinical staff may feel that inventory levels should be high, to avoid shortages; financial managers, however, hope to minimize inventory levels to hold down costs.

One of the most common ways to measure the performance of a commercial supplier or public warehouse is to calculate the service level provided to clients. Suppliers try to balance service level and the costs of holding stock. The single most important factor in establishing that balance is the average stock held by the supplier and, in particular, the safety stock.

Service Level to Operating Units

The *service level*, in its most representative form, is the percentage of individual items ordered from a supplier or warehouse that is issued from stock on hand. This is measured by counting the total number of items issued and dividing by the total number of items requested.

Service level = (# items issued ÷ # items requested) × 100

If twenty products are listed on a request, and ten units of each product are requested, there are 200 items on the order; if only 170 items were issued, the service level was 85 percent. When assessing the annual service level of a supplier, the key is the total number of items requested on all requisitions and how many of those items were supplied from stock on hand at the supplier's warehouse.

Some commercial suppliers (and public warehouses) are prone to making partial shipments. When an order is received, an initial shipment is made with part of the request; later, one or more additional shipments are made with the remainder of the order quantity. For purposes of measuring the service level, only the initial shipment after each order should count.

In some supply systems, it is too time-consuming to count all items requested and issued, and a count of line items (the number of different products ordered, disregarding order quantities) is used. This scheme makes it hard to decide how to count line items when only part of the request was shipped. Suppliers would argue that any of an item shipped should count as a full shipment for service-level measurement, but many clients would disagree. Systems have evolved to measure line-item service level in categories, for example, the percentage of line items that falls into the categories "none issued," "part issued," and "issued in full."

Other ways to measure service level include

▶ percentage of individual items or line items requested that are *delivered* within the promised lead time (this can be useful when delivery times vary);
▶ the value of all items shipped from stock as a percentage of the value of all items ordered;
▶ the percentage of full orders completely filled from stock. There are two variations—in one, either the whole order is shipped or not; in the other, performance is categorized as discussed for the line-item method.

Whatever measure is used, what is a reasonable service level? Many private-sector drug wholesalers promise 95 percent service levels to customers (although they do not always fulfill this promise). Is this level sufficient? The point to remember is that every percentage point decrease in service level by a supplier or warehouse represents a corresponding increase in shortages at the client facility. If a supplier promises a 95 percent service level, it is already expected that 5 percent of the requested items will not be shipped immediately (implying a potential 5 percent stockout at the receiving facility). If the level drops to 90 percent, then 10 percent of the items are not being shipped when they are needed. A public-sector drug supply system should strive for a 100 percent service level, at least for vital items; it might be reasonable to set lower goals for nonessential drugs and supplies.

Service level is directly determined by the average inventory level, and particularly by the average level of safety stock, held by the supply source. Figure 15.2 illustrates the typical relationship between safety stock and service level from a supply source (either commercial or public).

Note in Figure 15.2 that although the safety stock requirements increase as the service level increases, the relationship is not linear. As the service level increases above 80 percent, the amount of additional safety stock needed to produce a further increase in service level rises steeply. The amount of safety stock required to achieve a

99 percent service level may be double that required to achieve a 95 percent service level. For example, where a safety stock of 2,000 units is needed to achieve a service level of 95 percent, 4,000 units may be needed to raise the service level to 99 percent.

For both the supplier and the client, the balance between cost and service is really a matter of tradeoffs. For the client, if the supplier cannot or will not maintain adequate inventory levels to sustain an acceptable service level, it will be necessary to either change suppliers or increase safety stock levels at the receiving units. For the supplier, the tradeoff is between incurring higher inventory costs to maintain the promised service level or running the risk of shortage costs, as clients go elsewhere for service.

In commercial enterprises, safety stock levels are set using standard formulas using knowledge about demand patterns, inventory costs, sales income lost from stockouts, and other factors. If there is a stockout, it is normally accepted as the cost of tight inventory control. In public pharmaceutical systems, the cost of additional safety stock must be weighed against the potential adverse health and political impacts of stockouts.

When one designs or restructures an inventory management system, safety stock policy is an important consideration. The policy may differ at each level of the system, or between different facilities at the same level (depending on lead times and consumption patterns). The objective is to provide maximum service levels throughout the system with minimum necessary *total* safety stock.

Methods for Setting Safety Stock Levels

There are many ways of estimating the level of safety stock required to achieve specific service levels. All consider two major factors: average consumption and average lead time. Box 15.2 discusses simple methods for estimating safety stock needs. In most supply systems, more complex mathematical models for estimating safety stock needs will probably not provide any significant advantage over simple methods (see Section 15.9).

≡ 15.6 Inventory Control Models and Reorder Frequency

The ideal inventory control model is shown in Figure 15.3. In this ideal model, drugs are issued in response to demand; the stock on hand steadily declines until the point at which an order must be placed. The stock on hand consists of two components, the working stock and the safety stock (SS). In the ideal model, the supplier performs according to plan, the shipments arrive on time, the quantity ordered (Q_O) is received, and the

Figure 15.2 Safety Stock Requirements to Maintain Various Service Levels

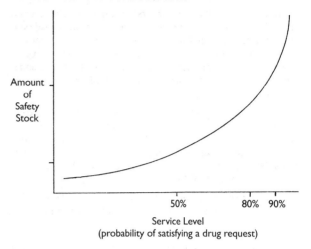

Amount of Safety Stock

Service Level
(probability of satisfying a drug request)

inventory level is back to its starting maximum point ($Q_O + SS$). Working stock varies from zero to the quantity ordered and represents the stock used to satisfy demand between deliveries. Note that in the ideal model, the average working stock is half of the order quantity:

$$\text{Average working stock} = {}^1\!/_2\, Q_O$$

The average inventory (I) or average stock on hand is the safety stock plus the average working stock:

$$I = SS + {}^1\!/_2\, Q_O$$

To reduce the average inventory and thereby reduce the inventory holding costs, either the working stock, the safety stock, or both should be lowered. When drugs are used at a constant rate, the line in Figure 15.3 representing stock on hand declines with a constant slope. Large, infrequent orders lead to high average inventory levels. The average working stock can be reduced by placing smaller orders more frequently. The average inventory can also be reduced by cutting the safety stock, but this increases the chance of stockouts.

As illustrated by the ideal model, any inventory control model used to manage purchasing must address three issues:

1. Safety stock—how much stock will be kept in reserve to prevent stockouts;
2. Reorder frequency—the period of time between each order for an item (also known as the procurement period);
3. Reorder quantity—the number of units specified when an order is placed.

Box 15.2   Estimating Safety Stock

The minimum safety stock needed to avoid a stockout is the quantity of stock used on average during the average lead time from the current supplier. This means that if an order is placed as soon as the stock level falls to the safety stock level, if demand is no greater than average during the lead time, and if the supplier delivers within the average lead time, a stockout will be avoided.

The most common method for estimating safety stock needs is to determine the average lead time for each item from the current supplier and the average consumption (per month or per week). If there were stockouts, consumption must be adjusted to what would have been used, as described in Chapter 14, Section 14.4.

The formula for setting the basic safety stock (SS) level is lead time (LT) multiplied by the average consumption (C_A):

$$SS = LT \times C_A$$

For example, if the average lead time is three months and the average monthly consumption is 1,000 units, the minimum safety stock would be 3,000 units.

Unfortunately, consumption patterns are not always smooth, and suppliers do not always deliver within the average lead time, so most supply systems increase the basic safety stock at least for critical items to cope with variations in consumption and lead time.

The simplest approach for coping with varying consumption and lead time is adding an arbitrary multiplier to the basic formula for safety stock; member countries in the Eastern Caribbean Drug Service pooled procurement system, for example, multiply the basic safety stock by 1.5 for vital items, to protect against stockouts.

Another simple way to adjust the safety stock for variable consumption is to review a one-year period and determine the maximum quantity consumed during the average lead-time period for the current supplier of the item and the average quantity consumed during that same lead-time period. For the example cited above, the average consumption during the three-month average lead-time period was 3,000 units; suppose that for any three-month period during the year, the highest consumption was 4,000 units. Using this method, the minimum stock level would be 3,000 units, and the additional safety stock allotment would be 1,000 units.

The information from lead-time analysis (see Chapter 41) can be used to predict the next lead time, as follows:

$$DD_E = DD_P + (OD \times OD\%)$$

where:

DD_E = expected delivery date

DD_P = promised delivery date

OD = average overdue period in days

$OD\%$ = percentage of orders overdue

Chapter 41 cites an eastern Caribbean supplier that had a contract lead time of 45 days but was late on 50 percent of shipments, with an average delay of 43 days. According to the formula above, this supplier has an expected delivery date of 66.5 days, calculated as:

$$DD_E = 45 + (43 \times 50\%) = 66.5$$

When calculating safety stock needs for products from this supplier, it would be safer to use a lead time of 66.5 days rather than 45 days.

When both consumption and lead times are highly variable, some commercial firms use a mathematical approach using the standard deviation of the average consumption and the average lead time to set safety stock levels (see Section 15.9).

Note that all these adjustments tend to increase inventory holding costs by increasing the safety stock level; therefore, it is important to monitor consumption and lead-time patterns continuously and adjust safety stock to the lowest levels compatible with current patterns. In a computerized inventory control system, this adjustment should be done automatically by the software.

As made clear in Figure 15.4, the policy on reorder frequency has a major influence on average stock levels and inventory holding costs, as well as on service level.

Different inventory control models based on reorder frequency have been developed to fit various situations. Two ways to classify these models are:

1. *Periodic versus perpetual review*: In periodic models, orders can be placed only at specified intervals, whereas in perpetual models, orders can be placed at any time.
2. *One-level and two-level:* In the one-level model, orders are placed at defined intervals, and the item is ordered at every interval. In two-level models, the user (or a minimum stock level) determines when to order and how much to order.

In drug supply systems, the most common inventory control models are

► annual purchasing—a one-level periodic review model, with the interval set at once a year;
► scheduled purchasing—a periodic review model in which orders are placed at prescribed intervals (such as weekly, monthly, quarterly, biannually), with both one-level and two-level variations;
► perpetual purchasing—a two-level model in which stock levels are reviewed each time stock is issued (or at least weekly) and orders are placed whenever stock falls below a minimum level.

Annual Purchasing

With annual purchasing (really a form of scheduled purchasing), procurement is done once each year for all items. Order quantities are normally calculated by large-scale quantification (see Chapter 14).

Once quantification is done, a tender or competitive

Figure 15.3 Ideal Inventory Control Model

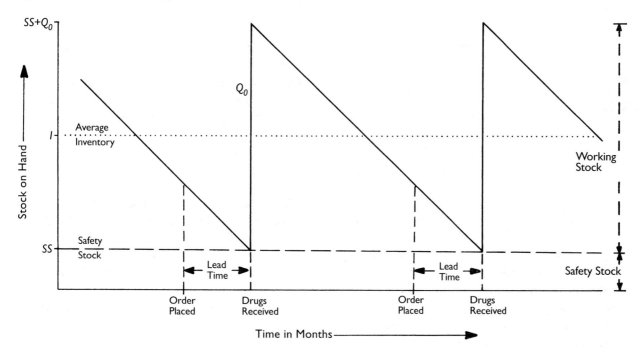

negotiation (see Chapters 13 and 16) is used to purchase the entire annual amount (or as much as can be afforded). Contracts with suppliers may provide that deliveries be spaced throughout the year if there are problems with local storage space, storage conditions, or security. In virtually all supply systems using annual purchasing, mechanisms exist to make supplementary purchases during the year. The main reasons that countries use annual purchasing include:

► Financial regulations and realities may dictate the choice.
► One single procurement can be easier to manage than more frequent purchasing, depending on staff capacities and availability of information.
► Drug purchase prices per unit are usually lower when large-volume purchases are made. This can be an important consideration when inflation and/or local currency devaluation is significant and progressive. In such cases, it is better to commit the funds at lower prices and higher exchange rates.
► Tradition and inertia may promote continuance of annual purchasing just because it has always been done that way.

There are several disadvantages with using annual purchasing as the sole purchasing model for the supply system:

► Actual consumption is often different from the annual forecast, leading to shortages and surpluses; expensive emergency orders are required to cope with shortages, and surplus stock may spoil or expire.
► Average stock levels and inventory holding costs are higher with this model (see Figure 15.4).
► Local suppliers that win annual tender contracts may find it difficult to cope with huge single deliveries.
► More storage space is required, unless deliveries from suppliers can be spaced throughout the year.
► It may be difficult to come up with the funds necessary to pay for the single annual purchase, particularly if hard currency is required.
► Workload in the procurement office and main receiving points is uneven.

In general, annual purchasing is best suited to new programs, where there is no existing system for inventory management. It may be mandatory in countries where there are limited local sources of supply and lead times from foreign suppliers average several months. Annual purchasing may also be preferred when donors support drug purchases. Even in systems that use mainly scheduled or perpetual purchasing, it may be best to purchase some items annually.

Scheduled Purchasing

In this periodic review model, specific ordering windows are determined, and regular orders can be placed only at

Figure 15.4 Impact of Reorder Interval on Average Inventory

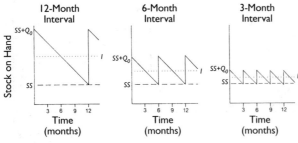

Key: I = average inventory Q_0 = order quantity   SS = safety stock

the scheduled intervals—for example, once each month, each quarter, every six months, or other interval. Orders are placed at the scheduled order date for quantities large enough to cover average needs until the next order is scheduled, plus stock needed during the lead time for that order (plus replenishment of safety stock, if needed).

One variation on this model is staggered review, in which the procurement office reviews one group of drugs (or drugs from one group of suppliers) at one interval, another group at the next interval, and so forth. In this manner, the workload in the procurement office and the financial requirements for drug purchasing are spread out during the year, while still limiting the number of orders placed to each supplier (which can be an important issue in supply contracts).

It is also possible to vary the ordering frequency according to ABC category, so that more expensive, faster-moving items are ordered more frequently and other items less frequently (this system is discussed below).

Scheduled purchasing with a review period of six months can operate in much the same way as annual purchasing, but shorter intervals require one of the options for calculating order quantities described in Section 15.9. Normally, an emergency ordering system is used when stock runs low between scheduled orders or when a supplier's shipment is delayed.

In scheduled purchasing, supply contracts can be negotiated anew at each interval, or longer contracts can be negotiated at the beginning of the year, with the provision that orders will be placed as needed at the specified ordering intervals (the estimated-quantity contract; see Chapter 16).

In most supply systems, it is customary to place a new order only after receiving a previous one. However, some programs use tandem ordering, with overlapping orders and different expected times of arrivals, if estimated lead times are reliable.

Scheduled purchasing has several potential benefits:

- An estimated- rather than fixed-quantity contract can be supported.
- Local suppliers may prefer a scheduled system, because it allows them to spread their demand out over the year.
- Inventory holding costs are less than with annual purchasing (see Figure 15.4).
- Less space is needed in warehouses than with annual purchasing.
- Items with variable demand can be purchased more frequently in smaller lots, reducing overstocking and costly emergency orders.
- The procurement unit can respond more rapidly to program needs and make better use of a limited drug budget.
- In many countries, it is easier to locate the funds and foreign exchange to make smaller, more frequent purchases.
- The procurement workload is fairly evenly spread over the year.

One potential difficulty is that when orders are placed late in the fiscal year, the purchasing cycle will not be complete before the end of the year. This may result in a conflict with regulations regarding spending time limits. Shortages due to poor forecasting or changes in demand are less likely with this model than with annual purchasing, but they can still occur with scheduled review periods three to six months apart.

If progressive inflation and devaluation are problems, an escalator clause may be required in annual estimated-quantity contracts; if a separate contract is negotiated at each ordering interval, prices are likely to increase throughout the year. In such cases, it may be best to procure as many essential items as possible, along with any items likely to increase in price, in the first part of the year.

Scheduled purchasing works most effectively when consumption patterns are relatively stable, at least for the duration of the period between orders. If there are wild fluctuations from month to month, perpetual purchasing would be preferable, assuming that it is logistically feasible.

Scheduled purchasing is probably the best choice as an alternative to annual procurement in countries that do not have immediate access to suppliers. The major requirements for managing scheduled purchasing are an inventory information system that can produce reliable information on consumption, stock levels, and outstanding orders, and the management and financial capacity to place all necessary orders according to the schedule.

Perpetual Purchasing

In this model, a perpetual inventory record is maintained for each item. The inventory position (stock on hand and on order) is reviewed on a regular basis (usually with every transaction, but at least weekly); whenever the stock position falls below a designated reorder point, an order is initiated. As will be discussed later, the order quantity may be predetermined or variable.

Safety stocks and average inventories are much lower with this model than with either scheduled or annual purchasing, but some safety stock is still needed. The chief advantage of perpetual purchasing over scheduled and annual purchasing is the ability to rapidly respond to sudden changes in consumption, because the inventory position is reviewed continuously and orders are placed frequently.

In some systems that use perpetual purchasing, orders are batched—that is, an order is not placed with a supplier until several different items are needed from that supplier. If batching is used, safety stock must be adequate to cover periods when a needed item is on hold for batching.

Perpetual purchasing is used by most hospitals and health systems in industrialized countries, where lead times for virtually all items are one or two days. In the United States, perpetual purchasing normally takes place in a prime vendor distribution system, whereby a commercial distributor supplies all contract items on short notice (see Chapter 6). This avoids the batching issue, because all or virtually all items are ordered from the same supplier.

If applied appropriately, perpetual purchasing produces an even workload for procurement, warehousing, and transport. Depending on the supply system's budgeting and financial policies, perpetual purchasing with frequent small orders may be useful in spreading cash requirements throughout the year.

In spite of the many benefits of a perpetual system, it is not suitable for all public-sector drug supply systems. There are several potential constraints. If lead times are not relatively short (one month or less), it will be difficult to use perpetual purchasing without maintaining large safety stocks (thereby defeating its purpose). If the supply system cannot maintain current and accurate stock records, the perpetual purchasing model will fail, because by the time transactions are posted, vital items may be out of stock. When it is necessary to obtain formal approval from the ministry of health or ministry of finance for each purchase and for foreign exchange permits, the time needed for approval may make perpetual purchasing awkward.

Perpetual purchasing is incompatible with fixed-quantity tenders. Therefore, if all drugs must be purchased by fixed-quantity tender, perpetual purchasing will not work. However, an estimated-quantity tender can readily accommodate the perpetual system (see Chapters 13 and 16).

The more frequent purchases in perpetual purchasing will drive up incremental purchasing costs and perhaps total purchasing costs, but any increase in incremental purchasing costs may be offset by decreased inventory holding costs. It may also be comparatively harder to fit perpetual purchasing into public health objectives and budgetary limits, because all the small purchases must be tracked for compliance with guidelines.

There are potential applications for perpetual purchasing in many drug supply systems even if the entire purchasing system cannot be converted to this method. For example, perpetual purchasing might be considered for fast-moving items that can be ordered at competitive prices from local sources. A perpetual system might be used by lower-level stores and facilities that order from a larger warehouse; this could be done whether or not the main warehouse uses perpetual purchasing, so long as the ordering cycles can be coordinated.

The main requirements for perpetual purchasing are

- ▶ stock records that are current and accurate;
- ▶ a computer with suitable software to manage an inventory of more than a few items (see Chapter 46);
- ▶ good access to and communication with suppliers and user units, with lead times of one month or less;
- ▶ ready access to funds, unless suppliers are prepared to wait for payment;
- ▶ an estimated-quantity contract that allows ad hoc orders, or a purchasing environment where formal contracts are not used.

Combinations of Annual, Scheduled, and Perpetual Purchasing

Although it may be simplest from a management perspective to establish one inventory control model for all drugs, this may not be the most cost-effective solution.

A thorough review of options may reveal that it would be best to purchase some drugs annually—for example, imported drugs in a country where local currency devaluation is a major problem, or low-priced, infrequently used drugs. Other drugs might be most effectively purchased through scheduled purchasing—for example, relatively slow-moving but regularly used items. High-volume drugs and very expensive drugs may be most

Figure 15.5 Value of Average Inventory by Service Level and Procurement Pattern

Procurement Pattern and ABC Category—Order Interval	Value of Inventory (Thousands of US$)				
			Service Level		
	99%	98%	95%	90%	85%
Pattern A A drugs—12 months B drugs—12 months C drugs—12 months	10,801	9,730	8,204	7,394	7,394
Pattern B A drugs—6 months B drugs—12 months C drugs—12 months	8,766	7,750	6,902	5,217	4,606
Pattern C A drugs—6 months B drugs—6 months C drugs—12 months	8,365	7,360	5,927	4,788	4,056
Pattern D A drugs—6 months B drugs—6 months C drugs—6 months	8,103	7,104	5,661	4,507	3,697
Pattern E A drugs—4 months B drugs—6 months C drugs—12 months	7,820	6,862	5,476	4,392	3,738
Pattern F A drugs—4 months B drugs—4 months C drugs—4 months	7,380	6,471	5,086	3,982	3,275

Source: Adapted from Quick 1982.

effectively purchased with a perpetual model, if logistically feasible.

ABC analysis can be used to examine the effect of variations in order frequency on average inventory value for Class A, B, and C items. Figure 15.5 shows the relationships among the average order interval, the average inventory level, and the service level for Class A, B, and C drugs in a large public-sector drug supply system. This projection is based on an average lead time of nine months (see Quick 1982 for details). Note the difference in average inventory value needed to maintain a 95 percent service level with the various permutations of order frequency for Class A, B, and C items.

Although the lowest average inventory cost is obtained in the example by increasing the frequency of ordering for all classes, this may increase the procurement workload and the costs of purchasing significantly, particularly if formal tenders are required. Changing the tender frequency for Class A items to twice rather than once a year, and the order quantity from twelve months' to six months' usage, reduces the average inventory value by almost half, while still maintaining the desired service level; this change should not increase the cost of purchasing to unaccept-

able levels (although a total variable cost analysis should be performed to check the potential impact).

Dear (1990) describes a reordering system that builds on ABC analysis, called ABC/FS. In this system, the A, B, and C items are further broken down into three categories—fast turnover (F), slow movement (S), and no movement in the past year (Class C items that might be reclassified as D for dead).

Using a mixed model of annual, scheduled, and perpetual purchasing, the purchasing office in this system concentrates on the fast-moving and expensive stock items, which have the most impact on inventory costs. Vital (V) and nonessential (N) classification can be combined with ABC/FS, with interesting implications for inventory management. For example, a Class A slow-moving item that is also a vital drug (ASV) might be accorded a higher safety stock than a Class A, fast-moving, nonessential item (AFN). An AFN item might be ordered only for specific patients as needed, or a class C, slow-moving, nonessential item (CSN) might be considered for nonstock status and ordered only as needed. Clearly, there are many different ways to use combinations of annual, scheduled, and perpetual purchasing, if the supply system can manage such flexibility.

≡ 15.7 Factors to Consider in Calculating Reorder Quantity

Once the basic inventory control model has been established, the final question is how much should be ordered at each order interval. This section examines the factors that must be taken into account; Section 15.8 shows how the factors are integrated into a reordering formula.

Factors in the Reorder Formula

Depending on the reorder formula used, any or all of the following factors may be essential variables.

Average Consumption. Sometimes called demand, the average consumption expected in the next purchasing cycle is the key variable that determines how much stock should be ordered. Future consumption is the great unknown of inventory management, so it is given special attention in this section. However, the other factors are equally important. Even if consumption is accurately predicted, stockouts will occur if the lead time is badly underestimated or if another factor is overlooked or miscalculated.

Lead Time. This is the time between initiation of a purchase order and receipt at the warehouse from the selected supplier. If there is a distinct trend in that supplier's performance, the average should be weighted toward recent performance with a moving average. However, if there is a fluctuating pattern—for example, two months, six months, two months, six months—it is best to apply lead-time analysis (Chapter 41) or calculate the standard deviation as discussed in Section 15.9 under "Mathematical Models for Reordering."

Safety Stock. Safety stock is the stock that should always be on hand to prevent stockouts. When lead times and consumption are predictable and stable, the reorder level and the safety stock level may be the same; however, when consumption patterns and lead times are highly variable, additional safety stock will be needed, as discussed in Section 15.5.

Reorder Level. The reorder level is the quantity of remaining stock that should trigger a reorder of the item. In the minimum-maximum ordering system, this is called the *minimum stock level.* The standard way to set the reorder level in a basic purchasing formula is to multiply the average lead time by the average quantity consumed during the lead time. This stock level may or may not be the same as the safety stock level, as discussed above.

Maximum Stock Level. In most reordering formulas, this level is the target stock level, which is the stock needed to satisfy demand until the next order after this one is received.

Stock Position. Stock position is the sum of *stock on hand* (working and safety stock) and *stock on order*, minus any *stock back-ordered* to clients. Overstocks may occur if there are already several months' worth of stock on hand or on order when a new order is placed. Stockouts may result if significant quantities from an upcoming order are on back-order to lower-level facilities and this is not factored into the reorder quantity.

Procurement Period. The procurement period covers the time until the next regular order will be placed. In a scheduled system, this might be in multiples of one month; in a perpetual system, it could be counted in days or weeks for the purposes of forecasting. Note that the quantity ordered plus the safety stock must cover the time until the next order is received, which is the procurement period plus the lead time.

Projecting Consumption

Ordering rationally requires forecasting future needs, the least predictable variable in a reordering formula. Three different methods can be used for forecasting consumption:

1. *Projective:* forecasts using past consumption to predict demand (in drug supply systems, the method most likely to produce reasonably accurate forecasts);
2. *Causal:* forecasts based on external factors such as market conditions, epidemics, changes in health system size and structure;
3. *Judgmental:* forecasts based on subjective estimates of purchasing staff and advice from other staff (the least demanding method, and often the least accurate, if used alone).

Generally, a reordering formula should be based primarily on projective forecasting, derived from average monthly consumption. The other methods can be used as appropriate to adjust actual purchase quantities. Unfortunately, although past consumption (past demand) is the best source of data for projection, there may not be a stable pattern or trend. In a series of observations of monthly consumption for a twelve-month period (called a time series), there may be several components in the observed consumption pattern:

Base rate: consumption that may be fairly stable from month to month;

Trend: a steady pattern of increasing or decreasing consumption, for example, increased usage due to gradually increasing patient attendances;

Seasonality: changes that are relatively predictable, such as increase in demand for chloroquine in the summer;

Cyclic demand: demand that ebbs and flows, for example, with a country's economic cycle;

Random noise: unexplained variations in demand; for example, in one month, one hundred bottles of amoxicillin suspension were consumed, with a pattern of thirty, ten, eighty, and twenty bottles in succeeding months, with no obvious reason for the variation.

It is relatively easy to adjust for a definite trend toward higher (or lower) use or seasonality (if it is predictable). Cyclic use patterns can also be dealt with if they are apparent. The real problem is random noise, and in many consumption patterns, random noise seems to be the dominant component.

Fairly complex mathematical models have been developed for smoothing forecasts—exponential smoothing, seasonal indexes, and other methods. Some of these models are discussed later in the chapter. Most incorporate factors such as trend and seasonality, while attempting to cope with random noise. However, these more complex models have limited value in most drug supply situations; the following methods of tracking average consumption (to forecast demand) are suitable for most drug supply systems:

Simple average consumption: the average monthly consumption over the past twelve months (or less, such as six months, if there are no seasonal changes in consumption);

Seasonal average consumption: the average consumption in the last comparable season or epidemic cycle for specific drugs;

Moving average consumption: the average monthly consumption in the most recent months—for example, the past two or three months.

The key variables in these methods are which months and how many months (or weeks or days) are included in the review period for which consumption is averaged. Note that consumption in the three methods is stated in monthly terms, but it could be daily or weekly for a perpetual system, or yearly for annual purchasing.

Whichever review period is used, if the item was out of stock for part of the period, it is essential to adjust the consumption to what it would have been if there had been no stockouts. One good method for doing this is described in Chapter 14, Section 14.4.

When consumption patterns during the year are fairly stable or there are unpredictable variations (random noise), simple average consumption provides adequate results, adjusting safety stock levels to cope with variations in consumption.

When there are big differences in seasonal demand, use of simple average consumption may produce stockouts in peak demand seasons (and simultaneously set stock levels too high in nonpeak seasons). Therefore, the seasonal average is used to adjust reorder and stock levels for each season. The review period is set to the number of periods in a season. For example, if there are four months in the malaria season, look at consumption patterns for chloroquine in the four-month malaria season last year rather than the past twelve months to predict needs for this year's season.

Moving averages are suitable for use when there is a definite trend in consumption up or down in recent months and there are reasons to expect the trend to continue. Both moving averages and seasonal averages fit well with scheduled purchasing, but they can be applied (with caution) to perpetual purchasing as well.

Integrating Experience and Other Factors

No matter how precise the reordering formula is, external factors may force an adjustment of the quantity suggested by a reordering formula. Most supply systems operate under a system whereby the reordering formula suggests quantities, but the purchasing manager makes the final decision. If the reordering formulas are appropriate, relatively few formula recommendations should be overruled by the manager (certainly fewer than 10 percent). However, if the manager knows about an external factor such as those cited below or believes that the formula is producing nonsense (perhaps reordering factors have not been properly entered), experience and local judgment should be the deciding factors.

The key is for the reordering formula to be understood and accepted by the responsible officials, so that managers are not looking for reasons to override suggested quantities. One way to ensure this acceptance is to involve operations-level managers in developing and approving the reorder formula that will be used. Examples of factors that might affect reorder quality follow.

Budget Status. Most supply systems operate under a specified budget ceiling. There are two basic approaches to budget management. In one, the supply system develops a purchasing budget for each item, specifying the quantity budgeted for the year. Then the orders during the year are tracked against this line-item budget. In order to increase the total annual quantity for any item, the quantity for another item must be reduced (or more funds must be located). In the other budget management approach, all procurement funds are lumped together, and orders are placed for whatever items are perceived to be needed until funds are gone. With either budgeting approach, managers need to monitor the items and quantities on each purchase order and cumulative purchases to make sure that the budget is not overspent.

Access to Funds. Even if funds are theoretically budgeted, they may not be available when it is time to place an order; if there are insufficient funds to purchase all the items suggested by the standard reordering formula, adjustments need to be made (see Chapters 14 and 41).

Pack Size and Minimum Order. The order quantity often needs to be adjusted so that even pack sizes are ordered. For example, if the formula suggests ordering 900 capsules, it might be possible to order nine bottles of 100 capsules. However, if the contract price is based on bottles of 1,000, the order would be placed for one bottle of 1,000. Similarly, if the formula suggests ten bottles of 100 capsules but the supplier's contract specifies a minimum order of twelve bottles, then twelve bottles must be ordered (such minimums should be avoided in supply contracts, if possible).

Expected Changes in Utilization. If a change is anticipated within the next purchasing cycle in the number of health facilities or in the formulary or essential drugs list, allowances need to be made in reordering schemes, particularly in annual and scheduled purchasing models.

Expected Price Increase. If it is known that prices will rise significantly for a drug or group of drugs before the next ordering cycle, it may be cost effective to order unusually high quantities if consumption patterns indicate that the higher quantities will be used before expiry (or loss or deterioration).

Rising Delivery Costs. If shipping costs are a major factor in total drug costs and they are expected to increase significantly, the approach is similar to the one used for rising prices. The drugs affected should be ordered in higher quantities, with the same precaution concerning capacity to use the entire quantity.

Quantity Discounts. Some suppliers routinely offer quantity discounts—for example, 10 percent off with a certain total monetary order, or one item free if twelve are ordered. In such cases, particularly for fast-moving items that will definitely be used, the reordering system should be flexible enough to take advantage of the discounts within funding limits. Again, the main limitation is the capacity to use the item before expiration or loss.

Excess Stock of Slow-Moving Products. If senior managers discover an excessive average inventory level, the temptation is to order a cutback in all purchasing. But this will only lead to shortages of fast-moving items, with no reduction for most of the problem stock. Strategies to promote the use of slower-moving items by substitution

for other drugs (as appropriate), close review of reorder levels and quantities, and close monitoring of the ordering procedures, without a purchasing freeze, are better alternatives.

Losses to Theft and Wastage. If there are significant losses, they need to be considered in the order quantity (see Chapter 14).

≡ 15.8 Standard Reordering Formulas
The previous section discussed factors that need to be incorporated into the reordering formula. This section looks at two approaches to the question of how much to order:

1. Minimum and maximum stock levels;
2. Consumption-based reordering formulas;

Minimum and Maximum Stock Level Formula
This formula is often used in scheduled purchasing, with set order intervals. Using this approach, one defines a theoretical maximum stock for each item to provide sufficient, but not excessive, stock to last from one order to the next, as well as a minimum stock level or reorder level that determines at what point an order should be placed. Safety stock may be included in the minimum stock level, or an additional quantity may be assigned to protect against variations in consumption and supplier performance.

Some supply system managers set the minimum and maximum stock levels arbitrarily for all items, but better inventory control is obtained with a flexible calculation for each item, based on standard reorder parameters:

- Average monthly consumption, adjusted for stock-outs (C_A);
- Supplier lead time (LT);
- Procurement period—time until the next order will be placed (PP);
- Safety stock—additional stock to cope with variability in consumption and lead time (SS);
- Stock on hand in inventory (S_I);
- Stock now on order from a supplier but not yet received (S_O);
- Quantity of stock back-ordered to lower levels (S_B).

The basic formula for setting the minimum stock level is the average consumption multiplied by the lead time, plus any additional safety stock. Time periods are usually expressed in months, and stock quantities, in basic units (see the glossary at the end of Chapter 13).Options for setting safety stock levels were discussed in Section 15.5; any safety stock needed in addition to the minimum stock level might be defined arbitrarily or by calculating the difference between average and maximum consumption. The equation for calculating the minimum stock (S_{MIN}) is:

$$\text{Minimum stock} = (LT \times C_A) + SS$$

Maximum (target) stock level (S_{MAX}) can be calculated as the minimum stock plus the procurement period multiplied by the average consumption; the equation is:

$$S_{MAX} = S_{MIN} + (PP \times C_A)$$

An example of minimum-maximum level calculations is a case in which the lead time for tetracycline capsules is two months, the average monthly consumption (adjusted for stockouts) is 1,000 capsules, and the additional safety stock allocated is 2,000 capsules. For a procurement period of six months, the following minimum and maximum quantities would be set:

$$S_{MIN} = (2 \times 1,000) + 2,000 = 4,000 \text{ capsules}$$

$$S_{MAX} = 4,000 + (6 \times 1,000) = 10,000 \text{ capsules}$$

When the stock level is found to be at or below the minimum level, the order quantity (Q_O) is calculated as the maximum stock plus stock back-ordered to clients, minus the sum of stock on hand and stock on order. The formula is:

$$Q_O = (S_{MAX} + S_B) - (S_I + S_O)$$

In the example above, suppose there are 3,000 tetracycline capsules in stock and another 2,000 on order. Since the tetracycline has been in stock, there are no back orders to health facilities. The quantity to order would be calculated as:

$$Q_O = 10,000 - (3,000 + 2,000) + 0 = 5,000$$

Some variation of this system is used in many different countries. As long as the minimum and maximum quantities reflect current lead times, consumption patterns, safety stock needs, and order intervals, this system works as well as any other basic reorder formula. The key is regular updating of the minimum and maximum levels. Otherwise, the original minimum and maximum levels will become obsolete, because average consumption and lead times change for many items. Then the formula will produce shortages of items that are moving faster than when the levels were set and overstocks of the items that are moving slower than before.

These problems are most likely to occur when the levels were set for each item by hand in one massive effort, with no formal plan for reviewing and updating the quantities. If there are several thousand items, at least one full-time worker is needed to keep the minimum and maximum quantities updated using a manual review system. Any supply system that uses this reorder formula to manage a large inventory would be well advised to obtain computer software that does the minimum-maximum quantity updating automatically, according to a formula similar to those above.

A supply system using the minimum-maximum method needs supplementary orders to cover situations in which the stock for an item has not sunk to the minimum when regular orders are placed but does so in the middle of the interval between orders, or when the order is not placed as soon as the reorder level is reached. In those situations, the stock will not last until the next regular order has been placed and received, unless safety stocks have been set very high.

One way to deal with emergency orders in a minimum-maximum system is called *modified optional replenishment* (MSH 1992b). With this system, there is a reorder level, which is the same as the standard definition for minimum level, as well as a second minimum stock level, which might be called the emergency warning level. If the stock position is above the reorder level at the reorder date, no order is placed. If the stock level falls to the emergency warning level between scheduled orders, an emergency order is placed.

Although the terminology can vary, this sort of emergency warning level can be useful in any supply system. Of course, emergency purchases must be closely monitored by managers. There may be some temptation to disregard the regular system and rely mostly on emergency orders (which can be ruinously expensive).

Consumption-Based Reordering Formula

This formula bypasses the step of setting (or calculating) minimum/maximum levels and instead calculates the proposed reorder quantity directly. The formula recommended here is basically the same as the formula for consumption-based quantification in Chapter 14 (except for the addition of back orders, which are normally not an issue in large-scale forecasting). The suggested next order quantity is calculated for each item based on the average consumption, lead time, desired safety stock level, stock position, and period of time to be covered by the purchase. The safety stock level in this formula serves a function equivalent to the minimum stock level in the previous formula, in that it is the level that warns of possible stockouts if an order is not placed. However, with this formula, an order quantity can be calculated at any time without waiting to reach the safety stock level.

Note that the variables are the same as those used in the maximum-minimum method; in fact, the proposed reorder quantity should be the same with both formulas, assuming the same variable values. This formula facilitates management of scheduled purchasing, because the formula always suggests an order quantity whenever there is not enough stock to cover the next procurement period, without regard to any predetermined reorder level. Another advantage with this formula is that when emergency orders are needed in a scheduled purchasing system, the same formula is used to compute emergency order quantity as would be used for a regular order.

This consumption-based re-ordering formula is suitable for perpetual purchasing, assuming that computer software is available that recalculates suggested order quantity on command, ideally after each transaction. Country Study 15.1 shows how scheduled purchasing is managed with this formula in the Organization of Eastern Caribbean States.

The variables in the recommended formula are

▸ average monthly consumption, adjusted for stock-outs (C_A);
▸ supplier lead time (LT);
▸ procurement period—time until the next order will be placed (PP);
▸ safety stock (SS);
▸ stock in inventory (S_I);
▸ quantity of stock now on order from a supplier but not yet received (S_O);
▸ quantity of stock back-ordered to lower levels (S_B).

In this formula, the basic minimum safety stock (which can be modified as discussed in Section 15.5) should be the lead time multiplied by the average consumption during the lead time. The formula is $C_A \times LT$.

The complete formula to calculate the quantity to order (Q_O) for each item (without considering intrasystem back orders) is the adjusted average consumption, multiplied by the sum of lead time and procurement period, plus safety stock, minus the sum of stock on hand and stock on order. The symbolic formula is:

$$Q_O = C_A \times (LT + PP) + SS - (S_I + S_O)$$

If the supply system uses back orders internally, and quantities are outstanding to operating units that must be filled when an order is received, the formula would add any outstanding back orders (S_B) to the projected demand requirements in the formula (as was the case for the minimum-maximum formula), yielding:

$$Q_O = C_A \times (LT + PP) + SS + S_B - (S_I + S_O)$$

Country Study 15.1 Scheduled Purchasing in the Eastern Caribbean

Scheduled purchasing is used in the Eastern Caribbean Drug Service (ECDS) pooled procurement program. Annual estimated-quantity supply contracts, with secondary supplier awards (see Chapter 16), are established through a restricted tender managed by the ECDS, a parastatal procurement agency serving the eight member countries of the Organization of Eastern Caribbean States. The supply contracts run from June 30 through July 1, based on annual estimates of need submitted by the eight member countries and compiled by the ECDS.

The countries use a scheduled purchasing system in which orders are placed every three to five months. The reorder quantity is calculated using the consumption-based forecasting formula; inventory is managed with computer software. Four of the countries use a special-purpose database program, INVEC-2 (see Chapter 46), and the others use commercial spreadsheets. The same reorder formula is used in both cases. Member countries are allowed four regular orders from each contract supplier during the year; some countries order from all suppliers at each interval, and others use a staggered method.

In this scheme, each country has a revolving drug fund at the Eastern Caribbean Central Bank; the country can order drugs only up to the value of the funds in its revolving account during any order interval. Emergency purchases are done when shortages occur due to delayed shipments, or when unusual demand depletes stock before another order is due to be placed with a contract supplier. If the primary contract supplier defaults, an order is placed immediately with the secondary supplier.

The contract suppliers that are located in the region allow more frequent orders in some cases, are frequently used as secondary contract suppliers, and are used as the primary source for emergency purchases.

For example, suppose (due to an epidemic of cholera) there are no tetracycline capsules in stock, and 2,000 are back-ordered to lower-level facilities. There is one outstanding order to the supplier for 3,000 capsules. The lead time for this supplier is two months, the average monthly consumption is 1,000 capsules, the safety stock is calculated as 2,000 capsules, and the procurement period is six months. The quantity to order is calculated as:

$$Q_O = 1,000 \times (2 + 6) + 2,000 + 2,000 - (0 + 3,000) = 9,000$$

≡ 15.9 Mathematical Models for Reordering

Many authoritative sources, including those cited in "References and Further Readings," agree that simple models such as those presented in Section 15.8 are preferable to more complex models in most situations. Objections to complex models include (1) that the refinements gained in controlling stock even in the best cases are not substantial in comparison to minimum-maximum and consumption-based formulas; (2) that in most cases, the information fed into the equations is only an estimate, leading to results that are not precise despite the air of precision lent by sophisticated calculations; and (3) that in many cases, staff do not understand the more complex models, do not trust the results, and make their own subjective determinations of order quantities and desired stock levels.

Mathematical models have been developed to address most aspects of inventory management. The most widely known of these models is the economic order quantity (EOQ), but others are worth mentioning, such as the economic order interval (EOI) and some of the mathematical approaches for smoothing forecasts of demand and lead time and for estimating safety stock requirements. EOQ and EOI are illustrated in some detail here, followed by brief discussions of some of the other models.

Economic Order Quantity (EOQ)

The EOQ concept has been around for more than fifty years and is widely applied in commercial firms that use a perpetual purchasing model. The basic idea is that there is an ideal order quantity for any item, which strikes an optimum balance between inventory holding costs and incremental ordering costs (see Box 15.3 and Section 15.10).

With its precise outputs, EOQ seems very sophisticated. It might appear that EOQ is exactly what is needed in all drug supply systems, or at least those that use perpetual purchasing. In fact, the need to order by package means that there will be some deviation from the true EOQ for many items. Another limitation is that the EOQ formula assumes that there is no lead time and that orders are received instantaneously. Since that is obviously not true, additional calculations are required to establish the appropriate safety stock level. This introduces uncertainty even if the basic EOQ calculation is exact.

The *Distribution Management Handbook* (Miller 1994) contends that EOQ is really the square root of two times a guess, times a scientific guess, divided by a precise guess, times management's guess. Nevertheless, the EOQ is still a reasonable choice for estimating order quantities in a perpetual purchasing system in which access to suppliers and funds is such that orders can be placed at any time. The quantities calculated using the model should, however, be treated as guidelines and not absolutes.

When other reordering formulas are used to manage inventory, it may be useful to calculate the EOQ periodically for high-use, high-value items (Class A) and compare the theoretical ideal order quantity with current practice.

Economic Order Interval (EOI)

A concept related to EOQ is EOI—the theoretical ideal interval for spacing orders placed for the EOQ. As is the case with EOQ, the EOI changes, depending on the values of the individual variables; with a much higher acquisition cost, the EOI decreases (more orders per year), and so forth. Also, like EOQ, the EOI formula produces recommendations that must be rounded.

Although EOI has its main application in systems that use EOQ to set the order quantity, EOI can be used in drug supply systems to check the theoretical ideal ordering intervals for scheduled purchasing and then to group items that would best be ordered monthly, quarterly, semiannually, and so forth. The EOI is also illustrated in Box 15.3.

Exponential Smoothing

Exponential smoothing is a common technique for coping with variation in consumption or lead-time patterns. In this technique, a smoothing constant (called *alpha*) is used to adjust the observed average consumption or lead-time values.

One application of exponential smoothing calculates the projected demand (D) by factoring in the average consumption from the three-month lead time (C_L), the consumption from the past month (C_A), and the smoothing factor alpha (α), which for these purposes is usually set between 0.1 and 0.2. The equation is:

$$D = C_L + [\alpha \times (C_A - C_L)]$$

If, for example, an item had averaged 150 units consumed per month over the last three months but 200 were used in the last month, the smoothed average using an alpha value of 0.1 would be:

$$D = 150 + [0.1 \times (200 - 150)] = 155$$

Clearly the difference between the simple average and the smoothed average would be greater with larger consumption values and with a higher alpha factor.

This is not a complex equation in itself, but choosing the value for the alpha factor is tricky (most authorities recommend trial runs using various values, then observing results and trying again). The higher the alpha, the more "adaptable" the forecast is to recent trends; however, the higher the alpha factor, the lower the reliability when there is a large random noise factor in the consumption pattern.

Standard Deviation of Consumption and Lead Time

The standard deviation of consumption and of lead-time can be used in mathematical models to adjust forecasts when there is considerable variation (random noise) in the consumption or lead-time pattern. Standard deviation is basically an estimate of how much an individual value is likely to vary from the average of all values in a series (see Rowntree 1981 for methods for calculating standard deviation).

The following equation illustrates how the standard deviation of lead-time consumption (SD_{LTC}) is calculated, for use in setting safety stocks:

$$SD_{LTC} = \sqrt{(LT \times SD_C^2) + (C_A^2 \times SD_{LT}^2)}$$

where

C_A = average monthly consumption
LT = average lead time
SD_C = standard deviation of consumption
SD_{LT} = standard deviation of lead time

For example, if consumption of an item averages 1,000 units per month with a standard deviation of 100, and the lead time averages three months with a standard deviation of 0.75 months, the average consumption during the lead-time period is 3,000 units, and the standard deviation of that lead-time consumption is calculated as:

$$\sqrt{[3 \times (100 \times 100)] + [(1,000 \times 1,000) \times (0.75 \times 0.75)]} = 769.74$$

Most values in any series of observations show a normal distribution pattern around the mean (average) value. (For example, in a population of men who average six feet in height, about half the men will be taller and about half will be shorter rather than exactly six feet.) It is a characteristic of normal distributions that the standard deviation times about two will encompass 95 percent of the values clustered above and below the average (see Rowntree 1981). This means that in our example, 95 percent of the time, the monthly consumption will fall within two times the standard deviation of monthly consumption.

This calculation could be used with any reordering formula to assign safety stock in order to theoretically achieve a 95 percent service level. For the example given above, $2 \times 770 = 1,540$ units would be needed as safety stock, in addition to average lead-time consumption. In a minimum/maximum formula, the minimum level would be 3,000 units ($C_A \times LT$), and the added safety stock would be 1,540 units. In a consumption-based formula, the total safety stock would be 4,540 units.

≡ 15.10 Identifying and Controlling Costs

The Total Variable Cost of Inventory Management

One goal of inventory management is to achieve a reasonable balance between holding costs on the one hand and

---

Box 15.3 Economic Order Quantity and Order Interval

EOQ

Although there are many variations, the most basic formula for the EOQ is:

$$EOQ = \sqrt{(2 \times U \times O) \div (H \times C)}$$

where: U = annual use, in units

O = incremental ordering cost

H = average holding cost (percentage of average inventory value)

C = projected net acquisition cost

Considering an example of dextrose bags for IV injection, assume a projected annual use of 25,000 bags at an average acquisition price of $2 per bag. Also assume that the estimated incremental ordering cost is $70 per order placed, and the average inventory holding cost is 40 percent. The calculation proceeds as follows:

Step 1: $2 \times 25,000 \times 70 = 3,500,000$ $(2 \times U \times O)$

Step 2: $2 \times 0.4 = 0.8$ $(H \times C)$

Step 3: $3,500,000 \div 0.8 = 4,375,000$ $([2 \times U \times O] \div [H \times C])$

Step 4: Square root = 2,091.65

This means that, according to the EOQ model, dextrose bags should be ordered in quantities of 2,091.65 bags. Before going further, the reader should consider what happens when the individual variables go up or down. For example, if the item's acquisition cost was $.20 (with all other variables the same), the EOQ would be 6,614.38 bags; if the price was $20, the EOQ would be 661.44 bags. If only consumption changed, annual use of 5,000 bags produces an EOQ of 935.41 bags, and annual use of 50,000 bags yields an EOQ of 2,958.04 bags. When incremental costs of purchasing go up, the EOQ goes up (to decrease the ordering frequency); as the holding cost percentage goes up, the EOQ goes down, to increase order frequency and decrease stock levels.

EOI

The formula for calculating the EOI uses the same variables as the EOQ but combines them as follows:

$$EOI = \sqrt{(2 \times O) \div (U \times H \times C)}$$

where U = annual use in units

C = projected net acquisition cost

O = ordering cost

H = holding cost

The EOI produces its result as fractions of a year (assuming that consumption is based on a year). For the EOQ example in Box 15.3, the EOI for orders of 2,091.65 bags would be 0.084 years, which converts to 1.004 months, 4.35 weeks, or 30.5 days. This is calculated as:

Step 1: $(2 \times 70) \div (25,000 \times 0.4 \times 2)$

Step 2: $140 \div 20,000 = .007$

Step 3: $\sqrt{.007} = 0.08366$ years

purchasing and shortage costs on the other. In order to maintain this balance, it is necessary to identify and quantify the relevant costs and examine how they interrelate. This analysis allows managers to see the "big picture" in the system and consider the impact of potential changes.

One way to compile information for analysis is called the total variable cost (TVC) of purchasing, which is the sum of all costs related to inventory management:

TVC = total drug acquisition cost + inventory holding cost + purchasing cost + shortage cost

Chapter 41 provides details on a method to compile and apply the TVC analysis. The manager's objective is to identify strategies that will minimize the TVC. If an intervention will reduce ordering costs but drive up inventory holding costs by an amount that produces a net increase in the TVC, it is not worthwhile. Alternatively, a strategy to increase ordering frequency might drive up the costs associated with purchasing, but the net savings in inventory control costs might be far greater than the incremental purchasing cost.

The typical annual inventory holding cost for a commercial firm is 25 to 35 percent of the average inventory value, but the percentage could be much higher for a public drug supply program. For example, during a multi-country assessment of inventory management practices in the Caribbean region, one country was found to have an *average* inventory of twelve months' consumption. The manager of this supply system was very proud of his stock levels, saying that he had no problem with stockouts. Of course, he had not given adequate consideration to the costs of holding inventory, which in this case equaled half of the entire annual drug purchasing budget.

Holding costs and purchasing costs basically oppose each other. Frequent ordering in small quantities drives up the average cost of placing an order (or managing a tender), because the procurement and accounting offices must go through all the steps on multiple occasions. However, more frequent orders should reduce average stock levels, and thus reduce holding costs. Annual ordering in large quantities tends to increase the average inventory level and holding costs but decreases the average annual ordering costs.

Usually there is an inverse relationship between shortage costs and holding costs, in that the shortage costs in a supply system are likely to be low when stock levels (and holding costs) are high, and vice versa.

Variable costs may be either stable or incremental. If the cost remains the same no matter how many transactions there are or how much inventory is involved, it is a stable cost. If the cost increases directly with the number of purchases or volume of inventory, it is an incremental cost. The difference is important when considering the potential impact of cost-saving strategies. By their nature, drug acquisition costs, many inventory holding costs, and shortage costs are incremental; most purchasing costs tend to be stable, but there are likely to be incremental components.

Structure of the Inventory Pipeline

To compile a total variable cost analysis, it is necessary to consider the structure of the supply system and to determine where variable costs are incurred. As discussed in Chapters 21 and 44, the inventory management system is similar to a pipeline, with warehouses and health facilities that function as reservoirs where stock is held. In order to ensure a continuous supply of drugs to patients, the pipeline must be filled; once filled, consumption must be matched by purchases.

One of the single most important decisions in terms of cost and efficiency of the distribution system is the number of storage levels in the system. Chapter 21 discusses options for selecting the best structure and considering set-up, operating, and inventory holding costs.

It is generally true that more levels of the supply system create higher inventory levels and inventory costs, but the increase is not always directly proportional. Ordering frequency, average supplier lead time, and policies for safety stock have a major impact on inventory levels. As shown in Figure 21.5 in Chapter 21, a supply system with three levels (regional stores, district stores, and health facilities) might have three times the inventory of a two-level system (district stores and health facilities). However, depending on the inventory management system's operating efficiency, the differences in inventory levels and costs between the two types of systems might be much lower or even greater than that shown in Figure 21.5.

Overstocking at health facilities and lower-level stores can have a disproportionate effect on the overall inventory costs. The large number of these units multiplies the impact of overstocking. When conducting an analysis of inventory costs or developing an inventory control policy, it is essential that the analysis consider costs at each level of the system and identify options for rationalizing order frequency and safety stock levels to achieve desired services with the lowest possible total inventory in the supply system.

Value of Stock Purchased and on Hand

The total expenditures on drug purchases, the quantity of stock on hand, and the value of that stock must be known in order to estimate inventory holding costs.

Drug Acquisition Costs. The total drug acquisition costs for a time period are the net expenditures for all drugs purchased, including the net unit price (including any discounts), shipping and insurance charges from the supplier to the initial warehouse, and import duties. This total is compiled from purchasing records and (if necessary) supplier invoices.

Calculation of the Inventory Value. The standard basis for valuing inventory is the original net purchase cost, as opposed to the selling price. There are four standard methods for determining the original purchase cost for all items in inventory: actual value, first in/first out (FIFO), last in/first out (LIFO), and average value. As discussed in Chapter 42, most drug supply systems are unable to accurately track actual value and should use either the average value or the FIFO method.

The key is that the method, once chosen, needs to be applied consistently from one financial year to the next; otherwise, year-to-year comparisons of holding costs and financial performance may be invalid.

Inventory Holding Cost

The inventory holding cost, also known as the *carrying cost*, is calculated as a percentage of average annual inventory value, which is obtained by adding the beginning inventory value for the financial year and the ending inventory value for the financial year and then dividing by two. Then the sum of the costs associated with holding inventory in the system is divided by the average annual inventory value, and the result is expressed as a percentage.

The inventory holding cost includes several components, many of which have both stable and incremental aspects:

Opportunity cost is the market value of funds tied up in inventory that could have been used for some other purpose. It is incremental—the higher the inventory value, the higher the opportunity cost.

Storage operating costs include warehouse staff salaries, warehouse rental or amortization costs, taxes, utility charges, building and equipment maintenance, and security. These costs are stable, unless more staff or storage space is added to handle an increased inventory volume.

Supplies for material management, such as packing material, are usually incremental costs—the larger the inventory volume and number of shipments, the higher the volume of supplies needed.

Transport costs are incurred each time the item is transferred from one level of the supply system to another. This cost consists of both stable components (staff and vehicle maintenance and depreciation) and incremental components (such as gasoline and tolls).

Deterioration and spoilage costs for drugs are more likely to occur with poor storekeeping practices, but there is some risk in all warehouses. In general, these costs are incremental—the higher the stock levels, the higher the costs of spoilage.

Expiry costs are often 3 to 5 percent of drug inventory each year. If this ratio holds, the costs are incremental as inventory value increases.

Obsolescence costs apply principally to equipment and spare parts, but changes in formulary lists and prescribing practices may make certain drugs obsolete. These may be viewed as stable costs; they do not necessarily vary with the inventory size or value.

Wastage costs due to theft and unexplained loss add considerably to the cost of carrying inventories. As noted in Chapter 14, it is not unusual to experience 10 percent in losses in public drug supply systems. These are likely to be incremental costs—the total loss increases as the average inventory rises.

Purchasing Costs

Purchasing costs are incurred with each tender for drugs and (less obviously) each time an order is placed.

Stable costs include the salaries and benefits of the normal complement of purchasing staff. Other stable costs are those for space, utilities, basic supplies, maintenance and depreciation, and communications.

Other purchasing costs are incremental; the more orders placed, the higher the total costs. These costs include forms and supplies, long-distance telephone calls and faxes, travel, and other expenses associated with the tender process, such as committee meetings. If staff, space, or equipment are added to deal with increased purchasing volume, this becomes an incremental cost.

Shortage Costs

Four types of costs are associated with stock shortages:

► The cost of an emergency purchase (usually at higher-than-normal prices);
► The loss of revenue if a client goes elsewhere to purchase the item;
► Increased morbidity and mortality due to shortages;
► Loss of goodwill—stockouts erode public confidence in the health care system.

These costs are difficult to quantify, but some estimates can be made. For example, revenue lost can be estimated if hospitals and regional warehouses order from the private

≡ Assessment Guide

Performance Indicators

As discussed in Chapters 4 and 36, indicators have been developed expressly for use in public-sector drug supply systems. Some of them should be considered as tools to measure inventory management performance, although there are no standards yet for the acceptable range of performance. They include

- average percentage of inventory variation in the stock record-keeping system, at a sample of warehouses and facilities;
- percentage of stock records that correspond with physical counts, at a sample of warehouses and facilities;
- percentage of a specified set of indicator drugs that are in stock at a sample of warehouses and facilities;
- average percentage of time out of stock for the set of indicator drugs;
- average lead time from suppliers and from warehouses to facilities.

Context for Inventory Management

- Are all supply system operations related to finished goods, or does the system also manufacture drugs?
- At what levels of the system are drug orders placed, either to suppliers or to other levels of the system?

Selection of Items for Stock Status

- How do managers and operations personnel determine which items should be held in stock and which (if any) should be ordered only as needed?

Costs Associated with Inventory and Purchasing Operations

- How is inventory valued, and what procedures are used to physically count stock and reconcile records?
- How many months' worth of stock is on hand at central storage facilities? At regional and district facilities? At hospital pharmacies, health centers, dispensaries, and other clinical facilities?
- What information is available on inventory values, operating costs of warehouses, operating costs of the purchasing department, and costs associated with shortages? If such information is available, how is it used?
- Are techniques such as ABC value analysis, VEN analysis, and total variable cost analysis used in formulating inventory management strategies? If so, in what areas?

Stock Records and Routine Reports

- What inventory records exist at each level of the health care system? How accurate and how current are the records? Do they supply the information needed for procurement and distribution decisions?
- If a computerized information system is in use, is it a general-purpose inventory management package or a special-purpose package developed for managing public-sector drug supply systems? Does it automatically calculate minimum and maximum quantities or consumption-based order quantities?
- What standard reports are produced on inventory status, procurement operations, and consumption patterns? How is the information used?

Safety Stocks and Service Levels

- How are safety stock levels calculated at each level of the system?
- What adjustments in safety stocks are made for variations in consumption and lead-time patterns?
- What percentage service levels are normally achieved by warehouses supplying lower levels of the system? What percentage service levels are provided by major suppliers to the system?

Purchasing Model

- How frequently are drug orders placed at each level that places orders? Is the same model used for all items?
- What percentage of orders are routine and what percentage are emergency orders?
- Are there any special factors that dictate the choice of inventory management strategies, such as government financial and administrative regulations, staff, existing management information systems, supplier access, or contract procedures?

Reorder Formulas

- What reordering formulas are used to determine purchase quantities? Is the same formula used at all levels and all facilities?
- What source data are used in the formulas?
- How much weight is given to the manager's experience and judgment? What other factors are considered?

sector when the CMS is out of stock. The total of those non-CMS purchases (adjusted for the difference between CMS and private-sector prices) is revenue lost to the CMS. The cost of emergency purchases is the difference between the total value of emergency purchases and the estimated value of the same quantity of the same items at regular contract prices. Shortage costs are largely incremental, in that as average stock levels and particularly safety stocks decrease, shortage costs increase. ■

≡ References and Further Readings

★ = *Key readings.*

★ Dear, A. 1990. *Inventory management de-mystified.* London: Chapman and Hall.

★ Dobler, D. W., and D. N. Burt. 1996. Inventory management. In *Purchasing and supply management,* 6th ed. New York: McGraw-Hill.

Downes, J., and J. Goodman. 1995. *Dictionary of finance and investment terms,* 4th ed. Hauppauge, N.Y.: Barron's Educational Series.

★ Miller, M. 1994. Inventory management. In *The distribution management handbook,* ed. J. Tompkins and D. Harmelink. New York: McGraw-Hill.

MSH (Management Sciences for Health). 1992a. Inventory concepts (trainer's and participant's guides). In *Managing drug supply training series.* Part 3. *Supply management.* Boston: MSH.

MSH (Management Sciences for Health). 1992b. Inventory management for procurement (trainer's and participant's guides). In *Managing drug supply training series.* Part 3. *Supply management.* Boston: MSH.

MSH (Management Sciences for Health). 1992c. Stock records (trainer's and participant's guides). In *Managing drug supply training series.* Part 3. *Supply management.* Boston: MSH.

Quick, J. 1982. Applying management science in developing countries: ABC analysis to plan public drug procurement. *Socio-Economic Planning Sciences* 16 (1): 39–50.

★ Rowntree, D. 1981. *Statistics without tears: A primer for non-mathematicians.* New York: Charles Scribner and Sons.

Warren, C., P. Fess, and J. Reeve. 1995. Inventories. In *Accounting,* 18th ed. Cincinnati, Ohio: Southwestern College Publishing.

★ Waters, C. D. J. 1992. *Inventory control and management.* Chichester, England: John Wiley and Sons.

| Part I | Part II | **Part III** | Part IV |
| Introduction | Policy and Legal Framework | **Drug Management Cycle** | Management Support Systems |

A Selection

B Procurement ▶ 13 Managing Procurement

C Distribution 14 Quantifying Drug Requirements

D Use 15 Inventory Management

16 Managing the Tender Process

17 Contracting for Drugs and Services

18 Quality Assurance for Drug Procurement

19 Small-Scale Local Production

20 Drug Donations

Chapter 16
Managing the Tender Process

≡ Summary

The primary function of a procurement office is to obtain the required items at the right time, in the correct quantities, and at the most favorable prices. The procurement office compiles a list of requirements, identifies potential suppliers, selects the most cost-effective supplier for each product, secures firm supply contracts, and makes sure that the suppliers and the health system comply with contract terms. Competitive tenders are recommended for most drug procurement in public-sector pharmaceutical systems, so this chapter focuses on the principles of efficient tender management.

In order to maximize the benefit of pharmaceutical purchases, corruption and favoritism in procurement must be minimized. It is equally important to avoid the appearance of favoritism, so the tender process should be as transparent as possible under national procurement laws.

A formal tender process includes drug selection and quantification, preparation of tender documents and contracts, notification and invitation to bid, formal bid opening, collation of offers, adjudication and supplier selection, award of contracts, performance monitoring of suppliers and clients, and enforcement of contract terms when necessary. Reliable suppliers are the cornerstone of effective procurement; tender adjudication and selection of suppliers is the critical step that determines the costs of drugs and defines the integrity of the procurement process. Adjudication should be based on formal written criteria and must be free from influence by special interests.

Accurate and timely information is critical at each stage of the process, and lack of effective information systems is a main cause of procurement delays and inefficiencies. The information system must be able to

- ▸ *produce information for quantification and tender documents;*
- ▸ *collate offers for adjudication;*
- ▸ *issue notifications of award and purchase orders;*
- ▸ *track order status and compliance with contract terms;*
- ▸ *manage communications with contract suppliers;*
- ▸ *track suppliers' performance for future tenders.*

≡ 16.1 Introduction to Tender Management

Many of the major policy and management issues relevant to pharmaceutical procurement were covered in Chapter 13. There are several types of procurement methods used to purchase pharmaceuticals, but the procurement method chosen for each drug should

- ▸ obtain the lowest possible purchase price for high-quality products;
- ▸ ensure suppliers' reliability, in terms of both quality and service;
- ▸ maintain transparency in the process and minimize the opportunity for illicit influences on procurement decisions;
- ▸ achieve these objectives with the least possible professional and clerical staff time and within the shortest possible lead time.

Figure 16.1 summarizes the most frequently used methods to purchase pharmaceuticals.

This chapter focuses on the management of competitive tenders. A well-qualified and experienced procurement manager, with access to high-quality market intelligence and communications facilities, can do well with negotiated procurement. However, in most public-sector programs, the majority of drugs should be purchased through competitive tenders.

Steps in the Tender Cycle

Once under way, the tender process becomes a cycle repeated each year in most programs. There are some situations in which tenders are conducted two or three times annually or, more rarely, every two years. The standard steps in the tender cycle are:

1. Determine the tender format and scope.
2. Define requirements—select and quantify drugs and supplies.
3. Select suppliers to participate in the tender.
4. Prepare and send tender documents.
5. Receive and open offers.
6. Collate offers for adjudication.
7. Adjudicate the tender.
8. Issue contracts to winning bidders.
9. Monitor performance and product quality.
10. Enforce contract terms as needed.

Each of these steps requires informed decisions about which of several possible procedures should be followed. In some countries, options may be limited due to laws and regulations, but even in these situations, the procurement program has several choices to make. The goal of this chapter is to provide information to help procurement managers make the best choices for their own situations.

Figure 16.1 Comparison of Procurement Methods

Procurement Method	Brief Description	Effect on Price	Procurement Lead Time	Workload for Procurement Office	Need for Evaluating Suppliers	Conditions Favoring Use
Open tender	Bidding is open for all interested suppliers	Usually lowest prices	Moderate to long	High	High	When many reputable suppliers are available and likely to be interested If prequalification is not feasible or not allowed by regulation or donor's provisions
Restricted tender	Participation of suppliers is limited to those who have registered with the government or who have prequalified	Favorable	Moderate to long	High	High	When substantial list of registered suppliers has been developed When capacity exists to manage prequalification and supplier monitoring
Competitive negotiation	The buyer approaches a small number of potential suppliers and bargains for specific price or service arrangements	Can be favorable	Short to moderate	Moderate	High	Experienced purchasing office with good access to market intelligence Low-price or small-volume items When special terms or specifications are required by the buyer for items not widely available Emergency purchases to supplement tender
Direct procurement	Purchase is made directly from a single supplier at the quoted price	Usually highest prices	Short to moderate	Low	High	Emergency purchases when negotiation is not possible Purchase of single-source drugs Low-price or small-volume items

≡ 16.2 Determining the Tender Format and Scope

Some countries have procurement regulations that determine the tender format for drug purchasing. The World Bank and some bilateral donors may mandate specific tender formats for procurement financed by loans or donated funds (see "References and Further Readings"). However, in many cases there is flexibility in structuring the tender; in those situations, options include

► restricted versus open tender;
► local or international scope;
► estimated or fixed tender quantities;
► split or single tender awards;
► primary/secondary contracts or rebids;
► required or optional use of local agents in international tenders;
► annual or biannual tenders versus multiple tenders during the year.

Restricted or Open Tender

One of the most important decisions to make is whether the tender will be restricted to known reliable suppliers or will be opened up to any supplier who is interested. This decision is required whether the tender is local or international.

A restricted tender with *prequalification* involves developing a list of registered suppliers based on past performance, references from previous clients, and documentation of product quality. Then, only those registered suppliers may participate in tenders. This avoids the necessity of trying to decide whether the lowest bidder should be awarded the contract. With prequalification, by definition, the lowest bidder should be qualified for the contract.

When prequalification works well, substandard suppliers are kept out of the tender process entirely. Prequalification is not beneficial if it protects favored suppliers from competition. In some countries, it is virtually impossible for a new supplier to survive the prequalification process, no matter how reliable the new supplier may be.

Prequalification can be extremely time-consuming, particularly if there is a policy to prequalify suppliers separately for each drug. As noted below, however, proper postqualification requires just as much time. The policy question is where the time should be allocated in the tender process.

An open tender with *postqualification* makes the tender available to all interested bidders. The suppliers and their offers are reviewed after they are received with respect to registration status, product quality, and past performance.

An open tender usually increases the pool of prospective suppliers (with the potential benefit of driving down prices), but it is no panacea. Drugs are unlike some other commodities, in that drug product quality is both crucial and difficult to ensure. Therefore, the success of open tenders with postqualification depends on the capacity of the procurement program to winnow out unqualified suppliers and poor-quality products after bids have been received, in some cases, from all over the world. The procurement office must go through a process similar to that used in prequalification. The difference is that there may be many more suppliers and products to screen. Moreover, bids are usually submitted with a time limit on price validity (see Chapter 17). It may be difficult to screen all suppliers and products after bid opening within the period of price validity. If there are delays, prices have to be verified, and in some cases, rebidding may be needed.

Finally, postqualification may also be used inappropriately to exclude qualified bidders, if someone in the procurement agency wants to tilt business toward favored companies.

The choice between restricted and open tenders should be based on the local situation. However, most successful private companies purchase supplies primarily from a selected list of reliable suppliers. Restricted tender with prequalification is a staple feature of many successful pharmaceutical procurement programs, such as group purchasing agencies in the United States and the Organization of Eastern Caribbean States. Prequalification is also recommended by the International Pharmaceutical Federation (FIP 1992).

In most procurement programs, the eventual goal should be tenders limited to registered, prequalified suppliers. Prequalification avoids wasting time on suppliers that do not perform according to contract and helps minimize the possibility of introducing substandard products. However, it is important to aggressively seek out potential new suppliers that may wish to become registered, in order to maintain competitive pressure on established suppliers.

If there is no information available locally on suppliers' performance and the probable time to develop a list of qualified suppliers is very long, it may be necessary to use postqualification for specific tenders. In these cases, it may be best to make the initial drug procurement from reputable international procurement agencies (see the list in MSH 1995) while systems, including a list of registered and qualified suppliers, are being developed.

International versus Local Procurement

The health system must decide if tenders will be open to international suppliers or limited to companies that are established in the country; this decision is necessary whether the tender uses pre- or postqualification.

At least for some items, an international competitive tender, whether open or restricted, almost always results in lower prices than a tender limited to the local market. For other items, such as parenteral solutions, where the shipping cost is high and the product cost is low, it may be cheaper to purchase locally, if there is a local manufacturing plant.

However, even if international procurement always offered better prices for all items, a country may have made a political decision to support local manufacturing. The government may believe that the cost benefit of international procurement does not outweigh the benefit of a strong local industry (although this need can be satisfied to some degree through local preference in international tenders).

The most common constraint on international procurement is drug registration. Countries with drug registration systems normally require that all drugs purchased through public tender be registered locally. Both restricted and open tenders can be limited to products registered in the purchasing country. This requirement may basically eliminate international procurement if the registration process is complicated and time-consuming.

Many countries are moving toward "harmonization," with virtually automatic registration if the product originates from a country recognized as having effective pharmaceutical regulatory systems. Some countries expedite or even waive registration for generic drugs for the public sector that are on the national essential drugs list.

Estimated- versus Fixed-Quantity Contract

There are two basic options for defining purchase quantity: the traditional *fixed-quantity, scheduled-delivery* purchasing contract, and the *estimated-quantity, periodic-order* contract.

The fixed-quantity contract specifies guaranteed quantities (with a small variation sometimes allowed) and delivery in either one large shipment or smaller separate shipments over the life of the contract. The purchaser accepts the risk that quantities for specific items may be too high (resulting in overstocks) or too low (resulting in shortages). If the purchaser actually needs more than the projected quantity (plus permitted variation), the price may be adjusted for additional quantities, depending on the contract.

With the second type of contract—the estimated-quantity, periodic-order (draw-down) system—the tender quantity is just an estimate. A contract price is negotiated for each drug, and members of the purchasing group order periodically from contract suppliers at the contract price throughout the contract term. Orders can be placed directly by group members or channeled to the supplier through the procurement office. Members order only the quantities of each item needed, regardless of the quantity stipulated in the tender estimate.

The supplier delivers to purchasers at the contract price throughout the term of the contract, regardless of the variation between projected and actual total quantity purchased under the contract. The supplier takes the risk that actual quantities will differ from those estimated: if the quantities are higher, it is not a problem (assuming the supplier has the necessary capacity), but if purchases are significantly lower than estimates, the supplier may not participate in future tenders. This system benefits the purchaser, because the purchaser's financial liability is limited to each order, and if demand changes, the purchaser is not burdened with unneeded stock or pressed to cover shortages.

Pharmaceutical tenders for most developing countries have been made for many years as fixed-quantity, scheduled-delivery tenders, and it might be expected that suppliers serving these procurement programs would resist the change to estimated-quantity contracts. However, in many countries, a surprising number of companies compete for estimated-quantity contracts and offer prices comparable to those seen in fixed-quantity tenders. The estimated-quantity, draw-down contract is used in the eastern Caribbean, in parts of the Zimbabwe tendering program, and in all group purchasing programs in the United States.

When the draw-down system is used, prices should be guaranteed for the entire period of the contract. If possible, prices should be negotiated as CIF (cost, insurance, and freight) or CIP (carriage and insurance paid), with no extra charges for freight and insurance (see Chapter 17). In highly inflationary environments, it may be necessary to tender more than once a year or to include an escalator clause effective after a certain number of months, based on inflation. When inflation is a severe problem, a guaranteed-quantity tender or a policy to make most purchases at the lowest contract price possible (that is, before an escalator clause takes effect) may produce the best results.

In countries where access to funds and foreign exchange is sporadic and uncertain, it may be necessary to tender on a periodic basis, as funds become available. This almost always requires a fixed-quantity, scheduled-delivery tender format.

Similarly, if most products must be imported and lead times are extremely long, fixed-quantity, scheduled-delivery contracts are best, because the draw-down system requires reasonable access to contract suppliers. It functions acceptably in the eastern Caribbean, with lead times of four to five months, but it would be difficult to manage where lead times are routinely greater than one year. One option is to limit tender participation to suppliers that can provide shorter lead times. This would likely produce a price increase but could potentially reduce waste.

In some situations, it might be best to combine the formats: negotiating fixed-quantity contracts for products that can be purchased most cost effectively in large single quantities, and using estimated-quantity contracts for other products.

Splitting Tender Awards

Some procurement programs routinely split contract awards among two or three suppliers, the rationale being to maintain capacity in several suppliers or avoid dependence on one supplier for a critical drug. However, any program that routinely splits tenders is almost certainly not getting the best possible pricing, and there is substantial opportunity for "bid rigging"—suppliers agreeing beforehand what bids will be offered, with the realization that all will benefit from a share of the pie.

There are circumstances in which split tenders are desirable. This is likely to be true when a country is making one huge annual purchase of essential drugs, the risk of supplier default is real, and the public health consequences will be severe if default occurs and the drugs are not available.

Primary/Secondary Contracts versus Rebids

When a supplier defaults, delays in receiving medicines have already occurred by the time the problem is understood. If contracts must be rebid through the entire tender procedure, it is likely that stockouts will result and/or high-priced emergency purchases will need to be made. A primary/secondary contract system can be useful in avoiding the delays in rebidding by providing an immediate option if the contract winner cannot perform. This sort of system is used in the eastern Caribbean and in many pharmaceutical purchasing groups.

In a primary/secondary system, two contract awards are made, with the primary award to the bidder offering the lowest price, and the secondary award to the second lowest bidder, provided it is a supplier that is expected to be able to supply under all conditions. The secondary contract should be used only when the primary supplier is unable to perform.

Primary/secondary awards are useful *only* if two requirements are met: the second lowest price is reasonably close to the lowest and thus worth locking in, and a reliable secondary supplier is prepared to accept that status and guarantee the price in case the primary supplier defaults. If either condition is not met, a secondary award is not worthwhile.

Some countries have regulations prohibiting these types of contracts, requiring that a new tender be made in the case of default. World Bank international competitive bidding (ICB) tender procedures call for rebids when a supplier defaults, but there is usually some flexibility for local purchasing and local competitive bidding in such cases.

Use of Local Agents in International Procurement

Multinational manufacturers and exporters are commonly represented in developing countries by local representatives. The decision to require, to encourage, or to avoid buying through local agents in international tenders affects the range of foreign suppliers, the efficiency of communication between the buyer and the supplier, and the choice of trade and payment terms. Major advantages and disadvantages of buying through local agents are listed in Figure 16.2.

Chapters 6 and 17 further discuss the potential for contracting with local distributors to provide warehousing and transport services.

Tender Frequency and Timing

Tender planning must take into account the time required for each step. The time required to develop a tender list, including drug selection and quantification, varies widely but may require two to six months even in established procurement systems. The time required to select suppliers for tender participation can also be long; in one African country it took more than one year for the first prequalification.

Preparing documents for tender usually takes at least a month once quantification is completed. The time spent waiting for tender offers depends on geographic scope (local versus international) and in some cases on regulations of the government or the funding agency. The minimum is likely to be forty-five days even in local tenders, and the average may be more like three months. Collation of offers is quicker with computerized systems, but at least one month should be allowed for this (in large tenders processed manually, the collation time may be three to four months). Adjudication and contract award are also faster in computerized systems, but again, one month should be allowed, and at least two months in manual

systems. Once contracts are awarded, the lead time between orders to the supplier and initial deliveries may be a month or less with local tenders, but international suppliers' lead times usually range from three months to one year or more.

Efficient procurement offices spread the tender workload throughout the year, with overlap from one tender cycle to the next; once contracts have been awarded for the first cycle, it is time to begin planning for drug selection for the next cycle. Frequent communication with clients and with suppliers is needed to make sure that the tender proceeds according to schedule. Figure 16.3 illustrates a typical tender cycle of fifteen months, with overlap.

The frequency of tendering should be attuned to the funding cycle and, for international tenders, to the availability of foreign exchange. It is not appropriate to tender once a year when funds, including foreign exchange, are released in monthly installments, because bids will expire before the funds for the actual awards become available.

≡ 16.3 Defining Needs

As discussed in Chapter 13, restricting the number of drugs on a procurement list can actually increase effective procurement volume for drugs that stay on the list. Selection of a restricted list of essential drugs can be better accomplished by a central agency than by a large number of health facilities. If selection is totally decentralized, the benefits of group purchasing will probably be lost. However, if the clients do not have real input into which drugs are selected, they will not feel that their needs are being served and will lose a feeling of ownership. This may result in direct purchases outside the tender contracts, undermining the integrity of the system. A balance needs to be struck.

Selection of Drugs for the Tender

The drug selection committee (see Chapter 10), which is often the formulary committee, should meet prior to each tender to finalize the list of drugs. If, for example, a tender is scheduled for June and quantification takes three months plus one month for clarification and tender document preparation, the drug selection committee would meet in January.

Requests for additions or changes to the procurement list should be compiled throughout the year by the procurement agency and/or the selection committee. Requests for additions to the list should be made in writing, with justification for the addition and (if applicable) the name of the product to be replaced. Technical staff of the procurement agency or drug selection committee should

Figure 16.2 Advantages and Disadvantages of Buying through Local Agents

Potential Advantages	Potential Disadvantages
1. *Speeds and improves communication.* Local agents may be authorized to make decisions without a special contact with the foreign supplier. When necessary, the local agent may be better able to contact the appropriate person at the foreign supplier's office.	1. *May slow and confuse communication.* If untrained, unmotivated, poorly supervised, or part-time, a local agent may lengthen and confuse arrangements with the foreign supplier. In addition, if the purchaser requires specific product information, a local agent may impede communication.
2. *Locates least expensive acceptable supplies.* In competitive tenders, it is in the interest of the local agents to locate inexpensive suppliers, including sources that might not otherwise have come to the attention of the purchaser.	2. *May increase cost.* Local agents may add as much as 15 to 30 percent to the visible cost, even though their commission is often much less than this. Higher unit prices are also paid for low-volume purchases through local agents, compared to direct purchase.
3. *Facilitates payment.* Local agents can sometimes accept local currency and allow deferred payment. Currency conversions can be troublesome, and some countries specify that payments be made in local currency to local agents.	3. *Serves as a source of black market drugs.* Licensed importers can be a major source of drugs for illicit use, and local agents need to be regulated through licensure and regular inspection of records and stocks.
4. *Expedites delivery.* Local agents often handle port clearing. When illicit commissions are required, local agents are better able to pay these fees and, by saving time, save money.	4. *May completely default on an order.* Local agents who are not financially stable may go out of business and disappear.
5. *Speeds receipt of emergency supplies.* Local agents often maintain stocks within the country, which speeds receipt of emergency supplies and may reduce the amount of warehouse space required.	5. *Attempts to increase drug consumption.* Local agents may employ detail men or company representatives to visit health system physicians to encourage product use, as well as to request new drugs.
6. *Affords greater legal recourse.* The presence of an in-country agent affords greater opportunity for legal action if the supplier defaults.	
7. *Introduces new products.* Occasionally, new products or formulations are introduced that are cost-effective alternatives to existing products. The agent is necessarily biased but may provide scientific articles in support of the product. Other information sources should be sought to supplement the introductory information provided by the agent.	
8. *May offer potential for prime vendor distribution.* In some countries, it may be possible to eliminate government warehousing and distribution costs by implementing a prime vendor contract with a local distributor that will warehouse and distribute drugs directly to public health facilities.	

compile information from the medical literature on the new product (and on the therapeutic category the product represents) for the selection committee. Many procurement programs require that for each addition to the list a similar product be deleted, unless the proposed addition represents a new therapeutic category.

Analyses of past procurements using methods such as VEN (vital, essential, nonessential), ABC, and therapeutic category analysis (see Chapter 41) should be compiled before the meeting of the drug selection committee to focus deliberations and help in rationally limiting the procurement list.

Once the selection committee has met, the procurement office develops a list of the approved drugs for quantification. In computerized procurement offices, this may take one or two weeks. Manual revision may take a month or more to allow for retyping, correction, and reproduction.

Quantification

As discussed in Chapter 14, it is the responsibility of the procurement office to produce a reasonably accurate estimate of drug requirements for each tender, but much of this responsibility can be decentralized. Quantification can consume considerable time in programs that are decentralized but involve multiple layers of review. With four levels of management authority (health area, regions/districts, provinces, and national), it may take six to nine months to develop a list of drug needs for procurement. If the quantification process extends to six months or more, a full year may pass by the time the drugs are actually received. In that time, needs may

Figure 16.3 Example of a Drug Procurement Timetable

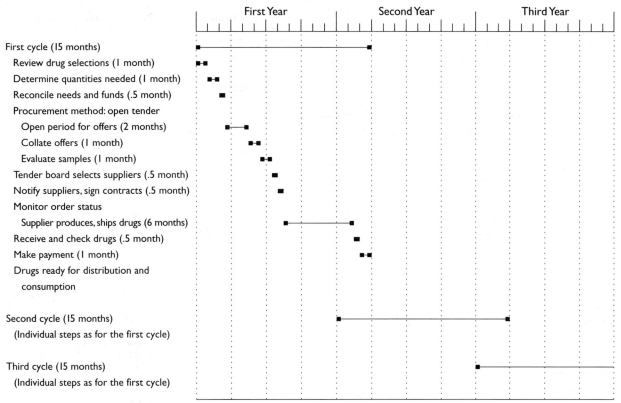

change, and money is wasted if the drugs purchased no longer match current needs.

One option for managing decentralized quantification is to have each management level with decision-making authority compile its own list. The list is then sent directly to the procurement office, which is responsible for comparing the list with past consumption, clarifying any questions directly with the client, and compiling the list for procurement. This avoids multiple layers of review at the district and province levels but increases the workload and responsibility of the procurement office.

Methods for large-scale procurement quantification—consumption-based, morbidity-based, and adjusted consumption—are discussed in Chapter 14. The choice of method is based largely on the type and reliability of data on drug usage, patient utilization, and morbidity patterns.

Countries should avoid making one major effort to quantify drugs and then relying on the same data for several years thereafter. No matter how accurate the original quantification may have been, given changes from year to year the earlier projections become increasingly unreliable guides to current procurement needs. One West African country did a major morbidity-based quantification in

1988 and was still using the same estimates in 1993, with adjustments based on the whim of the chief pharmacist. By 1993, the estimates did not match needs very well, and stockouts were rampant.

Once the quantification has been completed, the procurement committee should review and approve the list of drugs and the quantities proposed. It is important that the actual cost be estimated by the procurement office before the list is sent to the procurement committee for review, and definitely before the actual tendering is executed. If this is not done, the subsequent evaluation of tender offers may indicate that costs exceed funding.

≡ 16.4 Selecting Suppliers for Tender Participation

The selection of suppliers has a profound impact on the quality and cost of drugs acquired. Inadequate safeguards in supplier selection may result in the purchase of drugs that are ineffective, unsafe, or even deadly. As discussed in Chapter 13, hidden costs resulting from late deliveries, complete default on confirmed orders, losses due to poor packaging, or short expiration dates—common problems with unreliable suppliers—may raise the actual drug cost to several times the original contract cost.

New suppliers are constantly coming into the market, while others are changing to new fields, merging, or going out of business altogether. New companies may have difficulties with quality control and packaging for export during their first years of production but later become reliable low-cost producers. At the same time, a company long known for high-quality products and prompt service may become seriously deficient as a result of changes in management or regional distributors. A multinational company offering an attractive price may provide excellent service in one country and poor service in a nearby country, solely because of its choice of in-country representatives.

An efficient procurement office must therefore be able to maintain market intelligence so that reliable suppliers can be cultivated and unreliable ones replaced, whether the tender is restricted through prequalification or open with postqualification.

Types of Potential Pharmaceutical Suppliers

Government pharmaceutical factories, local private manufacturers, and foreign manufacturers are *primary* sources of pharmaceuticals, since these companies do the manufacturing themselves. Donors, international procurement services, independent foreign exporters, and local importers and distributors are *secondary* sources, since they obtain pharmaceuticals from manufacturers for resale. The seven principal classes of pharmaceutical suppliers are shown in Figure 16.4.

Drug Manufacturers. Drug manufacturers can be classified as *research-based* and *non-research-based* producers. The well-known multinational drug companies are research based in that their reputation and, to a large extent, their profitability depend on new drugs developed through research. These drugs are patented and vigorously promoted by brand name. Nevertheless, many such firms also produce a line of drugs that they sell by generic name at a lower price than their brand-name products. These drugs are often made on the same production line and sometimes in the same batch as the brand-name product. Quality standards are identical; only the packaging and appearance of the drug are different.

Non-research-based firms range from small, one-factory local companies to large local or international generic drug manufacturers. These manufacturers are often referred to as "generic drug houses," since they frequently market drugs only by their nonproprietary names. Although they may have less name recognition, many generic manufacturers produce products equal in quality to those of any brand-name company.

Figure 16.4 Locating Supply Sources

Sources of Pharmaceuticals	Means of Locating Suppliers
Primary sources	
Government production	Intragovernment negotiations
Local manufacturers	Locally publicized notice Direct inquiry to individual suppliers
Foreign manufacturers Multinational firms based in developed countries	Locally publicized notice (contact through local agent) Internationally publicized notice Direct inquiry through local agents Direct inquiry to home office
Firms in developing countries	Inquiry through national trade associations
Secondary sources	
Donations from bilateral aid programs, international agencies, and charitable organizations	Survey of government agencies to determine current sources Direct inquiry to local offices of UNICEF, foreign aid programs, religious and charitable groups, others Direct inquiry to home office of potential donors
International procurement services	Direct inquiry
Independent foreign exporters	As for foreign manufacturers
Local importers and distributors	As for local manufacturers

International Procurement Services. International procurement services are generally nonprofit companies or arms of international agencies. They provide services from one or more warehouses, and they vary with regard to selection of drugs, prices, means of quality assurance, payment terms, restrictions placed on the buyer, and nature and timeliness of service provided. Some well-established international procurement agencies are listed in the annual *International Drug Price Indicator Guide* (MSH 1995). Of the agencies listed as of 1995, only the International Dispensary Association (IDA) has its own manufacturing plants. Some procurement agencies, such as Crown Agents, are purchasing agents that must go through the sometimes lengthy process of negotiating prices with individual manufacturers and then arrange shipment from the primary supplier to the purchaser.

These agencies can play a valuable role in international tenders, providing competitive international prices for a range of products and access to small quantities of drugs—sales that may not interest primary manufacturers.

Their proposals should be evaluated by the same criteria used for other sources of supply, and they should specify the name of the manufacturer and the mechanism for quality assurance, like any commercial distributor.

Independent Foreign Wholesale Exporters. Independent foreign wholesale exporters—sometimes known as jobbers—purchase drugs from a variety of manufacturers for resale. There are many of these companies around the world that specialize in exports to developing countries. Most exporting countries exercise less strict control over jobbers than over manufacturers. Hence, it is essential to get the name of the primary manufacturer and to make sure that the distributor provides bona fide quality assurance documents and certifications from the exporting-country regulatory agency with each registration request, tender offer, and shipment. Forged certification documents have been received in some countries from less reliable foreign exporters.

Local Importers and Distributors. Local importers and distributors—also known as wholesalers—are often major forces in the local pharmaceutical market, both financially and politically. Like foreign distributors, these companies may not closely examine the quality of the products supplied by the manufacturers with which they work. In many countries, these companies have exclusive rights to represent certain manufacturers, and tender offers for these manufacturers' products come through the local distributor.

Locating and Contacting Qualified Suppliers

There are three basic ways of locating qualified suppliers: direct inquiries, advertisement of public tenders, and contacts with other procurement organizations and international agencies.

Direct Inquiries. Direct inquiries to local and foreign suppliers are the quickest means of attracting an offer. Direct inquiries to unknown suppliers are often necessary when establishing a purchasing system and in areas where current suppliers are unable to provide a specific drug at a reasonable price. Inquiries should be limited to countries that have established trade routes with the purchasing country and are known to enforce good manufacturing practices.

Public Tenders. Public tenders can be publicized through local newspaper notices, international notices, and direct mailings to known suppliers to attract a large number of bidders. Notices can be sent to international newspapers, trade directories, and journals with wide circulation; to foreign trade representatives in local diplomatic missions; to the country's diplomatic missions in supplying countries; and to government agencies responsible for foreign trade.

Programs that generally purchase only from registered suppliers may still publicize their intent to purchase through an international notice, in addition to contacting their registered suppliers directly. This is a safeguard to inform registered suppliers and may also arouse the interest of new suppliers.

Even when all foreign suppliers in a tender are represented by local agents, notice through international channels may be faster and more reliable than local agents in alerting foreign suppliers. Earlier notification allows suppliers more time to prepare offers and thus increases the probability of competitive offers.

Contacts with International Agencies. Contacts with international agencies may be one of the most effective ways for a procurement office with little international experience to identify potential suppliers. Local offices of the World Health Organization (WHO), the World Bank, or the United Nations Children's Fund (UNICEF) may be able to help establish communications with companies, trade associations, and procurement agencies, or with individuals who can suggest appropriate contacts. Procurement offices in other countries are usually willing to share information on reliable supply sources. International nonprofit procurement agencies may also be prepared to offer suggestions, although they exist primarily to offer services directly.

To know whether potential suppliers are offering good prices, procurement offices need a point of reference or sufficient experience in the market to make accurate cost estimates. One such reference for international prices for essential drugs, the annual *International Drug Price Indicator Guide* (MSH 1995), contains the latest catalog prices from several international procurement agencies and actual tender prices received by developing-country procurement agencies. Reference prices can also come from one of the nonprofit international procurement agencies such as UNICEF, Equipment for Charitable Hospitals Overseas (ECHO), or IDA, each of which provides a catalog illustrating its prices. The International Trade Centre in Geneva produces a comparative price list on raw materials used in pharmaceutical manufacturing, which is available on request.

Evaluating New Suppliers

When considering contract awards to previously unknown suppliers, it is important to establish how product quality will be assured. If the procurement office does not have a way to test products, it may argue against an award to a supplier that does not have strong references from reputable sources.

In addition to deciding whether a supplier is generally reliable, it must be determined which of the supplier's products are of acceptable quality. A supplier that is reliable in terms of quality assurance will probably be reliable for the full range of products, but this is not always the case. For example, some suppliers may produce good-quality liquids but not tablets or injections. There may be certain drugs with which the supplier has difficulty due to a lack of quality raw materials or a lack of certain equipment.

Some procurement programs establish a list of critical drugs for which there are quality issues and limit changes in suppliers for these products (see Chapter 18). It is certain that trying to qualify each supplier separately for each drug on the tender list will add substantial time to the pre- or postqualification process. In a West African country that decided to prequalify suppliers separately for each drug, the prequalification process for one tender took nearly eighteen months.

Procurement staff must develop a system of determining suppliers' reliability to eliminate suppliers that are substandard. There are two tasks: evaluating potential new suppliers (for pre- or postqualification) and rating the performance of past suppliers.

Evaluation of new (unknown) suppliers can be approached through

► formal registration;
► reference checks with past clients and international agencies;
► test purchases in small quantities;
► informal local information.

Formal Supplier Registration. Formal registration is the most thorough but also the most time-consuming method of evaluation. If the process is overly complex, it may discourage new suppliers. Formal registration is the norm when prequalifying suppliers for a restricted tender. If a local agent is involved, the registration process may provide useful information on the agent's reliability and relationship with the primary supplier.

Reference Checks with Past Clients and International Agencies. With an open international tender, bids may be received from any country in the world, and the procurement office will probably be unfamiliar with most of the bidders. Even with a restricted tender, new suppliers should be considered for registration. In both cases, it is critical to check the business references provided.

New suppliers that cannot provide references from other countries' procurement offices (or reputable international agencies) should be accepted with extreme caution,

if at all. If prices are sufficiently attractive, limited awards might be made on a trial basis (as described below). If a supplier has chronically failed to perform in past tender contracts, it is reasonable to assume that the pattern will continue and that the supplier should not be relied upon.

Purchasing offices that do not have international telephone and fax communications are at an extreme disadvantage in checking references for unknown suppliers. They run a real risk of awarding contracts to suppliers that will not perform reliably.

Test Purchases in Small Quantities. Some countries assess new suppliers by accepting offers on selected items when the prices and terms are favorable. They then monitor service and product quality and base future awards on performance. Products that present risks of poor bioavailability or for which timely delivery is crucial are usually not purchased from unknown new suppliers. For example, an unknown supplier might be awarded a contract for vitamin B complex but not for digoxin or benzylpenicillin. In practice, test purchasing is rarely used as the sole means of assessing a new supplier. It is generally used in conjunction with the other three methods: supplier registration, international reference checks, and local information gathering.

Solicitation of Local Information. It is important to solicit information from local agencies and individuals who may have had previous experience with a potential supplier. This is the least time-consuming, although sometimes the least accurate, method used to assess potential suppliers. The opinions of local pharmacists, physicians, and particularly industry representatives may be biased. A low-cost, high-quality supplier may be disqualified because of unsubstantiated negative information or opinions influenced by opportunities for personal gain.

Annex 16.1 shows information one should check when considering a new supplier. Sample registration forms used by the Eastern Caribbean Drug Service are available from ECDS or from Management Sciences for Health (MSH). Forms used by international nonprofit procurement agencies can be requested from the agencies.

Monitoring and Evaluating the Performance of Known Suppliers

Once a contract is awarded, monitoring the supplier's service and quality is the basis for decisions regarding future purchases. In many countries, this is done informally and without written records, which makes it difficult to assemble data for procurement committees to review. Successful purchasing agencies use a formal monitoring system, as described below in Section 16.9 on procurement information.

In general, suppliers that have performed poorly should be excluded from the next tender. Some procurement agencies give a probationary reapproval to suppliers that have had problems, such as too many partial shipments or excessive lead times, but offer high-quality products at competitive prices. If problems recur, they are then barred from the next tender. If a supplier's problems are sufficiently grave, it can be barred for a two-year period and then forced to go through reregistration. Annex 16.2 provides criteria for evaluating current or past suppliers.

Criteria for Rating Suppliers. Some procurement programs use a point system, assigning values to performance criteria such as those shown in Annexes 16.1 and 16.2. The relative weights of each category vary; for example, in some situations, the lead time may be very important and be given a high weight; in other situations, it may be a minor factor. In countries with strong regulatory control of the drug market, product quality may be given a low weight, because it is assumed that all registered products will be of acceptable quality.

Rating systems offer two options for ranking applications: in one, there is a minimum passing score; in the other, suppliers are ranked from top to bottom overall, and contract preference is given to higher-ranked suppliers when prices are equivalent. A supplier with a much higher rank might get the contract despite a competitor's offer of lower prices.

Another approach is to apply a yes/no screen for each criterion. If the supplier meets a minimum standard for each criterion, the application for qualification is approved; if the application fails to meet any of the minimum standards, the application is rejected.

Since ratings of supplier reliability and quality have a tremendous impact on the number and quality of suppliers that participate in a tender, the ratings must be as impartial as possible, with criteria written into the tender adjudication process. Ratings will always be subjective to some extent, so to ensure impartiality, the entire procurement committee, or at least a multiperson team, should be responsible for rating suppliers.

≡ 16.5 Preparing and Issuing Tender Documents

Once selection, quantification, and preparation of the tender list are completed, bid packages are sent out. For restricted tenders, they are sent to all prequalified bidders; in open tenders, they are sent to all interested bidders. The tender package typically includes the documents discussed below. (See "References and Further Readings" for sources of tender documents that can be adapted.)

The *invitation to bid* describes the procurement, the purchasing group that is soliciting offers, the conditions under which bids will be accepted, the address for submission, the date bids are due, and the dates to be covered by the contract.

The *instructions to bidders* cover how to submit documents, including how to state prices, dates of bid validity, what currencies to use, what documents are required in addition to bid forms, bid and performance bonds (if applicable; see Chapter 17), precautions against undue contact with procurement office staff, format for submitting offers, domestic preference (if any), criteria for bid evaluation, and procedures involved in adjudication, award, and notification. Forms should be appended for performance and bid bonds and for documenting domestic preference and value added, if applicable.

The *conditions of contract* discuss general conditions in the contract that will be signed with successful bidders and any special conditions applicable to the current procurement (see Chapter 17).

The *general technical specifications* provide information on good manufacturing practices (GMPs), pharmacopeial standards, nomenclature and description required for each product, shelf life and expiration date parameters, labeling instructions, packaging instructions, GMP and quality assurance certificates required, and other evidence of product quality to be submitted with the tender and with each shipment.

Specific pharmacopeial standards should be listed for each product; if any of a range of standards is adequate (*British Pharmacopeia, United States Pharmacopeia, European Pharmacopoeia*, or *International Pharmacopoeia*), this should be noted. If special packaging or labeling is required for a subset of products, this should be indicated on the schedule of requirements (see below), but a generic statement of packaging and labeling applied to all products should be included in the general technical specifications. Instructions about labeling (contents and language) and package inserts can be included in the technical specifications, unless there are specific requirements for a subset of products. These should be indicated on the tender list.

If all products are to be shipped to the same destination, on the same delivery schedule, by whatever means is most efficient and cost effective, this can be stated in the conditions of contract. If different instructions apply to certain products, this should be stipulated in the schedule of requirements.

The *schedule of requirements*, or tender list, provides a concise description of each product and the quantity required, along with any technical specifications unique to that item. If it can be printed with sufficient space for suppliers to enter offers, having suppliers use this space for bids greatly simplifies the collation of offers. Sufficient space should be provided so that the supplier can enter all relevant information, including the name of the original manufacturer.

The schedule of requirements should include the international nonproprietary name (INN), or generic name (for combination products, the name of each generic component), the strength in metric units for each component, the basic unit (tablet, capsule, vial, bottle), the package size, and the number of packages needed. Some tenders list both the total number of packages and the total number of basic units needed, to avoid misunderstanding and to allow for the possibility that a supplier may offer a different (but acceptable) package size representing the same number of basic units. The tender should specify whether the listed package sizes are the only ones acceptable; some procurement agencies request offers on all package sizes available.

Each unique product should have a separate inventory code number, used only for that product. This is useful in compiling product catalogs and is essential for computerized information systems. It can also be helpful in making sure that all parties are talking about the same item when clarifying issues with client facilities or with suppliers. For therapeutic category analysis, a supplementary code can be used to assign each drug product to a therapeutic category (see Chapter 41).

To simplify future procurements and make sure that all staff use the same terminology in procurement and tender functions, it is useful to compile all information about each tender product into a procurement catalog. With a computerized system, developing a catalog is simple; it is more difficult to update a product catalog manually, but it may be worth the effort to save time in compiling future tender lists.

≡ 16.6 Adjudicating the Tender

Tender adjudication involves several separate activities and stages:

► Prepare for adjudication during the open period.
► Receive and open bids.
► Collate bids for adjudication.
► Adjudicate offers and award contracts.

Preparing during the Open Period

The length of the open period (time between the invitation to tender and the closing date) varies from four to eight weeks. A longer open period lengthens the total lead time for obtaining drugs but may also increase the number of offers received. The procurement agency should prepare for receipt of documents, collation, and adjudication during the open period.

Some suppliers may request clarification as to product description, package size, pharmacopeial standard, labeling, or packaging requirements. If clarification is needed due to a mistake or omission in the tender package, it should be provided to all participating bidders. Similarly, if one supplier is given approval to offer a product or package that is similar to but not the same as that listed in the schedule of requirements, all bidders should be informed that such an exception is approved.

Receiving and Opening Tender Offers

To ensure confidentiality and to avoid accusations of price fixing or undue influence on decisions, the procurement agency must adhere strictly to the closing date. No bids should be opened before the date specified. A written record should be kept of all bids received, documenting the date received and the person who received the bid. The unopened bids should be stored in a locked, secure area until the closing date. The date of bid receipt should also be entered into the procurement management information system to track the response to tenders. If due dates are approaching and certain suppliers known to be reliable low-cost sources have not responded, the procurement agency can remind them of the approaching deadline by telephone or fax.

On the specified date, the bids should be formally opened, with at least one member of the procurement committee in attendance. Each opened bid should be logged in a ledger and numbered for future reference. It may be useful to write the number of enclosed pages on the outside of the tender envelope, to avoid confusion during adjudication.

Collating Offers for Adjudication

The first step in collating offers is to determine which offers, if any, are nonresponsive to tender conditions. Suppliers that have not met the basic requirements related to drug description, strength, pack size, quality requirements, and delivery date are nonresponsive. If required information has not been provided, the bid is nonresponsive. If the tender documents require the supplier's signed acceptance of contract terms and the supplier has not signed, the bid is nonresponsive.

Information from all responsive bids should be compiled in an adjudication report to allow side-by-side comparison of the offers. Nonresponsive bids should not be entered into the collated adjudication report, but the problems should be documented in writing for review by the procurement committee.

Prices must be converted to a common currency and adjustments made for differences in trade terms (for example, adding freight costs to those bids that do not include freight expenses). If local or domestic preference is considered in the adjudication, the adjudication report should separate offers eligible for the local preference margin, so that they can be fairly compared with offers that are not eligible.

Specific procurement programs such as INVEC-2, ECPRO-2, or Swedis or general spreadsheet programs (Lotus, Excel, or QuattroPro) are useful tools to simplify the collation of information and the preparation of an adjudication report. In a manual system, large charts can be used to list all products down the left side, with space for offers across, or a separate typed page can be used for each product, with spaces indicated to enter the supplier, the manufacturer, the price, and the lead time. Figure 16.5 illustrates an adjudication report prepared by a specialized computer program, INVEC-2.

Managing the Adjudication Process

The authority to adjudicate tenders and award contracts should be reserved to the procurement committee (or government tender board). Procurement office staff should assemble information for the tender board or procurement committee and make technical recommendations, but they should not have a vote in the contract decision.

As discussed in Chapter 13, the adjudication process must be free from influence by special interests; it should be open and transparent, with written rules for the process, including evaluation, award, any special criteria, and the appeal period for rejected bidders. Results of adjudication, including the winning bidder and the contract price, should be available to all participating bidders. In countries where drug procurement has fallen into disrepute, broadening participation in the procurement committee to make sure that it has final authority over all drug procurement and enforcing transparency in the tender process will help rebuild credibility.

Evaluation of Offers. This can be a quick process for restricted tenders. The procurement committee reviews the collated bid information and normally selects the lowest bidder for each product. Contracts are then developed.

For open tenders, supplier evaluation does not begin until bids are received, as adjudication is a two-stage process: ranking the bids according to standard evaluation criteria, and then beginning the postqualification supplier evaluation process. Once the postqualification analysis has been completed, the procurement committee meets again and determines whether the lowest evaluated bid should receive the contract. If not, the next lowest evaluated bid is considered, and so forth.

The procurement committee should carefully consider each item on the tender list and make an award for each item, unless no responsive bids were received. If the primary/secondary supplier system is used, equal care is needed in selecting secondary suppliers, since they will automatically be used if the primary supplier defaults.

Written bid evaluation criteria should be applied rigorously and without exception. Tender contracts should be awarded to the lowest bidder that has the capacity to supply products that meet the standards required (considering local preference, if applicable). This should be mandatory unless the lowest bidder has not performed in prior procurements.

In local tenders, the quoted CIF or CIP delivered unit prices are an adequate means of comparing costs. Terms offered other than letters of credit (such as deferred payment) may provide a substantial benefit and should be considered if stated in the evaluation criteria and in instructions to bidders.

Local and foreign suppliers may offer different trade terms (CIP to purchaser's warehouse, or CIF to purchaser's main port). To make these two prices comparable, CIF price must add all duties, fees, handling, and transportation costs to the purchaser's warehouse.

Delivery dates should be compared in terms of past suppliers' performance rather than promised delivery date. If the lowest acceptable bidder's expected delivery is beyond the required date, then the effect of a shortage must be considered in light of the cost of alternative treatments or of a special air shipment to cover the interim period.

Special Criteria. Special criteria are sometimes applied, such as a local preference margin calculated by adding a percentage to the value of foreign bids before they are compared with local bids. World Bank–financed ICB procurements allow local preference, to a maximum of 15 percent. Although pricing is the accepted means of granting local preference, some countries have accepted lower local standards of product quality. This is not recommended as a standard practice, but for some drugs that have a wide therapeutic margin—an example is multiple vitamins—it may not make an appreciable difference in therapeutic result if potency varies by 20 percent. For such drugs, it might be reasonable to relax quality standards in the tender specifications, but this should be done with great caution.

Figure 16.5 Sample Adjudication Report from INVEC-2

GMS197   Government Medical Store Tender

COMPARISON OF BIDS   **Printed: 12/02/97**

Product Code: 01002
Description : ACETAZOLAMIDE 250 MG TAB (PO) /TAB
Pack Size : 28 TABS
Qty Required: 10000 x 28 TABS

Comparison Unit: TAB

SUP. CODE	BIDDER'S NAME	COUNTRY OF ORIGIN	LEAD TIME	PACKS OFFERED	PACK SIZE	PACK PRICE	EXCH. RATE *	PACK PRICE (EC$)	<A>	<B>	<C>	ADJUSTED PRICE (EC$)	TOTAL BID VALUE (EC$)	COMPARISON UNIT VALUE (EC$)	REMARKS
(PHS/)	Phs Hospital Supply	PUERTO RICO	30 S	5,000	56 TABS	1.00USD	2.7169	2.72			C	2.72	13,584.50	0.0485/TAB	
FOU/	E. Foully & Company	BARBADOS	15 S	10,000	28 TABS	0.60USD	2.7169	1.63			C	1.63	16,301.40	0.0582/TAB	
NVP/	Novotec Ltd.	CANADA	56 S	10,000	28 TABS	0.70USD	2.7169	1.90			C	1.90	19,018.30	0.0679/TAB	
APO/	Aponics Inc.	MALTA	40 S	10,000	28 TABS	0.75USD	2.7169	2.04			C	2.04	20,376.75	0.0728/TAB	

Product Code: 01038
Description : DAPSONE 100 MG TAB (PO) /TAB
Pack Size : 100 TABS
Qty Required: 5000 x 100 TABS

Comparison Unit: TAB

SUP. CODE	BIDDER'S NAME	COUNTRY OF ORIGIN	LEAD TIME	PACKS OFFERED	PACK SIZE	PACK PRICE	EXCH. RATE *	PACK PRICE (EC$)	<A>	<B>	<C>	ADJUSTED PRICE (EC$)	TOTAL BID VALUE (EC$)	COMPARISON UNIT VALUE (EC$)	REMARKS
NVP/	Novotec Ltd.	CANADA	56 S	5,000	100 TABS	0.40USD	2.7169	1.09			C	1.09	5,433.80	0.0109/TAB	
FOU/	E. Foully & Company	BARBADOS	56 S	5,000	100 TABS	0.67USD	2.7169	1.82			C	1.82	9,101.62	0.0182/TAB	
APO/	Aponics Inc.	MALTA	40 S	500	1000 TABS	44.44USD	2.7169	120.74			C	120.74	60,369.52	0.1207/TAB	
(PHS/)	Phs Hospital Supply	PUERTO RICO	55 S	5,000	100 TABS	15.00USD	2.7169	40.75			C	40.75	203,767.50	0.4075/TAB	

Product Code: 02003
Description : AMPICILLIN 500 MG AMP (INJ) /AMP
Pack Size : 10 AMP
Qty Required: 4500 x 10 AMP

Comparison Unit: AMP

SUP. CODE	BIDDER'S NAME	COUNTRY OF ORIGIN	LEAD TIME	PACKS OFFERED	PACK SIZE	PACK PRICE	EXCH. RATE *	PACK PRICE (EC$)	<A>	<B>	<C>	ADJUSTED PRICE (EC$)	TOTAL BID VALUE (EC$)	COMPARISON UNIT VALUE (EC$)	REMARKS
FOU/	E. Foully & Company	BARBADOS	30 S	4,500	10 AMP	1.68USD	2.7169	4.56			C	4.56	20,539.76	0.4564/AMP	
NVP/	Novotec Ltd.	CANADA	56 S	4,500	10 AMP	2.16USD	2.7169	5.87			C	5.87	26,408.27	0.5869/AMP	
(PHS/)	Phs Hospital Supply	PUERTO RICO	30 S	900	50 AMP	11.25USD	2.7169	30.57			C	30.57	27,508.61	0.6113/AMP	
APO/	Aponics Inc.	MALTA	45 S	450	100 AMP	33.35USD	2.7169	90.61			C	90.61	40,773.88	0.9061/AMP	

* Use Exchange Rate as of Day of Bid Opening

Some programs try to maintain geographic and political dispersion of suppliers to protect against loss of a major supply source due to war, natural disasters, or international political problems.

Appeal Period for Rejected Bidders. Some countries allow an appeal period during which rejected suppliers may request reconsideration by the tender board. The appeal process varies greatly according to national regulations; the time to resolve appeals according to law may be less than a week or many months, but ideally, the appeal period should be no more than one month, to avoid delays in procurement.

≡ 16.7 Issuing Contracts to Winning Bidders

Once contract awards are made, contracts must be established with successful bidders (see Chapter 17).

A list of all contracts awarded, specifying for each item the supplier, price, and total value, should be made available to all responsive bidders; if necessary, the name of the successful bidder can be omitted from the public document.

If winning bidders decline to accept the contract, bid bonds (if used) are forfeited. In the primary/secondary system, the secondary supplier is contacted immediately. In other cases, the item must be rebid; depending on the volume, local competitive bidding may be the preferred method.

≡ 16.8 Monitoring Performance and Product Quality

The procurement office is responsible for monitoring performance and compliance with contract terms by suppliers and facilities that order drugs. The agency must actively track suppliers' lead time, delivery status, compliance with contract pricing and terms, shelf life, and packaging of products. In decentralized procurement systems, it is equally important to monitor facilities' performance. Are they ordering according to schedule, in reasonable quantities, and are they paying for their purchases according to the contract? Are total purchases roughly equal to estimated needs?

It is crucial to maintain an active program to ensure product quality before procurement and after receipt and distribution (see Chapters 13 and 18). Reports of problems from prescribers, dispensers, consumers, and purchasing managers must be recorded in the product and supplier files and reviewed as part of the monitoring and evaluation of suppliers.

There can be more latitude in considering new and unknown suppliers if there is access to reliable and rela-

tively inexpensive quality assurance testing. Unfortunately, this is not the case in many countries.

When testing is available, it is not necessary to test every drug from every supplier, but this should always be done for products that have been reported as suspect. Testing should be done periodically for random samples of drugs known to be subject to degradation in questionable storage conditions, drugs that have a low therapeutic index, and drugs received from suppliers of questionable or unknown reputation.

Chapter 17 discusses supply contracts and enforcement provisions. Enforcement is the key: there is no point in an elaborate contract unless it will be enforced when necessary. The reality is that unless substantial performance bonds are required as a condition of the contract (which may increase prices), there may be limited recourse in the case of problems with foreign suppliers other than canceling outstanding orders and withholding payment.

≡ 16.9 The Procurement Information System

The most important tool in the procurement office is its management information system (MIS). The MIS can be computerized or manual; computerized systems make it much easier to develop reports, and they speed up procurement processes such as prequalification and collation of tender offers for adjudication.

The greatest benefit can probably be realized with specialized computer software programs for procurement (see Chapter 46). However, even a simple word processor can drastically decrease the time needed to process tender documents and contracts, and commercial spreadsheet programs can accomplish most other tasks.

This section describes the information that should be tracked and used; the method of storing and retrieving the information is secondary. The information system includes several different types of records: on products, tendering and ordering, suppliers, clients, quality assurance, accounts receivable and payable for drug orders, and accounting records for the procurement office itself (see Chapters 42 and 45).

Product Records

Product files record the standard technical specifications for a specific item and the performance of past suppliers of the product. Detailed product records are particularly important when quality is critical. A sample product card for a manual system is shown in Figure 16.6. It is useful to produce a catalog of all items that can be used to compile quantification lists, tender lists, adjudication forms, and notices of awards.

Figure 16.6 Sample Product Card

Side One / Product Specifications

Generic name: PARACETAMOL		Category: ANALGESIC	
Trade names: CALPOL, PANADOL, TYLENOL			Code number: 02-4600
Form: TABLET	Dosage: 500 mg	Package size: 1,000 TABS	
Acceptable pharmacopeial standards: IP / USP / EP / BP			
Additional technical specifications: Standard specifications (Schedule A), plus: (1) Double-scored tablet, imprinted with unique identifiers (our logo) (2) Shrink-wrapped in packaging units of 10 x 1,000			

Side Two / Supplier History

Purchase Order Number	Supplier	Quantity	Unit Price	Date Promised	Date Delivered	Comments
085/97	GENERIX	5,000	20.25	01/98	02/98	
086/97	NOVAPHARM	10,000	21.80	01/98	12/97	
003/98	GENERIX	5,000	20.25	04/98		Revised Date 05/98
004/98	NOVAPHARM	10,000	21.80	04/98	03/98	
046/98	NOVAPHARM	15,000	23.00	07/98		

Figure 16.7 Sample Order Status Reports from INVEC-2

ITEMS ON ORDER (Sorted by Supplier/PO#/Description) -   14/02/97

SUPPLIER REQ #/PO NUMBER DATE ORDERED	<A>IR <S>EA	PACK SIZE	x	ON ORDER	P.O's PACK COST	ESTIMATED VALUE
GENETHICS LTD(GEN/)						
LUC-987/ 14/02/97						
01054 GRISEOFULVIN 500MG TAB (PO) /TAB	S	1000 TAB	x	7	48.75	341.25USD
02010 CHLORAMPHENICOL 1GM VIAL (INJ) /VIAL	S	100 VIAL	x	10	33.00	330.00USD
09001 BISACODYL 10 MG SUPP (RECT)	S	12 SUPP	x	150	1.50	225.00USD
Estimated Order Balance :				2,435.02 EC$		896.25USD
Estimated Supplier's Balance:				2,435.02 EC$		896.25USD
CARLISLE LABORATORIES LTD.(CAR/)						
LUC-988/ 14/02/97						
01002 ACETAZOLAMIDE 250MG TAB (PO) /TAB	S	1000 TAB	x	5	22.50	112.50USD
01006 ALBENDAZOLE OR MEBENDAZOLE 200MG TAB (PO) /TAB	S	500 TAB	x	6	13.00	78.00USD
01009 AMITRIPTYLINE 25MG TAB (PO) /TAB	S	100 TAB	x	10	0.55	5.50USD
01025 CARBIMAZOLE 5MG TAB (PO) /TAB	S	1000 TAB	x	3	9.00	27.00USD
Estimated Order Balance :				605.87 EC$		223.00USD
Estimated Supplier's Balance:				605.87 EC$		223.00USD
AN-MED INTERNATIONAL(ANM/)						
LUC-989/ 14/02/97						
01014 ATENOLOL 100MG TAB (PO) /TAB	S	100 TAB	x	10	1.39	13.90USD
01038 DAPSONE 100MG TAB (PO) /TAB	S	1000 TAB	x	10	4.30	43.00USD
01044 ERYTHROMYCIN 250MG TAB (PO) /TAB	S	1000 TAB	x	8	45.20	361.60USD
05005 CEPHALEXIN 25MG/ML SUSP (PO) 100 ML/BOTT	S	10 BOTT	x	10	15.60	156.00USD
Estimated Order Balance :				1,560.86 EC$		574.50USD
Estimated Supplier's Balance:				1,560.86 EC$		574.50USD
Estimated All P.O's Balance :				4,601.75 EC$		

ITEMS ON ORDER (Sorted by Description/Supplier/Date Ordered)

SUPPLIER	P.O.#	DATE ORDERED	<A>IR <S>EA	PACK SIZE	x	ON ORDER	P.O's PACK COST	ESTIMATED VALUE SUPP. CURR.	LOCAL CURR.
01002 (CAR/)	LUC-988	02/14/97	S	1000 TAB	x	5	22.50	112.50USD	305.65EC$
	Date Expected	03/07/97	Total IU on Order	5000 TAB					305.65EC$
ACETAZOLAMIDE 250MG TAB (PO) /TAB									
01006 (CAR/)	LUC-988	02/14/97	S	500 TAB	x	6	13.00	78.00USD	211.92EC$
	Date Expected	03/14/97	Total IU on Order	3000 TAB					211.92EC$
ALBENDAZOLE OR MEBENDAZOLE 200MG TAB (PO) /TAB									
01009 (CAR/)	LUC-988	02/14/97	S	100 TAB	x	10	0.55	5.50USD	14.94EC$
	Date Expected	02/14/97	Total IU on Order	1000 TAB					14.94EC$
AMITRIPTYLINE 25MG TAB (PO) /TAB									
01014 (ANM/)	LUC-989	02/14/97	S	100 TAB	x	10	1.39	13.90USD	37.76EC$
	Date Expected	02/14/97	Total IU on Order	1000 TAB					37.76EC$
ATENOLOL 100MG TAB (PO) /TAB									
01025 (CAR/)	LUC-988	02/14/97	S	1000 TAB	x	3	9.00	27.00USD	73.36EC$
	Date Expected	03/31/97	Total IU on Order	3000 TAB					73.36EC$
CARBIMAZOLE 5MG TAB (PO) /TAB									
01038 (ANM/)	LUC-989	02/14/97	S	1000 TAB	x	10	4.30	43.00USD	116.83EC$
	Date Expected	02/14/97	Total IU on Order	10000 TAB					116.83EC$
DAPSONE 100MG TAB (PO) /TAB									
01044 (ANM/)	LUC-989	02/14/97	S	1000 TAB	x	8	45.20	361.60USD	982.43EC$
	Date Expected	02/14/97	Total IU on Order	8000 TAB					982.43EC$
ERYTHROMYCIN 250MG TAB (PO) /TAB									

Figure 16.8 Standard Procurement Reports

Report Name	Contents
Reorder report	Suggested order quantities, sorted by item or supplier
Purchase orders pending	Outstanding orders, by item or supplier
Physical stock status	Summary list of quantities for all items in inventory, by name or code, with nearest expiry date
Stock detail report	List of all items in stock, with quantity by batch (lot number) and expiry date
Expired stock	All expired stock and stock without expiry date
Expiry risk	Stock at risk of expiry—stock quantity, expiry date, average use, and quantity and value of stock at risk
Out of stock	All items out of stock
Stock count form	Stock count list, by name, dosage form, location, or code
Inventory adjustment	List of items for which the stock count and records differ
Inventory variance	Changes made to stock balances outside normal process
Suppliers	List of all suppliers, with contact information
Accounts payable	Aged list of debts to suppliers
Facilities	List of all client facilities, with contact information
Accounts receivable	Aged list of debts from facilities
Summary of warehouse activity	Purchases and sales, year to date and month to date
Tender request	List of items needed, with specifications
Tender offers	Bid details for each tender offer
Adjudication report	Bids received by item, ranked by total cost (lowest to highest)
Tender award list	List of contracts awarded
Currency exchange history	Report on exchange rates by currency
Financial transactions	Financial transactions, by date and account code
Stock transactions	List of all shipments to facilities, by item or facility, with total value
Purchases/receipts	List of all purchases and other receipts, by item or source, with total value
ABC analysis	ABC analysis of warehouse consumption, and analysis for each client facility

Records Related to Tendering and Ordering

A record of each year's procurement, tracking the total quantity estimated and actually purchased of each item (along with the contract supplier and price), facilitates the estimation of future prices and is essential in assembling future quantifications and checking quantity estimates from clients in decentralized ordering systems.

An ongoing record of the order status and shipments pending can be made using separate folders for orders outstanding, orders received as partial shipments, and orders completed.

Another simple manual system uses a ledger to track each order (the order number, date ordered, date received, dates additional shipments were received, and dates payments were made), organized chronologically or by purchase order number. Systems that do not use purchase order numbers may find it difficult to keep track of outstanding orders.

A computerized information system can provide standard reports on order status, organized by product, purchase order number, or supplier. Figure 16.7 illustrates order status reports available from the INVEC-2 software program.

Records to Monitor Supplier and Facility Performance

Supplier performance monitoring has two components. First, there should be a system for monitoring lead time, compliance with contract pricing terms, partial shipments, remaining shelf life, compliance with packaging and labeling instructions, and compliance with other contract terms. This record should track the number and value of tender contracts awarded chronologically and the value of total purchases from the supplier by year. Second, there should be a file on each supplier, containing copies of all registration papers, references, special correspondence, complaints, and anecdotal information.

The facility performance monitoring system tracks total purchases compared with estimated quantities for each procurement cycle, purchases from noncontract suppliers, lead time for payment to suppliers (if that is the facilities' responsibility), compliance with deadlines for quantification, complaints about product quality and supplier service problems, and results of follow-up to complaints and requests for action.

Quality Assurance Records

A chronological record of all product quality complaints, with documentation as to the results of follow-up, should be separate but linked to a record that documents all quality assurance tests performed, the reason, and the results. These records should be linked to or entered into both product and supplier records.

Accounts Receivable and Payable

The procurement office should have a record of each order placed with contract suppliers, the dates payments were made against the outstanding amount, and the total amount still owed. A separate purchase order number for each purchase permits the records to be arranged by either purchase order number or supplier. Purchase order numbers should be included in every communication to the supplier: the initial order, the tender contract, and any subsequent communications.

If the procurement office is based in a warehouse that also sells drugs to clients, accurate records should be kept of amounts owed by clients and fees charged for procurement services. A separate transaction number assigned to each shipment or charge for services makes tracking easier.

Reporting

As discussed throughout this chapter, the procurement information system will be called upon to issue periodic reports for drug and supplier selection, quantification, and tender collation and adjudication, as well as status reports on orders or payments. Standard reports, such as those listed in Figure 16.8, are much more easily produced by a computerized information system, but even a manual system should be organized enough to produce the reports fairly regularly. ∎

≡ Assessment Guide

Quantitative Indicators

- ▶ Percentage by value of ministry of health (MOH) drugs purchased through a central procurement system;
- ▶ Percentage of average international price paid for last regular procurement (indicator drugs);
- ▶ Percentage by value of MOH drug purchases that are on the essential drugs list or national drug formulary;
- ▶ Percentage by value of MOH drugs purchased through competitive tender;
- ▶ Percentage by value of drugs purchased from local manufacturers;
- ▶ Average lead time for a sample of orders (calculated separately for all suppliers, local manufacturers, foreign suppliers);
- ▶ Average time period for payment for a sample of orders (calculated separately for all suppliers, local manufacturers, foreign suppliers).

Procurement Responsibility

- ▶ Is procurement managed centrally, or is authority decentralized?
- ▶ How much time is normally required to complete the following steps (and who is responsible for managing the step): selection, quantification, preparation of tender documents, tender adjudication, and contract award?
- ▶ Have the persons responsible for procurement been trained in this field?
- ▶ Is there a written procurement procedures manual? If so, do practices conform with the written procedures?
- ▶ What type of procurement method is normally used?
- ▶ Who determines the procurement method for a specific procurement?
- ▶ Are the methods based on law or written policies?
- ▶ How many different suppliers currently supply drugs to the health system?
- ▶ Are they bilateral aid programs, international procurement services, multinational companies, local import agents?

- ▶ Does a single supplier or small group seem to win most of the supply contracts for the system?
- ▶ Who is responsible for selecting potential suppliers?
- ▶ On what basis are the suppliers selected for tender participation?
- ▶ Is there prequalification of suppliers?
- ▶ Is a formal rating system used for evaluating suppliers' suitability?
- ▶ Are supplier selection criteria documented and closely adhered to?
- ▶ What role do local agents play in locating, selecting, and conducting business with pharmaceutical suppliers?
- ▶ Who has the authority to award contracts to suppliers?
- ▶ Are there written procedures for committee actions, and are they followed?
- ▶ What kinds of influences are brought to bear on the individuals who select the suppliers and award contracts?

Tender and Contract Methods

- ▶ Do tenders and supply contracts specify a fixed quantity and delivery schedule or an estimated quantity, with orders placed as needed?
- ▶ If both systems are used, what is the approximate percentage by value of drugs purchased under each system?
- ▶ What are the procedures for placing orders to suppliers?
- ▶ What is the average time required to get the order approved?
- ▶ Who approves the order?
- ▶ Is there an effective policy limiting MOH pharmaceutical procurement to drugs on the national drug formulary list or essential drugs list?
- ▶ For competitive tenders, does the schedule of requirements list drugs by generic name or brand name?
- ▶ Are any drugs or groups of drugs tendered by therapeutic group (for example, oral first-generation cephalosporin) instead of by individual drug in the group?

► Does the tender document specify pharmacopeial standards, WHO certification, specific packaging, specific labeling on package, specific labeling on individual dosage form, specific labeling language, delivery or order schedule, limit on back orders or number of partial shipments, minimum shelf life, replacement of goods damaged in shipment, samples submitted with bid?

► Are domestic companies allowed a local preference margin on bids? If so, what percentage?

► Is value added required for local preference? If so, what percentage is required, and how is value added determined?

► What is the usual basis for selecting the contract supplier? Is it the lowest price with no exceptions, the lowest price from a prequalified vendor, the lowest price of products deemed to be of acceptable quality, or some other standard policy?

► If product quality is a factor in tender awards, how is this determined?

► What circumstances prompt split tender awards, if any?

► Are secondary supplier awards routinely made in case the primary supplier fails to perform? If so, do secondary suppliers normally agree to honor original tender prices?

► What circumstances warrant switching to the secondary supplier?

► Are there constraints experienced in the use of secondary suppliers?

► Are bid bonds required?

► Are performance bonds required after contracts are awarded? If so, what are the usual amounts or percentage of procurement value required?

► Is a fee charged to vendors that request tender documents? If so, what is the amount?

► Does the tender contract provide for penalties if the vendor does not perform? If so, are these penalties enforced?

► Are contract terms to which suppliers are expected to adhere clearly specified?

► Do these terms provide sufficient protection from common difficulties such as late deliveries, inadequate drug labeling, short shelf life, and poor quality?

► Are trade terms, payment terms, delivery schedules, and payment methods clearly specified?

Payment to Suppliers

► Are there problems with timely access to procurement funds or foreign exchange? If so, how do they affect the procurement timetable?

► What are the usual payment terms for international purchases and for domestic purchases?

► What are the usual real lead times for payment for credit purchases (both international and local purchases)?

► What is the total debt owed to domestic vendors and to international vendors for drugs and supplies?

Procurement Information System

► Is there a systematic method for monitoring the status of outstanding orders and for providing information to other units regarding the status of outstanding orders?

► Do suppliers frequently refuse to supply an item for which they have won the contract, or do they default on an order?

► Are there frequent problems with suppliers' performance?

► What system is used to monitor the performance of suppliers and of health units that order drugs?

► What reports are prepared on performance, and how are these reports used?

► Are computers used in the tender management and procurement information system? If so, what kinds of software are used?

► Is the software and hardware suited to the purpose?

► Are personnel who use the computers trained in the use of the software?

► Does the computerized information system produce reliable information on consumption and performance?

► Is there a reliable system for maintaining and supporting the hardware and software?

≡ References and Further Readings

★ = *Key readings.*

ASHP (American Society of Hospital Pharmacists). 1991. ASHP guidelines for selecting pharmaceutical manufacturers and suppliers. *American Journal of Hospital Pharmacy* 48:523–24.

Broun, D. 1994. *Procurement of pharmaceuticals in World Bank projects.* Washington, D.C.: World Bank.

Cleverley, W. O., and P. C. Nutt. 1984. The effectiveness of group-purchasing organizations. *Health Services Research* 19:65–81.

Dorner, G., ed. 1992. *Management of drug purchasing, storage, and distribution: Manual for developing countries,* 3d rev. ed. Aulendorf, Germany: Editio Cantor Verlag.

★ FIP (International Pharmaceutical Federation). 1992. *FIP guidelines for drug procurement.* Amsterdam: FIP.

Hessou, C. P., and M. P. Fargier. 1994. Benin central purchasing office for essential drugs: A new experiment. *Essential Drugs Monitor* 18:8–9.

HID (Health Information Designs). 1988. *USAID handbook and field operations manual for pharmaceutical procurement in Latin America and the Caribbean.* Arlington, Va.: HID.

IDA (International Dispensary Association). 1994. *General purchase conditions of the International Dispensary Association— Non-profit procurement of medicines and medical supplies.* Amsterdam: IDA.

International Chamber of Commerce. 1990. *International rules for the interpretation of trade terms.* Paris: International Chamber of Commerce Publishing S.A., Cours Albert 1er, F-75008 (English-French).

McPake, B., and E. Ngalande-Bande. 1994. Contracting out health services in developing countries. *Health Policy and Planning* 9:25–30.

★ MSH (Management Sciences for Health). 1990. *Eastern Caribbean Drug Service procurement manual.* Boston: MSH.

MSH (Management Sciences for Health). 1992a. Procurement strategies (trainer's and participant's guides). In *Managing drug supply training series.* Part 1. *Policy issues in managing drug supply.* Boston: MSH.

MSH (Management Sciences for Health). 1992b. Supplier selection (trainer's and participant's guides). In *Managing drug supply training series.* Part 3. *Supply management.* Boston.

MSH (Management Sciences for Health). 1992c. Tendering and contracting (trainer's and participant's guides). In *Managing drug supply training series.* Part 3. *Supply management.* Boston: MSH.

★ MSH (Management Sciences for Health). 1995. *International drug price indicator guide.* (Updated annually.) Boston: MSH.

★ NEDP/MSH (Nigeria Essential Drugs Project and Management Sciences for Health). 1992. *Drug procurement procedures and documents manual.* Boston: MSH.

UNIDO (United Nations Industrial Development Organization). 1987. *A study to assist in improving management skills for procurement of pharmaceutical chemicals, their intermediates, and drugs (pharmaceutical formulations).* Vienna: UNIDO.

Westring, G. 1985. *International procurement: A training manual.* Geneva: International Trade Centre.

WHO (World Health Organization). 1995. *Use of the WHO certification scheme on the quality of pharmaceutical products moving in international commerce.* Geneva: WHO.

★ World Bank. 1993a. *Procurement technical note no. 4.3.2: Procurement of pharmaceuticals and vaccines.* Washington, D.C.: World Bank.

★ World Bank. 1993b. *Standard bidding documents for procurement of pharmaceuticals and vaccines.* Washington, D.C.: World Bank.

Annex 16.1   Criteria for Evaluating New Suppliers

Status
- ▶ Is the supplier a primary manufacturer or a distributor?
- ▶ If a manufacturer, does the supplier manufacture all products in-house?
- ▶ If the supplier does not manufacture all products in-house, who is the primary manufacturer for each product offered? Is it a known, high-quality manufacturer?

Quality Control
- ▶ Does the supplier use good manufacturing practices (GMPs)?
- ▶ Does the supplier have an on-site quality control laboratory or arrangements with an immediately accessible laboratory?
- ▶ What tests—chemical, biological, stability, accelerated stability, or others—are routinely performed during and after the manufacturing process?
- ▶ Are special tests performed for stability in tropical environments?

Inspection
- ▶ What official government agencies or reputable international organizations have inspected the manufacturing facilities?
- ▶ What are the results of the most recent inspections?
- ▶ What certification documents are available from the regulatory agency concerning the supplier's status and compliance with GMPs?

Personnel and Facilities
- ▶ What are the qualifications of key production and quality control personnel?

- ▶ What is the capacity of the supplier's plant(s)?
- ▶ Will the supplier have to subcontract portions of large awards?

Trade References
- ▶ What other local or foreign public procurement offices and hospitals buy from the supplier?
- ▶ How long has the supplier served the above groups?
- ▶ What is the experience of these customers with regard to the supplier's quality and service?

Financial Status
- ▶ Is the supplier financially stable?
- ▶ Will the supplier remain in existence for the entire contract period?

Corporate Associations
- ▶ Is the supplier a subsidiary, a parent company, or in some other way formally associated with any known supplier? If so, what is the reliability of the known supplier?
- ▶ Is the supplier producing certain products under a supervised licensing agreement with a known supplier?

Local Reputation
- ▶ How is the supplier regarded by knowledgeable physicians and pharmacists?
- ▶ Is any information available from public sources (such as newspapers or trade journals) concerning the supplier's performance locally or in other countries?

Annex 16.2 Criteria for Evaluating Current or Past Suppliers

Service

Participation Record
- Has the supplier attempted to alter or withdraw bids after submitting them?
- Has the supplier accepted an award of a bid and subsequently failed to deliver the product?

Response to Inquiries
- Has the supplier adequately responded to all inquiries from the purchaser within a reasonable period of time?
- Did the supplier provide regular information regarding the status of outstanding orders?

Delivery Time
- What was the supplier's average promised lead time? What was the actual lead time for the last procurement cycle?
- What percentage of shipments were late? How many days (weeks, months) late?
- What additional costs were incurred due to late shipments?

Adherence to Delivery Instructions
- Did shipments arrive under the proper shipping conditions (for example, cold storage for vaccines)?
- Did shipments arrive at the correct port?
- Did the supplier send full shipments as requested, or were there partial shipments? How many partial shipments on average?

Provision of Documents
- Did the supplier provide advance copies of documents according to contract terms?
- Did shipments arrive with all required documents correctly and completely filled out and signed?
- If required documents were omitted, how did the supplier correct the problem?

Packing and Labeling
- Did the supplier always ship the correct dosage form? Correct package size? Correct quantity in each package? Were short shipments frequent?
- Was labeling complete and adequate for proper use? Was it in the correct language?

Product Shelf Life
- Did all products shipped comply with contractual terms for remaining shelf life? If not, how many products were shipped with a shelf life less than that called for in the contract?
- Did the supplier promptly replace any items shipped that did not have an acceptable remaining shelf life or allow the return for credit or exchange of products nearing their expiration date (one standard is within three months of expiration date)?
- Did the supplier analyze samples of products approaching their expiration date to determine whether longer shelf lives can be applied to the products? Was there a charge?

Compliance with Contract Financial Terms
- Did all invoices comply with contract pricing terms? Were any problems promptly rectified?
- Were all shipments correctly insured and shipped according to financial terms in the contract?
- Were there any problems obtaining compensation or reimbursement for lost or damaged goods?

Information Available from Supplier
- Did the supplier make suggestions concerning ways in which the purchaser could reduce costs (for example, by combining or splitting orders or altering delivery schedules)?
- Did the supplier provide a printout of purchases and payments for use in reconciling accounts? Did the supplier provide information on purchases broken down by products and/or therapeutic categories?

Quality

Pharmaceutical Product
- Have complaints been received concerning product quality for this supplier? If so, what were the results of follow-up?
- Have products supplied conformed to specified pharmacopeial standards with regard to identity, purity, potency, physical appearance, dissolution, and other attributes? Have any products failed quality assurance testing conducted by the purchaser?
- Did the supplier provide requested batch analyses with each shipment?
- Did the supplier cooperate in making samples available and paying for quality control tests performed by independent quality assurance agencies? Were there documented product problems that the supplier refused to acknowledge and rectify?
- Did the products last throughout the period of their stated shelf life? Was any discoloration or disintegration reported?

Packaging Materials
- Were there specific examples of loss due to breakage or damage to packaging during shipments? If so, what was the extent or value?
- Did packaging meet standards appropriate to the climate of the purchasing country?
- Was external packaging sufficiently rugged to ensure arrival in the country in good condition?
- Did the external packaging protect the product from damage during transport within the country? For example, were vials sufficiently padded to withstand long trips on extremely rough roads?
- Was the immediate container able to withstand rough in-country transportation, heat, and humidity? For example, did pressure-sealed lids on tins shake loose on rocky roads?

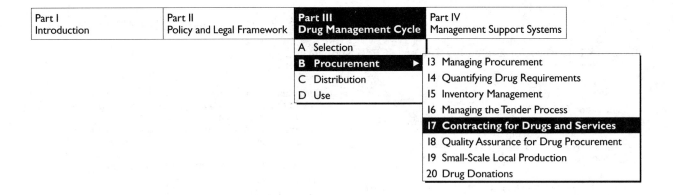

Part I Introduction	Part II Policy and Legal Framework	**Part III** **Drug Management Cycle**	Part IV Management Support Systems
		A Selection	
		B Procurement ▶	13 Managing Procurement
		C Distribution	14 Quantifying Drug Requirements
		D Use	15 Inventory Management
			16 Managing the Tender Process
			17 Contracting for Drugs and Services
			18 Quality Assurance for Drug Procurement
			19 Small-Scale Local Production
			20 Drug Donations

Chapter 17
Contracting for Drugs and Services

≡ Summary

A contract for goods or services is a legally binding document between a purchaser and a provider for a specified period of time. In the public sector, the purchaser is usually the government; the provider may be a private-sector company. Drug procurement agreements are by far the most common form of contract in essential drugs programs.

Some health systems contract out drug storage and transport services. Contracting out other services, such as port clearing, is also possible. Contracting out services can, in some cases, reduce program operating costs. The decision whether to contract out or to provide services in-house must be based on a careful analysis of costs, performance, and the capacity of the private sector to provide the goods and services in question. Contracting out is most likely to succeed when real competition takes place, the government is equipped to supervise the contract, and there are sufficient funds to pay the contractor.

This chapter considers

drug procurement contracts: *Careful specification and close enforcement of contract terms are mandatory for efficient procurement.*

warehousing and/or distribution service contracts: *Such arrangements reduce or eliminate the need to maintain government storage and transport infrastructure. In a* supply agency contract, *an autonomous private or parastatal agency operates warehousing and transport services on the government's behalf. In a* direct delivery contract, *the supplier delivers to regional or district stores and hospitals. Under a* prime vendor contract, *health facilities order from a contracted distributor and pay the manufacturer's contract price for the drugs plus a distribution fee.*

the service contracting process: *The process of contracting for services has four stages: (1) identify a service that could be provided by contract and establish the feasibility of contracting out; (2) prepare detailed tender specifications and contract terms; (3) short-list suitably qualified contractors, invite formal tenders, and appoint a contractor; and (4) monitor the contractor's and the government's performance.*

≡ 17.1 Overview of Contracts

A health system is responsible for ensuring a continuous supply of high-quality goods and services to its patients at an affordable cost. This does not mean, however, that the organization needs to manufacture the supplies or provide all the services itself. In most health systems, drugs and medical equipment are routinely supplied by private companies. Increasingly, the storage and distribution of these goods are also being contracted out. This chapter discusses

- ► contracts for drug procurement;
- ► contracts for the direct delivery of drugs by suppliers;
- ► contracts for nonsupply services such as transport;
- ► assessment and monitoring of the quality and cost effectiveness of contracts.

Contracting for services is also discussed in Chapters 22 (port clearing), 24 (warehouse construction), and 26 (transport and vehicle maintenance).

The essential first step in contract management is to decide whether an outside contract is needed. This decision has to be made by the authority whose budget will cover the cost of the contract. It is usually too expensive or impractical to produce supply items such as drugs and other health care goods in-house. In the case of services, however, this may not be so. The cost and performance of an in-house service as compared with a contracted service need to be assessed. This is not a one-time decision. Regular monitoring of the contracted service and annual comparison with an in-house alternative are necessary to establish whether contracting out remains the most cost-effective option.

A *contract* for the provision of goods or services is a legally binding document between a *purchaser* (or buyer) and a *provider* (or seller) for a specified period of time. In this context, the purchaser is generally the government or a public or private health care system, and the provider is a private-sector company or a parastatal. The responsibilities and interests of the purchaser and provider are defined by the contract terms and conditions.

The contracting process usually starts with the preparation of a *tender document*, which specifies the *technical requirements* of the goods or services required and the *terms and conditions* of the contract. Tenders are then formally invited and adjudicated. The service agreement becomes binding once a tender is accepted, a letter of acceptance is issued, and the contract is signed by both parties. If either party subsequently fails to comply with the contract, penalties are imposed. It is essential that the technical requirements and the contract terms and conditions be clear and comprehensive; if they are not, disputes may arise and the contractor may not perform as intended. Changes to a contract should be authorized only when

Figure 17.1 Contract Terms Must Be Fully Specified

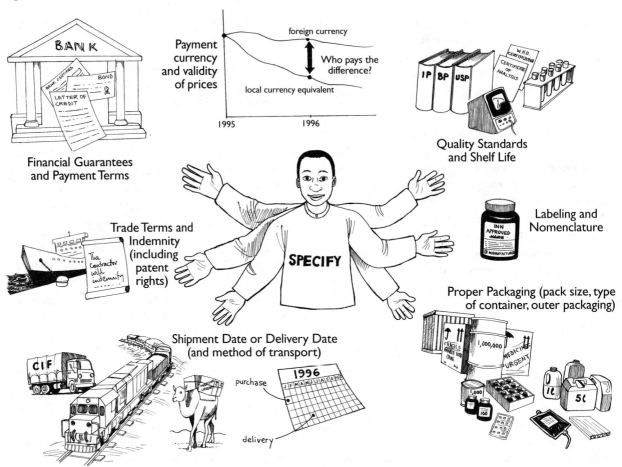

technical evidence supports the change or when the change is not significant.

Old service contracts should be reviewed to ensure that their terms and conditions are effective and that they comply with current legislation. Contracting out is not cost effective if the quality of the contracted service cannot be monitored and enforced. The assessment guide provides a checklist to guide the review process.

≡ 17.2 Critical Contract Terms in Drug Procurement

The discussion of tender management procedures in Chapter 16 introduced issues related to supply contracts. Tender specifications include many of the conditions of contract performance. Normally, by submitting a bid, the prospective seller agrees to the proposed contract terms (unless the seller stipulates otherwise in writing on the tender submission).

Although the tender documents specify the supplies and services expected, there should be a discrete written contract between the purchaser and the seller. The most critical

contract terms are discussed below (see also Figure 17.1).

Preparing an effective drug procurement contract is a specialized function requiring a great deal of care. Critical details include the specification of the drug, the quality standards required, the type of packing, the price and payment terms, and the last date of shipment. Failure by the supplier to comply with these requirements can cause substantial loss or extra expense to the buyer. From the supplier's perspective, if the procurement office places a verbal order and subsequently refuses to confirm it or fails to pay for an order as agreed, the supplier will suffer loss or added expense.

Trade Terms

Trade terms are used in drug supply contracts to define the division of costs and responsibilities during the shipment of commodities between the supplier and the buyer's stores. Trade terms were standardized by the International Chamber of Commerce in 1953 when it first published *Incoterms* (Downs 1992); these standards are reviewed and revised approximately every five years

Figure 17.2 Comparison of Common Trade Terms in the 1990 *Incoterms*

Category	Code	Code Meaning	Explanation
E / Departure	EXW	Ex works. Need to state a named place.	Seller pays for expenses at factory or warehouse. Buyer assumes all onward expenses.
F / Main carriage is unpaid	FCA (any cargo mode)	Free carrier. Need to state a named place.	Seller pays packing and delivery at the named point into the custody of the carrier and cleared for export.
	FAS (ocean freight only)	Free alongside ship. Need to state the loading port.	As above, with the exception that buyer pays for loading.
	FOB (ocean freight only)	Free on board. Need to state the loading port.	The same as FCA, but now for ocean freight use only.
C / Main carriage is paid	CFR (ocean freight only)	Cost and freight. Need to state the destination port.	Seller pays all expenses up to arrival at named port of destination, and buyer pays marine insurance.
	CIF (ocean freight only)	Cost, insurance, and freight. Need to state the destination port.	Seller pays all expenses up to arrival at named port of destination, including marine insurance.
	CPT (any cargo mode)	Carriage paid to. Need to state the destination port.	Seller pays freight and charges to named destination port. Buyer pays expenses from this port onward, including foreign customs clearance.
	CIP (any cargo mode)	Carriage and insurance paid. Need to state the destination port.	Like CPT, but the seller also has to procure and pay cargo insurance.
D / Arrival	DAF	Delivered at frontier. Need to state place.	Contract must define whether it is the seller's or the buyer's frontier. If it is the former, the buyer pays customs costs.
	DES (ocean freight only)	Delivered ex ship. Need to state port.	
	DEQ (ocean freight only)	Delivered ex quay. Need to state port.	
	DDU	Delivered duty unpaid. Need to state place.	Seller pays all charges up to delivery at place of destination, excluding duty and taxes. Buyer carries out customs formalities.[a]
	DDP	Delivered duty paid. Need to state place.	Like DDU, but seller also pays import duty. Buyer pays value-added tax (VAT).

Source: Adapted from Downs 1992.
[a] For DDU and DDP, seller and buyer must agree in the contract whose liability it is for rent or warehousing at the destination.

(International Chamber of Commerce 1990). Over the years, more precise definitions and new terms have been created to establish the exact point where the seller's costs and responsibilities end and the buyer's begin. However, old terms are still in common use, so it is important that both parties understand and agree on the contract terms. Figure 17.2. summarizes the trade terms most commonly used for government supply programs. It is advisable for procurement agencies to have a copy of the latest version of *Incoterms*.

The buyer usually specifies the applicable trade terms in the contract or tender document. The buyer must therefore understand the implications and the relative risks assumed by the buyer and the seller in case of loss or dam-

age with various trade terms. Of the terms listed in Figure 17.2, CIF (cost, insurance, and freight) and CIP (carriage and insurance paid) are generally preferable for drug supply tenders. These terms make it easier to compare tender offers fairly and to budget for the true cost of products on the tender list. In cost recovery programs, these terms also make it easier to determine the full replacement cost for each product. When using CIF or CIP terms, it is essential to specify precisely the final destination to which the cost of transport will be paid by the seller.

In many countries, transportation routes are limited, and economical delivery of goods from overseas requires a detailed knowledge of these routes. If the chosen supplier is unfamiliar with local trade routes but the procurement

Figure 17.3 Bid Comparison According to Currency Conversion Rate

Supplier	Tender Currency	Value of Bid in US$			
		On Date of Bid Submission	On Date of Bid Opening	On Date of Award	On Date of Payment
A	Deutsche mark	6.43	7.07	7.07	7.07
B	Yen	6.86	6.86	7.20	7.20
C	US dollar	7.14	7.14	7.14	7.14
D	Italian lira	7.57	7.57	7.19	6.84

Note: On the date of bid submission, supplier A offered the lowest price (US$6.43), but this was irrelevant, since supplier B had the most favorable price when the bids were opened (US$6.86). However, according to the IBRD guidelines, supplier A would ultimately be awarded the contract, since its bid was the lowest on the date of the award. Changes in parity subsequent to the bid award resulted in supplier D having the lowest bid at the time of payment. However, it would be purely speculative to attempt to anticipate changes in parity, which should be avoided in public procurement. Problems can be reduced by specifying or limiting the currencies that suppliers can use when bidding.

office is experienced, then FAS (free alongside ship) or FOB (free on board) terms may be preferable, with the buyer making separate arrangements for shipping and insurance. According to FAS terms, the seller pays for packing and delivery to the place of loading. The buyer pays loading costs plus export customs and documentation charges. Under FOB terms, the latter are paid by the seller.

In general, sea freight cost is about 10 percent and insurance about 1 percent of the FOB cost. Some buyers require that bidders give both CIP and FOB prices in order to determine whether shipping and insurance could be managed at a lower cost by the buyer. The eventual contract may also require that the FOB portion remain unchanged but that the CIP price be adjusted for actual freight and insurance costs. By this means, the buyer can collect data on actual freight charges and compare costs under the different trade terms.

Purchase Quantities

The buyer may request tenders for either fixed or estimated quantities (see Chapter 16). The contract terms should specify if estimated quantities represent a guaranteed minimum purchase or if there is no guarantee of quantities in the contract. The latter arrangement is standard practice in pharmaceutical group purchasing contracts in developed countries.

Exchange Rates and Price Comparisons

The International Bank for Reconstruction and Development (IBRD) guidelines suggest that price comparisons be based on the official rates of exchange prevailing on the day bids are opened, with the stipulation that if these rates subsequently change, the rates applying at the time of the award of contract should be used. Figure 17.3 illustrates how this rule would be applied to compare bids from four hypothetical suppliers (Westring 1985). Whether or not the IBRD guidelines are used, the method for bid comparisons should be stated in the contract terms.

The currency chosen for the comparison of bids can be a major influence on the award process. When bid evaluation is done in a currency with a high inflation rate, price differences at the time of bid opening and at the date of award can be substantial. In such circumstances, it is advisable to do the bid comparison in US dollars or another commonly accepted currency in international pharmaceutical trade, such as Swiss francs, German marks, Japanese yen, or British pounds.

Payment Currency

The contract must specify the payment currency. Generally, this is either a currency widely used in international trade (see above) or the supplier's or buyer's own currency. In the latter case, there is a speculative risk for the supplier if the local currency is not freely convertible or if the conversion rate fluctuates significantly. Many international suppliers either do not accept payment in local currency or include a "contingency factor" that increases prices.

When procurement offices can pay only in local currency, the need for a contingency factor may be avoided if the buyer is able to guarantee that payments will be converted into the supplier's currency at the exchange rate prevailing when the contract was awarded.

Validity of Contract Prices

The validity period is the period of time after contract signing during which contract prices apply. The length of this period depends on the type of tender and contract. If the tender specifies a specific quantity to be shipped at a certain time, the bid prices are normally valid until the final shipment has been received by the buyer and payment has been made. If the tender is based on estimated quantities with periodic orders, bid prices should be valid for a longer term. The standard in industrialized countries is one year, although shorter and longer terms are sometimes required. As discussed in Chapter 16, in highly inflationary environments, it may be necessary to tender more frequently or include a price escalation clause in the contract that adjusts prices for inflation at specific intervals (for example, quarterly). Such adjustments should be clearly specified; it may be useful to tie the adjustment to the actual rate of inflation as reported by the national central bank or other authoritative source.

Payment Terms

The contract must specify payment terms. Unless timely and secure payment is guaranteed, it is difficult to obtain the best prices. Many public-sector systems are either periodically short of funds or have a slow payment process. Suppliers generally require such supply systems to pay by irrevocable letter of credit, handed over before any shipments are made.

Letter of Credit. A letter of credit is an interbank document stating that a certain sum of money is available for the seller to claim from its bank as soon as it ships a consignment and presents the required documents (described in Chapter 22). A letter of credit generally involves a surcharge of 1 to 2.5 percent for the buyer. However, because it reduces the supplier's credit risk, this should facilitate a better contract price offer. Contract agreements often allow for some price fluctuations due to, for example, changes in freight and insurance costs. Accordingly, there may have to be a supplementary payment or refund at the time of delivery.

Deferred Payment (Commercial Terms). The buyer and the seller may contract for payment at the time of delivery (without a letter of credit), or payment may be deferred for a period of 30, 60, 90, 120, or 180 days. Both options are forms of credit buying, and the procurement agency must be careful not to contract for more supplies than it can ultimately afford. If a country defaults on deferred payment terms, it may subsequently be forced to pay solely by letter of credit.

Deferred payment allows the buyer to retain use of funds for a longer period. In addition, it enables the buyer to withhold payment if the supplier provides substandard or incomplete deliveries.

When tenders are being evaluated, the cost of payment options should be carefully compared. Suppose two suppliers quote the same price. Supplier A requires a letter of credit to be handed over when goods are cleared from the port. Supplier B allows a credit period of 120 days from receipt of goods until payment. If the annual interest rate in the buyer's country is 12 percent, then this credit period represents a 4 percent savings compared with supplier A's terms.

Quality Standards

The contract terms should state that all pharmaceutical products are to be manufactured in conformity with recognized pharmacopeial standards. The most commonly used standards in drug procurement are the latest editions of the *British Pharmacopoeia* (BP) or the *United States Pharmacopeia* (USP), but others, such as the *European Pharmacopoeia* (EA) or the *International Pharmacopoeia* (IP), may be appropriate in some circumstances. The major pharmacopeias include specifications for most pharmaceutical products, for both raw materials and finished products in their final dosage form, organized by generic (international nonproprietary name, INN), not by brand name.

As discussed in Chapter 16, the pharmacopeial standards should be specified in both the tender invitation and the contract. Suppliers should be required to state the pharmacopeial standard applicable to each product offered. The contract should specify that batch certificates and the World Health Organization (WHO) certificate of a pharmaceutical product must be supplied for each product (see Chapter 18).

Labeling and Nomenclature

Many otherwise identical drugs are marketed under several different brand names by multinational pharmaceutical corporations and by local enterprises (see Chapter 10). To avoid confusion in the selection, procurement, distribution, and use of drugs, it is strongly recommended that the contract terms require standard labeling for all products. General guidelines for labeling are as follows:

1. The language for labeling should be clearly specified in the contract.
2. All package labels should contain at least the following information:
   - generic name of the active ingredients;
   - dosage form (tablet, ampoule, vial);
   - quantity of active ingredient(s) in the dosage form;
   - number of units per package;
   - batch number;
   - date of manufacture;
   - expiry date (in clear language, not in code);
   - pharmacopeial standard;
   - instruction for storage;

▸ name and address of manufacturer;

▸ "not to be sold without a prescription" statement, if appropriate;

▸ "keep out of the reach of children" statement.

3. The label on each ampoule or vial should contain the following information:

▸ generic name of the active ingredient(s);

▸ quantity of the active ingredient;

▸ batch number;

▸ expiry date;

▸ name of manufacturer.

The full label (as specified in number 2) should appear on the immediate container.

4. Directions for use and precautions may be given in leaflets (package inserts). However, leaflets provide supplementary information and are not an alternative to labeling.

5. For products requiring reconstitution before use (for example, powder for injection), instructions should be on the label.

In some countries, unique identifiers are used to reduce theft and also to promote the essential drugs concept (see Chapter 39). However, such measures increase the cost of drugs.

Packaging

Proper packaging should be clearly specified in the tender documents and in the supply contract. General packaging guidelines are as follows:

1. If pack size is important, it should be clearly specified (for example, tablets and capsules packaged in amounts of 1,000; ampoules and vials packaged in amounts of 100).

2. Tablets and capsules should be packed in sealed, waterproof containers with replaceable lids that protect the contents against light and humidity. If individual packaging for tablets or capsules is required, this must be stipulated.

3. Liquids should be packed in unbreakable, leakproof bottles or containers.

4. Ampoules should preferably be one-ended and auto-breakable. Alternatively, packages should include an adequate supply of ampoule files to facilitate breaking. Light-sensitive products, such as ergometrine, should be packed in brown glass ampoules. Individual ampoules should be packed in plastic or in carton trays (five to ten ampoules per tray) with the trays packed (for example, in amounts of 100) in outer cartons.

5. Containers for all pharmaceutical preparations should conform to the latest edition of an internationally recognized pharmacopeia (such as BP or USP).

6. Outer cartons should be of strong, export-quality material able to withstand rough handling and the prevailing climatic conditions during transport and storage.

7. If the receiving warehouse is equipped to handle pallets (see Chapter 23), the contract should require that cartons be shipped on pallets. The preferred pallet size should be specified. Additional security against theft and water damage is provided if pallets are shrink-wrapped in clear plastic.

8. Each consignment must be accompanied by a detailed packing list, stating the number of cartons and the type and quantity of drugs in each carton. An outer carton should contain products with the same expiry date; this date should be printed on the carton as well as on the immediate containers. If required, outer cartons should also be labeled with a unique identifier (see Chapter 39) and/or a commodity code (see Chapter 23).

9. Upon delivery, packaging becomes the property of the buyer.

10. It is the supplier's responsibility to replace any packages and products found to be damaged at the point of delivery.

To ensure proper packing and labeling, it is advisable to instruct suppliers, particularly those that are new or unknown, to submit samples along with their bids. By assessing and visually checking those samples, problems due to poor packaging or labeling may be avoided. Packaging specifications for drug kits are discussed in Chapter 27.

Shelf Life and Expiry Date

Pharmaceutical products have varying shelf lives. The expiry date is specified by the manufacturer at the time of manufacture and can range from six months to over five years.

Supply contracts should specify the required minimum shelf life remaining for all pharmaceutical products. Because of the length of time required for local distribution, it is advisable to include a general condition that, at the time of arrival, at least two years of shelf life should remain. For products with a shelf life of less than two years, at least 75 percent of the shelf life should remain upon arrival.

As the same generic products from different manufacturers may have different shelf lives, suppliers should specify the shelf life for every product in their bids. This enables the procurement office to consider shelf life in the bid evaluation.

Bid Bonds and Performance Bonds

In international trade, it is sometimes difficult to be certain that suppliers are reliable. To encourage suppliers to live up to their obligations, financial guarantees may be required.

Bid bonds are earnest money or security deposits in the form of cash, certified check, bank draft, state bond, or other negotiable bank document that are provided by the potential supplier at the time a bid is submitted. This security (for example, 1 percent of the value of the offer) is forfeited if the successful bidder withdraws the offer or refuses to agree to the contract requirements. Bid bonds are refunded when the award is announced and all suppliers have accepted the contract terms. World Bank pharmaceutical standard bidding documents recommend the use of substantial bid bonds and performance bonds (World Bank 1993).

Performance bonds are security deposits in the form of negotiable fiscal documents that may be required at the time a contract is awarded. Their purpose is to guarantee that the supplier fulfills the contract obligations. An amount of 2.5 percent is often used for this purpose; deposits over 5 or 10 percent are rarely required. The deposit is separate from documentation involved in the letter of credit and is returned only after goods have been received in the country and are found to meet all contractual standards and to be of acceptable quality. The World Bank specifies a performance bond set at 10 percent of the contract value, posted as a cashier's check or irreversible letter of credit within 30 days of contract award. The bond is released once the contractual requirements have been fulfilled (World Bank 1993).

Both bid and performance bonds provide protection for the buyer against supplier default, but they are not common in the general pharmaceutical market. The potential financial risk may drive away many potential bidders, including reliable international companies. When the banking system of the purchasing country is poorly integrated into the international banking system, it may be difficult to retrieve the performance bond after the contract is completed.

The risk of supplier default can be reduced by inviting tenders only from suppliers of known reliability. Some drug procurement programs require financial guarantees only from new or previously unreliable suppliers.

Performance bonds are particularly unappealing to suppliers in a tender that calls for "draw-down" by purchasing group members, with orders placed throughout a contract period. In such cases, the supplier would presumably lose access to the performance bond funds for the entire contract period; most established pharmaceutical companies would not be interested in such a contract. Despite these reservations, performance bonds may be warranted in fixed-quantity open tenders with postqualification, where many bidders and suppliers may be largely unknown entities.

Shipment Date

For fixed-quantity contracts, the contract and the letter of credit (if used) should specify the last date by which the supplier is to ship the consignment. The implication of this is that the bill of lading (the standard shipping documentation) issued by the shipping company and signed by the master of the carrying vessel must be dated on or before the last date of shipment specified in the letter of credit.

The bank that holds the letter of credit is prohibited from accepting a bill of lading dated after the last date for shipment under the contract unless the buyer has agreed to the delay and the letter of credit has been suitably extended. If orders are covered by import licenses, an extension may also be needed from the appropriate office.

In contracts based on estimated quantities with periodic orders during the contract, the contract should specify the maximum number of days between the receipt of an order by the supplier and the shipment of goods.

Patent Provisions

In countries that recognize patent laws, most new drugs are covered by patent for periods ranging from two to seventeen years (see Chapter 10). During this period, other sellers are prevented from manufacturing and marketing the patented product without the consent of the patent holder.

Each country's policy regarding patent rights is governed by legal, political, and economic considerations, both local and international. Purchasing countries must decide which patent laws, if any, will be recognized in procurement. The simplest practice for buyers is to place the responsibility for observance of patent rights in the country of origin on the supplier. Contracts can stipulate that the supplier will indemnify the buyer against all claims that may arise on account of patent rights, trademarks, proprietary designs, or royalties.

Penalties for Default

The contract should specify the remedies available to each party in case of default by the other party, and the body of law under which disputes will be resolved.

Contracts with domestic suppliers are, of course, subject to the laws of the buyer's country. Contracts with international suppliers may also be written with that provision, but it is difficult to enforce local law on an international supplier that has no local operations. Even if a judgment is obtained, it may be impossible to retrieve damages.

Contracts are sometimes written with provisions that disputes will be resolved through arbitration, but this process is also unlikely to produce a favorable solution for a buyer that is injured through the default of an international supplier.

The contract should specify that the buyer will withhold payments in process and/or cancel any outstanding transactions in the event of supplier default. This remedy is suitable only in contracts in which there is some form of delayed payment and when the deliveries and payments are divided. If there is a single shipment with payment by letter of credit up front, payment will have been made by the time problems are discovered. Box 17.1 illustrates a typical contract for drug supply.

≡ 17.3 Contracts for Nonsupply Services

For many years, private companies have used outside contractors to provide specialized services at lower cost and with higher quality than the company can achieve in-house. It is increasingly common in many countries for governments to adopt the same policy.

Contracting out or *outsourcing* in health care has most frequently been used for nonclinical services such as equipment maintenance, laundry, and catering. There are many ways in which contracts might also be used in the public-sector drug supply system. Chapter 6 discussed various ways in which contracts may be used to manage pharmaceutical warehousing and distribution services to the public sector, extending in some cases to total service provision through the private sector. Chapter 22 points out options for contracting port-clearing services, and Chapter 26 discusses contracts for private-sector transport services.

Successful contracting out can tap private-sector expertise and efficiency yet still leave the government in overall control. In some cases, there may be additional development benefits. For example, a private transport firm that is awarded the contract to deliver drugs to remote rural locations may be able to offer local agricultural cooperatives a better price to carry their produce on the return trip. Contracting out can also reduce the cost to the supply system of wastage and losses due to theft, by making the contractor responsible for losses.

The main steps in contracting out nonsupply services are to

► identify a single well-defined service;
► carry out a feasibility study;
► specify the contract terms clearly and precisely;
► use a competitive tender to select the contractor;
► pay the contractor;
► monitor the contract.

When considering service contracts, the first step is to determine whether the private sector has the capacity to provide an adequate service. If the capacity exists, the next step is to calculate the cost of providing the service in-house and to establish, by means of a survey or formal tender, what the net cost of contracting or privatizing the service would be. If the private-sector service appears to be more cost effective and is able to provide at least the same level of service, it should be seriously considered. The answers to four other key questions may determine the feasibility and desirability of contracting for services (McPake and Ngalande-Bande 1994):

1. *Will real competition take place?* Are there multiple providers in the market, or is the service monopolized by one or two companies?
2. *Will competition actually promote efficiency?* When the background of the bidders is not known or when the service is new in the market, it may be difficult to assess the bidders' ability to meet the terms of the contract at the price and quality required. If a contractor fails to perform satisfactorily, the health service is left with an interrupted service and with the problem of finding an alternative supplier.
3. *Can the health system effectively supervise the contract?* Are there defined procedures for supervising contracts? Are these procedures included in the terms of the contract? Does the health system staff have the necessary skills, and is the information system able to provide indicators to monitor the contractor's performance?
4. *Will there be sufficient funding for the contract?* Budget constraints might make it impossible to fulfill payment obligations to contractors. For example, it may not be possible to release funds regularly or on time; this would likely lead to either suspension of services by the provider or less than optimal performance.

Before contracting out any service, a feasibility study should be conducted, and these questions should be answered.

Box 17.1 Sample Drug Supply Contract

Period of Contract. One year.

Trade Terms. Prices are CIF or CPT Warehouse Port Seatown unless otherwise specified; however, the invitation to tender requires that cost, insurance, and freight charges be listed separately, along with the total CIF price. The contractor is the *sole source of supply* for the duration of the contract.

Purchase Order. This is issued if there is an uncommitted balance in the country's drug account.

Assignment. The contractor shall not bargain, sell, sublet, or dispose of the contract without previous consent of the buyer.

Prices. The contract price is the maximum price of the item packaged and delivered for the duration of this contract and payable in US dollars.

Payment. Payment will be made by irrevocable confirmed letter of credit payable after forty-two days. All shipments will be inspected by an international inspection agency, and letter of credit is payable subject to submission of a clean report of findings.

Quality. All the products on this contract must: (1) meet the requirement of manufacturing legislation in the country of origin and be approved for use in that country; (2) be of USP or BP standard; (3) contain a lot or batch number and expiry date on the label of every dispensing unit; (4) be certified in accordance with the *WHO Certification Scheme for Pharmaceuticals Moving in International Commerce* (WHO Resolution 28.65B). This certificate should be issued by the health authorities of the country of original manufacture. Certificates of analysis shall be provided within one month of request for microbiological and pharmacological tests. Tests for each batch actually shipped should be sent as well and should reach this office before final arrival of the goods. Samples must be submitted in the case of a new supplier or new tendered item, product with changed presentation or formulation, or upon request by the buyer.

Labeling. Labels should be in English. All internal and external containers should be labeled with the INN for the active ingredient and should contain at least the following additional information: quantity of active ingredient, dosage form, number of units per pack, batch number, date of manufacture, expiry date, pharmacopeial standard, instructions for storage, name and address of manufacturer, directions for use.

Specifications. Supplies should conform to the specifications indicated in the tender document. No alterations, unless confirmed in writing, are acceptable.

Cold Storage. Items requiring cool storage and transport (for example, vaccines) should be shipped by air with proper insulating packing, ensuring product remains below 8°C for at least forty-eight hours. A written pre-advice with exact shipment details should be sent at least five days before the actual arrival of the consignment.

Performance Bond. The successful tenderer may be called upon, within one week after acceptance of the tender, to deposit with the buyer an amount equal to 2.5 percent of the total value of the contract. This amount will be forfeited if the contract is not completed within the time limit and to the satisfaction of this office.

Default. Should the supplier fail to
- deliver the supplies by the specified date or to the specified port; or
- replace, within one month, any rejected supplies; or
- comply with each and every other condition of this contract;

the government may do any or all of the following:
- after notice to the supplier, nullify this contract without compensation and obtain needed supplies from other suitable sources;
- recover from the supplier any losses sustained by this office resulting from supplier's failures;
- delist the supplier from the "preferred list of suppliers."

Delivery. Shipment shall be made as specified in the invitation to tender, unless an alternative delivery date has been agreed upon in writing. For each consignment the supplier shall send a shipment advice, clearly indicating date of shipment, name of the vessel, and estimated time of arrival in Port Seatown. No purchase order shall be completed by more than two (2) partial shipments. Payments for goods requested shall be made when total order is received in the purchasing country.

Indemnity. The supplier shall indemnify this government against all claims and shall bear the costs of defending such claims that are related to patent rights, trademarks, designs, and royalties.

Packaging. Supplies must be packed in immediate and external export containers, suitable to withstand rough handling in transit and storage under tropical conditions where humidity may be between 75 and 100 percent and temperatures between 25 and 30°C. On arrival at their ultimate destination, supplies should be free from damage. Containers should be sealed in a manner that makes tampering with the pack during transit easily detectable. The supplier shall be liable for all losses, damage, or expense due to insufficient or unsuitable packing. A clear packing list should be sent for all consignments, showing the individual content and including expiry dates of each carton.

Expiry Date. Unless otherwise specified, all items should have at least two years and/or 75 percent of their shelf life remaining from the date supplies are received by this office. Expiry dates should be clearly stated on all internal and external containers.

Unique Identifiers. All immediate and external containers should bear the words *Ministry of Health* together with the *WHO essential drug logo.* Application for exemption from this requirement should be made at the time offers are submitted.

Import Documents. The supplier is responsible for providing this office with all documents necessary for taking possession of supplies and clearing them. The supplier shall be held responsible for any expenses or losses incurred by incorrect, incomplete, or late provision of documents.

≡ 17.4 Feasibility Assessment

Contracting out may be one way of solving the problems of an unsatisfactory government-run service, but this is the case only if the process can be managed properly (see Country Study 17.1). If it is not, an unsatisfactory situation may be made worse. Senior health service managers are responsible for ensuring that a contracted service is feasible and cost effective, that the private sector can offer reliable tenderers that are able to provide good-quality service, and that the contract can be monitored effectively. This requires feasibility assessment, planning, implementation of the tender process, contract monitoring, and review.

Three main issues need to be considered to determine the feasibility of contracting out a service. First, the *cost* of the existing service must be compared with the cost of alternative forms of provision to determine whether contracting out is cost effective; second, the *capacity* of potential contractors to provide an acceptable quality of service must be assessed; and third, the service *performance* required must be clearly defined so that satisfactory tender documents can be prepared.

Comparative Cost

In the case of a new contract, the cost of the in-house service should be accurately assessed before tenders are invited. Figures can then be compared realistically with the cost of the tenders received (see also Chapter 21). Usually, two cost models of the in-house service are made, one including the capital cost of improving the service and the other excluding it. In addition, the potential cash benefits and out-of-pocket costs associated with privatization must be considered. On the one hand, income may be generated when buildings and equipment that are no longer needed are sold. On the other hand, severance payments may have to be made to workers whose jobs are eliminated. Another approach to this issue is to require the contractor to take over existing buildings and equipment and/or to absorb the existing workforce.

In the case of an existing contracted service whose cost effectiveness is being assessed, a suitable comparable non-contracted service in another health unit or province is needed to compare the cost of the in-house service with the price of the contract.

Standard cost-accounting methods should be used, and the cost per unit of service should be computed. Costs need to be assigned to each of the service units. This is sometimes difficult when such data are not routinely collected or compiled, or when all expenditures are categorized by line item and not by department or service. In such cases, a special study is required. After the data are

Country Study 17.1 Risks of Contracting Out Government Services

Zimbabwe. Since the mid-1950s, there has been a contract between the Ministry of Health (MOH) and a private hospital to provide hospital services to a district on a fee-for-service basis. McPake (1993) assessed the actual cost of contract services versus the price the government paid and the service cost of a similar public facility. Total recurrent costs in the public facility (for both inpatients and outpatients) were lower than in the contract service. Drug costs at the public facility were 26 percent of the drug costs from the contract services. Laboratory, X-ray, and operating room costs were more expensive per patient in the public facility, probably because the contract facility had higher productivity in this area and therefore reflected economies of scale. The fee-for-service nature of the contract and the lack of controls on the contract services provided resulted in 70 percent of MOH nonsalary recurrent expenditures for this district being used to pay this one contract. Lack of managerial capacity, poorly drafted contract terms, and no reviews of the cost effectiveness of this contract led to uncontrolled expenditures on secondary care for a small number of people.

Papua New Guinea. Using the same protocol as in the Zimbabwe study, Beracochea (1995) compared the cost effectiveness and quality of a public hospital with that of a contracted hospital managed by a nonprofit religious organization. The recurrent costs in the contracted hospital were 58 percent more than in the government hospital, but the outpatient costs per encounter were 15 percent less. The government hospital showed cheaper costs per X-ray and per operation but higher costs per lab test. Staffing levels, case mix, and economies of scale could explain these differences. When capital costs were included, the government hospital had much higher overall costs because of a recent development project that had upgraded its plant and equipment.

A second part of the study compared a government rural health center with a rural health center managed by a private company. The private health center was financed by a combination of user fees, fees for service to government, and contributions from a mining company. The government health center's cost per patient encounter was one-third the cost of the private one. Fewer staff and less equipment accounted for this difference. Poor definition of the contract terms had resulted in the private health center recruiting excessive numbers of staff and providing more types of services than envisaged in the original plan. In effect, it had grown into a district hospital without the government's consent but at its expense. It was not possible to measure revenue generated at the contracted health center through user fees or mining company contributions, and no reports were sent to the provincial authorities, who felt that they had no control over the contracted health center.

analyzed, the cost per unit of service is calculated (see Country Study 26.3 in Chapter 26).

Contracting out may be justified if potential contractors can provide good-quality service at a lower total cost. It is essential that the cost of the existing service be kept confidential; otherwise, tenderers may be tempted to underbid these costs without carrying out a proper analysis. They may then find that they are unable to provide an acceptable service at the bid price.

Private-Sector Capacity

A structured survey of private-sector capacity (see Chapter 4) can be used to assess the capacity and willingness of the private sector to provide the required service. The survey will help managers determine whether there would be competition for the contract and what options are available.

Performance Indicators to Compare Options

Performance indicators for the service need to be identified, for two reasons. First, it is essential to measure the performance of the existing service in order to establish where it succeeds and where it fails. Only by doing this can a realistic tender specification be prepared for the contracted alternative. Second, performance indicators are an essential component of contract monitoring; if the contractor cuts costs, it may be at the expense of quality. Once performance indicators for the type of service are identified, a checklist for their assessment is prepared. For example, indicators for the assessment of contracting out for the management of essential drugs warehousing and distribution might include

- total variable costs to the public sector (see Chapter 41);
- service level to lower-level warehouses and health facilities (see Chapter 15);
- availability of indicator drugs at pharmacies and health facilities;
- average lead time for receiving orders;
- average percentage of time out of stock for indicator drugs in facilities;
- number of complaints about short shipments or incorrect items shipped;
- number of complaints about damaged or poor-quality goods received.

≡ 17.5 Developing a Contract for Services

Once it has been determined that a contract is feasible, there are four major steps involved in developing a service contract:

1. Identifying qualified providers;
2. Developing and managing the tender for services;
3. Adjudicating and awarding contracts;
4. Monitoring performance.

Identifying Qualified Providers

A short list of contractors that are adequately qualified to tender for the contract should be drawn up. Depending on the size of the contract and local tendering regulations, this list may be prepared by informal inquiry, through structured interviews and inspections, or by means of a prequalification tender process. This step can be incorporated into the survey of capacity discussed above. Questions to consider include the following:

- Does the company have solid experience in providing this type of service?
- Is the company financially sound, and are its accounts satisfactory?
- Does the company have the necessary infrastructure and equipment?
- Are there sound management systems in place?
- Are there internal quality control measures?
- Does the company's management information system produce useful reports on services provided?
- Does the company have an adequate number of trained staff to handle the proposed contract?
- Can the company provide documentation of its performance according to the indicators deemed critical for the type of service?
- Are other clients satisfied with the service they receive?

Once a short list of qualified service providers has been prepared, the contract can be formally tendered.

Developing and Managing the Tender

After the decision to contract out a service has been reached, tender specifications and a service contract must be drawn up. This should clearly specify the duties of both contracting parties. The issues to be covered include

Scope of the service: This must include a detailed description of the service required and the anticipated workload. For example, in the case of a transport contract, there should be a full definition of the routes, the delivery points, the delivery schedule, and responsibility for loading and unloading. The contractor must agree to work as part of the national or provincial health system and to be supervised by the relevant authorities.

Performance standards and service quality: This section should define the performance and quality standards that have been set for the service, including matters such as service level, response rates, security measures, and maintenance standards. The duties of the contractor in maintaining and monitoring quality standards should be defined.

Contract management: This section should define the client's and contractor's responsibilities for overseeing the contract, assessing and monitoring performance, and reporting and payment procedures.

Staffing: The contract may specify how many workers should be assigned to the contract, although the contractor usually has total responsibility for the selection, discipline, and termination of staff. If extra staff or overtime are required, this will be at the contractor's expense. Contractors may try to cut costs by paying very low wages. This contributes to high staff turnover and poor service. If minimum wage legislation is in force, the contractor should be required to conform with it.

Staff qualifications: Where appropriate, staff qualifications and in-service training requirements should be specified.

Property rights over equipment: In cases in which the contractor takes over the service from the government, existing buildings, equipment, or vehicles may be used by the contractor. The contract should clearly define the ownership and disposal procedures for these assets. A detailed inventory should be attached to the contract describing the assets and their age, condition, and value at transfer. If the property is to be sold to the contractor, terms of reimbursement must be negotiated.

Payment terms: This section should define how payments are to be calculated and when they are to be made. If payments are to be linked to the exchange rate (or another index), the calculation method should be clearly defined. Generally, payment is made after a unit of service has been completed. This protects the government against the contractor's failure to perform. Payment in advance (for example, monthly or quarterly), based on estimated costs, is sometimes acceptable, however, especially when the contractor is a nonprofit organization. Three main payment mechanisms are used for nonsupply contracts:

1. *Block contracts* establish a fixed price for the entire contract. Such an approach may work for the service component of a central medical stores (CMS) management contract, where drugs and supplies are paid for separately, but not for more variable services such as transport.

2. *Percentage-of-turnover contracts* pay on the basis of a fixed percentage of turnover (for example, a percentage of the value of drugs managed or transported).

3. *Cost-per-quantity contracts* pay on the basis of some measure of the quantity of drugs handled (for example, drug transport may be charged per metric ton per kilometer or per cubic meter per kilometer).

Accounts and reports: The contract should define the reports necessary for effective management of the contract. These might include monthly accounting reports and reports of monthly deliveries.

Budget: The budget submitted by the contractor should be attached to the contract. It will help in the monitoring and auditing of the contract account and in budget planning.

Contract duration: The contract start and completion dates should be specified.

Contract review procedures: Contracts may specify a formal midcontract review, to allow problems to be overcome and procedures to be changed by mutual agreement. The health system should in any case review contract performance regularly.

Grounds for contract termination: The grounds and procedures for contract termination by either party must be clearly specified. These grounds should be fair to both parties and defensible in court in the event of a dispute.

Penalties for noncompliance with the contract: These penalties should be clearly defined. For example, the contractor could be penalized for late delivery or loss of drugs in transit. The government could be made liable for interest charges in the event of late payments.

Health system indemnity: The contract should indemnify the health system against any claims arising from delayed deliveries, injury to patients or staff of the system or the contractor, drug reactions, product defects, and similar problems caused by the contractor's negligence or inefficiency.

Insurance: The buyer's and the contractor's respective insurance obligations under the contract should be clearly defined. Items to be considered include fire and theft insurance and employer and public liability insurance.

Notices and communication: Procedures for communicating under the terms of the contract should be defined. Generally, all communication should be in writing.

Conducting the Tender

The steps for conducting a tender for services are similar to those in Chapter 16 (for drugs and supplies) and Chapter 25 (for construction). The key is to have a transparent process that is free from influence by special interests and to use written criteria to evaluate bids and select the contractor.

Monitoring the Contract

After the contract has been awarded, it must be monitored to ensure that *both* parties comply with its terms and conditions. A contract monitoring office should be set up to perform this task. The cost of running this office should be taken into account as part of the financial evaluation. The duties of the contract monitoring office include

- ► monitoring health system compliance with the contract conditions and correcting any health system performance defects that prevent the contractor from fulfilling the specified duties;
- ► monitoring the contractor's services to ensure that the standards specified in the contract are maintained and invoking penalty clauses if the contractor fails to achieve the required standards of performance;
- ► monitoring clients' satisfaction—for example, receiving stores should submit regular reports indicating whether the contractor delivers on time, listing any missing or damaged goods, and documenting other quality control and service problems (the contractor should be informed whenever problems occur);
- ► monitoring the contractor's activity reports;
- ► checking the contractor's invoices and certifying payments due under the contract;
- ► preparing an assessment of the contractor's overall performance before the contract is reviewed or renewed. ■

≡ Assessment Guide

Criteria for Assessing a Contract

► What is the purpose of this contract? Are there any documents attached that justify the decision to contract? Was an assessment made of in-house costs for the contracted service?

► What type of services or goods are being contracted? Are they nonclinical (storage, transport, food, linen, laundry, or catering services) or clinical (drugs, immunization patrols, anesthetic services)?

► Who prepared the terms of the contract?

► Does the contract comply with legislation?

► Who signed the contract? At what level was it tendered and signed (national, provincial, district, or local)?

► How were tenderers selected? How was the contract tendered? How many bids were submitted?

► How did bids compare with pre-tender estimates? How did the lowest bid compare with the assessment of in-house costs?

► Are required performance and quality standards and indicators defined? Are these sufficiently precise?

► Are payment terms clearly defined? Are they sufficiently precise?

► Is the contractor paid on time?

► What is the length of the contract period? Is it too short, too long, or indefinite?

► Is the contractor meeting contract standards? What are the penalties for performance failure? Have they been invoked? If yes, why?

► Has this contract been renewed? If yes, by whom and why?

► Has the contract been terminated? If yes, by whom and why?

► What is the cost of the contract? Are there any budget implications? What contract terms ensure accountability for the funds paid to the provider?

► Who monitors the contract? Is the provider required to submit any reports (accounting, productivity, and so forth)? Is the monitor required to prepare reports? Could any of these reports be located?

Source: Adapted from McPake 1993.

≡ **References and Further Readings**

★ = *Key readings.*

Beracochea, E. 1995. *Contracting out: The experience of Papua New Guinea.* Report submitted to the Public/Private Mix Network, Health Policy Unit, London School of Hygiene and Tropical Medicine.

Downs, D. E., ed. 1992. *Understanding the freight business,* 4th ed. Egham, England: Micor Freight UK.

International Chamber of Commerce. 1990. *International rules for the interpretation of trade terms.* Paris: International Chamber of Commerce Publishing S.A.

International directory of pharmaceutical companies. 1984. Surrey, England: PJB Publications Ltd.

McPake, B. 1993. *Contracting out in Zimbabwe: A case study of a contract between the Wankie Colliery Hospital and the Ministry of Health.* London: Health Policy Unit, London School of Hygiene and Tropical Medicine.

★ McPake, B., and E. Ngalande-Bande. 1994. Contracting out health services in developing countries. *Health Policy and Planning* 9:25–30.

Westring, G. 1985. *International procurement: A training manual.* Geneva: International Trade Centre.

★ World Bank. 1993. *Standard bidding documents for procurement of pharmaceuticals and vaccines.* Washington, D.C.: World Bank.

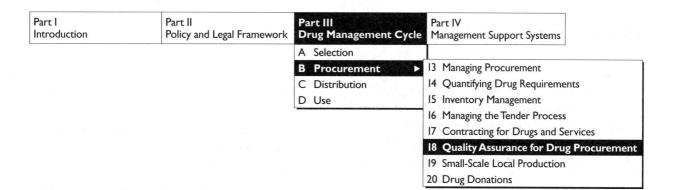

Part I	Part II	Part III	Part IV
Introduction	Policy and Legal Framework	**Drug Management Cycle**	Management Support Systems

Part III Drug Management Cycle

A   Selection
B   Procurement ▶
C   Distribution
D   Use

13   Managing Procurement
14   Quantifying Drug Requirements
15   Inventory Management
16   Managing the Tender Process
17   Contracting for Drugs and Services
18   Quality Assurance for Drug Procurement
19   Small-Scale Local Production
20   Drug Donations

Chapter 18
Quality Assurance for Drug Procurement

≡ Summary

The purpose of quality assurance in public drug supply systems is to make certain that each drug reaching a patient is safe, effective, and of standard quality. A comprehensive quality assurance program includes both technical and managerial activities, spanning the entire supply process from drug selection to patient use.

Established quality standards are published periodically in pharmacopeias. The most important characteristics of a drug product are identity, purity, potency, uniformity of dosage form, bioavailability, and stability.

Drug quality is affected by the manufacturing process, packaging, transportation and storage conditions, and other factors; these influences may be cumulative.

If a drug does not meet established quality standards, reaches its expiration date, or has been spoiled by local storage conditions, the possible consequences are

► *lack of therapeutic effect, leading to death or prolonged illness;*
► *toxic and adverse reactions;*
► *waste of limited financial resources;*
► *loss of credibility of the health care delivery system.*

A comprehensive quality assurance program must ensure that

► *drugs are selected on the basis of safety and efficacy, in a dosage form with the longest possible shelf life;*
► *suppliers with acceptable quality standards are selected;*
► *drugs received from commercial suppliers and donors meet specified quality standards at the time of delivery;*
► *packaging meets contract requirements and can withstand handling and storage conditions;*
► *repackaging activities and dispensing practices maintain quality;*
► *storage and transportation conditions are adequate;*
► *product quality concerns reported by prescribers, dispensers, and consumers are addressed and resolved;*
► *drug recall procedures are implemented to remove defective products.*

When establishing a quality assurance program, which should include training and supervision of staff members at all levels of the supply process and an effective information system, public officials must balance the costs of quality assurance procedures against the benefits of having safe, effective drugs.

≡ 18.1 Drug Quality

As in most manufacturing processes, the quality of a final drug product is determined by the raw ingredients, equipment, and technical know-how that go into producing and packaging it. Unlike a steel bolt or a tailored suit, however, a drug is a dynamic product whose color, consistency, weight, and even chemical identity can change between manufacture and ultimate consumption. A drug that passes all laboratory tests upon entry into a tropical country may be useless within a few months if the packaging, storage, and transportation conditions have been substandard.

The purpose of quality assurance in public drug supply systems is to make certain that each drug reaching a patient is safe, effective, and of standard quality. The quality of drug products is ensured by more than laboratory testing of drug samples, because a comprehensive quality assurance program includes both technical and managerial activities. Technical activities include evaluating pharmaceutical product documentation, performing or reviewing quality control laboratory tests, and monitoring product performance. Managerial activities include selecting suppliers, preparing contract terms, monitoring supplier

performance, and enforcing drug inspection procedures throughout the distribution network. It should be noted that quality assurance in drug supply is not the same as quality control in manufacturing (see Chapter 19, Section 19.2, for a discussion of the differences).

Defining and Assessing Drug Quality

There are many ways of defining and testing drug product quality. Established quality standards are published periodically in pharmacopeias, which provide detailed descriptions of drug characteristics and analytical techniques. Standards vary slightly from one pharmacopeia to another, so a particular drug product may meet the standards of one pharmacopeia and not quite meet those of another. When standards have not been established, as is sometimes the case for newly marketed drugs, analytical methods developed by the supplier are usually applied.

The major pharmaceutical manufacturing and exporting countries publish their own pharmacopeias, and on a regional basis, the European and Nordic pharmacopeias attempt to set common standards. The *International Pharmacopoeia*, published by the World Health Organization (WHO), and the US and British pharmacopeias are commonly used by public-sector pharmaceutical supply programs in developing countries.

One important limitation of the international and European pharmacopeias is that they do not provide specifications for individual dosage forms. The WHO *International Pharmacopoeia* (volume 4) has monographs for some essential drugs, and future publications are expected to have more monographs on finished dosage forms. The *European Pharmacopoeia* provides monographs for drug substances only. The analytical procedures in the *United States Pharmacopeia* (USP) tend to employ complex and expensive technology, which may be beyond the reach of many countries. The European Community, Japan, and the United States are engaged in ongoing efforts to harmonize pharmacopeial standards for drug registration. Until common standards are finally achieved, it is imperative that purchasers specify which pharmacopeial standards are acceptable.

For pharmaceutical procurement organizations, drug quality is assessed as product compliance with pharmacopeial specifications concerning its identity, purity, potency, and other characteristics. Uniformity of the dosage form, bioavailability, and stability are important characteristics that are also considered in the specifications.

Identity. The identity test should confirm the existence of the active ingredient(s) indicated on the label. This characteristic is generally the easiest to check.

Purity. Most drug products are made with ingredients added for bulk, consistency, or color that should not contain potentially harmful contaminants, significant quantities of other drugs (sometimes found when manufacturing plants are not kept clean), or microorganisms that could infect the patient.

Potency. The drug should have enough (but not too much) of the active ingredient. Harmful by-products of degradation must be absent or should be below defined limits. Most pharmacopeias specify a content range, such as 95 to 110 percent of the amount written on the label, rather than an exact amount. To ensure a long shelf life, manufacturers often produce drugs with the maximum allowable amount (for example, 110 mg rather than 95 mg). This provides a margin of safety for slight losses in potency over time.

Uniformity of Dosage Form. The consistency, color, shape, and size of tablets, capsules, creams, and liquids should not vary from one dose to the next. Any lack of uniformity may suggest problems with identity, purity, or potency. Problems with uniformity may not influence the safety or effectiveness of a drug, but they generally do influence the acceptability of a drug product to pharma-

Figure 18.1 Some Substances Exhibiting Potential Bioavailability Problems in Conventional Oral Forms

Aminophylline	Hydrochlorothiazide
Ampicillin	Iron sulfate
Carbamazepine	Isosorbide dinitrate
Chloramphenicol	Levodopa
Chloroquine	Methotrexate
Chlorpromazine	Methyldopa
Digitoxin	Nitrofurantoin
Dihydroergotamine	Phenytoin
Ergotamine	Prednisolone
Erythromycin	Prednisone
Estrogens, conjugated or	Quinidine
esterified	Rifampicin
Furosemide	Spironolactone
Glibenclamide	Theophylline
Glyceryl trinitrate	L-thyroxine
Griseofulvin	Warfarin

Source: WHO/EURO 1986.

cists, medical practitioners, and patients.

Bioavailability. Bioavailability refers to the speed and completeness with which a drug administered in a specific form (tablet, capsule, intramuscular injection, subcutaneous injection) enters the bloodstream. Generally, this depends on the other ingredients (solvents, binders, coloring agents, coatings) or the formulation (the way in which the ingredients are combined).

The comparative bioavailability of two drug products is particularly important when a product that is usually purchased from one manufacturer is replaced with a product of the same drug substance, in the same dosage form, and in the same amount, but manufactured by a different firm. Even though they contain the correct amount of active ingredient, preparations may not give the expected therapeutic result if the active ingredient is released too quickly, too slowly, or incompletely. Two drug products are said to be "bioequivalent" and may be used interchangeably if both are absorbed into the bloodstream at the same rate and to the same extent.

For a small number of drug products, studies involving human volunteers are required to establish bioequivalence. Figure 18.1 lists some drugs documented to have problems in bioavailability that require studies to determine the bioequivalence of products. Guidelines are available for the study of bioavailability, as well as specific bioavailability protocols for a small number of drugs (WHO/EURO 1986; NCM 1987; USP 1995).

If purchasing is done through established and reliable suppliers, the bioavailability of most brand-name and generic drugs used in primary health care is sufficient to ensure that the patient receives the intended effect from the drug product. It is important to decide which drugs have a potential bioavailability problem, since manufacturers

Figure 18.2 Drugs Found to Have Stability Problems under Tropical Conditions

Oral solids (tablets)	Oral liquids (syrups)
Acetylsalicylic acid	Paracetamol
Amoxicillin	
Ampicillin	**Injections/injectable**
Penicillin V	Ergometrine
Retinol	Methylergometrine

Sources: Sakolchai et al. 1989; WHO/UNICEF 1991; Hogerzeil et al. 1992, 1993.

cannot supply clinical studies for all products, and government procurement programs generally cannot perform bioequivalence testing. Where drug registration systems exist, manufacturers (suppliers) should be required to supply data on clinical studies whenever needed. Procurement agencies should also work with drug regulatory authorities (DRAs) in the country and use their information in making decisions.

Stability. A drug product must retain its properties within specified limits in order to be useful. The time that a drug's stability is under warranty is established by the manufacturer and, in some cases, by a country's DRA. This period ends with the product's expiration date. The stability of a drug product depends on the active ingredient, which can be affected by its formulation and packaging. Inadequate storage and distribution can lead to physical deterioration and chemical decomposition, reduced potency, and, occasionally, formation of toxic by-products of degradation. This is more likely to occur under tropical conditions of high ambient temperature and humidity.

WHO has published a list of drug substances that are less stable and thus require particular attention (WHO 1990). However, there are very few data on the stability of drug products under true field conditions. In recent years, several studies have examined the stability of a small number of essential drugs under tropical conditions of excessive temperature (over 40°C), high humidity, and inappropriate storage conditions (Sakolchai et al. 1989; WHO 1991b; WHO/UNICEF 1991; Hogerzeil et al. 1993). Figure 18.2 lists the drugs that have been found to have problems under tropical conditions.

Consequences of Poor Drug Quality

A poor-quality drug product is one that does not meet specifications. The use of poor-quality drug products may have undesirable clinical and economic effects, as well as affect the credibility of the health delivery system. Clinical effects can include prolonged illness or death or the inducement of toxic or adverse reactions. On the economic side, limited financial resources may be wasted on poor-quality drugs.

Lack of Therapeutic Effect May Lead to Prolonged Illness or Death. Poor drug quality can sometimes lead to serious health consequences—for example, the use of poor-quality cardiac drugs and medicines for seizures and asthma. With others, such as cold remedies and minor painkillers, a reduction of up to 50 percent in the content of the active ingredient has no serious consequences, although the best procurement policy is to require products that meet specifications.

Poor-Quality Drugs May Induce Toxic or Adverse Reactions. When some drug products expire or are exposed to adverse climatic conditions (for example, excessive heat and humidity in a tropical climate), they may undergo physical and/or chemical changes, which can result in the formation of possibly toxic by-products of degradation. Although fear of toxic drug degradation in tropical climates is prevalent, tetracycline is virtually the only common drug in which this occurs. Excessive active ingredients may also lead to toxic or adverse reactions.

A much more frequent problem is contamination with microorganisms, usually bacteria or fungi. The consequences can be quite severe, particularly in the case of injectable drugs. Contamination of creams, syrups, and other drugs in jars and tubes is especially common in tropical environments, but the consequences vary, depending on the type of organism and the drug involved. Errors in formulation and product contamination are uncommon with manufacturers who strictly comply with internationally accepted procedures and good manufacturing practices (GMPs). In practice, however, adherence to GMPs may vary from country to country or manufacturer to manufacturer. When contaminants are highly toxic or sensitizing or when toxic substances are inadvertently included in the product, the result can be catastrophic.

Poor Drug Quality Wastes Money. Ineffective care or the need to treat adverse drug reactions resulting from poor product quality leads to more costly treatments. Poor drug packaging casts doubts on product quality, leading to rejection by health personnel and patients. These products will then expire on the medical stores shelves, wasting limited financial resources.

Poor Drug Quality May Gravely Affect Program Credibility. Patients and providers may suspect the quality of drug products when therapeutic failure or adverse drug reactions occur. Changes in product appearance, such as discoloration, crumbling of tablets, hardening of oral suspensions, or changes in taste and smell, influence patients' perceptions. Patients may be discouraged from using health facilities, and worker morale may be affected, particularly if drug shortages are also common in the supply system.

Determinants of Drug Quality

The quality of a drug product coming off the production line is determined by the start-up materials, plant environment, manufacturing equipment, and technical know-how invested in developing and manufacturing the drug. The drug that ultimately reaches the patient, however, is further affected by packaging and by transportation and storage conditions.

These influences, especially factors in the manufacturing process, can be cumulative. For example, the selection of excipient substances used to give tablets bulk and consistency may not affect the color, texture, or chemical quality of a drug until the immediate container is opened in a hot, humid environment. Then, depending on the choice of ingredients, the tablet may remain firm and dry or become moist and crumble within a matter of days. Factory humidity during packaging may also have an important effect. If oral rehydration sachets are not packaged under very low humidity, moisture enters the sachet and may result in chemical changes in the mixture that make it difficult to use. Similarly, the amount of grinding, thoroughness of mixing, choice of packaging, maintenance of packaging equipment, and other factors can have an effect that may be immediately evident or may not appear until the drug reaches the point of consumption. Figure 18.3 summarizes these influences.

The dynamic nature of drug products and the cumulative effects of the production process, right through to packaging, handling, transport, and storage conditions, require quality assurance at all levels in the drug supply system.

Prevalence of Poor-Quality Drugs

Data from a WHO study (1995), summarized in Figure 18.4, indicate the extent of the drug quality problem, as detected by drug procurement programs that conduct laboratory testing of their products.

In recent years, national and international authorities have recognized the emergence of counterfeit drugs as a serious problem. These are both brand-name and generic drug products that are deliberately and fraudulently mislabeled with respect to identity and/or source. Counterfeit products may include drugs with the correct ingredients or with wrong ingredients, with an insufficient quantity of active ingredients or without active ingredients, or with fake packaging. Reports from some parts of sub-Saharan Africa suggest that counterfeit drugs may account for up to 70 percent of sales; these reports have not been documented and verified, but drug counterfeiting is an increasing problem in developing countries.

≡ 18.2 Practical Approaches to Quality Assurance

The procedures to establish a comprehensive quality assurance program can be divided into three categories:

1. Procedures to ensure that only drug products that meet current standards for quality are bought. These include
   ► careful product selection;
   ► careful supplier selection;
   ► certification of good manufacturing practices;
   ► batch certification (WHO-type certificate of a pharmaceutical product);
   ► inclusion of detailed specifications in the contract.

2. Procedures to verify that shipped goods meet the specifications. These include
   ► pre- and postshipment inspection;
   ► analytical drug testing.

3. Procedures to monitor and maintain the quality of drug products from the moment they are received until the drug is finally consumed by the patient. These involve
   ► proper storage and distribution procedures;
   ► appropriate dispensing;
   ► instructions to the patient on proper use of medications;
   ► product defect reporting programs.

Few drug management programs can effectively manage all the possible quality assurance activities for all the drug products that are procured. Consequently, realistic goals must be set to identify the combination of managerial and technical quality assurance activities that will be most effective under existing conditions. The critical elements in quality assurance for drug procurement are listed in Figure 18.5.

Setting Priorities in Quality Assurance

Since resources are limited, priorities for quality assurance activities should be targeted. The VEN (vital, essential, nonessential) method (Chapter 41) helps identify a small group of drugs that have the greatest health impact. Vital lifesaving drugs (antibiotics, cardiac medications, hormone replacement medicines, and intravenous solutions) warrant greater attention than other important but not lifesaving medications, such as those for fever and pain. ABC analysis (Chapter 41) can be used to identify those drugs that have the greatest budgetary effect if their quality is unacceptable. The choice of drugs to monitor closely is based on the following criteria:

Figure 18.3 Determinants of Drug Quality

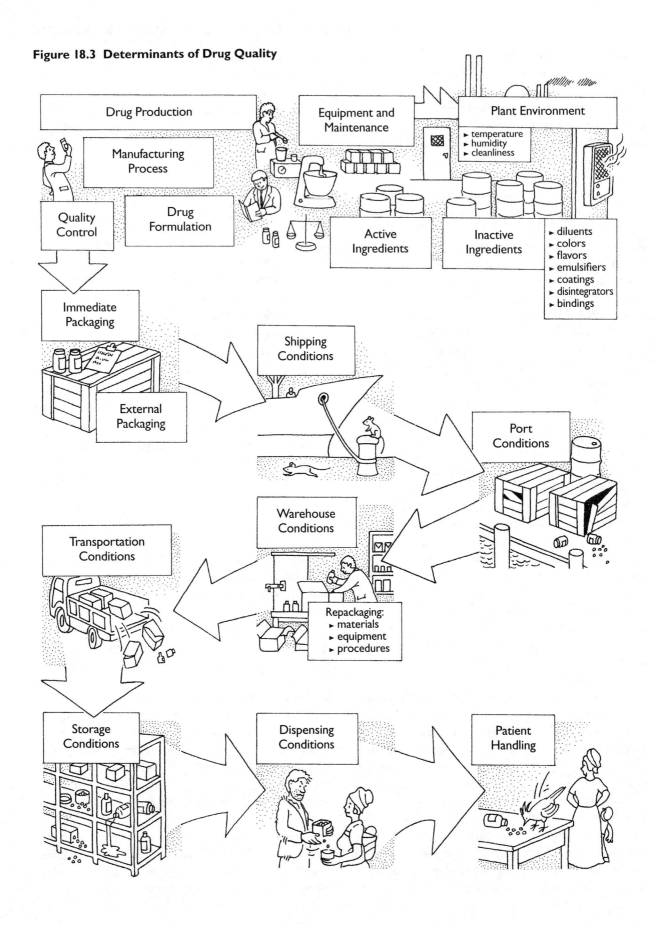

▶ Drugs with low therapeutic indices;

▶ Drugs with inherent bioavailability problems;

▶ Sustained-release preparations;

▶ Drug products from new suppliers and suppliers with problems in the past;

▶ Drugs that require stable dosage forms and appearance.

≡ 18.3 Obtaining Good-Quality Drugs

Obtaining drug products of good quality involves careful selection of suppliers and products, adherence to GMPs, reliance on appropriate pharmaceutical product and/or batch certificates, and detailed contract specifications.

Careful Product Selection

In many systems, therapeutic drug formulary committees first assess the safety and efficacy of selected drugs on the basis of evidence from clinical trials (Chapter 10). Specific product selection involves assessing the technical documentation provided by the supplier on pharmaceutical characteristics of the dosage form. Dosage forms that may offer longer shelf life include

▶ powders for reconstitution instead of injectable liquids;

▶ powders for reconstitution instead of oral suspensions;

▶ tablets instead of capsules.

Whenever appropriate, product-specific stability studies should also be requested from the manufacturer and critically reviewed. For a small number of drugs (certain heart, asthma, and seizure drugs, for example), studies that demonstrate bioequivalencey may also be necessary.

It is prudent to select products with packaging that can withstand rough transport and extreme climatic conditions, such as high heat and humidity. Plastic containers may be more appropriate than glass bottles for intravenous solutions, oral liquids, and disinfectants. Avoid metal tins that will rust. In some countries, unit dose or unit-of-use packages (blister packs) and containers with smaller quantities (for example, 100 tablets as opposed to 1,000 tablets) may be cost effective. These measures aim to avoid loss of product quality after the containers are opened, or as a result of frequent handling. The increased purchase costs should be weighed against the wastage that occurs with bulk containers, plus the costs of any repackaging.

Careful Supplier Selection

This is perhaps the most critical step in quality assurance (see Chapter 16). Suppliers can be selected competitively by restricted tender with prequalification, through open tender with postqualification, or, in some cases, through

Figure 18.4 Results of Quality Control Testing in Some Public-Sector Procurement Programs

Country	Number of Products Procured	Number of Samples Tested	Percent Passed
Ecuador	110	36	75
Fiji	400	5	Not available
Jamaica	250	51	80
Kenya	143	24	71
Malaysia	347	320	86

Source: WHO 1995.

less formal procedures. Standard procedures should include requiring certifications, gathering information on supplier reliability and product quality, inspecting product samples, and, if necessary, conducting laboratory testing of drugs with high potential for bioavailability or stability problems.

Contacts with DRAs and other purchasing groups (for example, the United Nations International Packing Centre [UNIPAC], the International Dispensary Association [IDA], the Eastern Caribbean Drug Service) and product-quality-testing laboratories can help with reference checks as well as exchanges of information on problem products. Publications by drug information services and professional organizations, such as the United States Pharmacopeia and the American Society of Health-System Pharmacists, provide information on the bioequivalence of drug products as well as on drug product recalls.

Information on suppliers' performance needs to be analyzed, and operational definitions and criteria must be developed and applied to assess the reliability of suppliers and avoid subjectivity. Lack of explicit definitions and criteria provides rejected suppliers with the opportunity to question the integrity of the procurement process.

For new suppliers, it is important to visually inspect samples of the drug product, packaging, and labeling. Some programs send samples for laboratory testing on a routine basis; others do so only when there are concerns about specific products. Although prepurchase testing may detect defective products, bear in mind that the samples are provided by the supplier, which will make every effort to ensure that the samples meet the standards. The samples may not, however, be representative of what will actually be sold or delivered.

Chapter 16 discusses the need for an information system that provides the procurement office and tender committee with feedback on suppliers' compliance with contracts. It is essential to keep a record of the condition of received goods, compliance with contract terms, and

Figure 18.5 Critical Elements in Quality Assurance for Drug Procurement

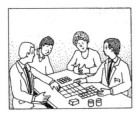

1. Product Selection (Chapter 10)
   ▸ products with longer shelf life (for example, powders for reconstitution rather than oral suspensions)
   ▸ avoidance of products with bioavailability problems, when possible

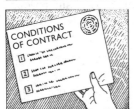

2. Supplier Selection (Chapter 16)
   ▸ supplier prequalification
   ▸ recent GMP inspection reports from national drug authorities
   ▸ formal supplier monitoring system
   ▸ limitation of purchases from new suppliers to noncritical products

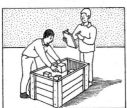

3. Product Certification
   ▸ GMP certificate from drug regulatory authority (prequalification)
   ▸ certificate of pharmaceutical products (WHO-type) for all new products, new suppliers
   ▸ batch certificate (WHO-type) for problem drugs only

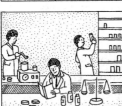

4. Contract Specifications (Chapter 17)
   ▸ acceptable pharmacopeial standards
   ▸ language, labeling requirements
   ▸ minimum shelf life
   ▸ packaging standards

5. Inspection of Shipments
   ▸ physical inspection of all shipments
   ▸ sampling for analysis of suspect products

6. Targeted Laboratory Testing
   ▸ therapeutically critical drugs
   ▸ drugs with known bioavailability problems
   ▸ new suppliers
   ▸ suppliers with quality difficulties in the past

7. Product Problem Reporting System
   ▸ system for reporting suspect or problem products

timeliness of delivery. This information, and that from the adverse drug reaction and product quality reporting system, should be considered when assessing offers and awarding supply contracts.

Product Certification

WHO has established GMPs for pharmaceutical products, similar to those enforced by the national drug control agencies in industrialized countries. They include criteria for personnel, facilities, equipment, materials, manufacturing operations, labeling, packaging, quality control, and, in most cases, stability testing.

In countries with effective drug control agencies, adherence to GMPs is enforced by a system of inspections and regulatory controls, often specific to individual drug dosage forms. A manufacturer may have acceptable standards for solid dosage forms but not for sterile injectable preparations. Recent reports of GMP inspections and drug recall histories can be obtained by writing to national drug control agencies. Often, a supplier must approve or at least expedite requests for performance reports from national drug control agencies, and failure to obtain such reports for the buyer makes past performance suspect. GMP reports can sometimes be obtained from other procurement programs or from international procurement agencies such as IDA, UNIPAC, or Crown Agents. Two additional resources, the Pharmaceutical Inspection Convention (PIC) and the Product Evaluation Report Scheme (PER), provide access to inspection information. Both of these were established by the European Free Trade Association (EFTA) in Geneva (see "Resource Organizations").

Buyers with pharmaceutical staff trained in GMP inspection may perform their own inspections of local manufacturers that are potential suppliers, if funds are available to do this.

As of December 1994, 138 national drug control agencies had agreed to participate in the WHO certification scheme on the quality of pharmaceutical products moving in international commerce. They agreed to certify that drug products are registered in the exporting country and that manufacturers' facilities have been inspected and comply with GMPs. However, a recent WHO study (1995) showed that very few importing countries actually request pharmaceutical product certificates for registration or for procurement purposes.

This certification scheme provides some assurance, based on inspection of the manufacturing facilities for GMPs by the competent authority of the exporting country. For the procurement office, it is an inexpensive means to help ensure the quality of purchased products. Through the certification scheme, the procurement office should be able to obtain the following information:

- ► Whether a product is licensed to be placed on the market in the exporting country, and if not, the reasons why;
- ► Whether the supplier manufactures the dosage forms, packages and/or labels a finished dosage form manufactured by an independent company, or is involved in none of these activities;
- ► Whether the manufacturer of the product has been inspected and the periodicity of inspection;
- ► Whether the certificate is provisional, pending technical review;
- ► Whether the information submitted by the supplier satisfies the certifying authority on all aspects of manufacture of the product undertaken by another party.

The reliability of the pharmaceutical product certificates issued under the WHO scheme and access to them depend largely on

- ► the reliability and responsiveness of the exporting country's authority;
- ► capability of the exporting country's authority to make adequate GMP inspections;
- ► capability of the importing country's authority to assess the authenticity or validity of the certificate of a pharmaceutical product submitted, especially when it is submitted through the manufacturer or importing agent.

Therefore, product certification under the WHO scheme is only as reliable as the agency performing it (see Country Study 18.1). Although national drug control agencies in the major drug-exporting countries are generally conscientious in their assessments, it may take some time to receive reports. Agencies in some countries have been found to be less reliable and responsive.

Batch Certificates

Reliable pharmaceutical manufacturers that actively attempt to comply with GMPs conduct batch analyses. Small local manufacturers that do not have their own quality control laboratories may contract quality control testing services from other manufacturers, private testing facilities, or national reference laboratories.

Some national drug control agencies provide individual batch certificates or certify the accuracy of the manufacturer's analyses. Laboratory analyses of samples from individual batches can also be obtained through international quality control organizations such as the Société Générale de Surveillance or the Service de Contrôle des Médicaments of the Belgian Pharmaceutical Association (see "Resource Organizations").

Some drug procurement offices request other certificates, such as the certificate of free sale, the certificate of origin, or the certificate of licensing status (see Figure 18.6). These certificates do not provide important information regarding compliance with GMPs, or results of laboratory testing of samples from individual batches. For this reason, the WHO-type certificate of a pharmaceutical product and batch certificate are preferred.

Drug Regulatory Authorities and the Procurement Market Today

In many countries, DRAs and procurement offices do not work together effectively, nor are integrated information systems in place. Ideally, when a DRA exists and drug registration is operational, procurement by government agencies should be limited to drugs registered by the DRA. Procurement offices should both seek information from the DRA and strive for closer cooperation with the authority. To facilitate registration of generic drugs, the evaluation and approval process should not be complicated. Clinical trial data are not normally required, resulting in the submission of an abbreviated application by the manufacturer or distributor. WHO recommends that all drugs on the public or private market in a country, whether they are imported or locally manufactured, be subject to the same standard of control, including drug registration.

The standard of control varies from country to country. In some exporting countries, drugs are registered and freely sold but not rigorously evaluated for efficacy. In other countries, which do evaluate efficacy, certain drugs may have been registered before evidence of efficacy was legally required. Moreover, in some countries, manufacturers may produce exclusively for export; the exporting country DRA may not closely scrutinize these manufacturing plants. Procurement offices still need to request certificates from the DRAs of the exporting country, as recommended by WHO.

Contract Specifications

Detailed specifications to help ensure that high-quality products are bought and received include

- ► name of the pharmacopeia reference standard to assess drug quality;
- ► language for the product label;

Country Study 18.1 Use of WHO Certification Scheme for Public-Sector Drug Procurement

An assessment of the use and effectiveness of the WHO certification scheme in drug procurement and registration systems was undertaken in 1993–94 (WHO 1995). (The fifteen importing countries participating in the assessment are shown in the table.) The assessment revealed that of these fifteen countries, only two (13 percent) were using the certification scheme as recommended by WHO by requesting a certificate of a pharmaceutical product during drug registration. Four (27 percent) were requesting the certificate in public-sector procurement. The others requested free sale certificates, GMP certificates, and certificates of analysis.

It was also found that most exporting countries have not standardized the text of their certificates and therefore do not issue a certificate of a pharmaceutical product as recommended by WHO. Reasons identified for the scheme not being used as recommended were

► poor understanding of the scheme among importing countries, and its difference from other certificates such as free sale and GMP certificates issued by exporting countries;

► lack of commitment by both importing and exporting countries, due in part to the voluntary and nonbinding nature of the scheme.

| | — WHO-Type Certificates — | | | | | |
Country	Product Certificate	Batch Certificate	Free Sale Certificate	GMP Certificate	Certificate of Analysis	Certificate of Origin
Benin					■	
Cameroon	■					
Central African Republic						
Ecuador			■			
Fiji	■	■				
Jamaica			■			
Kenya						■
Malawi					■	
Malaysia	■	■		■		
Myanmar	■					
Papua New Guinea	■					
Sri Lanka		■	■	■		
Tanzania	■	■	■	■		
Tunisia		■	■			■
Yemen		■	■	■		

Source: WHO 1995.

► minimum information required on the label (generic name, dosage form, strength, quantity, expiration date, manufacturer, batch number);

► additional information, such as the product registration number and date of manufacture;

► standards for packaging that will withstand the specific storage and transport conditions (for example, corrugated boxes with specifications for maximum size and maximum weight).

To reduce theft and resale, some programs may also require labeling and logos to indicate that the product is solely for distribution within a particular health care program (for example, Ministry of Health, Social Security Fund). Contract specifications are discussed in detail in Chapter 17.

≡ 18.4 Verifying the Quality of Shipped Products

The quality of products received needs to be verified as soon as possible after arrival, both by physical inspection of each shipment and by laboratory testing of selected products.

Inspection of Shipments

Regardless of other quality assurance procedures in use, each drug shipment should be physically inspected (see Figure 23.2). This means verifying adherence to contract specifications and order completeness, and also inspecting samples of all items to spot any gross abnormalities. Training competent receiving staff can be an economical means of ensuring drug quality as well as reducing losses due to supplier negligence or fraud.

Figure 18.6 Comparison of Certificates Used in Pharmaceutical Procurement

Type of Certificate	Uses	Limitations
WHO-type certificates		
Certificate of pharmaceutical product (WHO 1992 type)		
▸ Issued by DRA in exporting country	▸ Essential for product licensure	▸ Is only as reliable as issuing DRA
▸ Provides licensure status of product	▸ Ideally required for all new products	▸ Does not provide batch-specific information
▸ Provides inspection status of manufacturer	▸ Prequalification of suppliers	
	▸ Screening of new suppliers	
Statement of licensing status (WHO 1992 type)		
▸ Issued by DRA in exporting country	▸ Prequalification of suppliers	▸ Does not provide batch-specific information
▸ States that product is licensed	▸ Screening of new suppliers	
Batch certificate (WHO type)		
▸ Issued by manufacturer *or* DRA in exporting country	▸ Usually requested for antibiotics	▸ Issued by few DRAs
▸ Confirms that individual batches conform to specifications	▸ May be required for problem drugs	▸ Easily falsified
▸ Linked to certificate of pharmaceutical product		▸ May require additional expense
Non-WHO-type certificates		
Free sale certificate		
▸ Issued by DRA in exporting country	▸ Commonly used for licensure	▸ No indication that product has been evaluated for safety and efficacy
▸ Confirms product is sold in the country of origin		▸ No indication that product is registered for use in country of origin
GMP certificate		
▸ Issued by DRA in exporting country	▸ Prequalification of suppliers	▸ Only as reliable as issuing DRA
Analytic batch certificate		
▸ Issued by manufacturer	▸ Postqualification of suppliers	▸ Manufacturers' certificates may be falsified
▸ Contains results of analytical tests		▸ Does not necessarily conform to specifications approved at time of product licensure
▸ Not linked to certificate of pharmaceutical product		

Inspection in the exporting country before shipment can be arranged through an independent agency (for example, the Société Générale de Surveillance), for early detection of noncompliance with contract terms or defective products.

Laboratory Testing

Upon arrival, laboratory testing of batch samples may be undertaken routinely or "by exception." Most programs test random samples from only some of the batches. Testing "by exception" means that analyses are done only when a supplier or a particular drug product is suspect.

Laboratory testing is costly in terms of technical human resources, equipment, and reagents. Guidelines should target sampling to products that (1) have the greatest potential for bioavailability and stability problems, (2) are from new or questionable suppliers, and (3) have been the source of complaints. With new suppliers, a probationary period (for example, the first three shipments) is useful, during which their products are sampled with greater frequency. Suppliers whose failure rates are unacceptable are dropped from future tenders. Sampling from well-established suppliers is done much less frequently, often only for at-risk products.

Programs that require routine testing of samples for all products prior to distribution to health facilities often produce significant delays in product availability at the health facility level. The need for laboratory testing of products reported to have problems should be carefully assessed: many problems with quality are detectable on visual inspection and do not require a test. For example, verified observations of tablets that crumble before their expiry date, oral suspensions that harden, or injectable solutions that contain particles are enough to justify recalling the product without testing.

The tests that should be performed depend on the drug product and the reason for testing. Basic chemical analyses are done to verify the identity of the drug and to look for degradation, chemical contamination, or adulteration. WHO advocates a system of economical, less technically demanding, basic tests for commonly used drugs (WHO 1991a) that can be done in simple laboratories. A complete analysis of tablet and capsule forms includes tests for identity, potency, uniformity, disintegration, and dissolution.

Biological testing is more specialized and can be performed only in established facilities with staff trained to use microbiological and pharmacological methods. Microbiological tests include sterility tests for injectable drugs and eye preparations and microbiological assays of antibiotics and vitamins. Pharmacological tests include the pyrogen test, toxicity tests, hormone assays (for insulin and pituitary derivatives), and tests to determine the bioavailability of selected drug products.

Practical guidelines for establishing small and medium-sized testing facilities have been developed by WHO (1984). However, construction of a laboratory where one does not already exist should be considered with caution. It may not be cost effective for some countries to establish a sophisticated national drug control laboratory for a number of reasons, including

- low projected volume of work;
- insufficient financial resources for land purchase, facility construction, testing equipment, furniture, supplies, equipment maintenance, salaries, training, and other operating costs;
- lack of trained personnel, such as microbiologists, pharmacologists, laboratory technicians, and animal caretakers;
- lack of local capacity for maintenance and repair of equipment, difficulty in obtaining spare parts, irregular and unstable power supply.

WHO has supported regional quality assurance laboratories in Ghana, Jamaica, and Zimbabwe that have been underutilized. A recent WHO study (1993) identified the main causes of problems with the laboratories in Africa as

- lack of clear definition of roles;
- lack of prior feasibility studies;
- absence of a proper administrative framework, legal basis, and autonomy for the laboratories;
- lack of functional linkage between the laboratories and the DRAs of both host and user countries;
- deficiency in management, technical capability, human resources, training, equipment, reference materials, reference standards, guidelines, or procedures;
- inadequate financial resources and mechanisms to sustain the operation of the laboratories;
- lack of drug supply program funds to cover the cost of analysis;

- absence of information to potential users on the competence of the laboratories;
- lack of funds to support analysis and procedures for sample submission;
- problems of logistics for dispatching samples and receiving results.

In some countries, a college of pharmacy or an independent laboratory may have the required testing facilities. Also, many international quality control laboratories provide drug analyses at a relatively reasonable price. If analyses are performed by foreign laboratories, foreign exchange and billing problems may be reduced by requiring the suppliers to pay the laboratory directly, with the arrangement clearly described in the purchase contract. See Country Study 18.2 for descriptions of testing and other quality assurance procedures in several countries.

≡ 18.5 Maintaining Drug Quality
Maintaining drug product quality requires careful attention to storage and transport, as well as to dispensing practices and use.

Appropriate Storage and Transport
Procedures to help maintain drug quality begin with proper storage at the port and prompt release. Storage activities are discussed in Chapters 23, 24, and 25, and proper transport conditions are addressed in Chapter 26.

Appropriate Dispensing and Use
Inappropriate dispensing procedures contribute to drug product deterioration and contamination or medication errors. The following procedures help maintain the quality of drug products:

- Use only proper dispensing containers (for example, airtight containers, light-resistant bags or vials); the paper envelopes often used for end-user dispensing do not protect tablets and capsules.
- Require clear labeling of dispensed drugs and enforce procedures to label products with the patient's name, drug's name, strength, expiration date, and instructions for use and storage.
- Write dispensing information and instructions in the local language, avoiding the use of abbreviations, or use symbolic instructions.

The prescriber and the dispenser should counsel the patient on the proper use of medications, explaining *what* the drug is, *why* the patient needs it, *how* to take it, and *where and how* to store it until treatment is completed.

Country Study 18.2 Quality Assurance in Selected Countries

Bhutan. Drugs are procured by open tender from manufacturers in Bangladesh and India and from two international nonprofit suppliers. To reduce the number of questionable suppliers, WHO-type certificates of a pharmaceutical product are required. A performance rating system scores suppliers on three criteria: (1) delivery of the ordered quantity, (2) supply of products with minimum expiry date, and (3) delivery performance. Samples of drug products have been tested in Bangkok and Calcutta, with failure rates varying from 4 to 15 percent in different years. A manual inspection unit for IV fluids has been established at the medical supply depot. A fixed system of sampling and inspecting every batch has been established. The National Public Health Laboratory is being upgraded to test twenty commonly used drugs.

Costa Rica. In the mid-1970s, the Social Security Fund (CCSS) established a well-equipped, air-conditioned laboratory with the capability to perform chemical analyses for most drugs, biological analyses for antibiotics and vaccines, and pyrogen testing for injectables. In 1978, the laboratory was staffed and equipped to perform 400 tests per month but had been pushed to 600 per month. In the 1976–77 tender cycle, 79 of the 320 samples submitted from the bid were rejected (32.78 percent). Even after this screening, 292 of the 1,661 samples collected at the time of delivery were rejected (17.57 percent). In 1991, only 26 of 4,316 analyzed batches (2.2 percent) were rejected, possibly reflecting the effectiveness of prepurchase as well as postpurchase testing. The test results are used to qualify suppliers. In 1994, the product problem reporting program received three reports. One of the suspect products was confirmed to have suffered loss of stability.

Because of difficulties with suppliers, the CCSS instituted a requirement that quality control results be completed before payment is made. It takes one to four weeks for the laboratory to report test results. For tests of samples from a bid and samples taken from warehouse receipts, the CCSS pays for the first test performed but charges the supplier for any additional tests that are required.

Malaysia. The Government Pharmaceutical Laboratory (GPL) purchases pharmaceutical products by open tender. All imported drugs must be registered in Malaysia. A certificate of a pharmaceutical product and a GMP certificate are prerequisites for drug registration. In 1992, 100 percent of product license applicants provided a certificate of a pharmaceutical product either as a single certificate or as two separate certificates, free sale and GMP. Contact with certifying authorities is made directly. Sometimes, certificates are rejected because of noncompliance with the WHO format or content or because of a lack of signatures or designations of the certifying authority. In addition, batch analytical certificates are required for each batch of biological and blood products imported.

Since 1991, products purchased by the GPL are randomly selected for testing. In 1992, 320 samples were tested, out of which 132 samples (41 percent) failed. In addition, 132 samples of raw materials were tested in connection with tender offers. For raw materials, samples are collected at the time of bidding; for finished dosage forms, they are collected after receipt but before payment, and following complaints. Testing is done locally by the GPL quality control laboratory as well as at the National Pharmaceutical Control Bureau.

Organization of Eastern Caribbean States (OECS). The Eastern Caribbean Drug Service (ECDS) prequalifies and reviews suppliers annually for its restricted tendering process. The contract between ECDS and suppliers specifies labeling requirements, packaging, product dating, and pharmacopeial standards and requires certificates of analysis. Contracts are awarded annually after consideration of suppliers' previous performance, qualitative test results, and product-specific requirements. ECDS conducts routine quality testing on products from new suppliers, products with inherent quality problems, and suspect products reported by supplies officers. In the 1989–90 tender cycle, for 420 orders representing thousands of items, ECDS received thirty-four reports involving eighteen suspect products, which were tested at the Caribbean Regional Drug Testing Laboratory; only two failed to meet pharmacopeial standards.

Papua New Guinea. The majority of the products currently purchased by the Pharmaceutical Services Division (PSD) are from known suppliers whose products have previously been tested and with whom the PSD has had satisfactory results. For new suppliers, the PSD selectively requests a WHO-type certificate of a pharmaceutical product with the tender documents, except for well-established international manufacturers. In 1992, such certificates were obtained for only 3 percent of the products included in tenders. On delivery, products have to be accompanied by certificates of analysis.

Previously, product samples were tested with assistance from the national drug control laboratory in Canberra, Australia, for a fee of about US$40. Usually, the sample from the lowest bidder was tested first. Samples were also drawn randomly from goods received, since suppliers occasionally sent goods of different quality from the original samples. At present, however, no testing of drug samples is done, although there are laboratory facilities at the University of Technology in Lae.

Sri Lanka. Soon after the formation of the State Pharmaceuticals Corporation (SPC) to manage drug importation, both the public and the medical profession began to question the quality of some drugs. Hence, the SPC makes considerable efforts to ensure quality. It requires that a supplier register with SPC, provide a certificate of origin with each shipment, and bear the expense of testing by an independent laboratory chosen by the SPC. In addition, the SPC occasionally sponsors local studies of bioavailability. Because suppliers' own certificates of quality were often found to be unreliable, and an international quality control agency was not consistently responsive, the SPC developed a list of independent laboratories that they recommend to suppliers to perform the quality control checks.

Although a merit rating system was devised, it has not been implemented. The Tender Board, which decides on suppliers, relies on its own memory of experience with the company, the reports of board members who have inspected suppliers' facilities, and, to some extent, information from a registration system. The registration system is being used to ascertain bank references, trade references (such as large hospitals or government agencies in other countries that the board may contact for information on reliability and quality), and names of government agencies under whose authority the suppliers fall (and from which a confidential GMP and performance report may be requested).

Local testing is done at the National Drug Quality Assurance Laboratories for tender items, products manufactured locally, and products about which complaints have been made. Samples are selected at the time of bidding, after receipt and after payment, and following complaints. Samples are also sometimes sent to other laboratories, such as the Bureau of Pharmaceutical Laboratories in Kuala Lumpur, Malaysia, and the Medical Department in Oslo, Norway.

≡ 18.6 Monitoring Drug Quality

In spite of every effort, defective products occasionally slip through, and the quality of even the best-manufactured product may deteriorate. Furthermore, health personnel and patients alike may have erroneous perceptions of product quality, particularly when generic products are not well known and accepted.

Product Problem Reporting System

It is important to establish a national product problem reporting system for health workers to report suspected or confirmed problems with specific drug products. Figure 18.7 is a sample drug product evaluation form, which pharmacy staff and health care providers at all levels can use to report suspected lapses in drug or packaging quality. Standard procedures for product problem reporting should specify

- who should report the perceived product quality problem;
- how to fill in the reporting form;
- where and to whom the reporting form should be sent;
- what additional measures need to be taken, such as sending samples or information concerning the quantities involved;
- what follow-up information will be provided to the person or facility who reported the problem.

All reports should be carefully analyzed using laboratory testing as required, and appropriate actions must be taken. The reporter should be informed about the results and the actions taken, even if products are not defective, to encourage continued participation in the program. Product problem reports and results should be recorded to provide information for future procurement.

Product Recalls

Drug products found to be defective should be quickly recalled. The quality assurance unit should develop standard procedures for carrying out the recall. Rapid action helps avoid unnecessary exposure once the problem has been detected. Inventory control systems that track distribution to facilities by batch number greatly facilitate product recalls.

Recalls may be classified according to the degree of risk to the consumer: serious illness or death, temporary or mild illness, no adverse clinical effect. The level of recall is determined by both the degree of risk and the extent of distribution of the product and may be directed at the patient, health facility, or medical stores level.

After issuing a recall, the quality assurance program should monitor the progress of the recall to ensure complete compliance. The supplier should be notified and required to replace defective products. The procurement office should pursue other remedies specified in the contract, such as withholding payment until the defective products are replaced.

≡ 18.7 Personnel and Training in the Supply System

Central to the operation of most well-run drug supply systems is at least one qualified pharmacist with some training or experience in industrial pharmacy and procurement. Such an individual can be invaluable in establishing and overseeing quality control practices suited to local requirements. This person should participate in

- selecting drugs;
- setting technical specifications for drug contracts;
- reviewing supply offers and selecting suppliers;
- reviewing storage and transportation facilities;
- coordinating any drug quality testing and helping to train the inspectors who check drug shipments.

In some government systems, qualified pharmacists are employed at all levels, including the district hospitals, and they are expected to oversee local storage and transportation conditions. In addition, they report problems or questions concerning individual drugs to the main office. In other countries, locally trained dispensers are responsible for much of the day-to-day work and must be trained to detect and report quality problems.

In addition to pharmacists and pharmaceutical assistants, other staff members involved in quality assurance need training and supervision as a part of quality assurance efforts:

- In order to make informed decisions about supply sources and to monitor and promote quality assurance in their facilities, physicians, health administrators, and health system officials must know about the factors that influence drug quality.
- Port-clearing personnel should be trained to identify the categories of drugs requiring special storage and transportation conditions.
- Clerks responsible for inspecting drug shipments should receive formal training in inspection procedures.
- Drug inspectors must be familiar enough with drug labeling and packaging materials to determine whether contract conditions have been met with regard to the correct drug dosage, packaging, and labeling.

Figure 18.7 Sample Drug and Supplier Evaluation Form

Organization of Eastern Caribbean States
Eastern Caribbean Drug Service

DRUG & SUPPLIER EVALUATION FORM

Submitted by: _____

Country: _____ Date: _____

Sample Location
— CMS
— Other _____
(specify)

Address communications to:

ECDS
PO Box 3093
La Clery
Castries
St. Lucia

Telephone: (809-45) 25058/25895

Drug Description Generic Name, Strength, Form	Brand Name	Manufacturer or Supplier	Lot Number or Batch Number	Expiration Date	Comments

Suggested criteria for drug evaluation:
1. Physical characteristics • e.g., hardness, colour, mixing ease for reconstitution
2. Packaging • expiry date, lot or batch number, package insert
3. Labeling • language (English vs. French), legibility (esp. ampoules)
4. Patient acceptability • taste, colour, size of tablet, etc.
5. Health care provider acceptability • e.g., is the ampoule easy to break?

Guidelines for drug sampling:
1. Take samples from previously unopened containers
2. Minimum sample size: tabs/caps—200; injections—40 ampoules; liquids—400mL
3. Tabs/caps must be tightly packed in plastic/glass vial (DO NOT USE PAPER OR PLASTIC ENVELOPES)
4. Enclose COMPLETE LABEL (generic name, strength, quantity, manufacturer and supplier names, lot/batch number, expiry date, date of manufacture)
5. Print label legibly, and double-check lot number for accuracy.

IF A PROBLEM IS SUSPECTED, PLEASE SUBMIT COMPLETED FORM TO YOUR SUPPLIES OFFICER

Source: Organization of Eastern Caribbean States 1994.

≡ Assessment Guide

Quality Assurance Structures

► Are there stated policies and practices aimed at ensuring drug quality?

► Who is responsible for monitoring drug quality?

► In what laboratories is quality control testing done?

► Is there a formal system for reporting product quality complaints?

Quality Assurance Procedures

► Is the WHO *Certification Scheme on the Quality of Pharmaceutical Products Moving in International Commerce* used systematically?

► Are GMP inspections required for any local manufacturers?

► Is a physical inspection made of all drug products received?

► How many laboratory analyses were performed during the past year out of the total number of products or batches procured?

► To whom are results of analyses of suspected or confirmed defective products communicated?

► Are the test results of substandard drug products recorded for use in future procurement assessments?

► Is information on drug stability and problem drugs used in evaluating suppliers and drug products?

► Are storage conditions periodically evaluated at the ports of entry? At the central warehouse? At district and regional stores? In hospital pharmacies? At health centers and rural health posts?

► Do transport conditions significantly contribute to product deterioration?

► Do dispensing practices in the health facilities or pharmacies significantly contribute to product deterioration?

► Are the various levels of health workers adequately trained to carry out their respective roles in quality assurance?

Outcome of Quality Assurance

► In the previous year, how many reports were submitted on drug product problems?

► What number of drugs or batches failed quality control testing out of the total number of drugs or batches tested in the previous year?

► When local repackaging is done, the staff involved should be trained to assure drug quality.

► Finally, physicians, nurses, and paramedical personnel handling drugs throughout the health system need to know about the factors that influence drug quality and what they can do to ensure that the drugs dispensed to patients are safe and effective.

Quality assurance is a widely shared responsibility. Within the organizational structure of a supply system, responsibilities for the review and preservation of drug product quality at all levels need to be clearly established. If a drug becomes ineffective or unsafe by the time it reaches the patient, then all the other activities of the supply system have been in vain. ■

≡ References and Further Readings

★ = *Key readings.*

Hogerzeil, H. V., A. Battersby, V. Srdanovic, and N. E. Stjern-strom. 1992. Stability of essential drugs during shipment to the tropics. *British Medical Journal* 304:210–12.

Hogerzeil, H. V., G. J. A. Walker, and M. J. de Goeje. 1993. *Stability of injectable oxytocics in tropical climates. Results of field surveys and simulation studies on ergometrine, methylergometrine and oxytocin.* WHO/DAP/93.6. Geneva: WHO.

MSH (Management Sciences for Health). 1992. Quality assurance (trainer's and participant's guides. In *Managing drug supply training series. Part 3. Supply management.* Boston: MSH.

NCM (Nordic Council on Medicines). 1987. *Bioavailability studies in man: Nordic guidelines.* NLN publication no. 18. Uppsala, Sweden: NCM.

Sakolchai, S., et al. 1989. *A study of drug quality in primary health care drug provision system.* Bangkok: US Agency for International Development and Research Institute, Khon Kaen University.

Strom, B. L. 1987. Generic drug substitution revisited. *New England Journal of Medicine* 316:1456–62.

United States Pharmacopeia (USP). 1995. *National Formulary.* Vol. 18, Suppl. 2., *US Pharmacopeia,* 23d ed. Rockville, Md.: United States Pharmacopeial Convention.

WHO (World Health Organization). 1984. *WHO expert committee on specifications for pharmaceutical preparations.* 29th report. Technical report series no. 704. Geneva: WHO.

WHO (World Health Organization). 1986. *Accelerated stability studies of widely used pharmaceutical substances under simulated tropical conditions.* WHO/PHARM/86.529. Geneva: WHO.

★ WHO (World Health Organization). 1989. WHO certification scheme on the quality of pharmaceutical products moving in international commerce: Guidelines for use. *WHO Drug Information* 3:109–15.

★ WHO (World Health Organization). 1990. *WHO expert committee on specifications for pharmaceutical preparations.* 31st report. Technical report series no. 790. Geneva: WHO.

WHO (World Health Organization). 1991a. *Basic tests for pharmaceutical substances.* Geneva: WHO.

WHO (World Health Organization). 1991b. *Inland stability study (Sudan): Pilot study 1989–1991.* Geneva: WHO.

★ WHO (World Health Organization). 1992. *WHO expert committee on specifications for pharmaceutical preparations.* 32d report. Technical report series no. 823. Geneva: WHO.

WHO (World Health Organization). 1995. *Use of the WHO certification scheme on the quality of pharmaceutical products moving in international commerce.* Geneva: WHO.

WHO/DAP (World Health Organization/Action Programme on Essential Drugs). 1993. *Report of a meeting on the optimal use of regional drug quality control laboratories in Africa. Niamey, 8–12 November, 1993.* WHO/DAP/94.10. Geneva: WHO.

WHO/EURO (World Health Organization Regional Office for Europe). 1986. *Guidelines for the investigation of bioavailability.* Draft. Copenhagen: WHO/EURO.

★ WHO/UNICEF (World Health Organization/United Nations Children's Fund). 1991. *Study on the stability of drugs during international transport.* Geneva: WHO/UNICEF.

Resource Organizations

Crown Agents
St. Nicholas House
St. Nicholas Road
Sutton, Surrey SM1 1EL, UK

European Free Trade Association (EFTA)
9-11 rue de Varembé
CH-1211 Geneva 20, Switzerland
International Dispensary Association (IDA)
PO Box 37098
1030 AB Amsterdam, Netherlands

Service de Contrôle des Médicaments
Association Pharmaceutique Belge
Rue Archimède 11
B-1040 Brussels, Belgium

Société Générale de Surveillance S.A.
1, Place des Alpes
CH-1201 Geneva 1, Switzerland

United Nations International Packing Centre (UNIPAC)
UNICEF Plads
Freeport
DK-2100 Copenhagen 0, Denmark

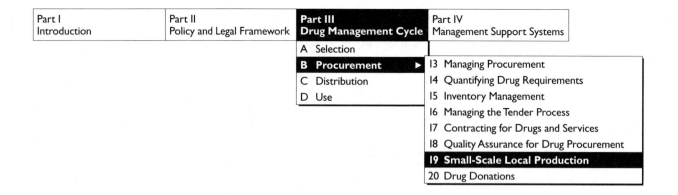

| Part I | Part II | Part III | Part IV |
| Introduction | Policy and Legal Framework | **Drug Management Cycle** | Management Support Systems |

A Selection

B Procurement ▶ | 13 Managing Procurement
C Distribution | 14 Quantifying Drug Requirements
D Use | 15 Inventory Management
| 16 Managing the Tender Process
| 17 Contracting for Drugs and Services
| 18 Quality Assurance for Drug Procurement
| **19 Small-Scale Local Production**
| 20 Drug Donations

Chapter 19
Small-Scale Local Production

≡ Summary

As discussed in Chapter 9, local pharmaceutical production can be conducted on a large scale (usually on a national level by the private-sector pharmaceutical industry or by the public-sector ministry of health). It can also be done on a small scale, perhaps at a regional or local level, by private nongovernmental organizations (NGOs) or not-for-profit mission organizations. This chapter focuses on small-scale local manufacturing and repackaging operations capable of producing nonsterile and sterile pharmaceuticals. It provides information to help program managers decide whether it is logical to begin small-scale local production and, if so, how to plan and carry it out.

In order to decide whether small-scale local production is a valid option, production capability and resources must be assessed. After a decision to produce pharmaceuticals locally is made, product selection and preparation, quality control, and pricing must be thoroughly studied and a plan of development established. When properly carried out, local pharmaceutical production and repackaging may significantly improve primary health care services.

Because of the multitude of difficulties encountered and the level of sophistication required, large-scale production is often not realistic in developing countries, at least when attempted by the public sector. Nevertheless, the need for some locally produced pharmaceuticals and laboratory reagents may exist, and if this need cannot be adequately met by an existing large-scale facility, hospitals (or associations of health care facilities) may have to produce what is needed on a much smaller scale. The rationale for local pharmaceutical production is to save lives that may be endangered by shortages of commercial products.

It was only in the last thirty years that the United States, under pressure from the pharmaceutical industry and strict government regulation, removed much of the preparation of simple pharmaceuticals (including IV fluids) from hospitals. The increased threat and expense of lawsuits played a major role in this decision to leave manufacturing in the hands of the pharmaceutical industry. In many developing countries, legislation still promotes the local production of pharmaceuticals. The long experience of high-quality, small-scale production by hospital pharmacies, which continues in many European countries even to this day, should not be forgotten in developing countries. However, quality must be assured.

Drug prices have skyrocketed in recent years, to the extent that some products that can be safely manufactured locally are simply not affordable if purchased and imported into developing countries, especially for the public health sector, with its meager resources. This means that some small-scale local production is likely to be cost effective in many countries, but it requires that management personnel ensure its safety and effectiveness. The experience of many countries confirms that this is possible, but the potential problems and risks should not be underestimated.

≡ 19.1 Overview of Small-Scale Local Production

There are several types of pharmaceutical production, with varying levels of complexity. This chapter is concerned only with the small-scale production of pharmaceuticals from existing raw materials that are usually imported (called secondary production in Chapter 9) and the packaging or repackaging of finished goods (called tertiary production) into smaller dispensing packs and course-of-therapy (COT) packages.

Small-scale production can be further divided into nonsterile and sterile production or compounding. Depending on the availability of qualified staff, adequate facilities, sufficient equipment, and all the other necessary resources, as well as a market for the final products, production may be very simple or quite sophisticated. A few examples of small-scale production, taken from the *Model List of Essential Drugs* (WHO 1995), are presented in Figure 19.1.

The following sections examine some of the management issues for each type of production, in order of increasing complexity.

Repackaging and Course-of-Therapy Packaging

Repackaging and COT packaging are relatively simple forms of local pharmaceutical production. They require the ability to provide adequate packaging, labeling, and control of the final product.

Repackaging is usually considered when the product can be purchased in bulk quantities at a favorable price and then repackaged locally, where labor costs are lower, and when local language labeling may be important. In addition to the cost savings, a more convenient package size can be made available to small health centers and individuals, as Figure 19.2 illustrates.

Many types of glass and plastic are used, with the choice often depending on what is being packaged. For instance, acids, solvents, and corrosive materials must be packaged

Figure 19.1 Examples of Pharmaceutical Products Suitable for Small-Scale Local Production

General Type of Production/ Use	Pharma- ceutical Dosage Form	Drugs with Potential for Local Production on WHO Essential Drugs List	Other Drugs with Potential for Local Production
Nonsterile/ Internal	Powders	Oral rehydration salts 27.9 g/l	Antacid powder mixture
	Simple solutions	Chloral hydrate syrup 2,900 mg/5 mL Chloroquine syrup 50 mg/5 mL Ephedrine elixir 15 mg/5 mL Iron solution 125 mg/5 mL Paracetamol syrup 125 mg/5 mL Phenobarbital elixir 15 mg/5 mL Piperazine syrup 500 mg/5 mL Promethazine syrup 500 mg/5 mL	Anticough/expectorant mixtures for adults
	Suspensions	Aluminum hydroxide suspension 320 mg/5 mL Barium sulfate suspension Chloramphenicol suspension 125 mg/mL Magnesium hydroxide suspension 550 mg/mL Metronidazole suspension 200 mg/5 mL Sulfadimidine suspension 500 mg/5 mL	Aluminum hydroxide + magnesium Trisilicate suspension Magnesium carbonate mixture (suspension)
	Emulsions		Mineral oil (liquid paraffin) emulsion
Nonsterile/ External	Ointments	Benzoic acid 6% + salicylic acid 3% (Whitfield's ointment) Dithranol ointment 1% Hydrocortisone ointment 1%	Coal tar and zinc ointment Menthol and eucalyptus ointment Sulfur ointment 10%
	Creams	Hydrocortisone cream 1%	
	Emulsions	Benzyl benzoate lotion (application) 25%	
	Pastes	Zinc oxide paste 25%	
	Powders		Zinc compound dusting powder
	Shake lotions	Calamine (zinc oxide 20%) lotion Thiabendazole 500 mg/5 mL	
	Solutions	Chlorhexidine solution 5% (for dilution) Coal tar solution 5% Gentian violet solution 0.5% Povidone-iodine solution 10%	Acriflavine (proflavine) solution 0.5% Antiseptic mouthwash Chloramphenicol eardrops 10% Ephedrine nasal drops 0.5%
Sterile/ Internal	Small-volume injections	Chlorpromazine injection 2.5% (25 mg/mL) Dextrose injection 50% Diazepam injection 0.5% (5 mg/mL) Gentamicin injection 4% (40 mg/mL) Lidocaine injection 1%, 2% Mannitol injection 2.5% (25 mg/mL) Promethazine injection 2.5% (25 mg/mL) Quinine injection 30% (300 mg/L) Sodium chloride injection 0.9% (normal saline) Sterile water for injection	Procaine injection 2% Quinine injection 5%
	Large-volume injections	Dextrose 5% in water Dextrose 5% in sodium chloride Hartmann's solution (lactated Ringer's solution) Sodium chloride 0.9%	CPD (ACD) solution (anticoagulant for transfusions)
Sterile/ External	Eye drops	Atropine solution 1% Gentamicin solution 0.3% Pilocarpine solution 2%, 4% Prednisolone solution 0.5% Tetracaine solution 0.5%	Argyrol (mild silver protein) solution 2% Astringent eyedrops

in glass, with lids that can be firmly closed. Fortunately, the majority of simple liquids, solids, and tablets can be packaged in rigid plastic bottles or resealable polyethylene bags of various sizes and thicknesses, usually with a write-on panel for the labeling or handwritten instructions to the patient. Section 19.4 gives further details on repackaging and quality control measures.

Nonsterile Production

Nonsterile production of topical ointments and oral or topical liquids is more difficult and complex than repackaging but less demanding than sterile production. If only nonsterile production is planned, resource requirements can be simplified. However, standard written instructions for batch preparation and packaging must be followed, and quality control must be closely monitored for each aspect of the process.

Every product requires a well-designed production control worksheet (also called a batch documentation sheet). It clearly specifies the production formula (the detailed recipe that the pharmacist must follow precisely) and the instructions for preparation. It includes spaces to verify packaging, labeling, and other control procedures. Figure 19.3 shows a sample pharmacy production and control worksheet.

The chief pharmacist of a facility is usually responsible for developing the master production formulas and instructions, as well as for training production staff. The staff should always work from photocopies of the master production and control worksheet, with a unique control number preassigned by the pharmacist in charge. Any changes to that formula, such as scaling down quantities to make a smaller batch, should be made only by a qualified pharmacist.

A pharmacy preparation, no matter how simple, should never be made from memory. The working copy of the pharmacy production control worksheet should be readily available or posted in the production area for easy reference and initialing of each production step and control procedure.

Sterile Production

Sterile production is the most demanding type, and it must be carried out in strict compliance with current good manufacturing practices (GMPs). Depending on need and capacity, sterile products that can be manufactured include eyedrops, small-volume injections, and large-volume injections (or parenteral products).

From a production process perspective, intravenous (IV) fluids are among the easiest products to make. The standard

Figure 19.2 Pharmaceutical Repackaging

Product Type	Name of Product	Bulk Package Size	Repackaged Size
Liquids	Denatured alcohol	20 L	500 mL
Solids	Talcum powder	50 kg	1 kg
Tablets	Aspirin 300 mg	1,000	100
	Aspirin 300 mg	1,000	12
	Cotrimoxazole 480 mg	1,000	10 (b.i.d. for 5 days)
	Mebendazole 100 mg	1,000	6 (b.i.d. for 3 days)

pharmacy production and control worksheet, including the sterility quality control aspects, is used (see Figure 19.3). From a technical perspective, however, the production of IV fluids is very demanding on resources and personnel. Special (often quite expensive) equipment, facilities, techniques, and quality control procedures need to be in place, along with the means to ensure continuous production with adequate reserves of ingredients and supplies, regular maintenance of equipment, and refresher training for production staff. The demands on supervisory personnel, who must ensure the high quality of the final product, are also much greater. Contaminated or incorrectly prepared IV fluids administered to very sick people can just as easily kill patients as help them.

If all the technical requirements are met, a highly motivated staff can produce high-quality sterile products that can have a major positive impact on health care (see Country Study 19.1).

≡ 19.2 General Technical Considerations

Although there may seem to be good reasons to produce certain pharmaceuticals locally, a feasibility study is essential before any production begins. Depending on the availability and quality of key resources, the pharmacy may be capable of undertaking only very simple production, or it may be able to manufacture a diversity of products of significant complexity.

The preproduction feasibility study must confirm that personnel, buildings, water and power supplies, equipment, and documentation (including production formulas) are already in place, or that a plan has been developed to produce them (see Chapter 9).

Personnel

Skilled employees are needed to ensure proper manufacture and quality control of pharmaceutical products and active ingredients. There must be sufficient qualified personnel to carry out all the tasks for which the manufacturer

Figure 19.3 Pharmacy Production and Control Worksheet

Ministry of Health
Department of Medical Supply

PHARMACY PRODUCTION AND CONTROL WORKSHEET

Name of the preparation: Sodium Chloride 0.9%

Control number: 97-03-20-A

Formula	Source of formula: USP/NF (1995), page 1418	Quantity	Raw Material Lot Number	Prepared by	Checked by
Sodium chloride		540.0 g	HCl 1052	AL	SD
Water for injection, freshly prepared	q.s. to make	60.0 L	—	AL	SD

Instructions:
1. Prepare all required equipment and packaging materials according to standard protocols.
2. Weigh the sodium chloride using a precision balance.
3. Mix and make the solution in a closed, graduated, stainless-steel mixing vessel.
4. Filter the solution under air pressure through a 0.45-micron prefilter and a 0.2-micron final filter into previously cleaned and sterilized bottles.
5. Stopper and cap the bottles.
6. Autoclave the batch immediately according to standard protocols.
7. After cooling, label the bottles.
8. Perform all the required quality control checks.
9. Hold in quarantine until batch is released by Quality Control.

Packaging
Done by: GL
Bottle used/size: DIN Class I 500 mL IV bottle
Closure Used: Chlorobutyl rubber stopper
Theoretical yield: 120 bottles
Actual yield: 115
Special storage required: None
Expiration date: 1 year
Checked by: TK

Quality Control / Sterile
Sterilizer used: Uniclave 88
Time: from 10:30 hour to 10:50
Temperature: 121°C Pressure: 1.2 Bar By: AB

Clarity Test:	Yes ✓	No	By: JR
Sterility Test:	Yes ✓	No	By: DA
Pyrogen Test:	Yes ✓	No	By: DH
Analytical Test:	Yes ✓	No	By: PR

Checked by: ML   Released from quarantine by: KK

Final Disposition of Production
Accepted: ✓
Rejected: Quantity added to inventory: 112   Received by: JB
Date: 3/28/97   Signature of pharmacist (or delegated person): R. L. Watt

Product Label
Made by: HE   Attached by: DW
Sample Label (attach below):

Sodium Chloride 0.9%

1,000 mL
Intravenous Infusion
310 mOsm/L
Store Below 25°C
Sterile and Pyrogen-Free
Do Not Use If Solution Contains Particles

Batch No: 97-03-20-A   Manufactured by:
Exp. Date: 3/20/98   Central Pharmacy
                              Sterile Production Unit

Country Study 19.1 The Role of Private NGOs in Providing Health Care Services in Zaire

Background. When Zaire became independent in 1960, there were no trained national doctors or pharmacists. Civil war then nearly destroyed the existing health infrastructure, which was rebuilt in the intervening years with the help of many NGOs and outside funding. Until 1980, the government provided many essential drugs needed by the public sector through its central medical stores or manufactured them in a national laboratory, supplemented by several production facilities operated by multinational firms and many private pharmaceutical warehouses. Nationalization of the pharmaceutical industry in the early 1980s, coupled with widespread mismanagement, led to the near total collapse of existing structures in a short time.

Development. In the 1980s, NGOs increasingly provided basic health care services, including procurement and distribution of essential medicines, as the government could not provide the services. An example was the creation of the SANRU primary health care project in 1981, which at its peak in 1991 was helping to coordinate health activities in the 306 health zones of Zaire (typically, each zone had a large referral hospital serving a population of about 100,000 people from 200 villages served by about twenty primary health care centers). One such zone was at Nyankunde, in the northeastern part of Zaire, with a full-service 226-bed mission hospital as well as a central pharmacy, training institutes, flying service, and communications network as part of the Evangelical Medical Center (CME) complex.

Pharmacy Role. The CME central pharmacy was expanded in 1983 to increase procurement of essential medicines by both importation and local production and to ensure distribution to twenty-eight satellite hospitals. The need for local production, and the lack of trained pharmacy personnel in many satellite pharmacies, led to the establishment in 1986 of a school for training pharmaceutical assistants, along with a community pharmacy to serve as a training site and retail outlet.

Long-Term Perspective. At its peak in 1991, the CME central pharmacy was producing nearly 100 different items (see the accompanying table), 75 percent of which were on the Zaire essential drugs list (the rest were miscellaneous laboratory solutions and CME "proprietary" medicines). Since 1991, hyperinflation (up to 13,000 percent), deteriorating infrastructure (less than 1,000 miles of potholed, semipaved roads for a country of 2,345,000 square kilometers), and continued political instability (many expatriates were forced to evacuate after riots and looting) have delayed a project to decentralize the pharmacy production to ten additional hospital-based local production units. In the meantime, the pharmacy and training facilities continue their functions with 100 percent Zairean personnel.

Central Pharmacy Production, 1991

Category of Pharmacy Preparation	Number of Different CME Preparations in Category	Total Quantity Produced in1991
Sterile		
Large-volume parenterals	5	4,468.0 L
Small-volume injectables	12	423.3 L
Eyedrops (and other drops)	20	54.5 L
Nonsterile		
Ointments	11	218.3 kg
Lotions	2	180.4 L
Powders	4	220.0 kg
Solutions	33	9,612.7 L
Syrups	5	989.5 L
Suspensions	4	675.9 L
Suppositories	1	306.0 units
Tinctures	2	482.0 L

is responsible, with individual responsibilities documented in written job descriptions. Employees must clearly understand their responsibilities and the importance of following all applicable good manufacturing practices (see "References and Further Readings").

There should be a qualified pharmacist responsible for managing all aspects of production. In practice, pharmaceutical assistants and other auxiliary personnel who have been specially trained by the pharmacist in charge of the production facility are often used. The chief pharmacist, in collaboration with other medical personnel, should select the products to be manufactured, order sufficient raw materials and packaging supplies, develop the appropriate batch formulas, and ensure the quality of the finished product and its final disposition.

Production personnel are the greatest source of contamination and error, and their initial training must be supplemented by regular refresher courses and periodic on-the-job inspections and evaluations. Work flow patterns must be developed to avoid contamination and mistakes. Personal hygiene—which includes hand washing, the wearing of proper clothing, and good clean-room techniques—must be stressed. Employees with infections and skin lesions should not be permitted to work in the production area. Outside traffic must be controlled, and the smallest possible number of workers should be used inside. Raw materials and packaging supplies should be stored away from the production area. Personnel should be motivated to follow written directions for all aspects of their work. Frequent turnover of staff should be avoided.

Supervisory and management personnel must ensure that GMPs and proper financial management and inventory control procedures are followed. To maintain effective quality control, analytical and inspection personnel who monitor the quality of products must be different from those who produce them. Finally, production personnel need to maintain close communication with the distribution unit to respond quickly to special production needs (in time of epidemic, for instance) and to avoid stockouts.

Buildings and Physical Plant

The production premises must be located, designed, constructed, adapted, and maintained to suit the scope of operations to be carried out. The layout and design must minimize the risk of errors and permit effective cleaning and maintenance to avoid cross-contamination and buildup of dust or dirt.

Since developing countries sometimes lack the financial resources to construct local production facilities that are equal to commercial pharmaceutical factories (usually the production is located in or associated with the hospital pharmacy), a balance must be reached between the ideal and the practical. Buildings can be simple but must be of adequate size for the work being done. The compounding area should be dust-free, which usually requires air-conditioning. Windows are needed for light; they should be barred for security.

The premises should be constructed and equipped to be easily cleaned and disinfected regularly, according to written procedures. The premises should be kept free from insects, pests, rodents, and other animals. Eating, drinking, and smoking should be confined to separate rooms, as should accommodations for changing clothes, washing, and toileting.

The number of buildings and rooms and the required room sizes will vary greatly, depending on a number of factors:

- General types of pharmaceutical production planned (nonsterile and/or sterile);
- Number of different pharmaceutical forms produced (external and internal liquids, powders, ointments, eyedrops, small- and large-volume parenterals, and so forth);
- Quantities of each pharmaceutical form produced (batch sizes);
- Volume of repackaging or COT packaging;
- Extent of pharmacy service provided (training center, central pharmacy distribution center supplying several satellite pharmacies, or a simple hospital pharmacy).

Separate rooms (or, in some cases, discrete work areas within a larger room) are needed for the following:

- Administrative activities;
- Dirty room for washing bottles (if reused);
- Nonsterile manufacturing;
- Sterile manufacturing clean room;
- Sterilizing and distilled water preparation (usually must be a separate room because of the substantial amounts of heat generated);
- Labeling and internal quality control;
- Storeroom(s) with shelving for raw materials, packaging materials, and finished products (including separate areas for flammable or hazardous products, refrigerated and frozen items, controlled substances, quarantined raw materials, and finished products awaiting quality control release);
- Shipping and receiving areas;
- Rest rooms/dressing areas (for men and women);
- Cafeteria/small kitchen with rest area for breaks;
- Maintenance workshop;
- Garage for vehicle and fuel storage;
- Classroom (may be combined with rest area);
- Adequate and convenient housing for staff and trainees (if an on-call system is used, and if visiting students are present);
- On-site (or access to external) laboratory facilities for microbiological and other quality control testing of raw materials and finished products.

Water Resources

The presence of an adequate potable water supply is fundamental. Unfortunately, production pharmacies in many developing countries do not have a municipal water supply, and where the service exists, the water must often be further treated before it can be used for pharmaceutical production. If water supplies are inadequate, alternative sources must be developed before production can start. The following sources have been used successfully:

- Rainwater;
- Surface water (lakes, rivers);
- Underground water (wells);
- Solar distilled water (small amounts, especially for eyedrop production).

Depending on the source, the season, the degree of contamination, and the volume needed, water from these alternative sources may require further pretreatment and laboratory test facilities to monitor its purity. Storage tanks, either underground with a pump or sufficiently above ground to provide adequate water pressure, are needed, along with the associated plumbing needed to bring the water to the production facility. Sewers and adequate wastewater removal must also be available.

Equipment

The location and design of equipment must minimize the risk of errors and permit effective cleaning and maintenance.

Electrical equipment specifications (voltage—110, 220, or 240 volts; number of cycles—50 or 60 hertz; and phases—single- or three-phase) and the total power consumed (watts) must be matched to the available supply, or electricity must be generated by local solar, hydroelectric, or diesel or gasoline generators. Voltage regulators and stabilizers may be needed to protect vital equipment.

All equipment used in manufacture or quality control should be regularly inspected, and operating and cleaning instructions should be kept near the apparatus. Weighing and measuring equipment should be calibrated regularly.

Telephones and fax machines are vital to communicate rapidly with suppliers and customers. Unfortunately, they are not always available or reliable in developing countries, particularly in rural areas. Advanced satellite communications systems are available and might be considered for large production facilities, if sufficient technical personnel exist for their installation and maintenance.

Documentation

Each production unit must have technical literature, including the current official national formulary and pharmacopeia (a legal requirement in some countries). References that document the formulas used in various countries (Reynolds 1996), production techniques (Gennaro 1995), and analytical, chemical, and physical tests should be available.

The source of the production formulas used should be referenced to the scientific literature and noted on the pharmacy production and control worksheet (see Figure 19.3). Batch size calculations and instructions must be verified by a pharmacist before manufacturing a new product. Unless the production pharmacist is well qualified, it is dangerous to experiment with new or modified formulas.

Product Quality

Three terms—quality assurance, good manufacturing practices (GMPs), and quality control—are frequently used interchangeably, but there are real differences, as the following sections illustrate.

Quality Assurance. Quality assurance may be defined as the sum of all activities and responsibilities intended to ensure that products meet all the applicable quality specifications in the final dosage form. Quality assurance must include an oversight and auditing component to deter-mine that procedures and systems are suitable and, if needed, to recommend appropriate changes.

Good Manufacturing Practices. According to the World Health Organization (WHO), GMPs are the part of quality assurance that ensures that products are consistently produced and controlled to the quality standards appropriate to their intended use and required by the drug regulatory authority. GMP rules are directed primarily at diminishing the risks, inherent in any pharmaceutical production, that cannot be prevented completely through the testing of final products. Such risks are essentially of two types: cross-contamination (in particular by unexpected contaminants) and mix-ups (confusion) caused by incorrect labels on containers or human error.

The pharmaceutical industry in the United States has been externally regulated only since 1963, when the Food and Drug Administration (FDA) first issued regulations describing the GMPs to be followed in the manufacture, packaging, and holding of finished pharmaceuticals. These regulations were significantly revised and updated in 1978, when the FDA proposed GMPs relating to the manufacture and control of large-volume parenteral products. Although never officially issued, these GMPs have become the guidelines used by the industry and the FDA in the manufacture, control, and inspection of all sterile products. Products that are not manufactured according to *all* the current GMPs are considered to be adulterated (not in compliance with GMPs).

Since 1968, WHO has attempted to standardize the GMPs of various countries into a single list (latest revision in 1992). These GMPs are applicable to local manufacturing in developing countries.

Although these GMPs are written for the pharmaceutical industry, when a pharmacy produces medicines locally, it should duplicate the standards that went into the manufacture of that product, not just those that apply to the final product. Obviously, hospitals do not have the same resources as the pharmaceutical industry, and the products they make are generally for local consumption, not commercial distribution. Nevertheless, a local pharmacy production unit should comply as far as possible with international GMPs, and should comply absolutely with GMPs adopted in the local production facility.

Quality Control. According to WHO, quality control is the part of GMPs concerned with sampling, specifications, and testing and with the organization, documentation, and release procedures that ensure that the necessary tests are carried out and that materials are not released for use, nor products released for sale or supply, until their quality has been judged to be satisfactory. Quality control is not confined to laboratory operations but must be involved in all decisions concerning the quality of the product.

Quality control of pharmaceuticals depends on meticulous adherence to written procedures in carrying out all operations. Quality must be designed into a product from the earliest stages; it cannot be ensured in the final product if GMPs were not present throughout the production process. Raw materials must be purchased from reputable suppliers and certified to conform to WHO standards of quality. Whether or not local quality control testing facilities exist, copies of the quality control analysis report of raw materials should be required from the supplier at the time of purchase.

Facilities and equipment must be designed so that the potential for cross-contamination of one product by another is eliminated. Material flow and personnel movements should be planned to reduce the potential for product mix-ups, and air and water provided for production must be adequate in amount and quality for the particular operations being performed. (For air quality, see WHO 1993.)

Figure 19.4 summarizes the interrelations among the three terms: quality control (QC) is a part of GMPs, which in turn are part of the total quality assurance (QA) system.

≡ 19.3 Feasibility and Cost Effectiveness of Local Manufacturing

In order to assess the feasibility of engaging in small-scale local manufacturing, issues involving product selection and market assessment, costs and cost recovery, and development planning must be examined.

Product Selection and Market Assessment

Assuming that the general technical considerations mentioned above can be met and sustained, the next step is to select the products that can potentially be manufactured, based on local demand versus availability.

The last step in this process is to determine the economic feasibility of local production. The purchase prices of the products can be obtained from commercial sources (such as tender catalogs). Then the actual costs to manufacture the same products locally must be calculated. Rarely should a product be made locally if it can be purchased at a lower net cost.

Real Costs

In the assessment of real costs, *all* costs to produce a product must be determined: raw materials, packaging supplies, staff salaries, equipment purchase and depreciation, space costs, utilities, shipping, and all other direct and indirect costs (see Country Study 19.2).

Figure 19.4 Components of Total Quality Assurance

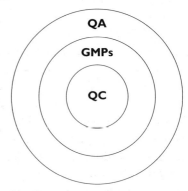

For example, the International Dispensary Association (IDA) calculated the cost of producing IV fluids in small batches of 30 liters using the equipment recommended in its booklet *Small-Scale Production of IV Fluids* (IDA 1992). The calculations were based on 250 batches per year of dextrose 5 percent in normal saline, reusing the bottles fifteen times but using a new stopper for every bottle produced, and depreciating the cost of new equipment over five years. The breakdown of costs was:

Equipment	US$.25/liter
Consumables	US$.30/liter
Bottles (complete)	US$.27/liter
Total	US$.82/liter

Shipping, insurance, and import duties on ingredients had to be added to this figure. Local costs for the building, personnel, water, and electricity (which cannot be usefully illustrated here because of their extreme variability) also had to be added. Note that even if equipment can be obtained as a gift, depreciation should be included in the sales price to build up enough capital to replace the equipment.

The larger the volume of production for a specific product, the lower the unit overhead cost. For this reason, reverse osmosis equipment, with its relatively high output, has often been chosen over the classic distillation equipment for the production of IV fluids.

Costs that are often neglected in calculating the total cost of local production include independent laboratory testing of the final products to ensure quality, when such testing is not possible in-house. If the government must inspect the production facility to ensure that it complies with current GMPs, these costs must also be added to the real production costs. Products that must be thrown away because of production mistakes, other waste, and losses to theft are additional hidden costs that must be included in the comparative cost analyses.

Cost Recovery

In order to sustain the production facility, it is often necessary to charge for manufactured products. Ideally, consumers would pay the full cost of products, which would be priced to allow for a small profit margin (25 to 33 percent) to pay for the replacement of supplies and ingredients. Since many of the facility costs are incurred in foreign exchange (for equipment, raw materials, and consumables not locally produced), if the cash receipts cannot be converted, some other financial mechanism will be needed to acquire foreign exchange. For this reason, sometimes it may be unwise to cancel production of marginally profitable products.

It may be necessary to devise a pricing strategy that allows a greater margin of profit on certain products with a rapid turnover, especially if they are cheap to produce (such as IV fluids), as a means of subsidizing other products with a slow turnover, such as certain laboratory solutions or eyedrops.

Make-or-Buy Assessment

When assessing whether a product should be manufactured locally, factors to consider besides cost include provision of local jobs and training, national or local pharmacy prestige, and more reliable access to products. In fact, a health system might choose to pay somewhat higher prices if the benefits of local production are significant.

Development Plan

It is advisable to start local production with the products that are the easiest to make, while also considering their potential impact on the quality of health care. Locally prepared COT (unit-of-use) packages or more convenient package sizes of imported bulk essential medicines are a frequent choice; usually it is cheaper to repackage products locally than to purchase COT packages.

Next, simple nonsterile solutions and ointments can be manufactured, since these products often consist primarily of water or other relatively inexpensive inactive ingredients.

Following this, IV fluid preparation and other small-scale sterile production of injections and eyedrops can be considered, if good quality can be assured, if the demand is sufficient, and if the products can be produced at a cost comparable to that of purchased products. A hospital pharmacy might consider production for several smaller health centers, in order to have batch sizes that are more economically justifiable.

The expansion of a local pharmaceutical production

Country Study 19.2 Local Infusion Production in Tanzania

Since 1978, the Infusion Units Project of the Evangelical Lutheran Church of Tanzania (ELCT) in Moshi has successfully installed over sixty local infusion units. In addition, the same appropriate technology has been successfully exported into neighboring developing countries such as Uganda, Zaire, and Madagascar.

As of August 1993, the project administrator estimated costs and savings as noted below (all figures are in Tanzanian shillings, with a value of about TSh200 per US$1 at the time, amended to reflect the 1993 cost of pyrogen testing).

Estimation of Production Cost (in TSh) of an Infusion Bottle (500 mL) for 1993

Additives (dextrose/salt)	30
Electricity	1
Kerosene/electricity for autoclave	2
Labels for bottles	2
Staff salaries	15
Service charge (maintenance, training)	10
Pyrogen testing	20
Depreciation, equipment spare parts, consumables (not detailed)	60
Total cost for the hospital	140

Estimation of Expenditure Reduction or Potential Profit (in TSh) on Sale of Infusions for the Hospital

► Basic information:

Sale price for the hospital's product:
200 to 300 (average, 250)
Market cost (with transport to the hospital)   440

► Potential hospital profit for production and sale of 10,000 bottles

10,000 bottles × (unit sale price − unit cost) = profit
10,000 × (TSh250 − TSh140) = TSh1,100,000

► Hospital cost savings with free distribution to patients: If the hospital gives locally produced infusions to inpatients, there will still be an expenditure reduction relative to purchase on the local market, where the price is TSh440 per bottle.

10,000 bottles × (open market price − production cost) = expenditure reduction
10,000 × (TSh440 − TSh140) = TSh3,000,000

Estimation of Expenditure Reduction for All Hospitals with an Infusion Unit in Tanzania

The total production of all forty-two producing units in 1992 was 698,703 bottles. Therefore, the *total savings* for all hospitals with an infusion unit in Tanzania in 1992 (compared to local purchase) amounted to:

698,703 bottles × TSh300 savings per bottle = TSh209,610,900 (US$1,048,055)

Source: Kamm 1995.

---

unit should be proportional to market demand, the resources available, and the cost of obtaining reliable products elsewhere.

☰ 19.4 Specific Technical Considerations

In addition to the general technical considerations mentioned earlier, the next three sections address issues of interest to technical managers responsible for the three types of local production.

Repackaging Operations

Consideration should be given to purchasing an electronic tablet-counting machine if the volume of work justifies the expense. It will greatly reduce the possibility of counting errors.

Generally, repackaged oral solid products are placed in resealable plastic bags of appropriate size. Plastic bags specifically made for drug dispensing are sufficiently impermeable to air and moisture to adequately preserve the repackaged product. For extra protection, COT packages can be placed inside a second larger bag or sealed container until needed. The local drug regulatory authority may provide guidance on an appropriate expiration date for repackaged drugs. If repackaging is done under true GMP conditions, and if containers meet pharmacopeial standards, the original manufacturer's expiry date might be retained. In the United States, expiry dates are normally set at one year after repackaging in a health facility.

Labeling is a critical aspect of repackaging. At a minimum, the generic name, strength, package size, expiration date, and batch number, as well as the name and address of the repackaging pharmacy, should appear on the label. COT labels should also have clear instructions to the patient in the local language. Self-adhesive labels that can be computer generated or printed using a small printing machine are recommended, although preprinted labels with a space to hand stamp a batch number and expiration date can be used.

Unless local experience shows differently, it is probably reasonable to give a one-year expiration date to repackaged products, assuming that repackaging is performed properly. In any case, expiration dates on repackaged products should never extend beyond the original manufacturer's expiration date (see Figure 19.5).

As in other types of production, there must be control records for each repackaged batch, with sufficient bulk products, packaging materials, and labels requisitioned and transferred to the production unit.

A unique batch number is assigned to each job. An easy system to remember consists of assigning the date, with the year written first, as the batch number, followed by a letter that indicates the job sequence on a given day. Thus, in the example shown in Figure 19.5, batch number 97-08-10-D means the fourth job planned on August 10, 1997 (note that the actual date of production may vary).

Well-kept records allow verification of all pertinent data, including the drug used, the packaging employee, the actual yield, and any observations, as well as a sample label. When the same product has been packaged repeatedly over a period of time, accumulated usage figures can be used to improve production planning. Note that the actual yield may not exactly match the theoretical yield because the bulk package is often filled by weight rather than actual count, or there may be breakage or spillage (which should be noted in the observations column).

Many repackaging operations reuse glass and sturdy plastic bottles for a number of liquids, or for various nonsterile and sterile production items. This is permissible, as long as the bottles are washed thoroughly, they do not leak, the old labels are completely removed, and a new batch label is produced every time. If a solution (iodine, for example) has permanently discolored a bottle, that bottle should be reused only for that particular product, if at all.

Nonsterile Compounding

As shown in Figure 19.1, a significant percentage of products on the WHO essential drugs list could theoretically be manufactured locally. When a new pharmaceutical production facility is opened, and until more experience is gained, it is best to begin with nonsterile products that have a large margin of safety and high turnover but are expensive to purchase as finished products (usually simple solutions and powder mixtures, for internal or external use).

Suspensions, emulsions, ointments, and creams are more difficult to formulate, but with proper equipment they can be made by most production facilities. Suppositories can be made without much difficulty if proper molding and packaging equipment is available. They are difficult to preserve in the hot climate of many developing countries, however.

It is very difficult to make tablets locally on a small scale. This operation requires specially trained personnel, highly sophisticated equipment, and ready access to raw materials and packaging supplies. It is rarely cost effective to make tablets in the relatively small amounts that are feasible in a local production facility. Capsules are also generally too difficult and expensive to make in the small batches normally made locally.

Additional technical details concerning the production of individual products must be left to other references (for instance, see Watt 1996).

Figure 19.5 Repackaging and Course-of-Therapy Packaging Control Sheet

Ministry of Health
Department of Medical Supply

REPACKAGING AND COURSE-OF-THERAPY PACKAGING CONTROL SHEET

Pharmacy Stock No: 1069

Name of Product: Aspirin Tablets 300 mg

Package Size: 12

Package Type: 60 x 80 mm resealable bags

Batch No.	Date of Production	Quantity Repackaged	Manufacturer	Mfg. Lot No.	Mfg. Exp. Date	Repack. Exp. Date	Theoret. Yield	Actual Yield	Repack. by	Checked by	Observations
96-12-15-A	12/15/96	5,000	Shanghai	XX03	3/98	12/97	416	415	HL	RW	
97-04-05-C	4/5/97	5,000	Shanghai	XX03	3/98	3/98	416	417	SD	RW	Note exp. date
97-08-10-D	8/14/97	5,000	Shanghai	YY72	5/2000	8/98	416	412	HE	RW	

PLACE SAMPLE OF EACH BATCH LABEL ON REVERSE SIDE   USE SEPARATE CONTROL SHEET FOR EACH UNIQUE PRODUCT

Country Study 19.3 Support of Small-Scale Production in Ghana

Use of twenty locally compounded pharmaceutical preparations was surveyed for twenty-seven church-related hospitals and health centers in Ghana by means of a questionnaire.

Estimated Quantity Needed per 10,000 Outpatient Consultations

Ointments
Gammexane ointment	25 kg
Ichthammol ointment	10 kg
Menthol liniment	40 kg
Sulfur ointment	20 kg
Whitfield's ointment	25 kg

Applications
Calamine lotion	50 L
Eusol solution	80 L
Gentian violet solution	20 L
Iodine tincture	25 L
Potassium permanganate solution	25 L

Mixtures
Antacid mixture	150 L
Antispasmodic mixture	50 L
Children's iron tonic	50 L
Cough mixture	250 L
Kaolin mixture	50 L
Oral rehydration solution	750 L

Various
Boric acid eardrops	1 L
Chloralhydrate	1 kg
Ephedrine nasal drops	5 L
Lysol solution	800 L

Seventy-eight percent of the hospitals and 19 percent of the health centers usually produced pharmaceutical preparations. Forty-one percent of hospital pharmacies were staffed by a hospital pharmacist and 33 percent by a pharmacy technician; three-quarters of the hospitals were producing IV fluids.

From the list, a standard formulary specifying composition and mode of preparation was developed; the total quantity of every raw material was calculated, based on a quantification estimate per 10,000 outpatient consultations; and combined production was established.

Most institutions collected their allocations from one of two distribution points within a month after arrival. The total cost was about US$150,000, and the average cost per estimated medical consultation was US$.02.

Country Study 19.4 Local Production by Ministries and Missions

In **Surinam**, the government-operated central production unit reduced its number of preparations from 200 to 70 after a reconsideration to make or buy. The nonsterile products include mixtures, syrups, disinfectants, ointments, nasal drops, and tablets. The sterile products include eyedrops, injectables, and IV fluids.

CHANPHARM, a church-operated drug supply unit in northern **Nigeria**, runs a considerable local production facility for its 315 member institutions, ranging from hospitals to health posts.

The Mission for Essential Drugs and Supplies (MEDS) in Nairobi, **Kenya,** offers technical and logistical support to over a dozen hospitals for IV fluid production.

The church-operated joint medical stores in **Uganda** produce a range of twenty-five sterile and nonsterile preparations. Technical and logistical support is offered for IV fluid production in thirty-one hospitals.

In **Ghana**, four central diocesan hospital pharmacies are supplying church hospitals with their own preparations. In 1992, the diocesan hospital pharmacy at Kumasi produced 9,000 liters of mixtures, 800 kg of ointments, 7,000 bottles of eyedrops, 10,000 vials of injectables, and 35,000 bottles of IV fluid. Similar production figures are reported by the sister project in Accra.

---

local production, using appropriate technology (Taylor 1989; WHO 1990).

The general technical considerations considered earlier apply here as well, but quality control must be more stringent, since these products are potentially more dangerous. The production facilities and personnel must conform to GMP standards for sterile pharmaceutical products (WHO 1992a, 1992b, 1993).

The four main threats in sterile production are:

1. Particles
2. Chemical impurities
3. Microorganisms
4. Pyrogens (fever-producing products from dead bacteria)

Preventive measures to be taken include

- maintaining a clean working environment;
- ensuring good aseptic technique by personnel;
- using pyrogen-free, high-quality, and properly stored raw materials;
- utilizing proper bottle-washing procedures;
- rinsing bottles with purified water prior to filling;
- using a new rubber stopper for each bottle;
- sterilizing the product immediately after filling the bottles;

IV Production and Other Sterile Compounding

Sterile products that can be successfully manufactured locally, such as IV fluids, small-volume injections, and eyedrops, consist primarily of purified water (see Country Studies 19.3 and 19.4). Injections consisting of powder to be reconstituted should not be locally made, since they often require special production facilities to avoid cross-contamination with other products. Due to the shortage of essential sterile eyedrops in many developing countries, much work has been done to encourage their small-scale

► employing a reliable autoclave;
► cleaning equipment immediately after use;
► drying equipment before storage.

Products packaged in injection vials with rubber stoppers (sometimes called serum bottles) are much easier to produce than those packaged in single-dose sealed ampoules. Products should be chosen for production based on cost-effectiveness considerations. In order to avoid contamination of the vial contents through multiple uses, multiple-dose products should contain a suitable preservative. Fortunately, the most common sizes of injection vials (10 mL up to 100 mL) have the same size rubber stopper and aluminum outer seal, which simplifies the procurement of packaging supplies.

For large-volume sterile production (using containers whose capacity exceeds 100 mL), the most important decision is the choice of water purification method, since the water is used in various preparations and to rinse bottles and other equipment. For a production unit to be economically justifiable, a minimum of about 10,000 liters per year, or at least one 30-liter batch per day, needs to be produced.

Since as much water is needed for rinsing operations as for actual production, the water purifying system should be able to produce at least 60 liters within the time of one batch run. Of the existing low-cost water purifying systems, only the reverse osmosis process can economically produce this much water in the required time. The alternative is to use more sophisticated and expensive distillation equipment and special high-temperature holding vessels (see Box 19.1).

Traditional stainless-steel distillers are durable but are being replaced with glass models because of GMP considerations. One such apparatus is the Schott distiller, which produces only 3 liters per hour and uses far greater amounts of electricity and water than reverse osmosis. At this rate, ten hours are required just to make enough water for a typical production batch, with nothing left over for rinsing equipment. In addition, the water distilled at the beginning of the process can be contaminated by bacteria by the time the last water is distilled ten hours later. This is the major drawback of small-capacity stills, because bacteria, which inevitably get into the product, have sufficient time to multiply unless the distillate is held at a very high temperature (80°C).

Risk of infection from bacteria can be controlled, because even solutions containing a significant bacterial load are sterilized when autoclaved. However, although all the bacteria have been killed, this sterile solution may still produce pyrogenic (fever) reactions, which are caused by the breakdown products of the dead bacteria. It is possible

Box 19.1 Comparison of the Two Principal Methods of Producing Purified Water

The United States Pharmacopeia (USP) accepts that purified water can be obtained either by distillation or by reverse osmosis (RO). Either of these methods produces water of extremely high quality, suitable for use in pharmaceutical production. According to the USP, the purified water can be used for the production of certain sterile preparations if it meets additional standards for purity, including ion content, as measured by conductivity. Water that does is then called water for injection (WFI). To achieve the low level of ions (particularly Na^+) required by the USP, RO water would have to be further demineralized by special mixed-bed exchangers, since the pretreatment water softening required by RO adds Na^+ to the feed water. This is not a major problem, however, since trace amounts of a physiological substance are involved, which field experience has shown are not harmful. When large quantities of water are needed, RO is preferred, since it is much more rapidly and efficiently produced, solving many of the problems inherent in sterile production taking place over many hours (multiplying of bacteria, allowing the formation of pyrogens when the product is terminally sterilized). All other factors are usually less important when one is choosing the best method to use for the preparation of purified water.

to remove all these bacteria by membrane filtration before sterilization, but the filled bottles must be sterilized immediately after filling. If these solutions are not sterilized within three hours after the production of the water, the chance of a pyrogen reaction is great.

Preparation of multiple small batches allows for much smaller and less expensive autoclaves and is usually preferable to making one large batch per day. Under no circumstances should the purified water, whether produced by distillation or by reverse osmosis, be kept for more than three to four hours without further sterilization or preservation. Speed is of the utmost importance in the sterile production area, and work flow patterns must be designed to facilitate rapid production while simultaneously minimizing the potential risk of contamination or error. As part of routine internal quality control, the environment in the clean room must be constantly monitored, and each bottle visually examined for particulate matter or other problems, such as cracks.

Appropriate reverse osmosis technology, conventional sterility testing, and simplified pyrogen testing using an indirect colony-counting method are described in the manual by Kamm (1995). A newer limulus test for direct pyrogen testing is specific and simple to perform. It is certainly the preferred method, if supplies can be obtained. *If basic sterility and pyrogen testing cannot be performed by a local laboratory, IV fluids should not be produced locally.* ■

≡ Assessment Guide

1. Review of Current Local Production

► For each local production facility, describe the following (if there is no current local production, go on to section 2):

  ► Type of facility and location
  ► Staff and training
  ► Size of the compounding area
  ► Building/production space
  ► Equipment used
  ► Climate control
  ► Source of conditioning, packaging materials
  ► Source of water
  ► Electrical supply
  ► Production records
  ► Quality control procedures
  ► Annual recurrent costs for:

    –Space
    –Utilities
    –Personnel
    –Packaging/supplies
    –Equipment
    –Maintenance
    –Overhead

  ► Clients
  ► Product recipes

► What type of pharmaceutical forms are produced?

► Attach a list of the products currently manufactured or compounded with the following information:

  ► Description (name, form, strength, route of administration)
  ► Pharmacopeial standard
  ► Manufacturer
  ► Manufacturing cost (actual or estimated)
  ► Quantity produced per year
  ► Selling price
  ► Is this product (or equivalent) also imported as a finished product? (If the answer is no, skip to the last bullet.)
  ► Cost of the imported finished product
  ► Selling price of the imported finished product
  ► Quantity imported per year

► Describe any problems or concerns.

2. Feasibility Issues

► Do local production facilities have to comply with GMP regulations or other similar regulations for the production, distribution, and investigation of drugs?

► Are there any special regulations in effect that govern local manufacturing by a hospital pharmacy? Are these regulations being adequately enforced?

► Is there any program for the inspection of local production facilities?

► How many inspectors does the drug regulatory agency have? How many inspections were made in each of the last three years?

► Do inspectors use a checklist for carrying out inspections?

► If the existing local production capability is insufficient or of poor quality, has a feasibility study been conducted to evaluate the market and available resources before local production is expanded?

► Have the results of the feasibility study been evaluated? Are sufficient personnel, buildings, water, power, equipment, and documentation present, or can they be obtained? What quality control facilities are available? Are they adequate for the products to be produced locally?

► Is there a need for COT or special packaging for local use? Are sufficient equipment, supplies, and personnel available to start this type of production? Is it possible to ensure that packaging, labeling, and quality control are adequate?

► What specific products (nonsterile and sterile) could be produced locally? Are they cost effective to produce? Is the production sustainable? (Is cost recovery in effect? Are funds available to purchase raw materials, packaging supplies, and spare parts?)

► Are production and control worksheets available for each product produced? Are repackaging and COT packaging and control worksheets available for each product?

► Are adequate maintenance facilities available for all the buildings and equipment?

► Are adequate training facilities and supervisory personnel available?

≡ References and Further Readings

★ = Key readings.

Bakker, P., H. van Doorne, V. Gooskens, and N. Wieringa. 1990. *Dermatologic preparations for the tropics*, Groningen, Netherlands: University of Groningen.

★ FIP (Fédération Internationale Pharmaceutique). 1993. *Guidelines for small-scale hospital production of large volume parenteral fluids in developing countries*. Amsterdam: International Pharmaceutical Federation, Netherlands Section of Hospital Pharmacists.

Gennaro, A., ed. 1995. *Remington's pharmaceutical sciences*, 19th ed. Easton, Pa.: Mack Publishing Company.

★ International Dispensary Association (IDA). 1992. *Small-scale production of IV fluids*. Amsterdam: IDA.

★ Kamm, G. 1995. *Manual for decentralized infusion production*. Moshi, Tanzania: Infusion Unit Project.

Liebsch, B., D. S. Nyamageni, S. S. Senya, and K. F. Steinhausen. 1988. *Tanzanian pharmaceutical handbook*. Dar es Salaam, Tanzania: Dar es Salaam University Press.

Monson, M. H., and P. E. Mertens. 1988. A system for making hospital solutions in the third world. *Tropical Doctor* 18:54–59.

★ Reynolds, J., ed. 1996. *Martindale: The extra pharmacopoeia*, 31st ed. London: Pharmaceutical Press.

Rhodes, D. 1988. *Good manufacturing practice*. Harare, Zimbabwe: Zimbabwe Essential Drugs Action Programme.

Taylor, J. 1989. *Manual for the local production of eye drops*, 2d ed. Bensheim, Germany: CBM.

Turco, S. 1994. *Sterile dosage forms*, 4th ed. Philadelphia: Lea and Febiger.

USP (United States Pharmacopeial Convention). 1995. *The United States pharmacopeia/the national formulary*. USP 23/NF 18. Rockville, Md.: USP.

Watt, R. 1996. *Manual for pharmacy workers in developing countries*. Unpublished. Coatesville, Pa.

★ WHO (World Health Organization). 1990. *The local small-scale preparation of eye drops*. WHO/PBL/90.20. Geneva: WHO.

WHO (World Health Organization). 1992a. *Good manufacturing practices for pharmaceutical products*. Technical report series no. 823. Geneva: WHO.

WHO (World Health Organization). 1992b. *WHO expert committee on specifications for pharmaceutical preparations*. Technical report series no. 823. Geneva: WHO.

WHO (World Health Organization). 1993. *WHO expert committee on specifications for pharmaceutical preparations*. Technical report series no. 834. Geneva: WHO.

WHO (World Health Organization). 1995. *The use of essential drugs: Model list of essential drugs*. Technical report series no. 850. Geneva: WHO.

Part I	Part II	**Part III**	Part IV
Introduction	Policy and Legal Framework	**Drug Management Cycle**	Management Support Systems

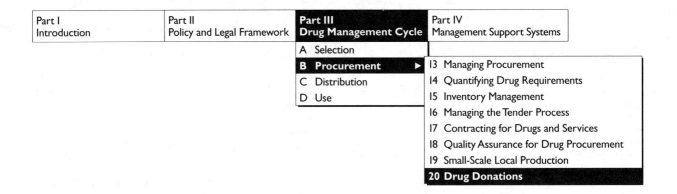

A Selection

B Procurement ▶

C Distribution

D Use

13 Managing Procurement
14 Quantifying Drug Requirements
15 Inventory Management
16 Managing the Tender Process
17 Contracting for Drugs and Services
18 Quality Assurance for Drug Procurement
19 Small-Scale Local Production
20 Drug Donations

Chapter 20
Drug Donations

≡ Summary

Most drug donations are given with the best of intentions but can nevertheless create problems at the receiving end. Often, donated drugs are not relevant to the needs of the recipient, or they arrive unsorted or close to expiry. They may be labeled with a brand name or in a language that is not understood. Many drug donations counteract government policies or violate national regulations of the recipient country.

Guidelines for drug donations are needed for a number of reasons. Donors and recipients do not communicate on equal terms, and recipients often need assistance in formulating their needs. Many donors do not understand the potential difficulties at the receiving end and need guidance. Drugs require special regulations because they are different from other donated items. Drug donations that occur without input from the recipient countries should be discouraged.

The three core principles for a useful drug donation are:

1. *A donation should be intended only to assist the recipient.*

2. *A donation should be given with full respect for the authority of the recipient.*

3. *Items that are not acceptable in the donor country for quality-related reasons are also not acceptable as donations: there should be no double standards in quality.*

These principles have been translated into a set of guidelines for drug donations. First, recipients should review and adopt these guidelines and present them officially to the donor community. Only then can they be implemented and enforced. Second, recipients should develop and publish administrative procedures for drug donations. Third, recipients should indicate to the donors, as clearly as possible, how they want to be helped, specifying the drugs they need, the quantities, and the priorities. Donors should inform the recipients well in advance which drug donations are coming, and when.

≡ 20.1 Introduction

In the face of disaster and suffering, there is a natural human impulse to reach out and help those in need. Donations of medicines are an essential element in alleviating people's suffering, and international humanitarian relief efforts benefit enormously from regular donations by private individuals, groups, and organizations. Unfortunately, many drug donations have caused problems instead of being helpful.

This chapter presents an overview of the problems encountered with inappropriate drug donations, describes a set of guidelines for drug donations, and offers some practical recommendations for recipients and donors.

≡ 20.2 Problems with Drug Donations

There are many different types of drug donations, and each has its own set of specific problems. The types covered in this section are

- drug donations in emergency situations;
- drug donations between governments as part of development aid;
- donations of returned drugs.

Drug Donations in Emergency Situations

A sizable disaster does not always lead to an objective assessment of the emergency medical needs, based on hard facts and past experience. Very often, an emotional appeal for massive medical assistance is issued. The term "medical supplies" in times of emergency has connotations that

often prevent an objective approach. Numerous examples of inappropriate drug donations have been reported (see Country Study 20.1). The main problems can be summarized as follows:

- Donated drugs are often not relevant for the emergency situation or for the level of care that is available.
- Health workers are not always familiar with the donated drugs.
- The drugs are often not registered for use in the recipient country and may not comply with local treatment guidelines.
- The drugs that arrive are frequently unsorted, difficult to identify, unknown in the recipient country, labeled with brand names, or labeled in a language that is not locally understood.
- The quality of the drugs does not always comply with standards in the donor country. Donated drugs may have expired or may expire before they reach the patient, or they may be returned drugs (half-finished packages that have been returned to the pharmacy, or free samples given to health professionals).
- The distribution plan often ignores normal administrative procedures. For example, the donation may not automatically be eligible for tax-free importation, resulting in high costs to the receiving agency; the distribution system may bypass the central government stores; or the value of the donated drugs may lead to a reduction in the government drug budget.

Country Study 20.1 Problems with Drug Donations

Armenia, 1988. After the earthquake, 5,000 tons of drugs and medical supplies worth US$55 million were sent to Armenia. This quantity far exceeded needs, and the handling, storage, and management of the drugs during the emergency were very demanding. It took fifty people six months to gain a clear picture of the drugs that had been received. It turned out that 8 percent of the drugs had expired on arrival, and 4 percent were destroyed by frost. Of the remaining 88 percent, 70 percent were finally sorted out. Of these, only 42 percent were relevant for an emergency situation, and only 30 percent were easy to identify. The main hindrance to identification was that the majority of the drugs were labeled only with brand names.

Burkina Faso, 1978. A 170-kg wooden crate with medicines was airlifted to a rural clinic in Burkina Faso. It contained 90 kg of drugs, half of which were expired upon arrival. Of the rest, 10 kg were useless or dangerous, 15 kg were usable but not really needed, and only 20 kg were of clear value. However, half of these were for use at a hospital and not really relevant for a rural clinic.

Eritrea, 1993. During the war for independence, despite careful wording of appeals, much time and energy had to be spent sorting drug consignments. Examples of inappropriate donations included seven truckloads of expired aspirin tablets that took six months to burn, a whole container of unsolicited cardiovascular drugs with two months to expiry, and 30,000 half-liter bottles of expired amino-acid infusion that could not be disposed of anywhere near a settlement because of the smell.

France, 1991. Pharmaciens sans Frontières collected 4 million kg of unused drugs from 4,000 pharmacies in France. These were sorted out in eighty-eight centers in the country. Only about 20 percent could be used for international aid programs, and 80 percent were burned. In view of the enormous investment in expensive human resources, the purchase of essential drugs under generic name would have been much more cost effective.

Guatemala, 1976. In the first week after the earthquake in Guatemala, 7,000 cartons of mixed drugs arrived. These were sorted by a group of forty pharmacy students at a rate of twenty-five to fifty boxes per day (it took about six months to finish the job). Only 10 percent of the drugs sent were sorted and labeled correctly and relevant to needs.

Guinea Bissau, 1993. In September, eight tons of donated drugs arrived; all were returned drugs collected from pharmacies in France, in quantities of between one and one hundred tablets. This donation contained 22,123 packages of 1,714 different drugs, which were very difficult to manage and greatly interfered with government efforts to rationalize drug supply and use.

Lithuania, 1993. Eleven women in Lithuania temporarily lost their eyesight after using a drug that had been provided through drug donations. The drug, closantel, was an anthelmintic that should be used only in veterinary medicine but was mistakenly given for the treatment of endometritis. The donation had been received without product information or package inserts, and doctors had tried to identify the product by matching the name on the box with the names on leaflets of other products.

Russia, 1992. Russian pharmaceutical production had fallen to below 5 percent of its 1990 level, and donations of drugs were welcomed. However, initial enthusiasm soured when the nature of some donations was discovered. Examples of donations included 189,000 bottles of dextromethorphan cough syrup, pentoxifylline and clonidine as the only antihypertensive items, triamterene and spironolactone as diuretics, and pancreatic enzyme and bismuth preparations as the only gastrointestinal drugs.

Sudan, 1990. A large consignment of drugs was sent from France to war-devastated southern Sudan. Each box contained a collection of small packets of drugs, some partly used. All were labeled in French, a language not spoken in Sudan. Most were inappropriate; some could be dangerous. These included contact lens solution, appetite stimulants, monoamine oxidase inhibitors (dangerous in Sudan), X-ray solutions, drugs against hypercholesterolemia, and expired antibiotics. Of fifty boxes, twelve contained drugs of some use. It would have been much better to have used the money spent on transport to purchase penicillin and other essential drugs in Kenya, which could then have been sent to Sudan.

Yugoslavia, 1994. Of all drug donations received by the WHO field office in Zagreb, 15 percent were completely unusable, and 30 percent were not needed.

Source: WHO/DAP 1996.

There are several underlying reasons for these problems. Probably the most important factor is the common but mistaken belief that any type of drug is better than nothing at all, and that expired drugs are good enough for people in need. Second, drug donations are often not based on an expressed need or cleared by the recipient before dispatch. Third, in many donor countries, donated drugs are tax-deductible (at full market price); this is why so many donated drugs arrive close to or past their expiry date and why they are not high-use, high-volume items. Drug donations initiated by pharmaceutical companies in exchange for tax breaks are particularly likely to be drugs that are not commonly viewed as essential.

Inappropriate drug donations create logistical problems because they must be sorted, stored, and distributed, sometimes using precious human resources and transport volume in disaster areas or war zones. Or they may pose an environmental threat if they have to be destroyed. Often, the total transport costs are higher than the value of the drugs.

Drug Donations as Part of Development Aid

Most of the problems noted above may also apply to large drug donations between governments given as part of development (commodity) aid. The situation is usually better than with emergency aid, however, as there is more

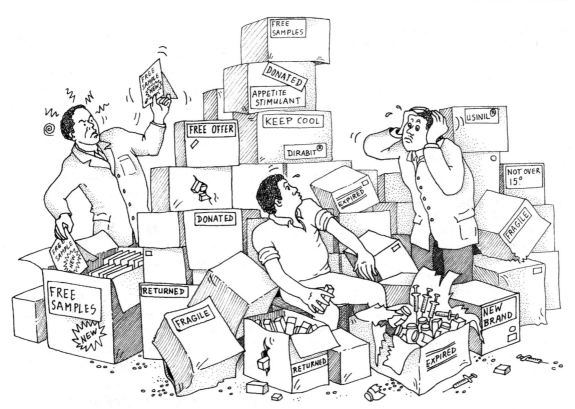

DONATIONS CAN THEMSELVES BE A DISASTER AREA

time to plan for the donations. Generally, the recipient is more involved in specifying what is needed.

The ideal situation occurs when the recipient country can indicate specific drugs and quantities needed, without any restriction on the selection and country of origin of the drugs. Unfortunately, this is rarely the case. The choice is often restricted to manufacturers or suppliers in the donor country. Even if the drugs are listed generically on the national list of essential drugs in the recipient country, the donated items are often brand-name products that may not be registered in the recipient country. The donation may then interfere with the implementation of national registration, quality assurance, and inspection schemes. If the selection of drugs is restricted by the donor, the donation may not be in accordance with national programs promoting standard treatment guidelines and rational drug use.

The same problems can also occur when drugs are imported as part of a barter (when goods are exchanged between countries without payment in hard currency). Here, the problem is that bartered drugs are usually selected from what happens to be produced in the exporting country, and the barter negotiations are carried out by staff of the ministries of trade and/or finance rather

than by pharmaceutical staff of the ministry of health. Although no currency exchange is involved, in the barter negotiations, the drugs are often valued at market value in the donor country and not at world market prices. Therefore, obtaining drugs through barter is often much more expensive in terms of opportunity cost than procurement by tender, despite the fact that no money is spent.

Donations of Returned Drugs
Many nongovernmental groups in developed countries collect unused drugs (returned drugs or free samples) and send these in emergency situations or, on a regular basis, to institutions in developing countries. At the receiving end, such donations can frustrate all efforts to manage and administer drug stocks in a rational way. Donating returned drugs is a clear example of double standards: in no developed country would the use of such drugs be permitted. In addition, these drugs are a problem for doctor and patient. The prescriber is forced to use countless different drugs and brands in ever-changing dosages; patients on long-term treatment suffer because the same drug may not be available next time. For these reasons, this type of donation is generally discouraged and even forbidden in

some countries. The immense effort required to sort the drugs is largely wasted because most of them are unusable.

The Need for Guidelines

The examples of inappropriate donations noted above constitute ample reason to develop international guidelines for drug donations. In summary, guidelines are needed because:

► Donor and recipient do not communicate on equal terms; recipients therefore need assistance in specifying how they want to be helped.
► Many donors mean well but do not realize the difficulties at the receiving end and need guidance.
► Drugs are different from other donated items, in that drugs can be harmful, they require labels and written information, they need adequately trained personnel to be used effectively, they may expire, and they may have to be destroyed in a particular way.
► Inappropriate donations frustrate the implementation of national drug policies and programs to promote rational drug use.

≡ 20.3 Chronology of Existing Guidelines for Drug Donations

In 1988, the Christian Medical Commission (CMC) of the World Council of Churches in Geneva was the first orga-

nization to issue guidelines for drug donations (CMC 1990; see Country Study 20.2). This carefully worded document was specifically intended to make more rational the many donations that are made to individual church-related hospitals by well-intentioned but ignorant groups of individuals. The guidelines are consistent with the World Health Organization (WHO) essential drugs concept and stress the need to use generic names, to provide the drugs in hospital packs, to limit drug donations to drugs on the national list of essential drugs or the WHO model list, and to send drugs with a shelf life of at least one year upon arrival in the recipient country. The document mentions tactfully that a financial contribution is usually more appropriate. Chapter 12 discusses similar CMC guidelines in relation to equipment donations.

In 1990, the WHO Action Programme on Essential Drugs, in collaboration with major international emergency aid agencies, issued a set of guidelines for donors that was included in *The New Emergency Health Kit* (WHO/DAP 1990). As with those of the CMC, these guidelines stress that donations should be based on a specific request by the recipient and should, in all cases, be cleared prior to dispatch. Minimum labeling and outside packaging information standards are also specified.

In 1994, the WHO office in Zagreb issued detailed guidelines for humanitarian assistance for the former Yugoslavia, where WHO acts as a clearinghouse for all donations of drugs and medical supplies (WHO 1994). The guidelines are specific for the situation, listing criteria for the acceptance of donations and for necessary documentation, labeling, and packaging.

The WHO Expert Committee on the Use of Essential Drugs has also discussed and endorsed a set of donor guidelines (WHO 1996). These are based largely on the earlier guidelines, but they add advice on quality assurance and specifically exclude the donation of returned drugs and drug samples.

≡ 20.4 Guidelines for Drug Donations

In 1996 WHO concluded a worldwide consultative process to develop *Guidelines for Drug Donations*, in close collaboration with the Office of the United Nations High Commissioner for Refugees (UNHCR), United Nations Children's Fund (UNICEF), the Red Cross, and nongovernmental organizations.

Core Principles

The first and paramount principle is that a donation should be intended only to assist the recipient, and all efforts should be made to maximize its positive impact.

Box 20.1 Guidelines for Drug Donations

These guidelines for drug donations, developed by WHO, reflect consensus among the major international agencies active in humanitarian emergency relief: WHO, UNHCR, UNICEF, International Committee of the Red Cross, International Federation of the Red Cross and Red Crescent Societies, Médecins sans Frontières, Churches' Action for Health of the World Council of Churches, and OXFAM.

There are many different scenarios for drug donations. They may take place in acute emergencies or as part of development aid in nonemergency situations. They may be corporate donations (direct or through private voluntary organizations), aid by governments, or donations to single health facilities. And although there are legitimate differences among these scenarios, the basic rules for an appropriate donation apply to all. The guidelines describe this common core of good donation practices.

The guidelines aim to improve the quality of drug donations, not to hinder them. They are not international regulations but are intended to serve as a basis for national or institutional guidelines, to be reviewed, adapted, and implemented by governments and organizations dealing with drug donations.

Selection of Drugs

1. All drug donations should be based on an expressed need and be relevant to the disease pattern in the recipient country. Drugs should not be sent without prior consent by the recipient.

2. All donated drugs or their generic equivalents should be approved for use in the recipient country and appear on the national list of essential drugs, or, if a national list is not available, on the WHO *Model List of Essential Drugs,* unless specifically requested otherwise by the recipient.

3. The presentation, strength, and formulation of donated drugs should, as much as possible, be similar to those commonly used in the recipient country.

Quality Assurance and Shelf Life

4. All donated drugs should be obtained from a reliable source and comply with quality standards in both the donor and the recipient country. The WHO certification scheme on the quality of pharmaceutical products moving

in international commerce (WHO 1992) should be used.

5. No drugs that were issued to patients and then returned to a pharmacy or elsewhere, or that were given to health professionals as free samples, should be donated.

6. After arrival in the recipient country all donated drugs should have a remaining shelf life of at least one year.

Presentation, Packing, and Labeling

7. All drugs should be labeled in a language that is easily understood by health professionals in the recipient country; the label on each individual container should contain at least the international nonproprietary name (INN, or generic name), batch number, dosage form, strength, name of manufacturer, quantity in the container, storage conditions, and expiry date.

8. As much as possible, donated drugs should be presented in larger-quantity units and hospital packs.

9. All drug donations should be packed in accordance with international shipping regulations, and be accompanied by a detailed packing list which specifies the contents of each numbered carton by INN, dosage form, quantity, batch number, expiry date, volume, weight, and any special storage conditions. The weight per carton should not exceed 50 kilograms. Drugs should not be mixed with other supplies in the same carton.

Information and Management

10. Recipients should be informed of all drug donations that are being considered, prepared or actually under way.

11. In the recipient country the declared value of a drug donation should be based upon the wholesale price of its generic equivalent in the recipient country, or, if such information is not available, on the wholesale world-market price for its generic equivalent.

12. Costs of international and local transport, warehousing, port clearance, and appropriate storage and handling should be paid by the donor agency, unless specifically agreed otherwise with the recipient in advance.

Source: WHO 1996.

This implies that all donations should be based on an expressed need by the recipient and that donor-driven donations are not advisable. The second principle is that a donation should be given with full respect for the authority of the recipient and be supportive of existing government policies and administrative arrangements. The third principle is that there should be no double standards: if the quality of an item is unacceptable in the donor country, it is also unacceptable as a donation (see Figure 20.1). The fourth principle is effective communication between the donor and the recipient.

If these core principles are adhered to, donations will usually be helpful rather than harmful, if the specific guidelines

on drug selection, quality, presentation, packaging, and labeling in Box 20.1 are followed.

Special Guidelines for Drug Donations in Emergency Situations

In emergency situations, it may not be practical to wait for a specific request from the recipient. In any case, however, all proposed donations should be approved by the recipient before they are sent.

In the acute phase of an emergency, or in the case of refugee populations without any medical care, it is better to send a range of drugs and medical supplies that is specifically designed for this purpose. The new emergency health

Figure 20.1 Four Core Principles for Good Drug Donations

1. A donation should be intended to assist the recipient.
2. A donation should respect the full authority of the recipient and support existing government policies.
3. There should be no double standards in quality.
4. There should be effective communication between the donor and the recipient.

kit, which has been widely used since 1990, contains drugs, disposable supplies, and basic equipment for a population of 10,000 for three months. Its contents are based on a consensus among the major international aid agencies (WHO, UNICEF, UNHCR, Red Cross organizations, Médecins sans Frontières, and OXFAM). It is permanently stocked by several major international suppliers (for example, UNICEF and IDA) and can be available within 48 hours.

From the recipients' point of view, a donation in cash for the local purchase of essential drugs is usually much more welcome than a donation in kind (assuming the local market is functional). Apart from being supportive of the activities of the local coordinating body, it is usually more cost effective and also supports local industry. In addition, local prescribers and patients are usually more familiar with locally available drugs. A donation in cash also avoids the problem of the coordinating body having to prioritize long lists of needs according to what might or might not arrive.

Special Guidelines for Donations as Part of Development Aid

When drugs are donated as part of development aid, there is usually more time available to specify needs and to follow guidelines on drug donations. Special care should be taken that the drugs and their specifications comply with the national drug policy and are in accordance with national treatment guidelines or common practice in the recipient country. Administratively, the drugs should be treated as if they were procured. This means that they should be registered for use in the country (probably through the same simplified procedure that would apply for government tenders). They should be entered into the inventory and distributed through the existing distribution channels. If cost-sharing procedures exist, the donated drugs should not automatically be distributed free of charge, and the donor should not insist on free distribution. A good example of a successful integration of donated drugs into the regular drug supply system in Mongolia is described in Country Study 20.3.

Country Study 20.3 Integrating Drug Donations into the Regular Drug Supply System in Mongolia

After the collapse of the former USSR, Mongolia became one of the countries where a large proportion of drug consumption is covered by drug donations. In this country, such donations are treated as regularly procured drugs.

Upon the arrival of a donation, all papers are sent to the Ministry of Health for clearance of the import. If the drugs are accepted, an import price is decided on by a special unit in the ministry. This price is normally equal to the last tender price for the same product or a price taken from the *International Drug Price Indicator Guide* (MSH 1995). Many donors are valuing their donations at a much higher price—for example, retail price in the donor country—but this is not accepted as a reference. If a product that is not on the Mongolian essential drugs list is accepted, it is given a price equivalent to that for a similar drug on the list, irrespective of the price in the donor country.

The value of the drug consignment is entered into the accounts of Mongol Emimpex, the state wholesaler. Each drug is then given a retail selling price by adding a 15 percent markup for the wholesaler and 23 percent for the pharmacist. These markups cover all expenses for control and distribution. The (assigned) import value is kept on a separate account and transferred to a fund controlled by the Ministry of Health for future drug procurement.

The main benefit of this system is that it is sustainable and not destructive to the existing drug supply system. It is well known that in many other countries uncontrolled sales of donated drugs take place, and the money is pocketed by health personnel. In Mongolia, the system is completely transparent. All drugs coming into the country are for sale, and the donors are assured that their import value goes back to the revolving fund.

The only drawback of the system is that even the most needy customers—patients or health institutions—have to pay for donated drugs, and they may not be able to do so. However, this would also be the case with normal drug procurement and has to be solved by health insurance systems or specific government support to the needy.

Source: WHO/DAP 1996.

≡ 20.5 Implementation of a Policy for Drug Donations

In managing drug donations, both recipients and donors need to act to ensure that appropriate donations are received and that good use is made of them.

Management of Drug Donations by the Recipient

Recipient governments must play a role in managing donations. No matter how disastrous the situation, failure to be involved may make things worse. National guidelines and administrative procedures need to be defined, and any requirements need to be specified in as much detail as possible.

Define National Guidelines for Drug Donations. It is notoriously difficult for recipients to refuse a donation that is already under way. For this reason, prevention is better than cure. The key point is that recipients should indicate to their (future) donors what kind of assistance they are likely to need and how they would like to receive it. If this information is provided in a rational and professional way, most donors appreciate it and will comply. Therefore, recipients should first formulate their own guidelines for drug donations on the basis of the CMC or WHO guidelines or the summary given above. These guidelines should then be officially presented to the donor community. Only after the guidelines have been presented and published can they be enforced.

Define Administrative Procedures for Drug Donations. It is not enough for recipients to adopt and publish general guidelines on the selection, quality, and presentation of donations. Administrative procedures need to be developed by recipients for defining needs, receiving donations, distributing, budgeting, and perhaps refusing or destroying some goods. Procedures need to be developed to carry out the following actions:

- ► Define needs;
- ► Prioritize among different requirements;
- ► Coordinate all drug donations;
- ► Decide what documentation is needed when a drug donation is being proposed, and who should receive these papers;
- ► Establish criteria for accepting or rejecting a donation;
- ► Coordinate reception, storage, and distribution of donated drugs;
- ► Agree on how donations are to be valued in budget and expenditure records;
- ► Agree on charging for donated drugs in the context of a public user fee program;
- ► Deal with donated drugs not registered or included in the national essential drugs list in the country;
- ► Dispose of worthless donations.

Specify the Needs for Donated Drugs. Recipients must also provide donors with as much specific information on drug needs as possible. This puts the onus on the recipient to prepare requests carefully, indicating quantities required and prioritizing the items. The more information given, the better. Openness about donations that are already in the pipeline, or anticipated, is helpful to donors. It is always greatly appreciated and pays off in the long run. Recipients are entitled to the same openness from donors with regard to drug donations that are in the pipeline.

Good Practices for Donors

Donors should always respect the four core principles listed in Figure 20.1. Donors should also respect the guidelines issued by the recipients and respond to the priority needs they have indicated. Donor-driven donations should be discouraged as much as possible. This is particularly applicable to donations that are initiated by international drug companies to obtain tax advantages, or donations of returned drugs or samples.

The public at large in the donor country is usually not aware of common problems with drug donations. It is therefore important that the government make some effort to create more public awareness of donors' responsibilities. The best moment for this is probably at the time of the public appeal through the media, when the government is requesting funds.

At the country level, it is usually recommended that the different donors choose a "lead donor" among themselves that coordinates the different actions among the donors and may also act as a central contact point in discussions with the recipient government.

As mentioned above, the recipient country should supply as much information on requested and approved donations as possible. But the donors themselves should also inform the recipient well in advance and in detail about which donations are coming, and when. This information will greatly assist the coordinating body in the recipient country in planning for the proper reception of the donations and in identifying the need for additional supplies. ■

≡ Assessment Guide

Indicators of Policy

- ▶ Is there a national policy on drug donations?
- ▶ What are the differences between the national policy and the WHO policy on drug donations?
- ▶ Is there a set of administrative procedures for managing drug donations?
- ▶ Do drug donations comply with the national list of essential drugs?

- ▶ Does the ministry of health have control over which drugs and supplies will be accepted?

Extent of Drug Donations

- ▶ What is the value of international aid received for drugs (cash and kind) compared with the value of the public drug budget spent?

Problems with Drug Donations

- ▶ What are the main problems with drug donations?

≡ References and Further Readings

★ = Key readings.

Arnold, P. J., and M. R. Reich. 1990. PVO pharmaceutical donations: Making the incentive fit the need. *Journal of Research in Pharmaceutical Economics* 2:49–70.

★ CMC (Christian Medical Commission–Churches' Action for Health). 1990. *Guidelines for donors and recipients of pharmaceutical donations*, 2d rev. ed. Geneva: CMC.

MSH (Management Sciences for Health). 1995. *International drug price indicator guide.* (Updated annually.) Boston: MSH.

WHO (World Health Organization). 1992. *WHO expert committee on specifications for pharmaceutical preparations.* Technical report series no. 823. Geneva: WHO.

WHO (World Health Organization). 1994. *Medical supplies donor guidelines for WHO humanitarian assistance for former Yugoslavia.* Zagreb, Yugoslavia: WHO.

WHO (World Health Organization). 1995. *The use of essential drugs.* Technical report series no. 850. Geneva: WHO.

WHO/DAP (World Health Organization/Action Programme on Essential Drugs). 1990. *The new emergency health kit.* WHO/DAP/90.1. Geneva: WHO.

★ WHO/DAP (World Health Organization/Action Programme on Essential Drugs). 1996. *Guidelines for drug donations.* WHO/DAP/96.2. Geneva: WHO.

| Part I | Part II | **Part III** | Part IV |
| Introduction | Policy and Legal Framework | **Drug Management Cycle** | Management Support Systems |

A Selection
B Procurement
C Distribution
D Use

Section C
Distribution

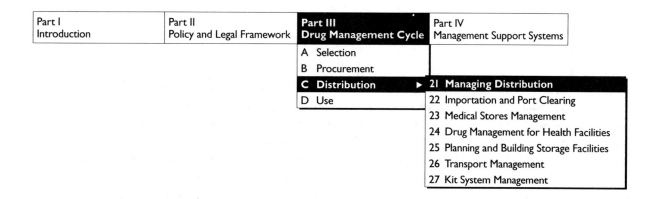

Part I	Part II	**Part III**	Part IV
Introduction	Policy and Legal Framework	**Drug Management Cycle**	Management Support Systems

A Selection
B Procurement
C Distribution ▶ **21 Managing Distribution**
D Use

22 Importation and Port Clearing
23 Medical Stores Management
24 Drug Management for Health Facilities
25 Planning and Building Storage Facilities
26 Transport Management
27 Kit System Management

Chapter 21
Managing Distribution

≡ Summary

Designing a system for storing and distributing drugs, medical supplies, and equipment is complex and important. Storage and distribution costs are a significant component of a health budget. Transportation costs can represent several times the value of the drugs distributed to remote locations.

Effective drug distribution relies on good system design and good management. A well-designed and well-managed distribution system should

- ► *maintain a constant supply of drugs;*
- ► *keep drugs in good condition throughout the distribution process;*
- ► *minimize drug losses due to spoilage and expiry;*
- ► *maintain accurate inventory records;*
- ► *rationalize drug storage points;*
- ► *use available transportation resources as efficiently as possible;*
- ► *reduce theft and fraud;*
- ► *provide information for forecasting drug needs.*

The distribution cycle includes the following steps:

- ► *port clearing*
- ► *receipt and inspection*
- ► *inventory control*
- ► *storage*
- ► *requisition of supplies*
- ► *delivery*
- ► *dispensing to patients*
- ► *reporting consumption*

There are four major elements of a distribution system:

1. System design *(geographic or population coverage, number of levels in the system, push versus pull system, degree of centralization);*
2. Information system *(inventory control, records and forms, consumption reports, information flow);*
3. Storage *(selection of sites, building design, materials handling systems, order picking);*
4. Delivery *(collection versus delivery, choice of transport, vehicle procurement, vehicle maintenance, routing and scheduling of deliveries).*

Whenever a new system is designed or an existing one is changed, cost analysis (comparing the total costs of using various options) can help ensure that limited storage, transport, and human resources are used effectively. There should be a program of performance monitoring to ensure that the distribution system works as intended.

Centralized distribution is not always the best option; some countries procure and distribute drugs regionally, and some use commercial supply systems, which often exist in parallel with public systems. Collaboration between private and public systems may occur at any level.

Operational planning and logistics skills are the key to developing a cost-effective distribution system. It is therefore important to have a logistics team staffed by qualified people.

The steps in planning a distribution system are as follows:

1. *Determine whether distribution operations should be carried out in the public or private sector.*
2. *Plan store locations and delivery routes:*
   - ► *Map the demand for drugs;*
   - ► *Locate supply entry points;*
   - ► *Rationalize primary storage points;*
   - ► *Plan primary distribution routes and locate intermediate stores;*
   - ► *Plan secondary distribution routes;*
   - ► *Size the stores.*
3. *Plan delivery schedules.*
4. *Establish staffing levels.*

In some countries, private or parastatal distribution companies can provide cost-effective alternatives for the storage and distribution of drugs, especially at the national and regional levels. Contracting out to such a company involves

- ► *assessing the cost of the existing system;*
- ► *preparing tender documents specifying service requirements;*
- ► *assessing the tenderers;*
- ► *signing the contract;*
- ► *monitoring the contractor's performance.*

Good communications are also essential to an effective distribution system.

≡ 21.1 Goals of Distribution Management

Storage and distribution costs are a significant component of the health budget. Transportation costs may exceed the value of the drugs distributed to some locations, especially in large countries with low population densities. Reducing these costs can mean that more money is available for drug purchases and for clinical care.

Health programs are frequently managed by well-qualified health personnel who lack logistics experience. *Logistics* is defined here as the "science (and art) of getting the right amounts of the right things to the right places at the right time" (Foster 1990, 207). Warehouse and transport managers, storekeepers, and drivers may have these skills but may have little influence on decision-making. The best way to use their knowledge and skills is to make them part of a logistics team to manage the system design process.

The primary management goal is to maintain a steady supply of drugs and supplies to facilities where they are needed while ensuring that resources are being used in the most effective way. A good distribution system is a *cost-effective* system.

A well-run distribution system should

► maintain a constant supply of drugs;
► keep drugs in good condition;
► minimize drug losses due to spoilage and expiry;
► rationalize drug storage points;
► use available transport as efficiently as possible;
► reduce theft and fraud;
► provide information for forecasting drug needs.

Senior management should regularly monitor the cost and performance of the distribution system as important indicators of the health care system's operations. Major alterations in the system should be introduced only after careful evaluation and planning, taking into account available human and material resources.

≡ 21.2 The Distribution Cycle

The distribution cycle begins when drugs are dispatched by the manufacturer or supplier. It ends when drug consumption information is reported back to the procurement unit. Figure 21.1 illustrates a typical public-sector drug distribution system and its interactions with the private sector.

The major activities of the distribution cycle are summarized in Figure 21.2. They include

Drug procurement (see Part III, Section B): The distribution sequence intersects the procurement process at the point at which drugs are available for delivery to the health facilities.

Port clearing (see Chapter 22): Unless the drugs are acquired locally or the international supplier takes responsibility for it, port clearing is the first step in making drugs available for distribution. Port clearing involves identifying shipments as soon as they arrive in port, processing all importation documents, completing any customs requirements, storing drugs properly until they leave the port, surveying the shipment for losses and signs of damage, and collecting the drugs as soon as they have been cleared. Port clearing may be managed directly or

through a separate contract with a port-clearing agent.

Receipt and inspection (see Chapter 23): Central stores staff must carry out a complete inspection of every shipment as soon as it is received from the port or local supplier. The shipment must be kept separate from other stock until this inspection has been completed. Inspectors should check for damaged and missing items and for compliance with the contract conditions concerning drug type, quantity, presentation, packaging, labeling, and any special requirements. Prompt and accurate inspection of all shipments is essential to ensure that suppliers fulfill their contracts. Insurance companies will demand an accurate record of any losses incurred before settling a claim.

Inventory control (see Chapters 15, 23, and 24): Establishing and maintaining effective inventory records and procedures are the basis for coordinating the flow of drugs through the distribution system and the primary protection against theft and corruption. The inventory control system is used for requisitioning and issuing drugs, for financial accounting, and for preparing the consumption and stock balance reports necessary for procurement. Record keeping must be sufficiently detailed to provide an "audit trail" that accurately traces the flow of drugs and funds through the system. This audit trail must be designed to satisfy the requirements of government auditors (and sometimes donor agencies) as well as program managers. An appropriate inventory management system should be adapted to suit the capacity and needs of personnel at all levels in the health program. Inventory records must be monitored regularly by supervisors to ensure accuracy and to avoid or detect losses.

Storage (see Chapters 23–25): Storage facilities may range from large mechanized warehouses at the national level to small wooden boxes sitting in health centers or carried by community health workers. Proper location, construction, organization, and maintenance of storage facilities help maintain drug quality, minimize theft, and maintain regular supply to health facilities.

Requisition of supplies (see Chapters 15, 23, and 24): Drug supply systems may operate under a push or a pull system (see Section 21.3). The forms and procedures for requisition are a key part of the inventory control system. They may vary from country to country and from one level to another within the same country. The requisition system may be manual or computerized, but it should always be designed to simplify distribution by facilitating inventory control, providing an audit trail for tracing the flow of drugs, assisting in financial accounting, and listing drugs issued.

Figure 21.1 Typical Public-Sector Drug Distribution System

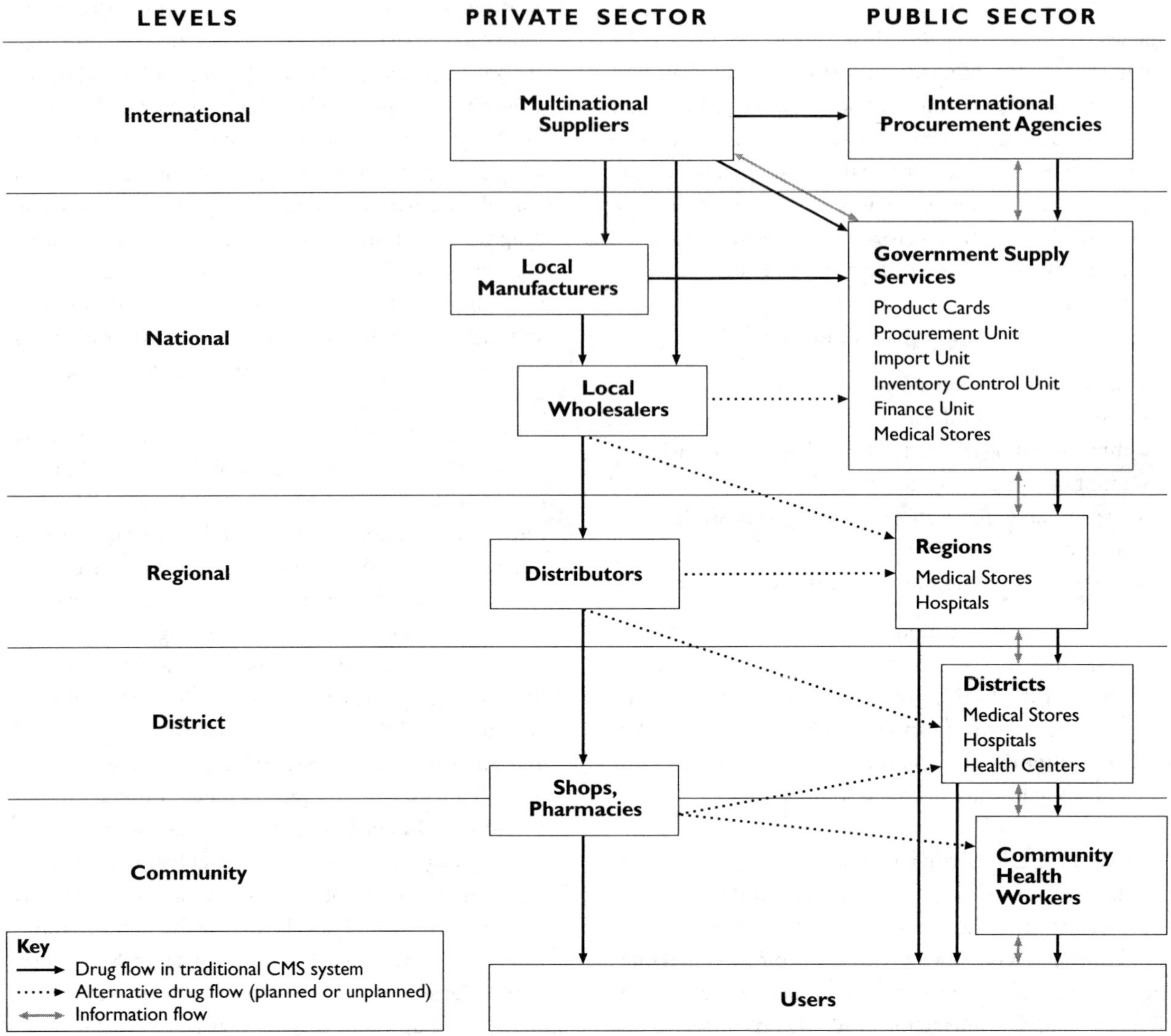

LEVELS	PRIVATE SECTOR	PUBLIC SECTOR

International
Multinational Suppliers → International Procurement Agencies

National
Local Manufacturers

Government Supply Services
- Product Cards
- Procurement Unit
- Import Unit
- Inventory Control Unit
- Finance Unit
- Medical Stores

Local Wholesalers

Regional
Distributors

Regions
- Medical Stores
- Hospitals

District

Districts
- Medical Stores
- Hospitals
- Health Centers

Community
Shops, Pharmacies

Community Health Workers

Users

Key
→ Drug flow in traditional CMS system
⋯▶ Alternative drug flow (planned or unplanned)
◀—▶ Information flow

Delivery (see Chapter 26): Drugs may be delivered by warehouses or collected by health facilities. Transport may involve air, water, railway, or on- and off-road vehicles. Cost-effective choices between public- and private-sector carriers need to be made. Transport managers should select methods of transportation carefully and schedule deliveries realistically and systematically, to provide punctual and economic service. Vehicle breakdowns; availability of fuel, lubricants, and spare parts; seasonal variations in access routes; safety along specific supply lines; and other local factors must all be considered in transport planning.

Dispensing to patients (see Chapter 32): The distribution process achieves its purpose when drugs reach hospital wards, outpatient clinics, health centers, or community

health workers and are appropriately prescribed and dispensed to patients.

Consumption reporting (see Chapters 14 and 15): The closing link in the distribution cycle is the flow of information on consumption and stock balances back up the distribution system to the procurement office for use in quantifying procurement needs. If adequate inventory and requisition records are kept, compiling consumption reports should be straightforward.

≡ **21.3 Distribution System Design**
Designing a distribution system requires systematic cost-effectiveness analysis and operational planning. Once the system is in place, regular performance monitoring is needed to ensure that the system functions as intended.

Figure 21.2 The Distribution Cycle

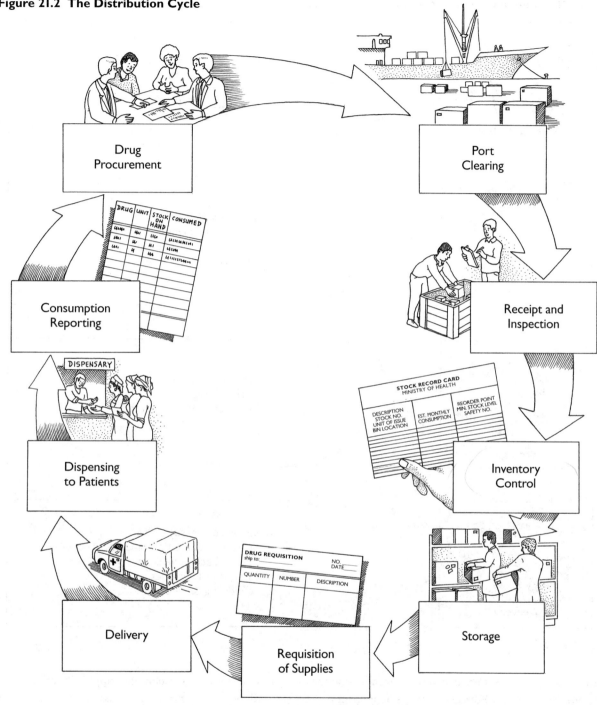

The major design characteristics for a distribution network (see Figure 21.3) are considered in detail in subsequent chapters and are mentioned only briefly here.

Basic Design Features

The basic characteristics of a distribution system include its degree of centralization, the number of levels in the system, and the geographic or population coverage. In a typical central supply model, drug procurement and distribution are coordinated at the national level. Drugs received at the central medical stores (CMS) are distributed to lower-level warehouses and onward to the health facilities. In a decentralized system, the districts or regions are responsible for receiving, storing, and distributing

Figure 21.3 Design Characteristics of Distribution Networks

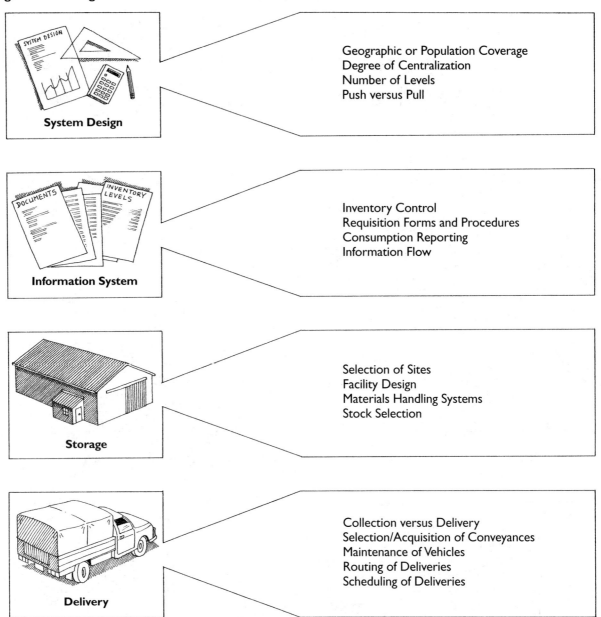

System Design
- Geographic or Population Coverage
- Degree of Centralization
- Number of Levels
- Push versus Pull

Information System
- Inventory Control
- Requisition Forms and Procedures
- Consumption Reporting
- Information Flow

Storage
- Selection of Sites
- Facility Design
- Materials Handling Systems
- Stock Selection

Delivery
- Collection versus Delivery
- Selection/Acquisition of Conveyances
- Maintenance of Vehicles
- Routing of Deliveries
- Scheduling of Deliveries

drugs; in some cases, they may also be responsible for procurement. Chapter 6 discusses various options for providing drugs to the public sector, some of which require in-house storage, and some of which eliminate part or all of supply system warehousing.

In designing a distribution system or redesigning an existing system, the following important steps have to be taken:

1. Determine the number of storage levels in the system.
2. Determine the location of storage sites.
3. Decide at which level of the supply system decisions will be made concerning orders.
4. Fix resupply intervals or frequency of placing orders.
5. Select a method for distributing drugs to user units.
6. Select an appropriate mode of transport.
7. Develop a set of feasible and economical delivery routes and work out a practical delivery schedule to service these routes.
8. Estimate operating costs and assess the cost effectiveness of contracting for storage and transport at one or more levels.

Figure 21.4 Comparison of Three-Level and Four-Level Distribution Hierarchies

Factors	Three-Level	Four-Level	Comments
Management complexity	Less complex	More complex	Four-level systems are more likely to have problems with transport, communications, and performance monitoring.

Set-up costs
  Buildings
  Equipment
  Vehicles
	Lower	Higher	In regions where clinical facilities are relatively numerous and/or widely dispersed, the costs of a four-level system may be justified.

Operating costs
  Personnel
  Utilities
  Fuel
  Expendable supplies
	Lower	Higher	The same observation as above.

Inventory holding costs	Lower	Higher	If a four-level system results in more dependable delivery, lower safety stock is needed, and inventory holding costs are not as high as expected.
Distribution of clinical facilities	Preferable with denser distribution	Often useful with sparser distribution	Distance can be measured in kilometers (miles), time, or transportation costs. Thus, an area that is small in square kilometers but is burdened with long travel times may benefit from a four-level system.

Quality of service
  Number of stockouts
  Ratio of interim and emergency
    to regular deliveries
	Variable, depending on the location of storage and clinical facilities and the reliability of transportation between facilities		Inventory control and delivery are harder to manage in extended systems, but with good management, such systems are more responsive to the needs of remote facilities.

Distribution Network

A public drug distribution system may require several layers of stores, each with distinct functions.

In a typical three-level distribution system, purchases are received by one or more *primary stores*, which generally serve a whole country or region and may or may not supply health facilities directly. The physical size of the primary stores is determined by national or regional demand for drugs and by the supply frequency. In some countries, this level has been eliminated, with direct delivery from suppliers to intermediate stores.

Drugs are distributed from the primary to the *intermediate stores*. Their size is determined by the demand of the area health facilities and the frequency of supply by the primary stores. Intermediate stores may be independent but are often on the site of a regional or district hospital. Intermediate stores distribute drugs to individual *health facility stores*. This would be a four-level system. Again, some countries eliminate both intermediate levels of store in favor of direct delivery to facilities from suppliers or a prime vendor (see Chapter 6).

Sometimes two layers of intermediate stores are needed, with first-level intermediate stores supplying second-level intermediate stores. For example, a regional store might supply district stores. Determining the optimum number of levels should be done individually according to program needs and resource constraints, weighing benefits against cost considerations. Some factors to consider in determining the number of storage levels are

► geographical factors
► population
► availability of storage space
► staff
► transport facilities
► political and other resource constraints

Figure 21.4 compares the three-and four-level systems in terms of management complexity, set-up costs, operating costs, inventory costs, and applicability according to location and density of clinical facilities. Three-level systems are easier to manage and may be less expensive to set up and operate. However, when clinical facilities are widely dispersed and travel times are long, the four-level system may provide better service and may even prove less expensive to operate when all costs are considered.

Figure 21.5 gives examples of four different distribution networks and shows how the quantity, and therefore the value of stock held in the system, tend to increase as more levels are added. Note that the relationships between costs and number of levels are not always as direct as shown in Figure 21.5—efficient inventory management in a CMS system might result in lower total inventory costs than would be found in a regional stores network with less efficient inventory management.

Figure 21.5   Comparison of Four Distribution Networks

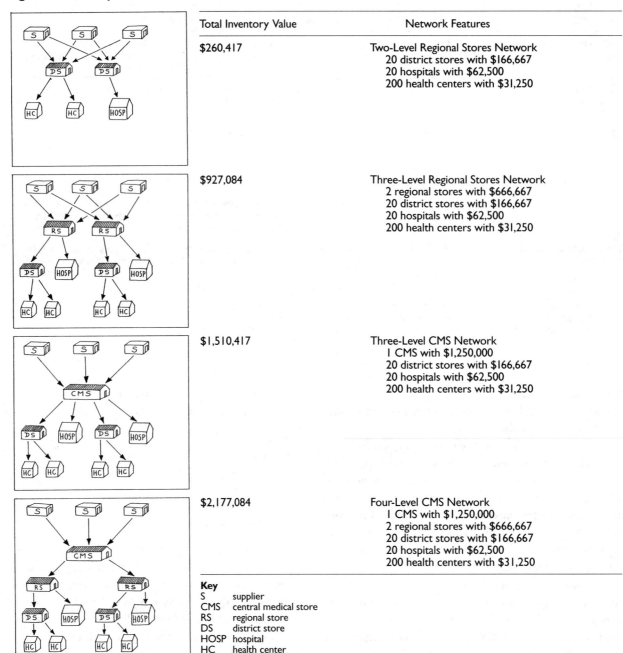

Total Inventory Value	Network Features
$260,417	Two-Level Regional Stores Network 20 district stores with $166,667 20 hospitals with $62,500 200 health centers with $31,250
$927,084	Three-Level Regional Stores Network 2 regional stores with $666,667 20 district stores with $166,667 20 hospitals with $62,500 200 health centers with $31,250
$1,510,417	Three-Level CMS Network 1 CMS with $1,250,000 20 district stores with $166,667 20 hospitals with $62,500 200 health centers with $31,250
$2,177,084	Four-Level CMS Network 1 CMS with $1,250,000 2 regional stores with $666,667 20 district stores with $166,667 20 hospitals with $62,500 200 health centers with $31,250

Key

S	supplier
CMS	central medical store
RS	regional store
DS	district store
HOSP	hospital
HC	health center

There is no foolproof method for establishing the optimal number of levels and facilities in the distribution system, but the following steps may provide a useful way of arriving at the best hierarchy for an individual country or program:

1. Diagram the existing distribution hierarchy (include all clinical and storage facilities and the supply lines connecting them).
2. Diagram three or four feasible alternative hierarchies (include patterns based on different linkages between existing facilities as well as patterns that require additional facilities).
3. For each of these alternatives, estimate as accurately as possible the values for the factors listed in Figure 21.4 (management complexity, set-up costs, operating costs, inventory holding costs, delivery times, and so forth). Total variable cost analysis is a good way to model these costs (see Chapter 41).

4. Select and implement the system that provides the best-quality service with available funds.

This systematic approach may identify previously unrecognized possibilities for improving distribution. Furthermore, the information generated can be used to substantiate requests to senior officials or external aid sources for additional funds, to implement a more costly, but more effective, plan.

Push and Pull Systems

An essential decision must be made as to which levels of the system will order drugs and which, if any, will passively receive drugs distributed from higher levels. The two basic alternatives are:

1. *Pull system*: Each level of the system determines what types and quantities of drugs are needed and places orders with the supply source (which may be a warehouse in the system or a commercial supplier). This type of system is sometimes called an independent demand or a requisition system.
2. *Push system*: Supply sources at some level in the system determine what types and quantities of drugs will be delivered to lower levels. A delivery plan is made at the beginning of a planning period, usually a year, and supplies are delivered according to the plan. This is also known as an allocation or a ration system—the best-known example in drug supply is the ration kit system (see Chapter 27).

When using a pull system, managers of operational units are expected to work out their own demand estimates and buffer stocks and submit requisitions to central stores indicating their requirements. In a push system, operational units are expected to supply certain stock and consumption information to the supply source, so that issuing officers can plan allocations.

As discussed in Chapter 27, pull systems are preferred whenever the capacity exists to manage them effectively. However, there are situations in which a push system is useful, such as disaster relief and when the supply pipeline does not function at all levels of the system. Conditions that tend to favor push and pull distribution systems are presented below.

Conditions Favoring a Pull System

► Lower-level staff are competent in assessing needs and managing inventory.
► Sufficient supplies are available at supply sources to meet all program needs.
► A large range of products is being handled.

► Field staff are regularly supervised, and performance is monitored.

Conditions Favoring a Push System

► Lower-level staff are not competent in inventory control.
► Demand greatly exceeds supply, making rationing necessary.
► A limited number of products is being handled.
► Disaster relief is needed, or the situation calls for short-term supply through prepacked kits (see Chapter 27).

Resupply Interval

Once the choice between a push and a pull system has been made, the next step is to select an appropriate resupply interval. This will determine whether deliveries are made to user units quarterly, monthly, weekly, or at any other time. If deliveries are made weekly, average stock levels will be low and the likelihood of stockouts will decrease, but transport costs will be very high. If deliveries are made only once a year, transport costs will be low, but the average stocks and storage costs will be high. See Chapter 15 for discussion of the relationship between delivery frequency and stock levels (and associated costs).

The optimum resupply interval needs to be worked out to suit individual program needs. Most public programs use intervals of one to three months. It is helpful to consider the following factors before making a decision:

► Storage capacity at each level of the system;
► Availability, order size, carrying capacity, and cost of transport;
► Seasonal factors that influence transport reliability;
► Staffing levels and competence of staff at each level of the system;
► Other factors, such as expiration dates, security against pilferage, and other locally relevant concerns.

Storage

Geographic distribution of population and health facilities determines where drugs are needed. Storage planning starts with an analysis of existing and future supply requirements to establish the type and quantity of drugs required by each facility and the overall volume to be handled by the distribution system. Suitable locations and sizes for the central and intermediate stores can then be determined. Store locations should be chosen to make the most cost-effective use of existing public and private transport networks (see Chapter 26).

Buildings can be renovated, purchased, rented, or built. The design of large storage buildings should take into account the storage conditions required for different products and the need to move large volumes of material efficiently. Stores at health facilities may consist of a simple storeroom with shelving. However simple the store, storage facilities should always protect against theft and damage by water, pests, or fire.

Well-sited stores are vital to the success of a distribution system. However, there is no such thing as a perfect site. There are often conflicting needs: a location may be conveniently close to a good road, but too far from the health centers it must serve. It is the responsibility of the logistics team to balance these needs. The following steps will facilitate the decision-making process.

Map the Demand for Drugs. Map the geographical distribution of drug demand. Where are the hospitals, clinics, and aid posts? Which ones serve the most people? Estimate the volume and weight of each facility's annual drug requirements using morbidity data, drug requisitions, and delivery records. Plan for expansion. Where are new or expanded health facilities likely to be located? How will this affect the geographical relationship between existing facilities and storage sites?

Locate Supply Entry Points. Most countries have a limited number of entry points capable of handling drug imports. These include major seaports and international airports, railway terminals, and cross-border customs posts. The logistics team should decide which points are the most appropriately located and best equipped for handling drug shipments. Some countries have several suitable entry points for drugs, and it may be efficient for drugs to be delivered through more than one port to more than one primary store. Multiple primary storage points may be justified in large countries or where physical barriers exist, such as mountain ranges or wide rivers without bridges.

Select Primary Storage Points. Review the location of the existing primary stores and consider whether they are well placed for current and future needs. The most suitable location for a primary store depends on geographic, demographic, and communications factors. A good choice is a point on the national transport network centered in the region with the highest population density. Using this location will help reduce overall transport costs. It is not essential for the primary store to be located in or near a major city. Although it may be administratively convenient, a city location may be logistically inefficient.

The location of in-country drug manufacturers and suppliers may affect the location of stores. Drugs received from these sources are generally delivered directly to primary or intermediate stores, and the transport portion of drug prices can be reduced if stores are located near a large concentration of local suppliers.

Plan Primary Distribution Routes and Locate Intermediate Stores. Good transport routes between the primary and intermediate stores (including any second-level intermediate stores) are crucial. These routes handle the largest quantities of drugs and must be reliable. Intermediate stores should therefore be located on good all-weather roads or close to railway stations or navigable waterways.

Depending on the volume of drugs to be delivered, a supply route that serves two or more intermediate stores on a circuit is usually cheaper than a route that serves only one. However, lengthy primary delivery circuits should be avoided where roads are bad, where overnight security is a problem, or where drugs may be at risk through long exposure to unacceptable temperatures (see Chapter 26).

Plan Secondary Distribution Routes. Secondary distribution routes link intermediate stores to health facilities. The planning of these routes requires detailed knowledge of rural road conditions, travel times, and available transport. Local input is essential. Drugs can be delivered from the intermediate store, collected from the intermediate store, or collected from a convenient health facility on a delivery circuit. The most practical solution for each health facility will vary.

Size the Stores. The previous steps establish which of the existing primary and intermediate stores are suitably located (or cannot be relocated) and where new stores are required. The volume of drugs to be held in each store can be estimated as described in Chapter 25. The maximum volume to be held depends on supply frequency: programs that receive single annual drug deliveries require larger primary stores than those supplied more frequently. Estimates for maximum stock levels must also take into account the safety stock volume. However, deliveries do not always arrive exactly on time, and consumption is not entirely predictable (as shown in Figure 21.6). Available storage capacity should always be greater than the calculated maximum stock holding to allow for emergencies and for program expansion.

The capacity of each existing store should be assessed. If the existing storage capacity is insufficient, five possible solutions are available:

1. Reorganize the store by changing the shelving layout or by introducing pallet racking (see Chapters 23 and 25).
2. Build or rent additional warehouse space. This option involves capital costs for warehouse construction or recurrent costs for warehouse rental.

Figure 21.6 Stock Volume in Store Design

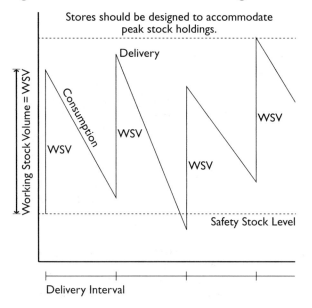

3. Increase the supply frequency to eliminate the need for additional storage space, probably at some increase in administrative costs. Suppliers may also charge extra for more frequent delivery. If the supply interval is already short, it may not be practical to decrease it.

4. Upgrade one or more underutilized lower-level stores to higher-level status.

5. If insufficient space at the primary level is the problem, consider holding larger stocks at the intermediate level, assuming the capacity exists. A system based on regular transfer of stock between stores at the same level should be avoided in most cases, because it is difficult to record such movements. However, some supply systems can manage redistribution, depending on the qualifications and motivation of the personnel involved.

Delivery Systems versus Collection Systems

The next important decision to be made concerns how supplies will be moved between the warehouse and the receiving facility. Basically there are two options: collection or delivery. In the case of a collection system, the receiving facility takes on the responsibility of collecting supplies from the warehouse. In a delivery system, the warehouse is responsible for delivering supplies with either in-house transport or a private-sector contract.

Each method has advantages and disadvantages; the choice should be based on individual program needs and constraints. General advantages and disadvantages associated with collection and delivery are shown in Figure 21.7.

Transport

Transport is frequently the least reliable link in the distribution system and is often a source of great frustration. Transport planning requires the selection of appropriate means of transport and the procurement and maintenance of vehicles or other conveyances. Issues to be considered include

- using private-sector alternatives
- planning transport system improvements
- acquiring and disposing of vehicles
- managing vehicle use
- maintaining vehicles
- maintaining drug quality during transport

Transport managers should make the best use of available transport through careful route planning and delivery scheduling, and they need to carefully consider private-sector alternatives; these issues are addressed in Chapter 26.

Delivery Schedules

Good planning is needed to ensure that each facility receives supplies regularly and on time. For example, an intermediate store may be responsible for forty clinical facilities with a delivery interval of one month. The total time required to supply all these facilities must not exceed one month. If analysis shows that a longer period is required to supply all facilities, then the delivery schedule must be changed or additional transport resources acquired. Figure 21.8 illustrates this concept.

When determining the appropriate delivery intervals for each store and health facility, consider the following factors:

Storage Capacity of Primary, Intermediate, and Health Facility Stores. Deliveries must never exceed the holding capacity of any store. This is more likely to occur with irregular or infrequent deliveries.

Increased Transport Costs per Unit Supplied for Deliveries to Small, Remote Facilities. An obvious solution is to supply these areas infrequently. The disadvantage is that this policy increases maximum stock levels at these facilities and may also increase the risk of stockouts.

Efficient Vehicle Usage. If delivery intervals are too frequent, vehicles may travel half empty. If delivery intervals are long, large vehicles will be needed. Vehicles owned by the health service may stand idle for much of the time.

Climatic Factors. It may be impossible to deliver to some facilities at certain times of the year. Delivery frequency and volume must be scheduled to work around interruptions caused by rainy seasons or other recurring climatic constraints.

Figure 21.7 Comparison of Delivery and Collection Systems

System	Advantages	Disadvantages
Delivery	► If proper delivery routes, order intervals, and delivery schedules are in place, the total cost of transport will be less. ► Deliveries of supplies can be combined with other important scheduled and compulsory visits to the field. Also offers an opportunity to supervise fieldwork. ► Drug selection, assembly, and packing operations can be scheduled and accomplished efficiently.	► Needs reliable transport facilities. Outright purchase or leasing of vehicles gives rise to high capital and operating costs. ► If the delivery route is long, there is the possibility of breakage and loss of quality. ► Security lapses may occur due to lack of a responsible officer accompanying goods in many instances. ► Health facilities may be closed when the delivery truck arrives, or there may not be a responsible officer on hand to receive supplies. ► The delivery truck may be in a hurry to get to the next destination, making it difficult to check for short shipments, damage, and other problems before the truck departs.
Collection	► Provides an opportunity for issuing personnel to meet people from the field and discuss common problems, and for field officers to meet and exchange ideas among themselves. ► Frees central-level staff from providing transport facilities to the field. ► Provides greater incentive to obtain supplies regularly, since the facility is responsible for collecting supplies. ► Allows field personnel to attend to other business in town. ► Offers the possibility of a greater choice of methods of transport. ► Allows for better checking, handling, and security of goods received.	► Takes up a lot of health facility staff time. ► Time may be wasted waiting for assembly of supplies, or supplies might not be ready for collection on the first visit. ► Total cost of transport may be high. ► Health center personnel may tend to increase the frequency of visits for various reasons.

≡ 21.4 Resources for Distribution Management

The Logistics Team

Transport and warehouse managers and other officers with responsibility for logistics often have low professional status, and their skills and experience are frequently undervalued, if not ignored. A first priority is to recognize the importance of logistics officers and transport managers. Their jobs and opinions must be taken seriously. A logistics team should be established to be responsible for the operational planning, implementation, and monitoring of the tasks described in this chapter. In large countries, regional teams may be more appropriate than a single national team. Team managers must stress the importance of improving drug availability and reducing distribution costs wherever possible.

Political pressures should be resisted (for example, a politician may want a store to be built in an inappropriate location for political reasons). If such problems are anticipated, it may be best if a senior, politically well-connected official without such an agenda leads the logistics team.

Staffing Levels

The logistics team must determine the staffing levels required to administer and operate the drug distribution system effectively. Are sufficient staff available? Are they appropriately trained? Are funds available to recruit and train additional staff, if necessary? No matter how well designed a distribution system is, it will not work unless there are enough suitably qualified staff members to run it.

Information Systems

Reliable management information is vital for coordinating the distribution network. Drug consumption information flows up and down the network. The information system consists of forms and procedures to record inventory levels, cost and sale prices, and receipt and issue of drugs. The system may be manual or computerized.

It is easy to visualize the one-way flow of drugs through the supply pipeline from CMS to regional or district stores and, finally, to hospitals, health centers, and community health workers. It is more difficult to understand and manage the complementary flow of forms and reports needed to coordinate drug distribution.

Figure 21.8 Planning for Monthly Requisitions and Deliveries

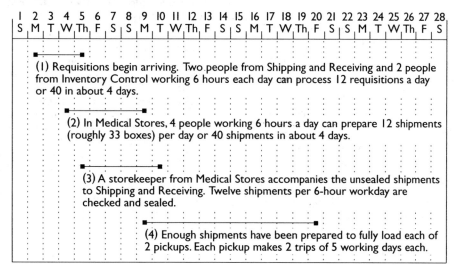

Forms, records, and reports form the core of the supply information system. Forms are documents that move from one unit to another, carrying specific information about drug needs, drug movements, and associated financial transactions. Copies of forms filed at various points in the distribution network form the audit trail to trace the flow of drugs and funds. Records may be maintained in computer databases, as card files, in ledgers, or in folders. Reports should be prepared regularly to summarize drug consumption and expenditures. Individual health facilities report to district offices, which report to regional offices, which report to the central office. Such reports are used to project drug needs, revise budgets, and assess drug use.

The forms shown in Chapters 23 and 24 can be adapted by any supply system to suit its requirements. Some forms may be usable as is, some may need modification, and additional forms may be required to suit special information needs.

When a new drug supply program is initiated or an existing one is revised, a complete information system should be established as part of the basic planning process (see Chapter 45). All necessary forms should be available, and all staff should be trained in the use of these forms before drugs start moving through the system. Without this type of preparation, the process of recording drug consumption and forecasting drug needs quickly breaks down.

Communications

Good communications are essential to a drug distribution system. Where reliable telecommunications networks and postal services do not exist, especially in rural areas, staff often have to travel long distances to deliver or collect reports and requisitions. These journeys should be combined with supervisory activities, but often they are not.

Good telecommunications reduce the need for travel, save staff time, and reduce wear and tear on vehicles. Maximum use should be made of the telecommunications resources available, and appropriate investments in communications technology should be made. Providing a facility with a radio transmitter or a fax machine may help avoid unnecessary travel costs.

≡ 21.5 Cost Analysis and Performance Monitoring

When you are designing or revising a distribution system, it is crucial to compile and analyze data on current operating costs and to model the potential cost impact of various alternatives. Total variable cost analysis, described in Chapters 15 and 41, is one method for analyzing costs and modeling alternatives in a supply system. This section gives an overview of the variable costs that apply to the distribution component of supply systems.

Cost analysis is not usually a continuous activity and should not be confused with performance monitoring (see Chapter 36), which should be carried out regularly using appropriate indicators to ensure that system performance is maintained.

The first tasks in an evaluation of options are to calculate the *in-house costs* of the distribution system and then to estimate the costs of other alternatives for comparison. In-house costs include storage space, stores operation, equipment, staff, holding and transport, administration and management, upgrading, and costs of contracting out (see Chapter 42).

Storage Space. This includes the annual cost of rent paid to private warehouse owners and the annual amortized cost of warehouses owned by the health care service.

Operation. These costs include local building taxes and utility costs (electricity, gas, water, and insurance).

Equipment. Included are annual amortized costs for equipment such as forklifts, for security equipment such as fire alarms and fire extinguishers, for specialized equipment such as cold rooms, for computer equipment used in stock control, and for other similar items. Costs should be amortized for items that are expected to have a useful life of more than one year.

Distribution Staff. Costs include overhead and wages paid to storekeepers, drivers, mechanics, and laborers.

Holding Stock (Carrying Cost). As discussed in Chapter 15, there is a real cost associated with maintaining stock in inventory. Sufficient inventory must be kept to protect against stockouts and to take full advantage of bulk purchasing agreements. Holding too much stock increases storage costs and locks up funds; a good distribution system balances these two factors.

Transport. Included are all distribution charges not covered by the supplier's contract, which may end at the factory gate, at the dockside, or at the client's own warehouse (see Chapter 22). Transport costs can include

► air freight or shipping;
► insurance;
► demurrage;
► port clearing;
► transferring goods between forms of transport;
► distributing drugs within the country;
► packing and unpacking.

If government vehicles are used for drug distribution, the costs include fuel, vehicle repair and maintenance, salaries and daily expenses for drivers, and vehicle amortization. If parastatal or private haulers are used, costs include fixed and variable transport charges.

In most cases, some costs (such as insurance and port-clearing fees) are outside the control of the drug program. However, freight charges depend on the volume and weight of the supplies ordered, as well as the fees charged by the shipping agent. Shipping costs are important considerations when evaluating drug tenders (see Country Study 21.1). It is easiest to compare costs from competing suppliers when prices are CIF (cost, insurance, and freight) or CIP (carriage and insurance paid) (see Chapter 17).

Administrative Overhead. Overhead comprises all admin-

Country Study 21.1 Evaluating Freight Costs

In a southern African country, free carrier (FCA) prices for vaccines from different sources were compared with the costs of the same vaccine at the port of entry, inclusive of air-freight charges. In several instances, there was no consistency between the FCA price and the delivered price. For example, the FCA cost of oral polio vaccine (OPV) from one Western European manufacturer was 13 percent higher than OPV from another Western European source. However, the more expensive vaccine was actually 13 percent *cheaper* at the port of entry. Similarly, the FCA cost of measles vaccine from a Japanese source was 2 percent higher than that from a North American source. At the port of entry, it was 31 percent more expensive.

Source: Feilden Battersby Health Systems Analysts 1995.

istrative costs incurred by, or allocated to, the distribution system.

Losses Due to Poor Management. Direct losses include

► damage from incorrect storage or transport conditions;
► theft of stock, whether by health workers or by outsiders;
► misdirection of stock;
► unnecessary supplies in stock;
► supplies that expire before they can be used.

There are also costs attributable to stock shortages. Extra costs are usually incurred when emergency purchases are made. When drugs are not available, it may be necessary to keep patients in the hospital longer, thereby increasing nursing costs and making beds unavailable for other patients. When patients cannot be treated properly, they may infect others. These indirect losses are difficult to calculate, but they could be estimated using techniques of cost-effectiveness analysis (see Chapter 3).

Upgrading. If additional expenditures are needed to bring an in-house distribution system to an acceptable level of efficiency, these costs must be compiled and included with other in-house costs for comparison with alternatives.

Contracting Out. Private storage and distribution costs should be estimated so that a comparison can be made with existing expenditures. This can be accomplished by assessing private-sector capacity (see Chapter 4) and conducting a nonbinding tender to determine the costs of private-sector services (see Chapter 17).

Collecting and Analyzing Cost and Performance Data

In order to calculate costs accurately, it is necessary to collect data from in-house accounting and reporting systems and from other sources (see Country Study 21.1). Data should be collected from natural cost centers; for example, if the system is organized on a regional basis, analysis of the costs by region will indicate how each region is performing.

Skilled staff are needed to design and carry out cost surveys, analyze data from survey questionnaires, and make useful deductions from imperfect data sets. The most informative survey collects field-based information from stock and vehicle maintenance records and from discussions with local staff. Chapter 4 discusses the management of an ad hoc assessment. Chapters 15 and 41 discuss data collection for total variable cost analysis. Chapter 36 addresses general principles of monitoring and evaluation, both valuable considerations when designing and implementing performance monitoring of the distribution system. In monitoring schemes, the same data should be collected from more than one source so that results can be cross-checked to assess the accuracy of existing record-keeping and reporting procedures (see Country Study 21.2).

≡ 21.6 Choosing between Improvement and Replacement

Most health services already have a drug distribution network, but needs and systems evolve. For instance, a program might begin by using drug kits and then wish to move to a requisition-based system, which is more complex and usually increases the number of individual items handled (see Chapter 27).

A distribution system may be outdated; storage points chosen long ago may not suit the present situation, and record keeping may be inadequate. Data may be inaccurate, not up-to-date, and not available in a clear, user-friendly form.

If the distribution system does not meet current needs, changes are necessary. The problems might be solved by improving the present system, but sometimes a complete and radical change is the best solution (see Country Study 21.3). Even a good system requires frequent minor adjustments to respond to changing needs.

The three examples below illustrate typical distribution problems and the types of action that may be appropriate to solve them.

Example 1. Poor Administration
Problems in this system include failure to comply with standard operating procedures, inadequate reporting of shortages by peripheral health facilities, and excessive losses due to theft.

Action: Review and strengthen supervision, administra-

Country Study 21.2 Performance Measurement

In an East African country, an analysis found that the value of warehouse stock according to the stock book was less than half of that assessed during visits to the warehouse. The finding that stock records were not accurate showed that the essential drugs program was not well managed and that it was impossible to monitor the program properly.

Selecting an appropriate measure of performance is important. In the same country, project staff proposed a simple indicator that could be used in rural areas of the essential drugs program. They suggested counting the number of community health workers (CHWs) supplied with drugs at least once per year. In this country, it was extremely difficult to make deliveries of essential drugs. If they had used a shorter period (such as one month) to measure performance, all CHWs would have scored zero, because for most of the year there are no deliveries. In this setting, choosing monthly deliveries as the indicator would fail to distinguish among the performance of the various health districts.

Source: Feilden 1991.

---

tive procedures, and reporting standards. It may be necessary to change personnel and/or provide incentives to improve performance.

Example 2. Seasonal Variations
Drug shortages occur because roads are closed during periods of heavy rain or snow.

Action: Review delivery intervals and delivery quantities to take account of predictable weather hazards. Deliver more supplies when the weather is good.

Example 3. Major Transport Problems
Major transport problems, such as lack of fuel or lack of vehicles in working order, arise.

Action: Are the causes of these transport problems local or general? Local problems may be solved by providing more spare parts or installing a fuel depot. General, widespread problems may be a sign of structural weakness, necessitating more radical solutions. Contracts with private-sector or parastatal organizations may be a more cost-effective way to manage all or part of the transport system.

≡ 21.7 The Private-Sector Option

Drug shortages are a common feature of government health services in many countries, even when legal and illegal private-sector vendors in the same countries provide a reliable supply of drugs. This is especially true in major towns and cities. This private availability in the midst of public shortage suggests that, in these countries,

Country Study 21.3 Replacing a Distribution System

In an eastern European country, a cold-chain study found that heat-labile vaccines provided by the World Health Organization Expanded Programme on Immunization (EPI) were stored at room temperature for extended periods. Vaccines were distributed by railway, and delivery took up to sixteen days. Toxoids were exposed in transit to high temperatures in summer and to freezing conditions in winter.

All EPI vaccines had formerly been manufactured, stored, and distributed by the state vaccine manufacturer. More recently, additional vaccines were donated from overseas. Responsibility for storage and distribution of these vaccines was imposed on the state vaccine manufacturer. The government made no payment for this service and provided no funds for additional cold-storage space.

It became clear that this confusing situation could not be resolved without significant reorganization and additional funding. An operational and cost-effectiveness study showed that the existing storage and transport system could not be improved within a reasonable period of time or at an acceptable cost. Several storage alternatives were investigated. Eventually, the parastatal pharmaceutical supply company responsible for imported goods was selected to provide the new national storage facility. This company had an established logistic capability and adequate storage space.

Government-run district vaccine stores are now being established. Suitable buildings have been selected and refurbished to standard specifications. A donor is providing cold-chain equipment.

To evaluate the most cost-effective way of transporting vaccines within the country, a study compared the existing railway-based system with possible road and air-road alternatives using different carriers. Although the air-road option was the cheapest, the Ministry of Health thought that it was not the best solution because it could not be controlled directly, and there were uncertainties over the future price of air transport. In the end, a road transport option was selected, using a refrigerated vehicle operated by the parastatal pharmaceutical distribution company.

A commercial storage and distribution contract will be drawn up with the parastatal, which will receive donated cold-chain equipment. The Ministry of Health will continue to purchase vaccines.

Source: Battersby 1992a, 1992b.

the private sector is able to distribute drugs more efficiently than the public sector.

As discussed in Chapter 6, there are alternatives in many countries to a government-run storage and distribution system. With a well-developed private sector, it may be possible and appropriate to contract out both storage and distribution to a private company. The first step should always be to identify local private-sector capacity. It is then possible to determine which combination of private and public systems is appropriate (Cairncross 1987). A contracted service can operate independently of the health service, or some combination of private and public systems may be appropriate.

In many countries, the private sector can offer a comprehensive and effective distribution service only to the regional or district level. In small or poor countries, there may be very few private-sector distribution companies, and when competition is limited, a contracted service may not be cheaper or better than the public sector (Bennett 1992).

Many formerly socialist economies have parastatal pharmaceutical distribution companies. Under the pressures of structural adjustment, these organizations are now forced to operate in the market economy (see Country Study 21.3). Parastatals can be well placed to provide distribution and transport services where a clear contractual (quasi–private sector) relationship between the parties incorporates performance targets and penalties for noncompliance.

Contracting out must be carefully considered, for managing it properly requires considerable staff time and expertise. In order to decide whether private provision of distribution systems is cheaper, the cost of the existing transport and distribution system must be assessed. Comprehensive tender documents must be prepared, specifying contractual arrangements and performance requirements precisely and unambiguously. It is then necessary to assess the capabilities and financial stability of the tenderers. Finally, after the contract is signed, the performance of the contractor must be carefully monitored. Contracting out is discussed further in Chapters 17 and 22. ■

≡ Assessment Guide

Drug Distribution System

- ► Which levels of the supply system order drugs from suppliers?
- ► Is distribution to lower levels done through a push or a pull system?
- ► Does the system include semi-autonomous vertical distribution components, such as EPI?
- ► How many levels are there in the distribution hierarchy? How many stores, clinical facilities, or pharmacies are at each level?
- ► What are the catchment populations of stores, clinical facilities, or pharmacies? Map the geographical distribution of each.
- ► Is the current distribution system based on collection or delivery?
- ► What volume of drugs is distributed to each store and each clinical facility or pharmacy per year? How often is each supplied? What is the physical capacity of each store? Is physical capacity ever exceeded? Map the current demand distribution.
- ► What changes in demand distribution are anticipated in the future?
- ► What mode of transport is used for each link in the distribution chain? What alternatives are available? What are the travel times and mileages for each link?

Supply Sources

- ► What percentages in terms of bulk, value, and number of items do overseas and in-country suppliers contribute annually?
- ► Which ports of entry are used by each of the overseas suppliers? Which ports clear imports most efficiently and with the least loss?
- ► Where are the in-country drug supply sources located?

Communications

- ► What methods of communication are available and actually used between each node in the distribution system (postal service, telephone, fax, radio link, physical visit)?

Performance Indicators

- ► Cost of stock held as a percentage of stock turnover;
- ► Percentage of health facilities submitting requisitions on time;
- ► Frequency of delivery;
- ► Number of items supplied out of total requested by clients (service level);
- ► Average stock position in months (quantity on hand and on order, divided by average monthly consumption);
- ► Stockout frequency for indicator drugs (see Chapter 41);
- ► Percentage availability of indicator drugs at each level;
- ► Quantity and value of expired items in stock;
- ► Losses due to damage and theft;
- ► Distribution costs per ton per kilometer;
- ► Vehicle availability and frequency of breakdowns;
- ► Vehicle fuel availability in different parts of the country (a good indicator of the transport system's ability to make deliveries);
- ► Mechanical breakdown frequency for vital temperature control equipment such as cold rooms and air-conditioners;
- ► Staff attendance rate and sick time used;
- ► Variation between actual and recorded inventory level;
- ► Currency of record maintenance;
- ► Supplier and warehouse lead time.

Monitoring and Evaluation

- ► Are there effective systems for monitoring and evaluating distribution system costs and performance? If not, which elements are missing?
- ► What is the annual operating cost of the distribution system as a percentage of drugs distributed? Are there significant regional variations?
- ► What are the costs of private-sector alternatives to in-house services?

Private-Sector Alternatives

- ► What private-sector drug distribution systems exist? Identify the location of private-sector pharmacies within catchment areas of clinical facilities or pharmacies.
- ► Who are the private-sector storage and transport providers? Assess whether they are capable of handling drugs and delivering services to areas where they are needed.

≡ Glossary

Bin card: Card that records receipts, issues, and balances held in the stores. The bin card is kept in the warehouse with the physical stock.

Card file: A stock record based on the use of cards stored in a file box or a plastic visible-edge record tray (Kardex).

Cold chain: A system of freezers, refrigerators, cold boxes, and other devices needed to maintain the proper temperature for vaccines from the point of manufacture to the point of administration.

Collection system: Drug distribution system in which the health facilities are responsible for providing transport of supplies from the warehouse to the health facility. Compare **delivery system**.

Delivery system: Drug distribution system in which the warehouse is responsible for providing transport of supplies from the warehouse to the health facilities. Compare **collection system**.

Demurrage: A charge assessed by shippers to purchasers that fail to unload and return containers. It can also apply when carriers are unable to off-load shipments due to delay through the fault of the purchaser.

Distribution system: A system of administrative procedures, transport facilities, storage facilities, and user facilities through which supplies move from a central point to the user facilities.

Double-shelf system: A system for stock control in which the stock of each item is physically separated onto two shelves. When the stock on one shelf is expended, the stock from the other shelf is used, and an order for replacement stock is placed.

First-expiry/first-out procedure (FEFO): A method of inventory management in which products with the earliest expiry date are the first products issued, regardless of the order in which they are received. This method is more demanding than FIFO (see below) but should be used for short-dated products such as vaccines.

First-in/first-out procedure (FIFO): A method of inventory management in which the first products received are the first products issued. This method generally minimizes the chance of drug expiration.

Holding costs: The costs of carrying inventory, usually expressed as a percentage of the average inventory. These include both the capital costs and the storage costs.

Imprest system: A form of periodic inventory control in which stocks are replenished up to a pre-established level. No running stock records are kept. The only stock control document is a preprinted sheet showing each item, its description, the unit of issue, and the imprest level. Generally used only at small facilities.

Inventory: The total stock kept on hand at any storage point to protect against uncertainty, permit bulk purchasing, minimize waiting time, increase transportation efficiency, and buffer against seasonal fluctuations.

Inventory control: The function of supply management that aims to provide sufficient stocks of drugs at the lowest costs possible.

Inventory models: Systems of inventory control that determine how much stock is bought and how often it is bought. See Chapter 15 for a discussion.

Inventory taking: A periodic activity in which a physical count is made of the stock and compared with inventory control records. Also known as physical stock count.

Issue: To distribute a specific amount of an item to an intermediary stocking facility or a health facility.

Lead-time demand: The number of units demanded and issued during the lead time.

Order picking: The systematic extraction of items from warehouse shelving to fill a client's order. Picking staff work from a picking list that defines the quantity and location of each item required.

Pallet: A transportable flat storage base, with or without sides, designed to hold goods and to permit handling by mechanical aids such as pallet trucks and forklifts.

Pipeline: The total storage capacity that must be filled in a drug supply system, including the central medical store, regional warehouses, district warehouses, and all regional facilities.

Pipeline analysis: The systematic diagramming of the supply system and calculation of the amount of stock held at each point in the system. The analysis determines the amount of stock actually needed and the amount of stock to be held at each storage point.

Prepacked kits: Also known as *ration kits* or *set packs*. An assortment of drugs and medical supplies to cover a set number of patient attendances, which are distributed unopened to health facilities.

Preventive maintenance: A series of maintenance and service activities performed regularly by a technician and/or operator and designed to prevent the breakdown of vehicles and other equipment. This is the least expensive form of maintenance.

Pull system: Drug distribution system in which each peripheral facility determines the drug quantities to be requisitioned from the procurement unit or warehouse. Compare **push system**.

Push system: Drug distribution system in which the procurement unit or warehouse determines what drug quantities are to be issued to the peripheral facilities. Compare **pull system**.

Receiving report: A document indicating when items were received, from whom, the total quantity in the shipment, the invoice price, and the amount of damaged or lost stock.

Routing: Determining the order in which facilities will receive their deliveries, based on the geographic location of facilities and an attempt to minimize delivery costs.

Safety stock: The buffer, cushion, or reserve stock kept on hand to protect against stockouts caused by delayed deliveries or markedly increased demand.

Service level: Most commonly defined as the percentage of items requested that are supplied, in the quantity requested, by a supplier or warehouse in one delivery. This term is sometimes used to describe the percentage of demand that is met from stock on hand.

Stock: Goods and materials stored for future use.

Stock count/physical inventory: The process of inventory taking, in which a physical count is made of all items in inventory and compared with the written record.

Stock numbers: Sequential numbers designating each item in inventory.

Stock position: All stock now available and soon to be available, including stock on hand and outstanding orders. This is sometimes called the *total inventory*.

Stock records: A generic term that applies to bin cards, Kardex records, stock ledgers, and computer files. These provide basic information for inventory management by recording all transactions for an item, including receipts, issues, orders placed, orders received, and stock losses.

Stocking cost: The cost of maintaining stock, including the capital and storage costs.

Stockout: Complete absence of an item that is normally expected to be on hand. In many cases, this can be misleading as an indicator, because a warehouse may always reserve a small stock—the warehouse is not literally out of stock, but there is a functional stockout because the warehouse will not issue the reserved stock.

Tachograph: A device that records comprehensive details of every journey and can provide a check on the accuracy of a driver's log.

Transshipment: Shipment of supplies to an intermediate location, from which they are forwarded by another means of transport to a facility.

Two-bin inventory control: Same as *double-shelf system*, except that two physically separate bins rather than shelves are used.

Unique identifiers: Techniques by which drugs can be identified as originating with the government supply system. Unique identifiers include labels with the program logo, reserved batch numbers, and imprinting of tablets and capsules.

Visual inventory system: A no-paper inventory control method in which the need to order is determined simply by looking at the inventory on the shelf. This system usually provides acceptable performance only in small facilities with a limited number of items in stock.

Working stock: That part of the inventory that is expected to be issued or consumed. It fluctuates between zero and the order quantity. The other component of inventory is the *safety stock*.

≡ **References and Further Readings**

★ = *Key readings.*

★ Battersby, A. 1985. *How to assess health care service logistics with particular reference to peripheral health facilities.* SHS/85.9. Geneva: World Health Organization.

Battersby, A. 1992a. *Distributing vaccines between Bucharest and the districts: Which mode of transport?* Report for UNICEF.

Battersby, A. 1992b. *Storing and distributing vaccines at national level: Which organisation?* Report for UNICEF.

Beenhakker, H. L., S. Carapetis, L. Crowther, and S. Hertel. 1987. *Rural transport services: A guide to their planning and implementation.* London: Intermediate Technology Publications.

Bennett, S. 1992. Promoting the private sector: A review of developing country trends. *Health Policy and Planning* 7(2):97–110.

Cairncross, S. 1987. The private sector and water supply in developing countries. Partnership or profiteering? *Health Policy and Planning* 2(2):183–84.

★ Compton, H. K. 1985. *Supplies and materials management,* 3d ed. Plymouth, England: Macdonald and Evans, and Institute of Purchasing and Supply.

Corbett, J. R. G. 1988. *Where there is no telephone.* Kinshasa, Zaire: Communauté Baptiste du Fleuve Zaire and Elim Church Zaire.

★ Creese, A., and D. Parker, eds. 1990. *Cost analysis in primary health care: A training manual for program managers.* WHO/SHS/NHP/90.5. Geneva: World Health Organization.

Dawson, J., and I. Barwell. 1993. *Roads are not enough: New perspectives on rural transport planning in developing countries.* London: Intermediate Technology Publications.

Dorner, G., E. Merck, C. G. Roepnack, R. Burchard, and FIP Industrial Pharmacists Section. 1992. *Management of drug purchasing, storage, and distribution: Manual for developing countries,* 3d ed. The Hague, Netherlands: Fédération Internationale Pharmaceutique.

Electrolux. 1983. *The storage handbook.* Singapore: Electrolux S.E.A. Pte., Ltd. (240 MacPherson Rd. #03-01/04, Singapore 1334).

Feilden, R. 1991. *Use of cost-effectiveness analysis in three countries in eastern and southern Africa.* Draft report for UNICEF Eastern and Southern Africa Regional Office.

Foster, S. D. 1990. Logistics and supply. In *Why things work: Case histories in development,* ed. J. B. Halstead and J. A. Walsh. New York: Rockefeller Foundation.

★ Johnson, J., and D. Wood. 1993. *Contemporary logistics,* 5th ed. New York: Macmillan.

McMahon, R., E. Barton, and M. Piot. 1992. *On being in charge: A guide to management in primary health care,* 2d ed. Geneva: World Health Organization.

★ MSH (Management Sciences for Health). 1992. Distribution and transport planning (trainer's and participant's guides). In *Managing drug supply training series.* Part 3. Supply management. Boston: MSH.

Osterblad, I. 1990. *A concept for procurement, storage, distribution of drugs* (unedited revised second draft). Geneva: World Health Organization.

Wolff, J., R. Cushman, F. Kweekeh, E. McGrory, and S. Binzen. 1990. *Beyond the clinic walls: Case studies in community-based distribution.* West Hartford, Conn.: Kumarian Press.

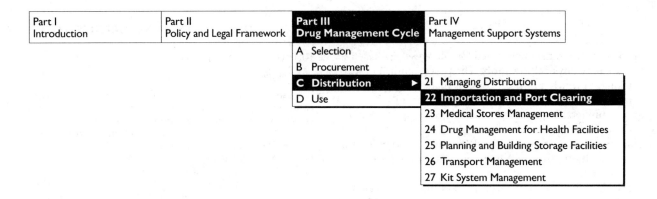

Part I	Part II	**Part III**	Part IV
Introduction	Policy and Legal Framework	**Drug Management Cycle**	Management Support Systems

A Selection
B Procurement
C Distribution ▶
D Use

21 Managing Distribution
22 Importation and Port Clearing
23 Medical Stores Management
24 Drug Management for Health Facilities
25 Planning and Building Storage Facilities
26 Transport Management
27 Kit System Management

Chapter 22
Importation and Port Clearing

≡ Summary

Port delays can be costly due to

- ► *reduced shelf life or, with vaccines, the possibility of complete loss of potency;*
- ► *increased theft;*
- ► *storage fees;*
- ► *stockouts, with emergency purchases made at high unit cost;*
- ► *cash flow problems caused by drugs being tied up in port.*

The port-clearing process consists of

- ► *identifying the arrival of shipments;*
- ► *locating the shipments;*
- ► *obtaining the documents needed for clearing;*
- ► *delivering goods to the warehouse.*

Expediting port clearing is an important function of the import unit, *requiring either a well-organized, paper-based*

activity monitoring system or a computerized information system.

Port clearing may be slowed by government customs and import regulations. Private companies are sometimes able to achieve more rapid port clearance than government agencies. There are two private-sector choices: either the supplier can be made responsible for the port-clearing process, or the task can be contracted out to a clearing and forwarding agent. Experienced and well-trained staff can significantly improve the port-clearing process. An analysis should be carried out to establish the most suitable method for managing port clearance.

Losses and damage in transit can be substantial. In order to recover insured losses, the import unit must press insurance claims systematically and speedily.

≡ 22.1 Managing Importation

This chapter discusses systems and procedures to improve the efficiency of port clearing. The port-clearing process is vital to the operation of a public drug supply program, whether it is performed by employees or contracted out.

In many countries, clearing drug consignments from ports is an inefficient and time-consuming activity that leads to many losses. Unlike products that are nonperishable or indestructible, drugs and medical supplies can be damaged by poor handling and storage conditions. They are also highly attractive to thieves. Thus, there is a critical need to clear drugs as quickly as possible after delivery to air, sea, and land ports.

Financial losses due to poor management of port clearing, such as those listed below, can be extensive and are often proportional to the delay in the port.

- ► Shelf life can be affected when products are kept in the port under incorrect storage conditions. In the case of vaccines and other heat-labile products, the product may be rendered unusable.
- ► The likelihood of theft is increased, especially when cartons are damaged by poor handling.
- ► Storage fees result from delays in clearing.
- ► Port-clearing delays result in longer delivery lead times. Unless funds are invested to increase safety stocks, stockouts may occur at storage and dispensing facilities, leading to extra expenditures on emergency purchases.
- ► Capital funds are tied up by port-clearing delays. This

worsens cash flow problems in programs operating a revolving drug fund.

In many countries, the efficiency and economy of port clearing are hindered by cumbersome or obsolete regulations and by the poor systems and procedures used by customs and port authorities. The resulting delays for importers are substantial, yet there seems to be no way to improve performance. The common practice adopted by private companies and individual importers is to obtain the services of a private clearing agent on a contract basis. An experienced agent has the best chance of negotiating the regulatory labyrinth in the shortest possible time.

≡ 22.2 Using a Clearing and Forwarding Agent

Importation and customs clearance is a specialized area of work. Unless the drug program already has an experienced team with clearing and forwarding skills, it is strongly recommended that a specialized clearing and forwarding agent be contracted.

If a private-sector agent is used, tenders for these services should be obtained from several companies, particularly if a large volume of business is involved. Tenderers should specify all charges and rates and clearly identify the duties they will perform (see Figure 22.1). Before an agent is appointed, it is important to obtain satisfactory business references from other clients. The agent's offices and warehouses should also be inspected to ensure that good business and

Figure 22.1 Contracting for Port Clearing

The following list includes the main features of a contract for port-clearing and forwarding services. Professional advice should be sought to ensure that terms and conditions are locally appropriate, legally enforceable, and realistic.

Scope of Work

- ► Dealing with customs formalities;
- ► Arranging clearance from the port or airport;
- ► Arranging transport to the agent's warehouse or the consignee's premises;
- ► Providing safe and secure warehousing prior to delivery, if required;
- ► Arranging for delivery to final destinations, if required;
- ► Specifying documentation to be provided by the supplier and by the consignee (for example, shipping advisory, bill of lading, air waybill, packing list).

Performance Standards

- ► Time periods allowed for each stage in the import and port-clearing process;
- ► Procedures for regular performance monitoring.

Service Requirements

- ► Reporting;
- ► Quoting for individual consignments;
- ► Payment arrangements;
- ► Penalties for poor performance;
- ► Security;
- ► Dealing with defective shipments;
- ► Restrictions on the subletting of services to other companies.

Payment Terms

- ► Port or airport charges itemized in detail;
- ► Agent's costs itemized in detail.

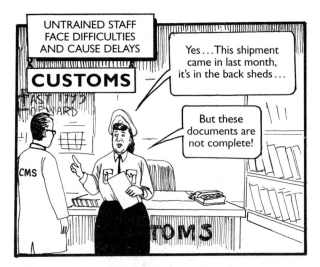

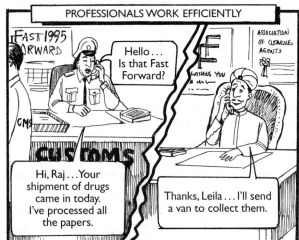

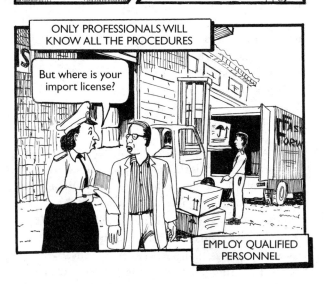

materials handling practices are observed. Drugs require special handling, and the agent should demonstrate the ability to deal with such items.

It is the duty of the clearing agent to understand local rules and practices and to help the recipient through the routines required. The agent should obtain documentation in advance of receipt in order to avoid storage charges and should also assist in obtaining relevant permits, waivers, or bonds.

The agent must take full responsibility for ensuring that the cargo is cleared and delivered with minimal delay and at the lowest cost. Even if this system is in place, it is important for the recipient to understand all the stages of the importation and port-clearing process.

≡ 22.3 Organizing an Import Unit

An alternative to contracting with a private-sector clearing agent is to organize an import unit in the supply system. This unit's responsibility should be specifically defined, and the responsible officials should be accountable to the drug supply program for prompt, reliable port clearance. The unit should have one or more experienced clearing agents on staff. Before the decision is made to organize an in-house import unit, its cost effectiveness

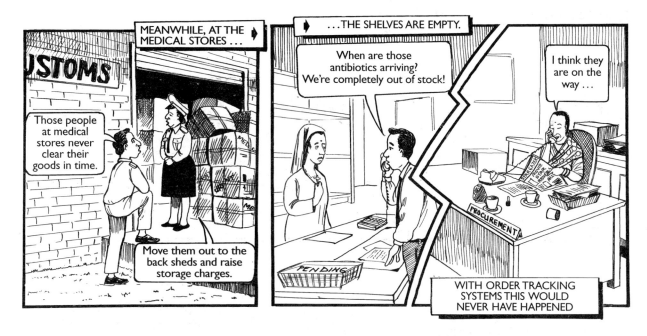

should be compared with a contract with a private clearing agent. Chapter 23 discusses the responsibilities of an import unit attached to medical stores.

≡ 22.4 The Port-Clearing Process

The most important steps in the port-clearing process are set out below. It is essential that shippers and their forwarding agents check port or airport conditions at each end of the journey. This includes establishing any limitations on the use and availability of containers and container handling equipment and the availability of refrigeration equipment to store vaccines and other heat-labile products.

Notify Buyer of Expected Arrival Date of Shipments

As soon as a consignment of drugs is shipped, it is the seller's responsibility to tell the buyer the name of the carrying vessel, aircraft, or vehicle and its expected time of arrival at the buyer's port. This is often done by telex or fax. The seller then dispatches to the buyer copies of all the documents mentioned in Figures 22.2 and 22.3. Once the buyer receives these documents, the local agents for the carrier can be contacted to obtain exact arrival details.

Locate Shipments

The shipper's local agent provides final details specifying the quay, airport, or land destination at which the shipment will arrive. Typically, a land destination will be a

customs bonded warehouse. Subsequently, the agent provides details of the specific port or customs warehouse to which the consignment will be cleared.

Obtain Documents Needed for Clearing

The port authorities require the original copies of the documents detailed in Figure 22.3 to permit clearance by the buyer. Along with these documents, the buyer prepares customs and port authority entries. Once these are completed, customs duties (if applicable) as well as port authority and other charges must be paid before the consignment of drugs is removed from the custody of the customs and port authorities.

Deliver to Warehouse

Except in the case of drugs requiring special storage conditions—for example, a cold room or a dark location—the consignment is kept in a general-purpose port or customs warehouse until delivery. The loading of the consignment onto trucks must be supervised by wharf officers. Drivers should be told precisely where the consignment is to be delivered.

≡ 22.5 Expediting Port Clearing

Port facilities in many countries are inefficient. Nevertheless, the port-clearing department or port-clearing agent can improve the situation by adopting better systems and procedures. Typical problems experienced by an import unit, and some methods for expediting work, are discussed below.

Figure 22.2 Processing of Import Documents

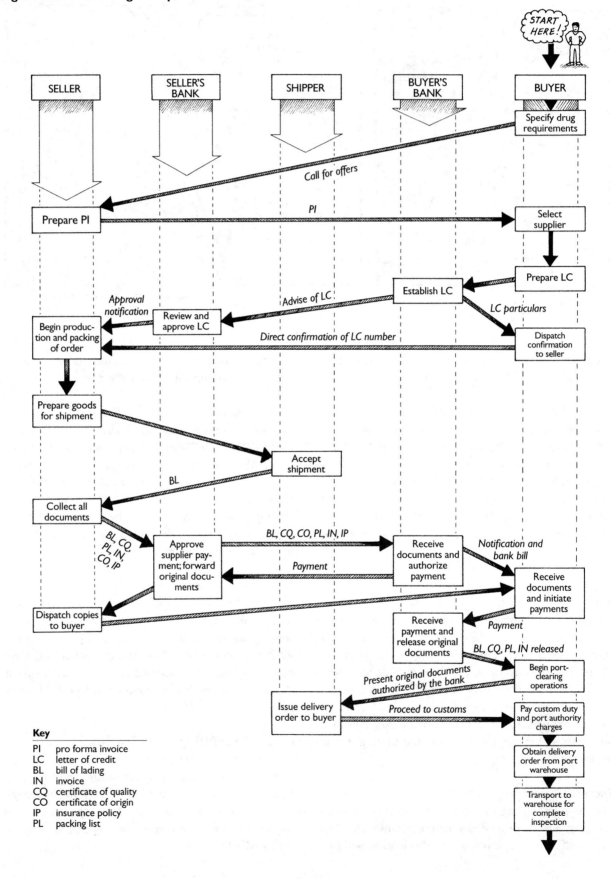

Key

PI	pro forma invoice
LC	letter of credit
BL	bill of lading
IN	invoice
CQ	certificate of quality
CO	certificate of origin
IP	insurance policy
PL	packing list

Figure 22.3 Documents Used in Port Clearing

Air waybill (AW). Document prepared by the shipper that provides details about the contents of the shipment, the route and carrier, and the shipping charges.

Bank bill (BB). A bill presented by the buyer's bank to the buyer that covers the total cost of goods received and any bank charges for processing the order (cable charges, interest on letter of credit, fees).

Bank guarantee (BG). In certain circumstances, the lack of necessary documents may make it impossible for the buyer to clear a consignment of drugs that has arrived at the port. In such instances, a bank guarantee from the buyer's bank can facilitate port clearing.

Bill of lading (BL). A document certifying that the goods are in the charge of the carrying vessel and dated on or before the last date for shipment as given in the letter of credit. The document is issued by the shipper and signed by the master of the vessel.

Certificate of origin (CO). Document stating that the product under consideration has been produced by the manufacturer in the country concerned. Such a certificate should be obtained from a national chamber of commerce or similar institute of the exporter's country.

Certificate of quality (CQ). It is the usual practice for a buyer to insist on certification from the supplier, such as batch certificates and a WHO-type certificate of a pharmaceutical product from the exporting country's drug regulatory authority (see Chapters 17 and 18).

Insurance policy (IP). Drug consignments are generally insured against damage, pilferage, and complete loss. The insurance policy indicates that a certain sum of money has been paid as a premium to cover the consignment of drugs. This document normally provides information about the nature and extent of coverage provided and the terms and conditions under which it is valid.

Invoice (IN). Document provided by the supplier indicating costs, freight, insurance, and any other payment due on the order.

Letter of credit (LC). An interbank document issued by the buyer's bank. It states that a certain sum of money is available for the seller to claim from the bank as soon as a consignment is shipped and the required documents are presented, as specified in the letter of credit. It becomes irrevocable when appropriated and numbered by the bank.

Packing list (PL). Prepared by the seller, this document describes in detail the contents of each package in a consignment of drugs, including drug strength, pack size, number of packs per carton, and number of cartons per package. This helps the buyer check whether drugs actually shipped are in accord with the packing list and the purchase contract.

Pro forma invoice (PI). Provided to the buyer by the supplier. It includes information such as the price of the product, shipping and insurance charges (if applicable), total value, a detailed description of the product offered, and terms of payment.

Use of an Activity Monitoring System

One of the biggest problems experienced by the manager of an import unit or port-clearing department is the supervision of staff engaged in clearing drugs at the port. Unlike the staff of other departments such as procurement and inventory control, many of the staff involved in clearing drugs have to spend much of their time outside the office. Hence, supervision, assignment of duties, and progress monitoring are difficult.

Under such conditions, it is helpful if the import manager maintains an information system that is capable of monitoring current port-clearing activities, causes of delays, and assignment of personnel. It should also expedite the clearing of urgently needed consignments.

Information and Documentation for Expected Consignments

Another major problem is lack of information on expected shipments. It is common for the import unit to spend a great deal of time checking with shipping agents to ascertain whether goods have arrived. In many instances, the import unit learns of the arrival of consignments only after the goods have actually landed. In some cases, high port storage charges have already been incurred by the time notification is received.

Excessive delays in port clearing and high port storage charges are usually caused by a breakdown of communication between the supplier and the purchasing department. As described in Chapter 17, the procurement contract should clearly specify the number of copies of invoices and shipping documents needed. One copy of the shipping document must be sent to the purchasing office by fax or other expeditious means when the shipment leaves the supplier's warehouse.

Often, the documents needed for clearing are not received on time from the supplier or too few copies are sent, resulting in additional delay and expense. To overcome this problem, it is important to maintain good communication among the supplier, the freight forwarder, the consignee, and all other parties. In addition, reports of supplier inefficiency should be incorporated into the general merit rating system of suppliers (see Chapter 16).

≡ 22.6 Pressing Insurance Claims

Once damaged goods or short shipments are identified, it is important to complete the insurance claim quickly. Recovery of insured losses depends on the existence of a conscientious, systematic routine for inspecting all shipments when they are accepted at the port or at the central warehouse (see Chapter 23). Consistent recovery of insured losses also depends on the assignment of qualified staff to claims processing. An effective monitoring system reduces the chance that claims will be forgotten or unduly delayed. This function should be part of the system used for monitoring the port-clearing process. ■

≡ Assessment Guide

Existing Arrangements

► Which air, sea, and land ports are used? What proportion of total supplies comes through each port?

► What is the average time to clear goods from each port?

Port Conditions and Clearance Procedures

► Are there cold rooms? Freezers? Locked warehouses? Fenced areas? Are drugs damaged by climatic conditions?

► What are the causes of recent port losses?
  – physical damage
  – theft
  – poor storage conditions
  – lost shipments caused by crowding or disorganized port management
  – delayed port clearance

► Who is responsible for port clearing?
  – central medical stores staff
  – ministry of health or government import unit
  – private import agents

► Do port-clearing staff know in advance when and where a shipment is due? Is this information used to speed port clearance? Do the same problems recur regularly?

► Are port-clearing staff trained in import documentation and port-clearing procedures?

► Does the import unit workload vary significantly throughout the year? If so, does this create any difficulties?

► Do port authorities assign priority to drug shipments?

► Do customs and import control regulations affect port-clearing efficiency? Do other agencies assist or impede port clearing?

► Are storage fees regularly incurred?

► Are there adequate procedures for receiving and checking drugs?

Private Clearing Agents

► Are private clearing agents available? Are they competent to handle drug shipments?

► How do charges for contracting with a private agent compare with the cost of existing arrangements?

Communications

► Does the import unit or agency have direct access to an overseas telephone line? Does it have a fax machine?

Monitoring and Evaluation

► What is the average time needed to clear shipments from the port?

► Are there effective systems for monitoring and evaluating import procedures? If not, which elements are missing?

► What is the annual cost of port losses as a percentage of the value of drugs received? Are there significant variations between ports? Why?

► If delays in port clearance are chronic, what are the causes?
  – poor procedures by the buyer
  – bureaucratic delays at the port
  – missing or incomplete documentation
  – lack of funds to clear goods

≡ **References and Further Readings**

★ = *Key readings.*

★ Downs, D. E., ed. 1992. *Understanding the freight business*, 4th ed. Egham, Surrey, England: Micor Freight UK.

★ International Chamber of Commerce. 1990. *International rules for the interpretation of trade terms* (in English and French). Paris: International Chamber of Commerce Publishing S.A. (Cours Albert 1er, F-75008, Paris, France).

Offitzer, K., ed. 1992. *Guide to starting your own import/export business.* New York: Citadel Press.

Wentworth, F., ed. 1970. *Handbook of physical distribution.* Epping, England: Gower Press.

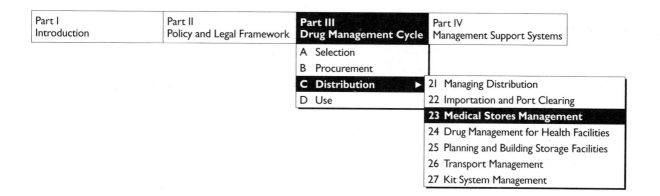

Part I	Part II	Part III	Part IV
Introduction	Policy and Legal Framework	**Drug Management Cycle**	Management Support Systems

A Selection
B Procurement
C Distribution ►
D Use

21 Managing Distribution
22 Importation and Port Clearing
23 Medical Stores Management
24 Drug Management for Health Facilities
25 Planning and Building Storage Facilities
26 Transport Management
27 Kit System Management

Chapter 23
Medical Stores Management

≡ **Summary**

This chapter discusses medical stores management at central-level stores and at regional- or district-level stores that are independent from health facilities. Medical stores management should assist the movement of supplies from source to user as cheaply and reliably as possible, and without significant wastage or theft.

The primary purpose of a store is to receive, hold, and dispatch stock. This process is controlled by an inventory control system, *which may be manual or computer based. The primary purpose of inventory control is to manage procurement and stock movements. The system should also be designed to provide information for performance monitoring.*

The following are characteristics of a well-managed stores operation:

► *The store should be divided into zones that provide a range*

of environmental conditions and degrees of security.

► *There should be an appropriate zone to suit every item to be stored.*

► *Stock should be arranged within each zone according to some orderly system.*

► *Stock should be stored on pallets on the floor, on pallet racks, or on shelves. Each of these systems requires specific types of handling equipment.*

► *Good housekeeping—cleaning and inspection, the disposal of expired and damaged stock, and the management of security—should be maintained.*

► *The management structure should be clearly defined.*

► *Staff should be appropriately qualified, trained, disciplined, and rewarded.*

► *To promote efficiency, staff should have good working conditions and facilities.*

≡ 23.1 Information for Inventory Control

The goals of medical stores management are to protect stored items from loss, damage, theft, or wastage and to manage the reliable movement of supplies from source to user in the least expensive way. Effective use of information is the key to achieving these goals.

The integrated process is known as *inventory control*. The purpose of an inventory control system is to ensure that the distribution system always contains the right goods in the correct quantities. A fully developed system has three key components:

1. An *inventory management system* to obtain the right goods and to monitor their intake and quality (see Chapter 15);
2. A *stock control system* to monitor the flow of goods within the system;
3. A *performance monitoring system* to check that the system is operating effectively.

Information is essential to management (see Chapter 45). Collecting, processing, and disseminating information are costly, but the cost of developing and maintaining an information system should be balanced against the costs of ineffective inventory control (see Chapter 15). The design of the information system is important, but its success depends primarily on well-trained, organized, and supervised staff.

Manual versus Computerized Systems

The information system must include data on products entering and leaving the warehouse, products in stock, products on order, and ways to monitor the progress of orders in the supply pipeline. Key elements of the system are well-designed forms and clearly defined procedures.

A decade ago, most public supply systems relied completely on manual stock records, but over the last few years, many programs have changed over to computerized systems. Even with computerization, however, it is good practice to maintain a manual system, such as bin cards, as a backup. There is a widely held belief that computerization solves the problem of inventory control. This is not true. A computer is not a substitute for trained staff; it is simply an additional tool for them to use (see Chapter 46). Both manual and computerized systems perform the same fundamental information processing tasks: data input, data storage, data processing, data retrieval, and data dissemination. The difference is that a computerized system enables some tasks to be accomplished more rapidly, accurately, economically, and flexibly. Nevertheless, data still have to be entered, manipulated, and interpreted by skilled and knowledgeable staff.

Procurement Information

The procurement cycle (Chapters 13–20) involves medical stores input at all levels of the distribution system. These activities are described below.

The medical stores unit provides the procurement unit with a list of the types and quantities of drugs needed. Once a supplier is selected and an order is placed, the procurement unit informs the medical stores unit about suppliers, unit prices, the quantities on order, the expected arrival dates of shipments, and other vital information.

The unit tracks information on inventory status, new shipments received and taken into stock, issues made to health facilities, expired drugs, damaged drugs, and audit data from physical stock checks.

The medical stores unit also keeps track of issues to individual health facilities, noting methods of transport, delivery times, and confirmation of receipts from user units. This tracking should generate information on the monthly and annual value of total issues, details of specific products, and how budget allocations are used.

After an order has been placed, its progress should be monitored until it is received at the central medical stores (CMS). A good monitoring system makes it possible to estimate realistic delivery times and to decide whether any supplementary or emergency orders are needed.

Both manual and computerized systems should identify milestones during the lead-time period, to facilitate communication with suppliers. Important milestones of procurement lead time are

- order initiating date;
- date of award to supplier (for tenders);
- letter of credit information;
- shipment information and date;
- arrival at port;
- port-clearing date;
- date of receiving report.

An effective supplier information system should include general information on suppliers and products, lead times, merit ratings, value of purchases, product quality, payment methods, and prequalification based on good manufacturing practices. Information about supplier performance should be compiled throughout the procurement cycle to assist in choosing future suppliers. Chapter 16 discusses the features of a procurement information system in more detail.

Stock Records
Stock records contain information about suppliers, customers, prices, stock receipts, stock issues, stock losses, and stock balances. These data are essential for planning distribution.

There must be a stock record (manual or computerized) for each item in the inventory. The stock record documents all transactions relating to an item. It may contain information about reorder level, reorder interval, reorder quantity, lead time, and estimated consumption rate. Many stores also maintain a bin card with each product

in the storage area as a duplicate record. In some stores, this is the most current and accurate record of inventory movement.

The design of stock cards and bin cards depends on the choice of inventory control system. For details regarding the design, selection, and use of different types of inventory control systems, see Chapter 15; examples of a stock record card and a bin card are provided in Annexes 23.1 and 23.2.

When a drug shipment is received at the CMS, it is inspected to ensure that it meets the specifications in the supply contract. If the shipment is satisfactory, the receiving section of the warehouse produces a receiving report (see Annex 23.3). This report brings the procurement lead-time period to an end.

Individual health facilities are the end-users of medical supplies. It is essential to maintain information from health facilities in order to monitor consumption, forecast drug requirements, and make other management decisions. Many medical stores information systems also keep general information on facility location, facility status, population served, method of distribution, delivery schedule, value of issues, and extent of current budget utilization.

Performance Monitoring and Reporting
Record-keeping and reporting systems should be designed to make the collection of data for routine monitoring as simple as possible (see Chapter 36). Stock records are a vital source of information on how effectively the distribution system is being managed. They provide detailed evidence of how products flow through the system and can be used to identify where problems are occurring so that corrective action can be taken. Regular reports on stock and order status, such as those described in Chapter 15, should be prepared by the medical stores and sent to the ministry of health, lower-level warehouses, and health facilities.

Communications
The medical stores must maintain effective communications with suppliers, with lower-level warehouses and health facilities, and with ministry of health managers. Periodic meetings with the staff of client facilities can help ensure good communications and a more effective supply system.

≡ 23.2 Flow of Stock and Paperwork
Stock, and the paperwork that accompanies it, should flow through the warehouse in an orderly manner. There are six stages to this process:

1. *Receiving.* Goods arrive in the receiving room and are inspected and entered into the stock recording system. Receiving reports are prepared.
2. *Storage.* Accepted goods are moved to their allocated storage positions in the warehouse, where they are stored in first-in/first-out (FIFO) or first-expiry/first-out (FEFO) order.
3. *Allocation of stock.* In most medical stores, the manager determines whether or not to allocate the complete quantities requested when a requisition is received. The decision depends on stock status and on a review of facility consumption patterns (and, in some cases, on budget status).
4. *Order picking.* An order-picking list is prepared (which may be the original requisition form rather than a separate list). Workers use this list to identify and collect the allocated items from the warehouse.
5. *Order assembly.* Individual orders are assembled and checked in the packing area. They are then packed for delivery. Delivery documentation is prepared.
6. *Dispatch and delivery.* The packed goods are loaded onto the transport and dispatched, accompanied by the necessary documentation, including a packing list recording all items and quantities. Ideally, an invoice showing drug unit costs and total value should accompany the shipment. Signed delivery notes are checked when the vehicle returns. If errors or damage has been reported, appropriate action is taken.

Formal and informal physical stock counts should be taken regularly to ensure that stock is being correctly handled and that losses and inaccuracies are properly accounted for.

Stock Receipt

Importation and port clearing are described in Chapter 22. The procedure outlined here assumes that these tasks are carried out by an import unit attached to the CMS. Port clearing may, however, be contracted to a clearing agent or made the responsibility of the supplier. In such cases, the goods are delivered directly to the CMS or are collected from the agent's warehouse. Final responsibility for inspection remains with the CMS.

With the exception of locally purchased items, multiple copies of the supplier's shipping documents and supplier's invoice should be received by the CMS before supplies arrive at the port of entry. This information is recorded on a manual or computerized form to track each purchase order. In addition, the import unit should record the arrival information. This advisory is clipped to the purchase order in the supplier's file to await the arrival of the shipment.

When notice of a shipment's arrival at the port is received, the necessary customs forms are completed. Often, it is necessary to visit the port to arrange for the release of the shipment.

Containers are inspected against the supplier's shipping document. The first part of the receiving report is completed (Annex 23.3). Any apparent damage and/or missing shipping cases are noted and reported to the port authorities and customs officials.

When the shipment arrives at the warehouse receiving area, contents should be quarantined until they have been checked (Figure 23.1). The receiving clerks systematically check the cases and their contents against the supplier's invoice. Discrepancies, variations, and damage are noted on the invoice. A prompt and thorough inspection based on predefined criteria is essential to quality assurance and as a precursor to any insurance claim. Figure 23.2 is a checklist with sample inspection criteria.

The annotated invoice is signed and dated by a senior staff member. Observations are summarized on the second part of the receiving report.

One copy of the receiving report is filed according to the purchase order number to which it corresponds. The other copy and the annotated supplier's invoice are passed to the stock control section. In some warehouses, a separate copy goes to the accounting department.

The items are then entered on their respective stock record cards (Annex 23.1). The new stock-on-hand totals are calculated, as well as the average cost per unit for each item. If a computerized system is used, receipts are entered into the system as prescribed in the software manual.

Stock Storage

After incoming stock has been checked and approved, it is formally released from the receiving area and moved to the warehouse to be stored in the appropriate zone. New stock may be stored on floor pallets, pallet racks, or shelves. If a fluid or semifluid location system is used (see Section 23.4), the exact location of each item must be recorded. If a bin card system is in use, receipts should be entered on the bin card when the items are transferred to the storage area.

Stock Control Using FIFO and FEFO

In order to avoid accumulation of expired and obsolete stock, items should be stored and issued on a FIFO or FEFO basis, according to the following guidelines.

The stock control system must record the expiry date

Figure 23.1 Checking Received Goods

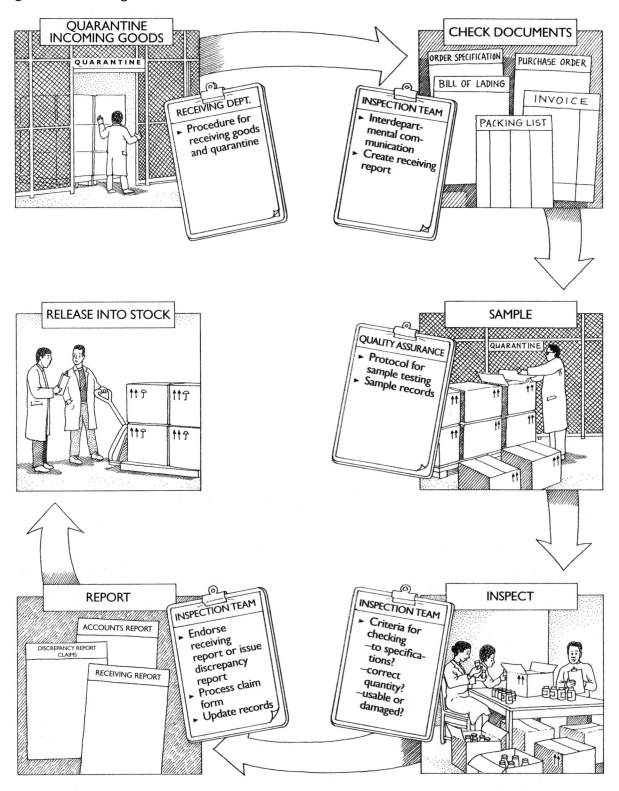

Figure 23.2 Inspection Checklist for Drug Receipts

All Shipments

Compare the goods with the supplier's invoice and original purchase order or contract. Note discrepancies on the receiving report. CHECK THAT:

❑ number of containers delivered is correct

❑ number of packages in each container is correct

❑ quantity in each package is correct

❑ drug is correct (do not confuse generic name and brand name)

❑ dosage form is correct (tablet, liquid, other form)

❑ strength is correct (milligrams, percent concentration, other measurement)

❑ unique identifiers are present, if required (article code, ministry of health stamp, other code)

❑ there is no visible evidence of damage (describe)

Take a sample for testing (if preacceptance sampling is a standard procedure).

Tablets

For each shipment, tablets of the same drug and dose should be consistent. CHECK THAT:

❑ tablets are identical in size

❑ tablets are identical in shape

❑ tablets are identical in color (shade of color may vary from batch to batch)

❑ tablet markings are identical (scoring, lettering, numbering)

❑ there are no defects (check for spots, pits, chips, breaks, uneven edges, cracks, embedded or adherent foreign matter, stickiness)

❑ there is no odor when a sealed bottle is opened (except for flavored tablets and those with active ingredients normally having a characteristic odor)

❑ there is no odor after tablets have been exposed to room air for twenty to thirty minutes

Capsules

For each shipment, capsules of the same drug and dose should be consistent. CHECK THAT:

❑ capsules are identical in size

❑ capsules are identical in shape

❑ capsules are identical in color (shade of color may vary from batch to batch)

❑ capsule markings are identical

❑ there are no defects (check for holes, pits, chips, breaks, uneven edges, cracks, embedded or adherent foreign matter, stickiness)

❑ there are no empty capsules

❑ there are no open or broken capsules

Parenterals

Parenterals are all products for injection (IV liquids, ampoules, dry solids for reconstitution, suspensions for injection). CHECK THAT:

❑ solutions are clear (solutions should be free from undissolved particles, within permitted limits)

❑ dry solids for use in injections are entirely free from visible foreign particles

❑ there are no leaking containers (bottles, ampoules)

and the date of receipt. Stock must be stored so that earliest-expiring or first-delivered batches are picked and issued first. When small quantities are involved, this can be achieved by placing the newly received stock at the back of the shelf behind the existing stock. When larger quantities are involved—for example, several pallet loads—the newly received items can be placed on the upper levels of the pallet racking. They remain there until the older stock has been issued. The picking stock is kept in an accessible position, assuming that orders are picked by hand in relatively small quantities. In warehouses where whole pallet loads are picked for distribution to lower-level stores, this is less of a concern, since mechanical transporters are used.

Newly arrived stock sometimes has an earlier expiry date than a previously received batch of the same item. If a FEFO system is used, this stock should be "promoted" so that it is issued before later-expiring stock. This is particularly important with products that have short shelf lives, such as vaccines.

Note that the system for stock rotation may be determined by the scheme for price increases, if drugs are sold to clients. If pricing is done on a FIFO basis, this system should also be used for stock management, except when newer stock will expire before it can be used under a FIFO rotation.

Order Allocation

Under a pull distribution system, lower-level stores and health facilities submit requests or requisitions for supplies. In most medical stores, a designated official is responsible for reviewing requisitions and allocating stock based on inventory levels at the requesting facility and in the issuing warehouse and on past consumption by the facility. The requesting facilities may have budgets that have to be considered in making allocations. Once the allocation has been made, the order can be picked.

Order Picking

The allocated quantities form the order-picking list. This list is passed to the storekeeper. In a large store—especially one that uses a fluid location system (see Section 23.4)—the picking list should specify the exact position of the items to be selected. In a small store, the storekeeper probably knows where everything is. The listed items are taken from stock in strict FIFO or FEFO order and transported to the packing area, where order assembly takes place.

If bin cards are used, the stock issued should be recorded on the bin card as it is pulled from the storage area.

Order Assembly

At the shipping location, the supplies are arranged in the order in which they appear on the requisition form (Annex 23.4). The order is double checked by the store-keeper or shipping clerk before the items are packed, sealed, and labeled for delivery. Some items, such as vaccines, require special packing and handling.

Order Dispatch and Delivery

With an in-house delivery system, supplies are generally distributed according to a fixed delivery schedule. The shipping clerk completes a delivery voucher (Annex 23.5). The voucher lists the number and type of the shipped packages. Their specific content is not identified unless the items require special handling, such as vaccines, loose items such as bulk germicides, and medical gas tanks. The voucher is signed by the driver, who takes two copies with him, together with two copies of the invoice or completed requisition form. The third copy of the delivery voucher remains bound in the delivery vouchers book, which is maintained by the shipping clerk.

When the delivery arrives at the receiving facility, the driver and the facility's receiving officer count and inspect the containers. Any apparent loss or damage is noted on the delivery voucher. The receiving officer and the driver sign both copies; each keeps one copy. Ideally, the received parcels should be opened and verified against the requisition form in the presence of the driver. Because of time constraints, however, this is not always possible.

The signed delivery voucher certifies that the driver has safely delivered the supplies. The receiving store retains the two copies of the completed requisition form. One is signed and dated and returned to the delivering store. Any differences between the contents of the delivery and the requisition form are reported on the form, and an investigation takes place.

The driver returns the signed copy of the delivery voucher to the inventory clerk, who signs and dates it and also signs and dates the permanent copy in the delivery vouchers book. That copy (now bearing the signatures of the driver, the receiving officer, and the inventory clerk, with the respective dates) is placed with the file copy of the completed requisition.

Some supply systems require that the receiving facility send a written notification of receipt. In such cases, the receiving facility should return a signed copy of the completed requisition to the CMS before the facility's next requisitioning date. The date of its return is entered in the register of requisitions (stores issues ledger) (Annex 23.6). If the receiving facility does not submit this "certified received" copy, the supplying store may refuse to fill the next requisition. The copy is filed in the individual requisitioner's file by date. If any discrepancies have been noted and subsequently verified, all relevant records, including the inventory card, must be adjusted. Again, all these records can be computerized, with file copies maintained.

Inventory Taking

The bin card (Annex 23.2) and the stock record card (Annex 23.1) and/or computer file provide a continuous record of each supply item in stock. The filed copies of the purchase orders and the verified copies of suppliers' invoices are used to document additions to the inventory.

The medical stores unit must regularly take actual counts of stock on hand to check that the stock balance on perpetual inventory records is correct. The government or stores audit office should also periodically certify that the recorded transactions and net totals are accurate. This audit exercise is carried out by examining procurements and requisitions and is verified by a physical stock count. As discussed in Chapter 15, the cyclic stock count is now preferred to the traditional annual count. This cyclic count is easier to manage and is more likely to allow reconciliation of discrepancies between records and physical stock.

Both active and safety stock in all locations should be counted as scheduled and compared with the numbers on the respective cards. Inventory verification, at every location where supplies are stocked, should be planned to

▶ enforce procedures and regulations designed to prevent loss and wastage;

▶ ensure that security measures are adequate;

▶ provide an additional form of evaluation that may reveal defects in the warehousing system;

▶ provide regular evaluation of storage conditions and the adequacy of storage facilities, layout, and stock arrangement;

▶ identify surplus, expired, and obsolete stock.

≡ 23.3 Zoning Stock within the Store

Drugs and essential medical supplies must be located in a part of the store with the correct combination of temperature and security. This initial zoning process is the most basic way in which supplies are arranged.

A zone can be a separate building or room, a locked cupboard, a refrigerator, a freezer, or a cold room. Figure 23.3 indicates several possible combinations and illustrates how to classify items according to their storage requirements. Thus, an item classified "2B" in this scheme would be stored at +15 to +25–30°C in a secure store.

Figure 23.3 Temperature and Security Zones

Category	A Normal security	B High security	C Flammable	D Corrosive
1 Uncontrolled temperature	■	■	■	■
2 +15 to +25–30°C (controlled humidity)	■	■		
3 0 to +8°C	■			
4 –20°C	■			

Notes: The +15 to +25–30°C zone is assumed to be air-conditioned and therefore humidity controlled. In temperate climates, this temperature range can be achieved without air-conditioning, but humidity control may still be necessary.

Cells marked ■ are commonly required temperature and security zones. Other combinations may be required for specific products. For example, zones "3B" and "4B" may be needed for vaccines if the vaccines have a black-market value—for instance, hepatitis B—or there is a particular problem with security for refrigeration equipment.

It is essential to follow the product manufacturer's storage instructions to the extent possible. If this is not possible, the product must be kept in the most suitable conditions available and used as quickly as possible. The product manufacturer should be consulted before violating recommended storage conditions to determine how long the product will remain safe and effective under the actual storage conditions.

If no specific storage instructions are given, "normal storage conditions" apply. Normal storage conditions for drugs have been defined as "storage in dry, well ventilated

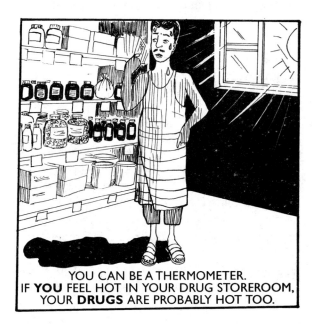

YOU CAN BE A THERMOMETER.
IF **YOU** FEEL HOT IN YOUR DRUG STOREROOM,
YOUR **DRUGS** ARE PROBABLY HOT TOO.

premises at temperatures of +15°C to +25°C, or, depending upon climatic conditions, up to +30°C" (WHO 1990). Each storage zone should have at least one thermometer, and temperatures should be recorded daily at the hottest time of day.

Storage at Uncontrolled Room Temperature

Many products can be be safely stored at uncontrolled room temperature. However, the temperature in the upper part of a store can exceed 40°C even in temperate climates. In cold climates, temperatures will drop below freezing in unheated stores. Such temperature extremes may damage some items. Chapter 18 discusses items known to be sensitive to extreme storage conditions (see Figure 18.2).

Storage at Controlled Temperature and Controlled Humidity

In hot climates, it is necessary to store many items in air-conditioned rooms. In humid climates, dehumidifiers are useful for preventing moisture damage. In cold climates, stores may need to be heated in winter to protect products that are damaged by freezing.

Cold Storage

The potency of vaccines, sera, test kits, and many other items depends on cold storage. Vaccines, in particular, must be kept at precisely controlled temperatures from the point of manufacture to the point of administration.

Cold-chain defects are a frequent cause of problems in immunization programs. The World Health Organization Expanded Programme on Immunization (EPI) publishes comprehensive advisory material on designing and implementing a cold chain. This material should be referred to for detailed technical advice. Figure 23.4 summarizes the requirements for an effective cold chain.

National and regional vaccine stores should be equipped with standby generators; ideally, district vaccine stores should have them as well. Having backups ensures that vaccines and other products are protected in the event of a power failure.

Secure Storage

Narcotics and other controlled substances should be kept in a secure room or in a safe. Ideally, a red warning light or warning bell that will activate when the door is unlocked should be fixed close to the store. The keys to the secure store should be kept in a safe.

Entry to the store must be controlled. No more than two assigned officers should have access. Typically, one should be the director of the store, the most senior phar-

Figure 23.4 Typical Requirements for an Effective Cold Chain

Level and Staff Functions	Management Activities	Supplies and Equipment Needed

National
Management
► National program coordination
► Epidemiology
► Logistics
► Transport management
► Training
► Procurement
► Budget and finance
► Data analysis
Central Store
► Storekeeping
► Delivery
Maintenance
► Equipment care and
  maintenance
	Program Planning
	► Demographic/epidemiological data
	► Administrative structures
	► Logistic systems
	Program Monitoring
	► Disease surveillance
	► Immunization coverage
	► Cold-chain and transport operation
	► Supplies usage
	► Program costs
	Supplies Management
	► Procurement, storage, delivery
	► Refrigeration monitoring
	► Transport management
	Independent Evaluations
	Staff Recruitment and Training
	Supervision of Operations
		Cold-Chain Equipment
		► +4°C cold room: twin refrigeration units,
		  recording thermometer, alarm
		► -20°C freezer room equipped as above
		► Icepack freezers and cold boxes *unless*
		  refrigerated vehicles are used
		► Standby power supply
		Working and Safety Stocks
		► Vaccines and injection equipment
		► Stationery and forms
		► Cold-chain monitor cards
		► Cold-chain equipment and spare parts
		Transport and Fuel
		Special Facilities
		Vaccine Control Laboratory (where feasible)

Regional/Provincial
Management
► Regional program
► Epidemiology
► Logistics and transport
► Training
► Data analysis and reports
Regional Store
► Storekeeping
► Delivery
Maintenance
► Equipment care and
  maintenance
	Program Monitoring
	► Disease surveillance
	► Immunization coverage
	► Cold-chain and transport operation
	► Supplies usage
	Supplies Management
	► Requisitioning, storage, delivery
	► Refrigeration monitoring
	► Transport management
	Staff Recruitment and Training
	Supervision of District Operations
		Cold-Chain Equipment
		► +4°C cold room *or* vaccine refrigerators,
		  thermometers, alarm
		► Vaccine freezers, thermometers, alarm
		► Icepack freezers and cold boxes *unless*
		  refrigerated transport is used
		► Standby power supply
		Working and Safety Stocks
		► Vaccines and injection equipment
		► Stationery and forms
		► Spare parts
		Transport and Fuel

District Management ► District program ► Data analysis and reports District Store ► Storekeeping ► Delivery Maintenance ► Equipment care and maintenance	Program Monitoring ► Disease reporting ► Immunization reporting ► Cold-chain and transport operation ► Supplies usage Supplies Management ► Requisitioning, storage, delivery ► Refrigeration monitoring ► Transport management Supervision of Health Facilities	Cold-Chain Equipment ► Vaccine refrigerators, thermometers, alarm ► Vaccine freezers, thermometers, alarm ► Icepack freezers and cold boxes ► Standby power supply Working and Safety Stocks ► Vaccines and injection equipment ► Stationery and forms ► Spare parts Transport and Fuel
Health Facility ► Giving immunizations ► Storekeeping ► Reporting ► Equipment care and maintenance	Supplies Management ► Requisitioning and storage ► Refrigerator monitoring ► Transport management Reporting of ► Disease incidence ► Immunizations given ► Refrigerator defects ► Transport mileage and defects ► Stock on hand	Cold-Chain Equipment ► Vaccine refrigerator with ice-making compartment and thermometer ► Cold boxes for outreach sessions ► Vaccine carriers Working and Safety Stocks ► Vaccines and injection equipment ► Stationery and forms Transport and Fuel

macist, or the most senior storekeeper (see also Chapter 39). Such precautions may also be needed for nonnarcotic drugs that are frequently stolen.

Flammables

Flammables, such as alcohol and ether, must be stored in special buildings or rooms. A separate building is best, because this greatly reduces the risk of a fire's spreading to the main store. The flammables store must be well ventilated and fireproof. It must be fitted with an "explosion hatch," which may be part of the roof or part of a wall.

Fuel must never be stored in or near a medical store. Fuel tanks should be placed inside a locked compound to prevent theft. There should be a continuous earth bank or low wall around the tanks. The area enclosed should be sufficient to hold the total volume of the fuel stored; this ensures that fuel is contained if there is a major spillage. If there is a fire, the risk of its spreading will be reduced.

≡ 23.4 Stock Location within a Zone

Within each zone, stock may be located in *fixed, fluid,* or *semifluid* locations. Fixed location systems are the simplest to manage, because each stock item is always stored in the same place. Fluid systems require sophisticated stock management, because the location of each stock item varies over time. Semifluid systems combine features of both systems.

Fixed Location

In a fixed location system, each stock item is allocated to specific shelves, pallet racking, or an area of floor. A fixed location system is like a house in which each family member has his or her own room. A room is left empty if the person is not at home.

For a fixed location system to work well, the store has to be large enough to accommodate the maximum possible level of stock for every item, including its safety stock. As stock is used up, the storage location is emptied and left vacant until a new shipment of the item is received.

With a fixed location system, stock administration is relatively easy. Goods can always be found in the same place. However, this system has certain disadvantages:

- ► Fixed location systems are inflexible. If there is a change in the quantity ordered or a change in packaging, the assigned location may become too large or too small.
- ► If a new item is ordered, there may be no place to store it.
- ► Theft may increase because all store staff are familiar with the locations of valuable items.
- ► Storage space may be wasted, because at times it is largely empty.

Fluid Location

In a fluid location system, the store is divided into many designated locations. Each location is assigned a code. Individual items are stored wherever space is available at the time of delivery. A fluid location system is like a hotel. Rooms are assigned only when guests arrive.

A fluid location system uses available space efficiently, but it requires sophisticated stock administration. Experience suggests that a store using a fluid location system can be 20 to 25 percent smaller than one using a fixed location system.

The administration of a fluid location system works as follows:

- ► The procurement unit provides information on the type, volume, and weight of goods arriving.
- ► The storekeeper assesses which locations will be empty when the new stock arrives and assigns a suitable location. These data are recorded in the stock control system.
- ► If insufficient space is available, other goods may be moved to create more space.
- ► The stock control location records are updated.

Fluid location systems require a classification system that allocates a unique code to each stock item. Also, the stock record for each batch of each item must always record the physical location of the item in the store. In a fluid location system, different batches of a particular item may be stored in several different places. For example, if item number 150-050-48 is 500 mg amoxicillin, 150-050-48: B1-B could be a batch of this product stored in aisle B, bay 1, cell B, and 150-050-48: C2-B another batch in aisle C, bay 2, cell B.

Semifluid Location

A semifluid location system is a combination of the previous two. It is like a hotel that has regular guests. Regular guests are always given the same room. Casual guests are given any room that is available.

In a semifluid system, each item is assigned some fixed space for picking stock. When an order is prepared, the order-picking staff know where to find each item. The remainder of the store is filled on the fluid location principle. When the picking stock runs low, the fixed locations are restocked from the fluid locations.

A semifluid location system is not as space-efficient as a fluid location system. However, picking stock is stored at a convenient height, and this eliminates the need for mechanical handling during order picking in stores that issue in relatively small quantities.

Another feature is that picking stock is always kept in the same place. Unlike a fixed location system, however, there is less risk that changing requirements will disrupt the system. If demand increases for a particular item, the picking stock can be replenished more frequently. As new products are introduced, it may be possible to subdivide picking bays to provide sufficient space.

≡ 23.5 Stock Classification

Items should be clearly organized within each zone of the store. This makes stock control, inventory taking, and order picking much easier.

In stores that use the fixed location principle, items can be physically organized in one of seven ways:

- ▶ therapeutic or pharmacological category
- ▶ clinical indication
- ▶ alphabetical order
- ▶ level of use
- ▶ dosage form
- ▶ random bin
- ▶ commodity code

In a fluid location system, clear organization and unique product identification are absolutely essential to the success of the system. Otherwise, items get lost. Coding by any one of the first four methods is inappropriate for a fluid location system, because the position of a particular stock item will vary over time. For example, if antipyretics are randomly distributed about the store in a fluid location system, it is not feasible to organize the store on the basis of therapeutic class.

However, therapeutic or pharmacological class, clinical indication, alphabetical order, and level-of-use classifications can still be used as a way of organizing the stock records, whatever stock location system is used. One of the advantages of a computerized stock control system is that records can be sorted in a variety of ways for different management purposes, for instance, according to therapeutic classes and also in alphabetical order.

Therapeutic or Pharmacological Category
Therapeutic or pharmacological classification may be an effective way of organizing drugs in smaller stores and in the dispensaries of small clinical facilities where the storekeeper is also the dispenser. It is not an advantage in larger stores.

Clinical Indication
A system based on clinical indication is similar to therapeutic category and may be convenient in small warehouses. All antihypertensives are together, as are all antidiabetics or other drugs with a common clinical indication. One problem is that many drugs have multiple clinical indications. A clinical indication system therefore requires a level of professional knowledge that stores staff are unlikely to have. If staff do acquire this knowledge, theft may become a problem.

Alphabetical Order
Alphabetical order (by generic name) is also attractive in peripheral stores that keep a small number of items. However, each change in the national (essential) drugs list

or in the level-of-use list requires a reorganization of the stores themselves and of the stock administration system. This method may not result in optimal use of available space.

Level of Use
In a level-of-use system, products used in only one level of facility are stored together. Storage according to level of use is an obvious way of organizing drug kits and equipment kits in higher-level stores. It is not a practical method for organizing individual items. First, more storage space is required because many commonly used items appear at more than one level. Second, distribution on a FIFO or FEFO basis becomes more difficult to achieve. Third, one of the other methods of organization is needed within each level of use to avoid chaos.

Dosage Form
A system based on dosage form is commonly used in smaller warehouses. Tablets and capsules are stored together, with separate areas for oral liquids, injections, creams and ointments, and topical liquids. Within each dosage-form area, products may be stored in a fixed, fluid, or semifluid manner and further organized by any of the other systems described in this section. The main advantages are that the forms are easy to recognize when receiving goods and this system allows optimal use of space.

Random Bin
The random bin is a unique storage space identified by a code. For example, a shelving unit can be divided vertically and horizontally into cells, each with a unique location code. A unit of shelving might be labeled "B," its bays "B1" and "B2," and its shelves "A," "B," and "C." A unique cell would be identified, for example, as B1-B (see Figure 23.5). This cell is called a *bin*.

The random bin storage method can combine the methods described above. For example, items are placed alphabetically within therapeutic classifications. Generic names are used throughout. If there is more than one brand of the same generic drug preparation, all are stored in the bin for that type.

Commodity Code
Commodity coding is an abstract organizational system. It offers maximum flexibility and can be used equally well in small and large stores.

This system is based on a unique *article code* combined with a unique *location code*. Examples of article codes include WHO technical specifications or UNICEF stock codes. Article codes can be designed to specify therapeutic class, clinical indication, level of use, or any other relevant data. In systems that use article coding and location coding, storekeeping staff do not need to have specific knowledge of pharmaceutical names and therapeutic uses.

Changes in the national drugs list can easily be introduced by assigning unique article codes to new products. Article coding works well in a computerized system. Tender contracts may require that only the article code be marked on the bulk packaging as well as on the smaller units of supply. This increases security but still allows the goods to be identified by those staff who have access to the coding key.

The location code is totally independent of the article code and is similar to the random bin principle. Suitable codes can be designed to incorporate any number of characteristics, including

- correct storage temperature for the product;
- correct security level for the product;
- whether or not the product is flammable;
- the building where the product is located;
- pack size;
- pharmaceutical form.

≡ 23.6 Stock Storage and Handling

Within each temperature and security zone, products must be stored so that they are easily accessible and protected against damage. There are four basic systems of storage: shelves, floor pallets, block-stacked pallets, and pallet racks. Direct storage of cartons on the warehouse floor should be avoided because their contents may be damaged by moisture. The choice of system depends on the following factors:

- Total quantity of products to be stored;
- Average volume of each product;
- Internal height of the storage building;
- Local availability of mechanical handling equipment and the skills to use and maintain it.

Pallets are generally used at the national and regional levels, where products are stored in bulk. At the district level and below, storage on shelves is most common. The fundamental rule for pallet storage is that there should be only one product line to a pallet. Pallets have the following advantages:

- They keep goods together and impose a disciplined method of storage.
- Large loads can be moved easily using mechanical handling equipment.

- Pallets are easy to transship because they do not require any unpacking and repacking.
- Pallets isolate goods from floors, which may be damp.
- If goods are supplied by the manufacturer on shrink-wrapped pallets, it is easy to see when tampering has occurred.
- Inspection for damage and for short shipments is easy to perform.
- When stock rearrangement is necessary, it is much easier to move pallets with mechanical handling equipment than it is to move a large volume of loose stock that has been placed on shelves.

Packaging Specifications

Appropriate packaging specifications reduce the risk of damage during handling (see Chapter 17). Floor pallets and pallet racks must be laid out to suit a selected pallet module. Pallets come in a range of sizes, and the size and weight of pallets affect the layout of the store and the choice of mechanical handling equipment. Whenever feasible, a standard pallet size should be adopted throughout the distribution system, and all suppliers should be required to conform to this specification.

Shelving

Storage on shelves does not require mechanical handling equipment and is a suitable choice when

- the volume and weight of individual items are too small to justify pallets;
- the internal height of a building is not large enough for multitier pallet racking and shelving can be used on its own or in combination with floor pallets or two-tier racking;
- manual goods handling is locally more reliable or economical than mechanical handling.

If shelving is used in a warehouse more than 4.5 meters high, it may be possible to install an independent mezzanine flooring system supporting a second tier of shelving. This can increase the available shelving volume by up to 100 percent, at the expense of some inconvenience in materials handling. Obviously, if this is done, high-quality construction is critical to avoid injury to staff and damage to stored goods.

Floor Pallets

Floor pallets are a good solution in warehouses with ceiling heights of less than 3 meters and in stores where the cost of pallet racking and forklift trucks cannot be justified. Many heavy or bulky items, such as rolls of cotton, drug kits, or large hospital equipment, require floor locations. Floors should be marked to indicate pallet and aisle positions.

Block-Stacked Pallets
Pallets containing light goods may be stacked on top of one another in blocks. Block-stacked pallets should be used only for items without expiry dates or with very high turnover, because the first-in items are at the bottom of the stack. Block stacking is a cheap and space-efficient method of storage, and no racking is required.

Pallet Racking
Simple pallet racks generally have two or three tiers. Two tiers of racking require a clear height of about 3 meters, and three tiers require a clear height of about 4.5 meters. It is possible to have several more tiers, but sophisticated mechanical handling equipment is then required.

The benefits of shelving and pallet racking can be combined. The bottom tier of racking may be used to store the working stock. This tier is at a convenient height for manual order picking. Alternatively, a special picking shelf can be placed immediately above the bottom tier of pallets. In both cases, the upper tiers can be used to store safety stock.

Load Handling
Each of the four storage systems described above requires suitable handling equipment and appropriate organization of stored goods. Correct handling equipment reduces the risk of injury to workers and damage to goods. Careful stock organization on shelves and pallets reduces unnecessary lifting and ensures easy access to goods during order picking.

Shelving. In order to reduce manual handling, goods should be transported to and from the shelves on trolley carts. Heavy items should be stored on the lower shelves. Whenever possible, other items should be organized so that frequently picked items are at waist height. Safety stock may be stored at a higher level.

Pallets. Loaded pallets can be moved only by using mechanical equipment. Hand-operated hydraulic pallet trucks and pallet lifts are suitable for floor pallets and for pallet racking up to three tiers high. Pallets stored at higher levels must be moved using powered forklift trucks. Figure 23.5 illustrates some typical storage and handling equipment.

≡ 23.7 Housekeeping
Housekeeping tasks for a store include cleaning and pest control, a regular inspection system, disposal of stock, precautions against fire, and strict security measures.

Cleaning and Pest Control
The store should be kept tidy and should be cleaned two or three times a week. Most warehouses have adequate personnel available for scheduled cleanups, and adequate cleaning equipment should be made available. Figure 23.6 illustrates good and bad stores management.

Pest control can be a difficult task, but to avoid possible contamination and physical damage to stock, it is necessary to keep insects, mice, and other pests out of the storage area. If needed, pest control measures such as poison should be implemented, with proper precautions.

Inspection
Senior staff should inspect the store regularly. The chief storekeeper must make sure that storeroom employees check the shelves and pallets daily for signs of theft, pests, or water damage and for deterioration due to climatic conditions. Storekeepers should open suspect containers and report problems to managers.

Disposal of Expired or Damaged Stock
Damaged or expired stock should be placed in a designated salvage area to await authority for disposal. A written record of all stock consigned to this area should be maintained. It is recommended that each item be valued at its acquisition cost. The responsible authority should be informed in writing that stock is to be written off. Disposal may be delayed if a committee decision is required, and substantial storage space may be needed for junk stock. Once destruction is authorized, the inventory control clerk must adjust the stock records. All drugs and other potentially toxic products should be disposed of in accordance with local regulations in a manner that does not pose a risk to public health.

Fire Precautions
Flammable trash, such as cartons and boxes, must not be allowed to accumulate in the store. Smoking must be strictly forbidden, with "No Smoking" signs posted throughout the store. Senior staff must obey the rule as strictly as junior staff, and penalties should be imposed on those who ignore the rules. A smoking area outside the warehouse should be designated. Management must ensure that fire-detection and fire-fighting equipment is regularly inspected and that staff receive adequate training in fire-fighting techniques and emergency action. There should be regular fire drills to reinforce that training.

Staff should check frequently for fire, but management is ultimately responsible. Night watchmen can serve the dual purpose of responding to fire alarms and protecting against theft.

Figure 23.5 Storage and Load-Handling Equipment

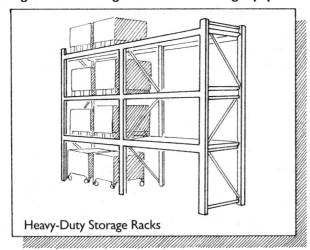

Heavy-Duty Storage Racks

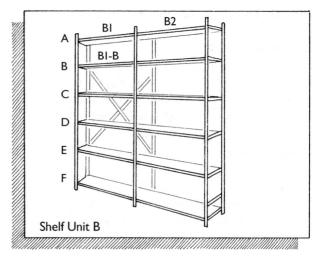

Shelf Unit B

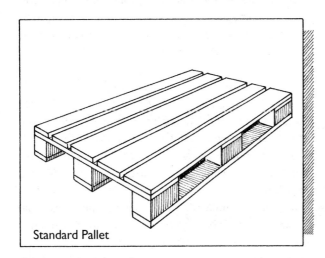

Standard Pallet

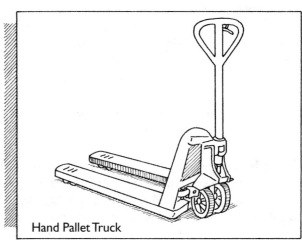

Hand Pallet Truck

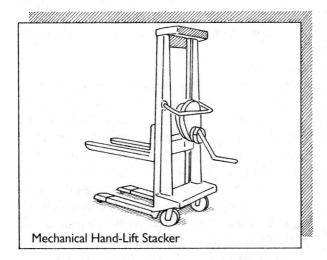

Mechanical Hand-Lift Stacker

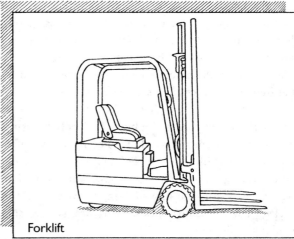

Forklift

Figure 23.6 Good and Bad Stores Management

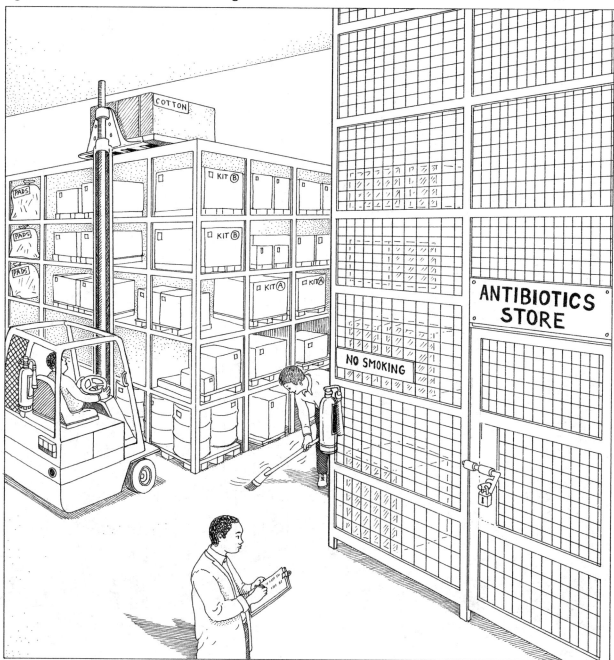

Security

Ideally, the chief storekeeper's office should have windows that overlook the loading bay, the compound entrance, and the store itself. A storekeeper who sits behind a closed door with the curtains drawn cannot observe what is happening on the site.

No vehicles should be allowed into the store compound unless they are authorized by the chief storekeeper or another senior staff member. A list of authorized vehicles should be prepared for the compound gate-keeper.

Pedestrian access to the storage buildings should also be strictly controlled. Visitors should report to the store-keeper's office and should not be allowed into the store area except on business. Business visitors should always be accompanied by a senior staff member. Visits by friends and family of staff should be discouraged. (See Chapter 39 for further discussion of security measures.)

Figure 23.6 Good and Bad Stores Management (cont.)

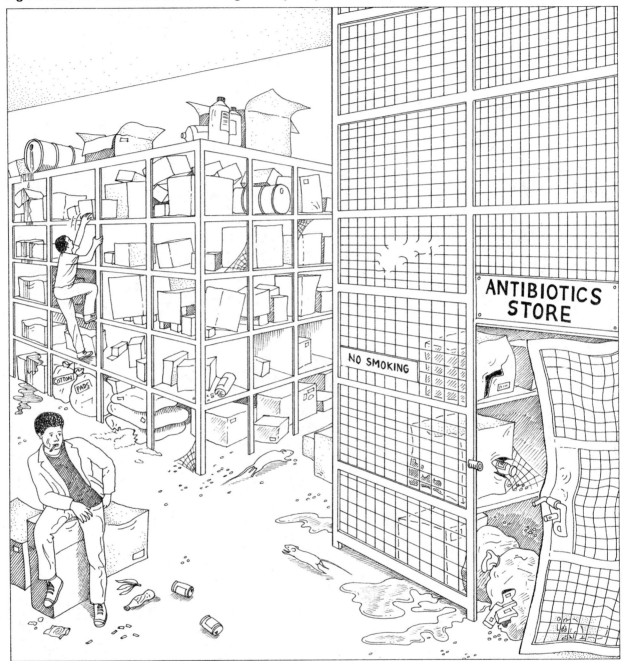

≡ 23.8 Organization and Management of the Medical Stores

This is a brief discussion of management issues; medical stores managers are encouraged to review Part IV of this book, which discusses management in detail.

The organization of a typical central medical store is shown in Figure 23.7. The organizational structure at an intermediate store is generally a compressed version of this structure.

Staff Training and the Medical Stores Procedures Manual

Every worker should receive appropriate job training. Most warehouse jobs are nontechnical, and in-service training and supervision of staff are likely to be the most effective approach. There should be a written procedures manual that covers

▸ general management policy;
▸ management structure;

Figure 23.7 Organizational Chart

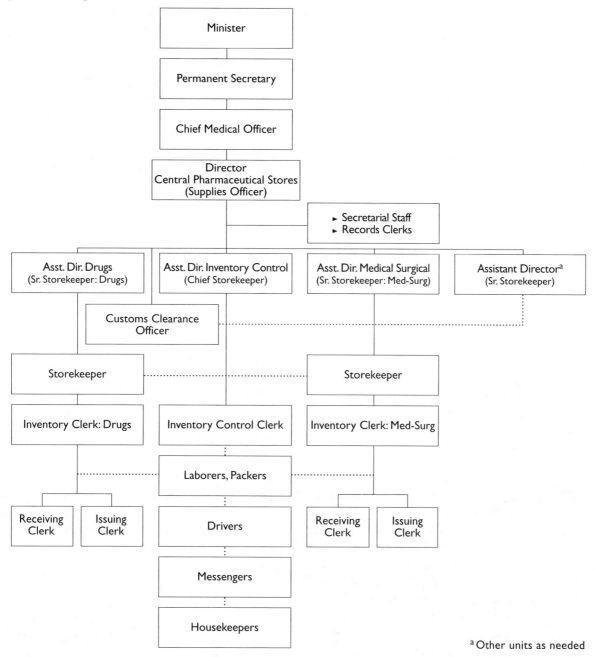

ᵃ Other units as needed

- job descriptions;
- reporting procedures;
- stock control and other record-keeping procedures;
- operational procedures;
- health and safety procedures.

The manual should include visual aids that clarify operations. These documents are normally used by the director and section chiefs to train new staff and to settle procedural questions. Figure 23.8 gives a sample contents list.

Each work area should have a copy of the manual.

The contents of the document should be reviewed and explained in group presentations. The manual should be available to every employee, and staff should be encouraged to use it in performing their duties.

Staff Supervision and Discipline
The supervisory hierarchy should be clearly described to all workers. Personnel problems should be solved at the appropriate level. Section heads who do not supervise their workers regularly and effectively should be replaced.

Figure 23.8 Contents of a Procedures Manual for a Central Pharmaceutical Supply System

Statement of Operational Policy

Organizational Staffing Pattern
- ► Central level
- ► Regional level
- ► District level
- ► Community level
- ► Lines of authority

Overview of Sequence of Tasks and Activities in Materials Management Process (with discussion of objectives of the process):
- ► Job descriptions (all personnel by level, each level treated separately)
- ► Logistics information system
- ► Flow chart of central, regional, and district information
- ► Supply operations forms (purchase order, receiving report, inventory card, requisition/issue form, issues ledger by item and facility, delivery voucher)
- ► Accounting system and procedures
- ► Inventory control system and procedures
- ► Security system and regulations
- ► Supply system administration
- ► Operating budget (utilities, salaries, maintenance, supplies, miscellaneous)
- ► Maintenance procedures (for buildings and equipment)
- ► Special operating instructions
- ► Cold-chain storage procedures
- ► Quality control procedures
- ► Shipping and packaging procedures

Positive feedback and encouragement are essential. Minor lapses in performance should be kept in perspective. Major problems, such as proven cases of theft or reckless driving, should be handled through established ministry regulations. Regular staff meetings can help maintain a sense of shared purpose and ensure that all staff members understand their responsibilities.

Career Development
Workers in the logistics system often have low status. They are frequently badly paid, work under poor conditions, and are not motivated. This results in low levels of performance.

An effective store relies on staff who want to perform their jobs correctly. When staff perform well, they should be rewarded and praised. Although it is difficult to do in many government supply systems, improving salary grades and promoting staff who show ability and commitment will help the organization retain good staff. Frequent transfers of personnel from one site to another should be avoided, if possible.

If stores staff are treated badly by management, they will look for other jobs, and their experience will be lost. A stores operation that relies on casual labor is more likely to suffer from theft, breakages, and distribution errors.

≡ 23.9 Staff Facilities
Good staff facilities encourage cleanliness, protect workers against occupational injuries, and contribute to good staff morale. Just as drugs are susceptible to damage from excessive heat or cold, staff performance and motivation suffer in these conditions.

Sanitary Facilities
Personal cleanliness is essential among workers who handle medical supplies. The store needs well-maintained sanitary facilities for staff and visitors. Sanitary accommodations should be located on the perimeter of the building to allow natural ventilation and keep the drains outside the building.

Staff Rest Areas
A separate rest area, with a kitchen and a pantry for preparing and storing food, improves staff morale and reduces fire hazards and the risk of vermin infestation in the warehouse. It also improves efficiency by segregating resting staff from working staff.

First Aid
There should be adequate first-aid equipment and dressings to treat workers who suffer injuries on the job. Emergency washing facilities should be provided in case a staff member comes into contact with a corrosive or toxic agent. It may be necessary to install emergency showers. Eye-washing sprays should also be provided. Local health and safety regulations should always be followed. ■

≡ Assessment Guide

General Description
► How are goods received and supplied?

► What facilities are served? How often is each supplied? What methods of transport are used?

Stores Management and Staffing
► Does an operations manual adequately describe procedures and responsibilities?

► Are staff positions described by category, listing posts approved and filled?

Receiving
► Are procedures for receiving and checking drugs observed? Are standard checklists used?

► What drugs were returned during the past year, and why?

► How are complaints concerning product quality handled?

Communications and Reporting
► What reports are regularly issued from medical stores, and for whom?

Stock Control
► What stock control system is used?

► Are random and periodic stock checks carried out? Is a stock auditing system in place?

► What percentage of stock records (and bin cards) correspond with physical counts?

Stock Management
► Is stock location fixed, fluid, or semifluid?

► Are drugs issued by FIFO or FEFO?

► What was the average stockout duration over the last year?

► How many expired drugs are in stock? What is their value?

► What was the value of inventory at the beginning and end of the last fiscal year?

Storage Conditions
► Are drugs zoned in correct combinations of temperature, humidity, safety, and security?

► How are drugs organized within each zone?

► Are vaccines stored and monitored in accordance with EPI recommendations?

► Is the store neat, and are effective pest control procedures in place?

Buildings and Equipment
► Is storage space too small, adequate, or excessive?

► Are the loading bay, receiving area, packing area, administrative area, staff rest area, and sanitary facilities adequate?

► What is the condition of roofs, walls, floors, ceiling, windows, doors, locks, burglar bars, and water supply and drainage installations?

► What storage systems are used (shelving, floor pallets, pallet racking)?

► What are the conditions of mechanical handling equipment, electricity supply, and telephones?

► Is there direct access to international communications?

≡ References and Further Readings

★ = Key readings.

Compton, H. K. 1985. Supplies and materials management, 3d ed. Plymouth, England: Macdonald and Evans, and Institute of Purchasing and Supply.

Electrolux. 1983. The storage handbook. Singapore: Electrolux S.E.A. Pte., Ltd. (240 MacPherson Rd. #03-01/04, Singapore 1334).

MSH (Management Sciences for Health). 1991. The family planning manager's handbook. West Hartford, Conn.: Kumarian Press.

MSH (Management Sciences for Health). 1992. Medical store management (trainer's and participant's guides). In Managing drug supply training series. Part 3. Supply management. Boston: MSH.

★ Mulcahy, D. 1994. Warehouse distribution and operations handbook. New York: McGraw-Hill.

PAHO (Pan American Health Organization). 1990. Guidelines for medical supplies distribution centers. Vol. 1. Regional and central centers: Planning, design, and construction. Washington, D.C.: PAHO.

WHO (World Health Organization). 1990. WHO expert committee on specifications for pharmaceutical preparations. TRS 790. Geneva: WHO.

WHO (World Health Organization). Forthcoming. Guidelines for establishing or improving national, regional and district vaccine stores.

WHO/UNICEF (World Health Organization/United Nations Children's Fund). 1993. Product information sheets, 10th ed. WHO/UNICEF/EPI.TS/93.1. New edition forthcoming. Geneva: WHO/UNICEF.

Annex 23.1 Stock Record Card

STOCK RECORD CARD

Generic Name: _Chloroquine_   Strength: _200 mg_   Dosage Form: _tab_

Code No.: _8022_   Unit of Issue: _tab_   Unit Price: _0.3400_

Class: _08:20_

Date	From Whom Rec./Issu.	Qty. Rec.	Qty. Issu.	Balance	Remarks	Signature
1/3/98	Inventory			100,000	Exp. 9/2000	
2/3/98	PHC I		5,000	95,000		
3/3/98	PHC II		6,000	89,000		
7/4/98	PHC I		10,000	79,000		
20/4/98	PHC III		5,000	74,000		
21/4/98	PHC I		3,000	71,000		
2/5/98	IDA	50,000		121,000	Exp. 5/2001	
7/5/98	PHC II		1,000	120,000		
8/5/98	HOSP		10,000	110,000		
8/7/98	HOSP		10,000	100,000		
15/7/98	PHC I		5,000	95,000		
31/7/98	PHC III		2,000	93,000		
3/8/98	PHC I		1,000	92,000		
30/8/98	PHC II		5,000	87,000		
30/9/98	PHC I		7,000	80,000		
5/10/98	PHC III		2,000	78,000		
8/10/98	PHC I		3,000	75,000		
1/11/98	HOSP		5,000	70,000		
7/12/98	PHC I		3,000	67,000		
15/12/98	PHC II		2,000	65,000		
1/1/99	PHC I		5,000	60,000		
13/1/99	PHC III		6,000	54,000		
14/1/99	PHC II		10,000	44,000		
2/2/99	HOSP		4,000	40,000		
3/2/99	HOSP		1,000	39,000		

Pharmacy _____

Fiscal Year	Mar	Apr	May	Jun	Jul	Aug	Sep	Oct	Nov	Dec	Jan	Feb	Usage	Exp.
FY: 97/98	11,000	18,000	11,000	0	17,000	6,000	7,000	5,000	5,000	5,000	21,000	5,000		
FY: /														

Annex 23.2 Sample Bin/Stock Card

Ministry of Health
Department of Medical Supply
BIN/STOCK CARD

Description: Paracetamol tabs 500 mg   Unit of issue: 1,000 tabs

Stock No.: 02-4600

Date 1998	Document/ Number	Received From/ Issued To	Units Received	Units Issued	Balance	Initials
Mar 5	BALANCE BROUGHT FORWARD				1,665	PF
5	IV 98534	PHC 42		10	1,655	RS
5	IV 98541	PHC 44		10	1,645	RS
6	IV 98543	HOSP 6		200	1,445	BJ
6	IV 98546	PHC 55		16	1,429	BJ
6	IV 98561	PHC 53		10	1,419	PF
6	IV 98562	PHC 52		12	1,407	BJ
6	IV 98565	PHC 54		10	1,397	PF
6	IV 98567	HOSP 7		150	1,247	PF
6	IV 98570	PHC 63		5	1,242	PF
6	IV 98572	PHC 64		5	1,237	BJ
7	IV 98573	PHC 66		5	1,232	RS
7	IV 98575	PHC 62		5	1,227	RS
7	IV 98574	PHC 68		5	1,222	RS
7	IV 98579	PHC 61		5	1,217	PF
7	IV 98601	PHC 65		5	1,212	PF
7	IV 98600	PHC 69		5	1,207	RS
7	IV 98603	PHC 67		5	1,202	PF
8	RN 98166	NOVAPHARM	10,000		11,202	BJ
8	IV 98605	HOSP 9		200	11,002	BJ
8	IV 98604	HOSP 8		200	10,802	BJ
8	IV 98609	PHC 71		10	10,792	BJ
8	IV 98611	PHC 75		12	10,780	RS
8	IV 98613	PHC 78		10	10,770	RS
8	IV 98614	PHC 72		15	10,755	RS

Annex 23.3 Receiving Report

Ministry of Health
Department of Medical Supply
Central Pharmaceutical Stores
RECEIVING REPORT

Supplier: Apotex Inc.

P.O. No.: DMS—116/97

Port of entry: Port St. Philip

Date received at port of entry: 05/12/98

Number of shipping cartons/containers: 3

Invoice No.: 686033

Carrier: Fast Forwarders

Date Cleared: 05/17/98

Certified that from external inspections, all containers appear to be suitable and without damage except as follows:

Nil

Gavaza H.	05/18/98
Clearing officer	Date

Certified that all items on the invoice and the purchase order (specified above) were received and, after inspection, released for removal to shelving except as follows (or as marked on the invoice):

Check Muvuro	05/22/98		Usopero M.	05/22/98
Receiving clerk	Date		Chief storekeeper	Date

Annex 23.4 Sample Requisition/Issue Voucher

Ministry of Health
Department of Medical Supply
REQUISITION/ISSUE VOUCHER

Requisition no.: PHC63-98-3-23

Health facility: Utano H.C.

Authorized by: Mukuru, DNO.

Date: March 4, 1998   Supply period: April   to   May 1998

Status of requisition:
☑ regular
☐ interim
☐ emergency

Item No. 1	Stock Number 1	Description 2	Unit of Issue 3	Stock on Hand 4	Quantity Requested 5	Quantity Approved 6	Quantity Issued 7	Amount ($) 8	Notes 9
1	02-0500	Aspirin tabs 300 mg	1000T	12	18	18	18	165.60	
2	02-2200	Chloroquine tabs 150 mg	1000T	3	5	5	5	61.00	
18	02-4600	Paracetamol tabs 500 mg	1000T	6	8	8	8	209.60	
19	02-4800	Phenoxymethyl tabs 250 mg	1000T	3	4	4	2	81.40	short
20	02-4850	Piperazine tabs 500 mg	1000T	1	1	1	1	11.20	

15:00 March 5, 1998	11:00 March 26, 1998
Hour and date requisition received	Hour and date shipment received

CLEARANCES:

Mutamba, SO	Kaeke, Dir.	Mhanda, PT	Mundandishe, PT
1. Shipping and receiving review	2. Director of medical stores	3. Inventory control unit	4. Medical stores
Mufawatamba, SO	Mugari	Tinoda, SRN	
5. Shipping and receiving	6. Driver or custodian accepts shipment	7. Recipient, acknowledgment of receipt of shipment	

Annex 23.5 Delivery Voucher

Ministry of Health
Department of Medical Supply
DELIVERY VOUCHER

Deliver to: Utano HC

Requisition no.: PHC 63-98-3-2R   Issue voucher no.: 98570

Received from Central Pharmaceutical Stores ___3___ sealed cartons and ___2___ containers described below:

3 x cartons

  1 x 5L disinfectant

  1 x bale of sanitary pads

for delivery to the above-named requisitioner/facility.

Mufawatamba	Mugari	09:00 Mar 26, 1998
Stores issuing officer	Driver/custodian of shipment	Date and time

Received by requisitioner from the above-named custodian of shipment, the containers and/or items stated above in good order, except as follows:

  1 carton damaged by leakage   Mugari

  1 container missing   Mugari

Tinoda (TINODA, SRN)	11:00 Mar 26, 1998
Receiving officer of requisitioning facility	Date and time

IF ANY DISCREPANCY IS RECORDED BY THE RECEIVING OFFICER, THIS DELIVERY VOUCHER IS TO BE INITIALED BY THE CUSTODIAN OF THE SHIPMENT AS WELL.

Annex 23.6 Sample Register of Requisitions

Ministry of Health
Department of Medical Supply
REGISTER OF REQUISITIONS
(STORES ISSUES LEDGER)

Stores Issue No.	Date	Requisition No.	Issue Voucher No.	Value of Issues ($)				Certified
				Drugs	Med-Surg.	Other	Total	
001	Mar 5	98-3-2R	PHC42 98534	2412.60	836.50	—	3249.10	Mariyacho
002	Mar 5	98-3-2R	PHC44 98541	2933.50	1078.50	—	4012.00	Mariyacho
003	Mar 5	98-3-4R	HOSP6 98543-45	28364.20	6517.60	937.50	35819.30	Mariyacho
023	Mar 8	98-3-2R	PHC75 98611	3545.30	948.60	—	4493.90	Zvinodura
024	Mar 8	98-3-2R	PHC78 98613	2266.40	592.30	—	2858.70	Zvinodura
025	Mar 8	98-3-2R	PHC72 98614	2947.70	876.10	—	3823.80	Zvinodura

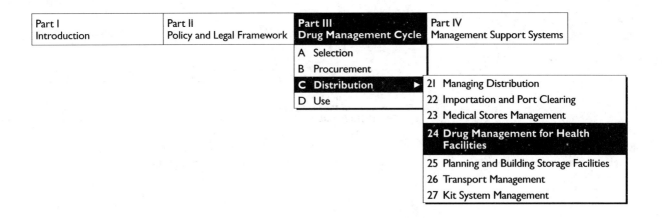

| Part I | Part II | **Part III** | Part IV |
| Introduction | Policy and Legal Framework | **Drug Management Cycle** | Management Support Systems |

A Selection
B Procurement
C Distribution ▶
D Use

21 Managing Distribution
22 Importation and Port Clearing
23 Medical Stores Management
24 Drug Management for Health Facilities
25 Planning and Building Storage Facilities
26 Transport Management
27 Kit System Management

Chapter 24
Drug Management for Health Facilities

≡ Summary

Managing drug supply at the facility level directly affects the quality of health care. If drugs are consistently unavailable, patients suffer and staff lose motivation. Everyone loses confidence in the health system, and patient attendance decreases. A constant drug supply promotes effective care, inspires confidence in the health facility, and contributes to job satisfaction and self-esteem among staff.

Every health facility, however large or small, needs to store and manage its drug stocks. There must be systems to ensure

  ▸ *secure storage;*

  ▸ *storage in correct environmental conditions;*

  ▸ *accurate record keeping;*

  ▸ *effective reordering;*

  ▸ *effective stock rotation and expiry monitoring;*

  ▸ *effective fire and theft prevention.*

Health workers and managers often believe that inventory control is possible only if and when resources are plentiful. This is not the case. Inventory control is about managing and using the resources available. There will be "sufficient resources" only if effective inventory control is implemented.

Good inventory control makes ordering and drug management easier. Essential drugs programs place a high priority on improving inventory control to ensure a reliable supply of essential drugs, vaccines, and other items at health facilities. To achieve this aim, staff need to be trained in inventory control, storage, and ordering procedures.

The choice of an appropriate inventory control method varies according to the type of facility, scale of operations, and staff capabilities. Despite these differences, the principles of effective inventory control remain the same.

≡ 24.1 Managing Drugs at Health Facilities

The purpose of inventory control at the facility level is to

  ▸ record the receipt and issuance of stock;

  ▸ maintain sufficient stock to last between deliveries;

  ▸ maintain stock at the lowest possible cost, and within budget limits;

  ▸ provide appropriate, safe, and secure storage;

  ▸ prevent expiry of drugs.

Benefits of a Successful Inventory Control System at the Facility Level

Maintaining a sufficient stock of items at a health facility has many benefits. Patients receive drugs promptly, and stockouts can be prevented even when deliveries are delayed. Supplies can be replenished at scheduled intervals, saving on administrative costs and transport time. Patients have confidence in the facility and seek help when they are ill. In addition, an effective inventory control system keeps track of and ensures accountability for supplies.

Problems Arising from Poor Stock Control

When inventory control fails, problems occur. A patient's condition may worsen because of a delay in treatment; a patient may even die if a lifesaving drug is out of stock. If drugs are not available in rural facilities, patients may have to make long and expensive journeys to obtain treatment. If drug availability at the secondary level is better than at the primary level, the community will lose confidence in

primary health care (PHC) and seek hospital treatment instead. When a drug is out of stock, a less suitable alternative may be prescribed. Frequent stockouts may establish or reinforce poor prescribing habits. Emergency orders, which are expensive for the purchaser and inconvenient for the supplier, may be required.

Staff commonly resist the implementation of inventory control systems. The reasons should not be ignored but brought out into the open for discussion. Common reasons for resistance are a perceived lack of time for record keeping or a feeling that "this is not my job." Lack of appropriate training may also play a major role in resistance to new systems.

Cost of Maintaining Stock

Stocking a new health facility can account for 25 to 50 percent of the facility's total annual budget. If stock is managed well, however, future expenses will be consistent with utilization. An efficient inventory control system saves money. Poor inventory control leads to wastage or increased costs for holding stock:

  ▸ Overstocking of certain items may tie up a substantial portion of the drug budget, leaving insufficient funds for other important, perhaps lifesaving, drugs.

  ▸ Overstocked drugs often expire.

  ▸ Poor storage conditions may result in spoiled stock (for example, dressings may be soaked by a leaking roof, or injectable drugs may lose potency if the storeroom is too hot).

► Poor stock records and poor security make theft easier.

► A change in prescribing policy or practice may make a drug obsolete. Without good inventory control, such changes may result in excessive wastage.

≡ 24.2 Managing the Storage Area

Good inventory control requires careful thought about the dimensions and design of the storage space, appropriate conditions for storage of different types of supplies, and the importance of stock rotation and systematic arrangement of stock, as well as attention to cleanliness, fire-prevention measures, and security within the store (see Figure 24.1).

Dimensions and Design of the Store

Storage should be located in a dry, weatherproof building. Stock should be organized and easily accessible on an adequate amount of good-quality shelving (most items in health facilities can be kept on shelves). Space and cold-chain equipment should be provided for the refrigeration of vaccines and other items. Temperature and humidity levels should be controlled within appropriate limits, and the space should be well ventilated. Drugs and medical supplies should be segregated from linen, food, and other nonmedical items. The building should be physically secure.

Sizing. Product and packaging innovations, as well as fear of HIV and hepatitis B infection, have increased the use of disposable medical sundries. This means that more storage space is needed. Designers of new facilities frequently underestimate storage requirements, and older facilities are often very short of space, with supplies stored in corridors and blocking work areas. There is often a lack of appropriate adjustable shelving and handling equipment.

It is more difficult to size hospital stores because they vary with the range of services offered and the organization of services. It is also necessary to consider stock levels and lead times in the estimate. However, the general rule is that *1 square meter per hospital bed* can be used for initial planning and costing, assuming that supplies are received every month. Guidelines on storeroom dimensions for small health facilities and hospitals are given in Figure 24.2 and in Chapter 25.

Receiving Bay. A weather-protected area designated for receiving supplies should be close to the storage area and preferably linked to it by a covered walkway. A pharmacy or medical stores department in a hospital may have its own delivery bay, which is often raised above ground level to facilitate unloading from large delivery vans. Smaller facilities have a single receiving bay providing access to ambulances and small delivery trucks. It may be necessary to designate one area of the actual storeroom as the receiving area, if there is no space for a separate receiving bay.

Storage of Supplies

Most drugs and medical supplies can be kept at uncontrolled room temperature. If the product has no special instructions, normal storage conditions apply. This means *storage in dry, clean, well-ventilated premises at temperatures of +15 to +25°C or, depending on climatic conditions, up to +30°C.*

Less stable drugs must be stored in specific conditions to maintain their effectiveness and prevent contamination. Storage instructions are product specific. Different brands of the same generic drug may have different storage requirements because their packaging or formulation differs slightly. The manufacturer's recommendations should be followed. The following categories of drugs require special storage facilities:

► Products that must be kept frozen (usually vaccines and sera);

► Products sensitive to heat that require refrigeration;

► Products that have a reduced shelf life at uncontrolled room temperature and need mechanical ventilation or air-conditioning;

► Flammable products that require separate, fireproof premises;

► Products prone to theft or misuse (see Chapter 39).

Items Needing Storage in a Controlled Environment. The usable shelf life of the following products may be reduced if stored at uncontrolled humidity or at room temperature in hot climates:

► Some injectable drugs (for example, adrenaline). Most injectable preparations are less stable than solid oral forms (tablets and capsules). Injectable preparations in solution are particularly unstable, whereas freeze-dried powder preparations (for reconstitution) are less degradable. Many injections must be protected from light as well as from heat.

► Intravenous fluids (particularly if purchased in plastic containers).

► Some suppositories, pessaries, creams, and ointments. These products may melt at temperatures greater than 30°C. Once this happens, it is not advisable to use them, because the active ingredient in the formula may become unevenly distributed.

► X-ray films and chemicals. Manufacturers typically recommend storage of X-ray film at a maximum of 21°C. Opened packages are also affected by humidity. A

Figure 24.1 Tips for Managing Stock in the Drug Storeroom

Security

Secure the drug storeroom
- double doors/double locks on entrance
- burglar bars on windows

Use extra precaution for "attractive items"

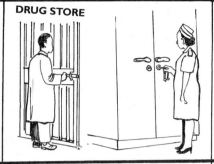

No lockable cupboards? Then improvise: secure using wire mesh, latch, and padlock

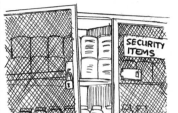

Bulk Storage

Store bulk off the floor

Allow air circulation

Limit the height of stacks to prevent crushing

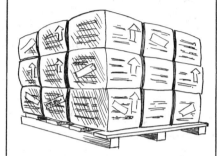

No pallets? Then improvise: construct a wood frame

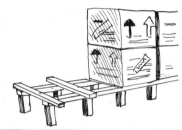

Orderly Arrangement

Provide sufficient shelving

Use a system for arrangement: by order code/drug category; alphabetic by generic name

Guard against spoilage: lightweight items higher up; heavy fluids, fragile items lower

Arrange neatly and label shelf for each item

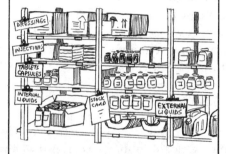

No shelves? Then improvise: support planks with bricks or crates; use strong cartons and other empty containers

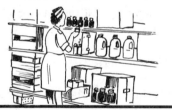

Accountability

Restrict access and check stock frequently

Maintain a stock card for each item if possible
- keep stock card next to item
- fasten stock card to shelf

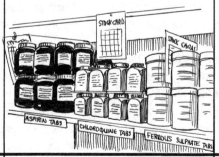

No stock cards? Then improvise: make your own or use a book

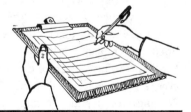

Stock Rotation

When receiving, place containers according to expiry date
- later expiry at back
- earlier expiry at front

When issuing
- take the container with the earliest expiry date

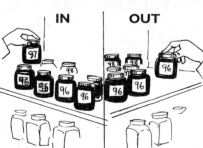

What about items without expiry date? Use FIFO

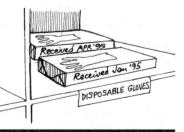

Figure 24.2 Guidelines for Storage Space Requirements

Demographic Feature	Supply Interval	Area Recommended
Catchment Area of Facility		
10,000	2 months	12 square meters
10,000	4 months	24 square meters
20,000	2 months	24 square meters
20,000	3 months	36 square meters
30,000	2 months	36 square meters
50,000	2 months	60 square meters
Number of Hospital Beds		
50	1 month	50 square meters
50	2 months	75 square meters
100	1 month	100 square meters

Source: Adapted from AHRTAG 1994.
Note: Requirements may vary considerably, depending on health care utilization rates. See AHRTAG 1994.

humidity range of 30 to 50 percent is advisable. X-ray film should be handled carefully to avoid staining, creasing, buckling, and friction.

► Products containing rubber, latex, cellulose, or some plastics. Condoms, most sterile disposable medical devices, and surgical products such as syringes, needles, and catheters require protection from excessive humidity, cold, and strong light. Any of these conditions may make products brittle, stained, malodorous, and unusable. Sterility cannot be assured if packaging is damaged.

In hot climates, these items should be stored in the coolest place possible, preferably with air-conditioning or air circulation fans. It is important to take account of the stability of drugs and the type of storage facilities available when preparing essential drugs lists (see Chapter 10).

Items Needing Freezing or Refrigeration. Vaccines, blood products, and some other drugs lose potency if kept, even briefly, at temperatures outside the recommended range. For these products, the cold chain must be maintained at every stage. (See Figure 23.4 and "References and Further Readings" for literature on cold-chain management).

All cold-chain equipment should meet World Health Organization (WHO) standards. Top-loading refrigerators and freezers are the most appropriate choice. Electric refrigerators of the ice-lined type have good "hold-over" characteristics in the event of a power failure. Front-loading types should be used only in places where the electricity or fuel supply is completely reliable, because they have very poor hold-over characteristics and temperature control.

It is essential to have a contingency plan in place *before* a refrigerator breaks down. Rural health facilities are often so small and so isolated that no other source of refrigeration is available. Larger facilities frequently have more than one refrigerator, and these can be used to store vaccines for short periods. Alternatively, an arrangement can be made to move the contents to a private refrigerator elsewhere in the community or to obtain a regular supply of ice packs until the defect is rectified.

It is also important to carry out routine monitoring and maintenance and to organize an effective repair system. The temperature in each appliance must be monitored and recorded routinely at least once a day. Any breakdown must also be recorded, including the period during which the drugs were exposed to uncontrolled temperatures. Drugs are then kept or discarded, depending on the program guidelines or the manufacturer's advice. Cold-chain monitor cards and devices in or on packages that change color or otherwise alert staff to potential damage assist in monitoring.

Freezing is as damaging as high temperatures for some items, including injectable contraceptives, ergometrine, insulin, adrenaline, and the DPT, DT, TT, and hepatitis B vaccines. Frozen toxoids can be detected by the "shake test." Recent evidence from eastern Europe shows that vaccines can freeze inside a refrigerator during winter months when heat in a building is inadequate. Refrigerators incorporating a heating circuit are now available to overcome this problem. Loss of potency in ergometrine injection has frequently been found in field studies and may also be detected visually. If the solution appears colored when compared with water, the injection has less than 90 percent of stated content and should be discarded.

Short periods at room temperature (during transportation or local distribution, for instance) are acceptable for many products (such as ergometrine and insulin), even though such exposure can, to some extent, reduce shelf life. Other items, such as vaccines, should always be transported in cold boxes.

Controlled Drugs. Narcotics (for example, pethidine injection, morphine preparations) and other specified drugs that may be abused are governed by special legislation and regulations that control import, export, production, supply, possession, prescribing, record keeping, and retention of documents. These drugs are sometimes called "dangerous drugs," a term more properly applied to all drugs.

The following security measures are suggested in the pharmacy and at each user level:

► A safe or reinforced, double-locked cabinet fitted with a light (preferably with a red bulb) that comes on when the door is opened;

▶ A special register recording details of each receipt or issue with two signatures, physical counting after each entry, and signatures at "handover-takeover";

▶ Independent audit (by supervisors and national drug inspectors).

Attractive Items. Some noncontrolled items are particularly prone to theft, abuse, or misuse. These include expensive drugs (cimetidine, praziquantel); certain antibiotics; psychotropics; equipment such as scissors, safety razors, and hypodermic needles; and sundries such as rolls of cotton. Such items should be stored in a separate locked area or cupboard, where they can be supervised.

These items require stricter record keeping and more frequent stock taking than other items. Periodic audits should be made of consumption (issues) against actual recorded use (outpatient registers, prescription records, or ward stock records) to expose any theft or misuse (see Chapter 39).

Flammables and Corrosives. Flammable liquids commonly found in health facilities fall into three categories, according to United Nations hazard classifications:

1. Flash point of -18 °C (for example, acetone, anesthetic ether);
2. Flash point of -18 to +23 °C (such as alcohols before dilution);
3. Flash point of +23 to +61 °C (for example, kerosene).

Bulk supplies of flammable substances require a separate outdoor store located away from the main buildings and pathways. Even small stocks of category-one flammables should be kept in an outbuilding designed specifically for that purpose (AHRTAG 1994). Fire-fighting equipment should be readily available.

A small working stock of flammables may be kept in a steel cabinet in well-ventilated premises, away from open flames and electrical appliances. The cabinets should be marked "highly flammable liquid" and bear the international hazard symbol. The cabinet shelves should be designed to contain spillage.

Corrosive or oxidant substances (such as trichloracetic acid, glacial acetic acid, concentrated ammonia solutions, silver nitrate, sodium nitrite, and sodium hydroxide pellets) should be stored away from flammables, ideally in a separate steel cabinet. Appropriate industrial-type protective gloves should be used when handling them.

Stock Rotation and Expiry Monitoring

The first-in/first-out (FIFO) rule ensures stock rotation and prevents wastage through expiry, assuming that newer stock has a later expiry date than older stock. New stock should be placed at the back of the shelf (or, if this is not possible, to the left-hand side). Stock should be issued only from the front or from the right-hand side. The expiry dates of drugs should be checked at the time of receipt. In the first-expiry/first-out (FEFO) system, the stock with the longest life should be placed farthest to the back (or farthest to the left); this system should be used when newly received stock expires before older stock.

Expiry dates should be noted on the stock record upon receipt. Stock nearing expiry should not be accepted unless it can be used before expiry. Facilities should regularly monitor expiry dates, and expired drugs should be removed immediately from stock. In most cases, they must be destroyed. There should be an agreed-upon procedure for disposal that protects public health. A written record is necessary, and in some countries a committee decision is required.

Health professionals sometimes have to decide whether to use an expired drug or withhold treatment. The drug may still be usable and could save a life, but an expired drug might actually kill a patient. Such decisions have ethical and legal consequences.

A group of experts discussed the issue in 1988 (WHO 1988). They concluded that there was no guarantee of a drug's effectiveness after the expiry date. They noted that in exceptional circumstances, when expired drugs might have to be used, it is vital to involve a pharmacist who is experienced in quality assurance and to inform the clinician. Drugs usually expire because they have been over-ordered, or if the FEFO rule has not been observed. In well-run stores where orders are placed regularly and stock is rotated, this should not happen. When it does, the supervisor should find out why and take corrective action.

Arrangement of Stock

Organizing stock systematically saves time when ordering or locating items and prevents stock from being lost. Chapter 23 discusses various systems for organizing stock (see Section 23.5). The systems most often used in health facilities are organization by therapeutic category, clinical indication, or dosage form, with products arranged alphabetically within those categories.

Treatment rooms and drug trolley carts should arrange drugs by therapeutic class (for example, antibiotics, antiasthmatics, or antihypertensives).

Liquids for internal use must be kept separate from those for external use throughout the supply chain, but particularly in treatment areas. Products for external use are often poisons. If kept with drugs for oral use, they

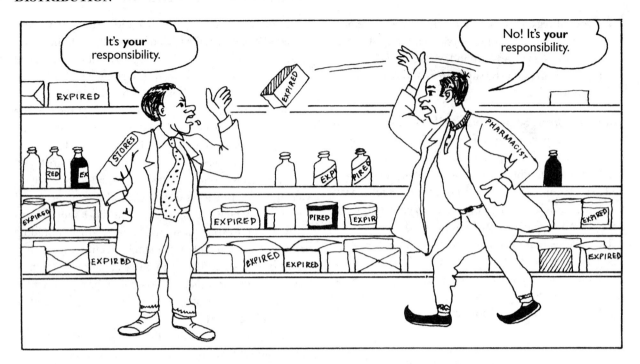

may be accidentally swallowed, which could be fatal. To avoid risk, it is important to observe the following labeling conventions:

► External-use products should be properly labeled according to the country's drug control legislation. Warning labels in red are recommended.
► All internal-use drugs should have black or blue printed labels.

Cleaning
A clean, tidy store is easier to manage than one that is dirty, untidy, and filled with waste. A cleaning schedule with clear designation of staff responsibilities should be established.

Fire Prevention
Fire-prevention measures should include a strict no-smoking rule, careful disposal of combustible waste materials, and careful handling of flammables. Fire-fighting equipment should be regularly checked and maintained, and staff should be trained with regular fire drills.

Security
Access to storage areas should be restricted for security reasons. All staff who handle supplies should be accountable for their actions. One or two trustworthy people should be responsible for keeping the keys, and one should be available on the premises at all times. The person in charge of the health facility is ultimately held responsible.

All storeroom windows should have burglar bars, and doors must be fitted with security locks. Work areas such as the pharmacy or dispensary should have double locks (see Chapter 39).

≡ 24.3 Inventory Control within Health Facilities
Every facility needs an inventory management system—and written procedures—to deal with ordering supplies, receiving and storing stocks, and recording and accounting for stocks.

In larger facilities, inventory management requirements are greater. At large hospitals, supplies are usually managed by pharmacists or other specialized staff. There may be separate facilities for the various activities and types of stock. At smaller facilities, such as health centers, activities tend to be integrated, and a single person may have multiple responsibilities. Even in a small facility, however, stocks of food and linen should be kept separate from medical supplies to maintain hygiene standards and to allow nonprofessional staff easy access to the food and linen.

Keeping Records and Ordering Stock
Chapter 15 outlines the principles of inventory management, which are equally relevant for small health facilities and large stores. Their application may be different, but the underlying methods are the same.

Keeping Records. The most important record is the stock card. The examples in Chapter 23 (see Annexes 23.1 and 23.2) contain most of the features that are likely to be required, but many variations are possible. At a minimum, there should be space for a description of the item and its stock number, the unit of issue (for example, 500-tablet jar, tablet, or mL), and expiry date, if applicable. Columns and rows to document receipt and issue of stock should appear below this standard information. In addition to the stock card kept next to the items on the shelf, there may be a stock ledger or stock book, which maintains a duplicate record of each transaction.

Ordering Stock. Most health facilities use a requisitioning system to order supplies. Staff must assess the rate at which individual items are used and have a clear understanding of the safety stock concept. Various methods of calculating order quantity exist, but *all* are based on monthly consumption. Monthly consumption can be determined from the stock card or from the monthly stock check.

Various ways of calculating safety stocks and order quantities are described in Chapter 15. One simple system of ordering for health facility use is the *imprest* or *topping-up system*. This system is particularly suitable for hospital wards and small health facilities that receive supplies frequently. In the imprest system, no running stock records are kept. The only stock control document is a preprinted sheet that describes each item and gives its stock number, unit of issue, and imprest level—the recommended maximum stock level for that item. The amount ordered is the difference between the stock on hand and the imprest level. In Zimbabwe, a modified imprest system has been developed, with a reorder amount based on three months' consumption established in advance; subsequent orders are always for that amount (see Country Study 24.1).

Another effective system is ordering based on consumption versus maximum stock levels, typified by the approach in Belize and Grenada (MSH 1991). The facility orders on a monthly basis, against a maximum stock level calculated as average monthly consumption multiplied by two. The monthly order quantity is then calculated as follows:

Quantity to order = (maximum stock − stock on hand) + (average monthly consumption × lead time)

Orders are sent to the issuing store on a requisition/issue voucher (see Annex 23.4). The facility and the issuing store should always keep copies of the requisition voucher or imprest forms. These should be compared with the stock cards to monitor consumption and prevent overordering.

Country Study 24.1 Zimbabwe Monthly Ordering System

In 1988, Zimbabwe introduced a nationwide system of inventory control using a requisition model as a central part of the Zimbabwe Essential Drugs Action Programme (ZEDAP). In the five years before the program, health services had rapidly expanded, demand had increased, and new branch stores in provincial capitals had improved distribution.

Medical stores personnel attended supply management courses either at independent training institutions in Zimbabwe or overseas. Personnel responsible for stock control at the larger facilities (central and provincial hospitals) had access to short courses in stores management at government training centers. At the health center and district hospital levels, however, staff had little or no training in supplies management. Training materials were developed, and these workers were all retrained in a new system of inventory control and ordering.

The inventory control system is based on monthly ordering. An item is ordered if the stock on hand is less than the reorder level, which is set at three months' consumption. The quantity ordered is the same as the reorder level (three months' consumption).

ZEDAP assessed the implementation of the inventory control system and the training program through periodic national surveys starting in 1989. The first assessment showed that a national inventory control system could not be taught through workshops alone. Only 52 percent of the facilities had started to keep stock cards, and 27 percent kept stock books. Consequently, alternative training strategies were developed, including on-the-job training and intensified support and supervision. Pharmacy technicians visited health centers frequently to help organize stocks in storerooms, verify stock records, and provide guidance on calculating minimum stock levels. The model of on-the-job training was chosen by the individual district and included attachment of health center nurses to the hospital pharmacy to work under the supervision of pharmacy technicians. By 1991, record keeping at the health center level was reaching target levels, stock cards functioned well, and stock-on-hand balances agreed with physical counts.

Storerooms were transformed by improved inventory control and ordering. Stock arrangement became excellent, and overstocking was reduced. Drug availability improved; figures for twenty-five essential items showed that increasing numbers of facilities met the target of 80 percent availability despite an average availability of 60 percent at central medical stores.

Inventory control systems have contributed to more efficient management of essential medical supplies in Zimbabwe, providing a positive example of the "pull system" applied at the primary health care (PHC) level. However, continuous support and supervision are essential to maintain functional inventory control systems at the PHC level. Where districts failed to provide continuity of support, inventory control systems were not as effective.

Source: ZEDAP 1994.

Receiving Stock

There should be a clear procedure for receiving stock. If goods are not checked into the store on arrival, chaos occurs. The person in charge should be responsible, whether or not he or she personally undertakes the task.

All deliveries should be formally received, whether inside or outside normal working hours. The number of packages delivered should be noted in a register and signed for by both the person receiving and the person delivering the goods.

Unpacking and Checking Stock

Supplies should be unpacked and checked next to the storage area, which may also be used for assembling stock for distribution. Two people should perform these activities, to provide a witness in case supplies are damaged or differ in type or quantity from what was ordered (or from what is shown on the packing list). Supplies should be individually checked using a checklist like the one in Figure 23.2 and their receipt recorded on the supply documents (packing list or returned requisition form). The copy of the original requisition form should always be compared with documents from the issuing facility to prevent later disputes.

The issuing store should be notified of any discrepancies (using a form like the one in Figure 24.3), including

- ► missing boxes or cartons;
- ► open boxes or cartons;
- ► missing items;
- ► quantity different from the one shown on the packing list;
- ► wrong items (items not ordered);
- ► damaged, broken, or poor-quality items.

Checking should be seen not simply as counting the units delivered but as part of the quality assurance system. This means visually inspecting the packaging, the integrity of containers, and the completeness and legibility of labels (approved drug name, strength, any special storage instructions, expiry date). The expiry date should be checked to ensure that there is adequate remaining shelf life (see Chapter 18).

Packaging is an important factor in maintaining the quality of drugs and other supplies when stability is a consideration. Good packaging protects the product from light and air. Packaging should be removed only after careful consideration of the impact on drug quality.

Finally, the delivery documents should be signed and filed for reference; they should usually be kept for a minimum of two years (or the time specified in regulations).

≡ 24.4 Distributing Stock from the Storeroom

Drugs need to be moved from the facility store to the places where they are used, such as treatment areas, wards, or outpatient facilities. The procedures are similar, whatever the size of the facility.

Small Health Facilities

Small facilities may not have a separate pharmacy, but they should have a drug storeroom or cupboard and a dispensing and treatment area. A working stock (often a single container) of common medications should be kept in the treatment area. Oral medication should be stored in a lockable trolley cart or cupboard. A small stock of common injectable drugs should be kept on a tray in the treatment room. There is usually a separate area for cleaning and dressing wounds, where an appropriate range of items should be kept on trolley carts and in lockable cupboards. These working stocks are replenished from the storeroom daily. It is critical that working-stock containers be kept closed except when they are actually being used, to avoid deterioration and loss of therapeutic value.

Hospital Pharmacy Departments

The movement and control of stocks are more complex in larger facilities where medical, surgical, and maternity care are provided. Separate stocks or storerooms may be needed. The hospital pharmacy should be responsible for restocking all drug storage areas and may also dispense to individual inpatients and outpatients. The volume of outpatient prescriptions may justify an outpatient dispensary separate from the main pharmacy.

The hospital pharmacy may have working stock from which it dispenses medications to inpatients and upon their discharge, to outpatients, and to wards, departments, and emergency trays. A "want list" should be compiled through the day, for daily replenishment from the storeroom. This responsibility should rest with a limited number of individuals on a rotational basis.

Prepacking for Outpatient Dispensing. To save time for both staff and patients in busy facilities with high prescription volumes, it is useful to prepack commonly dispensed oral medications in appropriate quantities for standard treatment courses. This packing can be done at quiet times of the day or week. Prepacking is also necessary when quantities smaller than the original pack are needed for ward stocks (see Chapters 19 and 32). In some countries, it may be cost effective to purchase commonly used drugs commercially prepacked in "unit-of-use"

Figure 24.3 Discrepancy Report

Ministry of Health
Department of Medical Supply
DISCREPANCY REPORT

Health facility: _Utano HC_   Date: _Mar 26, 1998_

1. Received by: _Tinoda SRN_   No. of cartons received: _3_

2. Witnessed by: _Jayuguru SRN_   No. of other containers received: _1_

DETAILS OF SHIPMENT

3. Issue voucher no./s: _98570_

4. Transporter: _DMS Driver_   Vehicle reg. no.: _25TCE176_

5. Name of driver: _Mugari_   Transporter shipment note: _MUG65_

6. List of cartons rcvd.: _3 cartons_   List of cartons not rcvd.: _1 container 5 Liter_

DETAILS OF DISCREPANCIES

7. Breakages (if any):

Issue voucher no.	Item Description	Code No.	Unit	Quantity Broken
98570	Chloroquine syrup	03-2500	Bottle 500 mL	2

8. Items missing:

Issue voucher no.	Item Description	Code No.	Unit	Quantity Missing
98570	Chlorhexidine solution 2%	04-1650	5 Liter	1

9. Items issued in error:

Issue voucher no.	Item Description	Code No.	Unit	Quantity Tampered With

10. Any other discrepancies/comments:

PLEASE CREDIT BREAKAGES AND RESUPPLY ANY MISSING ITEMS

---

11. Signature: _Tinoda (TINODA)_

   Office held: _SRN_

Figure 24.4 Items for an Emergency Tray at a Rural Health Center

3 x promethazine 50 mg/2 mL
3 x adrenaline 1:1,000
5 x aminophylline 250 mg/10 mL
10 x atropine 0.6 mg/1 mL
6 x chlorpromazine 50 mg/2 mL
2 x dextrose 50% 20 mL
3 x diazepam 10 mg/2 mL
1 x ½ Darrows and dextrose 200 mL
1 x Ringer's lactate 1,000 mL
2 x IV giving sets
2 x IV cannula 18G
2 x IV cannula 22G
2 x 23G scalp vein set
3 x 10 mL syringe with needle
3 x 2 mL syringe with needle
Rolls of cotton
Alcohol
Adhesive tape
1 x Dextrostix or Glucostix

Source: Zimbabwe Ministry of Health 1994.

Figure 24.5 Drugs Recommended for a General Ward in a Hospital

2 x atropine sulphate 0.6 g/mL
2 x hydrocortisone 100 mg
1 x IV potassium chloride 15%
2 x IM/IV promethazine 25 mg/mL
2 x 10 mL water for injection
3 x adrenaline 1:1,000
1 x IV aminophylline 250 g/mL
2 x IM/IV diazepam 10 mg
1 x IV digoxin 0.5 mg
2 x IM/IV furosemide 20 mg
2 x IV isoprenaline
1 x 5 mL lidocaine 2%
2 x IV propranolol 1 mg
1 x IM calcium gluconate 100 g/mL
1 x 20 mL IV dextrose 50%
1 x 50 mL sodium bicarbonate 4%

Source: Zimbabwe Ministry of Health 1994.

(course-of-therapy) containers. Important considerations when repacking drugs are:

► Use containers suited for maintaining drug quality.
► Avoid contaminating or mixing different batches of drugs.
► Label containers appropriately and assign a new "use-by" date (see Chapter 19).

Supplying Inpatients. As discussed in Chapter 38, there are three basic techniques for hospital drug distribution to inpatients: bulk ward stock, individual drug orders, and unit dose distribution. The bulk ward stock system is still used in many countries. The imprest or topping-up system is a common method for supplying wards with bulk stock. Empty containers are returned for refilling (the "full-for-empty" method) at weekly or twice-weekly intervals. Each ward should have a box that can be locked by both pharmacy and ward staff. Stricter security procedures for antibiotics, "attractive items," and narcotic drugs should be applied.

In a ward stock system, the pharmacy should provide a schedule indicating on which day each ward or department is to be supplied and specifying the category of supplies. It is essential that pharmacy, stores, and ward staff decide together about the types and quantities of drugs required, and that pharmacy staff monitor ward stock storage and record keeping (see Chapters 32 and 38).

Emergency Trays. A selection of drugs and equipment for emergencies should be placed in wards and outpatient departments. The contents should be recorded on a list and checked regularly. Whenever an item is used, it should be restocked immediately. The emergency tray should *not* be used for routine supplies. Figures 24.4 and 24.5 are examples from Zimbabwe. Figure 24.4 indicates contents of an emergency tray at a rural health center, and Figure 24.5 lists drugs recommended for a general ward in a hospital.

Supplying Community-Based Health Workers. Community health workers usually have a very limited selection of items. The topping-up system can be used to replenish stocks, as long as requirements are small and the health center is reliably stocked. A monthly supply interval is usually adequate.

≡ **24.5 Staff Training**

Staff who handle supplies should be trained in the following subjects:

► Setting up a storeroom and good storage practices;
► Use of stock control forms, including requisitions, stock records, and prescriptions;
► Cold-chain procedures, including the use and maintenance of refrigerators;
► Security and theft control.

Chapter 48 discusses the design and management of appropriate training programs for supply system staff. The *Managing Drug Supply* training series is available from Management Sciences for Health for use in training programs; volume 3 in the series is particularly concerned with aspects of supply management (MSH 1992). ∎

≡ Assessment Guide

See Chapter 15 for indicators of stock control performance.

Inventory Control System

- Is there a standard inventory control system at health facilities?
- Are stock cards or stock books used for every movement of stock in or out of the facility storeroom?
- Are drugs reordered according to a consumption-based system?
- Is the minimum or safety stock level set according to the frequency of delivery and average consumption?
- Are used stock cards, ledgers, or regulation books kept for a defined period?
- Do stock records correspond with physical stock for a sample of commonly used drugs?

Staff Training in Inventory Management

- Have the staff responsible for ordering, storing, or distributing drugs been formally trained in inventory management?

- Are procedures manuals for inventory management available in the health facility?

Stock Storage Facilities

- Have the stock storerooms been sized according to any formula?
- Is there a receiving area? Is there an unpacking area?
- Is there a discrepancy report form? Over the past year, has it been used?
- Is the storeroom dry, clean, well ventilated, and between +15 and +25°C?
- Is there a refrigerator? Is its temperature regularly recorded?

Storeroom Management

- When drugs or supplies are unpacked, are they stored according to FEFO or FIFO order?
- Over the past year, have expired drugs been used?
- Are there expired drugs in stock now?
- Are liquids for internal use kept separate from liquids for external use?

≡ References and Further Readings

★ = Key readings.

Africare. 1991. *Evaluation of the Sierra Leone essential drugs programme.* Prepared for the Sierra Leone Ministry of Health and UNICEF/Sierra Leone. Washington, D.C.: Africare.

★ AHRTAG (Appropriate Health Resources and Technologies Action Group). 1994. *How to manage a health centre store,* 2d ed. London: AHRTAG.

★ Battersby, A. 1983. *How to look after a health centre store.* London: Appropriate Health Resources and Technologies Action Group.

★ MSH (Management Sciences for Health). 1991. *Pharmacy inventory control operations manual, Belize Ministry of Health.* Boston: MSH.

MSH (Management Sciences for Health). 1992. *Managing drug supply training series.* Part 3. *Supply management.* Boston: MSH.

WHO (World Health Organization). 1984. *Report of a workshop on essential drugs: New management system of drug supplies to rural health facilities in Kenya.* WHO/DAP/84.2. Geneva: WHO.

WHO (World Health Organization). 1988. *Stability of drug dosage forms: Consultant group to the WHO Expert Committee on Specifications for Pharmaceutical Preparations.* WHO/PHA/ED/SPP/88.6. Geneva: WHO.

WHO (World Health Organization). 1991. *Guidelines on the storage of essential drugs in eastern and southern Africa: A manual for storekeepers.* HRH/91.14. Geneva: WHO.

Zimbabwe Ministry of Health. 1994. *Essential drugs list of Zimbabwe (EDLIZ).* Harare, Zimbabwe.

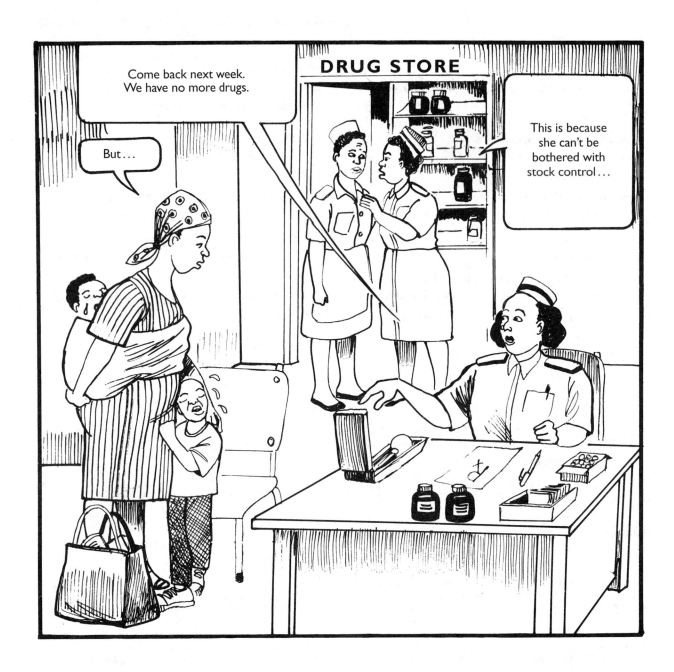

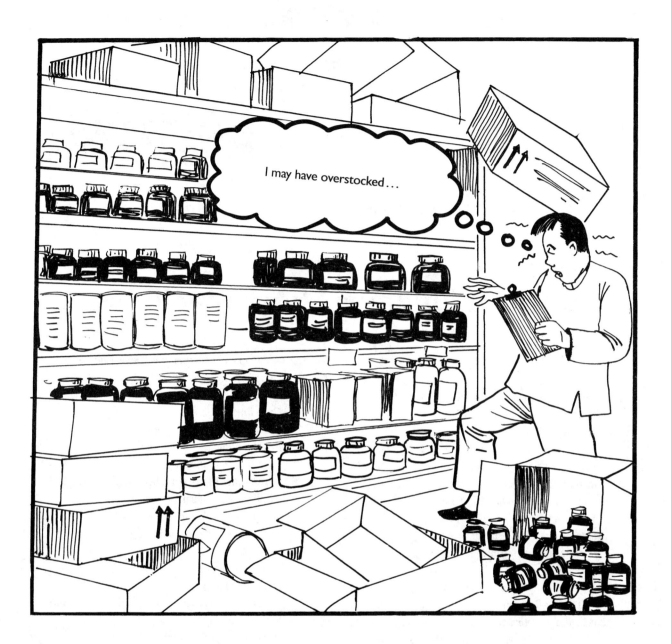

Part I Introduction	Part II Policy and Legal Framework	**Part III** **Drug Management Cycle**	Part IV Management Support Systems

A Selection
B Procurement
C Distribution ▶
D Use

21 Managing Distribution
22 Importation and Port Clearing
23 Medical Stores Management
24 Drug Management for Health Facilities
25 Planning and Building Storage Facilities
26 Transport Management
27 Kit System Management

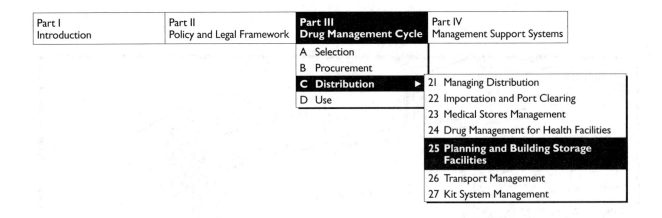

Chapter 25
Planning and Building Storage Facilities

≡ Summary

This chapter describes methods for obtaining effective storage facilities, a process in which supply system managers play a key role.

Storage facilities are of three basic types:
- Mechanized warehouses *rely on the use of mechanical handling equipment. They are appropriate where most goods are stored in bulk on pallets.*
- Manual warehouses *are appropriate where goods are stored in smaller quantities, mostly on shelves.*
- Storerooms *are fitted out with shelves, refrigerators, and a secure cupboard or safe. Every facility needs a location where drugs and medical supplies can be stored safely.*

Satisfactory storage accommodation may be obtained by reorganization *or* renovation *of an existing facility,* lease *or* purchase *of a commercial warehouse, or* new construction.

There are six stages in the procurement and construction process:

1. Inception
   - *setting up a project team*
   - *appointing consultants*

2. Feasibility
   - *carrying out a feasibility study*
   - *obtaining a budget allocation*
3. Site selection and acquisition
   - *selecting a site or building*
   - *obtaining the site or building*
4. Design
   - *preparing a detailed design brief*
   - *planning space and choosing equipment*
   - *designing the building*
5. Tender and project planning
   - *selecting a procurement method*
   - *drawing up a contract*
   - *conducting the tender process*
   - *planning the project*
6. Construction and commissioning
   - *managing the construction contract*
   - *commissioning the facility*

≡ 25.1 Types of Storage Facilities

Well-located, well-built, well-organized, and secure storage facilities are an essential component of a drug supply system. An effective building provides the correct environment for the storage of drugs and assists the efficient flow of supplies. Storage facilities fall into three categories: mechanized warehouses, manual warehouses, and storerooms.

Mechanized warehouses are designed around modern methods of storage and materials handling. A typical warehouse of this type has tiers of pallet racks. Mechanical handling equipment is used to unload and store goods received and often to load outgoing goods onto delivery vehicles. Mechanized warehouses can range from very simple buildings using manually operated handling equipment and manually operated stock control systems to highly complex operations that are entirely automatic and computer controlled. Mechanized medical warehouses are most likely to be primary stores at the national or regional level. Typically, they are located close to major transport routes.

Manual warehouses may also hold some stock on floor pallets, but most items are stored on shelves and are moved without mechanical assistance. Medical supply warehouses at the regional or district level are usually manual warehouses. They are often attached to a hospital, which they also serve.

Storerooms are needed in every health facility to store drugs and medical supplies safely. The smallest facilities may need only a drug cupboard, but most facilities require a room fitted out with shelves and refrigerators, along with a secure cupboard or safe for controlled drugs.

This chapter provides guidelines to help managers make rational choices about designing and constructing warehouses. There are six stages in the process: inception, feasibility, site selection and acquisition, design, tender and project planning, and construction and commissioning (see Figure 25.1).

This chapter is not a comprehensive technical manual and is not intended to be a substitute for the advice of a specialist. In most cases, specialist staff or outside consultants will be needed to deal with design and construction management issues. The day-to-day management of medical stores is covered in Chapter 23.

≡ 25.2 Inception Stage

From a consultant's standpoint, a good client (the supply system) should be knowledgeable and discerning. Most of the key decisions in a building project are made during the inception and feasibility stages, when client input is critical. These decisions fundamentally affect the cost and ultimate effectiveness of the project and should not be

Figure 25.1 Steps to Plan and Build a Storage Facility

Stages and Tasks	Principal Responsibility of:
Inception Stage	
State the aim of the project	Supply system
Establish the project team and appoint consultants	Supply system
Feasibility Stage	
Identify quantity and type of storage space needed	Project team
Review options for reorganizing existing warehouse space	Project team
Consider leasing or purchasing existing building	Project team
Determine whether a building is needed. If so:	Project team
► establish operational requirements and prepare outline brief	Project team
► assess financial, material, and personnel resources required	Project team
► contact relevant authorities	Project team
► establish outline budget and obtain budget allocation	Project team
► establish a program for the design and construction stages	Project team
Selection/Acquisition of Site Stage	
Short-list and evaluate potential sites and buildings	Project team
Select and acquire site or building	Supply system

ESTABLISH FEASIBILITY AND PROCEED WITH THE DESIGN

Design Stage	
Outline proposals	
Develop brief	Project team
Survey site or building	Project team
Prepare outline proposals showing main dimensions, allocation of space, and construction methods	Project team
Prepare cost estimates	Project team
Select suitable design	Project team
Obtain planning consent	Project team
Scheme design and detail design	
Design each room and fix sizes	Project team
Determine needs for storage and handling equipment	Project team
Decide on construction method and all materials	Project team
Make new cost estimate	Project team
Prepare and agree on final design drawings	Project team

THE DESIGN SHOULD NOT BE CHANGED AFTER THIS POINT

Production information	
Prepare production drawings, specifications, and bills of quantities, giving all information needed to construct the works	Project team
Select all fittings, fixtures, and equipment	Project team
Obtain approval from building regulations authority	Project team
Make final cost estimate	Project team
Tendering and Project Planning Stage	
Select method of building procurement	Project team/supply system
Prepare short list of contractors, or prequalification tender	Project team/supply system
Assemble tender documents and invite tenders	Project team/supply system
Analyze tenders and select the best	Project team
Make any changes required for cost reasons	Project team/supply system
Agree on contractor's program and procedures	Contractor/project team
Finalize insurances and sign the contract	Contractor/supply system
Tender for and obtain mechanical handling equipment	Project team/supply system

CHANGES BEYOND THIS STAGE WILL COST EXTRA TIME AND MONEY

Construction and Commissioning Stage	
Site work	
Supervise work on site	Project team
Hold regular progress meetings with contractor	Contractor/project team
Prepare valuations and make interim payments	Contractor/project team/supply system
Handover	
Witness tests, inspect the works, and list defects	Contractor/project team
Hold handover meeting and accept keys and building manual	Contractor/project team/supply system
Commissioning and defects period	
Commission building	Supply system
Check that the defects have been made good	Project team
Settle final account by releasing the retention sum	Contractor/project team/supply system

Source: Adapted from Mein and Jorgensen 1988.

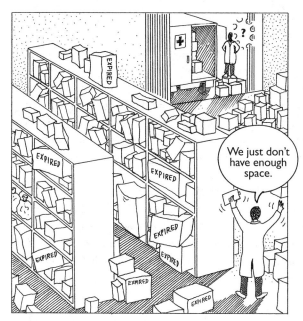 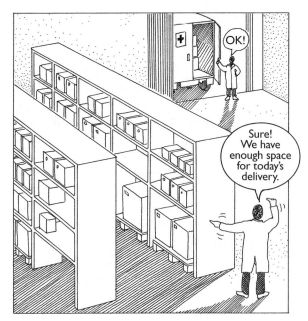

DE-JUNK OR EXPAND?

made casually. Particularly when resources are limited, careful feasibility planning is necessary to obtain effective warehouses at the lowest cost, while taking account of future needs.

The logistics team should be made responsible for establishing the most suitable locations for medical stores throughout the country, based on an overall analysis of the distribution system (see Chapter 21). Once a store location has been selected, the building procurement process can start. This process begins with a broad statement of the aims of the project. The subsequent steps are to

- ► establish a project team for the feasibility exercise;
- ► appoint consultants, if necessary;
- ► prepare a design brief and budget;
- ► consider the most cost-effective way to procure the required storage space (reorganization, renovation, rental, purchase, or new construction);
- ► obtain the budget allocation needed to implement the project.

Rebuilding from scratch may be more cost effective than renovation. Although renovating an existing building may appear to save money at first, this "saving" is often offset by lost opportunities for improving efficiency. Chances are that if the current structure is not adequate, a coat of paint will not make it so.

The Project Team

A project team should be formed as soon as the decision to obtain storage space has been made. The team should be directed by a senior drug program manager or health official. Its composition varies, depending on the size of the project and the project stage. The full team for the implementation stages of a large project such as a new central medical store (CMS) normally includes the lead consultant (usually an architect), the supply system representative, a quantity surveyor or cost consultant, a structural engineer, a mechanical services engineer, an electrical engineer, and a logistics and materials handling consultant.

A wide range of other people and organizations should be consulted. Broadly based consultation is essential to the development of an appropriate building design. Too often, a project design takes shape without adequate consultation between the people who are to work in the building and the specialists who are designing it.

Appointment of Consultants

If the project is complex, suitably qualified consultants should be appointed at the earliest possible stage for estimating building design costs, cost control, and logistics and materials handling. If the project is small and simple, professional consultants may be appointed after the feasibility stage, when alternative sites or buildings are being considered.

Building Design. Professional design assistance is essential to ensure that a building satisfies the design brief and is constructed in accordance with local building codes. There are various ways of procuring a design service.

In the *conventional* model, the architect is the leader of the project team. He or she is appointed by the client to prepare the design, specifications, and bills of quantities, in liaison with the engineering and cost consultants. In some countries, all other consultants work directly for the architect, and the cost of their services is included in the architect's fee. In other countries, each consultant is appointed separately by the client.

Once the contractor is hired, the architect monitors the building works and certifies the payments to be made to the contractor. Finally, the architect certifies when the building is complete and agrees on a final account with the contractor. The principal advantage of this model is that the architect acts as the client's agent throughout. This helps ensure that the finished building is completed to an acceptable standard.

In the *turnkey* model, the client hires a contracting company to provide a complete building product for a fixed price. The contracting company is responsible for appointing the design team, which prepares a scheme in accordance with a design brief agreed upon with the client.

In the *design-and-build* model, the client appoints an architect to prepare a design with an agreed-upon level of detail. The contracting company quotes a fixed price for building this design but is allowed to modify construction details to suit its own working methods. The architect has no executive authority on site but may continue to act as an observer for the client.

The principal advantage of the last two models is certainty about costs. The principal disadvantage is that quality control is largely in the hands of the contracting company, which has a vested interest in saving money and increasing its profit margin.

Cost Control. The quantity surveyor or cost consultant prepares preliminary cost estimates for the project. These estimates are updated as the design develops. This consultant may also contribute to the assessment of contractors' tenders, assist the architect in negotiating any variations in the contract with the contractor, and audit the final account.

Logistics and Materials Handling. If the project is large and complex and involves extensive mechanical handling equipment, the advice of a specialist is needed at an early stage. Without this advice, an accurate design brief cannot be prepared, and expensive mistakes may be made. Some architects have this expertise. Alternatively, advice can be obtained from a materials handling consultant or a supplier of materials handling equipment.

The appointed consultants should have relevant experience, the resources to manage the project, and a proven ability to complete satisfactory buildings on time and within the budget. The selection process should not allow corruption or favoritism; a formal tender helps minimize such problems. The client should draw up a list of qualified firms and invite each firm to submit a formal proposal for consideration by the project team. The proposal should set out the consultant's approach to the project and specify the fee that would be charged. Before making a final decision, the project team should visit the offices of the short-listed consultants, view some of their completed projects, and talk to other clients.

≡ 25.3 Feasibility Stage

The first task of the project team is to establish whether more space is really required. It may be possible to achieve the desired result by reducing the order interval or by reorganizing stock within existing buildings. If this is not possible, the feasibility study should establish the following:

- ► Type of store required;
- ► Approximate size of the store and site;
- ► Options for obtaining space;
- ► Short list of possible sites or buildings for the store;
- ► Staff recruitment and training implications;
- ► Outline budget or cost plan, including an assessment of operational and maintenance costs;
- ► Workplan for project completion;
- ► Site selection and acquisition for new construction.

Identify Type of Store Required

A *mechanized warehouse* is indicated if a large percentage of products will be received and stored on pallets. This type of warehouse requires powered forklift trucks and other equipment capable of moving pallets within the store. Pallets may be stored on the floor (pallet standing) or on pallet racks. Pallet racking makes the most efficient use of space. If pallet racking is chosen, the number of tiers determines the internal height of the store. This is a critical design decision that needs to be made at an early stage; it is dictated largely by the type of handling equipment used. A mechanized warehouse should not be considered unless there is an effective supply and service network for mechanical handling equipment. Preferably, there should be several sources of such equipment.

A *manual warehouse* is appropriate if the majority of products will be received and stored in packages that can be moved around by hand or with the assistance of trolleys. A manual store may also require some floor pallets. If pallets are to be handled, manual pallet trucks will be needed to off-load them from the delivery vehicles and move them around the store. Most items in a manual warehouse are likely to be stored on shelving units with a top shelf not more than 1.7 meters high. This means that the internal height of the store is not a critical factor.

Establish Approximate Size of Store and Site

The final size of the warehouse and the detailed site layout are established during the design stage. It is essential, however, for the project team to establish approximate sizes during the feasibility stage for three reasons:

- ► To short-list suitable sites or buildings;
- ► To establish a realistic design brief;
- ► To prepare a budget estimate.

Determining store size is complex, because the size of the store is affected by many factors. The most important factors are the volume of individual items, the maximum stock level for each item, and the way in which goods are stored (floor pallets, pallet racking, or shelves). Stock volume can be estimated from calculations based on volume of past shipments, by analysis of shipping volumes for specific items, or by item-by-item analysis.

Calculations Based on the Overall Order Value and Volume of Past Shipments. If the total value and volume of a shipment are known, it is possible to calculate the value per cubic meter of mixed drugs and other medical supplies and to use this figure as a basis for store sizing. Adjustments may have to be made for inflation if the data are drawn from different time periods. This method is most appropriate for calculating volumes at the CMS and other primary stores when a strict annual or periodic ordering system is used and the stock is "topped up" at known intervals.

Analysis of Shipping Volumes for Specific Items. For instance, one million aspirin, 300 mg, in tins of 1,000, in cartons, from a current supplier might occupy about 1.6 m³. A computer program (spreadsheet or database) can use this type of information for store sizing. This method is retrospective. It does not take account of differences in bulk for similar items from other sources.

Item-by-Item Analysis Using Average Volumes Taken from a Range of Suppliers. The World Health Organization (WHO) publication *How to Estimate Warehouse Space for Drugs* (Battersby and Garnett 1993) provides a method for doing this. Unfortunately, these guidelines do not cover nondrug items, and the calculations are tedious to perform without the aid of a computer. The worksheets in this document are based on a periodic inventory system but can be adapted to suit a perpetual inventory model.

The maximum net volume of goods to be stored is determined, taking account of maximum stock levels and allowances for future program expansion.

Whichever method of estimating stock volume is used, the store size and type are determined by

- ► maximum net volume of goods to be stored;
- ► how goods are to be stored and handled (floor pallets, pallet racking, or shelving);
- ► type of stock location system used (see Chapter 23);
- ► climatic conditions;
- ► area of ancillary spaces, including loading bays, cold rooms, packing areas, offices, sanitary facilities, and staff lounges.

Finally, the required site size is determined by

- ► size and type of store—a tall mechanized warehouse has a smaller "footprint" than a manual warehouse that would handle the same volume of inventory;
- ► space and clearance needed for ancillary buildings, including those for the storage of fuels and hazardous chemicals—safety considerations determine how far away from other buildings hazardous substances should be stored;
- ► access and parking for delivery and staff vehicles;
- ► access for fire engines and other emergency services;
- ► site area needed for future expansion.

Select Method of Obtaining Space

There are five ways of obtaining the necessary storage space:

1. Reorganize, renovate, or extend an existing health system warehouse. This can be the quickest and cheapest approach, if suitable buildings are available.
2. Lease a suitable commercial building. This has the advantage of speed and avoids a large capital investment, but there will still be fitting-out costs to suit the specific needs of a medical warehouse.
3. Buy a suitable commercial building. Again, this has the advantage of speed, assuming funds are available, but there will be fitting-out costs.
4. Build a standard building. Many countries have standard designs for health service buildings. Advantages of this approach are that design lead time is reduced, there is greater cost certainty, and the design should be proven. The disadvantage is that the performance of standard designs has often not been evaluated effectively. Poor designs may be perpetuated.
5. Build a purpose-designed building on an existing site, or obtain and develop a new site. This approach is likely to have the longest lead time and may be the most expensive, but this may not necessarily be so, especially if the government already owns the land. It should ensure the closest fit to the specified requirements.

Figure 25.2 Budget Outline for a Medical Stores Project

Name of Project: _____

Date of Budget: _____

Anticipated Construction Start: _____

Net Area: _____

Gross Area: _____

Capital Costs

1. Site acquisition: total cost + commission and fees
2. Construction
   a. Off-site work (roads, utilities)
   b. On-site work (roads, utilities, walks, paving, landscaping)
   c. Building (structure and works to 1.5 meters outside exterior walls)
   d. Fixed equipment (built-in counters, cabinets)
   e. Furnishings and equipment (movable equipment)
3. Professional services (surveys, soils analysis, planning, architecture, and engineering)
4. Miscellaneous costs (utility connection fees, plan approval fees, legal fees)
5. Inspection and testing (job inspection, material testing)
6. Contingencies (cost escalation contingency, construction contingency)
7. Financing (loan fee, interim and permanent financing costs, bond legal fees)

Recurrent Costs

8. Annual operational costs (staff salaries and overheads, insurance, equipment maintenance, security, communications, utilities)
9. Average annual maintenance costs (repairs and renewals)

Identify Possible Sites or Buildings

Once the sizes of the store and the site have been established, it is necessary to prepare a short list of suitable sites or buildings.

Identify Staff Recruitment and Training Implications

An assessment of personnel needs should be made at an early stage so that salaries and wages can be budgeted for and a recruitment and training program planned.

Establish an Outline Budget and Obtain a Budget Allocation

Funding may be obtained from government sources, donor agencies, or commercial sources. The cost consultant should prepare a budget for submission to the funding authority (see Figure 25.2). The budget should include estimated costs for site acquisition, consultants' fees, and construction costs. It should also include an assessment of annual operational and maintenance costs; if these items are not considered and budgeted for, the facility may not be sustainable. Once funding is approved, the implementation phase can begin.

Establish a Workplan

The feasibility stage ends with the preparation of a detailed workplan for the design phase, setting out the tasks and timelines for the participants. An outline workplan for the construction phase should also be prepared.

≡ 25.4 Site Selection and Acquisition for New Construction

When a budget allocation has been obtained, the project team should recommend the most suitable site or building from the shortlist.

Site Selection

In some countries, zoning laws completely prohibit development in some areas and allow only buildings of a particular type in other areas. Other regulations may limit the size and position of buildings on a chosen site. A suitable site must satisfy all the regulatory requirements, be economical to build on, have convenient access for vehicles and staff, be adequately served by utilities and communications, be secure, and have potential for future expansion. The Assessment Guide at the end of this chapter lists some criteria for site selection.

Site Acquisition

A site and/or the buildings on it may be purchased outright or leased on a long-term or short-term basis. Use of government land or outright purchase is the conventional route for government. Leasing may be a suitable method for an agency such as a nongovernmental organization (NGO) whose needs are limited in time. Whichever method is chosen, it is essential that the transfer of ownership or leasehold title be legally correct to avoid later disputes.

≡ 25.5 Design Stage

There are four stages in the design of a building. At the end of each stage, the project should be reviewed and a formal decision made to proceed to the next stage. The stages are:

1. *Preliminary proposals*: Preliminary design proposals are prepared and costed. An acceptable scheme is selected. If the building is to be procured on a turnkey basis, the contractor may be chosen at this stage.
2. *Schematic design*: The design is developed in sufficient detail to enable the client to approve basic spatial arrangements, materials, and appearance. A more detailed cost estimate is prepared. Mechanical handling equipment suppliers should be consulted where appropriate. At this stage, it may be necessary

to obtain formal permission to build from the relevant government authority and seek agreement on the scheme with the fire department. The layout of the building and basic method of construction should not be altered after this stage.

3. *Detailed design*: The construction details are worked out. The cost estimate is refined. Specialist subcontractors and suppliers (such as cold-room manufacturers) are consulted, and quotations are obtained. Formal application is made for approval under local building regulations. If there is to be a design-and-build contract, the contractor is typically selected during this stage. Major construction details should not be altered after this stage.

4. *Production information*: Final construction drawings are prepared, together with specifications and bills of quantities. These should be sufficiently detailed to enable contractors to tender for the project.

Client's Role

Executive responsibility for building design and monitoring of the construction contract rests with the project team. However, the client's representative on the project team has a project management role to play in the following areas:

▶ Attending meetings of the project team and monitoring progress;
▶ Developing the brief;
▶ Formally reviewing and approving the scheme as each design stage is completed (altering major decisions made at a previous stage is extremely disruptive and may cause delays and increase costs);
▶ Arranging payment of fees for planning and building control applications;
▶ Arranging payment of consultants' fees.

All of the project team, in turn, should ensure that the client is kept fully informed of progress and is provided with copies of drawings, correspondence, and other documentation.

Some of the general design features that should be considered during the design stages are outlined below.

Detailed Project Brief

The detailed project brief is the key design document. It should be developed in discussion with the people who will operate and use the building. The brief is not a fixed document. It will change and expand as the design develops in response to input from the client and from the project team. Typical elements of a brief are outlined in Figure 25.3.

Figure 25.3 Typical Elements of a Project Brief ("Functional Program")

Operational Brief
Inventory management and stock control systems and stores management procedures;
Description of major activities, including flow of goods and paperwork;
Type of stock to be accommodated;
Environmental and security (zoning) requirements for different types of stock (see Chapter 23);
Approximate volumes of stock to be accommodated in each zone;
Approximate throughput of store (maximum cubic meters per day received and dispatched);
Type of store required (mechanized, manual, or manual to be upgraded);
Schedule of male and female staff;
Types and number of delivery vehicles;
Number of staff and visitor vehicles to be accommodated;
Phasing and program expansion.

Site Development Brief
Site development restrictions;
Access and parking for vehicles and access for pedestrians;
Access for emergency services;
Site security and lighting, including gatekeeper's accommodation and barriers;
Landscaping;
Schedule of individual buildings (main store, flammables store, fuel store).

Building Accommodation Brief
Storage
Loading bay;
Incoming goods area (for checking, inspecting, sorting, unpacking, and palleting);
General storage areas (ambient, controlled temperature, controlled security);
Order assembly and dispatch area, including secure storage for assembled orders;
Handling equipment storage, including charging points for electric vehicles;
Ancillary storage (office consumables, packing materials, waste).
Administration
Detailed schedule of accommodation and facilities required for record keeping, communications, drug information, product testing, training.
Staff Welfare
Sanitary facilities and changing rooms;
First-aid room;
Lounges and cafeteria or lunch room.

Store and Site Planning

Storage buildings and site layouts should be planned to allow for future expansion with minimal disturbance to existing building elements, roads, and other physical infrastructure.

Storage buildings should be planned for maximum flexibility. The layout of shelving, racking, and ancillary spaces is certain to change during the life of the building. Buildings with widely spaced columns are easier to reorganize than those with closely spaced columns. Wide-span structures are more expensive to build, but their long-term advantages are likely to justify the extra expense in all but the simplest manual stores.

Stores that have a relatively square plan are generally cheaper to build and more efficient to operate than stores that are long and narrow. In a large store, cross aisles should be provided at reasonable intervals to reduce travel time from aisle to aisle. The most appropriate spacing depends on picking frequency. A rule-of-thumb is a cross aisle every 10 to 20 meters. When assigning storage locations, it is good practice to place slow-moving product lines in long aisles and fast-moving product lines in short aisles (see Figure 25.4)

Storage Methods

Goods can be stored in four basic ways: shelves, floor pallets (pallet standing), pallet block stacking, and pallet racks. The choice of storage method depends on the form in which goods arrive and how they are stored: in bulk on prepacked or store-packed pallets, or as smaller packages. The four methods are discussed more fully in Chapter 23. Figure 25.5 illustrates the major dimensional constraints of pallet racking. Figure 25.6 illustrates the major dimensional constraints of shelf storage.

Environmental Control and Energy Conservation

Opportunities for energy conservation exist in all aspects of warehouse design, construction, and operation, from site selection to equipment selection. A well-designed store can significantly moderate internal temperatures in a "passive" way. Passive design works with the site's microclimate by using trees for shade and shelter, correct building orientation for natural lighting and ventilation, and appropriate building materials and methods to control internal temperatures.

In hot, dry climates, good construction and nighttime ventilation can maintain daytime temperatures several degrees below ambient. In hot, humid climates, effective cross-ventilation is required. In cold climates, storage buildings should be well insulated. Mechanical systems such as air-conditioning need to be chosen with a view to future maintenance. Sophisticated systems may not be sustainable.

Adequate electrical lighting is required throughout the store. Some pharmaceuticals are affected by bright sunlight and fluorescent lighting, and stores should be designed to prevent such damage.

Special Storage Conditions

The building must provide specific storage conditions for different types of pharmaceuticals. See Chapters 18 and 23 for more details.

Ancillary Accommodations and Loading Bays

The design and sizing of ancillary accommodations should be carefully considered. These spaces include offices, staff rooms (for rest, recreation, and eating), sanitary facilities, changing rooms, receiving and packing areas, and storage space for pallets and other packing materials. Chapter 23 details these requirements.

The vehicle loading bay is a particularly important area. It is essential that it be protected from the weather and big enough to receive the maximum number of vehicles expected at any one time. In larger stores, the loading bay should be raised so that the floor of the vehicle is level with the floor of the warehouse. Dock-leveling devices are available to suit vehicles of different heights.

Guidelines for Security

Pharmaceuticals are small, valuable, and therefore prone to theft (see Chapter 39). The warehouse complex should be designed with security in mind.

- ► Unsupervised access from the loading bay to the store itself should not be possible. The main storage area where order picking takes place needs to be very secure.
- ► Ideally, the office area should have windows overlooking the loading bays and the warehouse access.
- ► The staff rest area, sanitary facilities, and changing rooms should not have direct access to the warehouse or from the outside.
- ► Visitors should have separate sanitary facilities.
- ► Staff parking should be well separated from the loading area.
- ► Adequate perimeter fencing and external lighting should be provided.

Mechanical Equipment Specifications

The storage systems and mechanical equipment needed to operate the store effectively, including shelving, should be specified in the design. Some of this equipment will be supplied and installed as part of the building contract, but some may be supplied under a separate "fitting-out" contract.

Fire Protection and Fire Fighting

All sections of the warehouse should have adequate fire-detection equipment and be well supplied with fire-fighting appliances. Smoke alarms are inexpensive to install and provide warning in case fire breaks out. The design should satisfy local building codes and the requirements of insurers in the following respects:

Figure 25.4 Options for Layout of Store Aisles

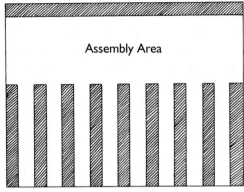

Very Frequent Access

Assembly Area

Frequent Access

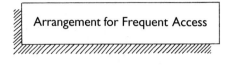

Arrangement for Frequent Access

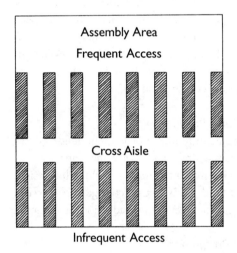

Assembly Area

Frequent Access

Cross Aisle

Infrequent Access

Combined Arrangement for
Frequent and Infrequent Access

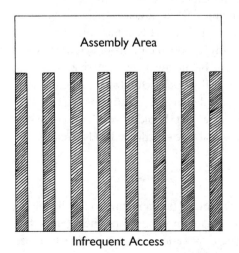

Assembly Area

Infrequent Access

Arrangement for Infrequent Access

Shelves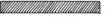

Figure 25.5 Pallet Racking: Dimensional Constraints

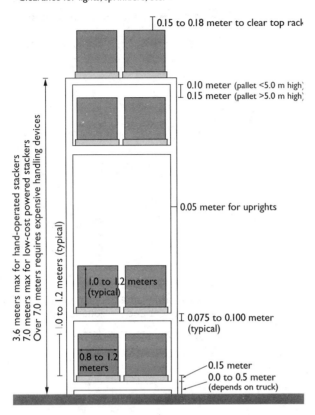

Clearance for lights, sprinklers, etc.

0.15 to 0.18 meter to clear top rack

0.10 meter (pallet <5.0 m high)
0.15 meter (pallet >5.0 m high)

0.05 meter for uprights

1.0 to 1.2 meters (typical)

0.075 to 0.100 meter (typical)

0.8 to 1.2 meters

0.15 meter
0.0 to 0.5 meter (depends on truck)

3.6 meters max for hand-operated stackers
7.0 meters max for low-cost powered stackers
Over 7.0 meters requires expensive handling devices

1.0 to 1.2 meters (typical)

Site and Building Layout and Construction
► Accessibility by the fire department;
► Adequate escape routes and emergency doors with locks that do not prevent staff from leaving the building in an emergency;
► Compartmentalized buildings to reduce the risk of fire spread;
► Noncombustible building construction.

Fire-Detection and Fire-Fighting Equipment
► Adequate provision of smoke alarms, heat detectors, and fire alarm sounders to ensure that fires are detected as soon as possible;
► Correctly positioned fire hydrants and hose pipes with an adequate and reliable supply of water;
► Correctly designed sprinkler systems (if a poorly designed system is set off by accident, water may ruin some stock; or if there is a fire, the system may soak stock that is well away from the core of the fire);
► Adequate numbers and types of fire extinguishers suitable for chemical fires (so staff can extinguish small fires before they spread).

Construction Standards
The method and standard of construction required should be agreed on as part of the brief-development process. These decisions are important because they affect the initial cost of the building and largely determine how long it will last and how much it will cost to maintain. The government may have standard equipment and construction requirements for all buildings of a particular type. Standardized requirements help simplify maintenance and reduce costs.

≡ **25.6 Tender and Project Planning Stage**
The tender stage marks the transition point between the design and construction phases. The three procurement routes described below illustrate a range of tendering possibilities. Variations exist, and the project team should recommend the most appropriate method.

Turnkey Procurement
In turnkey procurement, the tender documents consist of a *performance specification* or *schedule of requirements*. Tenderers are required to submit preliminary design proposals as part of their bid submissions. The successful tenderer then prepares a fully worked-out design for approval by the client before construction begins.

Design-and-Build Procurement
In a typical design-and-build procurement, tenderers are provided with design drawings and specifications. The tender submission is a fixed-price offer to build to the design. The successful tenderer is free to change construction details within the limits set in the tender documentation.

Conventional Procurement
In conventional procurement, tenderers submit bids based on a set of tender documents complete enough to enable the building to be constructed. There are variations on this method. In a "fast-track" contract, the contractor is appointed as early as possible in the design process and starts work on-site before the design work has been completed. The aim of this approach is to build more quickly by overlapping the design and construction stages.

Fast-track procurement should be considered only if all parties to the contract are experienced and extremely well organized.

The Contract
There should be a formal building contract for all building works, however small. Informal arrangements are recipes for disaster. There are various forms of contracts in use, ranging in complexity from a simple letter of agreement

Figure 25.6 Shelving: Optimal Layout with Ergonomic Considerations

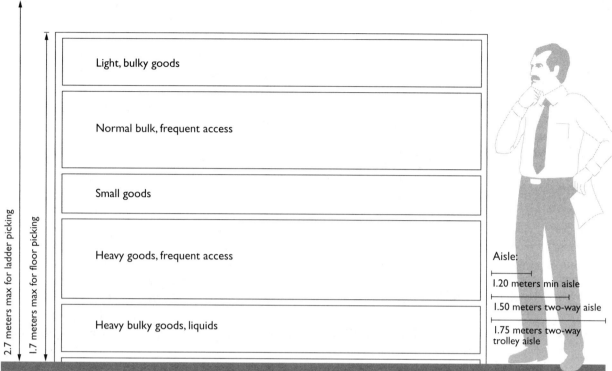

to a complex document. Contracts are often country or organization specific. A few are widely used internationally.

The contract is the legal agreement that commits the contractor to carry out work for the building owner according to the drawings, bills of quantity, and materials specifications within a specified time. A financial penalty may be imposed if the building is not completed on time. The contracting agency (client) agrees to pay the contractor a specified sum of money at agreed-upon stages during the course of the work or upon satisfactory completion. It is set out that the contractor has an obligation to rectify defects during a certain period after completion. The total contract sum may be varied if the nature or extent of the work changes. Under conventional procurement, the architect is the third party to the contract and can both represent the owner and act as arbiter in case of contractual disputes.

Tendering

A competitive tender is usually the best method of selecting a building contractor. Negotiation with one contractor may be applicable when there is only one contractor suitable for the job or when a government building agency (for instance, the ministry of works) is to undertake the project. In all other cases, the tender short list should be drawn up after careful screening. A list of each contractor's projects should be requested and verified. Commercial and bank references should be obtained. Completed projects should be visited, and it is helpful to talk with the architects and owners of these buildings to find out how the contractor performed.

Government clients generally have strict tendering procedures designed to prevent corruption and ensure accountability. There are three basic systems:

1. *Open tendering*: Under this arrangement, any suitably qualified contractor can submit a bid. Bids are then considered by the tender board.
2. *Prequalification tendering*: The contract is advertised, and interested contractors make formal prequalification submissions. The tender board meets and agrees on a short list of contractors. These are invited to submit bids, which are also considered by the tender board.
3. *Short-list tendering*: A short list of tenderers is drawn up by the project team or the client. Bids from this list are then considered by the tender board. This method is adopted by most private-sector and NGO clients. A minimum of three contractors should be invited, but the rules may require a larger number.

The tender instructions specify the date for the return of the bid, how it should be presented, and when bids will be opened. After the bid opening, the bids are analyzed by the project team, and the best one is selected. If cost reductions need to be made, these should be negotiated before the contract is signed.

Project Planning

Discussions are held with the successful contractor, and a construction program is worked out. All contractual matters, including the property and liability insurance obligations of the client and the contractor, are finalized and checked by both parties. If there is to be a performance bond, this is finalized (see Chapter 17).

The client finalizes funding arrangements so that payments can be made to the contractor on time and at the agreed-upon stages. The contract is then signed.

≡ 25.7 Construction and Commissioning

The contractual role of the client during the construction phase is largely confined to making payments to the contractor, approving any changes in the cost of the project, and attending formal site meetings. The contract supervising officer (usually the architect) is responsible for the day-to-day administration of the contract. The client should never issue direct instructions to the contractor; instructions should always be channeled through the supervising officer. The supervising officer should regularly provide the client with the following:

- Site meeting minutes;
- Reports on the contractor's progress and changes in the program;
- Reports on significant contractual or construction problems;
- Payment valuations;
- Details of changes to the design or specifications (variation orders);
- Details of changes in the cost of the project (cost reports).

In addition, the client must prepare to take over and commission the building. This means that staff must be allocated, recruited, and trained; equipment, furnishings, and stationery must be purchased; contract arrangements must be made with utility companies; and management systems for the new facility must be drawn up. Transport arrangements need to be established. These are demanding and time-consuming tasks, so adequate resources should be allocated.

Supervision

The supervising officer should carry out regular site inspections, preferably once a week, to ensure that the contractor is following the drawings and specifications. If the project is large, there may be a full-time site architect or a site monitor or clerk of works appointed by the client. The site monitor has no executive authority. His or her role is to act as the client's "eyes" on-site and to report to the client and the supervising officer.

Valuations and Payments

The contractor's work should not be paid for until it has been approved by the supervising officer. Any unsatisfactory work must be corrected before it is included in a valuation. Typically, valuations and payments are periodic (often monthly), based on a measurement of work actually completed. Alternatively, for simple projects, they may be made in defined amounts at defined construction stages (for example, 10 percent of the total contract sum when the floor slab has been laid). Payment is made against a certificate issued by the architect. A percentage (usually 5 to 10 percent) of the value of the certificate is retained by the client until the contractor has rectified all defects after the end of the specified defects liability period. The defects liability period usually extends for six or twelve months after handover.

Handover

The building is handed over to the client after the design team has fully inspected the completed building and witnessed satisfactory tests of the water supply, drainage, and mechanical and electrical services, and after the contractor has corrected any problems. A few outstanding items may remain to be finished, but the list should be short, and their completion should not interfere with the client's use of the building. The client should attend the pre-handover inspection and should not accept the building unless satisfied. The supervising officer then certifies that the contractor has achieved practical completion.

The contractor hands over all keys to the building and provides the client with instructions on the use of mechanical and electrical equipment. The design team provides a building manual containing a complete set of "as-built" record drawings (drawings revised to show changes made during construction) and general guidance on maintenance. The client's building maintenance officer should be briefed at this stage so that he or she gets to know the building during the defects liability stage.

≡ Assessment Guide

Is additional space really required, or can it be obtained by
- changing delivery intervals?
- reorganizing space within an existing warehouse?

If additional space is required, establish availability of funds and consider building procurement.

What type of warehouse operation is required?
- Mechanical? If yes, are the necessary equipment and servicing infrastructure available?
- Manual? If yes, will this decision unduly limit future program development?
- Manual, upgradable to mechanical? If yes, are funds available to ensure that the building is designed and built to be suitable for upgrading?

What is the most practical and cost-effective way to obtain additional storage space?
- Renovate an existing warehouse?
- Lease a commercial warehouse?
- Buy a commercial warehouse?
- Build a standard warehouse?
- Build a purpose-designed warehouse?

What is the most cost-effective method of building procurement?
- Conventional design service?
- Design and build?
- Turnkey package?

Compare short-listed sites or buildings against the following criteria:

Site Development Potential
- Will the relevant authorities allow the site to be developed as intended?
- Is the site large enough?
- Is the existing building on the site suitable, or will it have to be demolished?
- Is the site well drained? Is there any risk of flooding?
- Is the site protected from landslides, avalanches, and other natural hazards?

- Are ground conditions suitable for building economically?
- Can the site be developed at an acceptable cost?

Access
- Is the site close to the relevant transport links?
- Is the site well served by public transport? (Public transport is needed by stores staff.)
- Is the route to the site accessible year-round by all types of vehicles?
- Is there adequate access for vehicles and space for parking?

Utilities and Communications
- Does the site have a reliable main electricity supply?
- Does the site have a main water supply, borehole, or other reliable source of clean water?
- Is the water supply sufficient for fire fighting?
- Does the site have main drainage? If not, are ground conditions suitable for a septic tank or other autonomous system?
- Is there an existing standby generator? If so, is it powerful enough to supply the cold rooms and refrigerators in the new store?
- Does the site have access to reliable telephone and postal services?

Security
- Is the site likely to invite intrusion or vandalism?
- Can the site be properly monitored and supervised outside normal working hours?
- Is the site easily accessible by the fire department, police, and ambulance services?

Future Conditions
- Will access to the site and the security of the electricity, water drainage, and communications systems be adversely affected by future development in the area?

Commissioning

The client moves into the building and commissions it. At this stage, various "teething problems" can be expected. Some of these will be operational, and some will be caused by building defects. Building problems should be resolved by the contractor and the project team.

Defects Liability

During the defects liability period, the project team, the client, and the contractor agree on the final account. At the end of the defects liability period, the supervising officer inspects the building again and instructs the contractor to rectify any defects that have arisen. The contractor should be given reasonable access to the building to do this. When all defects have been corrected, a final certificate is issued, and final payment is released to the contractor. If there has been a major contractual dispute, the issue of the final certificate (and payment) must be delayed until this is resolved according to the terms of the contract.

Building or renovating a new medical stores facility is a major expense. The temptation to profit personally from the project by bribery or kickbacks is a reality that must be tackled head-on by the project team. There should be strict controls to prevent this. Advance payments should never be made to the contractor. The client should pay only for work that has been correctly completed and certified.

If the construction process runs into serious problems, there may be a dispute that the parties are unable to resolve. Arbitration is a method of settling such disputes without the need for legal proceedings. Informal hearings are held under the control of an arbitrator, whose judgment is final and binding on the parties to the dispute. This procedure is quicker and less expensive than judicial proceedings. However, arbitration may not be adequate if there are significant differences of opinion as to the quantity or quality of work performed. ■

≡ Glossary

Commissioning: The process of preparing a building for operation. This includes adjusting heating, ventilating, and air-conditioning systems; establishing security procedures; and training occupants.

Contract sum: The total amount payable by the owner to the contractor for performing the contracted work. Depending on the contract terms, this amount may be adjusted at the end of the contract to take account of variations that have been approved during construction.

Design-and-build procurement: In this method, the contractor takes responsibility for the detailed design and construction of a building based on an agreed-upon preliminary design.

Final account: A financial reconciliation prepared at the end of a building contract, in which the contract sum is adjusted to take account of all variations that have occurred during the construction process. (These variations include design changes by the client, design changes as a result of site conditions, claims for extra payment by the contractor for delays that are not his responsibility, and counterclaims by the owner for damages caused by the contractor's failure to keep to the program.)

Final certificate: A document issued by the architect or contract supervisor that states the amount of money owed by the client to the contractor (or vice versa) at the end of the contract.

Program or **brief**: A written statement of the owner's conditions and requirements for the project.

Record drawings: Drawings revised to show changes made during construction.

Retention: A sum (typically 5 percent) withheld from each payment made to the contractor during the course of construction. This money is usually released to the contractor after all defects have been rectified and the final certificate is issued.

Subcontractor: One who has a contract with the primary contractor to perform a portion of the work.

Turnkey procurement: A method in which the client hires a contracting company to provide a complete building product for a fixed price.

≡ References and Further Readings

★ = Key readings.

Battersby, A., and A. Garnett. 1993. *How to estimate warehouse space for drugs.* WHO/DAP/93.3. Geneva: World Health Organization.

Compton, H. K. 1985. *Supplies and materials management,* 3d ed. Plymouth, England: Macdonald and Evans, and Institute of Purchasing and Supply.

De Chiara, J., ed. 1990. *Time saver standards for building types,* 3d ed. New York: McGraw-Hill.

Electrolux. 1983. *The storage handbook.* Singapore: Electrolux S.E.A. Pte., Ltd. (240 MacPherson Rd. #03-01/04, Singapore 1334).

Falconer, P., and J. Drury. 1975. *Building and planning for industrial storage and distribution.* London: Architectural Press.

Johnson, J. C., and D. F. Wood. 1993. *Contemporary logistics.* New York: Macmillan.

★ Mein, P., and T. Jorgensen. 1988. *Design for medical buildings: A manual for the planning and building of health care facilities under conditions of limited resources.* Nairobi: Kenya National Federation of Co-operatives, Ltd. (with support from the Housing Research and Development Unit, University of Nairobi).

★ Mulcahy, D. 1994. *Warehouse distribution and operations handbook.* New York: McGraw-Hill.

PAHO (Pan American Health Organization). 1990. *Guidelines for medical supplies distribution centers.* Vols. 1–4. Washington, D.C.: PAHO.

WHO (World Health Organization). 1985. *Oral rehydration salts: Planning, establishment, and operation of production facilities.* WHO/CDD/SER/85.8. Geneva: WHO.

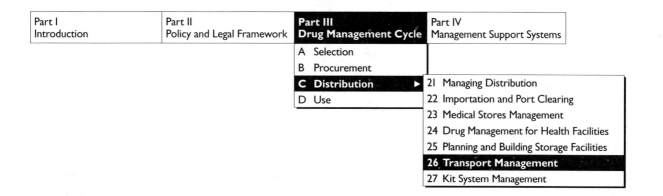

| Part I | Part II | Part III | Part IV |
| Introduction | Policy and Legal Framework | **Drug Management Cycle** | Management Support Systems |

A	Selection
B	Procurement
C	**Distribution** ▶
D	Use

| |
| 21 Managing Distribution |
| 22 Importation and Port Clearing |
| 23 Medical Stores Management |
| 24 Drug Management for Health Facilities |
| 25 Planning and Building Storage Facilities |
| **26 Transport Management** |
| 27 Kit System Management |

Chapter 26
Transport Management

≡ Summary

Unreliable transport for drug supplies is a major problem in many health care programs. Transport is difficult to plan and manage well. Politicians and senior program managers generally assign greater priority to other, more visible, aspects of health care delivery.

When planning transport system improvements, it is essential to

▶ *thoroughly review and understand the existing transport system;*

▶ *select suitable vehicles;*

▶ *ensure that vehicles are used for their intended purpose;*

▶ *maintain vehicles properly;*

▶ *replace vehicles before they wear out;*

▶ *provide funds for vehicle maintenance and replacement;*

▶ *consider alternatives, such as private-sector contracts.*

The costs of purchasing, running, and maintaining vehicles are high. If funding is inadequate, transport services will not be sustainable.

Transport services require effective management. This is particularly difficult to achieve in countries where transport is scarce. When there is a shortage of transport, health service vehicles are frequently misused for the personal benefit of health service staff. Strong management is necessary to eliminate abuses and to ensure that vehicles are used appropriately.

In many countries, the burden of managing transport and transport maintenance services can be reduced by contracting out these services to private or parastatal companies. Before this is done, existing operating costs must be accurately assessed so that a realistic cost comparison can be made. Transport contractors should then be carefully selected and monitored, and contract terms should be clearly drawn up and enforced.

Effective quality control procedures are needed to ensure that drugs are correctly packed to avoid damage.

≡ 26.1 Planning In-House Transport Systems

The existing transport system should be thoroughly reviewed to make efficient and rational use of existing resources. Current operating costs should be accurately assessed and compared with the projected cost of alternative systems. This section examines the issues that must be considered when planning improvements in a transport system.

Understand the Existing Transport System

It is necessary to have a clear understanding of the health system's purpose and organization and to understand the existing transport system and its problems. This requires an assessment of:

▶ Location and scope of transport needs of all warehouses and health facilities.

▶ Performance record of the existing drug transport system. A detailed inventory must be made of vehicles in use at every level in the distribution system, listing age, condition, operational status, and actual versus intended use. This is an essential starting point for any transport assessment and should be carried out thoroughly. The data collected may be used to determine whether the existing transport fleet, in its current state, is capable of satisfying program needs.

▶ Estimated costs for the repair of defective vehicles.

▶ Location and availability of spare parts, and vehicle servicing capacity.

▶ Location and availability of fuel.

▶ Geographical, climatic, and political factors that affect transportation.

▶ Population distribution. Transport costs per capita are much higher in sparsely populated areas than in areas of high population density. It is important to take this into account and to target funds in a balanced manner.

▶ The condition, capacity, and limitations of road, rail, and other transportation networks.

▶ Alternative transportation resources at every level. These resources include vehicles belonging to other government agencies, to nongovernmental organizations (NGOs), and to private-sector carriers. Vehicle sharing between programs is often a good option for reducing costs and improving reliability. Public transport should also be considered where suitable. Unconventional forms of transport such as bicycles may be highly cost effective, particularly in rural areas.

▶ The annual cost of the existing transportation system. A crude index of performance can be obtained by considering this cost as a percentage of the value of drugs delivered.

▶ Staff management issues related to transport.

If information is not already available, it should be collected using a structured survey (see Chapter 4). Total variable cost analysis is a good method for compiling cost data (see Chapter 41). Most information requires regular updating if it is to remain useful. Some data, such as vehicle breakdown reports, are required at monthly to quarterly intervals. Other data, such as road improvement information, need only occasional updating.

Plan Routes

Drug delivery routes should be planned at every level to make the best use of available resources. The following guidelines should be adopted:

► Arrange delivery routes and schedules so that vehicles start each journey fully loaded. It is inefficient to use a large vehicle to deliver small quantities of drugs. Unless full loads are being dropped off at a single delivery point, a delivery circuit may be cheaper to operate than a series of trips back and forth.

► Make maximum use of good roads. Shortcuts along poor roads may save fuel and time, but driving on good roads improves vehicle life.

► Use vehicles that are appropriate to the route. It is a waste of resources to use four-wheel-drive vehicles on surfaced roads.

► Arrange routes so that the vehicle can be parked in a secure compound during overnight stops.

► Plan routes to take account of fuel availability. If fuel is scarce, it may be necessary to carry fuel drums or to fit vehicles with long-range fuel tanks. This will reduce the space available for carrying supplies.

► Consult experienced drivers before deciding on the route. Drivers often have the best knowledge of local road conditions, fuel availability, weather, and security hazards. Their advice can be extremely valuable.

► Compare the costs of alternative combinations of routes and vehicles before making a final choice. Country Study 26.1 describes Zimbabwe's approach to vehicle selection. Transport cost assessment is described in Section 26.5.

Analyze Transport Alternatives

Major transport options are listed below:

► *Trucks, vans, and cars* are the most common means of transporting drugs, but there are many other forms of transport.

► *Air transport* is frequently used for delivering costly, heat-labile products, such as vaccines. Commercial air-freight charges are high, although packaging costs may be lower than with land transport. Theft may also be lower where airport security is good. In some

---

Country Study 26.1 Route Planning and Vehicle Selection in Zimbabwe

In Zimbabwe, drugs are distributed from five medical stores, where requisitions from health facilities are processed. They are distributed in three ways: (1) many health facilities receive their drugs by direct delivery; (2) other facilities' consignments are delivered to an intermediate drop-off point and require transshipment; and (3) provincial hospitals and other large facilities often collect drugs directly from the medical stores. A 1993 Zimbabwe Essential Drugs Action Programme (ZEDAP) survey showed that direct deliveries took an average of 7.3 days. Deliveries via drop-off points took an average of 12.9 days.

Delivery by medical store vehicles greatly increased between 1989 and 1993 and became the dominant mode of transport. During this period, delivery times were cut from an average of twenty-two days to an average of eleven days. Customer satisfaction increased.

The medical stores have been supplied with six-ton trucks towing five-ton box trailers that provide additional transport capacity. Typically, a trailer is loaded with supplies for one of the drop-off points. When it is empty, the trailer is left behind at the drop-off point. It is collected when the truck returns from making the other deliveries. Small transit stores are being built at the drop-off points to ensure security.

In some districts, camping trailers with a capacity of 750 kg are used. These trailers can be towed behind jeeps or pickup trucks and are used to deliver drugs in remote areas.

Source: Mogens Munck, ZEDAP 1994.

---

settings, such as countries with many islands, air transport may be the most cost-effective option for routinely transporting drugs. Light aircraft may be used to transport drugs and health workers to remote and otherwise inaccessible outposts and in emergency relief situations.

► *Boats* are appropriate in some areas with island communities, coastal settlements, navigable rivers, or large lakes. Drugs transported by boat must be packaged and stored to protect them against water damage.

► *Railways* are an excellent and cheap means of transport, provided the service is reliable. Rail transport is particularly suitable for bulk shipments between major depots. One disadvantage is that the supplies usually need to be transferred to another form of transport at the end of the rail journey. Transshipment increases the risk of theft and damage.

► *Private-sector trucking companies* can offer a cost-effective delivery service, especially between major population centers. This issue is discussed in Section 26.5.

► *Box trailer units* increase load-carrying capacity without the need to buy additional trucks. Small trailers, towed behind cars or pickup trucks, can also be used to transport drugs in rural areas.

► *Buses, minibuses, and other means of local passenger transport* can be used by health workers for transporting small quantities of drugs.

Many programs also use so-called intermediate transport (IMT) to augment the major transport mechanisms. Figure 26.1 compares the capacity and daily range of common IMT mechanisms.

Prepare Transport Plan

After the existing transport system has been analyzed and the transport alternatives assessed, the logistics team should choose among the various options and balance sometimes conflicting priorities. A detailed transport plan should then be prepared that describes how all warehouses and facilities will be served.

≡ 26.2 Vehicle Acquisition and Disposal

This section examines various methods of vehicle procurement, policy options for vehicle replacement, the process of selecting appropriate vehicles, and methods for disposing of broken or obsolete vehicles.

Select Method of Vehicle Procurement

There are four ways in which a health program can procure vehicles, boats, or aircraft: purchase, donation, lease,

Figure 26.1 Performance Characteristics and Relative Costs of Some Intermediate Forms of Transport

Vehicle	Max No. of People Carried[a]	Kg/m³ Supplies Carried	Max Speed (km/hr)	Max Range (km)	Route Limitations	Relative Cost[c]
Porter	–	25–35 0.25 m³	5	20	Unlimited	0–10
Standard bicycle	1	20[b] 0.25 m³	20	60	Reasonably flat	50–90
Load-carrying bicycle	1	25–100[b] 0.35 m³	10–15	30–40	Reasonably flat	60–100
Bicycle and trailer	1	150 0.5 m³	10–15	30–40	Reasonably flat, wide track	90–150
Bicycle and sidecar	1	150 0.4 m³	10–15	30–40	Reasonably flat, wide track	90–150
Tricycle	1	150 0.5 m³	10–15	30–40	Reasonably flat	150–200
Pack animal	–	50–200[b] Varies	5	20	Unlimited	Variable
Animal-drawn cart	Varies	500–3,000 Varies	5	20	Reasonably flat, wide track	100–180
Motorcycle	1	50–75[b] 0.25 m³	40–90	100–200	Steep hills	250–600
Motorcycle and sidecar/tricycle	1	200–300[b] 0.5–1.0 m³	30–60	80–150	Moderate hills, wide track	350–800
ATV (quad bike)[d]	1	50–75[e] 0.5 m³	30–60	60	Rough, hilly terrain	750–1,500
Single-axle tractor and trailer	Varies	1,500 Varies	15–20	50	Steep hills, wide track	1,500
Asian utility vehicle	Varies	500–1,000 2.0 m³	60	60	Steep hills, wide track	3,000

Source: Adapted from Hathaway 1985 and *WHO Technet News,* August 1989.
[a] Number of people carried with full load of goods.
[b] The maximum load weights for these IMTs are 50 percent of the values quoted by Hathaway (1985). Figures have been reduced to take account of the risk of damage to valuable commodities if unstable vehicles fall over when heavily loaded. In many cases, the volume carried, not the weight, is the limiting factor.
[c] Typical ranges are quoted. These are relative costs—no specific currency is implied.
[d] All-terrain vehicle, two-wheel-drive and four-wheel-drive.
[e] Payload given is without trailer. Trailers can be attached to ATVs.

or rental from the private sector. Contracting out transport to a private carrier should be considered as an alternative to procurement.

Purchase. Health programs generally purchase vehicles, which involves capital expenditure. Recurrent costs include vehicle insurance, servicing, and maintenance.

Donations. Vehicle donations are useful in some situations; in some countries, this is the main source of vehicles. There can be disadvantages, however. Donors may not fund insurance, servicing, and maintenance, and the health program will have to pay for these items. Donors may want to supply vehicles manufactured in the donor country, whether or not spare parts and maintenance skills are locally available. This can lead to serious problems. Careful analysis of the advantages and disadvantages should be carried out before soliciting or accepting vehicle donations. It is important to keep in mind that sustainability is the key issue, and donor agreements are of limited duration. The health system may not have the capacity to maintain vehicles; if it does not, the donated vehicles will have a limited life.

Lease or Rental. If an in-house transport system is to be maintained, the costs of leasing and purchasing should be compared. Leasing or rental companies provide vehicles on a short- or long-term basis and may also be able to supply drivers, for an additional charge. An advantage of leasing or rental is that additional vehicles can readily be obtained, and broken-down vehicles can be replaced as part of the contract agreement at no cost to the system.

Contracting Out. Private or parastatal trucking companies may have better transport management capacity than government agencies. Trucking companies are likely to be most competitive on the major routes. Contracting out the major routes means that the health service does not need to acquire and manage heavy vehicles, nor does it need to train drivers and maintenance staff for these vehicles.

Establish Vehicle Replacement Policy

Implementing a transport plan is only the first step; in-house transport systems quickly collapse if there is no vehicle replacement policy.

It is essential to review the transport plan regularly and to analyze vehicle operating costs carefully. Most important of all is to negotiate adequate funding to maintain the system. As vehicles get older, the cost of servicing and repairing them increases. Eventually they will have to be replaced. The balance between capital and recurrent expenditures therefore changes from year to year. This can pose a problem, particularly when many new vehicles are suddenly acquired from a donor. These vehicles will dete-

riorate at similar rates and will need to be replaced at about the same time.

There are four basic policy options for vehicle replacement:

1. A *target life* is set for each category of vehicle. All vehicles in a category are replaced when they reach this set age, regardless of mileage or condition.
2. A *target mileage* is set for each category of vehicle. All vehicles in a category are replaced when they reach this mileage, regardless of age or condition.
3. Vehicles are replaced, regardless of age or mileage, when they exceed a pre-set *maintenance cost*.
4. Vehicles are replaced when their *operational availability* (reliability) falls below a defined level. The aim should always be to operate a fleet with no breakdowns.

In practice, some combination of these four alternatives will probably be needed. For instance, a policy could be based on target life and mileage. Replacement occurs when one or the other of the two targets is exceeded. The chosen approach depends on the availability of funds and patterns of vehicle use. Commercial organizations have to operate their fleets as *profit* centers. Traditionally, government organizations and NGOs view their transport fleets as *cost* centers.

Figure 26.2 shows two graphs indicating the decline in resale value compared with the rise in maintenance costs over time. Graph A illustrates an idealized model for determining the best time to replace a vehicle. Using this model, vehicles are replaced as soon as annual maintenance costs exceed the capital value of the vehicle—in this example, after seven years. In practice, vehicle resale value is difficult to predict accurately over a long period, especially when operating conditions are harsh and the resale value of older vehicles is determined more by condition than by age. Moreover, maintenance costs do not rise in a smoothly increasing curve over time; rather, the maintenance cost curve is lumpy, as illustrated in Graph B, with peaks occurring whenever major components have to be replaced. Maintenance costs still exceed capital value after seven years, but by a smaller and fluctuating amount. Moreover, a significant proportion of these maintenance costs are fixed costs: preventive maintenance, tire replacement, and other costs that cannot be avoided, whatever the age of the vehicle.

The replacement policy should be reviewed regularly, based on an analysis of real data obtained from vehicle maintenance costs and operational reliability records. The operational costs of vehicle breakdowns should also be

Figure 26.2 Replacement Policy Graphs

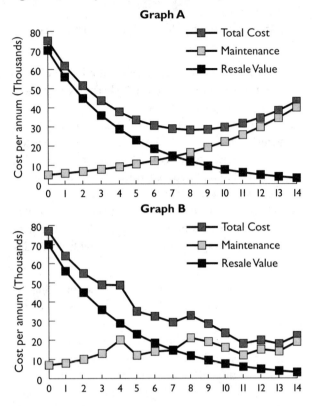

taken into account. These costs can be controlled to some extent by carefully planned preventive maintenance, but as vehicles become older, the risk of unforeseen failure increases.

The condition of every vehicle in the fleet should be reviewed annually and compared with its planned life span and replacement target. If a vehicle has to be replaced prematurely, it is important to understand why.

Transport plans should be adaptable to respond to changing circumstances. For example, when funds are short, a vehicle may be kept beyond its planned replacement life, provided the vehicle is reliable and spare parts are still available.

Select Appropriate Vehicles

Over the years, programs often acquire a random mix of vehicles from a wide range of manufacturers, which causes problems with maintenance and support. It is essential to select vehicles wisely, whether they are purchased or donated. Vehicle type, fuel, spare parts, temperature control, and need for refrigeration are critical issues.

Vehicle Type. Limit the variety of vehicles to simplify maintenance and enable vehicles to be interchanged within the distribution system. Choose vehicles that are in common use throughout the country. Nationwide avail-

ability of spare parts and maintenance capacity are the most important considerations in choosing a vehicle. If feasible, choose the same type of vehicles as other programs. This allows spare parts and servicing skills to be shared among programs.

Choose vehicles that are simple in design, easy to maintain, and suited to local road conditions. It is a waste of money to buy four-wheel-drive vehicles if they are to be used exclusively on paved roads. Choose vehicles that have interchangeable components, particularly items such as tires, batteries, engines, and transmissions. If an emergency arises, or if a vehicle is badly damaged, vehicles with interchangeable components can be used as sources of spare parts for others in the fleet.

If possible, choose vehicle manufacturers that do not change models frequently. This helps ensure the continuous availability of spare parts. In addition, it is easier to assess a vehicle's reliability if it has been sold for a number of years, and maintenance staff need less retraining.

Fuel. Diesel-powered vehicles are usually more cost effective than gasoline-powered vehicles. They are more expensive to buy and maintain, but they are more fuel efficient and may be more reliable and longer lasting. However, at temperatures below -5° to -10°C, diesel vehicles can be difficult to operate, unless fuel-line heaters or special low-temperature fuel is available. If fuel quality is a problem, select vehicles that can be adjusted to run on low-octane or adulterated fuel.

Accessories and Spare Parts. Every vehicle should have a tool kit, first-aid kit, and fire extinguisher. It is essential to purchase an adequate supply of spare parts, including oil filters, tires, and batteries. The quantity purchased will depend on future funding arrangements. If adequate funds for recurrent expenditures are ensured, the stock of spare parts can be renewed annually. If there is no assurance that such funds will be available, vehicles should be purchased with several years' worth of spare parts. This applies particularly to donated vehicles.

Temperature Control. Vehicles should be painted white to reduce internal temperatures during hot weather (where applicable). They may also need to be fitted with ventilator units. In India, unrefrigerated but insulated vehicle bodies have been used to control transport temperatures. Most pharmaceuticals should not be stored for prolonged periods at temperatures above 30°C. Even in temperate climates, this temperature can be exceeded when a vehicle is parked in the sun. Some drugs, vaccines, and blood products can be damaged by exposure to temperatures even well below 30°C. These items should be transported in cold boxes or refrigerated vehicles.

In very cold climates, blood products and some pharmaceuticals and vaccines need protection against freezing during transport. Goods compartments may need to be heated; alternatively, products can be transported for limited distances using vaccine cold boxes fitted with "warm packs."

Refrigerated Vehicles. Refrigerated vehicles are more difficult to maintain than conventional vehicles and should be considered only in countries with a good maintenance infrastructure. Choose vehicles that have independent body units. The refrigerated body lasts longer than the vehicle to which it is attached and may be transferred to a new chassis.

Refrigeration units that can be powered by an independent engine will continue to operate even if the vehicle itself breaks down. All units should have electrical backup power units for use during overnight stops, and suitable power outlets should be provided at the stopping points.

When refrigerated vehicles break down, the shipment can be exposed to unacceptable temperatures within a few hours. Ensure that adequate contingency plans exist for this hazard.

In countries with cold winters, refrigerated vehicles should be fitted with a heating circuit to prevent sensitive products from freezing.

Manage Vehicle Disposal

As a general rule, any vehicle that has been broken for six months should be disposed of. Most countries have committees that are responsible for deciding when to dispose of obsolete vehicles and equipment. However, this procedure is often cumbersome, and large numbers of broken vehicles are left to accumulate. These vehicles can be used to advantage in some countries. For example, they can be sold or dismantled for spare parts. The main constraint on sales is that proceeds usually accrue to the finance ministry rather than to the health ministry. Arranging for this money to be reallocated to the health service may be difficult.

≡ 26.3 Vehicle Use

This section examines the issues involved in managing vehicles efficiently, safely, and cost effectively and suggests ways to minimize system abuse.

Prevent Vehicle Misuse

In-house transport systems often fail because the system is abused. Government vehicles are frequently used for private purposes, particularly by drivers and senior managers, and especially in countries where vehicles and fuel are scarce or salaries are low.

It is difficult to plan and manage vehicle use and control misuse, but these activities are the key to sustaining a successful transport operation. Leadership and support are required from those people who have the authority to control negligent management practices.

The transport manager should control vehicle use, allocate transport resources, and be accountable for operational failures. Transport should be planned and managed to achieve the following goals:

► Allocation of transport resources to meet the needs of the organization rather than those of the individual;
► Prevention of unauthorized vehicle use;
► Assignment of the most appropriate vehicle and driver for each purpose;
► Use of alternatives, such as public transport, where appropriate and cost effective;
► Clear definitions of allowable uses by program staff and managers, to be respected by all users.

Regular users should prepare written schedules of their transport needs at least a month in advance. The transport manager can then prepare a plan that makes the best use of available resources. Time for preventive maintenance should be allocated in the plan. When possible, journeys should be combined so that vehicles travel full and do not make wide detours. A detailed weekly or monthly plan should be prepared and later compared with the actual course of events, with analysis and follow-up of discrepancies.

Methods of monitoring for abuses include:

► Check the mileage recorded on the odometer every week and compare this with the driver's official log.
► Install tachographs. These are legally required in European countries, but larger vehicles everywhere should be equipped with them. These devices record comprehensive details of every journey and can provide a check on the accuracy of the driver's log. The tachograph record also shows whether adequate rest stops have been taken.

Misuse of motorcycles, light vans, and other small vehicles is more difficult to control, especially when vehicles are allocated to facilities in remote areas. Staff may be encouraged to purchase motorcycles and other small vehicles from the health service at low cost; this reduces vehicle abuse, generates income for vehicle replacement, and gives staff an incentive to maintain vehicles properly. An approach adopted in Zimbabwe is to sell vehicles to health workers on extended repayment terms and then to pay a mileage allowance. The health worker is free to use the vehicle for private purposes but also has an incentive to maintain it. After five years, the vehicle becomes the worker's property.

When vehicle misuse is discovered, the problem must be dealt with firmly and quickly. Allowing an abuse to continue ensures that it will become part of the system.

Train Motorcycle Riders and Drivers

Well-trained drivers and riders have fewer accidents and better vehicle maintenance than those who are poorly trained. Driver-training modules are available from a number of sources (see "References and Further Readings"). A driver or rider should

► drive or ride carefully and without aggression toward other road users;
► be able to carry out preventive maintenance, minor servicing, and emergency repairs;
► be thoroughly knowledgeable about the routes and well informed about road and weather conditions and the location of service and refueling facilities.

Ensure Vehicle Security

Vehicle security is a serious problem in many countries. Vehicles are stolen for resale or for spare parts, and drugs may be stolen in transit. Precautions to take include:

► Keep vehicles in locked compounds or garages.
► Employ security guards.
► Plan delivery routes so that vehicles can be securely parked during overnight stops.
► Instruct drivers never to leave vehicles unattended during transit.
► Avoid driving at night, especially in countries where vehicles are poorly maintained or have no lights. Security problems are often worse after dark.
► Install burglar alarms and/or immobilization devices. Fit security deadlocks on cab doors and goods compartments. Where security is extremely difficult, it may be necessary to fit grilles around the cab interior.
► If long delivery trips are required, buy vehicles with sleeping compartments for drivers.
► Ensure that every vehicle is fitted with a fire extinguisher. Tools and spare parts should be carried so that the driver can make simple repairs without having to leave the vehicle unattended.

Ideally, all vehicles carrying valuable loads should have a second driver or a driver's assistant. On long journeys, a second driver is necessary to reduce the risk of the driver's falling asleep. If there is a breakdown or an accident, one person can guard the vehicle while the other gets help.

≡ 26.4 Vehicle Maintenance

Planned maintenance is an essential aspect of the transport system. It includes ensuring availability of spare parts, managing vehicle repair, and disposing of waste products.

Provide Spare Parts and Consumable Supplies

Vehicles cannot be serviced and repaired without an adequate supply of spare parts and consumables—lubricants, brake fluid, tires, batteries, and oil filters. If vehicles are not serviced, they quickly become unreliable.

It is the responsibility of senior logistics managers to emphasize that drug deliveries cannot be guaranteed without adequate funding for spare parts and consumables. Politicians and budget control officers must be persuaded to understand the importance of adequate recurrent funding or consider contract alternatives to in-house transport.

Manage Vehicle Maintenance

A consistently high standard of maintenance increases the fleet's reliability; this can be achieved only if the maintenance policy is clearly defined, enforced, costed, and monitored.

Vehicle maintenance can be divided into four levels:

1. *Preventive maintenance*, as defined in the manufacturer's service manual, includes lubrication, oil changes, replacement of oil filters and brake pads, tire changes, and other measures that keep the vehicle operating safely and efficiently. All these can be foreseen and planned for.
2. *Overhauls* involve the dismantling or replacement of major components, such as engines, clutch linings, or transmissions. The mileage at which a specific overhaul is required varies from vehicle to vehicle, but overhauls can be foreseen and planned for.
3. *Minor repairs* include replacement of broken headlights and minor body work. They do not require the tools or skills of a specialist. Many of these will be unforeseen but can be managed if parts are available.
4. *Major repairs* are needed in the case of crash damage or other unforeseen work that requires specialized tools and skills.

Preventive maintenance and minor repairs can be carried out in simply equipped workshops by relatively unskilled mechanics and require a small selection of frequently used spare parts and consumables. Preventive maintenance for every vehicle should be scheduled in advance as part of the management of vehicle use. Major repairs and overhauls have to be carried out in well-equipped workshops by skilled mechanics and require access to a comprehensive stock of spare parts.

A health program often needs a combination of maintenance levels. For instance, the health program can carry out preventive maintenance and minor repairs in its own workshops, and major repairs and overhauls can be contracted out to a central government workshop or a private garage.

The examples below indicate the range of options for organizing maintenance services. These options are based on the assumption that the health program is government run, but they are also relevant to NGOs.

Workshops Operated and Funded by the Health Program. The main advantage of this option is that workshops, maintenance staff, and the stock of spare parts are directly controlled by the health program. The main disadvantage is that transport maintenance services may be duplicated among government agencies, often when few trained staff are available. This duplication wastes funds and can result in maintenance units that lack proper staff or are too small to operate cost effectively. This is less likely to happen if only preventive maintenance and minor repairs are carried out.

Workshops Operated and Funded by Another Government Agency. A network of vehicle maintenance workshops operated by the ministry of works can be used to maintain all government vehicles. This is a traditional administrative solution. It can be satisfactory, provided that workshops are fully equipped, staff are well trained, and the government is committed to upgrading equipment and retraining staff as vehicle technology changes. A disadvantage is that the health program has no direct control over the quality of service, and there are no sanctions that can be applied if the service is unsatisfactory.

Privatized Government Maintenance Services. Workshop services owned and operated by government may be transferred or franchised to a parastatal organization or to a private company. Government agencies can then buy back the service at a rate that is periodically renegotiated. Privatization of government services has been widely advocated and has been adopted in many countries. Disadvantages include the possibilities of overcharging and corrupt and abusive billing and pricing practices.

Tendered Maintenance Contracts with Private Companies. An arrangement involving private maintenance contracts that run for one or more years has several advantages:

▶ The health program does not have to provide workshops or maintenance staff or hold stocks of spare parts. Capital investment is thus reduced, and the health program can concentrate on core activities.

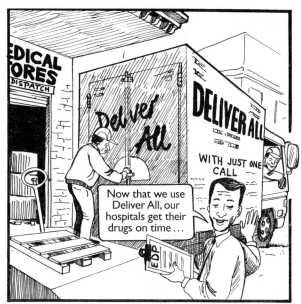

COMMERCIAL TRANSPORTERS MAY BE THE BEST CHOICE ON CERTAIN DELIVERY ROUTES

▶ Cost control may be better: the service contract can set a flat rate per year for maintaining each vehicle, which includes the cost of normal spare parts. Only unforeseeable items (such as accident repairs) need to be paid for, on the basis of individual invoices.

▶ Quality assurance clauses can be built into the contract. These can impose financial penalties whenever the service quality fails to meet set targets. Bonus payments to the contractor may also be justified if reliability exceeds target norms.

Contracts of this kind succeed only in countries with well-developed private vehicle-maintenance sectors. Tenderers must use sophisticated costing techniques if they are to offer realistic quotes, and they must have well-equipped workshops and reliable sources of spare parts and consumables. Government must have good monitoring, reporting, and accounting procedures. Otherwise, unsatisfactory service or corrupt practices may go undetected.

Private Workshops with Services Paid by Invoice. This option gives no cost certainty and no quality assurance. It should be used only for emergency repairs or when no other maintenance facilities are available.

Ensure Safe Disposal of Waste Products
Vehicle servicing produces toxic waste products. Oil, lubricants, tires, and batteries must be disposed of safely to avoid creating public health risks. The health program should require that the vehicle service organization

Figure 26.3 Comparison of Commercial Fleets, Government Fleets, and Mixed Fleets

Factor	Commercial Fleet	Government Fleet	Mixed Fleet
Government capital expenditure on vehicles	No	Yes	Yes, but reduced
Government expenditure on maintenance, insurance, wages, supervision, and per diems	No	Yes	Yes, but reduced
Flexibility to meet demand peaks	Yes	No	Yes
Fast transport beyond normal commercial routes	No	Yes	Yes
Security of drugs in transit	Should be good	Variable	Variable
Running costs	Lowest for large loads and long hauls	Lowest for stable requirements	Can provide an optimum mix

adopt a safe disposal policy that complies fully with local regulations.

≡ 26.5 Contracting Transport Services

This section examines the advantages and disadvantages of contracting out transport services to private transport companies. It also presents the costing decisions that need to be made and details procedures for selecting, working with, and monitoring contractors.

Private-Sector Transport Issues

Private transport companies in some countries can offer better and cheaper drug delivery service than the government is able to provide. These advantages are most likely to be gained in countries with a well-developed infrastructure and a good range of well-managed private transport companies. Where choice is limited, there may be insufficient competition to produce real cost savings.

Private carriers will probably be most competitive on routes between major population centers. On these routes, vehicles are unlikely to return empty, which lowers overall costs. Private carriers may be comparatively expensive when delivering to remote areas where return loads are unavailable, but this may not be true if there are existing delivery routes to these areas. The health program may be able to enter into a joint agreement with another agency that needs transport arrangements from the periphery to the center. Agricultural cooperatives are one possibility.

Whenever possible, drug deliveries should be organized so that the transport contractor is supplied with full loads. Low transport costs depend on maximum use of vehicle capacity. Contract transport may improve the security of drugs, providing the contractor is made responsible for any losses in transit.

Figure 26.3 compares the advantages and disadvantages of private-sector, government, and mixed transport fleets.

The above remarks relate principally to road transport contractors, but rail, air, and sea transport services may also be used for drug deliveries. The issues discussed below apply equally to these forms of transport.

Cost Assessment

A thorough cost analysis should be carried out before a decision is made to contract out transport services. A decision to introduce private-sector transport can have far-reaching implications. For instance, existing vehicles will have to be sold if they are no longer needed. If many vehicles are sold, government workshops may no longer have sufficient work to remain viable. Unless these issues are taken into account, the overall effectiveness and efficiency of the government transport operation may decline rather than improve. Country Study 26.2 provides an example of analyzing alternatives.

In-House Transport Costs

Any comparison of public- and private-sector transport alternatives requires a realistic assessment of public-sector vehicle operating costs. The annual operating costs for a vehicle are made up of the following elements:

Fixed Costs
► Amortized cost of the vehicle over its anticipated lifetime;
► Interest costs;
► Road tax;
► Insurance premium;
► Wages and overhead for the drivers.

Variable Costs, Based on Anticipated Annual Mileage
► Fuel;
► Preventive maintenance (filters, lubrication, brake pads, tires);
► Repairs and overhauls;
► Per diem payments to drivers for meals and accommodation.

Carrying Costs of Public-Sector Transport
► Cost of transport administration;
► Cost of parking and garaging.

Country Study 26.2 Contract-or-Buy Analysis in Zimbabwe

In Zimbabwe, the cost of running the drug delivery routes from the central medical stores (CMS) to the provincial stores using CMS vehicles was compared with the cost of using private-sector carriers. The results of the analysis were used to decide which routes should be contracted out to the private sector. The operating parameters and costs for CMS vehicles were as follows:

Payload of each truck	5 tons
Annual mileage of all vehicles	468,000 km
Fixed costs	$0.37 per km
Variable costs	$0.03 per km
Fixed + variable costs	$0.40 per km

These figures were used to calculate the cost of running each route using CMS vehicles and private carriers. Results are shown in the accompanying table. This table shows that for loads that are multiples of 5 tons, it is cheaper to use CMS vehicles. Although the cost differential decreases with increasing distance, this remains true even for destinations that are far away. The full cost advantage is obtained only if the trucks are hauling loads in both directions. An empty CMS truck costs the same per kilometer as a fully loaded one, but the private carrier does not charge for the return journey. If there is no load for the CMS vehicle to carry back, it becomes more economical to use hired transport to Gweru, Bulawayo, and Binga. The cost ratio in all three cases is less than 2.0.

					Ratio of Tariff Cost to Own Costs per 5 Tons	
Destination	Distance (km)	One-Way Cost of Using Own Fleet (US$0.40 per km)	Private-Sector Tariff (US$ per 100 kg)	Cost of Transporting 5 Tons	If full for return	If empty for return
Chinhoyi	110	44.00	2.94	147.00	3.35	1.67
Gweru	275	110.00	3.94	197.00	1.80	0.89
Masvingo	292	116.80	5.16	258.00	2.22	1.10
Bulawayo	439	175.60	4.73	236.50	1.36	0.67
Binga	880	352.00	7.69	384.50	1.09	0.55

Source: Mogens Munck, ZEDAP 1994.

Total variable cost analysis (see Chapter 41) can be used to compile cost data. Once these costs have been calculated, they can be used to assess the delivery cost per ton on specific routes. This cost can then be compared with quoted rates for alternative forms of transport. If the preliminary assessment indicates that private-sector transport is more economical, formal tenders to provide services should be conducted, as described in Chapter 17.

≡ 26.6 Maintaining Drug Quality

Transport managers are responsible for ensuring that drugs are not damaged during transit. It is essential that drugs be properly packed (see Figure 26.4).

The drug manufacturer's original outer packing should withstand normal handling and transportation. At the intermediate stores, this outer packing often has to be removed to allow the assembly of small consignments; these must be repacked for transport in strong cartons or reusable crates. Empty spaces in partly filled cartons or crates should be filled with newspaper, straw, wood shavings, or other loose material to stop the contents from rattling about and prevent cartons from being crushed. If mechanical handling equipment is available, loads may then be assembled onto pallets.

Pallets, cartons, or crates should be carefully and systematically loaded into vehicles on a first-in/last-out basis. They must then be held secure by straps, nets, or other means. The vibration caused by travel over rough roads can damage tablets and other breakable products; long delivery journeys over rough roads should be avoided whenever possible.

Delivery journeys in very hot or cold weather may damage temperature-sensitive products. Appropriate precautions must be taken, as discussed earlier in this chapter. Water damage during heavy rain can be avoided by ensuring that drugs are unloaded directly into a building and not left standing outside. ∎

Figure 26.4 Transporting Drugs Safely

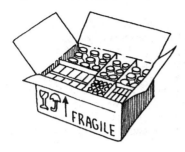
Fill voids in cartons with packing material

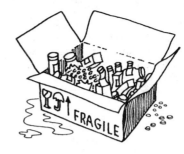
Prevent breakages

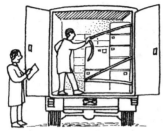
Load vehicles carefully and systematically first-out/last-in

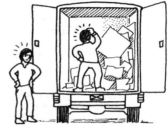
Save time when unloading
Prevent physical damage

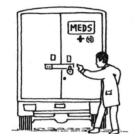
Secure vehicle doors

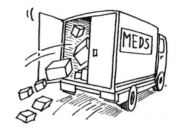
Prevent losses or theft

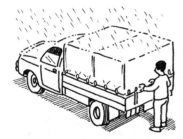
Protect supplies from sun or rain
Stay near the vehicle

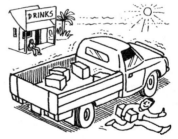
Minimize deterioration of drugs during transit
Guard against theft

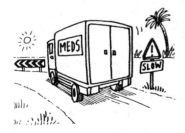
Start early in the day and drive with care, especially on hazardous roads

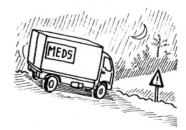
Avoid nighttime driving

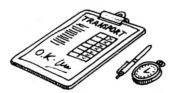
Ensure safe and timely delivery

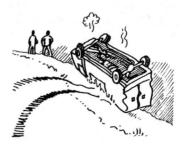
Prevent accidents

≡ Assessment Guide

Existing Transport System

► Does the program have a transport management department?

► What are the major transport problems?

► Who provides the transport budget? (Compare the transport budget with actual expenditures.)

► What types of vehicles are used? (List *all* types used and the source, model, quantity, age, mileage, condition, and location of each.)

► Are vehicles shared with vertical programs, such as EPI? Do availability and reliability vary among programs? If so, why?

► Do existing transport routes make effective use of vehicles?

► Is there a vehicle replacement policy? If so, how is replacement funded?

► Is there a policy for writing off broken-down vehicles? Is it implemented?

► Is there a preventive maintenance policy? Is it effective?

► What percentage of vehicles are in working condition? Describe by type and location of vehicle.

► Is there a policy to control and monitor vehicle use? Is it effective?

► Is there a driver training program? Is it effective?

► Is there a policy on transport security? Does it control losses?

► Are vehicles loaded correctly?

► What is the number of vehicles, compared to the number of drivers?

Transport Alternatives

► What are the transportation terms for overseas and in-country suppliers? Could these be changed to require direct delivery to lower-level stores?

► Which of the following modes of transport are available?
–program vehicles
–motor pool vehicles
–buses
–NGO vehicles
–intermediate forms of transport (IMTs)
–railways
–water transport
–commercial, government (including military), NGO flights

Private-Sector Transport Alternatives and Cost Comparisons

► Do vehicle rental and leasing companies exist? What are the charges?

► Are commercial carriers available? Are they capable of transporting drugs at rates equal to or lower than costs of in-house transport?

Maintenance Alternatives

► Are health program or other government workshops offered?

► Are there privatized government workshops?

► Are contracts with the private sector a possibility?

Monitoring and Evaluation

► Are there effective systems for monitoring and evaluating transport costs and performance? If not, which elements are missing?

≡ References and Further Readings

★ = *Key readings.*

Battersby, A. 1985. *How to assess health care service logistics with particular reference to peripheral health facilities.* WHO/SHS/85.9. Geneva: World Health Organization.

Chesher, A., and R. Harrison. 1987. *Vehicle operating costs: Evidence from developing countries.* Baltimore and London: Johns Hopkins University Press.

Dawson, J., and I. Barwell. 1993. *Roads are not enough: New perspectives on rural transport planning in developing countries.* London: Intermediate Technology Publications.

Hathaway, G. 1985. *Low-cost vehicles: Options for moving people and goods.* London: Intermediate Technology Publications.

★ MSH (Management Sciences for Health). 1992. Distribution and transport planning (trainer's and participant's guides). In *Managing drug supply training series.* Part 3. *Supply management.* Boston: MSH.

Riverson, J. D. N., and S. Carapetis. 1991. *Intermediate means of transport in sub-Saharan Africa.* Technical paper no. 161. Washington, D.C.: World Bank.

★ SCF (Save the Children Fund). 1993. *Using motor-cycles in development programmes: Guidelines for the management of motor-cycle fleets in demanding or harsh environments.* London: SCF Riders for Health.

★ SCF (Save the Children Fund) and TRANSAID. 1995. *Transport management.* London: SCF and TRANSAID.

Handbook no. 1: *An introduction to the role of field management in the provision and operation of transport.*

Handbook no. 2: *Managing your fleet.*

Handbook no. 3: *Fleet composition and size: Replacing or adding vehicles to the fleet.*

Handbook no. 4: *Competence and testing of drivers.*

Handbook no. 5: *Driver's responsibilities.*

UNICEF (United Nations Children's Fund). 1986. *Assisting in emergencies: A resource handbook for UNICEF field staff.* New York City: UNICEF.

WHO/EPI (World Health Organization/Expanded Programme on Immunization). 1991a. *Advanced driving for health.* Logistics for Health Technical Series. Geneva: WHO/EPI.

WHO/EPI (World Health Organization/Expanded Programme on Immunization. 1991b. *Guidelines for introducing motor-cycles into a primary health care program.* Geneva: WHO/EPI.

WHO/EPI (World Health Organization/Expanded Programme on Immunization). 1991c. *Riders for health: Manual for motor-cycle instructors.* Geneva: WHO/EPI.

WHO/EPI (World Health Organization/Expanded Programme on Immunization). 1992. *Monitoring vehicle use: A guide for national operations officers.* Geneva: WHO/EPI.

★ WHO/UNICEF (World Health Organization/United Nations Children's Fund). 1993 (revised regularly). *Product information sheets 1993/1994.* Geneva: WHO/UNICEF.

Part I Introduction	Part II Policy and Legal Framework	Part III **Drug Management Cycle**	Part IV Management Support Systems

A Selection
B Procurement
C Distribution ▶
D Use

21 Managing Distribution
22 Importation and Port Clearing
23 Medical Stores Management
24 Drug Management for Health Facilities
25 Planning and Building Storage Facilities
26 Transport Management
27 Kit System Management

Chapter 27
Kit System Management

≡ Summary

Drug kits contain selected drugs and medical supplies in pre-defined quantities. Emergency drug kits are well standardized and widely used by the main international relief agencies. Emergency kits prevent many common problems associated with drug donations. Ration kits provide standard quantities of essential drugs for routine use in rural health care at dispensaries and health centers, and sometimes at district hospitals.

A drug supply system based on ration kits has the following advantages:

  ► *Rational selection of a limited range of essential drugs;*
  ► *Simplified budgeting, procurement, storage, transport, and supply management;*
  ► *Reduced risk of theft;*
  ► *More reliable supply;*
  ► *More rational prescribing;*
  ► *Possible lower indirect costs.*

Ration kit systems have the following disadvantages:

  ► *Less flexible contents than in an open-order system;*
  ► *Difficulty adjusting the drug list to suit regional variations in morbidity;*
  ► *Possibility of stockouts and surpluses;*
  ► *Special management skills and additional space and staff required for kit packing;*
  ► *Lack of development of distribution and inventory control skills;*
  ► *Difficulty in monitoring expiry dates;*
  ► *Lack of fit in a cost-sharing system;*
  ► *Large payments when prepacked kits are procured;*
  ► *Higher direct costs.*

Ration kit systems should be considered when

  ► *drug supply to rural areas needs to be drastically improved;*
  ► *record-keeping and drug ordering capacities are limited;*
  ► *diversion and theft of drugs are common;*
  ► *drug needs are such that the number of different kits can be kept to a minimum.*

A kit-based system is a temporary solution to a logistics problem. A flexible system for distributing drugs should be instituted as soon as the necessary managerial capacity and administrative structures can be created.

≡ 27.1 Drug Supply Kits

Prepacked kits, also known as drug *ration kits*, contain an assortment of drugs and medical supplies. The drugs are packed centrally into sealed cartons and distributed unopened to the health facilities where they are to be used. Each kit is usually designed to supply a given number of patient attendances (for example, 1,000).

The kit system is a typical example of an *allocation*, or "push," system. Supplies are distributed on the basis of a centrally estimated need and not on the basis of a specific request. This is the opposite of a *requisition*, or "pull," system in which health units order supplies on the basis of demand (see Chapter 21).

The kit system has been widely used in emergency relief efforts. Since the early 1980s, several countries have adopted kit systems for the routine supply of essential drugs and supplies to rural health care facilities, usually monthly or quarterly. These two major uses of kits, for emergency situations and for regular supply, are discussed separately.

≡ 27.2 Kits for Emergency Situations

In acute emergencies, drugs and medical supplies are often a first priority. Needs are difficult to assess on short notice; many of the large international relief agencies therefore rely on ready-made kits that contain a selection of the most commonly needed items.

The most popular kit is the *new emergency health kit,* which is now generally recommended for basic health care immediately after a disaster. Many international and non-governmental organizations (NGOs) have agreed to use the same kit, and this has made it possible to maintain a permanent stock for immediate dispatch when an emergency arises. Thousands of kits are used every year in a variety of emergency situations. The kit contents and their intended use are described in a World Health Organization (WHO) information booklet (WHO/DAP 1990).

The kit measures about 4 cubic meters and weighs about 900 kg. It contains essential drugs, disposable supplies, and basic equipment for primary care up to the level of a health center. It can serve a population of 10,000 for three months (or about 10,000 consultation visits). The kit contains ten units for use by paramedical workers. It also contains a supplementary unit, with additional drugs and supplies for minor medical and surgical care at the health center level.

This new emergency health kit is adequate for the first phase of an emergency, when exact needs have not yet been established. Once it is possible to define needs more

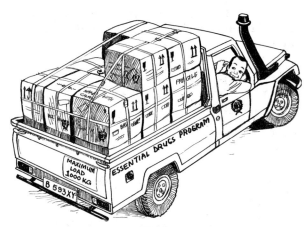

EACH NEW EMERGENCY HEALTH KIT IS
UNDER 1 TON, LESS THAN 4 CUBIC METERS,
AND FITS IN ONE TRUCKLOAD

> **Country Study 27.1 Emergency Drugs after the Armenian Earthquake**
>
> After the 1988 Armenian earthquake, which affected an area with a population of 700,000, international relief organizations sent over 5,000 tons of drugs and consumable medical supplies. However, because of difficulties with identification and sorting, 70 percent of these drugs could not be used immediately, 8 percent had expired on arrival, and 4 percent were destroyed by frost. Over the next six months, about 70 percent of the remaining drugs were sorted out by a group of fifty people. Only 42 percent of the drugs were relevant for an emergency situation. Only 30 percent qualified as easily identifiable and relevant for the medical conditions encountered. In the latter group were standard kits—easy to identify and suitable for emergency situations.
>
> In the disaster area, there was a dramatic lack of pharmacists and health workers, because they were devoted to organizing the warehouses and sorting the drugs. A supply system relying mainly on kits would have been more efficient than the chaotic item-by-item supply provided by the international aid effort. A more extensive kit supply system would have enabled immediate use of the drugs and better provision of medical aid to the population in need.
>
> *Source:* Autier et al. 1990.

precisely, some items in the standard kit may prove to be unnecessary, and other items may be insufficient or lacking. Most organizations then switch to other systems. Some of them—Médecins sans Frontières (MSF) or the Red Cross, for example—use different kits for the second phase.

MSF has about forty medical kits, consisting of different modules. These include an anesthesia module and modules containing dressings, surgical instruments, immunizations, intravenous infusions, and laboratory materials. The appropriate modules are dispatched after MSF field staff have assessed local needs. The Red Cross organizations use small kits to restock health facilities in emergency areas that are particularly busy. In addition to the hardware kit already available in these facilities, they may use a dispensary kit, a dressing kit, a pediatric kit, a sutures kit, an injection kit, and any others that are required.

The use of these kits prevents many of the problems with drug donations that were discussed in Chapter 18 (see Country Study 27.1).

≡ 27.3 Use of Ration Kits as a Distribution Strategy

In the early 1980s, the supply of essential drugs to rural facilities had become so unpredictable that several countries, including Kenya, Democratic Yemen, Tanzania, Uganda, and Bhutan, started to use ration kits for rural health care (see Country Study 27.2). The aim was to make a range of cost-effective essential drugs and supplies directly available to dispensaries and health centers, bypassing the district hospital. At that time, most of these programs were heavily supported by external donors; some of them still receive substantial external support.

The careful selection of drugs and the parallel development of treatment guidelines in the 1980s introduced the essential drugs concept to many national planners and rural health workers. The kit programs of the 1980s assisted in the dissemination of generic drugs and the promotion of the essential drugs concept in several countries.

In 1988–89, WHO carried out an evaluation of the use of kit systems as a distribution strategy. The experiences of ten countries that had used the system over a number of years were reviewed (Haak and Hogerzeil 1991, 1995). Of these ten countries, six claimed to have achieved national coverage (Bhutan, Kenya, Mozambique, Tanzania, Uganda, and Zambia). Figure 27.1 lists the countries where government kit programs were operating at the time of the evaluation. It also shows the types of health facility served and the number of drugs in each type of kit. Most kit programs aim at the dispensary and health center level of care; only a few countries include village health workers or district hospitals.

In eight countries, the kits were paid for mainly by donor funds. In seven countries, kits were packed by overseas suppliers; in three countries, both locally and internationally supplied kits were used. In Democratic Yemen and Zambia, local kits were packed in government facilities; in Kenya, this local packing was done in commercial facilities.

An analysis of the content of sixteen different kits for dispensaries and health centers identified twenty-one

Country Study 27.2 Kit Systems for Regular Drug Supply

The Uganda Essential Drugs Management Programme started in 1985 with two types of kits—one for health centers, which contained twenty-four drugs, and one for dispensaries, which contained twenty-three drugs. Based on information supplied by the kit users and obtained from field visits by program staff, the kit contents have been modified a number of times. At present, one universal kit, containing thirty drugs, is generally used. It is supplied to dispensaries, health centers, the outpatient departments of district hospitals in the public sector, and church-related health care facilities. Recently, a small supplementary maternity kit was introduced for health units providing maternity care.

The kits are paid for by a long-standing donor and are procured overseas. They are distributed free of charge within the public sector and at a reduced rate for church-related care. Treatment guidelines have been developed, and intensive prescribing and drug management training is part of the program.

This kit system has helped restore public confidence in rural health facilities. In the long run, the kit system will be replaced by a requisition system, with supplies being ordered from the newly autonomous central medical stores.

Figure 27.1 Countries and Types of Health Facilities Served by Drug Kits in 1988–89 and Number of Drugs per Kit

Country	Village Health Worker	Dispensary	Health Center	District Hospital	Mission Hospital
Angola		21	30		
Bhutan		49	68		
Democratic Yemen	8		24		
Guinea			29		
Kenya		22	30	40	
Mozambique	8	14	29		
Sudan	16	25	25	83	
Tanzania		34	35		
Uganda		28	28	28	28
Zambia	5		34		
Median number of drugs	8	25	30	40	28

Source: Haak and Hogerzeil 1995.

drugs that are used in at least two-thirds of the kits. These priority drugs are listed in Figure 27.2. These data are derived from stable kit programs and could be useful either as a starting point for new programs or for evaluation purposes.

The number of programs using kits for regular drug supply is declining. The main reasons for this are a reduction in long-term donor commitments, a general shift away from centralized public-sector funding for drugs, the incompatibility between kit systems and cost sharing, and an increasing desire to implement more flexible requisition systems.

≡ 27.4 Advantages and Disadvantages of Kit Systems

The benefits of a kit system depend greatly on the quality of the planning and on the initial kit design. Advantages and disadvantages need to be carefully weighed before a decision is made to adopt the kit approach (see Figure 27.3 and Section 27.6).

Potential advantages of a kit system are:

► Rational selection of a limited range of essential drugs and medical supplies;
► Simplified budgeting, procurement, storage, transport, and supply management, with reduced risk of diversion to hospitals and theft in transit;
► Scheduled supply intervals leading to more secure delivery to rural health units;

► Better and more equitable availability of essential drugs and medical supplies at the primary health care (PHC) level;
► Support for the development of treatment guidelines and prescriber training programs, contributing to more rational prescribing;
► Indirect savings.

Disadvantages are:

► Less flexibility in the selection of essential drugs for specific health problems in different regions, climatic zones, or types of health units;
► Resistance by senior prescribers due to limited range of drugs in the kit;
► Need for special management skills, space, and staff for central kit packing;
► Requirement that all funds be available at once;
► Lack of flexibility in the quantities of drugs, leading to stockouts or surpluses of certain items;
► Difficulty in supplying or returning individual items, which may lead to wastage due to expiry;
► Difficulty in monitoring expiry dates;
► Negative effect on development of supply management systems and skills for inventory control, quantification, ordering, and distribution planning;
► Added cost of kit packing;
► Difficulty in combining kits with a cost-sharing program.

Figure 27.2 Essential Drugs Most Frequently Included in Ration Kits for Health Centers and Dispensaries in Ten Countries

Drug	Quantities	
	Median[a]	Range
Acetylsalicylic acid 300 mg	3,000	1,777–15,000
Paracetamol 500 mg	1,000	200–2,000
Procaine penicillin inj. 3–4 MU	67	20–200
Ferrous salt + folic acid 60/0.25 mg	3,000	1,000–12,000
Gentian violet powder 25 g	8	2–50
Tetracycline eye ointment 5 g	70	20–300
Aluminum hydroxide 500 mg	600	300–2,000
Benzoic/salicylic acid ointment, g	300	100–2,000
Mebendazole, 100-mg tabs	400	100–3,000
Water for inj. 10 mL	700	233–2,000
Oral rehydration salts, powder for 1 L	200	20–600
Chloroquine 150-mg base	2,000	1,000–5,000
Lidocaine[b] 1–2%, inj. mL	90	10–160
Phenoxymethyl penicillin 250 mg	1,000	500–4,000
Epinephrine,[b] inj. 1 mg	5	2.7–10
Ergometrine,[b] inj. 0.2 mg	10	1–50
Metronidazole[b] 200–250 mg	500	125–4,000
Cotrimoxazole[b] 400/80 mg	1,000	250–5,000
Benzyl benzoate 25%, 1 L	1.5	0.3–2
Various disinfectants, mL	900	400–2,000
Diazepam,[b] inj. 10 mg	7	2–20

Source: Haak and Hogerzeil 1995.
[a] Median quantities per 1,000 patient attendances.
[b] Priority drugs for health centers only.

Country Study 27.3 Revolving Drug Fund and Kit Management in Guinea

The primary health care program in Guinea grew rapidly and included a cost-sharing system from the start. Initially, the information system for monitoring drug use did not function, and rural staff were not trained in drug management. A decision was made to introduce a kit system while keeping the cost-sharing system in place.

Although the kit contents were regularly modified, there were major disadvantages in combining the two systems:

► Cost sharing reinforced the need for good-quality care and availability of drugs.
► New kits were opened as soon as one item in the previous kit had run out. This resulted in an accumulation of half-used kits. The facilities then had no cash to purchase more drugs. Drugs could be procured only as part of a kit. Any "unsold" drugs remained in stock.
► Some drugs became heavily overstocked. However, a low-cost, efficient redistribution system, based on credits for future drug procurement, avoided large-scale waste of expired drugs.
► Management committees and health workers resented paying for kit drugs they did not need.

Although the content of the kits was reviewed several times, and standardized treatment was considered a priority, discrepancies between need and supply remained. After a few years, the kit system was abandoned and replaced with a requisition system using a limited drug list.

The inflexibility of the kit system is its most important problem. When kits are packed overseas (and they often are), it may take a year before a change in content reaches the rural facilities. In the meantime, there may be stockouts of certain items and surpluses of others. This problem is frequently perceived as serious, yet the WHO evaluation (Haak and Hogerzeil 1991) showed that in most long-term governmental kit programs (as opposed to emergency or incidental external kit projects), a stable kit content was reached in about two years. In the short term, the problem was sometimes solved by redistributing the accumulated drugs; in the long run, it was addressed by adapting the kit content. The latter is easier if the kits are packed within the country. In some countries, the problem was solved by changing to kits with a smaller number of commonly used drugs, with additional items being supplied through a requisition system.

The most serious problems of mismatch between need and supply have occurred in kit projects that were badly planned or operated in isolation from other supply structures. Some problems were directly related to poor performance by overseas suppliers.

Redistributing the accumulated surpluses is not always easy. When the same item has accumulated in most health units, redistribution does not make sense. However, most products that accumulated in the past were simple, commonly used, and very stable drugs. If they were supplied free, any surpluses could simply be taken back to the central store. In practice, surplus drugs are often returned to the nearest level operating with a requisition system, usually the district hospital. A special problem arises when the kit has been paid for, in which case returning surplus drugs may meet resistance, and some sort of credit system will have to be established. This is probably why kit systems and cost sharing do not go very well together. The combination was tried in Guinea, but the kit system was finally abandoned (see Country Study 27.3).

≡ **27.5 Cost Aspects of Kit Systems**

The direct costs of a kit system are higher than those of a regular requisition system, for the following reasons. Most international suppliers add 3 to 5 percent to the price for packing the drugs in ration kits. If kits are packed locally, labor costs may be a little less, but certain investments are needed (for example, carton boxes and a strapping device). If kits are procured ready-made, the number of potential suppliers is restricted, and there is less possibility to benefit from competitive prices for individual drugs. There is potentially some waste (estimated at an average of

Figure 27.3 Weighing Advantages and Disadvantages of Kit Systems

ADVANTAGES		DISADVANTAGES

Rational selection of a limited range of essential drugs and medical supplies

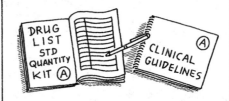

Less flexibility in the selection of essential drugs for specific health problems in different regions, climatic zones, or types of health units; resistance by senior pre-scribers due to limited range of drugs in the kit

Simplified budgeting, procurement, storage, transport, and supply management, with reduced risk of diversion to hospitals and theft in transit

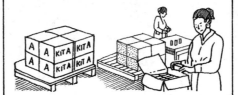

Need for special management skills; space and staff are needed for central kit packing; requirement that all funds be available at once

Scheduled supply intervals leading to more secure delivery to rural health units

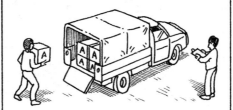

Lack of flexibility in the quantities of drugs, leading to stockouts or surpluses of certain items

Better and more equitable availability of essential drugs and medical supplies at the PHC level

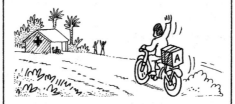

Difficulty in supplying or returning individual items, which may lead to wastage due to expiry; difficulty in monitoring expiry dates

Support for the development of treatment guidelines and prescriber training programs, contributing to more rational prescribing

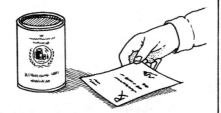

Possible slow development of supply management systems and skills for inventory control, quantification, ordering, and distribution planning

Possible indirect savings

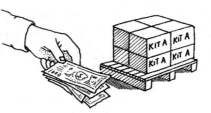

Added cost of kit packing; difficulty in combining kits with a cost-sharing program

4 percent) due to expiry of accumulating unused drugs (although it is not sure whether this is more than with most requisition systems).

Several factors may result in reduced indirect costs. Waste is reduced due to less pilferage during transport and less interception of drugs at the district level. A careful selection of kit contents implies that less money is wasted on items that are not cost effective, not needed, or inappropriate. Because of the regular supply, less safety stock is needed at the facilities. The regular availability of essential drugs reduces the number of patients who refer themselves to higher levels of care, where average treatment costs are higher. It is true that these advantages would also be achieved by a good requisition system, but the kit system has often been instrumental in realizing these improvements, although it is probably not needed forever to maintain them.

A pure cost comparison between a kit system and a requisition system also leaves out the many qualitative aspects that are not related to costs and are much more difficult to measure. The ease of supply management and the better availability of essential drugs at the primary care level may justify some extra costs. The limited time of health care providers can be used more efficiently. The quality of care may also improve, and lives may be saved. Some overstock (and potential expiry and waste) of cheap but lifesaving drugs such as oral rehydration salts and ergometrine injection can be justified (whereas overstock of an expensive but not lifesaving drug such as praziquantel cannot).

≡ 27.6 Conditions for a Successful Kit Program

A kit system is generally most useful when

- ► the objective is to improve the drug supply to rural areas;
- ► record-keeping and drug ordering capabilities are limited;
- ► requisitioned drugs remain at the hospital level and do not pass down the system;
- ► theft in the distribution system is common;
- ► drug needs are similar throughout the area, and only a few different kits are needed.

Before a kit system can operate properly, several conditions have to be met. First, drugs have to be selected (see Chapter 10), and quantities have to be estimated (see Chapter 14). Second, funding has to be secured, and this requires a real political and financial commitment to satisfying the health needs of the rural population. A third condition is a well-trained and dedicated management team. Finally, a program for training prescribers is essential. If the prescribers do not follow the treatment guidelines on which the kit contents are based, there will be a mismatch between drug supply and use, and patients' health may be at risk.

When should a kit system *not* be chosen? A kit system does not combine well with a cost-sharing program. A kit system is not needed when health facilities are close to the warehouse and when communications and transport facilities are good. Nor is it needed when there are no drug shortages in the public sector and there is already a well-managed and reliable requisition system. In situations in which there are management deficiencies but the capacity exists to overcome them, it may be better to develop a sustainable requisition system. A kit system may become very complicated if there are many different types of facilities or if there are considerable regional or seasonal variations in the incidence of health problems.

≡ 27.7 Implementing a Kit Program

Careful planning is required before a kit program is introduced (see Figure 27.4). Once a program begins, it is difficult to revise and may take a year or more to change. There are twelve steps to be taken.

Step 1. Assess the Supply System: Is a Kit System Appropriate?

The balance between advantages and disadvantages has been discussed. The situation should be carefully assessed (see Chapters 4 and 21) before choosing between a kit and a requisition system.

Step 2. Choose the Types of Health Unit to Be Supplied with Kits

A kit distribution system is usually most suitable for smaller, poorly managed, and poorly staffed facilities. In some cases, a mixed distribution system may be an appropriate choice. In a district hospital, for example, kits may be used in the outpatient department, and a requisition system may be used to supply additional drugs for inpatients. There is a growing tendency to reduce the number of different kits and to supplement a limited kit system with a simple requisition system.

Step 3. Prepare a List of Drugs and Other Items for Each Kit

Separate kits may be prepared for different types of health facilities, for example, one kit for dispensaries and one for health centers (see Chapter 10). Bulky products, liquid products, drugs needing cold chain, and drugs with short

Figure 27.4 Flowchart for Kit Program Planning

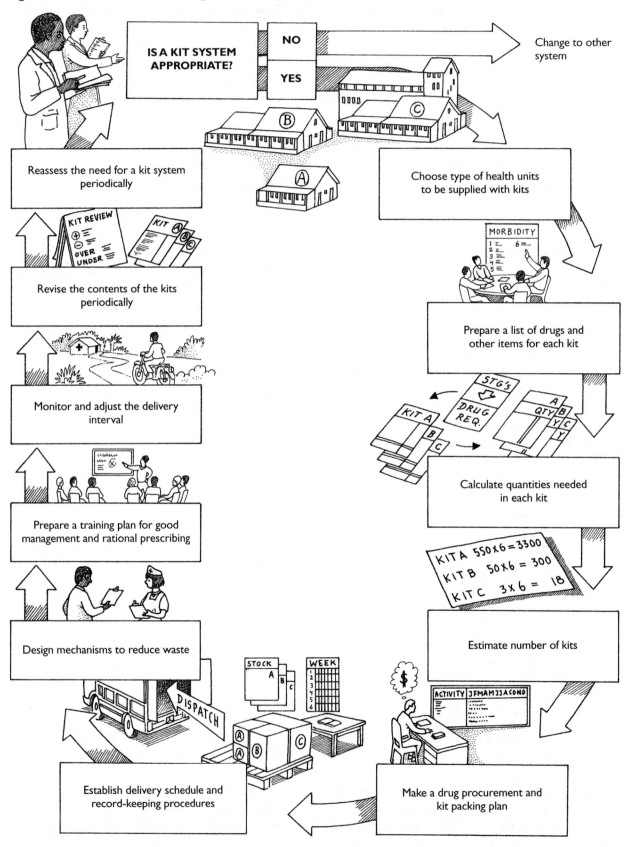

IS A KIT SYSTEM APPROPRIATE?

NO → Change to other system

YES

Choose type of health units to be supplied with kits

Reassess the need for a kit system periodically

Revise the contents of the kits periodically

Prepare a list of drugs and other items for each kit

Monitor and adjust the delivery interval

Calculate quantities needed in each kit

Prepare a training plan for good management and rational prescribing

KIT A 550 x 6 = 3300
KIT B 50 x 6 = 300
KIT C 3 x 6 = 18

Design mechanisms to reduce waste

Estimate number of kits

Establish delivery schedule and record-keeping procedures

Make a drug procurement and kit packing plan

shelf lives should be avoided whenever possible. If the kit system is being introduced following a long period of shortages, an additional starter kit may be designed that contains essential equipment to upgrade the facilities at the beginning of the program.

Step 4. Determine the Quantities of Drugs Needed in Each Kit

Usually, kits are designed for a certain number of outpatient consultations (1,000 to 5,000). Once this figure has been decided, the quantity of each item in the kit can be defined. Kit contents are normally intended to treat only the most commonly seen health problems, and it is assumed that all health facilities will see the same mix of problems per 1,000 attenders.

When a new kit program is to be started, the morbidity method is considered the best way to estimate requirements. This method helps determine both the type of drugs and their quantities, based on the expected number of attendances at a health facility (see Chapter 14). This first estimate can then be compared with the quantities used in other kit systems (see Figure 27.2).

In the first years of operation of the kit system, the consumption method can be used to adapt quantities to match actual consumption. Experienced kit suppliers can supply various kinds of kits and change kit contents with each order.

Step 5. Estimate the Number of Kits Needed

The quantity of each type of kit is determined by the number of health units served and the estimated number of attendances at each health unit. If a kit distribution system starts after a period when drug supplies have been reduced or absent, increased patient attendance should be anticipated and allowed for. Taking into account long delivery times, most orders cover a period of nine to eighteen months.

Step 6. Make a Drug Procurement and Kit Packing Plan

There are at least four ways to manage procurement and kit packing:

▶ Purchase prepacked kits from overseas;
▶ Purchase prepacked kits on open tender, from local and/or overseas suppliers;
▶ Contract a local company to pack all kits, using drugs purchased separately through local or international tender;
▶ Set up kit packing at national or regional medical stores.

The choice depends on cost, availability of staff, and availability of space at the medical stores. Prepacked kits are available through the United Nations Children's Fund (UNICEF), through international low-cost suppliers such as the International Dispensary Association (IDA), or from private companies. In some countries, such as Kenya, local suppliers compete in tenders for prepacked kits. Some programs begin by purchasing prepacked kits and concentrate on distribution and monitoring of consumption patterns. Once the system is operating well at the periphery, the feasibility of establishing packing operations at central or regional medical stores can be considered.

Kits are usually procured by tender (see Chapter 16). Tender specifications for each drug in the kit should be just as detailed as for individual drug tenders. In addition, the specifications should describe how the kit is to be packed and specify the quality of the outer carton, the method of strapping, kit labeling, and any other relevant features.

There can be significant problems in setting up a local packing operation. A kit cannot be packed until all items needed for the kit are available. If the supply of any item is delayed, the entire packing operation is held up, which may lead to stockouts at facilities. Because of this possibility, the period before drug expiry must be as long as possible.

Most programs pack or purchase kits in sturdy cardboard boxes sealed with tamper-proof tape or some other form of seal that will clearly reveal any attempt to open the box in transit. Lockable, reusable plastic containers are also available for locally packed kits. However, because kit distribution systems are used mainly where distribution conditions are difficult, it is unlikely that the containers will be returned to the central medical store.

One person should be assigned to check the contents of every kit to reduce the risk of theft during the packing process. A list of the contents should be made, signed, and dated, and a copy should be sealed into the kit. This list should also show the expiry date of whatever product is due to expire first, and that date should be marked on the outside of the carton as well.

Step 7. Establish Delivery Schedules and Record-Keeping Procedures

The delivery schedule depends on the average number of patient attendances at the facility. For example, when kits for 1,000 attendances are used, a facility with 200 to 300 attendances per month needs only one kit every three months.

A kit system simplifies record keeping but does not eliminate the need for it. At each level of the distribution chain, stock records should show the type, number,

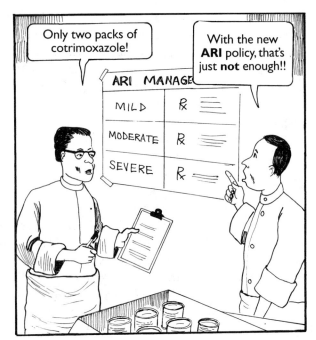

**KIT CONTENTS MUST KEEP UP
WITH STANDARD TREATMENTS**

source, condition, and value of each kit received and issued. A periodic stock count must be done. In short, a kit should be treated in the same way as any other item as far as stock keeping is concerned. At a rural facility, a tally card or ledger should keep a record of the number of kits received, opened, and in stock. As soon as a kit is opened, the contents should be entered into the item-by-item stock records at the facility.

Step 8. Design Mechanisms to Minimize Waste and Stockouts

Regular analyses of actual drug consumption should be made, particularly in the early stages of a kit program. A simple checklist should be prepared for supervisors. The following key information needs to be collected from rural facilities:

- Number of patient attendances per month;
- Recent kit delivery dates;
- The three drugs that are most often out of stock;
- The three drugs that accumulate most often;
- Proposals for changes in kit contents.

Information on actual deliveries and receipts should be collected and given to planners to assist in monitoring the program and in modifying distribution plans as required. Details of stockouts and surpluses, as well as any proposals for change, are particularly useful for adjusting the kit content.

Other mechanisms to prevent waste and stockouts are to

- allow individual requisitions for a few products whose consumption is variable (for example, antimalarials or drugs against schistosomiasis);
- create a simple system for returning unused stock;
- not use containers with more than 1,000 tablets;
- specify maximum possible periods before expiry for drugs received from suppliers;
- instruct kit packers to mark the earliest expiry date on the outside of the kit carton;
- keep supply intervals as short as possible.

Step 9. Prepare a Training Plan for Good Management and Rational Prescribing and Dispensing

Staff should be trained to use the standard treatment schedules on which the kit contents are based. As drug supply improves, training and retraining in rational prescribing and dispensing are essential to prevent misuse of the drugs.

Step 10. Monitor and Adjust Delivery Intervals

Any push system needs feedback, monitoring, and supervision if it is to operate effectively. Difficulties arise when a centrally planned delivery schedule is not regularly adjusted to conditions in the field, or when it is incorrectly assumed that planned distribution schedules are being followed. Receipt of the kits should always be confirmed. Stock levels at rural facilities should be reported regularly to spot any persistent stockouts or surpluses.

Step 11. Revise Kit Contents Periodically

The items and quantities in each kit should be reviewed regularly. In stable, long-term kit programs, it takes about two years to get a reasonable balance between supply and demand for the individual items in a kit. Even then, changing disease patterns and changing prescription patterns make it necessary to revise the kit contents periodically. The system can also be refined by adding other kits or by changing to a mixed system.

Step 12. Reassess the Need for a Kit System Periodically

At a certain stage, the program can change to other distribution methods, as described below.

≡ 27.8 Transition to Other Distribution Systems

After a kit system has been functioning regularly for some time, it is likely that drug supply conditions will improve.

Country Study 27.4 Transition from a Kit System to a Modified Optional Replenishment System in Cambodia

An international organization committed itself to organizing the central medical store in Cambodia in 1992. For the past five years, NGOs had been supporting a large number of facilities throughout the country and had delivered continuous training in drug management and rational prescribing. It was decided to introduce a three-phase drug distribution system:

1. *Basic kit:* This kit contained fourteen different drugs in quantities considered minimal for functioning.

2. *Complete kit:* This kit contained forty-three different drugs in much larger quantities than the basic kit. The quantities were not, however, adapted to each particular facility, so surplus accumulations and shortages often occurred.

3. *Modified optional replenishment system:* The initial maximum consumption per three months was set to be equal to the standard consumption multiplied by the expected number of attendances at each facility. These maximum levels were to be revised once a year.

The kit systems allowed the health facilities to operate, although the delivered quantities did not completely match the prescribers' needs. When the modified optional replenishment scheme began to function properly, it did a better job of meeting prescribers' needs. There was a reasonable level of procurement security at the central medical store.

Basic kits were supplied to health facilities, which had unqualified staff and no information on attendances and drug consumption. Complete kits were supplied only after a qualified person had been appointed and the facility's information system had improved. Finally, the modified optional replenishment system was introduced when certain minimum standards of infrastructure, management, and staffing had been achieved. The supply system was downgraded if a health facility showed signs of irrational drug prescribing or serious mismanagement of drugs.

This supply system was accompanied with a training program:

► The ministry of health published a standardized book on drug utilization.
► All responsible staff in the facilities' pharmacies were trained to use a standardized drug management system.
► Provincial medical and pharmacy supervisors were given the means and support to upgrade medical and managerial skills through continuous training and supervision.

Country Study 27.5 Drug Supply in the Solomon Islands: Changing from Kits to Order Systems

The Solomon Islands are located in the western Pacific region. There are very few roads, and travel is by canoe and small interisland cargo vessels. Over 95 percent of the population depends on the public sector for health services.

During the 1960s, drug kits were supplied to rural health centers every three months. The kit contents were standardized and matched to the catchment area of the facility. In the 1970s, a supplementary box with maternity supplies was added for those health centers providing maternity services.

Between 1978 and 1983, the expansion of services and increase in demand led to drug shortages. Provincial hospitals were supplied twice monthly with bulk supplies, and these hospitals began to supply health facilities with fast-moving items. An attempt was made to collect stock and consumption data, and these data were used to guide supply allocations.

Between 1983 and 1986, the clinic supply system was reviewed. A change was made from separate standard and maternity kits to a standard kit containing both drugs and maternity items and a supplementary kit that contained high-demand items. This arrangement allowed more flexibility to cope with the varying demands at different health facilities.

In 1986, the supply system was reviewed again. This review showed that large facilities were undersupplied, and small facilities were overstocked. Stock reporting was not used effectively to control supply. An experiment was undertaken in one of the more remote islands. Orders were delivered more frequently, and staff were allowed more freedom to order supplementary goods, even if they had received their regular supply. Staff responded enthusiastically, and with extra training, stock ordering improved. This led to fewer stockouts and less oversupply. Over time, other provinces in the country adopted the ordering system rather than continuing with a kit system.

The Solomon Islands case demonstrates that it is possible over time to convert from a push (kit) system to a pull (requisition) system, even in a country with extreme logistical challenges.

Source: ECHO (R. Skinner) 1994, unpublished.

More information on patient morbidity and drug consumption will be available to planners and to rural health staff. Policy-makers will get used to a limited range of essential drugs. Training of staff should have improved their management capacities. At this point, it may be possible to move to a more flexible distribution system.

Country Studies 27.4 and 27.5 illustrate how two supply programs moved through different stages.

Preparation for transition is mainly a matter of training. There should also be a reliable and complete information system. At a minimum, this should monitor the number of patients treated, drug consumption, and morbidity patterns. These data may also help determine whether sufficient management capacity exists to change to a requisition system based on real demand—a pull system—or to a more sophisticated push system. Three possible stages to an open-order system are outlined below.

Fixed Drug Allowance System

The first step may be to change from kits to a fixed drug allowance system. This system also defines the selection and quantity of drugs in advance. However, the goods are not physically packed in a kit and are not necessarily dispatched at the same time. Provided that feedback is available from the health facilities, this promotes a rapid and flexible response to changing needs.

Ordering within Defined Limits

The second step in the transition gives health workers some responsibility for ordering. Average drug consumption is calculated for each facility, and these data are used to define maximum and minimum stock levels for each item. Health workers are then taught to order their drugs within these limits.

Open Requisitioning from a Predefined List

The final stage in the transition makes health workers or pharmacy staff responsible for ordering the items and quantities they need from a predefined list, as described in Chapter 24. ∎

≡ **References and Further Readings**

★ = *Key readings.*

Autier, P., M. C. Ferir, A. Hairapetien, A. Alexanian, V. Agoudjian, G. Schmets, G. Dallemagne, M. N. Leva, and J. Pinel. 1990. Drug supply in the aftermath of the 1988 Armenian earthquake. *Lancet* 335:1388–90.

★ Haak, H., and H. Hogerzeil. 1991. *Drug supply by ration kits.* WHO/DAP/91.2. Geneva: World Health Organization.

★ Haak, H., and H. Hogerzeil. 1995. Essential drugs for ration kits in developing countries. *Health Policy and Planning* 10:40–49.

Moore, G. D. 1982. Essential drugs for Kenya's rural population. *World Health Forum* 3:196–99.

MSH (Management Sciences for Health). 1992. Kit distribution system (trainer's and participant's guides). In *Managing drug supply training series.* Part 3. *Supply management.* Boston: MSH.

WHO/DAP (World Health Organization/Action Programme on Essential Drugs). 1990. *The new emergency health kit.* WHO/DAP/90.1. Geneva: WHO/DAP.

≡ **Assessment Guide**

Use of Ration Kits

► Which levels of health care and what percentage of facilities receive ration kits on a regular basis?

► How does actual distribution compare with the annual distribution plan?

Description of Kits

► What are the kit contents, quantities, and intended number of patient contacts per kit?

► Are regional or seasonal kits in use? If so, what do they contain?

► What is the cost of each kit?

► What is the incremental cost for kit packaging versus open item procurement?

Financing, Procurement, and Distribution Management

► Who pays for the kits (government or external donor)?

► Are kits prepared and packed locally or internationally?

► Is kit distribution integrated with the regular drug supply system?

► On what basis are kits distributed (time interval, number of patient attendances)?

► Is there a procedure to order additional drugs or additional quantities?

► Which drugs are commonly out of stock before the next delivery of kits?

► What items are accumulating?

► What procedures are in place to deal with shortages? Are these procedures working?

► What procedures are in place to redistribute overstock? Are these procedures working?

Monitoring and Evaluation

► Is there an established procedure to update the contents of the kit? When was this update last done?

► Is supervision of the kit program integrated with general supervisory activities?

► What is the impact of the kit system on availability of drugs and supplies?

► What is the impact of the kit system on prescription patterns?

► Are mechanisms in place to check actual distribution of kits to rural facilities against the planned distribution schedule?

| Part I | Part II | **Part III** | Part IV |
| Introduction | Policy and Legal Framework | **Drug Management Cycle** | Management Support Systems |

A Selection
B Procurement
C Distribution
D Use

Section D
Use

Part I Introduction	Part II Policy and Legal Framework	**Part III** **Drug Management Cycle**	Part IV Management Support Systems

A Selection
B Procurement
C Distribution

D Use ▶ **28 Managing for Rational Drug Use**
29 Investigating Drug Use
30 Drug and Therapeutics Information
31 Promoting Rational Prescribing
32 Ensuring Good Dispensing Practices
33 Encouraging Appropriate Drug Use by
    the Public and Patients

Chapter 28

Managing for Rational Drug Use

≡ Summary

This chapter defines rational drug use and gives examples of irrational drug use and the adverse effects that can result. It considers factors underlying irrational drug use and possible strategies to address the problem.

Rational use of drugs requires that patients receive medications appropriate to their clinical needs, in doses that meet their individual requirements, for an adequate period of time, and at the lowest cost to them and their community.

Irrational drug use occurs with polypharmacy, with the use of wrong or ineffective drugs, or with underuse or incorrect use of effective drugs. These actions have an adverse impact on the quality of drug therapy and cost and may cause adverse reactions or negative psychosocial impacts.

A prescriber's lack of knowledge and experience is only one factor in irrational drug use. Other underlying factors can be found in the dispensing process, the patient or community, and the health system itself.

Strategies to address irrational drug use can be characterized as educational, managerial, or regulatory. Whichever method to change drug use is selected, the intervention is likely to contain the elements of focusing on key factors, targeting facilities with the worst practices, and using credible sources and communication channels. Personal contact (face-to-face meetings, for example) can sometimes be used to convey a limited number of key messages; these can be repeated and clarified using different media.

When implementing a strategy, the logical steps are to

- ► *identify the problem;*
- ► *understand the underlying causes;*
- ► *list possible interventions;*
- ► *assess available resources;*
- ► *choose an intervention;*
- ► *monitor and restructure the activity, as necessary.*

Interventions should be based on an understanding of the cause of the problem and on active strategies to change behavior. Experience indicates that the most effective interventions are those that

- ► *identify key influence factors;*
- ► *target individuals or groups with the worst practices;*
- ► *use credible information sources;*
- ► *use credible communication channels;*
- ► *use personal contact whenever possible;*
- ► *limit the number of messages;*
- ► *repeat key messages using different methods;*
- ► *provide better drug use alternatives.*

≡ 28.1 Definition of Rational Drug Use

The aim of any drug management system is to deliver the correct drug to the patient who needs that medicine. The steps of selection, procurement, and distribution are necessary precursors to the rational use of drugs.

The Conference of Experts on the Rational Use of Drugs, convened by the World Health Organization (WHO) in Nairobi in 1985, defined rational use as follows: *the rational use of drugs requires that patients receive medications appropriate to their clinical needs, in doses that meet their own individual requirements, for an adequate period of time, and at the lowest cost to them and their community.* Depending on the context, however, many factors influence what is considered rational. It may be rational, for example, for a drug seller to sell antibiotics without a prescription to earn enough income to survive.

This book uses the term *rational drug use* in a biomedical context that includes the following criteria:

- ► Correct drug;
- ► Appropriate indication—that is, the reason to prescribe is based on sound medical considerations;
- ► Appropriate drug, considering efficacy, safety, suitability for the patient, and cost;
- ► Appropriate dosage, administration, and duration of treatment;
- ► Appropriate patient—that is, no contraindications exist, and the likelihood of adverse reactions is minimal;
- ► Correct dispensing, including appropriate information for patients about the prescribed medicines;
- ► Patient adherence to treatment.

To conform with these criteria, prescribers should follow a standard process of prescribing, which starts with a diagnosis to define the problem that requires intervention. Next, the therapeutic goal should be defined. The prescriber must decide which treatment is required, based on up-to-date drug and therapeutic information, to achieve the desired goal for an individual patient. When the decision to treat the patient with drugs is made, the best drug for the patient is selected based on efficacy, safety, suitability, and cost. Then dose, route of administration, and duration of treatment are determined, taking into account the condition of the patient. When prescribing a drug, the prescriber should provide proper information to the patient about both the drug and the patient's condition. Finally, the prescriber should decide how to monitor the treatment, after considering the probable therapeutic or adverse effects of treatment.

The drug should then be dispensed to the patient in a safe and hygienic manner, making sure that the patient understands the dosage and course of therapy; then the patient takes the drug. Adherence occurs if the patient (and the community) understands and appreciates the value of taking specific drugs for specific indications (see Figure 28.1 on the drug use process).

≡ 28.2 Examples of Irrational Drug Use
Irrational drug use occurs in all countries. These include cases in which no drug is needed; the wrong drugs, or ineffective or unsafe drugs, are prescribed; effective and available drugs are underused; and drugs are used incorrectly.

No Drug Needed
Use of drugs when none is needed includes many nontherapeutic uses of pharmaceuticals. For example, in many countries, the majority of children suffering from minor upper respiratory infections are treated with antibiotics. Similarly, unnecessary and ineffective antimicrobials or antidiarrheals, instead of oral rehydration solution (ORS),

Figure 28.1 The Drug Use Process

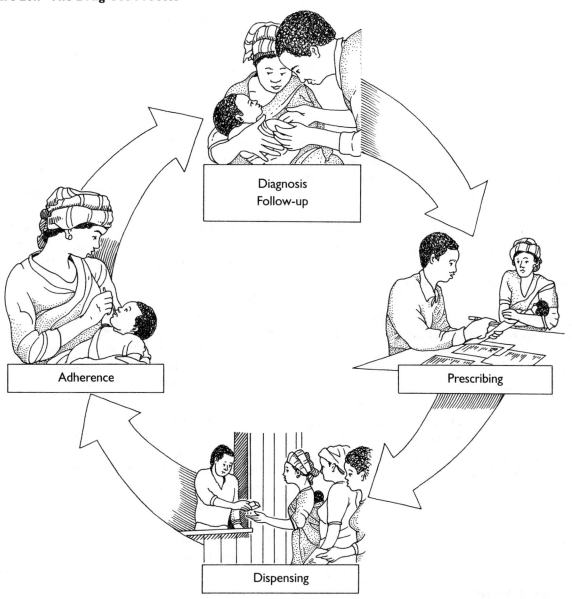

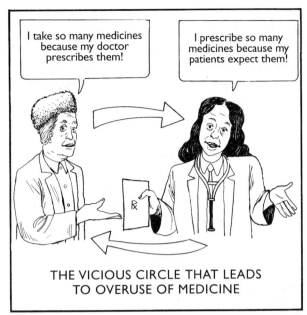

THE VICIOUS CIRCLE THAT LEADS
TO OVERUSE OF MEDICINE

Source: Teaching Aids at Low Cost.

are indiscriminately prescribed for many children with
acute diarrhea.

Wrong Drugs

In some countries, for example, many children with streptococcal pharyngitis are not properly treated with narrow-
spectrum penicillin. Instead, tetracycline, a drug that is not
recommended for the prophylaxis of rheumatic fever following streptococcal pharyngitis and that has serious side
effects for children, is usually prescribed.

Ineffective Drugs and Drugs with Doubtful Efficacy

Excessive and unnecessary use of multivitamin preparations or tonics is an example of this prescribing pattern.

Unsafe Drugs

The likelihood of adverse reactions outweighs the therapeutic effects when unsafe drugs are prescribed. Common
examples include the use of anabolic steroids for growth
and appetite stimulation in children or athletes. In many
countries, dipyrone (metamizol), a drug banned in most
developed countries, is used indiscriminately in both
health facilities and the community for a large variety of
minor ailments.

Underuse of Available Effective Drugs

In West Java, Indonesia, a study showed a few years ago
that ORS was prescribed for only a small proportion of
children with acute diarrhea. Regrettably, the underuse of

effective oral rehydration therapy for acute diarrhea in
children still occurs in many countries.

Incorrect Use of Drugs

Injectable preparations are commonly overused. Another
frequent incorrect use of drugs is giving a patient only one
or two days' supply of antibiotics rather than the full
course of therapy.

≡ 28.3 Adverse Impact of Irrational Drug Use

The inappropriate use of drugs on a wide scale can have
significant adverse effects on health care costs as well as on
the quality of drug therapy and medical care. Other negative effects are the increased likelihood of adverse reactions and patients' inappropriate reliance on drugs.

Impact on Quality of Drug Therapy and Medical Care

Inappropriate prescribing practices can, directly or indirectly, jeopardize the quality of patient care and negatively influence the outcome of treatment. The underuse
of ORS for acute diarrhea, for instance, can hinder the
goal of treatment: namely, to prevent or treat dehydration
and thus prevent death in children.

The likelihood of adverse drug reactions increases when
drugs are prescribed unnecessarily. Misuse of injectable
products in Indonesia, for example, has been implicated in
a high incidence of anaphylactic shock (see Country Study
28.1). Overdosage or underdosage of antibiotics and chemo-
therapeutic agents also leads to the rapid emergence of
resistant strains of bacteria or the malaria parasite.

Impact on Cost

Overuse of drugs, even essential ones, causes excessive
spending on pharmaceuticals and waste of financial
resources, by both patients and the health care system. In
many countries, expenditures on nonessential pharmaceutical products, such as multivitamins or cough mixtures, drain limited financial resources that could otherwise
be allocated for more essential and vital products, such as
vaccines or antibiotics. Inappropriate underuse of drugs at
an early stage of a disease may also produce excess costs
by increasing the probability of prolonged disease and
eventual hospitalization.

Psychosocial Impact

Overprescribing communicates to patients that they need
medications for any and all conditions, even trivial ones.
The concept that *there is a pill for every ill* is harmful.
Patients come to rely on drugs, and this reliance increases

the demand for them. Patients may demand unnecessary injections because during their years of exposure to modern health services they have become accustomed to having practitioners administer injections.

≡ 28.4 Factors Underlying Irrational Use of Drugs

Many interrelated factors influence drug use (see Figure 28.2). The health system, prescriber, dispenser, patient, and community are all involved in the therapeutic process, and all can contribute to irrational use in a variety of ways.

Health System

Factors affecting the health system include unreliable supply, drug shortages, expired drugs, and availability of inappropriate drugs. Such inefficiencies in the system lead to a lack of confidence in the system by the prescriber and the patient. The patient demands treatment, and the prescriber feels obliged to give what is available, even if the drug is not the correct one to treat the condition.

Prescriber

The prescriber can be affected by internal and external factors. He or she may have received inadequate training, or prescribing practices may have become outdated due to a lack of continuing education. The role models who are imitated may not prescribe rationally. There may be a lack of objective drug information, and the information provided by drug representatives may be unreliable. The temptation to generalize inappropriately about the effectiveness or side effects of drugs on the basis of limited personal experience is strong. Externally, a heavy patient load and pressure to prescribe from peers, patients, and drug company representatives all complicate prescribing decisions. Finally, profit may affect a prescriber's choice if the prescriber's income is dependent on drug sales.

Dispenser

The dispenser plays a crucial role in the therapeutic process. The quality of dispensing may be affected by the training and supervision the dispenser has received and the drug information available to the dispenser. A shortage of dispensing materials and short dispensing time due to heavy patient load may also have an adverse impact on dispensing. Finally, the low status of dispensers affects the quality of dispensing.

Patient and Community

The individual's adherence to treatment is influenced by many factors, including cultural beliefs, the communication

Country Study 28.1 Essential Drugs Program and Rational Use of Drugs in Indonesia

Indonesia is the fourth largest nation in the world in terms of population, with approximately 206 million inhabitants. The national essential drugs program was first adopted in 1979, immediately after the introduction of the essential drugs concept by WHO. A comprehensive national drug policy was first promulgated in 1983, with the aim of

- ensuring the availability of drugs based on the needs of the population;
- ensuring efficient and equitable distribution of drugs;
- ensuring rational and appropriate use of safe, efficacious, and high-quality drugs;
- promoting local production.

During the early years of the essential drugs program, efforts were understandably focused on ensuring the availability of essential drugs in health facilities rather than on the inappropriate use of drugs. Measures to promote rational prescribing hardly existed in the national essential drugs program in the 1980s. When a national drug utilization study was carried out in 1988, it turned out that inappropriate prescribing practices were common in health facilities throughout the country. A high proportion of drugs ended up being wasted through ineffective and sometimes harmful treatment. For instance, there was overuse of antimicrobials and injectable preparations throughout the country. Subsequent studies confirmed the existence of consistent patterns of inappropriate use of pharmaceuticals at various levels of health care.

These problems came to the attention of policy-makers, and in the late 1980s and early 1990s, training programs on the rational use of drugs were developed and implemented. A large amount of money from national and local government budgets has been spent on training activities. Questions remain, however, whether these training activities have had any significant impact on prescribing practices. Evaluations are needed for such a large-scale training intervention. Other approaches to improving prescribing have also been initiated in some districts, with some success. The next issue is how to incorporate the most effective approaches into the overall system and sustain them. Can they be replicated with similar success in other localities?

Experience shows that an essential drugs program will have an impact on prescribing if elements of rational drug use have been appropriately addressed. It probably would have been less complicated if these components had been considered at the beginning of the essential drugs program in Indonesia.

skills and attitudes of the prescriber and dispenser, the limited time available for consulting, the shortage of printed information, and community beliefs about the efficacy of certain drugs or routes of administration. For example, there may be a belief that injections are more powerful than capsules, or that capsules are more effective than tablets.

It is clear that although the knowledge and experience of the prescriber are important aspects of the interaction

Figure 28.2 Factors Influencing Prescribing

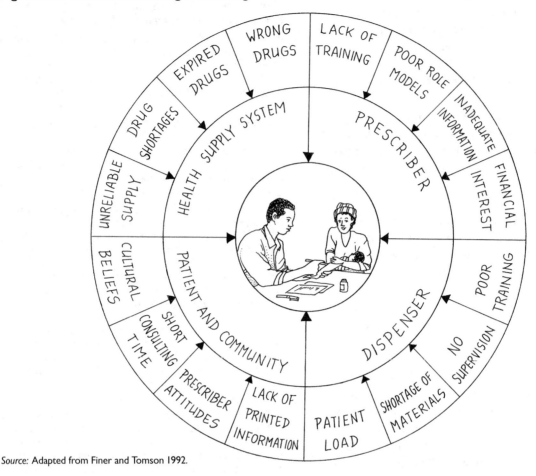

Source: Adapted from Finer and Tomson 1992.

between prescriber and patient, they are not the *only* factors. As discussed above, there are many causes for irrational drug use and many factors involved in the decision-making process.

These factors vary for each person and situation. This means that specific interventions to improve prescribing may work under some circumstances but not others. Due to the complexity of factors involved, it is unlikely that any single intervention will work in every situation.

≡ **28.5 Strategies to Improve Drug Use**

Before attempting to change drug use, the scale of the problem should be assessed and quantified. The underlying reasons for the problem behavior then need to be investigated. Quantitative and qualitative methods for assessing drug use are described in Chapter 29. *It is a mistake to intervene before understanding the reasons for a problem behavior.*

Whatever problem is being addressed, impartial drug and therapeutics information is needed. Such information

can serve as the basis for standard treatment guidelines or therapeutic standards. Information can be made available actively through drug bulletins or in a largely passive manner through drug information centers. Drug information is covered in Chapter 30.

Several choices exist for an intervention to change prescribing practices. These approaches can be characterized as educational, managerial, or regulatory. Whichever approach is used, the intervention should focus on specific problem behaviors and should target prescribers or facilities with a high incidence of the problem being addressed. Possible interventions are described in Chapter 31.

Once prescribing has been addressed, the next stage of drug use is dispensing. This crucial aspect of the provider-patient relationship is often neglected or delegated to an untrained person. Chapter 32 describes ways to ensure good dispensing.

The final stage of drug use occurs when the patient takes the medicines. The patient is more likely to take medicines as advised if he or she understands how to take the medicines and if there is general community awareness of rational drug use. Developing informational materials for patients and planning public education campaigns requires an understanding of cultural norms, values, and practices. Chapter 33 describes this process.

No matter which point in the drug use process becomes the focus of an intervention strategy, there are common characteristics of effective interventions:

Identify key influence factors: Why a person behaves in a certain way can be understood with the help of qualitative methods. Influences that can promote and prevent change can also be identified.

Target individuals or groups with the worst practices: The greatest impact is possible by focusing on these individuals or facilities.

Use credible information sources: Involve influential, respected authorities and ensure that materials are well referenced and authoritative.

Use credible communication channels: Communicating through existing, credible channels enhances the message and the acceptability of the content.

Use personal contact whenever possible: Face-to-face individual or small group meetings can communicate key messages most effectively.

Limit the number of messages: By confining the intervention to a few *key* messages, understanding is improved.

Repeat key messages using different media: People learn in different ways—some visually from text or graphics, some through spoken messages, and some through a combination of media. Repeating key messages using different approaches helps reinforce them.

Provide better alternatives: Whenever possible, give a positive message that encourages people to do something. Negative messages tend to alienate people. By stressing the positive, the negative behavior can be excluded. For example, *DO treat diarrhea with ORS. Antidiarrheals are not necessary.*

≡ 28.6 Developing a Strategy

Six steps to follow in developing a strategy to promote rational drug use are described below.

Step 1. Identify the Problem and Recognize the Need for Action

Within the facility, district, or country, there must be a consensus about the most important problems in drug use. Recognition of the primary problems may arise from an indicator survey, a disaster in which patients have been adversely affected, or an economic analysis of drug expen-

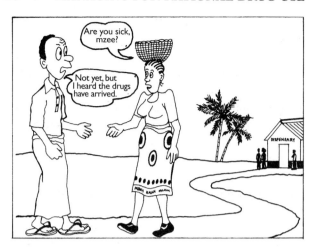

ditures. An effective response can be planned once all the involved parties, including prescribers, patients, and health service managers, recognize that there is a problem. If an influential prescriber or politician refuses to accept that a specific problem exists, it will be very difficult to intervene effectively. Thus, establishing a consensus that action is needed and securing support from all interested parties are important tasks.

Step 2. Identify Underlying Causes and Motivating Factors

As described in Section 28.4, many factors contribute to the irrational use of drugs. These factors must be investigated and understood before intervening. If this step has not been undertaken, the intervention is likely to fail. For example, a campaign to promote the use of generic drugs through posters will fail if the underlying reason for the lack of use is that the doctors do not know the generic names.

Step 3. List Possible Interventions

Educational, managerial, and regulatory interventions can be used to address the problem (see Chapter 31 for details).

Step 4. Assess Resources Available for Action

When deciding which intervention or combination of interventions to test, it is important to take stock of what resources are available. The most important limiting resource is usually human. *Who will implement the intervention?* and *Will that person have enough time to work on the intervention?* are questions that must be asked. Try to identify groups or individuals who would support the intervention. For example, generic manufacturers would support an intervention to popularize generics. Financial, transport, and material resources also need to be assessed.

Step 5. Choose an Intervention or Interventions to Test

Factors to consider when choosing an intervention include the effectiveness with which it addresses the underlying causes of the problem; its success rate in similar situations, areas, or countries; its cost; and whether or not it can be sustained with available resources. Whichever intervention is chosen, it *must* be tested before widespread implementation.

Step 6. Monitor the Impact and Restructure the Intervention

While testing the intervention, it is important to monitor related drug use as a way to evaluate its efficacy. For example, an intervention for banning antidiarrheals may lead to an increased use of antibiotics. On completion of the intervention, evaluate the results to decide whether or not it can be expanded to involve a larger population. An intervention's effectiveness in a small area with a limited number of people does not guarantee widespread success. Whenever possible, a combination or sequence of interventions should be used.

The remaining chapters in this section address the task of improving drug use. All these chapters should be reviewed before planning an intervention. ■

≡ Glossary

Adherence to treatment (also **compliance**): The degree to which patients adhere to medical advice and take medicines as directed. Adherence depends not only on acceptance of information about the health threat itself but also on the practitioner's ability to persuade the patient that the treatment is worthwhile and on the patient's perception of the practitioner's credibility, empathy, interest, and concern.

Clinical pharmacist: An individual trained in pharmacy, usually at the bachelor's degree level, who has had specialized training in the uses, side effects, contraindications, and dosages of medications for human use.

Clinical pharmacologist: A physician who has had specialized training in the uses, side effects, warnings, and dosages of medications for human use.

Course-of-therapy prepackaging: Prepackaging of drugs in sealed plastic bags, each bag containing a complete course of treatment for that drug, as established by standard treatment norms. The package usually contains a complete label with instructions for use.

Dispense: To prepare and distribute to a patient a course of therapy on the basis of a prescription.

Dispenser: A general term for anyone who dispenses drugs. Also specifically used to mean an individual who is not a graduate pharmacist but is trained to dispense medications, maintain stock records, and assist in procurement activities.

Drug use: The process of diagnosis, prescribing, labeling, packaging, and dispensing and of adherence to drug treatment by patients.

Generic substitution: Dispensing of a product that is generically equivalent to the prescribed product, with the same active ingredients in the same dosage form, and identical in strength, concentration, and route of administration.

Irrational prescribing: Prescribing that does not conform to good standards of treatment—for example, extravagant prescribing, overprescribing, incorrect prescribing, multiple prescribing, or underprescribing of medications.

Labeling: Placing written or symbolic instructions on the immediate container in which drugs are dispensed.

Pharmacology: The study of medicines and their actions.

Prescribing: The act of determining what medication the patient should have and the correct dosage and duration of treatment.

Standard treatment guidelines: Agreed-upon treatment practices for a diagnosed illness; may include more than details of drug treatment.

Symbolic labeling: A system of providing written instructions for patients using sketches and other graphic representations.

Therapeutic substitution: Interchange of one drug product with another that differs in composition but is considered to have similar pharmacologic and therapeutic activities, in accordance with written protocols previously established and approved.

≡ References and Further Readings

★ = *Key readings.*

★ Fabricant, S. J., and N. Hirschhorn. 1987. Deranged distribution, perverse prescription, unprotected use: The irrationality of pharmaceuticals in the developing world. *Health Policy and Planning* 2:204–13.

Finer, D., and G. Tomson, eds. 1992. *Essential drug information: The story of a workshop.* Stockholm: Karolinska Institute, Department of International Health Care Research.

HAI-Europe and University of Amsterdam Medical Anthropology Unit. 1991. *The provision and use of drugs in developing countries: A review of studies and annotated bibliography.* Amsterdam: Het Spinhuis Publishers.

Homedes, N., and A. Ugalde. 1993. Patients' compliance with medical treatments in the third world: What do we know? *Health Policy and Planning* 8:291–314.

MSH (Management Sciences for Health). 1994. *East and central African regional essential drugs programme training project, 1991–1994.* (Supported by Danida.) Boston: MSH.

★ MSH (Management Sciences for Health). 1995. *Promoting rational drug use.* Washington, D.C.: MSH.

★ Ross-Degnan, D., R. O. Laing, J. D. Quick, H. M. Ali, D. Ofori-Adjei, L. Salako, and B. Santoso. 1992. A strategy for improved pharmaceutical use: The international network for rational use of drugs. *Social Science and Medicine* 35:1329–41.

Soumerai, S. B., and H. L. Lipton. 1994. Evaluating and improving physician prescribing. In *Pharmacoepidemiology,* 2d ed., ed. B. Strom. Chichester, England: John Wiley and Sons.

Vance, M. A., and W. R. Millington. 1986. Principles of irrational drug therapy. *International Journal of Health Services* 16:355–62.

★ van der Geest, S. 1987. Pharmaceuticals in the third world: The local perspective. *Social Science and Medicine* 25:273–76.

Werner, D., and B. Bower. 1983. *Helping health workers learn.* New Delhi: Voluntary Health Association of India.

WHO (World Health Organization). 1987. *Conference of experts on the rational use of drugs, Nairobi: Report on the rational use of drugs.* Geneva: WHO.

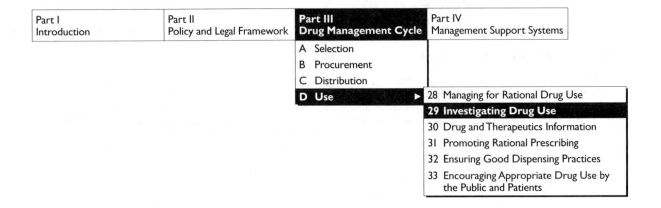

| Part I | Part II | **Part III** | Part IV |
| Introduction | Policy and Legal Framework | **Drug Management Cycle** | Management Support Systems |

A Selection
B Procurement
C Distribution
D Use ▶ 28 Managing for Rational Drug Use
29 Investigating Drug Use
30 Drug and Therapeutics Information
31 Promoting Rational Prescribing
32 Ensuring Good Dispensing Practices
33 Encouraging Appropriate Drug Use by the Public and Patients

Chapter 29
Investigating Drug Use

≡ Summary

Medical directors and clinicians, as well as policy-makers and managers, collect data to describe patterns of drug use, correct specific drug use problems, and monitor drug use over time. There are two basic ways to do this: quantitative methods, to measure what is being done, and qualitative methods, to provide information about why it is being done. Data on drug use can also be utilized to evaluate the impact of interventions.

There are many sources of quantitative data on drug use:

- *indicators for health facilities*
- *drug utilization review*
- *aggregate data*
- *private-sector drug use*

The most important source, however, is the drug use encounter, *the period of interaction between patient and health provider. To encourage consistency in drug use studies, the World Health Organization (WHO) and the International Network for Rational Use of Drugs (INRUD) produced a manual for investigating drug use in health facilities (WHO/DAP 1993). The manual defines core drug use indicators and provides a methodology for measuring these indicators.*

Private-sector practices can be examined by surveying private practitioners and investigating practices at retail drug sales outlets. Retail studies use methods such as interviews, stock or prescription surveys, observation of interactions with customers, or exit interviews. The simulated patient survey, consisting of visits to retail outlets by investigators posing as customers with specific health problems, is a particularly useful technique for studying retail practices.

Qualitative methods are useful for examining underlying feelings, beliefs, attitudes, and motivations. The most common qualitative techniques for studying drug use include focus group discussion, in-depth interview, structured observation of the process of care, structured questionnaire, and simulated patient survey. Each method has strengths and weaknesses and is appropriate in different circumstances.

One use of quantitative and qualitative methods is to gain a better understanding of the causes of problems before intervening to correct them. Outcome indicators for the intervention that are meaningful, reliable, and measurable must be selected. It is also necessary to randomly select appropriate study sites and a relevant comparison group and to measure outcomes before and after the intervention in both groups. Time series models may be used if an appropriate comparison group cannot be identified.

≡ 29.1 Reasons to Investigate Drug Use

Managers and policy-makers collect data about drug utilization for various reasons. These reasons can be grouped into three general categories:

1. To describe current patterns of drug use:
   - Measure consumption of particular drugs or therapeutic groups of drugs;
   - Compare use by individual health facilities or prescribers;
   - Decide whether drug use is clinically justified or cost effective;
   - Learn about the influence of prescribing on pharmaceutical costs.
2. To correct specific drug use problems:
   - Find out about the factors that cause specific problem practices;
   - Identify and correct problems in prescribing, dispensing, or patient use.
3. To monitor drug use over time:
   - Monitor quality of care within a health facility or geographic area;
   - Monitor the efficiency and cost effectiveness of prescribing.

A health manager who wishes to improve drug use proceeds through a cycle of activities (Figure 29.1) that includes (1) assessing current patterns of drug use, (2) defining standards of appropriate practice and identifying problems and their causes, (3) carrying out interventions to improve specific problems, and (4) evaluating improvements and monitoring subsequent practices. This process can be repeated to tackle increasingly complicated issues.

During the process of improving drug use, different kinds of data are needed. There are two basic ways to gather data: *quantitative methods* and *qualitative methods*. Quantitative methods are better for answering the question *What is happening?* Qualitative methods are suited for answering the question *Why is it happening?*

Quantitative methods are those used to collect data on such things as number of drugs prescribed, whether a patient receives an antibiotic, or the cost of antibiotic therapy. Quantitative data are used to create rates, averages, or

Figure 29.1 Identifying and Rectifying a Drug Use Problem: An Overview of the Process

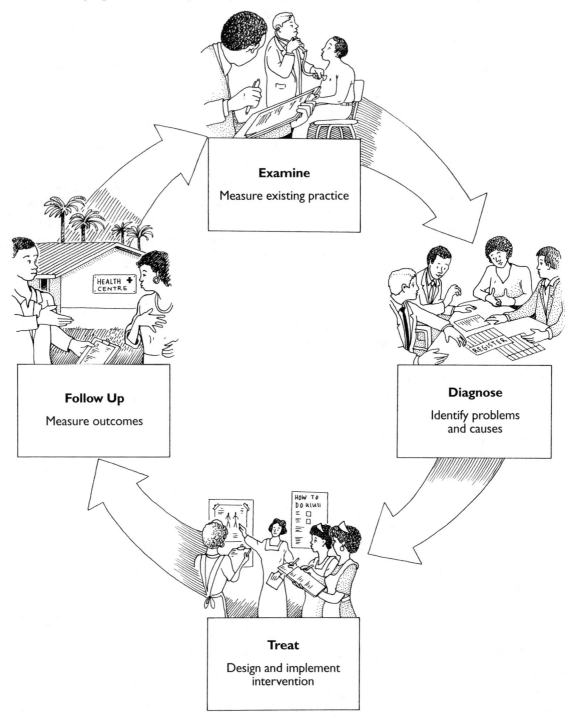

other summary measures to describe the nature and extent of a drug use practice.

Qualitative methods, often in the form of observations, descriptions, opinions, or discussions, are frequently used to describe the beliefs and motivations that underlie particular practices. *Without this information, it is difficult to determine why prescribers and patients act as they do, and therefore how their behavior can be changed.*

≡ **29.2 Data Sources and Measurement Issues**
Health managers often need to describe the use of specific drugs or drug classes or compare use among different

Figure 29.2 Sources of Quantitative Drug Use Data

Location of Data	Data Sources	Useful for Studying
Public-sector administrative offices, medical stores	For retrospective studies: ▸ Drug supply orders ▸ Stock cards ▸ Shipping and delivery receipts	Aggregate patterns of drug use and expenditures Comparative use of drugs within therapeutic classes Comparative use by different facilities or areas
Health facility clinical and medical record departments	For retrospective studies: ▸ Patient registers ▸ Health worker logs ▸ Pharmacy receipts ▸ Medical records For prospective studies: ▸ Patient observations ▸ Patient exit surveys ▸ Inpatient surveys	Aggregate patterns of drug use and expenditures Drug use per case, overall, and by group (age, sex, health problem) Provider-specific prescribing Characteristics of patient-prescriber interactions
Health facility pharmacies	For retrospective studies: ▸ Pharmacy logs ▸ Prescriptions retained in pharmacies For prospective studies: ▸ Patient exit surveys ▸ Patient observations	Aggregate patterns of drug use and expenditures Dispensing practices Characteristics of patient-dispenser interactions
Pharmacies and retail drug outlets	For retrospective studies: ▸ Prescriptions retained in pharmacies For prospective studies: ▸ Customer exit surveys ▸ Customer observations ▸ Simulated patient visits	Private-sector prescribing practices Drug sales without prescription Self-medication practices Characteristics of customer-salesperson interactions
Households	For retrospective studies: ▸ Family medical records ▸ Household surveys For prospective studies: ▸ Household drug audits ▸ Family medical care logs	Total community drug use Care-seeking behavior Self-medication practices Family drug use patterns Patient adherence to treatment

geographic areas, administrative units, or individual prescribers. Sources of data for such purposes differ, depending on the setting. A hospital administrator who wants to measure the use of expensive antibiotics requires different data than a program manager who needs to know how children in the community are treated for acute respiratory infection (ARI). Common sources of drug utilization data and their uses are outlined in Figure 29.2.

Characteristics of Drug Use Data
Drug data differ in scope and level of aggregation.

Scope. Data may describe public-sector practices (public facilities or administrative offices), private-sector practices (private practitioners, drug suppliers, or drug retailers), or community drug use (practices in the community, independent of setting). Data on public-sector practices are the most readily available, since these data flow out of routine record-keeping systems. Private-sector or community-based data are more expensive and time consuming to collect.

Level of Aggregation. Data on utilization may be aggregated to measure consumption of specific drugs or drug

classes or may focus on patient-specific use. Data on patient-specific use are usually more informative, although aggregate consumption data may be sufficient to answer many cost-related questions.

Retrospective studies can be conducted using data from routine record keeping or past studies. *Prospective studies* collect data, for example, from patient encounters. For retrospective studies, existing data, although potentially incomplete, are less expensive to use. They can also describe practices over a longer period of time. Prospective studies provide information about the treatment setting, diagnostic process, communication between health providers and patients, or the time of consultation and dispensing.

Drug Use Encounters: Basic Units
A *drug use encounter* is the period of contact between a patient and a health provider. Ideally, this encounter includes a number of components: history taking; the diagnostic process; selection of pharmacological and non-pharmacological treatment; prescription (and perhaps dispensing) of treatment; and explanations about treatment,

follow-up, or prevention. Drug use encounters that include one or more of these components occur in many settings, with health providers who range from highly trained medical specialists to itinerant drug sellers.

Critical data on drug use encounters include (1) identification of the specific setting, provider, patient, and date of the encounter; (2) patient age and gender; (3) signs and symptoms (patient complaint) or diagnosis (by the health provider); and (4) identification of drugs prescribed or sold, including brand or generic name, strength, and route (injection, oral, topical). Data on the total dose prescribed or sold (number of pills and duration of treatment) and the cost of the drugs dispensed are also valuable for specific purposes.

Studies in several settings have found that data collection forms need to allow for at least three diagnoses per encounter and at least ten drugs prescribed or sold. Data on total dose, duration of treatment, and drug cost are often difficult to collect accurately and can add substantially to the cost of data collection. Unless there are specific reasons to collect these items, such as designing an intervention, it is easier to limit drug-specific data to brand or generic name, strength, and route.

Measurement Issues

Problems in identifying, classifying, and quantifying drugs frequently occur when measuring drug use. With hundreds or even thousands of products on the market, many drug names are similar. The same drug is often available under different names and in many different dosages and forms. Identifying specific drugs and their ingredients, or grouping equivalent products, can be difficult and time consuming. Similarly, grouping cases according to health problem can be difficult in environments where record systems are imprecise and diagnoses are frequently uncertain. Some ways to handle these common problems have been developed.

What Is in a Drug? When deciding which drugs to place in specific groups, the following steps may be taken:

- Obtain a list of *generic drugs* such as the national essential drugs list or national formulary to use as the basis for developing the list of drugs and drug codes to be used in a particular study.
- If a system such as the Anatomical Therapeutic Classification (ATC) (WHO Collaborating Centre 1993a) or one of the other common systems is not used, develop a system of easy-to-recognize drug codes based on drug names and strengths (for example, "TET250T" for tetracycline 250 mg tablets). Coding systems are discussed in Chapters 10, 41, and 46.

- Use standard pharmaceutical references (MIMS, Martindale, USP–DI) to identify ingredients in brand-name drugs. Although expensive, the most useful single reference is probably Martindale. Organize the drugs identified into therapeutic classes or categories, as relevant for analysis.
- Count combination products as single drugs (because of the difficulty in deciding which ingredients count as separate products).

Which Drugs Belong Together? When attempting to place drugs in specific groups, it is useful to begin with an existing system of drug categories, such as the WHO list of essential drugs or the more elaborate ATC. If necessary, the drugs can subsequently be reorganized into more useful local categories. For classifying antibiotics, a commonly studied category of drugs, recommendations found in the WHO Collaborating Centre manual (1993a) can be used. Antibiotic creams, eye ointments, antibiotic-containing antidiarrheal products, and sulfa drugs can be included, but metronidazole and other antiprotozoals should be excluded (see Chapter 10).

How Many and How Much? The following procedures can be helpful when encountering problems in estimating the amounts of drugs dispensed or drug costs:

- Define the most common dispensing units (pills, milliliters, tubes, bottles) for every drug, and be sure that enumerators record these units consistently when data from drug encounters are coded.
- Identify any commonly used injections or liquids (for example, cough syrups) for which there may be inconsistencies in recording the correct basic unit (ampoule vs. mL, bottle vs. mL). Prepare a simple reference card for enumerators stating the correct units to be used for these drugs.
- For calculating drug costs in public-sector studies, use a single fixed set of unit costs (calculated per pill, per mg, per cc, based on bulk purchase prices) for all health facilities. This ensures that any variations in cost are attributable to drug selection and decisions about dosing.

Classifying Cases. When attempting to define reasons for treatment problems, it is important to develop explicit rules prior to data collection for classifying cases when only signs and symptoms are recorded and no diagnosis is made. In this way, health problems diagnosed as "malaria" can be distinguished from those recorded as "fever," or those diagnosed as "pneumonia" can be distinguished from "cough, fever, and difficulty breathing." When possible, use the WHO International Classification of Diseases (ICD-10) codes. Separate categories can be developed for classifying frequently repeated clusters of problems (ARI and otitis media, cough and fever).

Using Standard Treatment Guidelines. One issue that frequently arises in drug use studies is how to apply information from standard treatment guidelines to measure the quality of prescribing. Because clinical guidelines are usually not developed as management tools, using them to measure quality of care introduces a number of practical problems. In the developing world, clinical guidelines frequently exist in the form of standard diagnosis and treatment protocols. These standard protocols are most commonly intended for use in primary health care facilities, although some countries have developed standards for secondary and tertiary care facilities as well. How useful are these standard protocols in measuring the quality of pharmaceutical use?

Based on a given standard, some studies have tried to decide globally whether the use of drugs in a particular case is "correct" or "incorrect." In practice, this judgment is frequently difficult to make in a valid and reliable way. Local standard treatments may not be expressed in an explicit way that allows adherence to be accurately measured. Furthermore, standard guidelines are frequently difficult to apply for real patients with multiple health problems or problems that cannot be diagnosed accurately with available facilities.

A recommended approach for using standard treatments in drug use studies is to:

► Have local experts agree on explicit definitions of the standard diagnostic procedures and treatments for the health problems under study.
► Define one or more explicit aspects of these standards as separate indicators rather than trying to measure global adherence. Example: Was oral rehydration solution (ORS), which should *always* be recommended to treat diarrhea with mild dehydration, given or not? Was an antidiarrheal, which should *never* be recommended to treat diarrhea with mild dehydration, given or not? Was the recommended dose form of a drug used—for example, oral ORS rather than injectable intravenous saline solution? Was the appropriate amount of the drug used (daily dose times duration of therapy)?
► Concentrate on measuring adherence to the most unambiguous aspects of the standard.
► Analyze separately drug use encounters with only a single reported diagnosis or set of symptoms to be sure that the results are the same.

Unit of Analysis. Depending on the focus of a drug use study, it is possible to think of the patient, prescriber, or health facility as the intended unit of analysis. For community-based surveys or studies of patient-level factors such as ability to pay for drugs, the patient may be the appropriate focus. The individual prescriber may be the best unit of analysis for studies of specific prescribing practices or influences on prescribing. In many health systems, the health facility is the appropriate study unit to examine drug use in a geographic area or the reasons for differences in treatment practice.

Sample Size. When measuring drug use, the required sample size depends on which practices are being measured, how precise the measurements need to be, and the unit of analysis. There is usually a tradeoff between the costs of collecting data and greater uncertainty. People carrying out scientific research usually need more precise data with larger samples than managers or policy-makers who measure drug use to make decisions. Sample size must be planned accordingly.

Focusing on specific subgroups often improves one's ability to make good decisions. When possible, the sample in a drug use study should be stratified to compare key groups. Strata could be urban/rural, paramedic/physician, government/mission, or public sector/private sector. When possible, the sample size should be greater in groups that are likely to have poor practices, in order to learn more about the groups that are likely to be the focus of future interventions.

Ethical issues must be considered in any study that measures individual behavior. Managers in a health system may have the right to examine performance, but these efforts are likely to be more favorably received if they involve representatives of the practitioners whose performance will be investigated—their supervisors, for example. Studies from outside an administrative structure should always include appropriate efforts to obtain informed consent from prescribers and patients and to describe how the data will be used. Finally, emphasis should be placed on adequate and timely dissemination of findings for the benefit of those under study.

≡ 29.3 Measuring Drug Use: Quantitative Methods

Drug use encounters occur in many environments, including hospitals, health centers, private pharmacies or drug shops, and the home. In North America, hospital drug use is frequently studied by drug utilization review (DUR) (described in Chapter 38). Although many different methods are used to investigate drug use, this chapter

Figure 29.3 WHO Drug Use Indicators (Outpatient Facilities)

Core Drug Use Indicators

Prescribing Indicators
1. Average number of drugs per encounter
2. Percentage of drugs prescribed by generic name
3. Percentage of encounters with an antibiotic prescribed
4. Percentage of encounters with an injection prescribed
5. Percentage of drugs prescribed from essential drugs list or formulary

Patient Care Indicators
6. Average consultation time
7. Average dispensing time
8. Percentage of drugs actually dispensed
9. Percentage of drugs adequately labeled
10. Patients' knowledge of correct dosage

Health Facility Indicators
11. Availability of a copy of essential drugs list or formulary
12. Availability of key drugs

Complementary Drug Use Indicators
13. Percentage of patients treated without drugs
14. Average drug cost per encounter
15. Percentage of drug costs spent on antibiotics
16. Percentage of drug costs spent on injections
17. Prescription in accordance with treatment guidelines
18. Percentage of patients satisfied with the care they received
19. Percentage of health facilities with access to impartial drug information

Source: WHO/DAP 1993.

emphasizes the methods published by WHO (WHO/DAP 1993).

Studying Drug Use in Health Facilities Using WHO Indicators

Health managers and policy-makers often need to know about the quality of drug use in a group of health facilities. To simplify and standardize the study of drug use in these situations, the WHO Action Programme on Essential Drugs and INRUD produced the manual *How to Investigate Drug Use in Health Facilities* (WHO/DAP 1993; Hogerzeil et al. 1993). This manual describes in detail a set of reliable indicators to measure drug use and a standard methodology to collect the data for these indicators. The major points of the manual are summarized below.

The WHO manual defines twelve core and seven complementary drug use indicators (see Figure 29.3) that measure key aspects of drug prescribing, patient care, and availability of drugs and drug information at outpatient facilities. The *core indicators* are highly standardized and do not require national adaptation. Although not comprehensive, they provide a simple tool for quickly and reliably assessing a few critical aspects of drug use. With these indicators, results should point to specific drug use problems that need to be examined in more detail. All the nec-

essary data are collected from medical records or by direct observation at individual health facilities.

The manual also defines a set of *complementary indicators,* which are less standardized and require defining variables specific to the country or location. One important complementary indicator measures adherence to treatment guidelines. This indicator needs clear, explicit criteria to be reliable and informative.

To measure drug use, collect data from a sample of health facilities. The number of health facilities to include in the survey depends on the purpose of the survey. A regional or national drug use survey includes at least twenty facilities selected at random, with 30 drug use encounters sampled per facility, for a total of at least 600 encounters for the entire study. When the objective is to study drug use by individual facilities or prescribers in a sample, at least 100 prescriptions should be obtained at each health facility or for each prescriber. When possible, the prescribing data are based on one year of retrospective encounters, although prospective data can be collected if no retrospective data are available. Data on patient care and facility indicators are always collected prospectively.

Data from an indicator study can be presented in a variety of ways. The principal use of an indicator survey is to obtain a snapshot of current drug use practices to contrast with surveys from other areas or with "optimal" values for the indicators. Figure 29.4 presents selected results from twenty-one studies that used this basic methodology to study drug use. Both similarities and differences in drug use patterns are apparent. There is a relatively high number of drugs per case in Ghana and Nigeria (4.3 and 3.8); high injection use in Uganda, Sudan, Nigeria, Swaziland, Cameroon, and Ghana (36 to 56 percent); and low availability of essential drugs in Ecuador (38 percent). The rate of antibiotic use in primary care facilities was found to vary from 27 to 39 percent in Latin America, from 31 to 46 percent in Asia, and from 29 to 63 percent in Africa. By focusing attention on specific areas of concern, the indicators can help identify priorities for action.

Although a survey based on thirty encounters per facility mainly discerns overall patterns, it is also possible to contrast performance in individual health facilities. These facility-specific estimates can be unreliable because of low sample sizes, but interesting patterns often emerge (Figure 29.5). These estimates can show whether values of indicators are consistent or different across facilities and identify facilities that seem to have very low or very high values for specific indicators. Using qualitative methods, the reasons for these apparent differences can then be explored in more depth before designing interventions.

Figure 29.4 Selected Results of Studies Using WHO Indicators

Country	Number of Facilities	Number of Drugs Prescribed	Percent Antibiotics	Percent Injections	Percent Generics	Consulting Time (min)	Percent Who Know Dosing	Percent of Key Drugs in Stock
Africa								
Sudan	37	1.4	63%	36%	63%			
Malawi	72	1.8	34%	19%		2.3	27%	67%
Zimbabwe	56	1.3	29%	11%	94%			
Tanzania	20	2.2	39%	29%	82%	3.0	75%	72%
Nigeria	20	3.8	48%	37%	58%	6.3	81%	62%
Cameroon	20	3.0	51%	41%	58%			
Ghana	20	4.3	47%	56%	59%			
Uganda	127	2.4	53%	36%	86%	4.6	29%	
Mozambique	26	2.2	43%	18%	99%	3.7	82%	87%
Swaziland	20	3.0	54%	38%	63%	6.1	87%	92%
Asia								
Yemen	19	1.5	46%	25%				
Indonesia	20	3.3	43%	17%	59%	3.0	82%	
Bangladesh	20	1.4	31%	0%			63%	
Nepal	20	2.1	43%	5%	44%	3.5	56%	90%
Latin America and Caribbean								
Ecuador	19	1.3	27%	17%	37%			38%
Guatemala	20	1.4	27%	13%	72%			
El Salvador	20	2.2	32%	7%	72%			
Jamaica	20	2.4	30%	4%	40%			
Eastern Caribbean	20	1.9	39%	1%	49%			

Note: References available from Management Sciences for Health/INRUD.

Indicators can also be used to quantify the impacts of an intervention. In Yemen in 1989, researchers compared an essential drugs program area and a control area in which no program had been active. The number of drugs per patient in the project area was 1.5, compared with 2.4 in the control area; the percentage of antibiotics was 46 percent compared with 67 percent; and the rate of injections was 22 percent compared with 45 percent. In Uganda in 1994, a randomized controlled community-based trial was carried out in six districts, using the full set of WHO indicators as outcome measures. The study demonstrated that standard treatment guidelines plus prescriber in-service training resulted in significantly lower rates of overall drug use, injection use, and antibiotic use in comparison with controls; generally, provision of the treatment guidelines alone did not result in any significant changes.

Drug use indicator studies have also been undertaken on inpatients (see Country Study 29.1).

Finally, an indicator study can be a simple tool to motivate health personnel and policy-makers. For example, prior to a nationwide prescriber training program in Malawi, each of twenty-four district medical officers surveyed three health facilities in his or her own administrative area. This was a more effective strategy for educating and motivating them than randomly surveying twenty facilities for the whole country for a baseline survey. While carrying out this survey, participants not only learned basic skills for measuring key aspects of quality of care but also became familiar with ideas about standards of practice and how their own areas conformed to these standards.

The WHO indicators can be used to study drug use for specific problems such as diarrhea, malaria, or ARI. Such research can be undertaken after an indicator study by selecting a limited number of common conditions for secondary analysis. This secondary analysis may highlight inappropriate treatment of common conditions (for example, injectable chloroquine for malaria).

Using Aggregate Data to Measure Drug Use

To understand how drugs are used to treat specific illnesses, there is often no alternative to collecting patient-specific data. However, these data may be expensive or difficult to obtain. Aggregate data on drug consumption are often readily available from drug procurement records, warehouse or pharmacy stock receipts, or even records from drug importers or manufacturers. Sometimes aggregate data can be used to answer specific questions about drug use.

Examples of questions about drug use that might be answered using available aggregate data include:

What is the relative use of therapeutically substitutable products? For example, what is the relative use of aspirin

Figure 29.5 Comparison of Facilities in Indicator Studies in Uganda and Indonesia

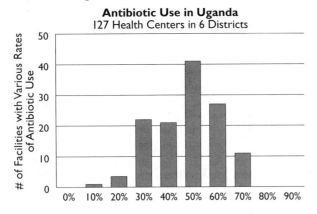

Antibiotic Use in Uganda
127 Health Centers in 6 Districts

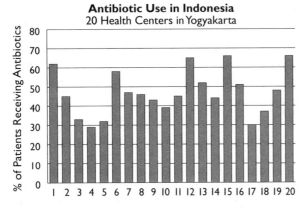

Antibiotic Use in Indonesia
20 Health Centers in Yogyakarta

compared with paracetamol, or chloroquine injections compared with chloroquine tablets compared with halofantrine tablets?

What is the per capita use of specific drugs or drug classes? For example, what is the per capita consumption of certain drugs that may be widely overused, such as benzodiazepines or cimetidine?

What proportion of the drug budget is spent on specific drugs or drug classes? For example, how much is spent on cephalosporins or on drugs to treat tuberculosis?

When one uses aggregate data, similar products may not share a convenient unit of comparison. If the primary focus is cost, all drug consumption data can be converted to monetary equivalents, using either actual or average purchase prices. However, if the focus is primarily clinical, this strategy will not work. Some researchers have established systems of therapeutic equivalence for particular drug classes, such as antipsychotic agents.

One widespread system to deal with product equivalence is the system of defined daily doses (DDDs) (WHO Collaborating Centre 1993b). A DDD is the "typical" dose of a drug used to treat the most common medical problem for which the drug is prescribed. The official DDD is usually the adult dose. Adjustments must be made to study pediatric drug use. Converting aggregate quantities to DDDs indicates roughly how many potential treatment days of the drug are procured or consumed. Drugs can then be compared on the basis of potential treatment days (see Figure 29.6). Because it is not known which diseases drugs are actually being used to treat or in what dosages they are prescribed, these comparisons are inexact. Nonetheless, it is possible to use these analyses to focus attention on important drug use problems.

The use of appropriate denominators is important in interpreting analyses of aggregate data. Often the information sought is not how much of a drug was used overall but how much was used per person, per visit, or per some other unit. The best denominator to use depends on the purpose of the analysis and the availability of data. Generally, the closer one can get to the population of concern, the better. For example, suppose the objective is to compare the use of ORS in one geographic area with its use in another area. One way would be to calculate packets of ORS used per child under five in each community. Another way would be to express utilization as ORS packets used per child visiting a health facility with a diagnosis of diarrhea, since this would control in part for possible differences in diarrhea incidence.

Reviewing Case Records

Useful information can be obtained from case records at hospitals or health facilities. The audit process can start with either a disease or a drug. Criteria are usually defined for correct and incorrect treatment of a disease or correct and incorrect use of a drug. Then case records of patients with the specified disease or who have received the drug are identified and reviewed, and the treatment of the disease is recorded and classified as correct or incorrect. The cost of the treatment can also be determined. When records are selected by drug, the use of the drug can be classified as correct or incorrect. For example, if watery diarrhea were the diagnosis selected for study, ORS would be the correct treatment. Antidiarrheals, antibiotics, and injections would be incorrect. If a drug such as procaine penicillin were the study drug, it would be correct to use it for tonsillitis, skin infections, otitis media, and pneumonia, but it would be incorrect to use this drug for parasitic infections such as worms or malaria.

When large numbers of records are surveyed, descriptive statistics can be generated, including the average number of drugs per contact, the average cost, and the percentage of patients receiving injections, antibiotics, or antidiarrheals. These indicators can be analyzed by specific diseases. A computer is required for studies in which a large number of records are surveyed and analyzed. A software package, PASS, has been developed to facilitate data entry, analysis, and report generation (see Chapter 46). Studies such as these can form the basis for interventions focused on specific disease management or drug use problems.

Surveying Private-Sector Drug Use

In many countries, most pharmaceuticals are prescribed and used in the private sector. Lack of access to data about private-sector drug use prevents managers and policymakers from addressing problems in this area. There are two basic strategies for examining private-sector practices: surveys among private medical practitioners, and surveys in retail drug sales outlets.

One direct way to find out about private-sector drug use is to ask private doctors and other healers who prescribe Western medicines to provide information about their own practices. Private practitioners are often willing to share information about their behavior if they feel that the reasons for collecting the data do not threaten them or their business. Private marketing companies in many countries have long collected these kinds of data from private doctors for use by drug manufacturers and distributors.

An alternative way to collect information about private-sector drug use is to survey retail outlets: pharmacies, licensed drug shops, over-the-counter drug sellers, and market vendors. Studies in many countries have found that persons selling drugs are often willing to explain what they know, to discuss their business, to have their interac-

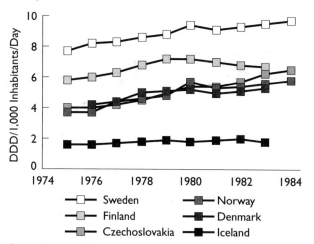

Figure 29.6 Using Defined Daily Doses to Compare Drug Use Patterns: Results from a Comparative Study of Insulin Use in Scandinavian Countries

Source: Dukes 1993.

tions with customers observed, and even to keep records of the drugs they sell. To receive this kind of cooperation, persons collecting data must carefully explain the reasons for a study, show drug sellers how they or their customers might benefit, and assure them of confidentiality.

Many different methods can be used to collect quantitative data in retail pharmacy establishments. Some methods and the types of information they are best suited to collect include

- ▸ *interviews with pharmacists or counter attendants*, to provide data about sales activity, knowledge and sources of information about drugs or clinical issues, and advising and sales practices;
- ▸ *surveys of drugs stocked or sold*, to measure product availability, retail cost, and sales volume;
- ▸ *surveys of prescriptions received*, to describe the patterns of private-sector prescribing;
- ▸ *observation of interactions with customers*, to examine customer demand, reasons for product selection, frequency of purchase without prescription, and communication about drugs;
- ▸ *exit interviews with customers*, to investigate knowledge about illness and drugs, care-seeking patterns, expectations, satisfaction with services, and reasons for product selection.

One method for studying retail drug use that deserves special attention is the *simulated patient survey.* This survey consists of visits to a sample of retail outlets by investigators posing as customers with specific types of health problems, for example, mothers of children with diarrhea

Figure 29.7 What Is Reported in Interviews May Be Very Different from What Is Done in Practice

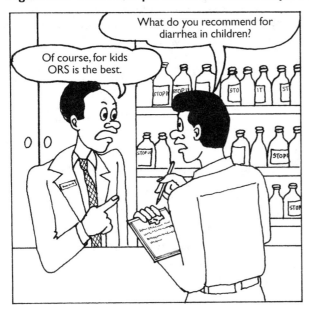
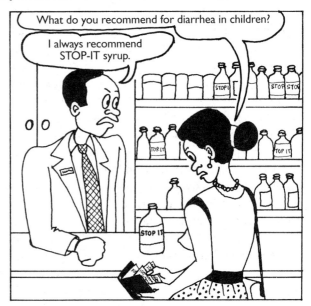

(see Figure 29.7). These investigators are trained to seek advice about treatment and to respond in a standard way to questions asked by the counter attendant. They usually buy whatever drugs are recommended to complete the transaction. After leaving the shop, they record details about questions asked about signs and symptoms; advice given about drugs sold; and other advice given about case management, prevention, or referral.

Examining Drug Use in the Community

Surveys of health facilities, private practitioners, or drug retail outlets furnish information about medication decisions for cases seen by these providers. However, these studies do not tell about drug use from the community perspective. For example, studies of providers tell nothing about times when people choose *not* to treat an illness, or about failure to use drugs due to lack of knowledge, economic or geographic constraints, or other factors. In the same way, these studies tell us little about the dynamics of care-seeking, the use of multiple health providers, or total drug consumption in a community. It is also not possible to learn how patients actually consume the drugs they receive.

To learn about community drug use, it is necessary to use techniques different from those discussed so far. In the past, community drug use studies have been carried out by medical anthropologists or sociologists, using extensive ethnographic or participant observation methods. The publication *How to Investigate Drug Use in Communities* (WHO/DAP 1992) describes a simplified methodology

that combines a household interview survey, surveys of drug distribution channels such as health centers or pharmacies, and qualitative investigations using focus groups or in-depth interviews.

The core of any quantitative study of community drug use is the cross-sectional household survey. These surveys should include a minimum of 100 to 400 households, depending on the desired precision of the results and available resources. The sample of households is drawn so that all important groups in the community are represented. Different types of information can be collected from the households, depending on the purposes and duration of the survey. These include

- ▶ knowledge about drugs and illness, including sources of community information about drugs;
- ▶ reported care-seeking and drug use behavior in general or during specific episodes of illness;
- ▶ illness diaries, in which respondents record all episodes of perceived illness, the actions taken to deal with these problems, any drugs received for the illness, and how they took these drugs;
- ▶ drug inventories, to identify the type and source of all drugs present in the household;
- ▶ health care and pharmaceutical expenditures;
- ▶ adherence (compliance), including purchase of prescribed drugs and actual patterns of drug consumption.

Understanding community attitudes about drug use is also discussed in Chapters 33 and 37.

Figure 29.8 Five Useful Qualitative Methods

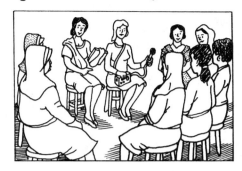

Focus Group Discussion
- 1.5- to 2-hour discussion
- guided by trained moderator
- group of 6 to 10 similiar respondents (age, gender, social status)
- focus on defined list of topics
- informal setting
- reveals beliefs, opinions, motives

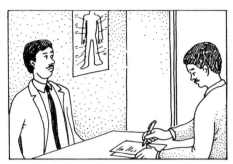

In-Depth Interview
- semistructured extended interview with respondent
- interviewer uses predefined open-ended questions
- usually covers 10 to 30 topics
- reveals attitudes, beliefs, knowledge

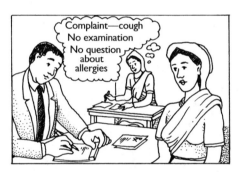

Structured Observation
- systematic observation of verbal and nonverbal behavior
- usually patient-provider interactions
- trained observers use structured recording form
- assesses actual behavior

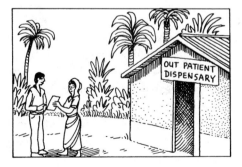

Questionnaire
- fixed set of standardized questions
- large sample of respondents
- respondents systematically selected to represent a larger population
- quantifies frequency of attitudes, beliefs, knowledge

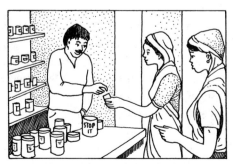

Simulated Patient Survey
- someone (the "simulated patient") poses as a patient or a relative of a patient
- simulated patient seeks care for specific health problem
- questions, advice, actions of health care provider recorded after encounter
- assesses actual behavior in a standardized way

Figure 29.9 Comparison of Qualitative Methods

Method	Key Points	Strengths	Weaknesses
Focus group discussion	Small; equal participation Homogeneous; shared point of view Informal; free interaction and open sharing of ideas Recorded; analysis at later time possible	Good at eliciting the beliefs and opinions of a group Richness and depth Easy and inexpensive to organize	Need for skilled moderator Beliefs and opinions expressed may not represent true feelings Potential bias in analysis
In-depth interview	Open-ended and in-depth questions Targets key informants or opinion leaders 5–10 interviews enough to explore important issues If target group is diverse, 5–10 held with each subgroup	Unexpected insights or new ideas Creation of trust between interviewer and respondent Less intrusive than questionnaire Useful with illiterate respondents	Time-consuming compared to questionnaires Data analysis can be difficult Bias toward social acceptability Need for well-trained interviewers
Structured observation	Data can be coded indicators or scales, list of events or behaviors, or diaries To count frequency of behaviors, at least 30 cases per group To understand typical features, a few cases in 5–6 settings may be enough	Best way to study provider-patient interactions, including patient demand, quality of communication, or interaction time Opportunity to learn about provider behavior in its natural setting	Threatening to those observed Observers must spend enough time to "blend in" Behavior may not be natural Need for skilled, patient observers Not useful for rare behaviors
Questionnaire	Fixed or open-ended responses Sample size depends on sampling method, desired accuracy, and available resources At least 50–75 respondents from each subgroup	Best method to study range of knowledge, beliefs, opinions, population characteristics Familiar to managers and respondents Required skills often locally available	Attitudes difficult to quantify Respondents may answer questions even if none apply Results sensitive to specific questions and wording Large surveys can be expensive
Simulated patient survey	Details of the condition are standardized Simulated patient purchases what is recommended Each facility should be visited by at least 5 simulated patients At least 20 facilities should be visited	Useful to compare knowledge and practices Identification of different practices for rich/poor, male/female, rural/urban	Ethical issues Need for simulators who can speak local language and are credible purchasers in the setting

≡ 29.4 Investigating the Reasons for Drug Use Problems: Qualitative Methods

The many factors that contribute to the irrational use of drugs are discussed in detail in Chapter 28. The best way to find out how factors such as knowledge, economic incentives, or attitudes and beliefs affect drug use and to identify the most important constraints to changing specific behaviors is to use qualitative methods. These methods have been developed by social scientists to investigate the causes of behavior.

Quantitative methods are used to describe drug use patterns or to pinpoint specific problems that need attention, but they are usually not good for understanding *why* these patterns or problems exist. Qualitative techniques are better suited to examine the feelings, beliefs, attitudes, or motivations that underlie an observed problem. They are helpful in exploring the causes of a problem, constraints to changes in behavior, and opportunities for correcting the problem.

Qualitative methods are based on talking to people at length and in depth or observing their behavior. When used in a formal way, these methods often involve highly trained interviewers or observers directed by an experienced social science researcher. Increasingly, however, managers and policy-makers are using qualitative methods to rapidly assess the causes of a problem. Managers themselves do not need to know how to carry out qualitative research but only what these methods are and when they may be useful.

Five useful techniques for collecting qualitative data on drug use are focus group discussions, in-depth interviews, structured observation, questionnaires, and simulated patient surveys. These methods are outlined briefly in Figure 29.8, and their strengths and weaknesses are compared in Figure 29.9. Anyone interested in knowing more should obtain a copy of the manual *How to Use Field Methods to Design Drug Use Interventions* (MSH/INRUD 1995).

How can qualitative methods be used to design an

Country Study 29.2 Combining Interviews, a Simulated Patient Survey, and Focus Groups: Results from the Kenya Drug Sellers Project

To discover the extent and causes of problems in diarrhea treatment in Kenyan pharmacies, a team from the Ministry of Health Control of Diarrhoeal Diseases Programme carried out a series of studies of private pharmacies in Nairobi and several smaller towns before designing a training program for counter attendants. These activities followed a model described in the *Guide for Improving Diarrhoea Treatment Practices of Pharmacists and Licensed Drug Sellers* (WHO/CDD 1993).

The team carried out a survey of pharmacies to find out basic information such as who worked in the pharmacies, what products they stocked, and how many customers with diarrhea sought treatment each week. Counter attendants were interviewed to find out what they knew about diarrhea and the drugs to treat it, what they said they recommended to treat the last case of childhood diarrhea they encountered, and where they got their information about drugs and health.

In order to contrast what drug sellers actually recommended with what they said they recommended (see the accompanying graph), the team also sent local women to these pharmacies a few days later to present a standardized case of simple watery diarrhea. The women recorded what questions they were asked, what they were sold, and what advice they were given.

After reviewing the results of these two methods, the team held focus group discussions with counter attendants and in-depth interviews with shop owners to explore the reasons for observed problems and factors that might motivate drug sellers to change their practices. For example, counter attendants were asked to comment on their perceptions of ORS, a prod-

uct that the survey showed they were quite familiar with, yet which was seldom sold to investigators.

Based on all this quantitative and qualitative information, the team designed a training program that emphasized key messages about the need to treat diarrhea with food, fluids, and ORS and the potential dangers of antidiarrheals. The messages and materials also appealed to counter attendants' desire to be better health professionals, which focus groups revealed was very strong. After a brief (two- to three-hour) interactive training session, it was found that the sales of ORS during a second round of simulated patient visits had doubled in comparison to control areas, and the sale of antidiarrheals had fallen by about 40 percent.

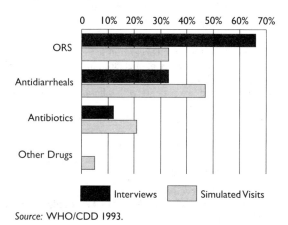

Source: WHO/CDD 1993.

intervention? Country Study 29.2 describes how the managers of the Control of Diarrhoeal Diseases Programme in the Kenya Ministry of Health used questionnaires, a simulated patient survey, and focus groups to explore the nature and causes of problems in diarrhea treatment in private retail pharmacies before they designed an intervention to train pharmacy attendants. Based on the combined results of these methods, they were able to design targeted printed materials and training messages that proved to be effective in changing drug sales and patient counseling behavior.

≡ 29.5 Using Data to Design Interventions
The best understanding of the origins of problems can often be obtained by using quantitative and qualitative methods together.

Proceeding from Problem Definition to Intervention Design
As illustrated in Figure 29.1, the first step in improving drug use is to measure existing practices and identify spe-

cific problems. This is usually done quantitatively, for example, by carrying out an indicator study. After narrowing attention to specific problems, it is necessary to understand why they occur—the motivations and constraints—and then to suggest possible actions to correct the problems. The objectives of this process are to

- describe the problem in *greater detail;*
- evaluate the *feasibility* of an intervention to correct the problem;
- direct the proposed intervention to specific patients, providers, and behaviors (*targeting*);
- define *intervention messages* that can motivate changes in behavior;
- choose the best *format and specific activities* for an intervention.

Interventions implemented without gathering this information are likely to fail. Explicit questions should be formulated to guide this process. The goal is to identify a practical strategy to change behavior. Only questions that can help in the design of a better intervention should be

---

Country Study 29.3 Improving Diarrhea Treatment in Pelotas, Brazil

A review of health center records in Pelotas, Brazil, found that there were problems in treating diarrhea in children. Prior to launching an educational intervention for physicians to improve practices, the study team used patient exit interviews, in-depth interviews of physicians and patients, and observations of treatment episodes to answer questions in five areas:

To Describe the Problem in Greater Detail
- Are practices the same in facilities managed by the municipality, the university, and the state government?
- Is lack of correct knowledge about diarrhea or its treatment a common problem among physicians and patients?
- Is there a lack of knowledge about the causes and correct diagnosis of diarrhea? About the need for ORS? About the dangers of specific antidiarrheals? About the efficacy of antibiotics or antiparasitics?
- How do physicians think other physicians manage diarrhea?

To Decide Whether an Intervention Is Feasible
- How much do patients' expectations influence physicians' treatment choices?
- How satisfied are patients with different kinds of treatment for diarrhea?
- How important is patients' satisfaction to physicians?
- Do physicians feel that patients are capable of learning about diarrhea and its treatments?
- Would physicians or other staff have time to counsel patients about diarrhea or other health problems?

To Target the Intervention
- How often do mothers ask directly for specific types of treatment?
- Are there nonverbal ways that mothers influence physicians' decision-making?

- How do physicians respond when asked for certain treatments?
- Do physicians feel a group identity with colleagues at the health center?
- To which respected peers do physicians turn with questions about treatment?
- How often do physicians approach colleagues with medical questions?

To Define Specific Intervention Messages
- How important to physicians is the self-image of being a knowledgeable scientist or powerful healer?
- When physicians have changed their practices in the past, what has caused them to do so, and how do they feel about these changes?
- What do physicians think about prototype materials developed to promote correct diarrhea treatment practices?

To Decide on the Format and Style of the Intervention
- How do physicians get information about new health problems or drugs?
- Do they ever attend continuing education sessions, and are these useful?
- Do they read any journals (which ones)?
- Do they learn about drugs from drug package inserts, advertisements, or drug company representatives, and is this information valued?
- How do physicians respond when presented with summaries of the practices of their health center in relation to similar facilities?
- How do physicians feel about different models for continuing education: group seminars, visits by medical experts, visits by pharmacists?

---

asked. For example, imagine that a survey finds that 64 percent of patients treated in one district receive injections, but that this varies from 11 to 93 percent in the twenty facilities studied. Questions to be answered during the investigation process might include:

- Are injections given more frequently to adults or to children, and are they given more often for specific health problems? (*greater detail*)
- Do facilities with low and high injection use differ in number of staff, percentage of staff who are paramedics, patient volume, distance from the district center, frequency of drug stockouts? (*greater detail, targeting*)
- Do mothers expect to receive injections for their children, and do they tend to go to prescribers who give injections more frequently? (*targeting, feasibility*)
- Are health providers and patients aware that injections can transmit hepatitis and AIDS, and that they can cause anaphylactic shock? (*intervention messages*)

- How do prescribers react when they are shown data from the indicator study on their use of injections in relation to their peers? (*intervention format and activities*)

Asking focused questions keeps the process oriented toward intervention design. The optimal number of questions depends on how much is already known about the problem and the target group. Country Study 29.3 lists the questions that guided the diagnostic process in an educational intervention to improve diarrhea treatment by physicians in a city in southern Brazil.

After asking a set of specific questions, a manager or policy-maker must choose quantitative and qualitative methods to answer them. As described above, each method has strengths and weaknesses. Often it is best to try to answer the same question using different methods. For example, suppose one objective is to determine whether patient demand for injections helps explain why they are given so frequently. One way to do this is to observe a sample of clinical encounters to see how many times patients indicate verbally or nonverbally that they prefer injections. Patients can also be interviewed to see if they are satisfied with their treatment or if they plan to go elsewhere to look for different treatment. Finally, in-depth interviews or focus group discussions with prescribers can explore their feelings about patient demand and their perceptions about whether it affects their practice.

Combining Results to Design Interventions

Each quantitative or qualitative method addresses the subset of diagnostic questions it is well suited to answer. At the end of the process, these separate inputs must be combined to design an intervention. One strategy to integrate data efficiently is to hold a *synthesis meeting* of everyone involved in the investigation process.

If everyone at the meeting is not familiar with all the studies, the first activity should be to present separate reports on each study. Each report should briefly cover the specific study questions addressed, the methods used, the results, and the conclusions. Written summaries of findings and tables or graphs should be distributed. Discussion of specific findings can take place after all the reports have been presented. Sometimes findings from two methods are complementary, but sometimes the results contradict each other. If the findings suggest important issues for discussion, these issues should be listed as they are raised and covered later in the integrated discussion.

After systematically answering all the questions, the participants in the synthesis meeting should have a good idea of the general content of an intervention that might be effective. The specific behaviors to focus on will be more apparent, as will the specific target groups of prescribers or patients likely to gain the most from the intervention.

The synthesis meeting should then direct its attention to designing an intervention. The process of synthesizing data to draw conclusions about intervention design can be difficult. Before attempting this synthesis, the group should be familiar with what is known from experience with the different intervention models presented in Chapter 31.

≡ 29.6 Evaluating Interventions

Research has shown that interventions are most effective when they target specific problem behaviors. A training program discouraging polypharmacy as a general problem is likely to have less impact than training that targets specific commonly overused drugs or specific health problems in which polypharmacy is common. Interventions can target several problems at once. For example, an intervention to improve pneumonia treatment might combine training for health workers in how to use a standard ARI treatment protocol with community-based education about case recognition and care-seeking. Interventions can also have unintended outcomes. For example, interventions that address the overuse of injections might unintentionally cause a decrease in immunizations.

Selecting Appropriate Measures

Interventions should be evaluated by looking for both intended and unintended changes in specific outcomes. For all the outcomes of interest, indicators that are meaningful, reliable, and measurable must be selected. When choosing the most useful outcomes to measure, consider the following:

► Select the key behaviors targeted by the intervention and the most likely substitute behaviors.
► Select outcomes that can be clearly and explicitly defined.
► Select outcomes that can be reliably measured, preferably using routinely collected data.
► Focus on several important outcomes rather than measuring all possible changes.
► Measure more than one dimension of success, especially if some changes are secondary—for example, changes in prescribing that follow changes in knowledge about specific drugs.

Using Basic Principles of Research Design

Managers carry out interventions because they think that they will work, but they sometimes give insufficient attention to evaluating their impacts. Techniques for designing research on health services and evaluating interventions are covered in detail in other books. But every evaluation should include the four basic steps described below:

Step 1. Select the Correct Study Unit. Because the behavior of patients and prescribers is affected by other people, the correct study unit is often the health facility. In some interventions that involve changes in administrative procedures, the correct study unit may be the district.

Step 2. If Possible, Randomly Assign Study Units to Intervention and Comparison Groups. An appropriate *comparison group* is the most important feature of a good evaluation (see Figure 29.10). Random assignment of study units to intervention or comparison groups is not always possible. If it is not, choose a comparison group that is as similar as possible. In situations in which everyone will receive a particular intervention, it may be possible to compare early recipients with those who have not yet received the intervention.

Figure 29.10 Importance of a Comparison Group

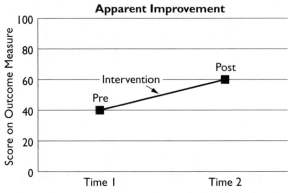

This figure shows an apparent improvement in outcome score from about 40 measured at Time 1 to more than 60 at Time 2. With information only from the group that received an intervention between these two times, it is tempting to conclude that the intervention caused the improvement in outcome scores.

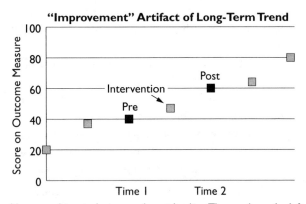

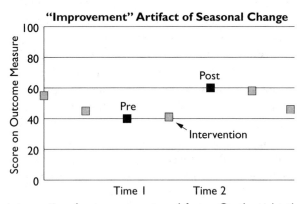

However, this conclusion can be misleading. The graph on the left shows that the intervention group has actually been experiencing a steady improvement in scores before, during, and after the intervention due to some external factor. On the right, the outcome seems to be seasonal, and it happened to be measured at a low point in the cycle at Time 1 and a high point at Time 2.

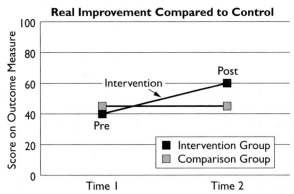

Only by using a comparison group can one guard against many possible incorrect conclusions about the effects of an intervention. Any reasons for change in outcomes outside of the intervention itself should affect both groups equally. Changes in the two groups can be compared to estimate the intervention's impacts.

***

Step 3. Measure Outcomes Before and After the Intervention in Both the Intervention and the Comparison Groups. With at least two measurement points, it is possible to examine both equality at baseline and change in practices. Data must be collected in the same way in the comparison and intervention groups, since the process of being observed often causes changes in behavior.

Step 4. Measure Impacts over Time. Short-term impacts

Figure 29.11 Using Interrupted Time Series

Time series are a powerful method for investigating drug use. Data that are routinely collected in many health systems about the use of different types of drugs can easily be displayed as time series. It is also possible to look at patient-specific information on drug treatment in sample medical records. In most cases, these series are made more stable by dividing by a meaningful denominator, such as rate per 100 attendances or proportion of total antibiotic expenditures.

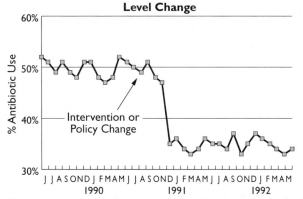

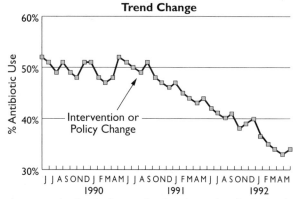

The figure on the left shows a sudden reduction in the level of antibiotic use following an intervention. The figure on the right shows a reduction in the trend rather than a drop in the level.

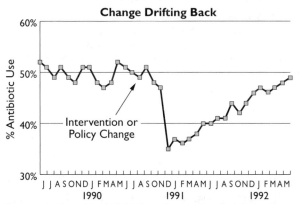

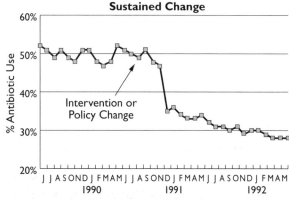

Frequently there is a drift back to the previous baselines after an intervention, as shown in the figure on the left. In some cases, there may be a level change, which can be sustained or increased over time, as shown in the figure on the right.

Time series techniques allow one to assess the individual and cumulative effects of interventions over time.

---

often disappear unless they are reinforced. To know whether an intervention really works, look at short- (one month), medium- (six months), and long-term (one year or more) impacts.

Sometimes it is not possible to identify a good comparison group, for example, after a change in national pharmaceutical policy or for an intervention in a single health facility. In these situations, interventions can be evaluated through *time series* (see Figure 29.11). This method can be used to compare patterns of drug use before and after the intervention. Time series models are usually useful only under certain conditions:

► The data must be consistent for the entire time period. For example, if the data come from a hospital,

there should be no major changes in hospital personnel or services. If the data are from a sample of health facilities, the analysis should be limited to facilities that have reported consistently.

► Each time point should represent an equal length of time (for example, one week or one month).

► There should be at least six to twelve time points preceding the intervention and the same number of time points after the intervention for a reliable examination of underlying trends.

The techniques described in this chapter have been used by researchers for many years. In a number of countries, essential drugs program managers have also used these methods to guide their decision-making (see Country Study 29.4).

By using simple quantitative survey methods to estimate the size of the problem and qualitative methods to understand the reasons for the problem behavior, a manager can rationally plan his or her program to maximize the probability of success. Spending a relatively small amount of time and money to investigate before taking action is likely to save time and money in the future. ∎

Country Study 29.4 Investigative Surveys Undertaken as Part of National Essential Drugs Program Management

In **Indonesia**, multiple studies have been undertaken utilizing aggregate consumption data, indicator studies, and intervention studies. These have been used to guide national programs and World Bank–supported regional activities.

In **Kenya**, an indicator study was undertaken in five regions as part of the overall planning management and evaluation of the essential drugs program.

In **Malawi**, a national drug use indicator survey was undertaken in every district, covering seventy-two facilities, before national training on standard treatments.

In **Nepal**, simulated patient studies have been used to investigate practices of drug sellers to assist in designing training programs to improve their practices.

In **Uganda**, researchers studied the effect of training prior to redesign of training programs.

In **Zambia**, a study was performed in the capital in which different training methods were evaluated by detailed record review, using DUR techniques.

In **Zimbabwe**, an indicator-based baseline survey was performed before the first national policy and planning workshop. This survey is repeated every two years, and it was expanded to include urban facilities and the private sector.

≡ Assessment Guide

When assessing a country's or program's capacity to investigate drug use, two main areas should be considered:

- Results of previous studies;
- Technical capacity to undertake drug use investigations.

Previous Studies

- Have any studies been performed on community drug use using the WHO/DAP manual *How to Investigate Drug Use in Health Facilities*? If yes, what were the results?
- Have any special studies been undertaken to investigate specific drug use problems (such as injection use)? If yes, what were the results?
- Have any routine surveys such as census or household surveys included questions on drug expenditures or use?
- Are pharmaceutical consumption data easily available for the public or private sector?

- What are the prevalent attitudes that will have a positive or negative effect on the use of health services and drugs?

Technical Capacity

- Are any social scientists involved in studying drug use or health-seeking behaviors?
- Are there local experts who could assist in quantitative or qualitative surveys?
- Is there a unit within the ministry of health that is dedicated to health systems research?
- Do the medical training schools undertake field research or offer student training in the field?
- What types of records are available in the public and private sectors that would facilitate research on drug use?

≡ References and Further Readings

★ = *Key readings.*

Dukes, M. N. G., ed. 1993. *Drug utilization studies: Methods and uses.* World Health Organization (WHO) regional publications, European series, no 45. Copenhagen: WHO.

★ Hogerzeil, H., V. Bimo, D. Ross-Degnan, R. O. Laing, D. Ofori-Adjei, B. Santoso, A. K. A. Chowdhury, A. M. Das, K. K. Kafle, A. F. B. Mabadeje, and A. Y. Massele. 1993. Field tests for rational drug use in twelve developing countries. *Lancet* 342: 1408–10.

★ MSH/INRUD (Management Sciences for Health/International Network for Rational Use of Drugs). 1995. *How to use field methods to design drug use interventions.* Boston: MSH/INRUD.

Quick, J. D., and H. M. Thuo. 1994. Adoption of WHO drug use indicators in hospital (letter). *Lancet* 343:237.

Riegelman, R. 1996. *Studying a study and testing a test: How to read the medical literature.* 3d ed. Boston: Little Brown.

Smith, P. G., and R. H. Morrow. 1991. *Methods for field trials of interventions against tropical disease: A toolbox.* New York: Oxford University Press.

Varkevisser C. M., I. Pramanathan, and A. Brownlee. 1991. Designing and conducting health systems research projects. In *Health systems research training series.* Vol. 2, Pt. 1. *Proposal development and fieldwork.* Ottawa: International Development Research Centre (PO Box 8500, Ottawa, Ontario, Canada K1G 3H9).

WHO/CDD (World Health Organization/Control of Diarrhoeal Diseases Programme). 1993. *Guide for improving diarrhoea treatment practices of pharmacists and licensed drug sellers.* WHO/CDD/93.43. Geneva: WHO/CDD.

WHO Collaborating Centre for Drug Statistics Methodology. 1993a. *Guidelines for ATC classification,* 4th ed. Oslo: WHO.

WHO Collaborating Centre for Drug Statistics Methodology. 1993b. *Guidelines for DDD,* 2d ed. Oslo: WHO.

★ WHO/DAP (World Health Organization/Action Programme on Essential Drugs). 1992. *How to investigate drug use in communities.* WHO/DAP/92.3. Geneva: WHO/DAP.

★ WHO/DAP (World Health Organization/Action Programme on Essential Drugs). 1993. *How to investigate drug use in health facilities: Selected drug use indicators.* WHO/DAP/93.1. Geneva: WHO/DAP.

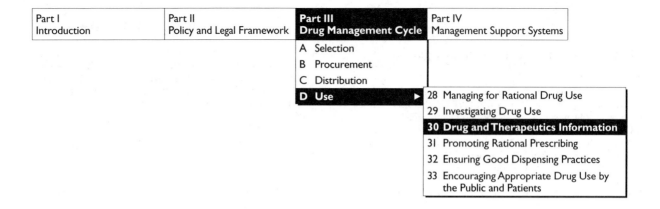

| Part I Introduction | Part II Policy and Legal Framework | **Part III Drug Management Cycle** | Part IV Management Support Systems |

A Selection
B Procurement
C Distribution
D Use ▶

28 Managing for Rational Drug Use
29 Investigating Drug Use
30 Drug and Therapeutics Information
31 Promoting Rational Prescribing
32 Ensuring Good Dispensing Practices
33 Encouraging Appropriate Drug Use by the Public and Patients

Chapter 30
Drug and Therapeutics Information

≡ Summary

Prescribers, pharmacists, and patients all require information on drugs. The sources of this information can be classified as primary (articles or papers on original research), secondary (reviews of the primary literature), and tertiary (formulary manuals, standard treatment manuals, textbooks, and review articles, or drug product information approved by drug regulatory agencies). Promotional literature has limited utility, as it provides biased information designed to promote sales of commercial products.

The skills required to evaluate drug information sources can be provided by a drug information center (DIC); ideally, there should be one in every country. A DIC can be established in an accessible hospital or university department. The center should provide information proactively as well as respond to queries. The center requires trained staff with access to both text and computer information sources.

The activities of such a center include sending staff out to provide information; developing, producing, and disseminating a drug bulletin based on modern communication principles; and teaching.

Funding the center may be difficult, but diversified funding should be sought whenever possible. Funding from drug companies may appear to affect the center's impartiality and should generally be used only for capital projects. Other problems that may affect the center include

▸ *inadequate information sources;*
▸ *lack of acceptance;*
▸ *inadequate communication systems;*
▸ *lack of political will to establish or sustain the center.*

≡ 30.1 Drug Information

Access to clinically relevant, up-to-date, user-specific, independent, objective, and unbiased drug information is essential for appropriate drug use. Prescribers, dispensers, and users of medicines all need objective information. A health care system can provide access to the highest-quality medicines, but if those medicines are not properly used, they may have negligible benefits or even adverse effects. Although access to good drug information does not guarantee appropriate drug use, it is certainly a basic requirement for rational drug use decisions.

Drug information comes in many forms (written and audiovisual material, computer disks, and CD-ROMs, for example), and the need for drug information varies among different types of health care providers and patients. For example, physicians and pharmacists need access to the full range of information about generic and brand-name drugs, indications and contraindications for use, drugs of choice and therapeutic alternatives, dosing, precautions for use, drug interactions, side effects, adverse effects, clinical features and treatment of overdose, availability, and cost of a course of treatment. Patients need basic instructions for using prescribed and self-care medicines. In addition, patients and the general public increasingly expect, and are being provided with, more comprehensive drug information (see Chapter 33).

Identifying and accessing the sources of different types of drug information are important activities for a drug management program. When limited funds do not allow the program to provide systemwide access to necessary

information resources and individual practitioners are unlikely to be able to purchase information themselves, a centralized drug information service should be considered.

The primary role of a DIC is to give clear and definitive information on essential drugs and promote their rational use. A secondary role of the center is to keep up-to-date with pharmacological and therapeutic literature and disseminate relevant information when it becomes available.

≡ 30.2 Sources of Drug Information

Information sources fall into three classes. *Primary* sources are the foundation on which all other drug information is based. These include journal publications on drug-related subjects, such as reports of clinical drug trials, case reports, and pharmacological research. A list of primary information sources appears in Annex 30.1.

Secondary sources function as a guide to or review of the primary literature. Secondary sources include review articles, meta-analyses, indexes (*Index Medicus*), abstracts (*International Pharmaceutical Abstracts*), and combinations of abstracts and full-text reprints.

Tertiary or *general* sources present documented information in a condensed format. Examples include formulary manuals, standard treatment manuals, textbooks, general reference books, drug bulletins, and drug compendia. It is advisable to obtain the most current edition available when using secondary or tertiary sources.

All information sources have limitations, and drug information providers should use them with care.

Evaluation of Information Sources

Evaluating information sources is an important skill (see Figure 30.1). The *Guide to Good Prescribing* (WHO/DAP 1994b) contains a useful section on assessing literature. *Studying a Study and Testing a Test* (Riegelman 1996) is a valuable primer on evaluating medical literature.

Primary Sources. Evaluating primary literature is difficult. The most reliable evidence comes from reports on randomized controlled trials. Proper evaluation of these trials requires considerable experience, and systematic reviews of combined trials (meta-analyses) may be necessary. This work is being undertaken by the Cochrane Collaboration (see Box 30.1).

In judging primary literature, one cannot assume that the results of a study or a research paper are valid simply because it has been accepted for publication. However, it is useful to consider the source of a study or paper when one seeks to determine its quality. There are a number of respected medical and pharmacy journals whose high standards for acceptance and publication make it unlikely that a research article containing erroneous data or misrepresented information would survive the editorial and review process. Annex 30.2 lists some English-language journals that have strong editorial policies and peer review processes that include conflict-of-interest disclosure requirements to minimize the possibility of biased or unsupportable conclusions being reported. There have been cases, however, in which highly respected journals have published inappropriate articles. One way to monitor such problems is to read the letters to the editor published in journals. If questionable conclusions survive the peer review process, some reader will undoubtedly write to the journal editor and state his or her observations or concerns. Reputable journals readily share this type of correspondence, often allowing the authors of criticized articles the opportunity to respond.

Information published in journals without a strong review process needs to be more carefully screened. "Throw-away" or controlled-circulation publications, provided free of charge by a special-interest group (a drug manufacturer, for example), require careful scrutiny to determine what biases, if any, exist.

Secondary and Tertiary Resources. Secondary information resources are essentially derivations of the primary literature. Some review articles summarize the results and conclusions of a number of reports from the primary literature (usually with comments by the reviewer). A relatively recent type of review article, the meta-analysis, combines and analyzes the results from several reports (see Box 30.1).

Figure 30.1 Evaluating Information Sources

Questions to ask when reviewing original clinical articles include:

▶ In which journal was the article published? What is the reputation of the journal? Is it known to have high standards for the acceptance of articles? Are articles peer reviewed?
▶ Who is the author, and what is his or her affiliation?
▶ Does the article report the results of a properly designed clinical study, or is it based on case reports or observations? If a clinical study, what was the sample size, and how were participants selected? Were there controls? Was the study prospective or retrospective? Is the report adequately referenced?
▶ Are reasonable conclusions drawn?
▶ Who funded the study? Is there any potential for conflict of interest?

Questions to ask about bibliographic, abstracting, or indexing services include:

▶ What journals or information resources are covered by the service, and are these resources the ones that are essential for the particular purpose?
▶ What is the lag time between the publication of a journal and its inclusion in the service?
▶ How easily can the service be used? Are key words indexed? Are there subject headings?
▶ If abstracts are provided, who develops the abstracts, and how accurately do they reflect the primary source?

Questions to ask about consensus-generated documents include:

▶ How is consensus defined, and how are the individuals participating in the consensus definition process selected?
▶ How good is the consensus-generation process?
▶ Are references provided and accessible?
▶ Is the consensus process open to public review and comment?
▶ Is the information based on evidence published in peer-reviewed literature, or is it simply a compilation of use patterns reported as being accepted by the medical community?
▶ When was the consensus document published, and how frequently is the information updated?
▶ Who published the information, and what kind of reputation does the publisher have?

Questions to ask about secondary and tertiary references written by individuals or groups of individuals include:

▶ Who is the author, and what are his or her qualifications?
▶ Who is the publisher, and what is its reputation?
▶ Who paid for the development of the information? Does it come from a special-interest group? If the publication is reporting proceedings from a conference, who organized the conference, and do the organizers have a special interest?
▶ Has the information been peer reviewed? How good is the peer review process?
▶ When was the information developed, and how current is it?
▶ Are references included in the article, or is it possible to access the references by other means?

Bibliographic, abstracting, or indexing services provide listings or compilations of published articles. Some list the addresses of the principal authors; others contain abstracts of articles, along with key words or subject headings to help users find the articles or references they are looking for. Examples of such services include *Medline, Current Contents, International Pharmaceutical Abstracts, Index Medicus, Excerpta Medica*, and the *Iowa Drug Information Service* (which also includes full-text reprints of articles). Different systems cover different journals and may, for instance, omit letters to the editor. There is a lag period between initial publication of a primary source and its inclusion in such secondary sources. It is important, therefore, not to rely entirely on one secondary source.

Drug bulletins can be valuable in helping prescribers and supply system managers to determine the relative merits of new drugs and keep up-to-date. Drug bulletins can have a variety of sponsors, such as government agencies, professional bodies, university departments, philanthropic foundations, and consumer organizations. They are published in many countries, sometimes free of charge, and many are highly respected because of their unbiased information. Examples in English are *Drug and Therapeutics Bulletin* (United Kingdom), *Medical Letter on Drugs and Therapeutics* (United States), and *Australian Prescriber* (Australia). *Prescrire international* is available in both French and English. National drug bulletins are appearing in several countries, including Bolivia, Cameroon, Malawi, the Philippines, and Zimbabwe. The main advantages of national drug bulletins are that they can select topics of national relevance and use the national language.

Tertiary references, written by individuals or groups, are often developed with the input of consultant reviewers and may be widely peer reviewed. In general, the more thorough the peer review process is, the more sound the information is likely to be. In many countries, the most widely available tertiary resources are formulary manuals and standard treatment manuals produced by the health system. These important resources are discussed in Chapter 11. Drug bulletins (national and international) and textbooks such as those listed in Figure 30.3 are also tertiary sources.

Probably the most widely accepted secondary and tertiary information sources are those that report the consensus of experts, a process that involves a high level of scrutiny and feedback. A consensus statement is the closest one can come to agreement among experts. In most instances, consensus is defined as having addressed and considered all dissenting views so that, at a minimum, all disagreements have been publicly stated and considered. Examples of consensus documents include the *Antibiotic Guidelines* developed by the Victoria (Australia) Depart-

---

Box 30.1 The Cochrane Collaboration

The Cochrane Collaboration was established in 1992 in England to support a systematic up-to-date review of all relevant randomized control trials (RCTs) of health care. The collaboration is based on the ideas of Archie Cochrane, who pointed out in 1972 that because resources are limited, they should be used to provide *equitably* those forms of health care that have been shown in properly designed evaluations to be *effective*.

The Collaboration encourages reviewers to join a review group, which systematically studies all reports of RCTs of a treatment for a specific problem. Often the group uses a technique known as meta-analysis, in which the results of a number of different RCTs are combined to get around problems of small sample sizes.

The Cochrane Collaboration, based in centers in England, Canada, Denmark, the United States, Italy, and Australia, produces a database of systematic reviews, maintains a register of people interested in specific areas, and promotes collaborative reviews internationally.

The Collaboration publishes the reviews in both a hard-copy and a computerized format so that people in drug information centers can share the information. The Cochrane Collaboration is also interested in recruiting people to join groups to undertake reviews of subjects. The planned end result of this work is the publication of information about the interventions that have been shown to be effective when tested in RCTs.

The UK Cochrane Center can be contacted at National Health Service, R & D Program, Summertown Pavilion, Middle Way, Oxford OX2 7LG, England. Telephone: 44-865-516300. Fax: 44-865-516311. E-mail: cochrane@vax.ox.ac.uk.

---

ment of Health and Community Services, *Pharmacological Treatment of Heart Failure*, developed by the Swedish Medical Products Agency, *Management of Cancer Pain*, developed by the US Agency for Health Care Policy and Research, the *United States Pharmacopeia–Drug Information* database, and *Oncology Guidelines* from Zimbabwe.

Manufacturers' Promotional Information

Drug information provided by manufacturers is secondary or tertiary information. This type of information is so commonly available and frequently used, however, that it warrants a separate discussion.

The type and quality of information provided by drug manufacturers vary considerably from country to country, depending on governments' regulations and ability to enforce them. Information that may or may not be approved by a country's regulatory agency, textbooks, and journal reprints are among the materials companies usually provide. In materials sponsored by a pharmaceutical company, only favorable views of the sponsor's products may be presented, and the materials may not furnish adequate information for good prescribing decisions. Sales representatives may provide only partial information about products they are promoting. In practice, governments often have difficulty controlling what information is provided by companies. In the United States, where controls are fairly tightly enforced, the Food and Drug Administration (FDA) frequently orders manufacturers to withdraw and correct misleading materials. Some European countries also have tight controls. A multinational lobbying organization, MaLAM, monitors misleading advertisements (see Box 30.2), as does Health Action International. The World Health Organization (WHO) has developed ethical guidelines for drug promotion (see Box 30.3).

This does not mean that manufacturers' information is universally bad and should not be used at all, as manufacturers can supply very timely and useful drug information. However, health care professionals or patients utilizing manufacturer-supplied information need to recognize that the source of the information is biased and make a judgment about its value (see Figure 30.2).

Product inserts and labeling provided by drug manufacturers do not necessarily reflect all current accepted uses of a drug. In many instances, the indications on a product's approved labeling do not match how that drug is routinely used in medical practice. Once a medicine is approved for marketing and used for one indication, subsequent clinical trials and experience may show that it is useful for other indications as well. Changes in product labeling to reflect this new information need to be authorized by the drug approval agency. Often this is not done for years after the new use is first reported in the medical literature. In some cases, new information is never added to a product's approved labeling because it is not economically advantageous for the drug company to go through the approval process. In cases in which a drug's generally accepted uses go beyond its government-approved labeling, the drug information specialist or health care professional has to rely on the medical literature for help in judging which uses are appropriate and which are inappropriate.

Many health professionals regularly use references that compile approved product labeling provided by pharmaceutical manufacturers, or brief descriptions of product availability and use based on product labeling. In the United States, the most common reference of this type is the *Physicians' Desk Reference* (PDR), which provides the full product labeling for drugs selected by the respective pharmaceutical companies. In the United Kingdom, the Association of the British Pharmaceutical Industry (ABPI)

Box 30.2 Drug Information: Medical Lobby for Appropriate Marketing

The Medical Lobby for Appropriate Marketing (MaLAM) was formed in 1983 in Australia. In 1995, it had over 1,000 members in thirty different countries. The aim of MaLAM is to use the influence of doctors to encourage drug companies to provide sufficient, accurate, and consistent information so that correct decisions can be made about prescribing and dispensing drugs.

The organization works by targeting a different example of misleading advertising each month. An editorial board writes a letter questioning the assertions in an advertisement. Copies of this letter are then distributed to MaLAM members, most of whom are doctors. After these members review the letter, they may request a copy of the company's response from the appropriate official at the drug company. In a review published in *Lancet* in 1989, ten international companies were asked to justify claims about seventeen products. Seven companies cited a total of sixty-seven references, none of which was deemed to justify the claims.

MaLAM has acted as a stimulus for groups to start monitoring the advertising of pharmaceuticals and other medical products. In Sri Lanka, medical students who are MaLAM members meet regularly to review advertisements.

MaLAM has also influenced multinational corporations to modify their promotional practices, for example, in relation to the marketing and sale of antidiarrheal drugs intended for use in children.

MaLAM can be contacted through MaLAM Canada, PO Box 158, Station D, Toronto, Ontario, Canada M6P358. Telephone: 416-964-7186.

Data Sheet Compendium is commonly used; and in many other countries, the country-specific or regional edition of the *Monthly Index of Medical Specialties* (MIMS) provides brief information on products marketed in that country or region. The limitations of these types of publications must be kept in mind, particularly in regard to the drugs and information omitted. These are *not* comprehensive information sources; manufacturers pay to have selected products included.

≡ 30.3 Setting up a Drug Information Center

A drug information center is a vital part of efforts to rationalize drug use. In a small country with limited means, this may mean a small office in the national hospital where a shelf of books and WHO publications is kept, and where a hospital pharmacist is responsible for answering queries. Ideally, however, countries should develop formal drug information centers (DICs) as part of their national health programs. A DIC should work closely with the national essential drugs program and be involved in the production of national drug-related materials.

Box 30.3 WHO Ethical Guidelines for Drug Promotion

Since 1967, WHO has been concerned about improper pharmaceutical advertising. In 1985, participants at the Nairobi meeting on the rational use of drugs suggested that the 1968 criteria needed updating. A new statement on ethical criteria for medicinal drug promotion was adopted in 1988. In 1994, the World Health Assembly repeated its concerns about drug promotion and called for further action to be taken.

Promotion of pharmaceuticals should support the national drug policy. The criteria state that advertisements should be consistent with the approved scientific data sheet and should be fully legible. Advertisements to the public should be for nonprescription drugs only. Medical representatives should have appropriate training and should present information in an accurate and responsible manner. They should make available to prescribers and dispensers complete and unbiased information on products. Medical representatives should *not* offer inducements to prescribers or dispensers.

Under the criteria, free samples may be provided in modest quantities to prescribers. The criteria also state that *provision of free samples of nonprescription drugs is difficult to justify from a health perspective.* When a pharmaceutical company sponsors a symposium or scientific meeting, its involvement should be clearly stated in advance at the meeting and in any publications.

The criteria recognize that postmarketing surveillance is important but cautions that it should not be misused as a disguised form of promotion. The criteria also define standards in packaging and labeling, patient information, and promotion of exported drugs.

Many countries and some companies have adopted these criteria as a guide for marketing practices, but others have not, since WHO depends on member countries to implement the standards.

Copies of the ethical criteria are available from WHO offices and have also been published in full in the WHO *Essential Drugs Monitor* no. 17 (1994).

Figure 30.2 Questions to Ask about Manufacturer-Supplied Information

- ► Has the information been approved by the country's drug regulatory body?
- ► Are references to the medical literature provided or available? Do they come from peer-reviewed journals?
- ► Was the information unsolicited, or was it provided in response to a request or question?
- ► Does the information contain negative references to the use of other medicines that might be substitutes or therapeutic alternatives to the drug in question? If so, are such negative references warranted?
- ► Do the claims for the drug's effectiveness appear overly positive or sensational?
- ► Is the information balanced with the negative outcomes related to the use of a medicine (such as side effects or adverse effects)?
- ► Are cost comparisons included?
- ► Does the information included in the product insert or the labeling reflect current medical practice and standards?
- ► Is the package insert dated and periodically updated?

Philosophical Commitment

A DIC should be both reactive and proactive. Reactive, or passive, duties include providing information for people who call or come to the center with questions. Although this is an important function, it certainly should not define the limits of a center's activities. A center's impact will be greater if it functions proactively by reaching out with drug information for people who need it, in a format that is convenient and effective.

A drug information service should be built on a cooperative model, involving all health care disciplines and utilizing existing resources to the greatest extent possible. It should be driven by the needs and expectations of its users but should also work to create demand and raise expectations.

Site Identification

Ideally, a DIC is centrally located, in or adjacent to a major hospital or other major health care facility. Location within a hospital, university, or other academic institution provides a network of medical disciplines that will support and enrich the work, allowing better access to drug information and to libraries, research facilities, and academic and educational activities. Possible alternative sites include a facility within or adjacent to a medical or pharmacy association or a relevant governmental agency (such as the ministry of health, drug regulatory authority, drug approval unit, or quality control laboratory).

A secure space of approximately 32 square meters in one or two rooms allows for office work space, storage of references, placement of communications equipment, and space for visitors to use the DIC's resources. It may be

To be successful, a DIC requires a stable location and environment, a philosophical commitment to providing needed drug information, physical space to house the center, basic information references, staff, equipment to support information access and dissemination, and communication equipment.

A drug information center and a poison control center are two different services, although they are often combined. Poison control is usually an emergency service requiring rapid telephone response. The drug information service deals with both urgent requests for therapeutic information and requests that require a more detailed review and synthesis of information.

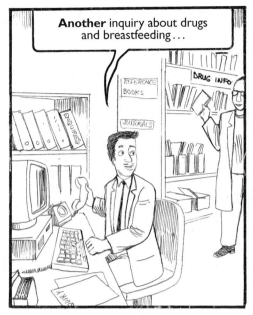
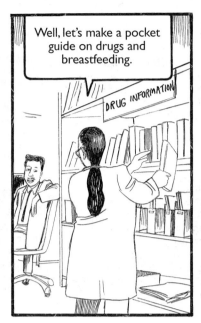
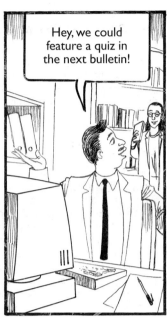

DRUG INFORMATION SHOULD BE RESPONSIVE TO CLIENTS' NEEDS

necessary to involve several institutions in the support of a DIC. In Zimbabwe, for example, there is a mutual agreement that the DIC at the university provides services on behalf of the Ministry of Health. In turn, the government covers some recurrent expenses.

Staffing and Equipment Requirements

A DIC needs dedicated staff who will not be diverted to other activities and duties and who can provide dependable coverage for the center's stated business hours. This translates into one or two full-time employees, including a full-time clinical or hospital pharmacist who specializes in drug and toxicologic information or in clinical pharmacology, toxicology, and drug information. Additional staffing may be required if activities other than information provision are part of the center's mission.

The training and experience of the staff must be clinically based. The user population for any information service is primarily clinicians, and expertise in pharmacotherapy is essential to communicate effectively with them. When an appropriately trained person is not available, every effort should be made to train someone to fill the position. Other relevant professionals—medical, paramedical, or nonmedical—and specialists in information communication techniques may be required to provide specific information and services. When specialists are not available but nonspecialist doctors are, it may be possible to appoint a doctor with some training in clinical pharmacology to head the center.

A typist is typically employed by a DIC, but ideally, the center should have a qualified secretary and clerical staff to help establish, maintain, and update the information system. Arrangements for maintenance and cleaning of the equipment and facilities of the center should also be made.

Proper photocopying, communications, and computer equipment is important in establishing a viable drug information service. A computer, CD-ROM drive, printer, and appropriate software programs are highly desirable, as access to electronic drug and therapy databases is growing rapidly. However, small centers can provide important drug information services using basic texts and other printed references.

Access to fax equipment and a telephone line for fax use are necessary. If computerized access to electronic databases at other sites and to clients (such as hospitals) is anticipated, a modem connection and dedicated telephone line will also be necessary. As services of the DIC increase, two telephone lines may be needed. Electronic communication through networks such as HealthNet and E-DRUG is likely to become more important in the future (see Chapter 46).

If the service operates on a twenty-four-hour basis but the center does not provide facilities for staff to be at the center while they are on call (by rotation), an answering machine is necessary to provide the name and telephone number of the consultant on call. A suitcase or other portable container can be used to carry the basic literature when DIC personnel are on call.

Figure 30.3 Basic References for a Drug Information Library

Latest editions of:

American Medical Association (AMA) drug evaluations
American Hospital Formulary Service (AHFS) drug information
British National Formulary
Drug availability reference (specific for the country or region)
Ellenhorn and Barceloux, *Medical Toxicology: Diagnosis and Treatment of Human Poisoning*, or another clinical toxicology or poisoning text
Goodman and Gilman, *The Pharmacological Basis of Therapeutics*, or another basic pharmacology text
Gosselin, Smith, and Hodge, *Clinical Toxicology of Commercial Products*
Index Nominum: international drug directory
Martindale: The Extra Pharmacopoeia
National formulary or essential drugs list
Price reference (specific for the country or region)
Textbook of internal medicine (such as Harrison's *Principles of Internal Medicine* or the *Oxford Textbook of Medicine*)
Tropical medicine reference (in countries where appropriate)
United States Pharmacopeia–Drug Information (USP–DI)

Basic Information Resources

The latest editions of the textbooks listed in Figure 30.3 could form the core of a basic library for a DIC, along with journals and newsletters (see Annex 30.1), WHO materials, and computer databases. Although the most flexible and efficient of these resources are the computer databases, cost may limit their availability. Print resources, if kept up-to-date, can adequately cover basic information needs; some of them can be obtained free of charge from WHO (see Figure 30.4). The *Essential Drugs Monitor*, produced by WHO/DAP, provides a regular review of publications related to drug use.

Although subscriptions to medical and pharmacy journals and newsletters are expensive (the equivalent of a year's salary in some countries), some basic subscriptions should be considered if the funds are available. Because acquiring and updating information is costly, establishing a link to a medical library is very important. The addresses of organizations that produce widely accepted drug newsletters or bulletins, which are inexpensive and useful sources of information, can be obtained from the International Society of Drug Bulletins (ISDB). See Box 30.4 and the *Essential Drugs Monitor*, no. 19 (1995).

Electronic databases that are available on CD-ROM are becoming essential resources for well-equipped DICs. Databases that should be considered include

- Medline on CD-ROM;
- British National Formulary;
- DrugDex;
- Poisindex;

Figure 30.4 WHO Basic Information Resources

WHO Pharmaceutical Newsletter
WHO Drug Information
Essential Drugs Monitor
WHO Model Prescribing Information
WHO Technical Report Series

- USP Drug Information;
- Martindale: The Extra Pharmacopoeia;
- AHFS Drug Information;
- International Pharmaceutical Abstracts;
- Embase;
- Iowa Drug Information Service (also available on microfiche, which is less user-friendly but more complete).

Many donors and organizations such as the United States Pharmacopeia (USP) and the British National Formulary (BNF) are seeking ways of making information available at a reasonable cost (see Annex 30.2).

≡ 30.4 Managing a Drug Information Center

A DIC should provide a variety of services, from responding to patients' and doctors' queries to proactive efforts such as publishing newsletters or drug bulletins, participating in clinical activities, and organizing formulary and treatment guideline committees (see Country Study 30.1). DIC staff are also likely to be involved in training health professionals and regularly evaluating the performance of the center's staff. Although DICs tend to be small units, it is important that each one have a well-developed annual plan.

Proactive Outreach

Health care professionals in both the public and private sectors often have little time or funds to spend on drug information resources. A DIC can fill this gap, but the service must be effectively marketed.

Drug information professionals need to work to build credibility and improve perceptions of their accessibility and value to health care. This can be done by

- building alliances with the most influential clinicians, providing them with particular information they request and involving them as consultants and reviewers;
- ensuring that they are readily accessible by telephone or in person;
- making an extra effort to find answers for clinicians who have raised unusual drug-related questions;
- participating in national essential drugs list (EDL)

Country Study 30.1 Building from the Basics: A New Drug Information Service in Nepal

A drug information unit (DIU) was recently established within Tribhuvan University Teaching Hospital in Nepal to provide independent drug information to hospital staff and to teachers and students at Nepal's Institute of Medicine. The DIU is run by two clinical pharmacologists and one pharmacist. It is located in an easily accessible area within the main hospital building, close to the hospital library.

Drug-related questions may be presented to the DIU by telephone, in person, or in written form. A standard record of each question is kept for future reference. Questions put to the DIU during its first three months came from all major departments. The most frequently asked questions, in decreasing order, concerned drug indications, adverse drug reactions, drug use in pregnancy, and drug dosage. Answers were provided verbally or in writing.

In addition to its query-answering service, the DIU publishes the bimonthly *Drug and Therapeutics Letter*, with brief reviews on drug and therapeutics topics. The whole bulletin can be read in fifteen minutes. It is distributed to doctors and postgraduate students and to other hospitals in Kathmandu, and it is also displayed in the wards and the library. The hospital pays all production and distribution costs; there is no drug company sponsorship or advertising.

For consumers, the DIU produced a wall poster in Nepali on basic dos and don'ts about medicines, which was posted throughout the hospital. DIU staff are also involved in the development of the hospital formulary.

The most frequently used reference in the DIU is *Martindale: The Extra Pharmacopoeia*. Other frequently used books include the *British National Formulary*, Goodman and Gilman's *The Pharmacological Basis of Therapeutics*, and Harrison's *Principles of Internal Medicine*. Medline searches are done in some cases.

The USAID-supported Rational Pharmaceutical Management Project provided reference books, a computer and printer, and the USP–DI database to start the center. The DIU hopes to acquire more books, journals, databases, computers, and other equipment over time.

Source: Annual report 1995.

committees, hospital drug committees, and standard treatment guidelines (STG) committees;

► preparing short, problem-oriented, practical bulletins on drug use problems specific to the country, district, or hospital;

► making patient rounds with doctors and other clinical staff;

► providing in-service training to health facility staff;

► making short presentations to outpatient groups;

► making presentations to community organizations.

Drug Bulletins

The development, production, and dissemination of newsletters or drug bulletins that address relevant drug information issues often help develop the market for a DIC. These periodicals should promote rational drug therapy and appear at regular intervals, ranging from weekly to quarterly, depending on their purpose and on the capacity of the DIC. Drug bulletins should provide impartial assessments of drugs and practical recommendations, based on a comparison of treatment alternatives and on the consensus of the main specialists in the field.

Drug bulletins are more likely to be effective if they comply with the following principles (see Figure 30.5):

Understand the reasons for prescribing behavior: As mentioned in Chapter 31, providing information alone does not change undesirable behavior. Understanding the reasons for the behavior is a necessary first step to developing appropriate messages.

Be oriented toward decisions and actions: Prescribers need information that is immediately useful in their daily work.

Emphasize and repeat only a few key messages: If too many ideas are brought up in the bulletin, none will be absorbed. A few messages that are the focus of the bulletin and are repeated are more likely to be retained.

Figure 30.5 Example of a Credible Drug Bulletin

Use of color (red in original)

DRUG INFORMATION PROGRAM

Beth Israel Hospital
330 Brookline Ave.
Boston, MA 02215
(617) 735-4255

Harvard Medical School
643 Huntington Ave.
Boston, MA 02115
(617) 732-1840

PHARMACOKINETICS IN DAILY PRACTICE (third in a series)

Headline

ORAL METRONIDAZOLE:
A First Consideration
in Anaerobic Infections

Oriented to action

Beth Israel Hospital

Credible sources

Harvard Medical School

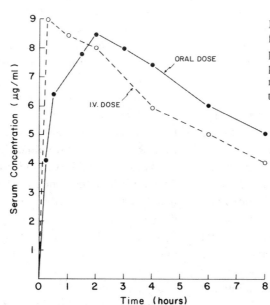

Metronidazole may well be the drug of first choice in the treatment of many patients with anaerobic infections. Surprisingly, the oral form of this agent reaches serum levels quite comparable to those achieved with intravenous use.

Repetition

Attractive graphics

Oral metronidazole achieved the same serum levels as the intravenous preparation when 500mg was administered via each route in a crossover study. Data from Mattila et al.[1]

Well-referenced authority

Oral versus intravenous use
Unlike most commonly used systemic antibiotics, **metronidazole is almost completely absorbed when given orally.** As a result, comparable serum levels are attained with either oral or intravenous therapy using the same dose and interval (see graph).[7] Patients with a variety of serious anaerobic infections, including intra-abdominal abscess, peritonitis, endomyometritis, and pelvic abscess have been successfully treated by the oral route with metronidazole.[8,10] **Intravenous therapy offers no advantage in patients able to take and absorb oral medication.** Patients begun on intravenous metronidazole because of impaired g.i. function may be switched to the oral form of the drug as soon as their clinical status permits feeding.

Brief and simple text

Capture attention with headlines and visually appealing illus-trations: An effective bulletin grabs the reader's attention with attractive graphics that emphasize key messages.

Keep text brief and simple: Although readers of the bulletin may be well educated and knowledgeable, a bulletin should provide immediately accessible information.

Reference the best research and have respectable sponsorship: The bulletin should be affiliated with a credible organization or institution such as the medical society or medical school. Key messages in each issue should be supported by a few well-chosen and respected references. It is better to have three references to the *Lancet, New England Journal of Medicine, British Medical Journal,* or *Journal of the American Medical Association* than twenty references to unpublished reports.

Be relevant: Materials in the bulletin should relate to clinical issues that affect the target audience and should discuss drugs that are available in the audience's country or health system.

The ISDB (see Box 30.4) produces a regular newsletter, organizes annual courses for international editors of bulletins and newsletters, and provides a forum for the exchange of high-quality information and ideas related to promoting effective dissemination of information.

Training

Training in the management of a drug information center or service is necessary for key personnel, as is training on drug information retrieval, literature evaluation, publications development, and sustainability planning and funding. A large drug information service should ideally have a career structure similar to those of academic or educational institutions. All staff members should have the opportunity for additional training and advancement within their own capabilities. When appropriate, professional staff should be encouraged to undertake relevant research activities. Recommendations on education and training requirements for establishing a center in a developing country have been published by the Drugs and Toxicology Information Service (DATIS) in Zimbabwe (Kasilo and Nhachi 1993).

Evaluation

Ongoing monitoring and evaluation is particularly important for services like a DIC, where resources are limited and it is essential to get the most out of the available funding. Monitoring should be built in from the start and document the questions asked, responses provided, references used, complaints and compliments received, timing of

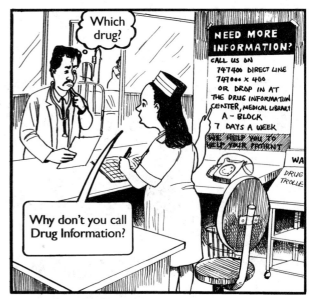

A DRUG INFORMATION SERVICE MUST BE ADVERTISED TO POTENTIAL USERS

responses, and services provided (such as new drug evaluations). The queries should be analyzed, and the results documented in the annual report. In addition, periodic input from users of the drug information service should be sought through personal contacts, questionnaires, or focus groups.

This information can help the center's manager make good decisions about future programs and budgeting. For example, if a certain inquiry has been made several times by different individuals, the question may be a good topic for an article in the drug information newsletter or bulletin. If the same complaint about DIC service is made repeatedly, perhaps a review of the center's operations is in order. If a certain textbook or database is not frequently used, perhaps it should be replaced by another one.

Sources of Help

Funding for the establishment of a DIC may come from government resources, donors supporting essential drugs projects, professional associations, university or other training programs, nongovernmental organizations, or a coalition of several of these groups.

A number of national and international professional organizations have programs that focus on providing help to developing countries. For example, the Pharmacy Information Section of the International Pharmaceutical Federation attempts to link DICs in developed countries with counterparts in developing countries. Such collaboration between centers in developing and developed countries is very valuable, enabling the exchange of information and staff for teaching and training. The ISDB is also a useful channel for support.

Funding Issues

The source of funding may affect how the unit functions. No matter how it is financed, the integrity of the unit is paramount. No special interests should be able to influence what information is or is not given out.

It may be possible to obtain initial capital funding from the sources listed above. These organizations often provide funds for the purchase of items such as computers, furniture, or photocopiers. For sustainability, it is wise to purchase a two- or three-year maintenance contract for such equipment as part of the initial capital costs.

Obtaining an adequate level of recurrent funding, particularly for staff salaries and journal or CD-ROM subscriptions, can be more difficult. Therefore, while the center is being established, every effort should be made to secure recurrent funding. For example, if a donor provides the start-up capital, the government may be persuaded to commit funding for a full-time pharmacist at the center. If there is a hospital located near the center, it could be a source for long-term funding. In some countries, it is possible to implement user fees; this should be done gradually, after the DIC has been accepted by users.

Drug companies may be willing to support such a center, but this should be considered cautiously. If drug information critical of a sponsoring company's product is disseminated, support may be withdrawn. In general, funding from a drug company should be used for discrete projects, such as replacement of a photocopier.

Drug information professionals in developing countries inevitably become fund-raisers to maintain activities. For example, in Cameroon, a consortium of donors was mobilized to share support for the drug bulletin.

Problems and Possible Solutions

Service from DICs can be hampered by numerous problems, ranging from lack of readily available information and adequate communication systems to financial and human resource limitations and lack of acceptance or interest on the part of the community or policy-makers. Here are suggestions for dealing with these difficulties.

Incomplete Sources of Readily Available Information. The time lag before new information becomes widely available is a weakness that is difficult to overcome. Combining sources and linking with other reference centers by fax or E-mail can help.

Lack of Acceptance of the DIC as a Source of Reliable and Relevant Information. Involving influential clinicians in the development and review of outreach materials and providing prompt, efficient, and relevant responses to queries will improve users' perceptions.

Limitations in Financial and Human Resources. Planning for financial sustainability must start with the initiation of drug information services. External support may be available, but only for the start-up period. Efforts can be made to lobby for basic operating expenditures through the ministry of health's recurrent budget. Local professional associations and universities may also be approached for support.

Inadequate Communication Systems, Especially in Developing Countries. Communication limitations hamper the establishment of information networks in many countries, but these systems are improving rapidly worldwide. Linking to HealthNet (see Chapter 46) may improve communications capacity.

Lack of Political Will on the Part of Policy-Makers to Establish Drug Information Centers. Inviting policy-makers to visit the centers and lobbying for recognition of the value of information can be helpful, particularly as real examples of information failures can be used to demonstrate the need.

Although these kinds of problems are common, so is the realization of the need for DICs in all countries. As users in more countries become accustomed to the benefits of DICs, the demand for such services will grow and generate increased interest in establishing and supporting them. ∎

≡ Assessment Guide

Drug Information Center

► Is there a drug information unit or center? If so, how is it funded and staffed?

► Does the drug information unit or center (or another independent body) provide regular information on drugs to prescribers and dispensers?

► How many issues of independent drug bulletins are published each year?

► What percentage of prescribers receives copies of independent drug bulletins?

► What level of financial support did the drug information center receive?

► How many queries did the drug information center respond to in the past year?

► What current information resources are available? Which are most frequently used?

Local Drug Information Resources

► Has a national essential drugs list or formulary been officially adopted and distributed country-wide?

► Is there a national publication (formulary bulletin or manual), revised within the past five years, that provides objective information on drugs?

► Is there a national therapeutic guide with standardized treatments for common diseases?

► What percentage of advertisements violates regulations on the ethical promotion of drugs, and how many sanctions have been implemented?

► What percentage of prescribers has direct access to a (national) drug formulary?

≡ **References and Further Readings**

★ = Key readings.

Association Mieux Prescrire. *Prescrire international* (quarterly newsletter). Paris: Association Mieux Prescrire (Boîte Postale 459, 75527 Paris Cedex 11, France).

Consumers' Association. *Drug and therapeutics bulletin* (fortnightly newsletter). London: Consumers' Association (14 Buckingham Street, London WC2N 6DS, England).

Gong, S. D., M. Millanes, and K. B. van Repir. 1992. Drug information pharmacists at health care facilities, universities, and pharmaceutical companies. *American Journal of Hospital Pharmacy* 49:1121–30.

Herxheimer, A. 1991. Drug bulletins are part of the scientific literature. *Current Contents Life Sciences* 34:4–9.

Herxheimer, A., C. S. Lundberg, and B. Westerholm. 1993. Advertisements for medicines in leading medical journals in 18 countries: A 12-month survey of information content and standards. *International Journal of Health Services* 23:161–72.

★ Kasilo, O. M. J., and C. F. B. Nhachi. 1993. Recommendations on education and training requirements for establishing a drug and toxicology information center in a developing country. *Journal of Clinical Pharmacy and Therapeutics* 18:365–69.

Ohman, B., H. Lyrvall, T. C. Alvan, and F. Sjoquist. 1992. Clinical pharmacology and the provision of drug information. *European Journal of Chemical Pharmacology* 42:563–68.

★ Riegelman, R. 1996. *Studying a study and testing a test: How to read the medical literature.* 3d ed. Boston: Little Brown.

USP (United States Pharmacopeia). 1996a. USP–DI Vol. 1. *Drug information for the health care professional.* Rockville, Md.: United States Pharmacopeial Convention.

USP (United States Pharmacopeia). 1996b. USP–DI Vol. 2. *Advice for the patient: Drug information in lay language.* Rockville, Md.: United States Pharmacopeial Convention.

WHO (World Health Organization). 1992a. Drug information centers. *WHO drug information* 6:106.

WHO (World Health Organization). 1992b. *Provision and dissemination of drug information: Report of a consultative group.* WHO/DMP/PROV/93. Geneva: WHO.

WHO/DAP (World Health Organization/Action Programme on Essential Drugs). 1994a. *Essential Drugs Monitor,* no. 17. Geneva: WHO.

WHO/DAP (World Health Organization/Action Programme on Essential Drugs). 1994b. *Guide to good prescribing.* WHO/DAP/94.11. Geneva: WHO/DAP.

WHO/DAP (World Health Organization/Action Programme on Essential Drugs). 1995a. *Essential Drugs Monitor,* no. 19. Geneva: WHO.

WHO/DAP (World Health Organization/Action Programme on Essential Drugs). 1995b. *How to set up a drug information centre in a developing country.* Geneva: WHO/DAP.

Annex 30.1 Primary Information Sources

Medical and Therapeutic Journals
Annals of Internal Medicine
British Medical Journal
Journal of the American Medical Association
Lancet
New England Journal of Medicine

**Drug and Toxicology Information and
Pharmacology Journals**
British Journal of Clinical Pharmacology
Clinical Pharmacology and Therapeutics
European Journal of Clinical Pharmacology
Human and Experimental Toxicology
Journal of Toxicology and Clinical Toxicology
Medical Toxicology and Adverse Drug Experience

Pharmacy Journals
American Journal of Hospital Pharmacy
Annals of Pharmacotherapy
Clinical Pharmacy
DICP—Annals of Pharmacotherapy
Journal of Clinical and Hospital Pharmacy
Journal of Clinical Pharmacy and Therapeutics
Pharmaceutical Journal UK

Journals in Specific Areas
American Journal of Emergency Medicine
Annals of Emergency Medicine
British Journal of Obstetrics and Gynaecology
Critical Care Medicine
Journal of Antimicrobials and Chemotherapy
Journal of Infectious Diseases
Journal of Paediatrics and Child Health

Essential Drugs Lists and Therapeutic Formularies
British National Formulary, updated every six months
Essential Drugs List for Zimbabwe, Ministry of Health,
  Republic of Zimbabwe (1994)
The WHO Model Lists of Essential Drugs: The Use and
  Selection of Drugs. Technical Report Series 615, 641, 722,
  770, 850 (1977, 1979, 1983, 1985, 1988, 1992, 1995), World
Health Organization, Geneva
WHO Model Prescribing Information: Drugs Used in
  Anesthesia, Parasitic Diseases, Mycobacterial Diseases,
  Sexually Transmitted Diseases, Skin Diseases

Annex 30.2 Useful Addresses

Royal Pharmaceutical Society of Great Britain
1 Lambeth High Street
London SE1 1JN, England

United States Pharmacopeial Convention, Inc.
12601 Twinbrook Parkway
Rockville, Md. 20852, US

Victorian Medical Postgraduate Foundation, Inc.
Chelsea House, 3d floor
55 Flemington Road
North Melbourne VIC 305, Australia

World Health Organization
Action Programme on Essential Drugs
Publications Office
1211 Geneva 27, Switzerland

Part I Introduction	Part II Policy and Legal Framework	**Part III** **Drug Management Cycle**	Part IV Management Support Systems

A Selection
B Procurement
C Distribution

D Use ▶

28 Managing for Rational Drug Use
29 Investigating Drug Use
30 Drug and Therapeutics Information
31 Promoting Rational Prescribing
32 Ensuring Good Dispensing Practices
33 Encouraging Appropriate Drug Use by
the Public and Patients

Chapter 31
Promoting Rational Prescribing

≡ Summary

The ultimate goals of studying and intervening in drug use practices include

- ▸ *improvement of quality of health care through effective and safe use of pharmaceuticals;*
- ▸ *improvement of cost effectiveness of health care through economic and efficient use of pharmaceuticals.*

Before attempting to intervene to change drug use practices, underlying reasons for problem behaviors must be understood. Interdisciplinary collaboration involving health and social science experts is of utmost importance in this task.

Strategies to improve rational prescribing can be characterized as educational, managerial, and regulatory.

Educational strategies include

- ▸ *training of prescribers (formal and continuing education, supervisory visits, group lectures, seminars, workshops);*
- ▸ *printed materials (clinical literature and newsletters, treatment guidelines, drug formularies, flyers, leaflets);*
- ▸ *approaches based on face-to-face contact (educational outreach, patient education, influencing opinion leaders).*

Managerial strategies include

- ▸ *approaches to selection, procurement, and distribution (limited procurement lists, drug utilization review and feedback, hospital and regional drug committees, cost information);*

- ▸ *prescribing and dispensing approaches (structured drug order forms, standard diagnostic and treatment guidelines, course-of-therapy packaging);*
- ▸ *financing (price setting, capitation-based budgeting).*

Regulatory strategies include

- ▸ *drug registration;*
- ▸ *limited drug lists;*
- ▸ *prescribing restrictions;*
- ▸ *dispensing restrictions.*

An intervention should be focused on a specific problem behavior and targeted at the facilities or people that have the greatest need for improvement.

Interventions should be carefully selected with regard to efficacy, feasibility for implementation in the existing system, and cost. Before wide-scale implementation of an intervention, it is imperative to evaluate its effectiveness and cost in the existing health setting.

Programs to ensure rational use of drugs should be an integral part of health and medical care services. The responsibility for promoting rational use of drugs belongs to decision-makers, administrators, and clinicians. It is also the responsibility of health care professionals, consumers, educators, and pharmaceutical companies.

≡ 31.1 Improving Prescribing: A Conceptual Framework

Inappropriate prescribing is a manifestation of irrational drug use behavior when drugs are not prescribed in accordance with guidelines based on scientific evidence to ensure safe, effective, and economic use. The underlying reasons for such practices on the part of prescribers and consumers need to be understood and addressed in any intervention.

Qualitative methods of research are useful in understanding why inappropriate prescribing behaviors occur (see Chapter 29). This approach makes it possible to design interventions relevant to a particular situation that form part of a systematic cycle directed at improving the quality of patient care. Most of the strategies for improving prescribing practices are mutually supportive. A comprehensive policy should aim at influencing prescribing behavior at all levels of the system, focusing on the priority problems and targeting the prescribers involved.

The first step in improving prescribing practices is to identify the nature and scope of the problem. This may be

done through a prescription survey, review of drug management data, or observation of a particular practice or event. If further investigation confirms that the observed behavior is a significant problem in the health system, an effort should be made to define the underlying causes clearly. This process is described in Chapter 29. A package of interventions is then planned, focused on specific problems and targeting specific actors: prescriber, patient, and community. Inputs from the target audience are important when formulating the package of interventions, as different sets of interventions may be applied to address inappropriate prescribing practices and prevent them from recurring. Each intervention must be monitored and evaluated to assess its impact. Evaluation of impact needs to be directed at the specific prescribing pattern or prescribing behavior that the intervention is designed to affect. Clearly ineffective interventions can be dropped, and those that are partially effective can be revised to improve their efficacy. Effective interventions can then be incorporated and, if required, replicated on a wider scale in the health care system. The complete cycle of drug use

Country Study 31.1 Investigating a Problem in Malaria Treatment in Ghana

In Ghana, patients who were given chloroquine for malaria were not responding to treatment. The community referred to this as "Go Slow." When this problem came to the notice of the health authorities, it became important to establish whether there was chloroquine-resistant malaria in the country. It was discovered that a majority of the patients had not received adequate treatment for their malaria. Most had received a single injection of chloroquine daily for three days. A formal questionnaire was administered, and a prescription study was conducted at selected health facilities. This study revealed that an average of 92 percent of patients with malaria attending health centers were given injections. Children were being overtreated, whereas adults were undertreated according to the standard treatment guidelines of the Ministry of Health, despite the fact that the questionnaire showed that prescribers had adequate knowledge of malaria treatment.

Focus group discussions were held with the prescribers to ascertain why their practice differed from their knowledge. Their responses indicated that the problem was related to factors in the health system (lack of supervision, peer influence), to patient factors (self-medication, patient demand for a particular form of treatment), and to sociocultural factors (the way the community views prescribers, the community's perception of the power of injections, the presence of quack doctors, and the ready availability of drugs without prescription). The proposed interventions included educating the prescribers and the community on the appropriate use of antimalarial drugs.

Figure 31.1 Intervention Strategies to Improve Drug Use

Educational Strategies

Training of Prescribers
- ▶ formal education (preservice)
- ▶ continuing education (in-service)
- ▶ supervisory visits
- ▶ group lectures, seminars, and workshops

Printed Materials
- ▶ clinical literature and newsletters
- ▶ treatment guidelines and drug formularies
- ▶ illustrated materials (flyers, leaflets)

Approaches Based on Face-to-Face Contact
- ▶ educational outreach
- ▶ patient education
- ▶ influencing opinion leaders

Managerial Strategies

Selection, Procurement, and Distribution
- ▶ limited procurement lists
- ▶ drug utilization review and feedback
- ▶ hospital and regional drug committees
- ▶ cost information

Prescribing and Dispensing Approaches
- ▶ structured drug order forms
- ▶ standard diagnostic and treatment guidelines
- ▶ course-of-therapy packaging

Financing
- ▶ price setting
- ▶ capitation-based budgeting

Regulatory Strategies
- ▶ drug registration
- ▶ limited drug lists
- ▶ prescribing restrictions
- ▶ dispensing restrictions

Source: Adapted from Quick et al. 1991.

interventions was described in Chapter 29, and the required actions for each step are depicted in Figure 29.1. An example from Ghana dealing with a drug use problem in malaria treatment is described in Country Study 31.1.

≡ 31.2 Characterizing Interventions

A wide range of interventions is available to address irrational prescribing (see Figure 31.1). These can be categorized as preventive or curative. Preventive approaches ensure that the prescriber starts off prescribing in an appropriate manner. Curative interventions attempt to reverse a pattern of irrational prescribing. As is often true in medicine, it is far easier to prevent than to cure prescribing problems.

Interventions can be characterized as:

Educational: Prescribers are *persuaded* by providing information or knowledge to them. These strategies may be implemented in the form of face-to-face education or training, seminars, and provision of written materials. A single-shot educational intervention without follow-up and monitoring is usually least effective and the impact, if any, is not sustainable.

Managerial: Prescribers are *guided* in the decision-making process, through limiting lists for routine procurements, drug utilization review and feedback, supervision and monitoring, provision of treatment guidelines, and monitoring of their use of the guidelines.

Regulatory: Prescribers are *forced* to restrict the decision-making process in prescribing. These strategies include generic policies, prescribing and dispensing limitations, and withdrawal of questionable drugs from the market. These strong strategies are often unpopular with prescribers or consumers and may also bring about unintended effects, such as a change to other inappropriate prescribing practices.

Many interventions have a limited impact over time, and although temporary improvement may occur, prescribers may revert to their previous behavior if the intervention is not followed up. When interventions of different types are combined, the impact is likely to be synergistically increased.

Irrational prescribing is a universal problem. Considerable experience indicates which interventions are effective in high-income countries and in particular public health care systems, but these interventions cannot always be transferred to other settings. Therefore, it is important that a range of interventions be considered. Those that succeed in one country may not succeed elsewhere. Health care organizations, local communication channels, level of education, and other factors all influence the effectiveness of specific strategies in specific environments.

≡ 31.3 Focus and Target of Interventions

For an intervention to be effective, it needs to be focused to achieve a specific goal and targeted at those prescribers who have a particular prescribing problem. For example, in a training intervention, a general lecture on pharmacology is unlikely to be effective in changing prescribing. A clearly focused presentation on the correct treatment of simple diarrhea—encouraging oral rehydration solution (ORS) and discouraging antidiarrheals, antibiotics, and injections—is far more likely to achieve the desired results.

Quantitative surveys frequently find that there is considerable variation among facilities. For example, a survey in Tanzania found that antibiotic use varied between 20 and 70 percent (Figure 31.2). Most facilities fell within the range of 20 to 40 percent. Only three facilities showed over 50 percent antibiotic use, and seven had over 40 percent use. These high users would be the facilities to be targeted for any intervention. Both the potential impact and the cost effectiveness of the intervention would be greater in these facilities.

≡ 31.4 Educational Interventions

Educational interventions are the most common and are often disappointing in their limited impact. Although the basic training of prescribers is essential for promoting rational use of drugs, educational components often need to be combined with managerial and regulatory interventions. See Chapter 48 for discussion of various types of training programs.

Training of Prescribers

Prescribers make many decisions concerning drug use. Their training occurs in formal and informal ways throughout their careers.

Formal Education (Preservice). In general, prescribers are either doctors or trained paramedical staff. The training of these two groups differs in content and approach. Doctors control the use of scarce drug resources not only through

Figure 31.2 Facility-Specific Percentage of Patients Receiving Antibiotics

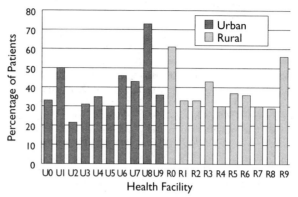

Source: WHO/DAP 1993.

their own prescribing practices but also through their influence as instructors, supervisors, and trendsetters for the often larger force of paramedics. Thus, sound training of doctors in good prescribing practices can have a significant effect on the rational use of drugs.

The curricula of most health personnel training institutions contain segments that deal with drug treatment. Because prescribing is often not taught in these curricula, students often learn prescribing from what they see during clinical "model" practices. For doctors and paramedical personnel, training on drugs and how to use them should cover:

Basic pharmacology: Principal mechanisms of drug action, metabolism, absorption, distribution, and elimination. In basic pharmacology, students gain knowledge about interactions between drugs and living systems at the theoretical level.

Clinical pharmacology: Study of the different classes of drugs with regard to clinical efficacy, risks, clinical pharmacokinetics, drug-drug interactions, drug-disease interactions, drug-genetics interactions, the concept of clinical trials, and pharmacoeconomics. In clinical pharmacology, students learn how to use drugs properly and rationally at a more practical level.

Therapeutics: The use of drugs to treat disease. Therapeutics is the practical application of basic and clinical pharmacology. It has traditionally received less attention than pharmacology in prescribers' formal education.

In the last decade, a number of educational programs have been developed to improve the teaching of pharmacotherapy. The World Health Organization (WHO) Action Programme on Essential Drugs has developed a manual (WHO/DAP 1994) for undergraduate medical students on the principles of rational prescribing, intended for use in developed and developing countries. This *Guide to Good Prescribing* presents students with a normative model for pharmacotherapeutic reasoning. First, the students are taught to generate a standard pharmacotherapeutic approach to common disorders, resulting in a set of first-choice drugs, called "P(ersonal)-drugs." In the course of developing their P-drugs, the students are taught to consult existing national and international treatment guidelines, national formularies, pharmacology textbooks, and any other source of drug information. Then they are shown how to apply this set of P-drugs to specific patient problems using a six-step problem-solving routine: (1) define the patient problem; (2) specify the therapeutic objective; (3) verify the suitability of your P-drug; (4) write a prescription; (5) inform and instruct the patient; and (6) monitor and/or stop the treatment.

The rationale behind this approach is that at some time in the course of their studies or early in their careers, medical students develop a set of drugs that they will use regu-

larly from then on. However, this choice is often made on irrational grounds, such as the prescribing behavior of their clinical teachers or peers, without really considering the alternatives or knowing how to choose among them. The manual not only helps students select P-drugs in a rational way but also teaches them to consult, understand, and use existing treatment guidelines in an intelligent way. For example, it teaches the students how to verify, for each individual patient, whether their P-drug is the most appropriate choice in this individual case and, if necessary, how to adapt the drug, dosage form, dosage schedule, or duration of treatment. The training has been field-tested and evaluated in seven medical schools, with a proven impact on the students (Country Study 31.2).

In addition to the safety and efficacy of a drug, other important considerations for students include the use of generic names and attention to cost, supply logistics, and the effects of transportation, storage, and drug quality on the availability and stability of drugs.

Experience shows that students usually learn about prescribing from their clinical tutors. The value of medical faculty trained in clinical pharmacology should not be underestimated. However, the task of incorporating and implementing the teaching of rational drug use into the curricula is not solely the responsibility of clinical pharmacologists. This should become the concern and responsibility of staff from various disciplines involved in training, particularly clinicians.

In addition to giving increased attention to clinical pharmacology, medical faculties should increase their students' awareness of the importance of pursuing drug information throughout their clinical training and practice. As part of their training in clinical pharmacology and therapeutics in Yogyakarta, Indonesia, medical students also learn to critically assess drug information and advertisements as well as reports of clinical trials published in a local medical journal. This has proved helpful in improving their knowledge, skills, and critical attitudes.

Paramedical staff are commonly the first point of contact for patients in most rural areas and in some health facilities in urban areas. Improper use of medicines by these health workers can be dangerous and wasteful, whereas prompt and appropriate use of medicines can save lives and prevent patients from becoming more debilitated. Paramedics and nurses in a number of developing countries are not legally allowed to prescribe. In reality, however, they see and prescribe for the majority of patients arriving at the health centers. No formal continuing education for paramedics can be developed, because legally, paramedics are not meant to be formal prescribers.

Figure 31.3 Excerpt from a Standard Treatment Manual

	10. Gastrointestinal Conditions	83
Management		
	ADULTS	CHILDREN
Ascaris Lumbricoides (roundworms)	Levamisole 2.5 mg/kg as a single dose OR Mebendazole 100 mg BD x 3 days OR Albendazole 400 mg STAT	Levamisole 2.5 mg/kg as a single dose OR Mebendazole 100 mg BD x 3 days OR Albendazole 200 mg STAT for children under 2 yrs
Hookworm	Levamisole 2.5 mg/kg as a single dose OR Mebendazole 100 mg BD x 3 days OR Albendazole 400 mg STAT	Levamisole 2.5 mg/kg as a single dose OR Mebendazole 100 mg BD x 3 days OR Albendazole 400 mg Albendazole 200 mg STAT for children under 2 yrs + ferrous sulphate
Trichuris Trichiura (whipworms)	Mebendazole 100 mg BD x 3 days Albendazole 400 mg STAT	Mebendazole 100 mg BD x 3 days Albendazole 200 mg STAT for children under 2 yrs
Strongyloides Stercoralis	Albendazole 400 mg BD STAT x 3 days OR Thiabendazole 25 mg/kg x 3 days	Albendazole 400 mg BD STAT x 3 days OR Thiabendazole 25 mg/kg x 3 days
Enterobius Vermicularis (pinworm)	Mebendazole 100 mg BD x 3 days Levamisole 2.5 mg/kg as a single dose REPEAT AFTER 10 days	Mebendazole 100 mg BD x 3 days Levamisole 2.5 mg/kg as a single dose REPEAT AFTER 10 days
Taenia Saginata (beef tapeworm)	Niclosamide 2 gm; 1 gm before breakfast, 1 gm 1 hr after breakfast	Niclosamide 2 gm; 1 gm before breakfast, 1 gm 1 hr after breakfast
HOOKWORM	Anemia develops if iron intake is slow and infection is significant. If patient fails to respond to therapy, consider other cause; for example, blood loss, poor adherence to treatment	

Prevention
Appropriate prevention depends on the particular worm. In general:
• safe water provision
• handwashing and trimming of fingernails
• frequent changing of undergarments and sheets
• use of latrines.

Source: Ministry of Health, Government of Kenya 1994a.

Many countries find it useful to limit paramedics to a specific drug list and provide a pocket drug reference manual based on this list. Medical workers are encouraged to use the manual rather than depend on recall for selecting drugs and drug dosages for all but the most frequently treated conditions. Figure 31.3 illustrates the content and format of a pocket-sized drug reference manual used in Kenya. These workers do, however, need to be taught to diagnose so that they can use the appropriate treatment guidelines.

Formal training in pharmacology and therapeutics provides a sound basis for paramedics to prescribe standard drugs and to understand the uses of new drugs that are added to their drug lists. An example of the curriculum used for such a training program in Tanzania appears in Chapter 48.

Continuing Education (In-service). Once their formal training is completed, prescribers develop their own prescribing practices, which are then influenced by whatever

drug information and commercial pressure they receive, the diagnostic facilities available to them, the expectations of the community, and drug availability. Continuing education provides an opportunity for them to keep informed on changes in the use of drugs.

In some areas, local associations of physicians or auxiliary medical workers have identified their need for continued training in therapeutics and have participated in seminars and other medical meetings designed to keep them up-to-date with current drug information. Government health programs sometimes sponsor presentations for health personnel. In many countries, however, continuing education is not available for most prescribers, including those in teaching hospitals. Even when it does occur, it is often dominated by promotional messages from pharmaceutical companies that sponsor the events and are necessarily biased in favor of their products. Most prescribers are not trained to evaluate such information critically and tend to accept whatever they are told. They

> **Country Study 31.3 Improving the Rational Use of Drugs for Acute Diarrhea in Indonesia: Testing Different Educational Methods for Prescribers**
>
> In many health facilities in Indonesia, most episodes of acute diarrhea are still inappropriately treated with ineffective antimicrobials and antidiarrheals, even though therapy using oral rehydration solution (ORS) has been widely accepted as an effective treatment for acute diarrhea in children.
>
> In an attempt to improve the rational use of drugs in treating acute diarrhea, an innovative strategy of educational intervention was undertaken, employing small group face-to-face training of prescribers at the health center. The goal was to increase the use of ORS and reduce the use of non-rehydration medications. The impact of this approach on prescribing practices was evaluated and compared with a conventional method of educational intervention based on a formal seminar for prescribers and with a control group who received no training. The formal seminar included lectures, handouts, and large group discussions.
>
> The study was carried out in six districts in Yogyakarta, Indonesia, with fifteen health centers randomly selected from each district. Prior to the intervention, focus group discussions involving prescribers and consumers in each district were conducted to investigate the underlying motivations for drug use in acute diarrhea. The findings of this qualitative study were used to develop intervention materials and were specifically addressed during the intervention session.
>
> The small group training was carried out at each health center, utilizing an interactive discussion involving eight to twelve prescribers from the center. A trainer from the district health office, whose routine task was supervision and monitoring of the health centers, led the discussions. These normally lasted for two hours and focused on the appropriate management of children with acute diarrhea. Underlying motivations for inappropriate use of drugs were discussed and addressed.
>
> The prescribing practices for acute diarrhea were collected and evaluated three months before and three months after the interventions. Both large and small group teaching interventions were effective in reducing the use of antimicrobials and antidiarrheals. However, the small group face-to-face training was less costly in terms of implementation and was preferred by the prescribers. Furthermore, it could be implemented in the existing supervision mechanism of the health centers. When the two groups were compared eighteen months after the intervention, the health centers receiving small group interventions had sustained the improvement, but those receiving large group interventions had not.

must also deal with the enticement of gifts and incentives proffered by drug company representatives.

Like their physician counterparts, paramedical staff tend to become more routine in their prescribing habits once they have been practicing for several years, and this may lead to illogical prescribing. Regular teaching and monitoring by senior paramedical staff or medical officers, with attention to the medical workers' prescribing habits, is essential.

Rational prescribing among paramedical staff can be promoted by

▸ requiring them to keep a brief listing of patients seen and diagnoses made;
▸ devising and making available a limited list of specific drugs with which paramedics must be familiar;
▸ ensuring regular monitoring and supervision, with frequent on-site refresher training.

Supervisory Visits. Personal supervision and case review are often difficult or impossible. Therefore, in many programs, if paramedical staff keep a list of patients seen, with diagnoses and treatments prescribed, their prescribing habits can be quickly reviewed, and suggestions for improved drug therapy can be made. In-service refresher courses and discussion of cases by paramedical staff can be organized locally, using the health center as a base and the visiting doctor as educator. In this way, supervision can be educational and supportive, not punitive.

Group Lectures, Seminars, and Workshops. Lectures, seminars, or workshops given to a relatively large number of people are the most widely practiced activities for continuing education. They may be effective in improving prescribers' knowledge but are likely to be ineffective in changing prescribing behavior. When such seminars are focused on *specific* prescribing behavior, however, improvements can occur. A study in Indonesia (Country Study 31.3) compared large group seminars with on-site small group teaching. Both were found to be effective, but the small group seminars had a longer-term effect.

Printed Materials

Printed materials carrying new information that is immediately relevant to the prescriber may help bring about a change in prescriber behavior. In general, however, printed materials may increase prescriber knowledge but rarely affect actual performance when used alone.

Printed materials are most useful when they are used in combination with other intervention strategies, especially those that involve active interaction between the party providing and the party receiving the information.

Clinical Literature and Newsletters. Many prescribers claim that they obtain information about therapeutics from medical journals. Unfortunately, many journals report research results that may not be directly applicable to daily practice. In addition, journals may overwhelm the prescriber with more information than can be digested, making it difficult to decide about the best prescribing choices.

Medical newsletters, such as *The Medical Letter* or *Drug and Therapeutics Bulletin,* focus on a limited number of topics and provide summarized information in a form that is more immediately useful to the prescriber. Such information often compares and contrasts clinical choices and costs and provides recommendations about "optimal" treatments.

Treatment Guidelines and Drug Formularies. In many countries where an essential drugs list has been developed, treatment norms or guidelines have also been published (see Chapter 11). Such manuals are relatively inexpensive to produce and have several advantages over material from the drug industry and sources from outside the country. They are not biased by commercial interest, include only those preparations available in the country, recommend doses that are appropriate for the local population, and provide special warnings that are relevant to local genetic, environmental, and epidemiological factors.

Consulting physicians and medical school faculty may oppose the preparation and distribution of reference manuals, fearing that they will lead to "cookbook" medicine. This fear seems to be largely unfounded, and physicians in the most prestigious medical schools in developed and developing countries are writing and promoting such handbooks. The Zimbabwe program has been particularly successful in involving all levels of health workers in the development and use of such guidelines (see Country Study 48.3).

Illustrated Materials (Flyers and Leaflets). Commercial drug companies frequently use short, colorful, attractively printed materials to convey promotional messages. These materials usually contain only one or two ideas that are repeated in different ways using text, drawings, tables, and charts. This type of material is often used in conjunction with face-to-face educational outreach or focused meetings.

Approaches Based on Face-to-Face Contact

The most effective means of changing behavior has consistently been face-to-face contact. The drug industry uses this method through its representatives because it works!

Educational Outreach. One of the methods found to be effective in improving prescribing practices after completion of training is targeted outreach education. The efficacy of this approach has been demonstrated by the marketing of pharmaceutical companies, whose salespeople promote their products on a one-to-one basis to carefully targeted prescribers.

In this method, principles of communications theory and behavioral science are combined with conventional educational techniques to provide information to physicians about drugs that are often used inappropriately and to promote their replacement with more therapeutic alternatives. This may be done by trained educators or opinion leaders and can be incorporated into the existing supervision system of health care services.

Principles of educational outreach include

► focusing on specific problems and targeting the audience of prescribers;
► addressing the underlying causes of the prescribing problems: misleading beliefs, poor knowledge, false perceptions;
► allowing an interactive discussion and involving the targeted audience;
► using concise and authoritative materials based on credible scientific information;
► giving sufficient attention to solving practical problems encountered by prescribers in real settings.

The face-to-face approach should focus on a specific problem. One such intervention in the United States aimed to reduce the use of an oral cephalosporin, cerebral and peripheral vasodilators, and propoxyphene. The interventions consisted of face-to-face education plus printed materials; printed materials only; and a control group. The group receiving face-to-face education reduced its use of the targeted drugs. This change was maintained for at least nine months after the beginning of the intervention. In Indonesia, face-to-face education given to a small group of prescribers at health centers has been effective in both improving the appropriate use of drugs in acute diarrhea and reducing the use of nonrehydration medications such as antimicrobials and antidiarrheals (see Country Study 31.3).

Patient Education. Patient or consumer education plays an important role in promoting rational use of drugs. Inappropriate prescribing patterns may derive from the demands or misconceptions of patients, although these demands are often exaggerated by prescribers to justify their prescribing habits.

One way to educate patients about the rational use of drugs is through individual communication during the contact between prescriber and patient. This communication often cannot take place, however, because of the limited time available and the heavy patient load. In health facilities in developing countries, the average patient contact time is often only one to three minutes—too short for effective communication. Another reason may be the

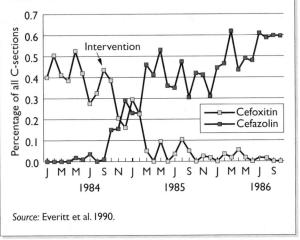
prescriber's unwillingness to communicate with patients or a lack of skill or interest in doing so. Prescribers are often not adequately trained in patient communication or are not sensitive to its importance. In Indonesia (Country Study 31.4), a project has been developed with mothers' groups to educate the community about drugs.

Consumer education is carried out in many countries through mass campaigns via radio, television, or pamphlets and other printed materials (see Chapter 33).

Influencing Opinion Leaders

The attempt to train students in good prescribing practices can be frustrated by the environment in which they learn. For example, if a physician refers to drugs by their brand names during clinical training, the students will copy this practice and any other poor prescribing habits the physician may exhibit. Young doctors who have to prescribe according to the wishes of their senior colleagues can also pick up poor prescribing habits. One way of dealing with this situation is to identify the opinion leaders who influence the prescribing patterns of students and doctors in the establishment. Improving the prescribing practices of these leaders, as illustrated in Country Study 31.5, will indirectly influence those of the younger doctors and students.

≡ 31.5 Managerial Interventions

Managerial interventions frequently require considerable effort to initiate and maintain. However, they can produce a sustained impact with small risk of adverse or unexpected consequences.

Selection, Procurement, and Distribution

Drug use can be influenced by aspects of drug management such as selection, procurement, and distribution. When the people responsible for these activities are consulted and informed, they are likely to cooperate in supporting rational prescribing.

Limited Procurement List

The most common managerial intervention is selecting a limited list of drugs that will be routinely purchased. Other drugs may be made available but require special approval (see Chapters 10 and 13).

Drug Utilization Review and Feedback

Drug utilization review (DUR) is a tool to identify problems in the medication use process: drug prescribing, dispensing, administration, and monitoring. As problems are identified, strategies are developed and implemented to improve the use of drugs. If actions are successful, the result will be improved patient care and more efficient use of resources.

The approach to developing a program varies, but there are nine important steps to follow:

Step 1: Establish Responsibility for the DUR Process. The pharmacy and therapeutics (P&T) committee (or its equivalent) usually takes responsibility for the DUR program.

Step 2: Establish the Scope for Each Study. A DUR focuses on the areas that show the most potential for improvement. A DUR may study one medication (such as ranitidine), a therapeutic class (H$_2$ antagonists), or a particular age group or diagnosis (patients over 65 years old with duodenal ulcers). DUR might focus on one step in the medication use process, such as prescribing, or include other aspects, such as drug labeling or drug administration. Pharmacists, nurses, and physicians are a major source of suggestions for focusing DUR studies. Formal mechanisms for identifying problem areas include adverse drug reaction reporting, medication error reporting, or ABC and VEN analysis (see Chapter 41). DUR usually focuses on drugs or therapies that are high use, high cost, high risk, or problem prone. Figure 31.4 is a decision matrix for selecting DUR studies to undertake. The higher the score, the more likely that this should be the problem to be studied.

Step 3: Establish Criteria or Indicators, Including Benchmarks or Thresholds. Criteria usually include the following components:

Uses: appropriate indications, treatment of underlying conditions, appropriate treatment of symptoms in treating underlying diseases;

Selection: efficacy (comparative), safety, cost (total), duplicative therapy;

Dosing: indication-specific dosing (age, diagnosis), indication-specific duration, dosing intervals;

Interactions: disease, food, drug, laboratory;

Preparation and dispensing;

Administration;

Monitoring: clinical, laboratory;

Outcome: therapeutic, safety.

Thresholds or benchmarks are established for each indicator to define the expectations or goals for complying with the criteria.

Step 4: Collect and Organize Data. Data collection forms can be developed based on the criteria and configured into simple yes-or-no or fill-in-the-blank questions. Depending on the complexity of interpretation required, the data collectors may or may not need a medical background. Data collection for hospital-based DUR studies is usually carried out by pharmacists, nurses, or medical records personnel. In hospitals where computers are used, the data collection may simply require printing a report from the computer databases.

The most common data sources are patient charts. Other sources are dispensing records, medication administration records, and laboratory reports. It is important not to collect too much data but to focus on specific indications related to the problem.

A cumulative report should include data from at least thirty patients or at least 5 percent of the expected volume (whichever is greater).

Step 5: Analyze Data. The data need to be tabulated and

Figure 31.4 Selection Matrix for Drug Utilization Review

Medication/Health Problem	High Use	High Cost	High Risk	Problem Prone	Total Score
Paracetamol	1	0	0	0	1
Acute respiratory infections	2	0	1	1	4
Ceftriaxone	1	2	0	0.5	3.5
Warfarin	0.5	0	1	2	3.5
H₂ antagonists	1	1	0	1	3
Surgical antimicrobial prophylaxis	1	1.5	0.5	1	4

reported in a standard format for comparison with benchmarks.

Step 6: Develop Conclusions. The P&T committee reviews the results of the data analysis and develops conclusions regarding reasons for differences between results and benchmarks.

Step 7: Make Recommendations. The P&T committee recommends actions required to improve knowledge or change behavior. The committee may recommend a more focused study or a focus group to understand the issues more clearly.

Step 8: Take Action. Implementation of recommendations must be part of every DUR.

Step 9: Follow up. Did the intervention achieve its objectives? Whenever an intervention is undertaken, there should be follow-up to assess the impact of actions taken and determine whether further action is required. Such action may include refining the criteria and thresholds or reanalyzing the causes of deficiencies and developing a new action plan.

Country Study 31.6 is an example of a DUR in a community hospital in the United States. Country Study 31.7 includes an example of a DUR in Kenya. The Kenya example is a variation of the methodology in Country Study 31.6 and a more appropriate application for that environment.

A self-monitoring program on drug usage at health centers, utilizing the WHO/INRUD drug use indicators, has been designed and implemented in a district day-to-day health management system in Gunungkidul District, Indonesia (Figure 31.5). With this program, prescribing indicators at the health centers are collected monthly. Prescribing data, based on these indicators, from different health centers are compared by the district health office and then fed back to the prescribers. The evaluation shows that such monitoring and feedback significantly improved prescribing patterns, reducing polypharmacy and the use of antibiotics and injectable preparations. The average

Country Study 31.6 Drug Utilization Review at a US Hospital

At a small community hospital on the West Coast of the United States, the P&T committee is responsible for a DUR program that evaluates four to six drugs or drug therapies per year. In December 1993, the committee received a report from the quality assurance coordinator noting that the rate of postoperative infections for abdominal surgeries was significantly higher than the national average. The pharmacy director informed the committee of his observation that ceftriaxone was often used for these patients, a costly and inappropriate choice. The committee decided to undertake a DUR for abdominal surgery wound infection antibiotic prophylaxis.

The health problem met all indications for a DUR: high use, high cost, high risk, and problem prone. The chief of surgery was a member of the P&T committee. He concurred with the committee that the criteria should be developed from recently published recommendations in *The Medical Letter*, which included drug selection, dosing, and timing of administration. The accompanying figure is a summary of the DUR study. The table illustrates the benchmark targets for each indicator, the actual percentage of compliance based on quarterly data collection, and the conclusions, recommendations, actions, and follow-up.

Abdominal Surgery Wound Infection Antibiotic Prophylaxis

Collection period: January–December 1994
Total Number of Cases: 162

Date of report: January 1995
Number of Cases Reviewed: 120 (74%)

Criteria	Benchmark	Indicator: % Compliance per Quarter			
		1st	2nd	3rd	4th
1. Antibiotic selection (per *Medical Letter*)	100%	70%	85%	94%	100%
2. Correct dose (per *Medical Letter*)	95%	65%	90%	94%	97%
3. Preop dose 0–2 hours prior to surgery	95%	30%	52%	89%	94%
4. Postop dose only for dirty surgery	98%	78%	89%	82%	91%
5. No postop infection	96%	90%	93%	96%	100%
6. No adverse reactions to drugs	97%	97%	100%	87%	97%

Conclusions

Criterion 1. Surgeons are selecting antibiotics that are not considered the drug of choice for the indicated procedure.

Criterion 2. Surgeons are prescribing unnecessarily high doses of antibiotics.

Criterion 3. Preop doses are delayed: current procedure is for pharmacy to send drug to operating room rather than preop area. Turnaround time for dispensing from pharmacy often delays drug administration.

Criterion 4. Surgeons order postop antibiotics for patients who do not meet criteria for dirty surgery.

Criterion 5. High rate of postop infections may improve with compliance with criteria.

Recommendations

1. Send letter to all surgeons with the following information:
   (A) current postop infection rate versus national average,
   (B) criteria and recommendations from *The Medical Letter*,
   (C) results of the DUR data collection,
   (D) estimated cost impact of inappropriate drug selection and unnecessary drug use.

2. Remove cefoxitin from formulary due its disadvantages of short half-life and relative cost of therapy as compared with cefotetan.

3. Change procedures to administer preop doses in the preop area rather than the operating room. Instruct in-service nursing and pharmacy staff on new procedures.

4. Add approved antibiotics to floor stock in preop area for emergencies.

Actions

1. The chief of surgery informed the surgery committee about the DUR and the criteria in February 1994.

2. A letter was sent to all surgeons in April 1994.

3. Cefoxitin was removed from the formulary.

4. New procedures for administration were adopted in June, and staff in-service training began in July 1994.

5. Antibiotics were added to preop floor stock in July 1994.

Follow-up

Criterion 1. Met benchmark in 4th quarter. The education of surgeons contributed to an improvement in antibiotic selection.

Criterion 2. Met benchmark in 4th quarter. The education of surgeons contributed to an improvement in antibiotic dosing.

Criterion 3. Changes in procedures, floor stock, and in-service training of staff improved the timing of preop antibiotics but still not meeting benchmark. Benchmark is unrealistically high due to multitude of contributing factors for emergency procedures. Lower the benchmark to 93 percent.

Criterion 4. Education decreased unnecessary postop antibiotic prescribing for a short time; then surgeons began to return to old practices. P&T sent individual letters to specific surgeons, and the practice improved in the last quarter of the year, but still not meeting benchmark. Report cases of noncompliance to surgery committee for peer review and recommendations.

Criterion 5. Postop infection rate gradually improved throughout the year, meeting and exceeding the benchmark.

Criterion 6. Allergic reactions increased in the 3d quarter due to the change in floor stock procedures and preop nurse failing to screen for patient allergies. Previously, the pharmacy screened for allergies prior to dispensing. Nurses received in-service training for allergy screening, and the allergic reaction decreased in the last quarter, meeting benchmark.

Country Study 31.7 Antibiotic Use Review

Antibiotics represent one of the most widely prescribed forms of drug therapy. In some cases, the antibiotics prescribed may be inappropriate or too expensive. To ensure that antibiotics are prescribed appropriately and rationally, pharmacists have to review antibiotic usage periodically. The aim of antibiotic use review (AUR) is to determine the pattern (rates and costs) of antibiotic usage in a particular setting. The results of an AUR program are often communicated to those concerned individually, through a memo, or through a general bulletin showing the norm and peer comparisons. The starting point of an AUR program is the formation of criteria by the drug and therapeutics committee (DTC). Prescriptions are checked for appropriateness of dosage, therapeutic indication, duration of treatment, and so on, according to the criteria. Deviant cases are recorded. AUR studies can be set up such that various clinicians, wards, and facilities can be compared.

The steps for performing an AUR are:
1. Select the subjects of the program.
2. Draft criteria and standards that define acceptable quality of care for subjects selected in Step 1.
3. Obtain endorsement of the criteria and standards from the DTC.
4. Evaluate the quality of services in question using the criteria and standards.
5. Identify deficiencies in quality (if any).
6. Analyze the causes of deficiencies.
7. Formulate a plan for eliminating deficiencies.
8. Implement the plan.
9. Re-evaluate the quality of services, as in Step 4.
10. If usage is not acceptable, reanalyze the causes of deficiencies and devise a new plan for their elimination.

The worksheet for an AUR for amoxicillin is shown in the accompanying table, which considers ten patients from one prescriber in Kenya.

Review Criteria from DTC	#1	#2	#3	#4	#5	#6	#7	#8	#9	#10
Indications[a]	Tonsillitis	Otitis media	Urethritis	Bowel sterilization	Severe gram-negative meningitis	Boils/abscess	Severe cystitis	Surgical prophylaxis	Pneumonia	Severe wound infection
Appropriate indication?	Yes	Yes	Yes	No	No	Yes	Yes	Yes	Yes	Yes
Amoxicillin dosage[b]	250 mg tds	250 mg tds	250 mg tds	1,500 mg bd	500 mg tds	250 mg tds	500 mg tds	250 mg tds	250 mg tds	500 mg tds
Duration (usually 5 days)	5 days	7 days	7 days	1 day	10 days	7 days	5 days	5 days	5 days	7 days
Cost per capsule (Ksh.)	30	30	30	30	30	30	30	30	30	30
Total cost[c]	470	650	650	380	1,800	650	920	470	470	1,280

[a] Acceptable indications are:
  ► Upper/lower respiratory tract infections
  ► Genitourinary tract infections
  ► Septicemia
  ► Surgical prophylaxis
  ► Skin and soft tissue infection
  ► Osteomyelitis
  ► Peritonitis
[b] Acceptable dosage is usually 250 mg tds. Dosage may be doubled in severe cases.
[c] Total cost for usual dosage for 5 days = KSh.470. This includes dispensing fee of KSh.20.

Source: Ministry of Health, Government of Kenya 1994b.

Calculations
1. Calculate the frequency of inappropriate prescribing:
   $2/10 \times 100 = 20\%$
2. Total costs due to inappropriate prescribing:
   $380 + 1,800 = KSh.2,180$ (a loss).
(NB: Only drug costs are considered; drugs prescribed inappropriately are viewed as a waste.)

Summary and Comments
1. For patient #4: bowel sterilization would require a long-acting sulfonamide or neomycin tablets.
2. For patient #5: for severe gram-negative meningitis, patient would need a cephalosporin.

number of drugs per prescription decreased from 4.2 to 3.1, and antibiotic and injection use also declined dramatically. The drug use indicators (WHO/DAP 1993) can themselves be used at the local level for self-audit and feedback, as illustrated in Figure 31.6.

Hospital and Regional Drug Committees
Drug and therapeutics committees play an important role in improving prescribing practices at the national and regional levels, as well as at the district and institutional levels (see Chapters 11 and 38). Their role has expanded in some settings from selecting drugs for formularies to

► reviewing drug requisitions and revising them to fit budget allocations;
► determining which drugs should be made available to each type of health facility (if this is not determined at the national level);

Figure 31.5 Antibiotic and Injection Use in Gunungkidul District, Indonesia

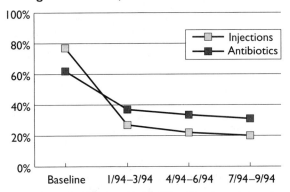

Source: Gunungkidul District Health Office, Yogyakarta, Indonesia.

▶ developing standard treatment norms for the common illnesses treated in the area or institution;

▶ establishing prescribing limitations aimed at controlling irrational drug use (for example, limiting certain antibiotics to use only under the recommendation of a consultant);

▶ limiting the amount dispensed at one time to curb abuse of particular drugs and reduce waste;

▶ reviewing antibiotic resistance patterns and revising guidelines for antibiotic use;

▶ stimulating drug education activities among hospital staff;

▶ supervising and monitoring prescribing practices.

Cost Information

Drug cost is an underappreciated aspect of prescribing. Expensive newer drugs are frequently used when comparable well-established and cheaper ones are available for the same condition. Several different mechanisms have been used to encourage physicians and paramedical staff to consider cost in their drug selections. These include using cost bar graphs, drawing up facility drug budgets, and printing prices in drug manuals and on requisition forms.

Cost Bar Graphs. In many countries, diagrams or charts showing side-by-side comparisons of prices for alternative drugs have been circulated (for examples, see Figures 31.7 and 31.8). The intention is not to mandate that practitioners always choose the least expensive drug but rather to encourage them to take cost into consideration.

Facility Drug Budgets. In health programs that receive budgetary funds for drug procurement, specific drug budgets may be allocated to individual districts, hospital areas, or health centers. When annual estimates of drug needs are made, or when regular requisitions for drugs are prepared, the expected acquisition cost of the drugs is

Figure 31.6 Drug Use Indicators Can Be Used for Self-Audit and Feedback

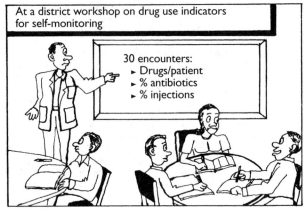

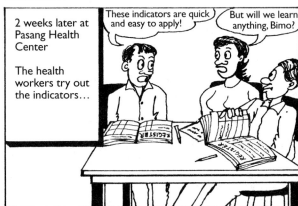

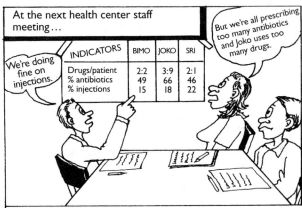

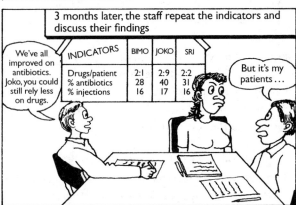

Figure 31.7 Excerpt from Government Stores Catalog in Zimbabwe

Code	Description	Unit	Price
25/0307	Aminophylline 25 mg/mL IV	Am/10 mL	0.50
25/0495	Amphotericin B 50 mg	Vial	16.89
25/0504	Ampicillin 500 mg	Vial	0.78
25/0584	Ascorbic acid 100 mg/mL	Am	0.18

compared with available funds. If reductions in drug requests are necessary—and they usually are—the medical practitioners at the hospital or health center can participate in making the choices. This puts the decision-making closest to the point of drug use. In some settings, this level of involvement by practitioners has helped create a cost consciousness that makes even their daily prescribing more cost effective.

Printing Prices in Drug Manuals and on Requisition Forms. Even when practitioners are not required to make their drug use conform to a specific budget, cost consciousness can be promoted by including recent drug prices in therapeutics manuals, drug lists, and other forms used in prescribing or requisitioning drugs. This measure alone may accomplish little, but in combination with some of the other measures described in the preceding pages, it may be quite helpful. Again, physicians and paramedical staff need not be required to pick the least expensive drug in all cases, but the price list may encourage them to make inexpensive choices.

Prescribing and Dispensing Approaches

Managers can guide the prescribing and dispensing process by intervening at crucial points of the process.

Structured Drug Order Forms. For drugs that are frequently prescribed in hospitals, such as antibiotics, standard forms can be devised to optimize correct drug use. The prescriber is provided with a drug order sheet containing a preprinted list of preferred drugs and dosage regimens for key drugs. Such forms have increased the cost effectiveness of prescribing for hospital inpatients in the United States. For example, the form for antibiotics would specify correct standard dosages and an antibiotic review after 72 hours.

Standard Diagnostic and Treatment Guidelines. Specific guidelines can be abstracted from formulary and therapeutics manuals (see Chapter 11). Guidelines for common conditions such as postoperative pain, hypertension, diabetes, and various forms of cancer can be agreed upon by the staff. Patients are treated in a standard manner according to the protocols. This approach has many benefits. Garnering agreement to follow the institutional guide-

Figure 31.8 Comparative Daily Cost of Injectable and Oral Antibiotics

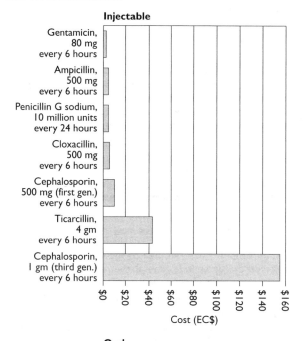

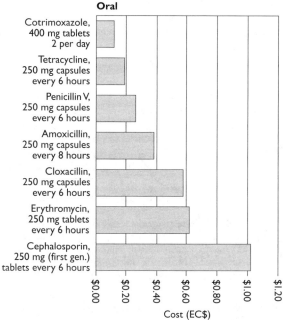

Source: Organization of Eastern Caribbean States, Eastern Caribbean Drug Service 1993.

lines may be time-consuming, but the active involvement of prescribers in this process can lead to significant changes in clinical practice. These guidelines can also be used as the basis of DUR and procurement lists.

Course-of-Therapy Packaging. Course-of-therapy (COT) packaging, often in the form of blister packs, has been widely used for oral contraceptives and, more recently, for

Country Study 31.8 Unintended Effects of Drug Restrictions

In the United States, poor patients' health care costs are covered by the Medicaid program. This program is administered by the states in different ways.

In 1992, New Hampshire decided to limit Medicaid outpatients to three drugs per month; another state, New Jersey, chose not to place limits. Researchers studied the drug use patterns and hospital and nursing home admissions for patients who had been taking more than three drugs per month.

As expected, there was a 35 percent decrease in the number of drugs per patient, but there was an increase in the dosages of the drugs prescribed. The unexpected outcome was a 120 percent increase in nursing home admissions and a 20 percent increase in hospital admissions.

After eleven months, the three-drug limit was withdrawn and replaced with a $1 copayment scheme. Admission rates and medication levels returned to the levels that existed before the drug limit. In general, the patients who were admitted to nursing homes were not discharged.

In retrospect, the behavior of the physicians who admitted their patients to nursing homes was quite rational. There were no drug limits for inpatients, and patients could continue to receive their medications by entering nursing homes. Thus, Medicaid saved a little on drug costs, but the cost of extra admissions outweighed these savings.

The monthly proportion of patients in nursing homes is shown in the accompanying graph.

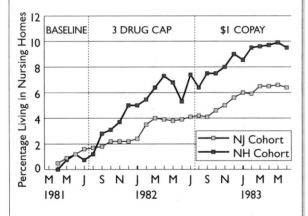

Source: Adapted from Soumerai et al., *New England Journal of Medicine* 1991; 325:1075.

tuberculosis therapy. Although such packaging adds to the cost of drugs, there are gains in convenience for both the dispenser and the patient. Comparative prices should be obtained before switching completely to COT; in many markets, there is a 10 percent or higher average difference between bulk and COT packaging. Prepacks (described in Chapter 32) are a form of COT packaging.

Financing

Setting prices and changing the way fees are collected can affect the way drugs are used.

Price Setting. The price charged for drugs can be used to encourage more rational use of them. For example, in cost-recovery programs, V(ital) drugs (see Chapter 41) can be sold at less than their real costs, and N(onessential) drugs can be sold at greater than their real costs. This cross-subsidization can encourage the use of vital effective drugs while discouraging the sale of nonessential, less effective drugs. Charging for a course of therapy rather than for each individual treatment (injection, tablet) encourages the patient to complete the prescribed therapy. Generic drugs are usually cheaper than their brand-name counterparts, making their use rational from a cost standpoint. Pricing incentives such as preferential markup on generics and reference pricing can be used to encourage generic substitution. (See Chapter 6 for more information on pricing policies.)

Capitation-Based Reimbursement. When a payment to health care providers is made by a third party, drug costs are better controlled with a fixed per capita payment as compared to a per visit or per drug reimbursement. But caution is needed to ensure that needed drugs are not underprescribed.

Drug Sales by Prescribers. If the health worker receives the profit on drug sales, as occurs in Japan and in some Bamako Initiative projects, there is an inducement to overprescribe. Although prescribers may deny this, the findings are consistent across cultures and countries: prescribers who benefit from drug sales prescribe more than those who do not.

≡ 31.6 Regulatory Approaches

Regulatory approaches aim to enforce decisions that are intended to improve prescribing. These methods are frequently used but sometimes have unintended or unexpected outcomes, which may result in extra costs or adverse patient consequences. Such effects have been noted in the United States (Country Study 31.8) with the use of a limit on the number of monthly prescriptions patients could receive. This study, however, does not rule out the use of carefully structured caps.

Drug Registration

Most countries have drug regulations that limit drug sales in the country to registered drugs. In countries where drug registration is enforced, it limits the types and numbers of drugs available for prescribing. An effective registration process helps keep dangerous and ineffective drugs off the market. The requirements for registering new drug substances are stringent in some countries. In others, however, the facilities for assessing new products are not readily available, and monitoring and enforcement are unreliable.

Limited Drug Lists

Limited drug lists can be a managerial intervention, as described earlier, or a regulatory intervention, in which case certain drugs are completely banned. Limited drug lists (formularies) have been used since the early 1970s to control costs and promote rational use in public- and private-sector pharmaceutical programs. In some cases, governments have gone farther, banning certain drugs or drug classes from both public and private markets. Limited drug lists are the main mechanism to prevent the use of dangerous, ineffective, and unnecessarily expensive drugs. However, the danger exists that when safe but relatively ineffective drugs (such as kaolin for diarrhea) are withdrawn from the list, they may be replaced by effective drugs (metronidazole, for example) used inappropriately. This occurred in one country when antidiarrheals were banned. Metronidazole use increased from 10 percent to 65 percent in cases of watery diarrhea.

Prescribing Restrictions

In theory, once a drug is registered, it can be prescribed by all medically qualified prescribers. Health authorities often restrict paramedical staff to a limited number of drugs on the national essential drugs list. These limitations are imposed to cut down on wasteful prescribing and inappropriate use of expensive drugs. At the health facility level, the use of expensive or powerful drugs may be limited to the more experienced prescribers. In some hospitals, the use of third-generation cephalosporins is restricted to specialist prescribers. Prescriptions by junior staff have to be countersigned by the specialist. In some settings, the junior prescriber can prescribe such drugs only for 24- to 48-hour use; any extension requires the authorization of the specialist. Prescribing limitations may take the form of drug registration, limited drug lists (essential drugs lists), drug formularies, or prescribing and dispensing privileges by level of use (facility level and competence level of prescriber). Another possible restriction is to limit the number of drugs prescribed to two or three per patient. However, this restriction is easily evaded by issuing two separate prescriptions.

Dispensing Limitations

Limiting the amount of drugs to be dispensed has been applied in some countries to control wasteful or potentially dangerous dispensing. Examples of this approach follow.

- ▶ One Asian country established a system of three- and five-day limits for all outpatient prescriptions, except those for chronic diseases. Most antibiotics are given for five days, and all other medicines for acute illnesses are limited to three-day courses.

- ▶ In South America, one large rural health program established a system of prepackaging drugs in unit-of-use plastic bags containing the minimum amount of drug needed for one course of therapy.

- ▶ The government-supplied university hospital in one Southeast Asian country put dispensing limits on items that may be abused, tend to be prescribed indiscriminately, or are potentially dangerous. Maximum dispensing quantities have been established for codeine, diazepam, vitamin C tablets, and vitamin B complex, among others.

Such limitations can have adverse effects on the treatment of some diseases. For example, antibiotic treatment for typhoid typically requires more than five days. Patients with chronic diseases such as epilepsy or diabetes are forced to visit health centers frequently and may end up missing treatments. Therefore, when setting restrictions on duration of therapy or dispensing quantities, exceptions must be built in to cover chronic diseases and exceptional cases.

≡ 31.7 Developing an Intervention Strategy

When a problem has been identified and quantified and its causes have been determined, an intervention needs to be selected. A wide range of possible interventions has been indicated in Sections 31.4, 31.5, and 31.6.

Selecting an Intervention

The first step in selecting an intervention is to clearly define the problem to be solved. The behaviors specific to the particular health problem, as well as factors causing variability in performance, need to be identified. It is also important to assess the beliefs and motivations of the prescribers that may contribute to the observed behavior. These assessments may require further studies involving qualitative investigational methods. Once the problem has been defined, a package of interventions can be considered.

Cost effectiveness has to be considered in the selection process. The implementation of the selected interventions needs to be carefully designed. The use of a control group enhances the detection of differences. Key outcomes must be defined beforehand. An evaluation of the impact versus the cost of the intervention is also necessary. The outcome of the intervention must be fed back to the participants to reinforce the changes that have occurred.

Figure 31.9 Framework for Formative and Intervention Studies

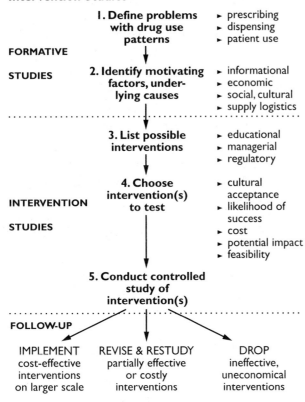

Source: Quick et al. 1991.

Figure 31.10 Combined Intervention Strategy: Prescribing for Acute Diarrhea in Mexico City

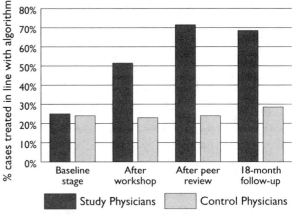

Source: Gutierrez et al. 1994.

The selection of an appropriate intervention should consider its

likely effectiveness: What intervention is most likely to be effective in addressing the specific drug use problems and their underlying causes? Are there any previous studies or documented experiences about this specific intervention?

feasibility: Is the intervention feasible to implement, taking into account the existing health care system and the available personnel?

cost: What is the cost of the intervention? Can it be borne by the available resources?

potential impact: If the intervention is effective, what impact will it have, and what will be its magnitude? Can beneficial impacts outweigh the cost and possible adverse effects?

unintended effects: What are the possible adverse effects of the intervention?

The framework for formative and intervention studies is described in Figure 31.9. The selected intervention, however, must be formally tested in a well-designed experiment before implementation).

Combining Interventions

Interventions can be combined. This approach was taken in Mexico, where the treatment of diarrhea was unsatisfactory. The first intervention was an educational workshop, which improved prescribing from 24.5 to 51.2 percent compliance with a treatment norm. This was followed by a managerial intervention, peer review, which further improved prescribing to 71.6 percent compliance with the same norm. There were only minor changes in the control group (see Figure 31.10). After eighteen months, the improvement had been maintained.

It is usually more effective to combine different types of interventions. A mixture of large group education and small group education, combined with audit and feedback, is more likely to produce sustained changes than is a repetition of the same intervention. In general, regulatory interventions should be carefully structured, and active surveillance is essential to detect unexpected or unintended effects. Many countries do not have the capacity to monitor or enforce regulations, limiting the effectiveness of regulatory approaches.

Social Marketing of Interventions

Implementing interventions without taking into account the level of understanding and acceptance of the prescribers or consumers carries the risk of failure or unintended effects. For instance, a policy of prescribing generic drugs is in place in public health facilities in many countries. When prescribers are not well informed about the advantages of generics, they may not comply with generic prescribing, and they may transfer their negative perceptions to their patients, which, in turn, further jeopardizes the implementation of the policy (see Chapter 10). Withdrawing popular

---

≡ Assessment Guide

Indicators of Prescribing Quality
- ► Average number of drugs per encounter;
- ► Percentage of drugs prescribed by generic name;
- ► Percentage of encounters in which an antibiotic is prescribed;
- ► Percentage of encounters in which an injection is prescribed;
- ► Percentage of drugs prescribed from the essential drugs list or formulary;
- ► Average consultation time;
- ► Prescription in accordance with treatment guidelines;
- ► Percentage of patients treated without drugs;
- ► Percentage of patients satisfied with the care they received.

Indicators of Prescription Costs
- ► Average cost per encounter;
- ► Percentage of drug costs spent on antibiotics;
- ► Percentage of drug costs spent on injections.

Educational Interventions
- ► Is there an official continuing education system on rational use of drugs for prescribers and dispensers?
- ► How many training sessions on drug use were given for prescribers in the last year?

- ► What percentage of prescribers surveyed attended at least one training session in the last year?
- ► Out of all the training sessions organized in the past three years, what percentage was related to drug use?
- ► Is the concept of essential drugs part of the curricula in the basic training of health personnel?

Managerial Interventions
- ► Is there a national therapeutic guide with standardized treatments?
- ► Do hospital drug and therapeutics committees undertake drug utilization studies? What results are available?
- ► What kinds of managerial interventions have been tried? Were their effects evaluated?

Regulatory Interventions
- ► At what levels of the system are limited drug lists used?
- ► What other regulatory interventions have been used?
- ► What evaluations have been undertaken of the impact of regulatory changes?

Note: Chapter 29 contains additional indicators and measures for assessing prescribing and the effect of interventions to promote rational prescribing.

---

drugs from the market without giving proper information to the public can create confusion and anxiety for consumers, especially for routine users of the drugs. Whenever regulatory or managerial action is taken, informational and educational approaches need to be incorporated for prescribers as well as consumers and patients.

Evaluating the Impact of an Intervention

Evaluation of whether an intervention has caused the desired effect—that is, improvement in prescribing behavior in a cost-effective manner—is often neglected. An intervention strategy is often implemented without prior field testing to prove that it works in the existing system and is effective in influencing prescribing practices. Many countries have implemented countrywide training programs without proper design and evalua-

tion. In these cases, the waste of resources in terms of funds, time, and energy will only further increase the burden on health care services. Some health managers falsely assume that if any intervention program takes place the desired goals have been accomplished. Yet the production and dissemination of treatment guidelines to health care facilities, for example, does not necessarily mean that prescribers will use the guidelines or improve their prescribing practices.

Evaluation of impacts should be regarded as an important component of any intervention strategy. The following points should be considered in making an evaluation:

- ► An evaluation plan should be devised when planning an intervention. Before implementing a program on a wide scale, it is imperative to do a field test to find out whether the evaluation can be implemented feasibly in the existing health care setting and whether it is effective in influencing prescribing practices.

► Evaluation of the impact of an intervention program should focus primarily on the indicators targeted by the intervention messages. Secondary indicators can also be selected, as appropriate. Depending on the objectives and scope of the intervention, evaluation may include relevant aspects such as knowledge of the targets, changes in perception about a specific practice of interest, the process of care, and cost of prescribing.

► Apart from relevance, the selection of indicators for impact evaluation should take into account reliability and feasibility of collecting data from the existing system.

► The evaluation of any intervention should use appropriate design and methodology, with adequate sample size, sampling, and use of control groups.

► It is always desirable to measure the long-term sustainability of the impact of any intervention. Changes in prescribing behavior and practice observed immediately after an intervention often return to their baseline levels after a longer period of time. Experience shows that changes in prescribing usually return to pre-intervention levels after six months unless there is a continuation of the intervention messages. The use of time series analysis may be particularly useful in showing effects over time.

Measurements of drug utilization, including measurements of the impact of intervention strategies, are discussed in more detail in Chapter 29. ■

≡ References and Further Readings

★ = Key readings.

Avorn, J., and S. B. Soumerai. 1983. Improving drug-therapy decisions through educational outreach. *New England Journal of Medicine* 308:1457–63.
★ Denig, P. 1994. *Drug choices in medical practice: Rationales, routines, and remedies.* Groningen, Netherlands: University of Groningen.
Everitt, D. E., S. B. Soumerai, J. Avorn, H. Klapholz, and M. Wessels. 1990. Changing surgical antimicrobial prophylaxis practices through education targeted at senior department leaders. *Infection Control in Hospital Epidemiology* 11:578–83.
Gutierrez, G., H. Guiscafré, M. Bronfman, J. Walsh, H. Martinez, and O. Muñoz. 1994. Changing physician prescribing patterns: Evaluation of an educational strategy for acute diarrhea in Mexico City. *Medical Care* 32:436-46.
★ Hogerzeil, H. V. 1995. Promoting rational prescribing: An international perspective. *British Journal of Clinical Pharmacology* 39:1–6.
Hogerzeil, H. V., G. J. Walker, A. O. Sallami, and G. Fernando. 1989. Impact of an essential drugs program on availability and rational use of drugs. *Lancet* 1:141–42.
Landgren, F. T., K. J. Harvey, M. L. Mashford, R. F. Moulds, B. Guthrie, and M. Hemming. 1988. Changing antibiotic prescribing by educational marketing. *Medical Journal of Australia* 149:595–99.
Ministry of Health, Government of Kenya. 1994a. *Clinical guidelines for diagnosis and treatment of common hospital conditions in Kenya.* Nairobi.
Ministry of Health, Government of Kenya. 1994b. *Good management of hospital drugs and supplies manual.* Nairobi.
OECS/ECDS (Organization of Eastern Caribbean States/Eastern Caribbean Drug Service). 1996. *Regional formulary and therapeutics manual.* 4th ed. Castries, St. Lucia: OECS/ECDS.
★ Quick, J. D., R. O. Laing, and D. Ross-Degnan. 1991. Intervention research to promote clinically effective and economically efficient use of pharmaceuticals: The international network for rational use of drugs. *Journal of Clinical Epidemiology* 44 (suppl 2): 57S–65S.
Ross-Degnan, D., R. O. Laing, J. D. Quick, H. M. Ali, D. Ofori-Adjei, L. Salako, and B. Santoso. 1992. A strategy for promoting improved pharmaceutical use: The international network for rational use of drugs. *Social Science and Medicine* 35: 1329–41.
Soumerai, S. B. 1988. Factors influencing prescribing. *Australian Journal of Hospital Pharmacy* 18:9–16.
Soumerai, S. B., and J. Avorn. 1990. Principles of educational outreach ("academic detailing") to improve clinical decision making. *Journal of the American Medical Association* 263: 549–56.
Soumerai, S. B., T. J. McLaughlin, and J. Avorn. 1989. Improving drug prescribing in primary care: A critical analysis of the experimental literature. *Milbank Quarterly* 67: 268–317.
★ Soumerai, S. B., J. D. Quick, and Y. Tawfik. 1987. Changing the unchangeable: Principles and experiences in improving prescribing accuracy. *World Pediatrics and Child Care* 3:287–91.
Soumerai, S. B., D. Ross-Degnan, J. Avorn, T. J. McLaughlin, and I. Choodnovskiy. 1991. Effects of Medicaid drug-payment limits on admission to hospitals and nursing homes. *New England Journal of Medicine* 325:1072–77.
WHO/DAP (World Health Organization/Action Programme on Essential Drugs). 1993. *How to investigate drug use in health facilities: Selected drug use indicators.* WHO/DAP/93.1. Geneva: WHO/DAP.
WHO/DAP (World Health Organization/Action Programme on Essential Drugs). 1994. *Guide to good prescribing.* WHO/DAP/94.11. Geneva: WHO/DAP.

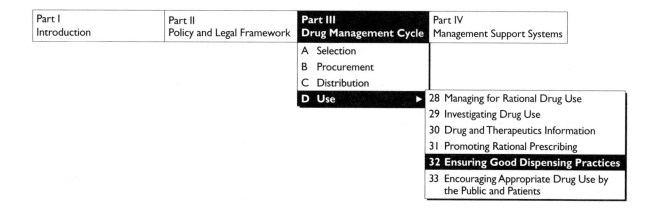

Part I	Part II	Part III	Part IV
Introduction	Policy and Legal Framework	**Drug Management Cycle**	Management Support Systems

A Selection
B Procurement
C Distribution
D Use ▶

28 Managing for Rational Drug Use
29 Investigating Drug Use
30 Drug and Therapeutics Information
31 Promoting Rational Prescribing
32 Ensuring Good Dispensing Practices
33 Encouraging Appropriate Drug Use by
    the Public and Patients

Chapter 32
Ensuring Good Dispensing Practices

≡ Summary

Good dispensing practices ensure that an effective form of the correct drug is delivered to the right patient, in the prescribed dosage and quantity, with clear instructions, and in a package that maintains the potency of the drug. Dispensing includes all the activities that occur between the time the prescription is presented and the medicine or other prescribed items are issued to the patient.

A safe, clean, and organized working environment provides a basis for good practice. Dispensing must be performed accurately and should be done in an orderly manner, with disciplined use of effective procedures. Care should be taken to read labels accurately. The dispenser must count and measure carefully and guard against contamination of medicines by using clean equipment and avoiding handling of medicines.

Staff who dispense must be qualified or trained in the knowledge, skills, and practices necessary to dispense the range of medicines being prescribed. Their performance should be regularly monitored.

Prepackaging medicines can improve efficiency in dispensing. Safety in dispensing can be improved by routine procedures for checking before issuing medicines to patients.

Cost factors inevitably lead to the use of packaging that is less than ideal. The solution must be the best compromise between cost and the risk of waste, with regard to maintaining standards of cleanliness and effective treatment.

Labeling is also affected by cost. Labels should contain information about the medicine and its correct use. The style and language of labeling should be appropriate to the needs of the patient.

Ensuring patients' understanding of how to take their medicines is a primary responsibility of dispensers. Dispensers should check understanding by asking each patient to repeat instructions.

Good records are a sometimes neglected but essential part of dispensing; they facilitate good management and monitoring of services provided.

Dispensing refers to the process of preparing and giving out medicine to a named person on the basis of a prescription. It involves the correct interpretation of the wishes of the prescriber and the accurate preparation and labeling of medicine for use by the patient as advised. This process may take place in a public or private clinic, health center, or hospital or in a shop or community pharmacy setting. It is often carried out by many different kinds of people with a variety of training and backgrounds. No matter where dispensing is done or who does it, any error or failure in the dispensing process can seriously affect the care of the patient.

Dispensing is one of the vital elements of rational drug use. Within rational drug use programs, efforts have often been concentrated on ensuring rational prescribing habits, overlooking the dispensing and actual patient use of drugs.

It is commonly assumed that dispensing is a simple, routine process that cannot go wrong. Yet all the resources involved in patient care up to the point of dispensing may be wasted if dispensing does not result in the named patient receiving an effective form of the correct drug, in appropriate packaging, and with the correct dose and advice (see Figure 32.1).

This chapter considers the factors that influence the process of dispensing and are therefore important in ensuring "correctly dispensed" medicine.

≡ 32.1 Dispensing Environment

Dispensing environments must be clean, because most drug products are taken internally, making it important that they be hygienic and uncontaminated. The environment must also be organized so that dispensing can be performed accurately and efficiently. The dispensing environment includes

- staff
- physical surroundings
- shelving and storage areas
- surfaces used during work
- equipment and packaging materials

Staff involved in dispensing must maintain good personal hygiene and should wear clean protective clothing.

The physical surroundings must be maintained as free of dust and dirt as possible. Although the dispensary must be accessible to patients, care should be taken to locate it in a protected place and not beside, or open to, a road or other area where dust, dirt, and pollution are common.

Maintaining a clean environment requires a regular routine of cleaning shelves and a daily cleaning of floors and working surfaces. There should be a regular schedule for checking, cleaning, and defrosting the refrigerator. Spills should be wiped up immediately, especially if the liquid spilled is sticky, sweet, or attractive to insects and flies. Food and drink must be kept out of the dispensing area, with the refrigerator used strictly for medicines.

Figure 32.1 Good Dispensing/Bad Dispensing

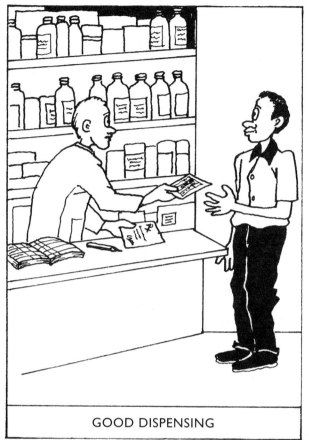

GOOD DISPENSING

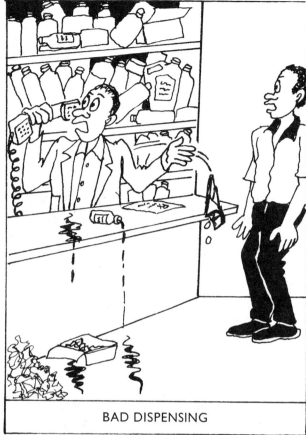

BAD DISPENSING

Dispensing equipment is used for measuring liquids or counting tablets or capsules. Uncoated tablets normally leave a layer of powder on any surface they touch, which can easily be transferred to other tablets or capsules counted on the same surface. This is called *cross-contamination* and could be dangerous if the contaminating substance (for example, aspirin or penicillin) is one to which a patient is sensitive. It is essential to clean any equipment used for different products, both between uses and at the end of the day.

The dispensing environment must be organized to create a safe and efficient working area. There should be sufficient space to allow for movement by staff during the dispensing process. However, the distance that a dispenser must cover during the dispensing process should be minimized to maintain efficiency.

Stock containers and prepacked medicines must be stored in an organized way on shelves, preferably according to dosage forms (for example, tablets and capsules, syrups and mixtures) and in alphabetical order. All stock containers in use must be clearly and accurately labeled to ensure the safe selection of the correct preparation and

to minimize the risk of error (see Figure 32.2).

In addition, a system of stock rotation should determine which items are to be used first, on either a first-in/first-out (FIFO) or first-expiry/first-out (FEFO) basis. Recommended storage conditions relating to temperature, light, and moisture should be followed as closely as possible to maintain product quality. Stock bottles must be kept closed except when actually in use.

A limited range of preparations will be used with the greatest frequency, and these "fast movers" can be placed in the most accessible areas for the convenience of dispensers.

≡ 32.2 Dispensing Person

A superficial look at dispensing suggests that it is a process of supplying goods to a patient on the basis of a written order, and that it can be done successfully by anyone who can read the prescription, count, and pour. As a result, dispensing is often delegated to any staff member who has nothing else to do, who then performs this function without any training or supervision. This situation is irrational and dangerous.

Figure 32.2 Illustration of a Stock Container Label

```
                 Tablets

              PARACETAMOL
                 500 mg


            Batch no. 9312101
        Date of Manufacture: 12/96
           Expiry Date: 11/99
```

One major difference between supplying medicines and medical supplies and supplying other goods is that with medicines the patient usually does not know the correct use, and is unable to judge the quality, of the product he or she receives. Therefore, responsibility for the correctness and quality of medicines supplied lies entirely with the person dispensing them, and the patient must rely on the dispenser's ability. Consequently, in most countries, professional pharmacists are legally responsible for the distribution of medicines to the general public. In many countries, however, a shortage of qualified pharmacists or trained dispensers is an obstacle to achieving this level of control.

In addition to reading, writing, counting, and pouring, the dispenser, or dispensing team, needs additional knowledge, skills, and attitudes to complete the dispensing process, including:

- ▶ knowledge about the medicines being dispensed (common use, common dose, precautions about the method of use, common side effects, common interactions with other drugs or food, storage needs);
- ▶ good calculation and arithmetic skills;
- ▶ skills in assessing the quality of preparations;
- ▶ attributes of cleanliness, accuracy, and honesty;
- ▶ attitudes and skills required to communicate effectively with patients.

The level of training needed for the particular dispensing task is determined by the range of medicines dispensed and the extent to which calculation and preparation are required.

Dispensing personnel must receive an appropriate level of training that allows them to correctly dispense the range of medicines prescribed. This is true of both the private and the public sectors (see Country Study 32.1). At a basic health facility, where a limited range of medicines is used and the number of patients is small, the training can be basic, highly structured, and based on existing health care knowledge from previous training. Dispensing assistants

Country Study 32.1 Training of Drug Retailers and Wholesalers in Nepal and Kenya

Nepal. The Division of Drug Administration of the Government of Nepal has offered a three-week (eighty-hour) training course for drug retailers and wholesalers since 1981. Approximately 2,800 have passed the course examination and are registered "professionalists," which permits them to sell all groups of drugs. The course provides basic information on the nature of drugs and their handling and storage, as well as the action and correct use of commonly issued drugs. The third edition of the *Handbook for Drug Retailers and Wholesalers* was published recently. The handbook forms the basis of the course content (eight units in all) and is retained thereafter as a reference.

Kenya. The Kenya Control of Diarrhoeal Diseases Programme, with WHO support and in collaboration with a number of local institutions and consultants, carried out a training intervention in ninety urban pharmacies located in five towns in Kenya. This followed a background assessment that showed considerable discrepancy between stated and actual practices in treatment advised and products sold for childhood diarrhea. Training was face-to-face as well as through four types of printed materials. In the short term, the training resulted in improved knowledge and practices in giving advice and making sales related to the treatment of childhood diarrhea. In some areas, significant changes were seen (growth of sales of oral rehydration solution and decrease in sales of antidiarrheal preparations).

with this level of training may be employed at higher levels (for example, a district hospital) but work under the guidance and supervision of trained pharmacy staff, such as a pharmacy technician. Dispensers in community pharmacy shops should also be trained in the basics of good dispensing practices and the care of medicines.

Where graduate pharmacists are scarce, they are more effectively employed as trainers and supervisors rather than technicians performing the routine tasks of dispensing.

≡ **32.3 Dispensing Process**

The consistent and repeated use of a good dispensing procedure is vital in ensuring that errors are noticed and corrected at all stages of the dispensing process. The term *dispensing process* covers all the activities involved, from receiving the prescription to issuing the prescribed medicine to the patient. There are five major areas of activity (see Figure 32.3):

1. Receive and validate the prescription.
2. Understand and interpret the prescription.
3. Prepare items for issue.
4. Record the action taken.
5. Issue medicine to the patient with clear instructions and advice.

Figure 32.3 The Dispensing Cycle

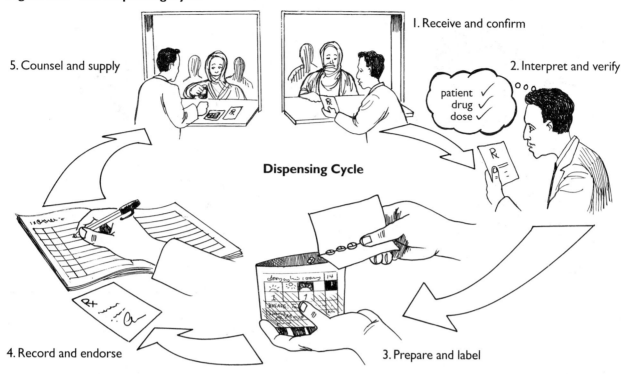

Step 1. Receive and Validate Prescription

Upon receiving a prescription, the staff member responsible should confirm the name of the patient. This is particularly important when the clinic is dealing with a large crowd of people and when there is any risk that staff or patients may mix up prescriptions. Cross-checking the name and identity of the patient must also be done when issuing the drugs.

Step 2. Understand and Interpret Prescription

Interpreting a prescription must be done by a staff member who can

- read the prescription;
- correctly interpret any abbreviations used by the prescriber;
- confirm that the doses prescribed are in the normal range for the patient (noting sex and age);
- correctly perform any calculations of dose and issue quantity;
- identify any common drug-drug interactions.

It is assumed that the prescription will be in written form. Verbal orders for drugs should be given only in exceptional and emergency situations. In such cases, the order should be repeated back to the prescriber to ensure accuracy, and written confirmation should be supplied within an agreed-upon period. If the person dispensing the medicine has any doubt about what is required by the prescriber, he or she must check with the prescriber. Illegible writing by prescribers may be a popular joke, but it has serious implications when many drug names are confusingly similar. *Checking a prescription may save a life* (see Country Study 32.2).

Any calculations should be double checked by the dispenser or counterchecked by another staff member. An arithmetical error could be fatal.

Step 3. Prepare Items for Issue

Preparation of items for issue is the central part of the dispensing process, and it must include procedures for

---

Country Study 32.2 Dispensing Errors Cost Lives

A patient had been given a prescription for an antacid—something beginning with "D" and ending in "l." The prescription was poorly written, but the dosage of two tablets four times a day was correct. The dispenser at the shop was not quite sure about the drug name but knew of a new drug just on the market with a trade name that began with "D" and ended with "l," and so dispensed it. That was how glibenclamide tablets (brand name Daonil) were dispensed at a level eight times the recommended daily dose, and the patient died of hypoglycemia. The prescriber who wrote out the prescription had the antacid Diovol in mind, but the handwriting was unclear. Although it is easy to see how this tragedy occurred, the fact remains that it should not have happened.

Figure 32.4 Writing Drug Labels

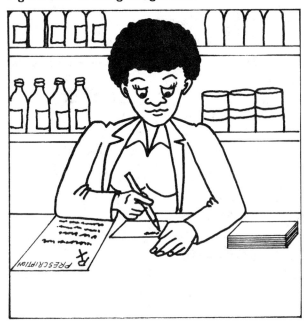

Figure 32.5 Selection from a Shelf: Read the Label Every Time

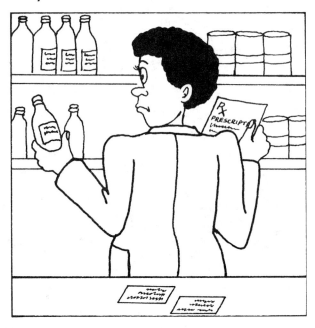

self-checking or counterchecking to ensure accuracy. This part of the process begins once the prescription is clearly understood and the quantity has been calculated. It is good practice to write the label at this point in the process as a form of self-check (see Figure 32.4).

Select Stock Container or Prepack. A good dispenser selects the item by reading the label and cross-matching the drug name and strength against the prescription. Most well-trained staff deliberately read the container label at least twice during the dispensing process (see Figure 32.5). A poor dispenser selects according to the color or location of the container, without consciously reading the label.

Another dangerous practice that should be discouraged is having many stock containers open at the same time. In this situation, drug selection is frequently made according to appearance only, which could lead to errors. In addition, medicines continuously exposed to the air eventually deteriorate in quality. Open and close containers one at a time.

Measure or Count Quantity from Stock Containers. Liquids must be measured in a clean vessel and should be poured from the stock bottle with the label kept upward. This avoids damage to the label by any spilled or dripping liquid (see Figure 32.6).

Tablets and capsules can be counted with or without the assistance of a counting device (see Figure 32.7). The most important rule to follow is that *the dispenser's hands must not be in direct contact with the medicine.* Using the hands is bad practice for both hygienic and drug quality reasons. Counting should be done using one of the following:

- ► Clean piece of paper and clean knife or spatula;
- ► Clean triangular tablet counter;
- ► Lid of the stock container in use;
- ► Any other clean, dust-free surface.

Immediately after measuring or counting, the stock container lid should be replaced and the stock container label should be rechecked for drug name and strength.

Pack and Label Medicine. Tablets or capsules should be packed into a clean, dry container, such as a bottle, plastic envelope, cardboard box, or paper envelope. All these are satisfactory in a dry climate. During the rainy season or in humid climates, however, cardboard or paper will not protect tablets and capsules from moisture in the air, which can quickly ruin drugs and make them unfit for use. Capsules and sugar-coated tablets are the most vulnerable.

Liquids require clean bottles and effective caps or closures. Under no circumstances should two liquid medicines be mixed together for dispensing. They may interact chemically and become ineffective or dangerous. In many situations, suitable containers for dispensing liquids are difficult to obtain, and a policy of prescribing solid-dose preparations whenever possible is recommended.

Labeling should identify the drug name and strength (even if the patient cannot read) and clearly indicate the dose to be used (both amount and frequency) and the quantity dispensed. The method by which this information is communicated varies according to legal requirements, container and label facilities, and the needs and

Figure 32.6 Position Label Upward When Pouring Liquids

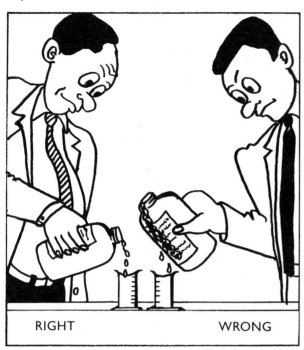

RIGHT   WRONG

Figure 32.7 Counting Methods

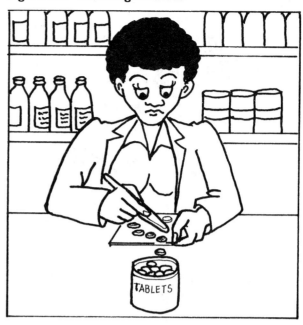

abilities of the patient. The ultimate objective is a fully written or printed label. Symbols may have to be used to indicate the amount and frequency of dosage (see Section 32.5). It is better to label envelopes and paper packaging for solid-dose medicines before packing the medicine. If auxiliary labels (see Section 32.5) are available, the appropriate ones should be affixed to the dispensing package.

At this point, the dispensed preparation should be checked against the prescription and against the stock containers used. This can be done as a self-check, but it is valuable to have the final check done by another staff member.

Step 4. Record Action Taken

Records of issues to patients are essential in an efficiently run dispensary. Such records can be used to verify the stocks used in dispensing, and they will be required if there is a need to trace any problems with medicines issued to patients.

Three different methods can be used to keep a record of medicines dispensed. *When a prescription is retained*, the dispensing staff should initial and annotate the prescription and either file it or enter the details into a record book when they have time. *When the prescription is returned to the patient*, details of the medicines dispensed must be entered into a record book before the items are issued to the patient. The date, the patient's name and age, the medicine name and strength, the amount issued, and the dis-

penser's name should be entered into the register. *When computers are used in the dispensing process*, the computer program should retain the information, which can then be recalled to generate summary reports.

Step 5. Issue Medicine to Patient with Clear Instructions and Advice

The medicine must be given to the named patient, or the patient's representative, with clear instructions and any appropriate advice about the medicine. The amount of detailed advice that should be given about possible side effects varies from patient to patient. Verbal advice is important, because both illiteracy and poor labeling may be problems.

Apart from emphasizing the dose, frequency, length of treatment, and route of administration, the priority is to give the patient information that will maximize the effect of the treatment. Advice should therefore concentrate on

- ▶ when to take the medicine (particularly in relation to food and other medicines);
- ▶ how to take the medicine (chewed, swallowed whole, taken with plenty of water);
- ▶ how to store and care for the medicine.

Warnings about possible side effects should be given with care. Common but harmless side effects (nausea, mild diarrhea, urine changing color) should be mentioned to prevent a frightened patient from stopping the treatment. More serious side effects should be mentioned only

Figure 32.8 Ensuring Understanding

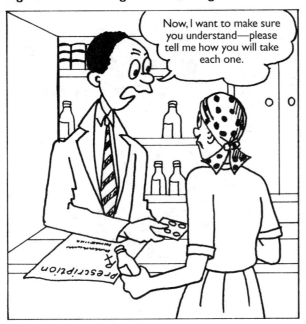

Figure 32.9 Check Routines, Prevent Mistakes

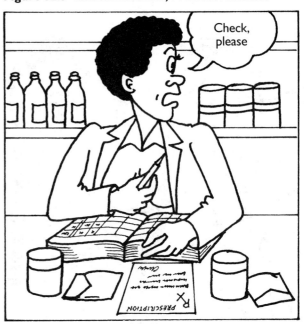

with the agreement of the prescriber, who needs to take those risks into account when prescribing the medicine.

Every effort must be made to confirm that the patient understands the instructions. This can be difficult if someone is collecting items for a patient or for several patients, particularly if the same medicines are prescribed in different dosages. Whenever possible, the staff member dispensing the medications should have the recipient repeat back the instructions (see Figure 32.8).

Every patient must be treated with respect. The need for confidentiality and privacy when explaining the use of some types of medicine must be recognized, and efforts should be made to structure medicine collection so that advice to patients can be as individual as possible. The person receiving the instructions may be feeling ill, and the success of the treatment rests on the accuracy of the dispenser's communication with the patient.

≡ 32.4 Promoting Efficient Management in Dispensing

Good dispensing practices are under the greatest threat when there is a crowd of patients demanding immediate attention. The need for speed must be balanced with the need for accuracy and care in the dispensing process. At this point, the patient's care, or even life, is in the hands of the dispenser. In dispensing, accuracy is more important than speed.

One good way to reduce the dispensing time and improve safety is to prepackage and label commonly used medicines. This process also distributes some of the dispensing workload to less busy hours. See Section 32.6 for a more detailed discussion of prepackaging.

Another way to prevent staff from making errors when working under pressure is to organize the work so that more than one individual is involved in the dispensing process for each prescription. This introduces a system of counterchecks, which is a wise precaution in most situations (see Figure 32.9).

Useful techniques to ensure quality in dispensing include

► *maintenance of records* on what drugs and products have been issued;

► maintenance by the pharmacy department of a *daily list of drugs in stock* to inform prescribers which drugs are available, thereby ensuring that only these drugs are prescribed;

► a *two-prescription system*, whereby two separate prescriptions are written: one for drugs available in the pharmacy, and one for those that are not but can be ordered; this helps avoid rewriting of prescriptions;

► *efficient staff scheduling* to make the best use of available staff—more staff at peak hours, enough coverage to keep one window open during lunch, starting and ending times coordinated with patient flow;

► participation by the pharmacy staff in *hospital committees* to identify and resolve patient flow, communication, and other problems.

Regular inspection using a checklist may improve dispensing in a health facility (see Figure 32.10).

≡ 32.5 Packaging and Labeling of Drugs

When the drugs have been collected from the shelf, they must be packaged so that they can be stored by the patient and labeled to ensure patient understanding.

Containers for Dispensed Medicine

The purpose of a medicine container or packaging is to preserve the quality of the medicine up to the time of use, as well as to provide a surface for attaching or writing a label with identifying details and instructions for use. The container should not affect the quality of the medicine in any way or allow other contaminants to do so.

In the ideal situation, such a container would match the standard criteria laid down in textbooks and international standards. These describe the nature and color of the container and its closure (cap or top), as well as the requirements for good labeling. Since many health systems cannot meet this ideal for financial or logistical reasons, it is important to seek the best possible solution, keeping in mind basic principles. Figure 32.11 compares various options, as does the booklet *Low Cost Medicine Packaging* (Vogler 1990).

Labeling of Dispensed Medicine

When there is a shortage of suitable containers, the labeling of medicines is frequently inadequate or even nonexistent. As a result, dispensed medicines are often used incorrectly and do not provide the intended treatment. *Studies have shown that even in countries with the most sophisticated labeling practices, only about 50 percent of medicines are taken as intended by the prescriber.* Despite these discouraging statistics, labeling is important, and efforts should be made to provide information about the nature and contents of the preparation, the dosage regime to be followed, and the identity of the intended patient (see Figure 32.12). This is important even if the patient is illiterate, since another family member may be able to read the instructions.

In some countries, small auxiliary labels are available with preprinted instructions such as "Shake well before using" or cautions such as "May cause drowsiness." Where available they should be routinely used.

Prepackaged medicines should always be labeled with the name, strength, and quantity of the preparation and, where there are established courses of therapy, the dosage regimen. Such a label should leave a space for the patient's name to be added.

Self-adhesive labels are unlikely to be available, but labels can be inserted into containers or stapled onto bags for

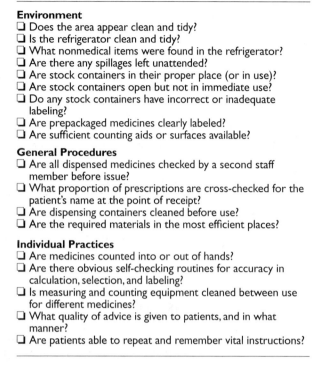

Figure 32.10 Sample Inspection Checklist

Environment
- ❑ Does the area appear clean and tidy?
- ❑ Is the refrigerator clean and tidy?
- ❑ What nonmedical items were found in the refrigerator?
- ❑ Are there any spillages left unattended?
- ❑ Are stock containers in their proper place (or in use)?
- ❑ Are stock containers open but not in immediate use?
- ❑ Do any stock containers have incorrect or inadequate labeling?
- ❑ Are prepackaged medicines clearly labeled?
- ❑ Are sufficient counting aids or surfaces available?

General Procedures
- ❑ Are all dispensed medicines checked by a second staff member before issue?
- ❑ What proportion of prescriptions are cross-checked for the patient's name at the point of receipt?
- ❑ Are dispensing containers cleaned before use?
- ❑ Are the required materials in the most efficient places?

Individual Practices
- ❑ Are medicines counted into or out of hands?
- ❑ Are there obvious self-checking routines for accuracy in calculation, selection, and labeling?
- ❑ Is measuring and counting equipment cleaned between use for different medicines?
- ❑ What quality of advice is given to patients, and in what manner?
- ❑ Are patients able to repeat and remember vital instructions?

tablets and capsules. Such instruction labels may be preprinted, or the process can be simplified by having rubber stamps made for the common regimens (for example, "one to be taken three times a day"). These should be written in the local language. If paper envelopes are used as containers, the instructions can be stamped onto them directly.

Where there are high levels of illiteracy or where research has proved that written labels are not effective, consideration should be given to the use of pictorial or graphic labels, as illustrated in Figure 32.13. Before any large investment is made in printing such labels, however, they should be pretested to make sure that they communicate effectively. Picture language can be very culture specific.

The use of computers and printers to produce labels for dispensed medicine is now common in many countries. The software is designed for use on desktop personal computers, and these can be considered if they are available and affordable. Using computers can be very attractive and efficient, but the need for a continuous supply of computer paper or labels, as well as for a consistent electricity supply, must be considered.

≡ 32.6 Course-of-Therapy Prepackaging of Medicines

Prepackaging of medicines for dispensing is valuable if the following conditions apply:

Figure 32.11 Packaging Materials for Drug Dispensing

Category of Packaging*	Package Characteristics	Examples
Tablets/capsules		
Desirable	Clean, dry, plastic or glass container with tightly sealing cap or seal	Blister packages, plastic sachets, tightly sealing plastic or glass containers with screw or snap cap
Acceptable	Clean, dry container that provides protection from dirt and moisture	Zip-lock plastic bags, glycine paper, hinged-lid boxes, sifter-top boxes, tight-top tins
Undesirable	Unclean absorbent paper, cotton, cardboard containers with no provision for closure	Unsealed plastic bags, paper bags, newspaper or other printed paper
Liquids (oral and topical)		
Desirable	Clean, dry, light-resistant glass container with tightly sealing cap	Amber or opaque bottle with screw cap
Acceptable	Clean, dry plastic or glass container with tight-fitting cap	Glass or plastic bottle with tight-fitting cap
Undesirable	Unclean paper, cardboard, metallic, or plastic (not formed) container with no provision for closure	Previously used liquid-containing cartons, plastic-lined paper bags, plastic bags
Liquids (otic and ophthalmic)		
Desirable	Clean (preferably sterile), light-resistant glass or plastic container with a dropper incorporated into a tightly sealing cap or a top fitted with dropper with a protective sleeve	Amber dropper bottle, opaque plastic dropper bottle
Acceptable	Clean, dry plastic or glass container with tight-fitting cap and a clean plastic/glass dropper (separate)	Glass or plastic bottle with tight-fitting cap, glass or plastic dropper with protective container (cardboard, zip-lock, plastic, or paper)
Undesirable	Anything other than above	Anything else
Creams/ointments		
Desirable	Clean glass or porcelain wide-mouth jar with tightly fitting lid or collapsible plastic or metal tube	Wide-mouth jar with well-closed lid, cream or ointment tube with cap
Acceptable	Clean glass or porcelain jar with lid	Glass or porcelain jar
Undesirable	Anything other than above	Anything else

* Desirable: Packaging should meet listed requirements for period greater than 30 days.
  Acceptable: Packaging should meet listed requirements for up to 30 days.
  Undesirable: Packaging provides no protection from dirt, moisture, or other contaminants, thus permitting rapid deterioration or contamination.

► Large numbers of patients come for medicines at the same time.

► A few medicines are prescribed frequently, and in the same quantities.

► The type of packaging used will provide protection from the atmosphere until the patient uses the medicine.

► It is possible to label the package with the drug name and strength.

► Prescribers are involved in the selection of packaging quantities and agree to prescribe the chosen quantities.

Benefits of Course-of-Therapy Prepackaging
Course-of-therapy prepackaging has many advantages:

► Safer, easier, and faster distribution of drugs with less room for error, which frees the dispenser from routine counting chores and allows more time for communication with patients;

► Improved credibility among users, due to the attractiveness and cleanliness of the package, which can be comparable to that of commercial drugs;

► More accurate and efficient prescribing by all health workers because of the standard treatments chosen for prepackaging;

► Possibility for routine prepackaging to be done by untrained staff following clear procedures and subject to appropriate quality checks and controls;

► Easier and more accurate recording of inventory, with better control over drug supplies and more accurate consumption data.

Importance of Controls in Prepackaging Process
Prepackaging of drugs is technically a "manufacturing" process, which must be done under strict controls reflecting good manufacturing practices (GMPs). In particular:

► Only one kind and strength of medicine is prepacked at a time in one work area or on one surface.

► The supervisor checks beforehand that the "prepacker" has the correct labels and that the number of labels and containers is the same and corresponds to the number of tablets or capsules to be prepacked. For example, to prepack in amounts of 20 from a bulk container of 1,000 tablets, the packer requires 50 containers and 50 labels.

► The supervisor checks the product at the end of the process.

► A written record is kept of the details (name, strength,

Figure 32.12 Dispensed Drug Label

Tetracycline tablets 20

250 mg

One to be taken four times a day

Daniel Piri 3/3/96

Figure 32.13 Pictorial Labeling

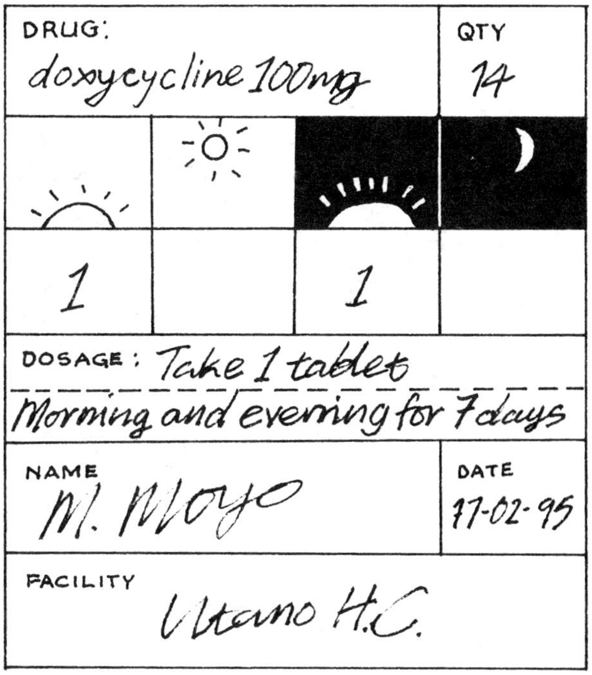

batch number, expiry date) of the preparation to be packed, the number of packs produced, the date packed, the name and signature of the packer, the name and signature of the supervisor, and the internal batch number for the prepackaged product.

Precautions and Quality Checks

Prepackaging is repackaging, and the legal responsibility for the quality and labeling of the newly packed medicine is transferred from the original manufacturer to the repacker. Therefore, the quality of the product must be checked before and after prepacking. Package seals must also be checked on a regular basis to ensure that they close tightly and will protect the prepackaged medicine adequately.

The amount to be prepackaged depends on rate of use and the climatic conditions. In humid climates or during the rainy season, only an amount sufficient for a few days' needs can be prepacked, especially if the new packaging cannot be tightly closed. Prepackaging is a waste of time and resources if the product becomes unfit for use. Chapter 19 provides more information on procedures for repackaging.

≡ 32.7 Aids in Counting Tablets and Capsules

Aids for counting tablets and capsules include triangular tablet counters, pan weighing scales, and electronic tablet counters.

Triangular Tablet Counter

A triangular tablet counter is an equilateral triangle made of wood, metal, or plastic with raised edges along two sides. Metal or plastic is preferred because these surfaces can be easily cleaned or washed between uses for different products. The tablets are counted by counting the number of rows of tablets and then pouring them into the container using a raised edge as a guide (see Figure 32.14).

This simple device is good for counting small quantities of round compressed tablets, regardless of their size. The smaller the tablet, the more tablets can be counted at one

time. With care, the triangle can be used for sugar-coated round tablets. It is also useful as a surface on which to count any tablet or capsule, making the transfer to a container a simple process. The key for the number of rows and number of tablets is shown in Figure 32.14.

Pan Weighing Scales

Scales can be particularly useful when counting tablets or capsules during prepackaging. The balance must be free to move, and the pans must be clean. The required number of tablets or capsules is counted and placed on one of the scale pans. Equal quantities of the same tablet or capsule can then be counted by adding to the other scale pan until a balanced position is reached.

Electronic Tablet Counter

When prepackaging is done on a large scale, as in a teaching hospital for both ward and outpatient department use, the use of an electronic counter may be justified (Country Study 32.3).

≡ 32.8 Pharmacy Personnel

The availability of qualified pharmacy personnel varies widely throughout the world, and the status given to different levels of trained pharmacy staff is equally varied. These facts reflect the indeterminate role of trained pharmacy personnel in health care services.

Drugs play such a prominent role in the provision and cost of health care that it is surprising how often the management

Figure 32.14 Tablet Counter in Use

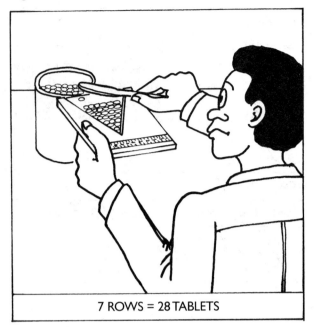

7 ROWS = 28 TABLETS

Key

Rows	4	5	6	7	8	9	10	11	12	13
Tablets	10	15	21	28	36	45	55	66	78	91

Country Study 32.3 Tablet-Counting Machine in Nepal

Patan Hospital in Kathmandu, Nepal, is a 138-bed hospital providing inpatient and outpatient services. In 1991, a study of outpatient dispensing was performed. On average, 34,000 tablets were dispensed per day. Seventy-five percent of these were in prepacks. Meeting this demand required between three and five pharmacy assistants prepacking continuously.

To address this problem, a tablet-counting machine was purchased. The electronic counter counts tablets or capsules into containers or dispensing bags. Since its installation, the machine has been used every day and has had no mechanical problems over a period of three years. The machine has freed up the staff to talk with patients and cope with the increased workload.

of this resource is left to untrained and nonspecialized staff. It is important to appreciate the potential value of an appropriately trained pharmacy workforce.

There are three recognized cadres of pharmacy staff: pharmacists, pharmacy technicians (or technologists or auxiliaries), and auxiliary or assistant staff. The first two normally receive their training in the formal educational sector.

Chapters 47 and 48 discuss in detail aspects of human resources and training related to drug management.

Pharmacists

In most countries, a pharmacist is a professional who is registered with the appropriate national board or society after having obtained a university degree in pharmacy, frequently followed by a year of supervised work or apprenticeship.

Pharmacists are employed to practice in four main areas: drug control administration, hospital pharmacy, the manufacturing industry, and community (retail) pharmacy. The first two areas usually fall into the public sector, and the latter two into the private sector, although an industry may be owned and operated by the public sector. Along with their practices, many pharmacists are also involved, either full-time or part-time, in teaching, training, and research.

The role of pharmacists in drug supply has altered sig-

nificantly in the last twenty years. It can be summarized as moving from the care of pharmaceuticals (being product centered) to pharmaceutical care (being patient centered). A decrease in the need to compound medicines and an increase in the complexity and potency of available manufactured finished products have resulted in a change from concern about the preparation of drugs to involvement in the use of drugs by patients.

The training of pharmacists in industrialized countries reflects this change by providing more clinical and patient-oriented teaching, which prepares pharmacists to be participating members of the clinical team in hospitals and primary health care. Pharmacists are increasingly involved in deciding on and designing treatments, and they are recognized by health professionals and the public as experts in the field of drugs. The expertise and potential contribution of pharmacists to public and private health care have yet to be appreciated by those countries that seek to provide an effective drug supply without an adequate and trained pharmacist workforce.

Pharmacy Technicians

Pharmacy technician training is normally a government-recognized vocational course provided on a full- or part-time basis through technical colleges or health training institutes. The length of training may vary according to the national education system. In most developing countries, courses are two to three years, whereas a course can be one year or less in industrialized countries. All courses emphasize practical skills and experience in dispensing medicines, and work experience is commonly a significant portion of the course. Basic teaching is given in pharmacology, pharmaceutics, microbiology, and related subjects. There is always a need to revise and update course content to meet job requirements.

≡ Assessment Guide

Dispensing Indicators

► Average dispensing communication time. This measures the time the dispenser actually spends explaining how the drugs should be taken.

► Percentage of prescribed drugs actually dispensed. This is primarily a stock indicator.

► Percentage of drugs prescribed adequately labeled. Packages should contain at least patients' names, drug names, and when the drug should be taken (dose and frequency).

► Patients' knowledge of correct dosage.

Dispensing Regulation

► Is there a licensing system to regulate the sale of drugs (wholesalers, pharmacists, retailers)?

► Are pharmacists legally allowed to substitute generic drugs for brand-name products?

► Is there an official checklist for carrying out inspections in different types of pharmaceutical establishments?

Dispensing Training

► At each level in the health care system, who is responsible for the dispensing of drugs? What training do these individuals have in the principles and practices of drug dispensing?

► How much supervision do these individuals receive? What type of pharmaceutical training is available in the country? Are there standardized education curricula for pharmacy personnel? Are experience requirements for dispensers spelled out and reasonable, given the numbers and geographical distribution of individuals meeting, or eligible for meeting, these requirements?

See also the checklist in Figure 32.10.

Pharmacy technicians are important members of the pharmaceutical care team, and they constitute the largest group of trained pharmacy personnel in many countries. Their training qualifies them to work effectively in dispensing and drug supply activities. They have enough training to be involved in decision-making and supervision of other staff, and individuals with experience can be given significant responsibility.

Insufficient planning has been directed to developing attractive and rewarding career structures for pharmacy technicians so that those with experience and ambition can fulfill their potential.

Country Study 32.4   Training Pharmacy Assistants in Transkei, South Africa

In Transkei, South Africa, eighteen pharmacists are responsible for managing pharmacies in twenty-seven hospitals, a central medical store, three polyclinics, and over 279 health centers. Due to the shortage of pharmacists, most pharmacies in hospitals and other facilities are managed by pharmacy assistants.

Pharmacy assistants have eight years of basic education and receive on-the-job training. A formal training program was developed to supplement the on-the-job experience. The nine-week course was spread over thirty weeks and included stock management, dispensing practice, and related issues such as maintenance of the cold chain, supplies, and pharmaceutical terms. A manual was produced to serve as a training and reference resource.

Auxiliary or Assistant Pharmacy Staff

Auxiliary staff complete a relatively short on-the-job training program to assist pharmacists and technicians in the routine work of dispensing and drug supply (see Country Study 32.4). Such training should be oriented to the tasks of the work environment. Assistant staff should follow written protocols and need to be supervised in their work, especially if the products of that work are given directly to patients. They should not be expected to interpret prescriptions on their own. Their supervisors should recognize that, with experience, these assistants can develop high skills in particular areas. ■

≡ References and Further Readings

★ = Key readings.

Jama, A. S., L. Heide, and A. Peterson. 1985. Colour coding of labels for essential drugs. Tropical Doctor 15:195.
Royal Pharmaceutical Society of Great Britain. Updated semi-annually. Appendix: Standards of good professional practice. In Medicines, ethics, and practice: A guide for pharmacists. London: Royal Pharmaceutical Society of Great Britain (Lambeth High St., London SE1 7JN, England).
Vogler, J. 1990. Low cost medicine packaging. London: Appropriate Health Resources and Technologies Action Group.
★ WHO (World Health Organization). 1990. The role of the pharmacist in the health care system. Geneva: WHO.
Zimbabwe Ministry of Health. 1987. ZEDAP training unit: Dispensing drugs. Harare, Zimbabwe.

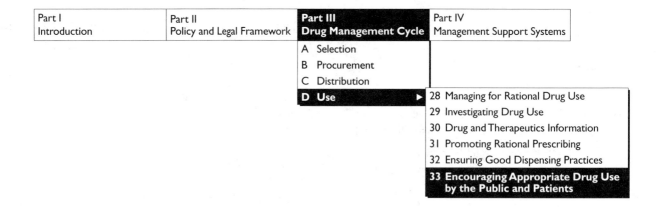

Part I	Part II	**Part III**	Part IV
Introduction	Policy and Legal Framework	**Drug Management Cycle**	Management Support Systems

A Selection
B Procurement
C Distribution

D Use ▶

28 Managing for Rational Drug Use
29 Investigating Drug Use
30 Drug and Therapeutics Information
31 Promoting Rational Prescribing
32 Ensuring Good Dispensing Practices
33 Encouraging Appropriate Drug Use by the Public and Patients

Chapter 33
Encouraging Appropriate Drug Use by the Public and Patients

≡ Summary

Although prescribers play an essential role in the choice of medicines, the role of the patient is equally important. Public knowledge, attitudes, and perceptions regarding the use of medicines influence the decision to seek health care, from whom, and whether to follow the proposed treatment. In some countries, most medicines, including prescription drugs, are bought directly over the counter, often from unauthorized sources, and often in response to aggressive commercial marketing.

There is a need for public education in the use of medicines. Relevant strategies, based on known facilitating factors and possible constraints, must be developed and implemented.

Six steps toward more effective education programs are:

► *Investigate the situation.*
► *Plan activities.*
► *Develop materials.*
► *Test and revise the materials.*
► *Implement activities.*
► *Evaluate the activities.*

It is important to develop programs in collaboration with the people whose drug use patterns have been targeted for change, taking into account the cultural and social context in which beliefs and practices have developed. All educational materials must be pretested on the target audience.

≡ 33.1 The Need for Public Education about Appropriate Drug Use

Although the prescriber's role in promoting rational drug use is important, the patient and the cultural context in which therapy is selected cannot be ignored. The knowledge, attitudes, and education of the public in relation to disease etiology and treatment are critical determinants in the decision to seek health care, the choice of provider, the use of medicines, and the success of treatment.

Patients are actively involved in the therapeutic encounter and treatment. It is the patient who decides whether to go ahead with a treatment or not, a choice often influenced by the views of family, close friends, and the community. In many developing countries, an entire social network's collective knowledge and experience may be mobilized in the therapeutic decision. People make a series of decisions before a treatment is self-chosen or adopted:

First: People who are ill have to believe that their health status has deviated from the norm, that there is something wrong with them. To some extent, this perception is culturally defined. In the case of children, the knowledge and experience of the mother are critical determinants.

Second: People or care-givers of children have to decide whether this alteration of health status is significant enough for them to seek help or whether the symptoms will go away without treatment.

Third: Once they decide that help is needed, people choose where to seek help: a hospital, primary health care center, private physician, pharmacist, market vendor, traditional healer, relative, or some other member of the community. They may decide, erroneously or not, that the symptoms are minor or that they have sufficient familiarity with the required treatment to take care of themselves, with either a modern pharmaceutical or a traditional remedy. An example from the Philippines is given in Figure 33.1.

Fourth: Once they have a prescription or have received a recommendation for products from a pharmacy, patients decide whether to buy the drugs, whether they are going to buy all or some of the items recommended, and which drugs to buy. Cost considerations may require a choice of which items to buy and which to ignore.

Fifth: Patients decide whether and when to take the medicines, how to take the medicines, whether to continue if side effects occur or symptoms disappear, and what to do with medicines that remain unused.

Without public education in the appropriate use of drugs, people lack the skills and knowledge either to make informed decisions about how to use drugs (including when not to use them) or to understand the role of drugs in health care. Public education provides individuals and communities with information that enables them to use medicines in an appropriate, safe, and judicious way. Inappropriate drug use has serious health and economic consequences for both individuals and the community. Appropriate drug use by patients and consumers is an *integral* part of successful national drug policies.

The Alma Ata declaration states that "*people have the right and duty to participate individually and collectively in the planning and implementation of their health care,*" a principle that should be a cornerstone of national public health and hence of drug policy. Public information and education on drug use are considered by the World Health Organization (WHO) to be key elements in national drug policy. Yet despite the progress by some countries, drug use education for the public is seldom allocated the necessary

Figure 33.1 Community Drug Distribution Channels: An Example from the Philippines

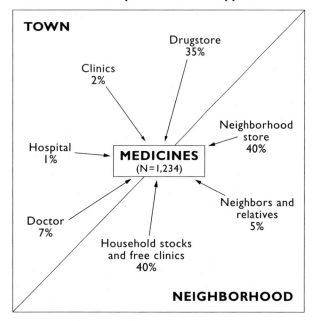

Source: Hardon 1991, reprinted with permission.
Note: The total from the figure is 98 percent due to rounding.

human and financial resources. It is frequently treated as a marginal activity or one to be tackled only when the other elements of drug policy are in place.

Problems

Irrational drug use has been well documented and includes overuse, underuse, and inappropriate use. Various factors contribute to these problems: lack of adequate regulatory systems, shortages of essential drugs and availability of nonessential drugs, lack of objective drug information for prescribers and consumers, poor communication between prescribers and patients, exclusion of patients from the information needed to become partners in therapy, and the considerable influence of drug promotion on both prescribers and consumers.

Most developing countries have public health problems of drug misuse, including

- ▶ widespread availability of "prescription" drugs from itinerant peddlers, market stalls, or nonlicensed drugstores;
- ▶ increasing incorporation of Western medicines into the local culture, leading to their adoption by traditional practitioners who are untrained in their use and by the community for self-medication;
- ▶ deregulation and the expansion of the private sector as a source of drugs, with a corresponding commercialization of drug supply and promotion.

Benefits

Improving public understanding about medicines will not resolve all these issues, but—together with other activities to promote rational use—will contribute to the development of better drug use.

At an individual level, the benefits of improved public understanding include

- ▶ better appreciation of the limits of medicines and a lessening of the belief that there is a pill for every ill;
- ▶ more balanced partnership between consumer-patients and health care providers;
- ▶ more critical attitude toward advertising and other commercial information, which often fails to give objective information about drugs;
- ▶ better understanding of how to take medicines when needed.

At the community level, the benefits include

- ▶ more understanding and support for drug policy and measures to rationalize drug use;
- ▶ more economic use of drugs and less waste of resources;
- ▶ improved confidence in health services and health care providers;
- ▶ increased success of measures to deal with public health problems.

Education is needed at a general level to give people a better understanding of what medicines are, how they act in the body, their risks and benefits, and their role in health care. At a more specific level, education is needed to tackle particularly serious problems of misuse. Campaigns for the wiser use of specific drugs (for example, in diarrheal disease control programs) have proved effective in reducing morbidity and mortality and in cutting down on needless expenditures.

≡ 33.2 Principles of Public Education in Appropriate Drug Use

The following principles should guide public education in appropriate drug use:

- ▶ Drug use should be seen within the context of a society, community, family, and individual. Public education on drugs should recognize cultural diversity in concepts of health and illness or notions about how drugs work. The different expectations surrounding Western and traditional medicines need to be considered, as do preferences for injections or for tablets of a particular color because they are considered more potent. Social factors such as poverty, disadvantage, and power relations can also influence drug use.

► Education in the appropriate use of drugs should be integrated into school curricula.

► Public education should encourage informed decision-making by individuals, families, and communities on the use of drugs and on nondrug solutions.

► Public education should be based on the best available scientific information about drugs, including their efficacy and side effects.

► To facilitate informed choices on drug use, public education should be accompanied by supportive legislation and controls on drug availability.

► Nongovernmental organizations (NGOs), community groups, and consumer and professional organizations have important roles to play in public education programs and should be involved, when possible, in the planning and implementation of education activities.

► Effective public education about drugs requires a commitment to, and an understanding of the need for, improved communication between health care providers and patients. This should be reflected in appropriate educational and training curricula for providers.

≡ 33.3 Developing Public and Patient Education Strategies

Strategies to encourage appropriate drug use by the consumer can be public or patient centered, but they should always be culturally specific. A public-centered approach provides the community, or target populations within the community, with information on the role of medicines and on how to make appropriate health-seeking decisions at times of illness. A patient-centered approach focuses on how a patient who has received a prescription or drug can be encouraged to adhere to the prescribed treatment. Strategies in both categories are discussed below. (The term *adherence [nonadherence] to treatment* is used in this chapter instead of the more common *compliance [noncompliance]*, which carries an inappropriate judgmental connotation.)

≡ 33.4 Public Education in Appropriate Drug Use

Effective communication involves a *process* (see Figure 33.2) that evolves and is modified as new information on its effectiveness and areas for improvements become evident.

Public education can aim to influence people's thinking in many ways, including

► organizing campaigns to promote the values and benefits of essential drugs;

► empowering the consumer to understand what a correct prescription should look like and to know what questions to ask a health care provider;

► providing young people with a general information base about the action and use of medicines on which they can draw as adult consumers;

► targeting a particular public health problem related to medicine use, such as home injections and the reuse of needles;

► working through commercial pharmacies to offer information on specific drugs and treatment categories, as in the comprehensive information programs developed by the National Corporation of Swedish Pharmacists and the Pharmaceutical Society of Australia.

Providing information is much easier than changing behavior. Many studies show that knowledge does not necessarily influence action. Changing people's behavior generally requires a long-term strategy undertaken after a careful analysis of the situation and identification of priority problems, with knowledge of the societal context in which the strategy will be carried out. Identification of target groups and pretested, culturally specific materials are necessary. These materials should always be evaluated for their impact not only on knowledge acquired but also on actual behavioral change.

The steps shown in Figure 33.2 are discussed below.

Step 1. Investigate

Investigation is the foundation for the communication process. It should address the following issues:

Information already available: Information about the problem can be gleaned from reports of studies or from annual reports of organizations working in related fields.

New information needed: If it is not already available, information is needed on sources of drugs and on how health services and drugs are used in the community. The more data obtained on audience characteristics, the better: demography, socioeconomic and literacy status, language patterns, community decision-making and leadership processes, characteristics of prescribers and users, and local beliefs and practices relating to disease etiology and the use of medicines are all useful.

Communication networks: What sources of information about drugs are most credible to the target audience, including nonmedical sources? What channels of information reach users most effectively? Do mass media channels play a role?

Figure 33.2 Six Steps toward Effective Communication

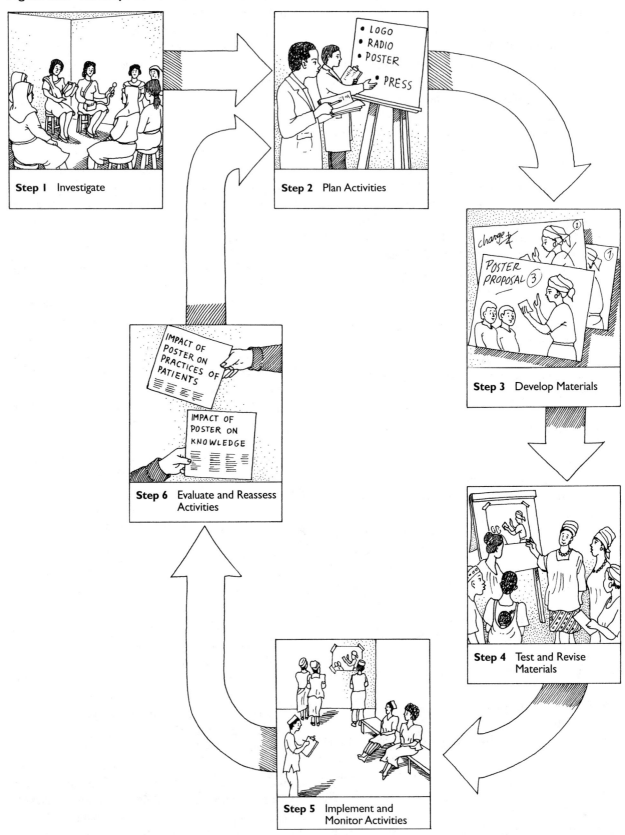

Communication development: What resources exist in research, education and training, production and distribution of information, and social mobilization?

A combination of quantitative and qualitative research methods can be used to obtain the necessary data. *Quantitative methods*, such as household surveys, provide useful information on levels of knowledge and on the practices and beliefs prevalent in a population: they measure *what* is happening. *Qualitative methods*, such as focus group discussions and in-depth individual interviews, yield substantial information about specific behaviors, as well as the reasons and motivations underlying them: they explore *how* and *why* things are happening. These methods, described in Chapter 29, generate many ideas and provide language for communication materials.

Step 2. Plan Communication Activities

Initial research and prioritization of problems define the behaviors to be adopted or changed or knowledge to be acquired, as well as constraints and facilitating factors that will affect the planning process and the feasibility of possible objectives. The target audience may be the entire population in the case of a broad-based national program; more often, it will be a subsection of the community such as schoolchildren, mothers of young children, the elderly, community leaders, or women's organizations.

The communication plan defines objectives and outlines how they are to be reached. It should include the elements discussed below.

Realistic and Well-Defined Communication Objectives. These objectives should focus on specific problems and target the people exhibiting the problem behavior. General campaigns may raise awareness, but they are unlikely to result in significant behavioral changes. Country Study 33.1 discusses problems with drug use in one state of Mexico and the strategies used to address them.

Approaches to Change. Approaches can include either a "campaign" approach of short, high-intensity programs that focus on single issues (for example, injection misuse) or longer-term, sustained efforts integrated with other primary health care and educational activities (such as a literacy reader on drug use, lesson outlines for the primary or secondary school curriculum, or routine health center education sessions).

The communication strategy may use a persuasive or social marketing approach to influence the target audience. Social marketing, often criticized as a top-down approach, can be an effective communication strategy, particularly in specifically targeted campaigns that take into account com-

---

Country Study 33.1 Michoacan, Mexico, Holds a Campaign to Promote the Rational Use of Drugs

Given evidence of overuse of medications by the general population, overprescription of medications by doctors, and unethical drug promotion, a nongovernmental organization in the Mexican state of Michoacan embarked on a short but intense educational campaign. Prescribers, government officials, community members, students, the media, and communication experts participated in planning the campaign.

This campaign targeted the general public as well as prescribers and medical students. The materials developed included posters, leaflets, press articles, slides, radio and television programs, and posters for doctors. Many of the printed materials were displayed at points of prescription; others were used during three-day seminars held at the local medical school. The mass media broadcasts lasted for three months, with increasing intensity just before the medical school conferences.

Feedback after the campaign was very positive. Medical professionals and students expressed increased awareness of the problems. The pharmacology curriculum of the local university was revised. Articles published in the local and national press suggested a significant change in general knowledge about rational drug use.

Source: WHO 1996.

---

munity needs, perceptions, and values. Alternatively, giving people the information and problem-solving and decision-making skills necessary to make their own decisions is ideal in the long run but much more difficult to implement and evaluate. With disadvantaged groups, it can also involve "consciousness-raising" and promoting awareness that they can become empowered to make decisions and control their own lives. For example, consumers can be encouraged to act with authority and ask questions of the health care provider (see Figure 33.3).

Communication Channels to Deliver Messages. Ideally, a communication program should combine channels, including interpersonal channels, to maximize exchange. Each channel has its own strength: what matters is that it be cost effective and appropriate to the audience and the message. Possibilities include

- printed materials—posters, leaflets, textbooks, comics;
- mass media and audiovisual media—radio, television, newspapers, videos, tapes;
- interpersonal (or face-to-face) encounters—health workers, schoolteachers, community leaders, shopkeepers, community organizations;
- folk media—community theater, puppets, singing groups, and other folk media (important traditional channels in many countries).

Figure 33.3 Questions for a Consumer to Ask about a Prescription: An Example from the Philippines

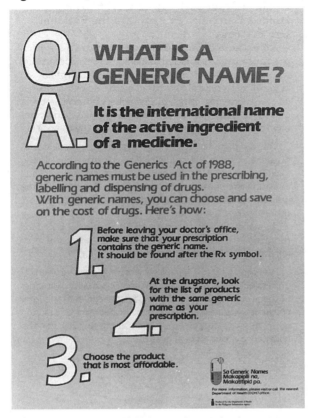

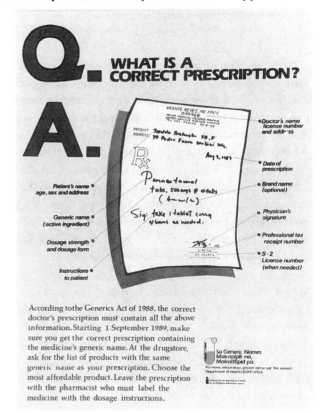

Source: Department of Health, Philippines. Reprinted with permission.

Collaborating Institutions. Collaborating with a wide range of institutions—NGOs; consumer organizations; women's, youth, or social solidarity organizations; development agencies such as WHO and the United Nations Children's Fund (UNICEF); and professional associations—enhances visibility, potentially increases impact, and promotes rational use concepts and the national drug policy. Religious groups provide a substantial proportion of health care and are potential partners in many countries.

Monitoring and Evaluation (see Steps 5 and 6 below). Milestones (for example, number of manuals produced or number of workshops completed) can be used to chart progress toward the objectives of the communication plan.

Timetable, Budget, and Source of Financing. For each activity, the plan should define when it is to occur, who is responsible for it, and the funding source. A common method of displaying such information is a Gantt chart (see Chapter 35).

Step 3. Develop Communication Materials
The research undertaken in the previous steps provides data for prioritizing areas of intervention, approaches,

communication channels, and messages to be conveyed. It should also provide insight into the cultural context of behavior and beliefs and indications of useful language and expressions.

Step 4. Test and Revise Materials
Materials should always be pretested on the target audience to answer the following questions:

► Does the target audience understand the materials?
► Do they feel that the materials apply to them?
► Do they find the materials attractive?
► Is there anything offensive or culturally inappropriate?
► Is the message convincing? If not, why not?
► Based on audience response, do changes need to be made in the message or its format?

Pretesting materials is *essential* and often produces surprising results. A picture may be completely misunderstood, particularly if it uses a stylized design in a society that is relatively inexperienced in interpreting graphic images. For example, a poster in Central America initially showed four boxes illustrating the correct sequence for mixing oral rehydration solution (ORS). The sequential numbers included in each box were interpreted by the target audience to mean that one cup of water was to be added to the packet, two corners torn off, three packets emptied into the bottle, and the bottle shaken four times.

Step 5. *Implement and Monitor Activities*

It is important to make sure in advance that all materials will be ready at the start of the program, channels of distribution have been organized, and everyone involved is fully informed about program goals and strategies.

Once the program starts, a clear system of monitoring should assess whether

- target audiences are receiving program materials and messages;
- target audiences are using the materials and understanding the messages (in the case of radio programs, this might include a program log with transmission times and tapes and listener interviews to determine whether the messages were understood);
- the program is on schedule (if not, why not?);
- delays in program implementation will have implications for future planned activities.

Step 6. *Evaluate and Reassess Activities*

An evaluation to determine whether program objectives were met should also distinguish between *knowledge acquisition* and *behavior change*. One may occur without the other, but most educational interventions target both. Pre- and postintervention quantitative research can help measure impact on behavior, and it is useful to define some clear quantitative indicators, such as the percentage of respondents who self-treat a specific condition correctly or who never reuse disposable syringes. Measures that can be used to determine impact include

- exposure to project messages and materials;
- proportion of knowledge change;
- change in consumer satisfaction;
- change in drug sales patterns;
- proportion of reported behavior change;
- use or adaptation of the program by other groups as a model in developing their own projects.

When possible, compare results with those from a control group not exposed to the intervention (see Chapters 29 and 31).

Reassessment of procedures requires feedback on:

- What problems were experienced in developing and implementing the program?
- What factors outside the project (for example, change

of legislation, increase or decrease in available drugs, support from the ministry of health) contributed to its success or lack of success?
- What factors within the project contributed to its success or lack of success?
- What improvements could be made?
- What are the most important lessons to be learned for the future?

Fully documented communication activities are easier to monitor and evaluate, so future program planners can learn from the experience. Even when communication activities are carried out on a large scale, it is often very difficult, particularly in developing countries, to obtain reports of them. This leads to unnecessary duplication, loss of experience gained, and waste of resources.

In summary, the steps outlined above are valid for small educational interventions or national programs. Even if resources are sufficient only for a small-scale educational intervention, it is still important to know *why* people act as they do: no human behavior takes place in a vacuum; it is always "rational" within a given personal framework. Many beliefs about health care do not match a biomedical model, and recognition of both strengths and weaknesses of local traditions is needed. It is always necessary to use the credible channels of communication in a community to provide information. Materials must be pretested, since the perception of professionals will not be the same as that of a layperson whose formal education may be limited or nonexistent. Above all—and particularly when resources are limited—it is necessary to prioritize interventions in terms of the risk the problems pose to public health, and then focus on the major problem behavior and target the main risk groups.

≡ 33.5 Patient Education in Appropriate Drug Use

Patients' nonadherence to prescribed treatment is a global problem. Some studies have found nonadherence rates of over 50 percent, even in life-threatening situations. Causes include

- inappropriate attitudes and poor communication skills of providers;
- patients' fear of asking questions;
- inadequate consulting time;
- lack of access to printed information in simple language, such as patient leaflets or adequate labels;
- inability to pay for prescribed drugs;
- complexity and duration of treatment, particularly in cases of chronic disease.

Attitudes and Communication Skills of Providers

Numerous studies point to patient dissatisfaction with health care providers' attitudes. Common descriptions, particularly of prescribers in the public sector, include the adjectives cold, uninterested, rude, aggressive, abrupt, and authoritarian. Although such descriptions do not fit many dedicated and skilled practitioners, inappropriate attitudes toward patients are sufficiently well documented to indicate a significant problem. Research also shows that prescribers' and dispensers' communication skills are often weak: they tend to use complex terminology that patients cannot easily understand; they frequently lack knowledge of behavioral theory and practice; and they may have limited awareness of the scale, problems, and causes of patient nonadherence to treatment. The low priority given to communication skills in medical, paramedical, and pharmacy schools undoubtedly contributes to this situation.

Fortunately, some medical and pharmacy schools—notably in Australia, Canada, and Europe—are beginning to include communication techniques in their basic curricula, teaching behavioral theory and using role playing, and sometimes video as learning tools. Audiovisual feedback to students markedly enhances their acquisition of such skills, and basic communication training should be an integral part of any prescriber's or dispenser's education and refresher training.

Adherence to treatment is linked to the clarity of the prescriber's explanation: patients often feel that instructions are stated unclearly or not at all. The timing and clarity of a message powerfully affect how it is received, understood, and retained. Patients remember best the first instructions presented; instructions that are emphasized are better recalled; and the fewer instructions given, the greater the proportion remembered. Thus, a message must not only be clearly stated; it must also be organized and delivered in a way that allows the patient to attend to and process the information completely.

Although adherence to treatment depends on a patient's acceptance of information about the health threat itself, the practitioner must also be able to persuade the patient that the treatment is worthwhile. Adherence to treatment is linked to the patient's perception of the practitioner's friendliness, empathy, interest, and concern. Finally, in most circumstances, it is essential not only to specify the precise actions to be taken (for example, taking two pills twice a day) but also to suggest how that action can be inserted into the daily routine (for example, taking them at breakfast and dinner).

Patients' Fear of Asking Questions

Patients often hesitate to ask providers to clarify either their basic health condition or the treatment proposed. This hesitancy can be linked to fears of appearing foolish, to differences in social status and language, or to nonencouragement by providers. A more fruitful patient-provider interaction can be encouraged by increased sensitivity on the part of providers, active involvement of consumer organizations in promoting such interaction, and specific campaigns to empower patients. (See examples from Australia and the United States in Figures 33.4 and 33.5.) Consumer organizations are also campaigning to promote more fruitful patient interaction with doctors.

Inadequate Consulting Time

Providers sometimes attribute lack of interaction with patients to the pressures of work. In some hospital departments or busy practices where consultation time is extremely limited, this is clearly a problem. If a patient is accorded only one or two minutes of consulting time, more harm than good may occur. The cost to the patient is high in terms of time, travel, and drug expenses. Many health centers and outpatient departments see all their patients during a few morning hours. One possibility to consider is extending this period so that each individual can receive more time with the prescriber and dispenser. Another possibility is to train staff to make better use of the time available and to ensure that patients don't fall into an "information gap": if the provider does not have the time to explain the treatment to the patient and ensure that the instructions are fully understood, the dispenser or nurse should be trained to do this. Staff must be encouraged to understand that effective communication with patients is not an unrealistic ideal but a core aspect of clinical practice.

Availability of Printed Information

Adherence to treatment may be increased by the availability of printed information in simple language. In Sweden, all pharmacies must have patient information sheets available on each medicine. In the United Kingdom, the Association of the British Pharmaceutical Industry has published guidelines for drafting patient information leaflets. The United States Pharmacopeia publishes several drug-specific and disease-specific leaflets, in addition to its annually revised volume of authoritative drug information for patients (USP 1996), which is also available on CD-ROM. Such leaflets need well-written text, effective graphic design, large print size, and clear layout to enhance legibility; a question format may stimulate consumer involvement (see Figure 33.6).

Figure 33.4 Talking about Prescriptions: An Example from Australia

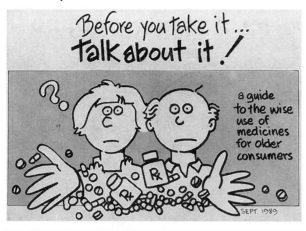

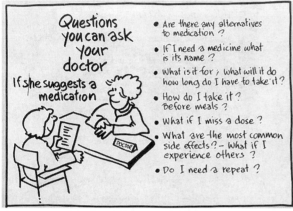

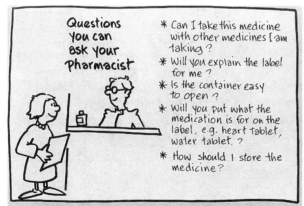

Artist: Greg Gore. Published with permission of the Australian Consumers' Association.

In many parts of the world it is not feasible to produce leaflets for individual patients. High rates of nonliteracy in some countries also limit the value of such information. Yet simple instructions for the most commonly used and misused drugs could be printed on inexpensive paper a few inches square, and many countries have produced standard treatment guidelines and formularies for health

care providers. In some countries, such as Nepal and the Philippines, materials are produced for nonprofessional drug sellers (see Chapter 32, Country Study 32.2).

Simple booklets for display in retail outlets and health centers can provide consumer information on the most common drugs. Even nonliterate patients can obtain information from such publications with help from family or community members. Public access to sources of impartial drug information is particularly important in view of the trend toward privatization of drug supply.

Pictograms can provide reinforcing information about medicines. A setting and rising sun or moon to represent different times of the day for taking medicine have been used in a number of countries, although an evaluation in Bangladesh found that dispensers had to be trained in their use. The United States Pharmacopeia–Drug Information (USP–DI) has developed a series of pictograms for use on drug labels (see Annex 33.1). Each country needs to develop its own symbols reflecting culturally known objects. Pretesting is important, as patients need to understand the symbols without explanation. Canada provides one successful example of the wide use of pictograms, although not for drug use. In the early 1970s, a set of 225 public information signs were developed and are now well known and widely used as a matter of public policy. Standardized road signs are another example of the use of pictograms.

Unaffordability of Drugs

Many providers have little or no knowledge of the cost of the drugs they prescribe. Prescribing a needlessly expensive brand-name drug when a much cheaper generic version of equal quality is available has consequences for the health sector, the community, and the individual patient. When part of the cost is borne directly by the patient, the drug may not be purchased at all because the patient cannot afford it. When more than one drug is prescribed (in some countries, the average number of drugs per prescription is five to six), the patient may be able to afford only one or two of the products listed and may choose the less important, relatively cheaper ones, such as vitamins, or buy only a partial treatment.

Providers need to know the approximate prices of drugs they prescribe, select the cheapest available drugs that are compatible with quality and therapeutic needs, and keep the number of products prescribed to a minimum. If more than one drug is prescribed, the provider should indicate the most important ones to the patient.

How can issues of cost be brought home to prescribers? Some countries, for example, Sri Lanka, have issued wall

Figure 33.5 Talking about Prescriptions: Examples from the United States

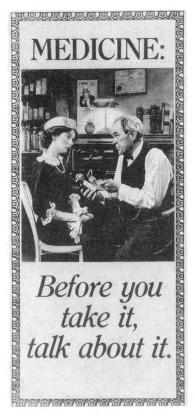

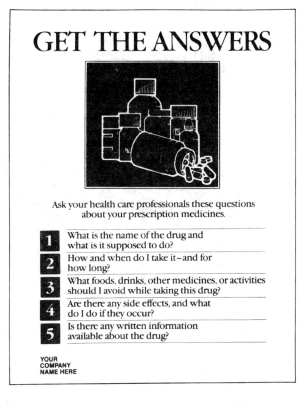

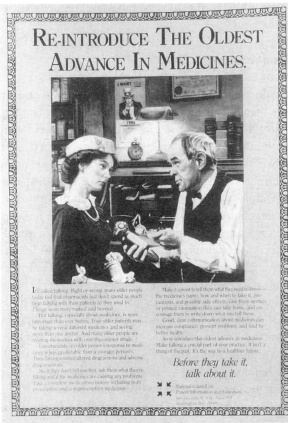

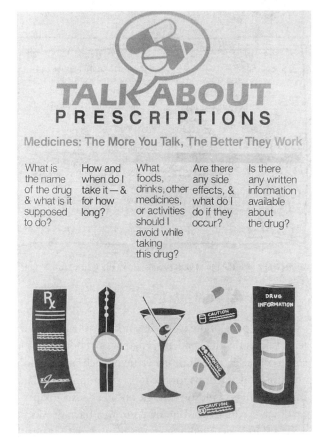

Source: Artwork courtesy of National Council on Patient Information and Education, Washington, D.C. Reprinted with permission.

posters for physician consulting rooms showing comparative costs of products in certain drug groups. Others publish price information in formularies and treatment guidelines. Australia conducts cost-awareness campaigns for prescribers for those drug groups in which huge differences exist.

Complexity and Duration of Treatment

The longer and more complex the treatment, the greater the likelihood that the patient will not follow it. Adherence to short-term treatments (less than two weeks) can be improved by clear instructions, special "reminder" pill containers and calendars, and simplified drug regimens (see Figure 33.7). Adherence to long-term treatments is more difficult to achieve. Although no single intervention is useful on its own, combinations of clear instructions, follow-up of nonattenders, patient self-monitoring, social support, cues for when to take the drugs, rewards, and group discussions are useful.

≡ 33.6 Facilitating and Constraining Factors

Public education activities are affected both positively and negatively by many influences (see Figure 33.8), which vary according to the level of development and health care infrastructure.

Factors that can facilitate public education are increased awareness of the need for drug education, including political will; knowledge of the factors underlying people's health-seeking behavior; and expanded coverage by mass media.

Factors that can constrain public education include a lack of coherent policies on both drug use and public education; commercial interests; professional interests; weak infrastructure; lack of resources; and economic, social, and cultural influences.

Facilitating Factors

Facilitating factors stimulate, provide, or promote a fertile environment for public education. Identifying these factors can improve public education campaigns.

Increased Awareness of the Need for Public Education on Drugs. Public interest in and demand for drug information have increased over the past decade. This awareness has been accompanied by the concept of the right to know and increasing expectations that individuals should take an active role in health care decisions. These changes have been stimulated by the democratic process, the growth of organized consumer and public-interest groups, and the movement for individuals to take more responsibility for their own health care. Awareness of the level of

Figure 33.6 Standard Drug Information for Consumers

What is _____ (insert product name)?
Why use _____?
When should _____ be/not be used?
What precautions should be taken?
  ▸ by children
  ▸ during pregnancy
  ▸ when breastfeeding
  ▸ while driving or operating machinery
  ▸ if taking other medicines
How should I take _____?
What should I do if I miss a dose?
What should I do if I take too many tablets?
What undesirable effect might _____ cause?
How should I store _____?

patient nonadherence to treatment regimens and of inappropriate forms of self-medication has also grown.

Increased networking allows public education experiences to be shared among government health services, NGOs, and community-based groups, so groups can learn from the experience of others.

As a response to both regulatory requirements and consumer pressures, some pharmaceutical companies are moving toward the provision of improved and user-friendly written patient information. Some professional bodies (notably pharmacists) in Europe, the United States, and Australia are developing training programs for their members to promote communication skills and interaction with consumers.

Knowledge of Social and Behavioral Theory. Research in the last decade has greatly expanded the knowledge base underlying health- and medicine-seeking behavior, particularly its cultural dimensions. Anthropologists have studied how drug consumption is culturally mediated (van der Geest, Hardon, and Whyte 1990).

Expanded Coverage by Mass Media and Information Technology. Recent advances in communication technology have created powerful mechanisms to convey educational messages. In the last decade, many people have gained access to radio and television, opening up new opportunities to reach large audiences, including nonliterate populations, with health-related messages.

With new information technology, some health professionals and patients have greater access to information from on-line databases and electronic mail (see Chapter 46). This has many potential benefits, including rapid access to objective information and low-cost sharing, pooling, and comparative evaluation of different methodologies.

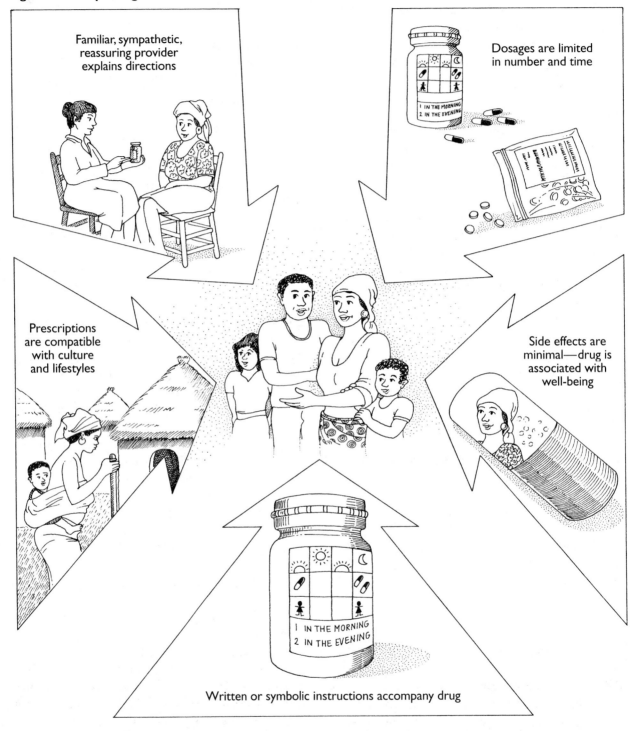

Figure 33.7 Improving Adherence to Treatment

Familiar, sympathetic, reassuring provider explains directions

Dosages are limited in number and time

Prescriptions are compatible with culture and lifestyles

Side effects are minimal—drug is associated with well-being

Written or symbolic instructions accompany drug

Constraining Factors

The factors that inhibit the implementation of public education strategies need to be recognized and evaluated, as solutions vary according to the particular situation of each country. The successes and failures of others can help in developing a framework for effective action (see "References and Further Readings").

Lack of Coherent Policies for Both Drug Use and Public Education. Many countries need to strengthen their national policies on drug use and to incorporate public education in them. Without a clear policy, it is difficult for public education to take place in a cohesive manner and be adequately supported. A fragmented approach can confuse the public with conflicting and competing messages.

The weak state of public education on drugs in many countries is partly the result of a lack of political commitment to public education in general. Within health services, public education is often given a low priority and is consequently poorly financed and staffed. Sometimes this void is filled by NGOs, which usually depend on donor agencies for funding that can be withdrawn or reallocated. In some instances, public education on drugs is considered a sensitive issue, because it may lead to community challenges of commercial and other vested interests. To improve the situation, a multisectoral approach involving key actors outside the health sector is crucial.

Commercial Interests. Commercial interests do not always match public interest. Particularly in developing countries, where control of drug promotion may be nonexistent, weak, or unenforceable, industry may contribute to inappropriate drug use by conducting promotional activities based on inaccurate information.

Professional Interests. Resistance to change within professional groups can constrain public education. Prescribers tend to hold influential and powerful positions, and they may not perceive the need for, or the importance of, public education. In turn, they often do not fulfill their professional role of providing advice on the appropriate use of drugs on either a personal or an organizational basis.

Public education can appear to conflict with existing values and power relationships, for example, by leading the public to challenge the traditional prescriber-patient relationship. Professional groups may oppose public education if they perceive it as a threat rather than a challenging opportunity arising from a new relationship with the community.

Weak Infrastructure. Lack of infrastructure within the health system for implementation of drug policies, including public education, can be a major constraint. Any effort to educate the public on appropriate drug use can be undermined if necessary drugs are inconsistently available in the public sector yet readily at hand in the private sector. Consumers then face the dilemma of reconciling public educational messages that motivate appropriate behavior with the reality of the marketplace.

Lack of Resources. Effective public education requires sufficient funding and the allocation of trained staff to enable targeting of population groups through appropriate strategies. Public education on drugs requires an extensive program to train health workers and other field staff in communication skills and appropriate drug use.

Social, Economic, and Cultural Factors. Lack of involve-

Figure 33.8 Factors That Facilitate or Constrain Public Education

Facilitating Factors	Constraining Factors
Increased awareness of need for drug education, including political will	Lack of coherent policies on both drug use and public education
Knowledge of factors underlying people's health-seeking behavior	Commercial interests Professional interests Weak infrastructure
Expanded coverage of world's population by mass media	Lack of resources Economic, social, and cultural influences

ment and participation of the target groups often leads to problems. Support for public education programs may be prematurely withdrawn because of a failure to recognize that bringing about behavioral change is a slow and long-term process.

A need exists for public and patient education in appropriate drug use. Such programs—whether run by government, development organizations, NGOs, community groups, or professional bodies—merit support and encouragement. Public education should form an integral part of both national drug policy and prescriber training. Policy-makers, professional bodies, prescribers, dispensers, and educators have important advocacy and technical roles.

A coalition of resources improves the chance of success and expands capacity and reach. Smaller-scale programs can provide valuable experiences to be shared, and they may later serve as development models for more comprehensive strategies. Finally, and perhaps most critically, health care practitioners must be convinced of their core educational role. They must be taught how to perform that role effectively and work to alter the all-too-common perception of patients as passive recipients of treatment.

When planning a campaign for promoting generic use (Chapter 10) or a national drug policy (Chapter 5), or when starting cost recovery (Chapter 44), similar communication elements can be included. These may involve a good logo, radio spots, a flyer or visual aid, a public poster, and possibly folk media (Figure 33.9). Although every element is not needed in every campaign, using these components helps vary the way in which the message is conveyed.

≡ 33.7 Communications for Essential Drugs Programs

Careful planning is needed for campaigns to promote new programs, such as expanded generic use (Chapter 10), a national drug policy (Chapter 5), or a cost recovery

Figure 33.9 Hints for Selecting Communication Methods for Public Education Programs

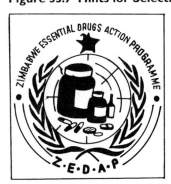

A Good Logo
- is simple, not cluttered
- is immediately understandable and explicit, not abstract
- is related to the key program benefit; a symbol of a key idea
- gives the idea of results
- is easily reproducible
- works in different sizes and settings
- dramatizes the overall tone of the change approach
- is positive and uplifting

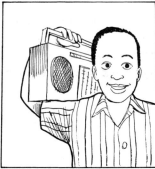

An Effective Radio Spot
- presents one idea
- begins with an attention getter
- is direct and explicit
- repeats the key idea at least two or three times
- asks listeners to take action
- makes the audience feel part of the situation
- maintains the same tone as the overall change approach

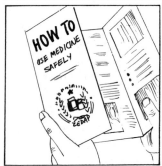

A Useful Flyer or Visual Aid
- carries the information most likely to be forgotten
- uses visuals, not only words, to tell the story
- shows people doing key behaviors
- uses attractive images
- is concise
- maintains same tone as overall change approach
- is organized so that it favors a logical action sequence
- is designed for easy use as a visual aid
- matches graphic and language skills of specific audience

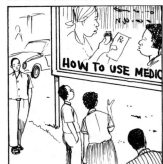

An Effective Public Poster
- dramatizes a single idea
- attracts attention from at least 10 meters away
- uses visuals to carry message
- is memorable
- models the behavior whenever possible
- shows the product's benefit to audience
- is consistent with tone of overall change approach

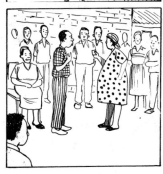

Folk Media
- use local drama groups and musicians; often powerful vehicles for sharing health-related messages
- include traveling health fairs with puppet shows, musical acts, distribution of printed materials, and appearances by local celebrities
- stimulate interest in national and local programs, for example, through fairs that travel from village to village

Source: Adapted from Rasmuson et al. 1988.

≡ Assessment Guide

Public Education Indicators

► Are there public education campaigns on drug use?

► Is drug education included in the primary and secondary school curricula?

► What materials have been produced for public education activities? How were these materials pretested? What evaluations of public education campaigns have occurred?

► What percentage of the public health or drug budget is allocated to public education?

► What amount is spent on public education campaigns on drug use, and what percentage does this represent out of the total amount spent on public health education campaigns?

Drug Promotion Regulation

► Are there controls on drug promotion based on regulations and consistent with the WHO ethical criteria for medicinal drug promotion?

► How many advertisements violated regulations on the ethical promotion of drugs out of the total number of advertisements monitored?

► How many sanctions were implemented for advertisements in violation of regulations, and what percentage of the total number of violations identified resulted in sanctions?

---

program (Chapter 44). The communications elements described in Figure 33.9 can be used in such campaigns.

A simple, clear logo should be developed to identify all printed materials from the campaign. An effective radio spot or audio cassette that communicates a key message may be useful to reach nonliterate community members. A flyer or pamphlet can be prepared to provide ongoing information. Posters that convey a single idea can also be created, but graphics that are understandable in the particular culture must be chosen. A recent innovation in some countries has been the use of folk media, such as drama and songs, to convey key campaign messages. ■

≡ References and Further Readings

★ = *Key readings.*

General

Hardon, A. 1991. *Confronting ill health: Medicines, self-care, and the poor in Manila.* Quezon City, Philippines: Health Action International.

van der Geest, S., A. Hardon, and S. R. Whyte. 1990. Planning for essential drugs: Are we missing the cultural dimension? *Health Policy and Planning* 5:182–85.

Resource Materials

Most of the materials listed below are available free of charge to people in developing countries. This applies in particular to publications from the WHO Action Programme on Essential Drugs (DAP), UNICEF, the Academy for Educational Development, and Health Action International (HAI). A comprehensive international information base on drug education programs for the general public is being developed by WHO/DAP.

Planning Public Education Programs

Hubley, J. 1993. *Communicating health: An action guide to health education and health promotion.* St. Albans, England: Teaching Aids

at Low Cost (TALC, PO Box 49, St. Albans, Herts AL1 4AX).

Explores the role of communication in improving people's health and discusses strategies for health education, health promotion, and empowerment of families and communities. Good chapter on pharmaceuticals.

Rasmuson, M. R., R. E. Seidel, W. A. Smith, and E. M. Booth. 1988. *Communication for child survival.* Washington, D.C.: Academy for Educational Development, US Agency for International Development.

Presents a systematic consumer-based methodology for bringing about positive changes in health practices and includes numerous case studies and descriptions of health communication projects in developing countries.

United States Department of Health and Human Services. 1989. *Making health communication programs work: A planner's guide.* NH publication no. 89-1493. Washington, D.C.: US Government Printing Office.

A developed country perspective but still useful from a structured planning viewpoint.

WHO (World Health Organization). 1987. *Communication: Planning, management, and appraisal of communication activities.* Geneva: WHO.

WHO/CDD (World Health Organization/Diarrhoeal Diseases Control Programme). 1987. *Communication: A guide for managers of national diarrhoeal disease control programmes.* Geneva: WHO/CDD.

A good manual that is also valid for planning communication programs on controlling noncommunicable diseases.

WHO/DAP (World Health Organization/Action Programme on Essential Drugs). 1994. *Public education in rational drug use: Report of an informal consultation.* WHO/DAP/94.1. Geneva: WHO/DAP.

Outlines the rationale and principles of public education in drug use and identifies strategies for the development of DAP's activities in this area.

WHO/DAP (World Health Organization/Action Programme on Essential Drugs). 1996. *Rational drug use: Consumer education and information.* WHO/DAP/MAC 8/96.6. Geneva: WHO/DAP.

★ Zimmerman, M., N. Newton, L. Frumin, and S. Wittet. 1989.

Developing health and family planning print materials for low-literate audiences: A guide. Washington, D.C.: Program for Appropriate Technology in Health.

An excellent introduction to the development and testing of print materials, articulating principles valid for all communication programs.

Drug Promotion and Marketing

Chetley, A. 1993. *Problem drugs*, 2d ed. Amsterdam: Health Action International.

HAI (Health Action International). 1992. *Promoting health or pushing drugs?* Amsterdam: HAI.

Lexchin, J. 1994. *Pharmaceutical promotion in the third world.* Penang, Malaysia: International Organization of Consumers' Unions.

★ WHO/DAP (World Health Organization/Action Programme on Essential Drugs). 1994. *Essential Drugs Monitor,* no. 17.

Issue on drug marketing. Contains reports of recent studies, action to take, and full text of the WHO ethical criteria for medicinal drug promotion.

Studies of Community Knowledge, Attitudes, and Practices Regarding Use of Medicines

WHO/DAP (World Health Organization/Action Programme on Essential Drugs). 1994. *Selected annotated bibliography on essential drugs*, 3d ed. WHO/DAP/94.5. Geneva: WHO/DAP.

Detailed list of articles available from WHO/DAP, 1211 Geneva 27, Switzerland.

Patient Education Materials

Association of the British Pharmaceutical Industry. 1988. *Patient information advice on the drafting of leaflets.* London: Association of the British Pharmaceutical Industry (12 Whitehall, London SW1A 2DY, England).

International Medical Benefit/Risk Foundation. 1993. *Improving patient information and education on medicines.* Geneva: International Medical Benefit/Risk Foundation (12 rue Jean-Calvin, CH-1204 Geneva, Switzerland).

USP (United States Pharmacopeia). 1996. USP-DI Vol. 2. *Advice for the patient: Drug information in lay language.* Rockville, Md.: United States Pharmacopeial Convention.

Materials from National Education Campaigns on Rational Drug Use

Australia: Campaigns on drug use and the elderly and the wise use of medicines; also a school education kit using videos, TV spots, brochures, and posters. For further information, contact National Director, Australian Pharmacy Self Care Programme, National Secretariat, PO Box 21, Curtin, ACT 2605, Australia.

Philippines: Posters, leaflets, and TV spots. For further information, contact Director, Bureau of Food and Drugs, Alabang, Muntinlupa, Metro Manila, Philippines.

United States: Campaign on medicine: "Before you take it talk about it." Posters, leaflets, radio spots, information folders, activity sheets. Annual newsletter for "Talk about Prescriptions Month." For further information, contact Executive Director, National Council on Patient Information and Education, 666 11th Street, NW, Suite 810, Washington, D.C. 20001.

Annex 33.1 Pictograms for Use on Drug Labels

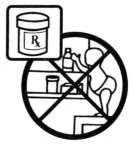
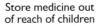

Store medicine out of reach of children

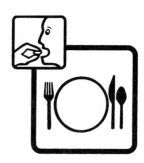

Take with meals

Do not take with meals

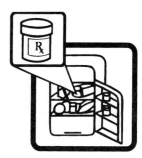

Store in refrigerator

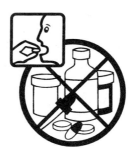

Do not take other medicines with this medicine

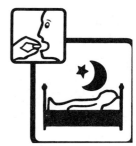

Take at bedtime

Source: Copied from United States Pharmacopeia–Drug Information. © 1989, the USP Convention, Inc. Reprinted with permission.

Part IV
Management Support Systems

Part I	Part II	Part III	Part IV
Introduction	Policy and Legal Framework	Drug Management Cycle	**Management Support Systems**
			A Organization and Management
			B Financing and Sustainability
			C Information Management
			D Human Resources Management

Section A

Organization and Management

Part I Introduction	Part II Policy and Legal Framework	Part III Drug Management Cycle	**Part IV** **Management Support Systems**	
			A Organization and **Management** ▶	**34 Managing Drug** **Programs**
			B Financing and Sustainability	35 Planning for Drug Management
			C Information Management	36 Monitoring and Evaluation
			D Human Resources Management	
				37 Community Participation
				38 Hospital Drug Services
				39 Security Management

Chapter 34
Managing Drug Programs

≡ Summary

Although management means different things in different contexts, all managers are responsible for the accomplishments of their organization. They must balance their time among the three activities of crisis management, routine administration, and long-term program development. They are called upon to fulfill the roles of

▸ *leader: providing direction, motivating staff, maintaining liaison with other organizations;*

▸ *communicator: maintaining networks of formal and informal contacts, disseminating information, serving as spokesperson;*

▸ *decision-maker in four areas: resource allocation, program change and development, problem-solving, and negotiation.*

Effective managers require technical, analytical, and people skills. They set priorities based on the urgency, relevance, impact, and future consequences of competing issues. They follow systematic processes for decision-making and problem-solving. Necessary skills can be acquired and practiced through formal management training programs.

Important concepts of modern management include

▸ *total quality management (TQM), with a focus on continuous improvement of services and use of teams to achieve common objectives;*

▸ *management by wandering about (MBWA), or maintaining frequent contact with programs and staff;*

▸ *participatory management, involving staff in planning, decision-making, and problem-solving;*

▸ *managing for performance through the use of management by objectives (MBO), the joint setting of performance targets, and periodic assessment of progress.*

Improvements in drug supply involve change. To manage change effectively, managers must understand internal and external change forces, sources of resistance to change, use of force field analysis, and principles for successful change management.

The management process, which is at the hub of the drug management cycle, consists essentially of three basic functions:

▸ *planning (see Chapter 35)*

▸ *implementation (see Chapters 40–48)*

▸ *monitoring and evaluation (see Chapter 36)*

Managers devote most of their time and energy to implementation. When new management systems are needed, they are often best introduced in phases.

≡ Managers are charged with using human, financial, and other resources to achieve results. Directors of medical services, chiefs of pharmacy divisions, heads of essential drugs programs, administrators of mission health services, and executives of pharmaceutical companies all have different roles and responsibilities but share one thing in common: they are all managers. Managers plan, implement, monitor, and, in the end, are responsible for the accomplishments and shortcomings of their organizations.

Part IV of this manual, "Management Support Systems," is concerned with the knowledge and skills required to manage organizations, finances, information, and people. The preceding sections on selection, procurement, distribution, and use presented the technical core of the drug management cycle. Management support systems form the hub of this cycle (Figure 34.1). This chapter describes basic management functions, the characteristics of a successful manager, and aspects of planning, implementation, and monitoring.

≡ 34.1 What Is Management?

Health staff frequently comment on management: "The last director was a great manager." "That program was very badly managed." "That NGO is really well managed." "There's no management in that office." But what is management?

Management has existed since people began working together to raise crops, to defend themselves, and to protect themselves from nature. Yet there is no single definition of management; it means different things in different contexts and can be described in a variety of ways (McMahon et al. 1992; Ivancevich et al. 1994).

Management is achieving results through people: Management is a commitment to achieve objectives. This requires a variety of resources, the most important of which is people. Coordinating, leading, and motivating the work of other people is the core of successful management.

Management is using resources efficiently: Resources are always limited. Good managers are able to make the best use of available resources to achieve the objectives of the organization or program.

Management is a profession and a career: In the past, many people became managers by accident. Today, health professionals make a career of management and often receive specific training in health administration,

Figure 34.1 Drug Management Cycle

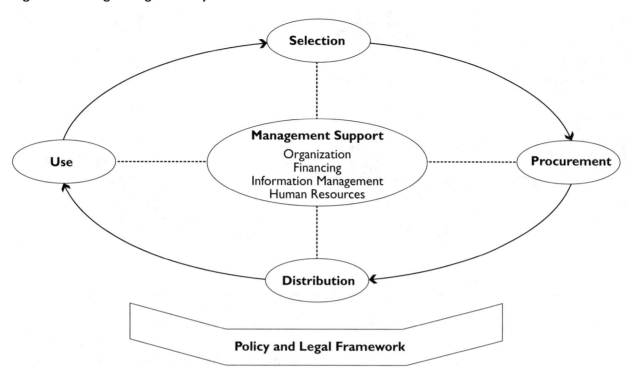

personnel management, information systems, and other aspects of management. Like law and medicine, management comprises a body of knowledge and operational concepts.

Management is a resource: The resources required to run a program are sometimes described as the three Ms: money, man (or woman) power, and management. Management is a critical resource, the absence of which can result in considerable waste of the more tangible resources.

Management is an art: Good management involves creativity, good judgment, and intuition. Although some people have a talent for management, most people learn the art of management through experience, good role models, or formal management training.

Management is a science: Good management decisions and actions depend on the ability to systematically gather information, logically analyze relationships, and draw conclusions.

≡ **34.2 What Makes a Successful Manager?**

Many people rise to positions of responsibility in organizations with no formal training in management. Some are successful, others are not. What makes a successful manager? Certainly the realities of local politics, economics, human resources, and infrastructure development have a great deal to do with success or failure. Within these con-

straints, however, success lies in the tasks, roles, skills, and qualities of the manager.

Management Tasks

In most programs, the manager's day is filled with three quite different types of activities:

1. Crisis management
2. Routine administration
3. Long-term program development

Crisis management—or "fighting fires"—can consume entire days or sometimes entire weeks: an overdue proposal to a donor, a shipment of emergency drugs stuck at the port, an outbreak of meningitis in one part of the country, a break-in at the regional store in another part of the country. Many such crises are actually preventable through better management of the other two activities, but learning to respond quickly and decisively—and not to overrespond— is an important part of becoming an effective manager.

Routine administration includes the whole range of day-to-day activities involved in receiving reports, managing staff, making decisions, and generally conducting the business of the program. These activities are necessary but can often be managed more efficiently through delegation, improved time management, and other skills described in the management chapters of this manual.

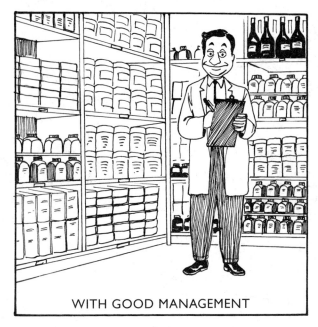

WITH GOOD MANAGEMENT

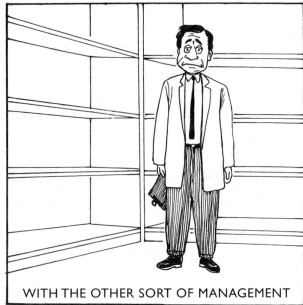

WITH THE OTHER SORT OF MANAGEMENT

Unfortunately, many managers are so consumed by the first two tasks that there is little time for long-term program development. Ironically, failure to plan and implement needed changes often increases the number of fires and makes even routine administration less efficient and more time-consuming than it should be. Outside advisers are sometimes effective not because of any special skill but because they are freed from fire fighting and routine administration to concentrate on program development.

An effective manager is able to balance his or her time among the three tasks, responding promptly to crises and efficiently handling routine administrative work while still attending to the long-term growth and development of the program or organization.

Managerial Roles

A role is a set of expectations placed on anyone in a position of responsibility by the people around that person. A manager plays many roles, but the most important are those of leader, communicator, and decision-maker (Mintzberg 1975). When a manager fails to perform these roles effectively, staff grumble, work stalls, and the program suffers.

Leader. The role of leader involves giving clear direction to the organization and motivating staff with a sense of purpose. It also involves interactions with other leaders in the organization, with local professional and community organizations, and often with international and donor agencies. Finally, leadership involves a ceremonial or figurehead role: presiding at official functions, honoring long-serving staff, immunizing the one-millionth child.

Communicator. The role of communicator establishes the manager as the central focus for receiving and disseminating information. A good manager builds a network of formal and informal contacts who help monitor changes, opportunities, problems, or misunderstandings that may affect the program. Networking is especially important in formalized relationships, such as those between ministries (finance and health, for example) or between programs and their donors. Building a wide network of contacts is also extremely valuable in managing multicultural or multilingual relationships, in which it may not always be clear what messages are really being communicated.

Communication also involves disseminating information to staff members so that their work is aided by what the manager has learned. Insecure managers trying to protect their jobs sometimes purposefully withhold relevant information from subordinates. Sadly, by failing to help subordinates in their work, the manager increases the chances that the program will perform poorly, which in turn reflects badly on the manager. Feedback also improves the quality of information submitted to the manager.

Finally, the manager's role as communicator involves serving as a spokesperson and presenting program needs and activities to higher officials, to donor organizations, or to the community.

Decision-maker. Leadership and communication set the stage for the manager's role as decision-maker. Managers are called upon to make decisions in four areas: resource allocation, program change and development, problem-solving, and negotiation. Deciding on the allocation of drugs, money, people, vehicles, or other resources is often sensitive. Program plans and priorities help support and justify decisions, but a manager's good judgment is always required.

As opportunities present themselves, managers must make decisions about change and development within their organizations and negotiate with senior officials, donors, or staff about objectives, deadlines, financing, and staff assignments.

Accepting Managerial Roles. Many health professionals assume managerial roles quite naturally, often without conscious awareness of the roles they are playing. Others become aware of role expectations but resist them: they avoid providing leadership, fail to communicate effectively, and defer decisions. Resisting management roles makes progress difficult for the manager and for those around him or her.

Managerial Skills

A health system manager requires a number of skills:

▶ *Technical skills:* pharmacy, medicine, accounting, epidemiology, or other skills related to a specific job;

▶ *Conceptual and analytical skills:* ability to synthesize information, understand the prevailing circumstances, and use planning techniques to move the program forward;

▶ *Decision-making skills:* using conceptual and analytical abilities to identify and select among options and adjust decisions based on experience;

▶ *People skills:* understanding, motivating, and directing people; building teams and improving group effectiveness;

▶ *Financial skills:* budgeting, assessing value for money in people and projects, negotiating, adhering to budgets, and coping with constraints;

▶ *Communication and research skills:* listening, reading, writing, running meetings, and making public presentations;

▶ *Computer skills:* proficiency in using word-processing, spreadsheet, and other relevant software to improve productivity.

These skills do not come simply from being placed in a management position; they require awareness, willingness to learn, training, and practice. The first step is to assess personal strengths and weaknesses. The next step is to identify opportunities to develop skills that are weak or lacking.

Those concerned with drug management policy are increasingly recognizing the need to support formal

Figure 34.2 Ten Qualities of an Effective Manager

1. Provides clear direction
2. Encourages open communication
3. Coaches and supports people
4. Recognizes staff for good performance
5. Follows up on important issues and provides feedback
6. Selects the right people for specific assignments
7. Understands the financial implications of decisions
8. Encourages creativity and new ideas
9. Gives staff clear-cut decisions when they are needed
10. Consistently demonstrates a high level of integrity

Source: Adapted from Ivancevich et al. 1994.

training in management. Management training needs to be included in continuing education programs, donor-assisted development projects, and wherever else the opportunity exists.

Qualities of a Successful Manager

Mastering management tasks, roles, and skills is essential. But before managers can organize others' work, they must organize their own. What are the qualities of a effective manager?

One study of organizations identified ten qualities of a successful manager, regardless of age, sex, type of business, size of organization, or working environment (Figure 34.2). These qualities reflect attitudes, habits, and behavior patterns. They are not concrete skills such as suturing a wound or compounding a topical skin preparation, but they do require continual awareness and practice.

≡ 34.3 Setting Priorities

Managers are constantly making choices about how they and their staff use time. Devoting time to one problem or decision means that another must wait. Even the best manager cannot handle all decisions and all problems at the same time.

Some managers try to take each problem in the order presented, giving it as much time as it takes and then moving on to the next problem. These managers become too involved in the details of each problem and end up trying to "micromanage" their programs and people.

Effective management means setting priorities. Which decision should be made first, and which problems should be solved first? How much time and effort should be put into a specific problem or decision? What tasks should be delegated to other staff?

To set priorities, managers can ask themselves several questions about each issue (decision, problem, activity) that demands their time and attention:

Urgency: Many issues seem urgent, but which ones really have an absolute deadline or time limit?

Relevance: Which issues are most central to long-term strategic plans and goals?

Impact: Which issues are likely to have the greatest impact on major program activities?

Future consequences: Which issues present the greatest threat to or the greatest opportunity for the future of the program?

Growth tendency: Which issues will get worse if not addressed sooner rather than later?

In general, issues should receive low priority if they are not urgent, are not likely to have a significant impact on future activities, or are not likely to become worse if left unattended.

An important principle for setting priorities is *management by exception*. With this approach, the manager expects staff to handle all decisions, problems, and activities, except for those that are of special importance, have long-term consequences, or are in some way unusual. This allows the manager to focus on those issues that really need his or her attention. Management by exception is similar in some ways to the 80-20 rule in ABC analysis (see Chapter 41). It is a principle that helps managers focus on the most important areas. Management by exception can be applied to a variety of management tasks:

► Program development efforts should focus on the key aspects of drug policy implementation that present the greatest difficulties.

► Routine reports should be reviewed to identify districts, facilities, or activities that are doing exceptionally badly (so that corrective action can be taken) or exceptionally well (so that they can be acknowledged and learned from).

► Follow-up supervisory visits should be made to regional depots, districts, or health units that are known from routine reports or other information to be having the most problems.

Management by exception and the key priority-setting questions apply mostly to the allocation of human resources. Chapter 35 discusses priority-setting for financial and other tangible resources as part of the planning process.

≡ 34.4 Decision-Making and Problem-Solving

Successful management requires prompt, thoughtful responses to the problems that inevitably arise when plans are put into action. Some managers are very good at both decision-making and problem-solving; others defer decisions, avoid problems, or make impulsive responses that prove to be ill advised.

Seven-Step Process

Although they are different in some respects, decision-making and problem-solving can both be approached through a seven-step process:

1. Review the basic objective.
2. Define the decision to be made or the problem to be solved.
3. Assess the situation; determine the cause of the problem.
4. Identify alternative solutions.
5. Compare the alternatives using defined criteria.
6. Select and implement the best decision or solution.
7. Follow up and adjust.

Common Mistakes

Decision-making and problem-solving can go wrong at any of the seven steps, but there are some common mistakes that lead to bad decisions or unworkable solutions:

Losing track of the original objective or solving the wrong problem: The basic problem must be clearly identified. Managers may be presented with a problem of inadequate financing for drugs when the real problem is that the procurement unit is wasting money by not following the essential drugs list. Or considerable time and money may be invested in renovating and reorganizing the central warehouse to improve the supply system when the real problem is that staff are not adequately motivated or trained.

Failure to properly assess the situation or the causes of the problem: If the causes of a problem are thoroughly understood, the solution is often obvious. It is therefore important to identify what additional information is needed to adequately understand the situation. With a stockout of penicillin, for example, the manager needs to know whether it is because the drug was not ordered, not shipped, not delivered, or consumed more rapidly than expected.

Failure to identify all relevant alternatives: Managers who act too quickly may achieve poor results because they have not considered the options. Similarly, managers who avoid decisions and problems may do so simply because they have not made the effort to identify reasonable alternatives.

Lack of clear criteria for selecting among alternatives: If it is clear what is to be accomplished, then the criteria for

Figure 34.3 Comparison of Traditional and Modern Managers

Traditional Manager

- ► acts as authoritarian figure, critic
- ► is concerned about structure and procedures
- ► tries to succeed alone
- ► pushes staff to focus on manager's needs and concerns

- ► gives little feedback
- ► is critical; discourages individual initiative
- ► uses threats to control staff
- ► uses one-way, top-down communication
- ► is secretive
- ► knows all the answers
- ► holds decision-making authority; makes decisions single-handedly
- ► decides not only what should be done but also how it should be done
- ► resists change as a threat
- ► is concerned with punishing people for doing a bad job
- ► creates fear, which discourages staff from asking questions and making suggestions

Modern Manager

- ► acts as facilitator, coach
- ► is concerned about objectives and results
- ► succeeds through the success of the team
- ► encourages staff to focus on the program's needs and concerns
- ► gives positive feedback and constructive negative feedback
- ► is supportive; coaches staff to take initiative
- ► uses encouragement and support to motivate staff
- ► uses two-way communication
- ► shares information
- ► recognizes the expertise of other team members
- ► involves staff in decision making

- ► allows staff to participate in deciding what should be done and defining how they can best do it
- ► welcomes change as a source of improvement
- ► helps people do a better job
- ► creates a sense of security; staff ask questions and make constructive suggestions

Source: Adapted from Ivancevich et al. 1994; Rees 1991.

choosing among alternatives should be clear. Sometimes cost is a major factor; sometimes time is.

Failure to follow up and adjust: Things seldom work out exactly as expected. Managers must be willing to adjust their actions based on experience. Lack of follow-up or stubborn unwillingness to adjust to experience can waste resources.

One effective way for managers to improve decision-making and problem-solving is to ask staff to go through these steps themselves before coming to the manager. They should present the manager not only with a question or a problem but also with a list of alternative courses of action, a recommended course, and the reasons for the recommendation. The manager can then make the final decision. With staff doing the basic problem-solving, it is likely to be a better decision, and one that requires much less time and effort.

Managers who maintain control by being the only source of answers and solutions may resist this approach. But as the quality of decisions—and with it, program performance—improves, the manager will soon appreciate the benefits of the new approach.

≡ 34.5 Modern Management Methods

Over the last few decades, some new management concepts have emerged: total quality management, management by wandering about (MBWA), participatory management, and managing for performance. The role of the manager has also changed.

The Traditional versus the Modern Manager

Traditionally, managers were seen as authoritative figures who received all information, made all decisions, and gave orders to subordinate staff for implementation. They managed through power, discipline, and rigid control. Many public- and private-sector senior officials and managers continue to function as traditional managers.

The growing complexity of modern organizations and the increased understanding of how people function have led to a different concept of the modern manager. Figure 34.3 contrasts the attitudes and style of traditional and modern managers.

Total Quality Management

Total quality management (TQM) is a philosophy and a set of concepts and techniques that have been adopted by many successful organizations. It focuses equally on the quality of the results and on the quality of management. The fundamental commitment is to continuous improvement of services for beneficiaries, clients, or customers. Achieving continuous improvement requires a manager with a modern outlook, the plan-do-check-act (PDCA) cycle, teamwork, and management by fact.

PDCA Cycle. The PDCA cycle (Berry 1991) lies at the core of efforts toward continuous improvement of national drug policy implementation and essential drugs program management (Figure 34.4). The steps of planning and doing often go quite smoothly. But many implementation efforts fail at the third point in the cycle by not checking results through systematic monitoring. An even

Figure 34.4 The PDCA Cycle for Continuous Improvement

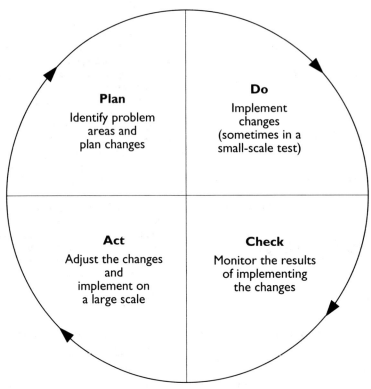

Source: Adapted from Berry 1991.

greater problem is the failure to use monitoring results to adjust the plan (act) based on experience.

Adhering to the PDCA cycle is especially important for new initiatives. Efforts by the government of the Philippines to promote generic drug use (see Country Study 5.1) have continued to progress because the ministry of health not only planned and implemented the new policy but also checked the reactions of doctors and pharmacists and then acted to overcome specific sources of resistance and provide additional information to doctors.

Teamwork. Another important aspect of modern management is teamwork. Some would-be leaders try to achieve success on their own, but sooner or later, every director, chief, or supervisor learns that managers cannot manage alone. The manager and staff should work as a team.

A team is a group of individuals working together to achieve common objectives. An effective team interacts openly and works together efficiently to produce the desired results: *together everyone accomplishes more.* Factors that influence teamwork include commitment to a common goal, team composition, team dynamics, and team leadership.

A commitment to common goals and objectives is vital to the success of a team. Difficulties often arise because the team has never reached consensus on its goals. Planning can become an effective team-building exercise.

There are several different types of teams, depending on the team members and the purpose. Senior-level divisional or department heads or program managers within a division may meet weekly or monthly. Such groups can and should function as teams. Within a program, the program director or manager generally has several senior staff members who are responsible for different units or functions. At the level of the health unit, the medical director and chief administrator, along with other senior health and administrative staff, should form an effective team. These are all examples of groups that are in continuous existence and should always strive to work as a team. In addition, task-specific working groups may be established to solve a specific problem, to develop new procedures, or to plan major changes. The existence of such teams is time-limited, making good teamwork especially important.

Team dynamics are important. Although individual team members take responsibility for specific assignments and deadlines, there must also be a feeling that "we are in this together." This implies a level of participation among team members in questioning, planning, and decision-making. Blaming individual team members for undesirable outcomes undermines the collective sense of responsibility for success.

Effective teams maintain individual self-esteem by respecting differences among team members; by criticizing only ideas, not people; and by ensuring that each person's contribution is heard. Mutual trust is also necessary; dishonesty or betrayal of confidential information can undermine this trust. Conflicts among team members will inevitably arise, but such conflicts should be quickly identified and resolved (see Chapter 47).

Perhaps the most important element in good teamwork is good leadership. An effective team leader has the characteristics of the modern manager outlined in Figure 34.3. The team leader succeeds by helping the team succeed. The team leader must serve as facilitator, communicator, and coach. The team leader must ensure that the objectives of the team are clear and that the sense of shared commitment and constructive team dynamics exist.

Management by Fact. Continuous improvement in a program's activities requires hard data, not personal bias or unfounded assumptions. Management by fact involves rationality, candor, and unbiased information.

Rationality implies that planning and decision-making are logical, structured, and oriented toward the goals of the organization. Managers who are inexperienced, insecure, or easily pressured by outside forces often make reactive, reflex decisions that are not based on fact and are not oriented to either immediate objectives or long-term goals.

Staff cannot help a program manager make the best decisions if the manager is not candid about the state of the organization. Candor—frankness and directness in communicating about the real situation—is important between managers and staff, as well as among different departments. The central stores manager cannot make plans for handling an unusually large delivery if the procurement manager does not inform him that such a delivery is expected.

Closely related to openness among managers and staff is accuracy in the information provided to managers. Good management decisions depend on up-to-date, unbiased information. Managers who punish staff for providing bad news eventually find that staff are telling the manager only what he or she wants to hear.

Management by Wandering About

Formal communication occurs through policy statements, memoranda, reports, meetings, and formal instruction. It follows the organizational structure: managers communicate downward to their staff, and staff report upward to managers. Formal communication is useful for gathering some types of information and for decision-making, but it has its limitations.

Effective managers regularly get out of their offices. They use informal communication to learn what is really happening. The director of medical services who makes frequent visits to districts and health facilities rather than staying at headquarters; the essential drugs program manager who regularly gets around to all regional stores and to local training courses on rational drug use rather than occupying himself with paperwork at the office; the hospital chief nursing officer who is frequently on the wards, in the operating room, or in the outpatient area rather than staying in her office—all these people are managers who stay informed, keep their staffs informed, and are therefore better able to run their programs or departments.

This active approach to communication is called *management by wandering about* (MBWA). MBWA is essential to successful management because it results in direct contact between the manager and staff. The importance of keeping in touch with people in the organization cannot be overemphasized.

Through MBWA, managers learn about real problems and often about potential solutions. They have a better understanding of the strengths and weaknesses of the organization. In turn, the staff become more familiar with the constraints that management faces and are better able to make useful contributions to the program.

Participatory Management

An important feature of increased decentralization is greater *participatory management*, that is, involving more people in planning, decision-making, problem-solving, and other management processes. This kind of management takes time and requires a manager who can facilitate staff involvement rather than simply direct staff work. It also risks increasing rather than decreasing conflict, and initially, staff may act only in their own self-interest.

More importantly, participatory management also brings more information, creativity, and experience to planning and decision-making, often resulting in better conclusions and better implementation efforts. Participatory management works best when

- managers are clear about the focus and limits of participation;
- the topic is important and relevant to the program and the staff;

► the topic is one that can be realistically addressed by the group;

► staff have the necessary education, training, and experience;

► managers and staff share common values;

► staff do not feel threatened by participating.

Staff who are brought into participatory planning, decision-making, or problem-solving will become frustrated and disillusioned if the task is an unrealistic or impossible one, if they feel misled about the extent to which management will accept the results of the participatory process, or if they believe that management is not listening to and valuing their contributions.

Although participatory management can improve the quality of plans and decisions, a high level of participation is not always advisable. Participation should be limited when time is short, when the decision is a minor one, or when the decision involves significant conflicts of interest among staff.

Managing for Performance

Setting clear objectives, as described in Chapter 35, is essential to program and project management. Implementing these plans through individual staff members' actions requires an additional step.

Management by objectives (MBO) is a participatory process in which managers and individual staff members set objectives to be used to periodically assess performance. Human resources management, including staff motivation and supervision, is considered in Chapter 47. MBO provides the link between overall implementation activities and individual staff performance.

MBO has been used around the world for over three decades. Ideally, staff members should first be asked to draft their own *performance targets* or objectives, in line with the program's overall goals and objectives, which are then reviewed and finalized with the supervisor. The last and most important step is to periodically assess progress toward achieving these targets.

Performance targets or objectives should be written, specific, measurable, appropriate to the individual or unit, realistic, and time-bound. They may specify performance levels for ongoing activities or plans to complete new tasks. Examples of individual performance targets within an essential drugs program would be:

► For the training officer: to develop one new unit for an ongoing continuing education program on rational drug use;

► For the chief supplies officer: to undertake random stock and record checks at least weekly;

► For the district pharmacist: to submit quarterly returns indicating consumption rates for individual drugs, overstocks, shortages, and other critical information.

Progress should be reviewed by the individual staff member or unit and supervisor on a regular basis. The review should assess progress toward each target, identify implementation problems, make any required changes in the targets, and suggest additional inputs required to achieve the targets.

≡ 34.6 Managing Change

Improvements in managing drug supply involve changes in policy, organizations, and individuals. Successful development is in many respects the management of change, and an organization that does not change eventually fails.

Change occurs at different levels and magnitudes, from restructuring the entire supply system to simply introducing a new dispensing register, or from launching a comprehensive national drug policy to changing generic labeling requirements. Strategic planning may lead to major changes, whereas annual workplans generally involve smaller operational changes.

Effective management of change depends on an understanding of change forces, resistance to change, and principles for successful change management.

Change Forces

Forces for change may come from within or outside the organization. Internal forces include pressure from individuals genuinely seeking to improve the program, from ambitious individuals pursuing their own ends, or from individuals and groups who are dissatisfied.

Sources of external pressure for change can include parts of the government or society, groups working globally, or specific donors. Such external pressure may arise from economic factors, political forces, or philosophical differences. External pressure may also arise from trends toward democratization, decentralization, or privatization.

Managers who do not recognize and respond to change forces risk being overwhelmed by them. Many directors of medical services and program managers have lost their positions because they failed to appreciate the need for change and did not exert leadership in managing change.

Resistance to Change

Resistance to change is a normal human response. Common sources of resistance to change include:

Personal self-interest: People who perceive a threat to their status, power, or personal finances are reluctant to change.

Vested interests: Those who are benefiting from the current situation resist change.

Bureaucratic inertia: Bureaucracies develop a structure, policies, and procedures of their own: "We've always done it this way." The response to change can be to subvert it with innumerable delays, diversions, and other barriers.

Habit: People resist change in organizations, but they also resist changing themselves. Most people find comfort and safety in the familiar.

Fear and uncertainty: Change generally involves risk. Although things are supposed to get better, they could become worse if the change is unsuccessful.

Conformity and peer pressure: If new warehouse procedures or computerization of procurement systems is seen as a threat to jobs, coworkers may pressure colleagues to undermine the changes.

Rejection of outsiders: Changes are sometimes designed, proposed, or advocated by "outsiders" and may bring in new managers or staff. Changes associated with outsiders are often resisted, regardless of the potential benefits of the changes themselves.

Understanding the sources of resistance to change can help identify ways to reduce this resistance, described later in the section on principles for managing change.

Force Field Analysis

To plan for change, it is useful to identify forces that favor or support change and forces that oppose change. Force field analysis is a technique for identifying *driving forces*, those forces that push toward an objective, and *restraining forces*, those that stand in the way. The balance of these forces determines the point of equilibrium.

Implementing change or solving problems involves unbalancing the forces and shifting the equilibrium. There are three steps (see Box 34.1):

1. *Diagnosing:* identify all driving and restraining forces.
2. *Unfreezing:* find ways to reduce restraining forces, strengthen driving forces, or find new driving forces.
3. *Redefining:* re-establish the equilibrium at the new target point.

Force field analysis uses a brainstorming technique, which is ideal for management teams. It enables a logical, systematic review of any problem or change situation, facilitates a comprehensive discussion of factors and possibilities, and is a highly participatory planning method that enhances teamwork.

Principles for Successful Change Management

Success depends on the magnitude and circumstances of the change as well as on the organizations and people affected by it. There are several principles for being an effective change manager:

Know oneself: Managers should recognize their own reactions to change and their strengths and limitations.

Learn how others feel: Using both direct and indirect channels of communication helps managers assess reactions to change and adjust the change process.

Know the organization: Any organization has both a formal structure of reporting relationships and informal channels of influence. Understanding the organization, often with the help of others, is important to planning and managing change.

Generate "ownership" through participation: The seeds of success or failure for change are sown even before the change has been fully planned or implemented. Involving potential supporters and implementers early in the process generates a sense of ownership.

Share the credit: Part of generating ownership involves sharing the credit. Leaders who capture the credit for themselves are likely to find themselves alone at a critical point in the process.

Look for win-win strategies: Change is more likely to succeed if every interest group benefits in some way. Generic drug substitution can benefit both customers and retail pharmacists if the pharmacist is allowed to make a little more money on a much less expensive drug.

Develop a sense of timing: People often expect and want policy and program changes when the leadership changes. New governments and new managers provide an opportunity for change.

Share information and educate: Much of the resistance to change comes from fear and uncertainty. This can be reduced by clear and open communication with staff.

Facilitate and support: Fear and anxiety can also be reduced if managers listen, show concern, and support staff in their effort to understand and adapt to change.

Be persistent: Change does not happen immediately. Successful change often occurs slowly, step-by-step. A gradual approach, with occasional retreats (two steps forward, one step back), is sometimes the best way to succeed.

Use force sparingly: Threats of firing, reassignment, loss of privileges, or other forms of coercion may be necessary to manage specific individuals or groups. Such measures should be used selectively, and only when other approaches have not worked; threats that are not carried out soon become hollow.

Box 34.1 Force Field Analysis

Force field analysis is a technique for analyzing the forces in an environment that can drive or restrain a change. Force field analysis involves the following steps:

1. Write the objective at the top of a flip chart.

2. Draw a line down the middle of the sheet.

3. Brainstorm and list on the right-hand side all the restraining forces: those factors in the situation that will have a negative influence on the achievement of the objective.

4. On the left-hand side, list all the driving forces: those that will have a positive influence on the achievement of the objective. (It is important to put down only those factors that are actually present in the current situation, not what would be desirable in the future.)

Once the force field has been fully set out, strategies for creating change can be developed.

5. Draw a line under the list in the left-hand column and write "Action Points."

6. Analyze the array of forces that has been constructed. Consider how the positive ones can be strengthened or augmented and, more importantly, how the negative ones can be eliminated or counteracted. The questions to be asked at this stage are:

► Can any of the restraining forces be reduced?
► Can any of the driving forces be strengthened?
► Can any new driving forces be found?

7. In light of the foregoing analysis, list action points that will be helpful in achieving the objective.

In the accompanying figure, the objective is to move from a current level of 50 percent drug availability (vertical bar on the left) to a level of 75 percent drug availability (bar on right). The first step is diagnosis—identifying driving and restraining forces. Here are some of the forces that might come out:

Driving Forces	Restraining Forces
Political pressure to solve drug problem	Interference in procurement process
New drug management leadership	Order quantities incorrect
Up-to-date essential drugs list	Lax storage and distribution system
New training on rational drug use	Overprescription by health workers

Driving and Restraining Forces

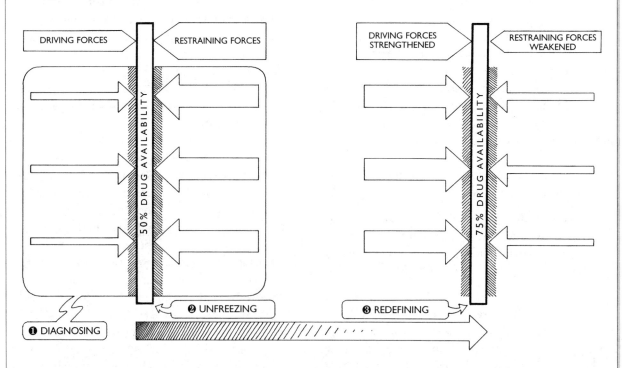

Source: Fisher 1991.

These techniques are useful in overcoming resistance to change and in managing change only when a manager has a clear sense of direction and purpose.

≡ 34.7 The Management Cycle

All management activities can be distilled into three basic functions, which together form the management cycle (Figure 34.5): planning, implementation, and monitoring and evaluation.

Planning

Planning is the process of analyzing the current situation, assessing needs, establishing goals, setting objectives and targets, and determining the strategies, activities, responsibilities, and resources needed to achieve the objectives. Well-formulated plans form the basis for all major decisions regarding the use of human, financial, and other resources. Planning also establishes the basis for monitoring and evaluation.

In health programs, there are three main levels of planning, which differ in purpose, time frame, and level of detail:

1. *Strategic planning:* long-term development planning concerned with the overall effectiveness and direction of the program or organization. It establishes or confirms a common vision of what the organization or program is meant to achieve. National development plans, national health policies, and national drug policies are forms of strategic planning.
2. *Program planning:* medium-term planning (three to five years) that specifies major objectives, activities, and resources needed for a specific program or organization. Essential drugs program master plans and most large, multiyear project proposals are forms of program planning.
3. *Work planning:* short-term planning (usually six to twelve months) that lists for each major objective the specific target outputs, required tasks, individual responsibilities, schedule, and budget. Work planning also includes operational planning such as that required to produce a national formulary manual, renovate a medical store, or conduct a major educational campaign on rational drug use.

To maximize the chance of success, it is essential that those who will be involved in implementing a plan be involved in formulating the plan. For strategic plans, this may mean senior ministry or program officials. For annual workplans, this may mean only the staff of the units involved.

Chapter 35 describes in detail the planning process, the three levels of planning, and various planning methods.

Implementation

Implementation is the process of carrying out a plan by organizing and directing the work. It involves managing people, money, information, and other resources to achieve the intended results, as described in Parts I–III of this manual. Implementation requires skills in priority-setting, decision-making, and problem-solving.

Monitoring and Evaluation

The last step in the management cycle is monitoring and evaluation. Although closely related, monitoring and evaluation are two distinct activities.

Monitoring. Monitoring is the process of observing implementation activities and comparing actual performance with plans. By focusing on achievement of objectives, monitoring helps the manager maintain direction through supervisory visits, routine reporting, sentinel reporting sites, and special studies. Objective indicators help track performance against targets.

Monitoring is an integral part of implementation, and it should contribute to improved performance. It involves communicating plans and targets, reviewing progress, and using monitoring results to take prompt action. Actions may include providing corrective feedback, reallocating staff or other resources, adjusting plans and targets, or requesting additional information.

Evaluation. Evaluation is a periodic assessment of progress toward achieving long-term objectives and goals. Whereas monitoring is concerned with whether activities are being implemented as planned, evaluation is concerned with the overall relevance, effectiveness, efficiency, sustainability, impact, and future of the program. Evaluation builds on information gathered for monitoring purposes, but it requires additional information. Evaluation methods are also useful in pharmaceutical sector assessment for project planning (see Chapter 4).

Chapter 36 describes monitoring and evaluation methods, the use of indicators, common pitfalls, and ways to use the monitoring system to improve performance.

≡ 34.8 Implementation Strategies

Implementation is the process of putting plans into action, and it requires most of a manager's time and energy. Good planning is essential, but the true test of a plan is in its implementation: organizing people, money, information, and other resources to achieve the planned objectives.

Figure 34.5 The Management Cycle

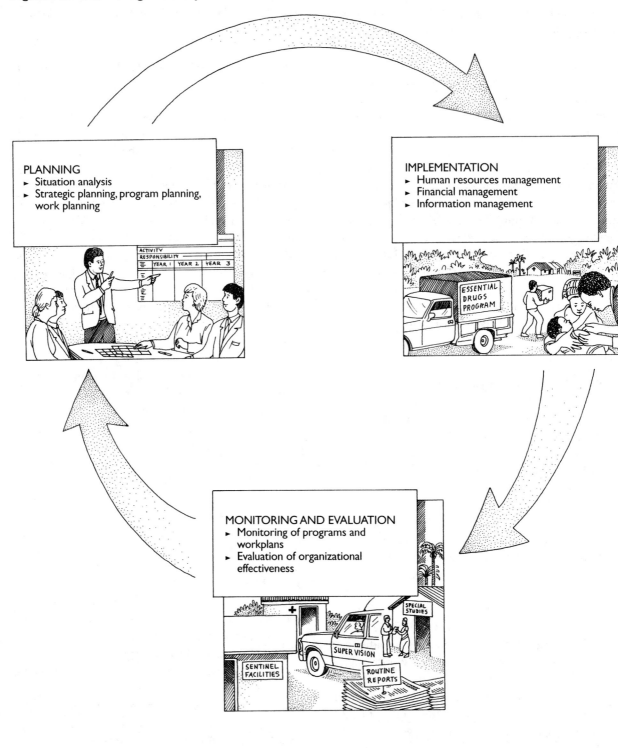

PLANNING
► Situation analysis
► Strategic planning, program planning, work planning

IMPLEMENTATION
► Human resources management
► Financial management
► Information management

MONITORING AND EVALUATION
► Monitoring of programs and workplans
► Evaluation of organizational effectiveness

Specific aspects of implementation are covered in other chapters of this manual, including:

Organizational structure for drug supply (Chapter 6): alternative models for drug supply, centralization versus decentralization of drug supply systems;

Personnel management (Chapter 47): staff selection, job descriptions, support and supervision, communication, delegation, motivation, and discipline;

Financial management (Chapter 42): budgeting, cash planning, costing, accounting, financial control and reporting;

Information management (Chapter 45): information needs, information systems, and use of information for decision-making.

Management Development

Improving the performance of essential drugs programs often means developing and implementing new management systems or strengthening existing ones and developing the capacities of staff. Examples include the process for selecting essential drugs and publishing the results; the committee structure, procedures, and forms used for tendering and other procurement activities; the inventory control system and delivery schedule for distribution; and the collection procedures, recordkeeping, and banking procedures needed for a revolving drug fund.

Effective management systems are rarely developed by people sitting behind a desk, and management systems never implement themselves. Too often, new management systems are designed in isolation and implemented without adequate testing. To effectively strengthen or develop management systems, four key steps are necessary:

Step 1. Assessment of needs: What are the management needs? The procurement system for a program that buys drugs only from a few established international low-cost suppliers is likely to be quite different from one that buys through open international tender.

Step 2. Interactive system design and testing: In an interactive design process, those responsible for developing new systems work closely with operational staff. For example, new district systems can often build on innovations developed by an individual district or several health facilities. Procedures, recording systems, or reporting forms can be tested and revised at selected sites.

Step 3. Implementation training: Training based on general management concepts often has limited impact. But implementation training is an indispensable part of management development and should be as practical

as possible and include a visit to facilities that have already implemented the new systems.

Step 4. Focused supervision: Training alone will not ensure implementation of new systems. Considerable follow-up supervision, focused on those units that are having the greatest difficulty, is often needed.

Country Study 34.1 describes the application of these steps to strengthen management systems and management performance in Kenya's user fee program.

The concept of interactive system design is especially important. Staff tend to resist changes or centrally designed systems that fail to consider local needs or practical constraints. Most importantly, experienced operational staff have clever ideas and solutions of their own to contribute. Interactive system design should not be seen as a totally democratic process in which everyone's ideas are adopted. Instead, it is a creative but pragmatic process in which the most demonstrably useful ideas are incorporated into the final design.

Phased Implementation

When new management systems, reporting forms, or other major changes are introduced, it is often advantageous to implement changes in phases rather than at all levels and all sites at the same time. For example, introduction of a new standard treatment manual or ordering system would begin with a national workshop for key staff from provincial hospitals, followed several months later by provincial-level workshops for key district staff within the province. Finally, each district would hold workshops for its staff.

The advantages of phased implementation are that

► it is more practical than introducing changes at all levels and all sites at the same time;

► it allows some real-world testing and revision of new systems before national implementation;

► for changes that may have political implications, such as the introduction of user fees, it allows the public to adjust to new ideas and provides some flexibility in the timing of expansion to other levels;

► it allows time for training and follow-up at one level before moving to the next level;

► if new systems have become fully functional at the initial level, facilities at this level can serve as training sites for the next level;

► senior medical and administrative staff at one level who have become familiar with the new system become more effective advocates and supervisors at the next level.

Country Study 34.1 Management Development and Phased Implementation: Kenya's User Fee Program

The Kenya Ministry of Health (MOH) introduced a new user fee program in December 1989 as part of a comprehensive health financing reform. The program was introduced simultaneously at all facilities, which did not permit testing of fees and systems, proper training of staff, or adequate supervision. Implementation was weak, and when problems emerged, they were so widespread that the MOH was unable to take corrective action. In September 1990, the outpatient registration fee, which had been the major revenue source, was suspended. Inpatient, laboratory, X-ray, and other fees remained in place.

In 1991, the MOH initiated a program of management improvement in anticipation of gradual introduction of outpatient drug and treatment fees. New management systems were developed in steps.

Assessment of Management Needs. Through a series of field visits beginning in early 1991, specific requirements and constraints were identified. New systems were needed to address such issues as location and staffing of cash collection points, collection records that were straightforward but provided adequate cross-checks, methods for issuing and recording waivers, and pharmacy records to ensure that drugs dispensed equated with fees received.

Interactive System Design. From mid-1991, staff from the MOH and the project began working with the eight provincial hospitals to develop practical systems to meet the management needs identified. Several hospitals had developed innovative methods for handling different aspects of user fee management. These methods were incorporated into the evolving national system.

A group of hospital pharmacists adapted and field-tested long-established antibiotic registers to serve as general drugs and revenue registers. These new registers included spaces for recording and making daily tallies of payments and exemptions.

In late 1991, a national workshop with clinical, administrative, pharmacy, and nursing staff was held to review system design experience. Following this, an operations manual was prepared to document the new system.

Implementation Training and Follow-up Supervision. The operations manual became the basis for workshops and follow-up supervision, first at the provincial level, then at the district level. Over a one-year period, workshops were reinforced by follow-up supervisory visits, and the new management systems were effectively implemented at most of the eight provincial hospitals. Revenue collection increased dramatically at these hospitals, and improvements in the quality of care were noted. These hospitals then became training sites for the districts within their respective provinces.

Finally, in mid-1993, districts were provided with a simplified operations manual for introducing systems at health centers to manage drug fees, laboratory fees, and other treatment fees. Training of health center staff at district headquarters involved firsthand observation of user fee management systems at the district hospitals.

Phased Introduction of Drug and Treatment Fees. Having laid the foundation with improved collection and expenditure procedures, the ministry began phased introduction of drug and treatment fees. The new fees were introduced at the national hospital in April 1992, at provincial hospitals in July 1992, at district hospitals in January 1993, and at health centers in July 1993. Phased introduction of the new fees allowed health staff, politicians, and the public to adjust gradually to the new fees.

Thus, over the three-year period, a user fee program that had run into initial implementation problems strengthened its management systems, increased revenue generation, and successfully introduced drug and treatment fees through a phased approach to management development and implementation of changes.

Phased implementation may start at the central level and move to the provincial or state, district or regional, and local levels; it may also be geographical, completing the introduction of new systems in one area, province, or state before moving to the next. ∎

≡ Assessment Guide

Managerial Roles, Skills, Approaches

► Do managers balance their time effectively among crisis management, routine administration, and long-term program development?

► To what extent do managers fulfill the roles expected of them with regard to leadership, communication, and decision-making?

► Do the individuals in management positions have needed skills (technical, conceptual, analytical, decision-making, people, communication, computer)? If not, are they willing to learn? Have opportunities for management training been identified?

► Do managers set priorities based on the urgency, relevance, impact, future consequences, and growth tendency of issues? Do they manage by exception?

► To what extent do managers use a systematic process for decision-making and problem-solving?

► How frequently do managers have contact with operational staff? Do they involve staff in planning, decision-making, and problem-solving?

► Do managers and staff jointly set performance targets and use them to monitor performance?

► Which of the following management practices or techniques associated with total quality management are used—the plan-do-check-act cycle, teamwork, management by fact?

► Do managers follow principles for successful change management? Do they understand internal and external forces for change and sources of resistance to change? Do they use force field analysis?

Management Cycle

► Do management processes employ the three separate functions of planning, implementation, and monitoring and evaluation?

► What levels of planning take place—strategic planning, program planning, work planning?

► Does the planning process involve staff who are responsible for implementation?

► Are new management systems designed with input from operational level staff? Is implementation phased? Are staff trained in the use of new systems?

► Does regular monitoring take place? Are monitoring results used to make corrective adjustments?

► Are evaluations focused on the program or project's relevance, effectiveness, efficiency, sustainability, and impact?

≡ Glossary

Activity: An action aimed at achieving a particular objective.

Audit trail: The series of records and forms that compose the information system, and the cross-referencing of these forms to allow the flow of drugs and funds to be traced. Used in evaluating system performance and in tracing losses.

Critical path method (CPM): A planning method that uses a network model to arrange and schedule project activities; sometimes referred to as PERT-CPM, due to similarities with the project evaluation and review technique (PERT).

Delegation: The assignment by a manager of an activity, task, defined scope of authority, or responsibility to a staff member under the manager's supervision.

Evaluation: A periodic assessment of progress toward achieving long-term objectives and goals. Monitoring and evaluation are the third phase in the management cycle.

Force field analysis: A highly participatory planning technique employed in change management, which is used to identify driving forces, those forces that push toward a particular change, and restraining forces, those that stand in the way.

Gantt chart: One of the earliest types of project control charts—also called an activity-time chart, chronogram, or schedule of activities and responsibilities—that is usually included in a workplan. As a clear, concise summary of planned activities, it is useful for communicating plans to staff, checking financial and other resource requirements, and monitoring progress.

Goal: The general aim toward which the organization or program is striving.

Implementation: The second step in the management cycle; the process of putting a plan into action by organizing and directing the work. It involves managing people, money, information, and other resources to achieve intended results.

Indicator: Criterion used to measure changes, directly or indirectly, and to assess the extent to which the targets and objectives of a program or project are being attained. Indicators should meet the criteria of clarity, usefulness, measurability, reliability, validity, and acceptance by key stakeholders.

Indicator drug: One of a small number of representative drugs, also known as tracer or index drugs, selected to be used with performance indicators to assess the performance of a drug supply system.

Information system: The system of records kept at offices, storage facilities, and clinical facilities; forms that are used to communicate supply needs, consumption data, and other information about the system; reports that summarize the data from records and forms for planning and evaluation purposes; and procedures that coordinate the use and flow of these documents.

Logical framework approach (LogFrame or LFA): One methodology used by many donors to identify, plan, implement, and monitor projects.

Management by exception: A technique in which the manager expects staff to handle all decisions, problems, and activities, except for those that are of special importance, have long-term consequences, or are in some way unusual.

Management by objectives: A participatory process in which managers and individual staff members set objectives to be used to periodically assess performance.

Management cycle: The process consisting of the three interconnected functions of planning, implementing, and monitoring and evaluating.

Mission (or mission statement): A brief general description of the type of organization, its main purpose, and its values.

Monitoring: The ongoing process of reviewing the degree to which program activities are completed and objectives are being met, to allow for corrective action to be taken during implementation. Monitoring and evaluation are the third phase in the management cycle.

Objectives: Results that a program or workplan seeks to achieve. A well-formulated objective fits the SMART mnemonic: *s*pecific, *m*easurable, *a*ppropriate to overall objectives or goals, *r*ealistic in terms of available resources, *t*ime-bound (there is a deadline).

Operating costs: One of three components in drug supply costs, also termed recurring costs; includes all items that are routinely included in the annual operating budget.

Participatory management: The process of involving staff in management processes in order to bring more information, creativity, and experience to planning, decision-making, and problem-solving, often resulting in better conclusions and better implementation efforts.

Performance target: An objective or desired standard of performance for an individual or unit that is written, specific, measurable, appropriate to the individual or unit, realistic, and time-bound; is in line with overall program goals and objectives; and is used to periodically assess progress.

Planning: The first step in the management cycle; the process of analyzing the current situation, assessing needs, establishing goals, setting objectives and targets, and determining the strategies, responsibilities, and resources needed to achieve the objectives. Three levels of planning are strategic, program, and work planning.

Program plans: Medium-term plans (three to five years) that specify major objectives, activities, and resources needed for a specific program or organization; examples include master plans and multiyear project plans.

Project evaluation and review technique (PERT): A planning method that uses a network model to arrange and schedule project activities; sometimes referred to as PERT-CPM, due to similarities with the critical path method (CPM).

Rapid assessment procedures (RAP): Procedures that rely on qualitative methodologies, such as in-depth interviews, structured observation, focus group discussions, or small random sample surveys, to assess a specific implementation activity.

Revolving fund: A fund for which initial capital is provided by government appropriation or bilateral donation but is then intended to be self-sustaining, with all expenditures being replaced from monies collected for the fund.

Sentinel sites: Selected units or facilities from which more detailed information is collected for monitoring purposes, on a more frequent basis, than from other units.

Strategic plans: Long-term development plans concerned with the overall effectiveness and direction of a program or organization.

Strategy: A broad plan of action for fulfilling a program's basic purpose and achieving its main goals.

Supervise: To oversee; to provide direction; to guide and instruct with immediate responsibility for performance.

SWOT analysis: Analysis undertaken in the course of strategic planning that consists of an assessment of the internal *s*trengths and *w*eaknesses of an organization or program, as well as external *o*pportunities and *t*hreats.

Targets: Measurable, time-limited, intermediate progress points toward objectives; also called milestones.

Task: Specific work to be performed as part of an activity and within a certain time.

Total quality management (TQM): A philosophy and a set of concepts, techniques, and management practices characterized by a fundamental commitment to continuous improvement of services for beneficiaries, clients, or customers.

Workplans: Short-term plans (usually six to twelve months) that list for each major objective the target outputs, required tasks, individual responsibilities, schedule, and budget.

≡ References and Further Readings

★ = *Key readings.*

Adenika, F. B. 1992. *Principles of essential drugs management.* Ibadan, Nigeria: Shaneson C.I.

★ Amondo-Lartson, R., G. J. Ebrahim, H. J. Lovel, and J. P. Ranken. 1984. *District health care.* London: Macmillan.

Berry, T. H. 1991. *Management: The total quality transformation.* New York: McGraw-Hill.

Brown, L. D. 1993. Assessing the quality of management (user's guide, module 7). In *Primary health care management advancement programme.* Geneva: Aga Khan Foundation.

Fisher, F. 1991. *Guide for managing change for urban managers and trainers.* Nairobi: United Nations Centre for Human Settlements (Habitat).

Hilton, M., L. M. Franco, G. Murphy, and M. Francisco. 1993. Problem-solving (manager's guide). In *Primary health care management advancement programme.* Geneva: Aga Khan Foundation.

Ivancevich, J. M., P. Lorenzi, S. J. Skinner, and P. B. Crosby. 1994. *Management quality and competitiveness.* Burr Ridge, Ill.: Richard D. Irwin.

★ McMahon, R., E. Barton, and M. Piot. 1992. *On being in charge,* 2d ed. Geneva: World Health Organization.

Millar, M. 1993. Assessing the quality of management (facilitator's guide, module 8). In *Primary health care management advancement programme.* Geneva: Aga Khan Foundation.

Mintzberg, H. 1975. The manager's job: Folklore and fact. *Harvard Business Review* 53(4):49–61.

Peters, T. J., and R. H. Waterman. 1982. *In search of excellence.* New York: Warner Books.

Rakich, J. S., B. B. Longest Jr., and K. Darr. 1985. *Managing health services organizations,* 2d ed. Philadelphia: W. B. Saunders.

Rees, F. 1991. *How to lead work teams: Facilitation skills.* San Diego, Calif.: Pfeiffer and Company.

★ Reynolds, J., M. Francisco, and S. Gearon. 1993. Better management: 100 tips (manager's guide). In *Primary health care management advancement programme.* Geneva: Aga Khan Foundation.

★ Williams, R. B., ed. 1985. *Hospital pharmacy management primer.* Bethesda, Md.: American Society of Health-System Pharmacists.

Part I	Part II	Part III	Part IV
Introduction	Policy and Legal Framework	Drug Management Cycle	**Management Support Systems**

A Organization and Management ▶

34 Managing Drug Programs

35 Planning for Drug Management

B Financing and Sustainability

C Information Management

D Human Resources Management

36 Monitoring and Evaluation

37 Community Participation

38 Hospital Drug Services

39 Security Management

Chapter 35
Planning for Drug Management

≡ Summary

Planning, the first step in the management cycle, is the process of assessing needs, establishing goals, setting objectives and targets, and determining the strategies, responsibilities, and resources needed to achieve the objectives. Three levels of planning differ in purpose, time frame, and level of detail:

Strategic planning is concerned with an organization's or government agency's fundamental purpose, takes a long-term perspective, and involves policy-makers and senior officials. A national drug policy, for example, may result from a strategic planning process. Strategic plans should be written and officially endorsed. They are most useful when

- *current strategies are not working;*
- *the political or social environment changes dramatically;*
- *there is a new initiative or restructuring of programs;*
- *there is a crisis.*

Program planning follows from strategic planning and focuses on medium-term objectives. For each objective, a program or project plan should specify targets, responsibilities, schedule, and budget. It is best implemented through opera-tional workplans. Essential drugs programs, for example, should have program plans.

Work planning is usually undertaken annually and should involve staff who will be responsible for implementation. Workplans generally specify major tasks, measurable outputs, individual responsibilities, timing (at least to the month), budget, and source of funds for each activity or task. Gantt charts are often included and are useful for monitoring.

Some project planning methods and tools that can be helpful include the critical path method (CPM) and project evaluation and review technique (PERT), the logical framework approach (LogFrame), and various computer software packages.

Plans may fail to achieve their intended objectives when

- *planning is unrealistic or overly ambitious;*
- *existing commitments have not been considered;*
- *implementers have not been involved;*
- *there is inadequate support, funds, staff, or time;*
- *planning is undertaken for the wrong reasons or at the wrong level;*
- *implementation is not regularly monitored.*

≡ Planning is a part of every person's life. Without plans, life would be chaos. Similarly, every organization and every program needs to plan. A good plan begins with the present situation and asks where the organization or program is going, how it will get there, what resources are needed, and how progress can be measured. Planning is an essential tool for effective work, not a limit on what can be done.

Planning is the first step in the management cycle described in Chapter 34. A well-formulated plan provides direction for an organization and is necessary to coordinate implementation efforts, staff activities, and financial operations.

≡ 35.1 The Planning Process

Planning is the process of analyzing the current situation, assessing needs, establishing goals, setting objectives and targets, and determining the strategies, responsibilities, and resources needed to achieve the objectives. Before reviewing in detail the different levels of planning, it is useful to consider the reasons for planning.

Why Plan?

It is always possible to find reasons not to plan: "We're too busy; we have no time for planning." "We have no drugs and no money; there's nothing to plan with." "Whatever we plan is changed by the higher-ups." But good planning is essential to the success of any program or organization. When time or money is limited, planning is even more important.

Planning is a *process*, not simply the creation of a *product* (the plan). The planning process, as well as the result, are important for achieving at least five purposes:

1. *To clearly identify long-term goals:* Is the program addressing the right goals and objectives? It is easy to continue doing the same things in the same way. But are these the best things to be done and the best way to do them?

2. *To assess current needs and problems:* What is the current pharmaceutical sector situation? What are the most pressing problems?

3. *To ensure wise use of available human and financial resources:* Good planning helps coordinate the use of limited resources and avoid duplication. A plan that has been agreed on becomes a commitment of available resources and gives managers more control and a basis to say yes or no to unexpected requests.

4. *To obtain additional resources:* A good plan with clear objectives is useful for building support from senior officials, board members, and others in authority for

obtaining additional staff or funding, and it is usually essential for donor or other external support.

5. *To provide a basis for evaluating effectiveness:* Without a stated plan, it is difficult to assess what the program is achieving.

Levels of Planning

Organizations engage in three levels of planning that differ in purpose, time frame, and level of detail: strategic planning, program planning, and work planning (Figure 35.1).

Strategic Planning. Strategic planning or development planning is concerned with the overall effectiveness and direction of the organization. This level of planning begins with a clear statement of the ultimate aim, mission, or vision for the organization. It ends with specific strategies for achieving this mission. Strategic planning takes a long-term perspective, usually five years or more; is less detailed than program or operational planning; and is carried out relatively infrequently.

Program Planning. Program planning focuses on clearly defined medium-term objectives (up to five years) within the program's overall long-term goals. It specifies major activities that address the objectives, responsibilities (usually by unit, not by individual), and time frame (usually by year or quarter, not by month). This is usually the time frame and level of planning for development assistance projects. In such instances, program planning can also serve the needs of project planning. In the context of essential drugs, program plans are also called *master plans.*

Figure 35.1 Levels of Planning: The Planning Pyramid

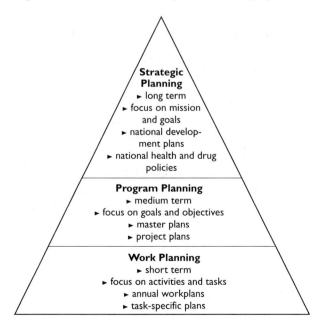

Strategic Planning
► long term
► focus on mission and goals
► national development plans
► national health and drug policies

Program Planning
► medium term
► focus on goals and objectives
► master plans
► project plans

Work Planning
► short term
► focus on activities and tasks
► annual workplans
► task-specific plans

Generally, program plans should be tied to activity-specific budgets.

Work Planning. Work planning or operational planning is short-term planning (usually one year or less). Typically, this means annual workplans that specify all major activities, individual responsibilities, time frame (detailed at least to the month) and often activity-specific or task-specific budgets. Operational planning covers specific tasks such as producing a national formulary manual for the first time, renovating a medical store, or carrying out a major public education campaign on rational drug use.

Planning Questions and Terms

Whether preparing a strategic plan, a program plan, or a workplan, people engaged in the planning process address four key questions:

1. Where are we now?
2. Where do we want to go?
3. How will we get there?
4. How will we know when we have arrived?

Planning terminology varies considerably among organizations, countries, and programs, even though the questions are similar. What is a "goal" to one person is an "objective" or a "target" to another. Since there is no universally agreed-upon terminology, there are no right or wrong definitions. For consistency, however, this manual follows generally accepted international terminology (WHO 1984) and uses planning terms as defined in the following paragraphs, which the reader can adapt to the local setting.

1. Where Are We Now? All planning begins with an *assessment* of the current situation and needs. Chapter 4 describes pharmaceutical sector assessment and different methods for conducting an assessment.

2. Where Are We Going? Statements of intent describe the expected *outputs* of a plan. This can be done in four levels of breadth and detail:

Mission: The mission, or mission statement, is a brief general description of the type of organization, its main purpose, and its values.

Goal: Goals define the general aims toward which the organization or program is striving. In an essential drugs program, for example, one goal might be, "To ensure that safe, effective, affordable essential drugs are available at all public health institutions."

Objectives: Objectives are results that the plan seeks to achieve. A well-formulated objective can be defined by the SMART mnemonic:

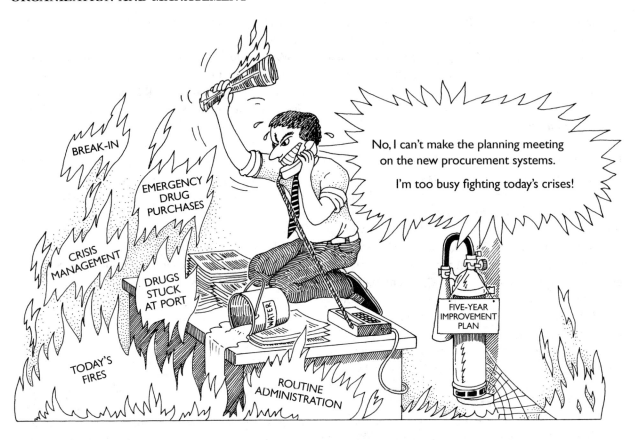

► *Specific*—to avoid differences of interpretation;

► *Measurable*—to enable monitoring and evaluation;

► *Appropriate*—in relation to overall objectives or goals;

► *Realistic*—in terms of available resources;

► *Time-bound*—in terms of deadlines.

Sometimes it is useful to distinguish general objectives (which may not fit all SMART criteria) from specific objectives (which should fit the SMART criteria). A general objective might be, "To ensure that all drugs used in government facilities are prescribed according to national treatment guidelines." Within this general objective, a specific objective could be, "To achieve at least 75 percent compliance with national treatment guidelines in government health centers by the year 2000."

Targets: Targets, or milestones, are measurable, time-limited, intermediate progress points toward objectives, for example, "By 1998, achieve at least 50 percent compliance with national treatment guidelines." Targets may also apply to process objectives, for example, "Train 600 clinicians (about 33 percent of an estimated 1,800 clinicians) in rational drug use."

3. How Will We Get There? Methods for achieving specific objectives and targets can also be described in different levels of breadth and detail:

Strategy: a broad plan of action for fulfilling a program's basic purpose and achieving its main goals, for example, "Promote rational prescribing through strengthening formal education, continuing education, and supervision."

Activity: a specific action aimed at achieving a particular objective, for example, "Conduct a workshop on rational prescribing."

Task: specific work to be performed as part of an activity and within a certain time, for example, "Prepare session notes and overhead transparencies at least four weeks before workshop."

The *inputs* for achieving the desired objectives and targets are people, time, and money. Plans should therefore describe responsibilities, schedules, and budgets, with the level of detail depending on the type of plan.

4. How Will We Know When We Have Arrived? A key function of management is monitoring and evaluation linked directly to the planning process. Monitoring is a continuous process that focuses on the implementation of specific activities and the achievement of targets. Evaluation occurs intermittently and focuses on achievement of objectives and long-term goals.

Achievement of goals, objectives, and targets should be monitored informally on an ongoing basis. Formal review of program plans should happen at least annually. Progress on workplans should be reviewed monthly or quarterly.

Indicators help measure changes directly or indirectly and assess the extent to which the targets and objectives of a program or project are being attained (WHO 1984). As described in Chapter 36, indicators are an integral part of monitoring and a useful contribution to evaluation.

Who Should Plan?

The test of a plan is in its implementation; to maximize the chances of success, those involved in implementing a plan should be part of formulating it. Therefore, it is important to establish the planning team at the outset. For strategic planning, this usually consists of policy-makers and senior staff. For program and work planning, it should include all key people in the unit concerned.

Planning can be top-down or bottom-up. In *top-down planning*, major discussions and decisions start at the top. Situation assessment and other planning data may be provided by operational units, but setting goals, identifying options, and choosing among options all happen at the senior level. In *bottom-up planning*, the process starts with each operational unit carrying out its own planning exercise and developing a plan that is then merged with others and revised to form the overall plan.

Bottom-up planning is most appropriate for operational and project planning, in which the purpose and major goals are already clear. Top-down planning may be more appropriate for strategic planning, in which the basic mission and goals must be defined, but top-down planning still requires input from lower levels.

Planning is too important to be left to planners or outside advisers alone. Nonetheless, planning units and health information units may play important roles, as they are usually adept at gathering and analyzing data and presenting the results. Although national planning ministries often maintain population, economic, and other forecasts to estimate program growth, they are not experts on drug management and cannot fully assess alternative drug management strategies and solutions.

Local or international expert advisers can make important contributions. They can provide a neutral outside perspective, skills in organizing and in analyzing perspectives from other countries, and suggestions of practical alternative strategies that might otherwise be missed. At the same time, expert advisers may have their own agendas and may be unfamiliar with the circumstances of the program.

Good Plans and Good Opportunities

Good managers are always reviewing their basic goals, assessing the current situation, considering current strategies, and monitoring the impact of their programs. The most effective managers always have a long-term strategic perspective in mind and are constantly watching for, and making the most of, development opportunities.

It is important, therefore, to adapt plans to changing circumstances and opportunities. Most enlightened senior officials and donors would prefer to hear that plans should be changed to make better use of limited time and money rather than be told that by faithfully following the original plan, opportunities were missed and resources were wasted.

≡ 35.2 Strategic Planning

Strategic planning is concerned with developing a shared vision of mission or fundamental purpose. It is concerned with the overall effectiveness and direction of the program. Fundamentally, strategic planning asks the question: Is the program or organization *doing the right things*? In contrast, program planning is more concerned with the question: Is the program or organization *doing things the right way*?

Specific questions that a strategic thinker asks are:

► What are the basic values of the organization?
► Who is meant to benefit from our services?
► Are the stated goals the correct goals?
► Are the strategies for achieving these goals the most appropriate for the circumstances?
► Is the structure of the program or organization well suited to the goals?

For example, is the correct goal to provide free drugs for all patients? Or is it to ensure access to drugs for all patients, with only the poorest receiving free drugs and others paying a reasonable fee? Is a large, centralized government supply system the best way to supply drugs to government health facilities?

When is a strategic plan needed? A strategic planning exercise is most needed and most useful in the following situations:

When current strategies are not working: Program directors or their superiors often accept perpetually marginal or poor results simply because "we've always done it this way" or "nobody has thought of a better way." Strategic planning provides a mechanism for finding better ways. For example, if the current strategy of centralized supply is failing to ensure a regular supply of drugs, the best solution may not be a project to renovate central medical stores but a strategic planning exercise to consider restructuring the supply system.

When the political or social environment changes dramatically: Changes in government or replacement of senior ministry officials may offer the opportunity or result in the demand for change. The pharmaceutical sector may be affected by prevailing national trends such as decentralization, civil service reform, or privatization. Strategic planning can help restructure a program to adapt to such trends and take maximum advantage of opportunities for improved program performance.

When there is a new initiative or restructuring of programs: The development of a new essential drugs program, the integration of essential drugs and family planning commodities, or the creation of a division of pharmaceutical services all provide opportunities and challenges for senior officials and program managers. A strategic plan can help them respond to such changes.

When there is a crisis: Not all crises create the need for a strategic plan, as some are short-lived and do not reflect underlying deficiencies. But a major currency devaluation, a national disaster such as an earthquake or flood, or a debt crisis may have long-term consequences that mandate new approaches.

A national drug policy (see Chapter 5) represents a government effort to articulate new goals and strategies for the pharmaceutical sector and often results from what is effectively a strategic planning process.

Strategic planning involves several steps, which are outlined in Figure 35.2. Different authors may describe these steps differently, but the basic ideas are similar.

Step 1. Create the Guiding Framework

Who will organize the work of the planning team? Who will be on the planning team? Who else will be consulted, and how will they be consulted? Why is a strategic plan being sought, and how will it be used? All these questions must be answered in establishing the guiding framework for strategic planning.

In long-term strategic planning, it is essential that policymakers and senior officials be involved. Even if much of the background work and organization are done by operational staff, the key decision-makers must be involved at the beginning to help establish goals, review strategic options, and endorse the final plan.

The planning process lays the groundwork of support for implementation and requires identifying the key stakeholders, or those individuals and organizations with an

---

Figure 35.2 Steps in Strategic Planning for Drug Management

Step 1 Create the Guiding Framework
  ▸ *Create the planning team.*
  ▸ *Identify stakeholders: the community, patients, beneficiaries, health staff, national government, politicians, ministry of health, essential drugs program, suppliers (local industry, overseas suppliers).*

Step 2 Establish the Mission of the Organization or Program
  ▸ *Clarify mission, long-term goals.*

Step 3 Assess the Current Situation and Environment
  ▸ *Identify strengths, weaknesses, opportunities, and threats within the current program or organization.*

Step 4 Establish Specific Goals

Step 5 Identify Strategic Options
  ▸ *Question everything about current structures and operations.*
  ▸ *Think creatively.*

Step 6 Use Defined Criteria to Select Specific Strategies
  ▸ *Decide who chooses.*
  ▸ *Establish criteria for choice based on information and facts.*
  ▸ *Avoid bias and reflex reactions.*

Step 7 Transform Strategies into Action Plans
  ▸ *Prepare the strategic plan.*
  ▸ *Prepare program, project, operational plans.*

Step 8 Assess Impact and Adjust Strategies

Source: Adapted from Helfenbein et al. 1994.

---

interest in the drug sector: ministry of health, treasury, other ministries, the pharmacy division, the essential drugs program, health facilities, health care providers, international agencies, bilateral donors, development banks, local industry, overseas manufacturers, pharmaceutical suppliers, patients, the general public, local communities.

Having identified the stakeholders, the next question is: How will they be involved? As full participants? As contributors to selected parts? As commentators to draft plans? Chapter 5 describes different ways in which advice can be sought in formulating a national drug policy.

Finally, responsibilities for the planning process must be assigned, a timetable established, and a budget prepared.

Step 2. Establish the Mission of the Organization or Program

Every organization or major program should have a mission statement or statement of purpose that addresses at least two questions: *Why does the program or organization exist?* and *Who are the beneficiaries?* Policy-makers and program managers may assume that they know why there should be national drug policy or why an essential drugs program exists. But it is useful to ensure that there is agreement on the long-term goal or mission that underlies the policy or the existence of the program.

The mission statement for a church-sponsored essential drugs supply service in East Africa states, for example:

"The Mission for Essential Drugs and Supplies (MEDS), aims to provide the Church Health Units throughout Kenya with a reliable source of Essential Drugs and Supplies, of proven quality, at affordable cost, combined with appropriate training in Clinical Diagnosis and the Rational Use of these drugs."

This statement, which clearly describes the purpose and intended beneficiaries of MEDS, is made available to all MEDS staff members and the health units it serves. It mentions the quality of services, the source of funding (there will be a cost to health units), and the services provided (training as well as drug supply).

A discussion of the purpose of a program is needed to formulate a mission statement and create a shared vision among the leadership and senior staff. For example, the following alternative mission statements for a national essential drugs program have very different implications for the management, financing, and operation of the program:

► The purpose of the national essential drugs program is to ensure the availability, accessibility, and quality of drugs to all members of society.
► The purpose of the national essential drugs program is to provide high-quality essential drugs to ministry of health facilities, with emphasis on ensuring access for the poor and medically needy members of society.

Mission statements may also include value statements such as: "The national essential drugs program is based on the belief that provision of a limited list of low-cost, high-quality essential drugs is a highly cost-effective health care intervention." Mission statements need to be communicated publicly and should be reviewed periodically to ensure that they remain appropriate.

Step 3. Assess the Current Situation and Environment

Systematic assessment, as described in Chapter 4, means documenting what is going well and what is not going well. Increasingly, this process involves objective indicators that allow comparison of pharmaceutical sector structure, process, and performance with targets, over time, and with other countries. These indicators are important and should be included in any planning process. In the context of strategic planning, however, situation assessment is much broader, in that it looks at the environment of the pharmaceutical sector—the context in which the program is working.

SWOT analysis is a useful method for assessing the internal and external environment. A SWOT analysis considers internal *s*trengths and *w*eaknesses of the organization or program, as well as external *o*pportunities and *t*hreats.

For example, a particular essential drugs program may have internal strengths that include a well-established drug selection process, an efficient procurement office, and a program of regular workshops on rational drug use. Internal weaknesses may include poor central and regional storage facilities and unreliable transport. For the same program, a growing private-sector distribution network may provide external opportunities for contracting out storage and transport functions. But decreasing government revenues due to an economic downturn may represent an external threat to the program. In this example, the SWOT analysis might suggest maintaining the government's role in selecting, procuring, and promoting the rational use of drugs but decentralizing warehousing, contracting out distribution, and encouraging local financing.

Step 4. Establish Specific Goals

The goals of a program or organization should follow from its mission and the functions central to achieving that mission. A strategic plan for the pharmaceutical sector may have goals related to drug availability in government health facilities, rational drug use, drug quality, access to drugs in the private sector, the role of nongovernmental organizations (NGOs) in expanding access and rational drug use, control of drugs on the market, and local production. Examples of two goals are shown in Figure 35.3.

Step 5. Identify Strategic Options

Perhaps the most serious mistake in strategic planning is to think only of familiar strategies or those that have been tried in the past. The greatest benefit from planning often comes from identifying practical new options. To generate new ideas, a number of strategies can be useful:

► *Talk to people* with relevant experience and *listen* to what they suggest. Ministries of health, private health care providers, mission health services, and various NGOs work under very different circumstances, yet many of the problems they face are similar. Strategies that have been successful for one may be useful to another, perhaps with modifications or adaptations.
► *Learn about other programs* from published reports, project evaluations, or other local sources and from international agencies such as the World Bank or the World

Figure 35.3 Key Elements of a Strategic Plan for an Essential Drugs Program

Mission (overall goal): Improve the health of the population by ensuring the availability and proper use of essential drugs for the treatment, prevention, and diagnosis of common health problems at government health facilities.

Goal: Drug availability—ensure that safe, effective, high-quality essential drugs are available at all times at all government health facilities.

General Objectives:
▸ Financing—ensure that financial resources are adequate to meet basic drug needs.
▸ Procurement—obtain a regular supply of drugs at favorable prices.
▸ Quality assurance—ensure that procured drugs meet recognized standards of quality and that quality is maintained through the distribution chain.
▸ Central storage—ensure that drugs are properly stored, with minimal expirations or other losses.
▸ Delivery—ensure timely delivery of drugs to health units.
▸ Storage at health units—ensure that drugs are properly stored, with minimal expirations or other losses.

Goal: Rational use—ensure that drugs are rationally prescribed, correctly dispensed, and appropriately used by patients.

General Objectives:
▸ Selection—maintain an up-to-date list and information on safe, effective, affordable essential drugs.
▸ Prescribing—ensure that drugs are prescribed according to local standard treatment guidelines.
▸ Dispensing—ensure that drugs are correctly identified, labeled, and packaged and that patients are clearly instructed on drug use.
▸ Patient use—ensure that patients consume drugs as prescribed and do not use drugs in an unsafe manner.

Health Organization (WHO) Action Programme on Essential Drugs or independent organizations such as Management Sciences for Health.

▸ *Visit other programs* through study tours or by arranging short visits as part of regional conferences. Often the most useful lessons—both positive and negative—come from the experiences of neighboring countries. Although some question the benefit of study tours, when the right people are sent to the right places for the right reasons, study tours can be extremely effective in opening up thinking to new ideas and stimulating alternative views of the future.

▸ *Brainstorm within the planning team.* Brainstorming helps groups be more creative at all levels of planning, decision-making, and problem-solving. Proven to be highly successful in a wide range of organizations and cultures, brainstorming is neither a free-for-all nor a formal discussion. Chapter 48 gives specific guidelines.

▸ *Bring in outside expertise.* Local or international advisers

can be costly but may offer practical suggestions and important ideas that might otherwise be difficult or impossible to obtain.

In short, to identify strategic options, it is important to think creatively and to question everything about current structures and operations.

Step 6. Use Defined Criteria to Select Specific Strategies

Once the full range of options has been identified, the most promising ones should be selected for further consideration and carefully evaluated. Final judgments should be based on information and facts, not on unfounded biases or reflex reactions.

Who should be involved, and how should choices be made? Senior officials and those most central to the implementation process should participate in selecting specific strategies using established criteria against which each option can be assessed. Commonly used criteria are:

▸ *Potential impact:* If the strategy is successful, how large an impact can be expected? For example, would shifting to international competitive bidding reduce prices by 40 to 50 percent, or by only 5 to 10 percent? Whenever possible, the potential impact should be expressed in terms of cost savings or other financial benefits.

▸ *Political feasibility:* Successful development is in large measure a political process. Judgments must be made about expected political support and opposition.

▸ *Technical feasibility:* Local infrastructure development, available human resources, and even the state of pharmaceutical science influence technical feasibility. For example, a demand-based pull system for supplying health centers, although theoretically less wasteful than the push system, may not be feasible when most staff have only minimal education. It may become feasible, however, as the general level of education and experience rises.

▸ *Financial feasibility:* Many good ideas are presently unaffordable. Financial feasibility may relate to recurrent operating costs or initial development costs (see Chapter 42) and may depend in part on donor interest.

▸ *Cost effectiveness:* Cost effectiveness (see Chapter 3) relates the cost of a particular strategy to its effectiveness or potential impact. Usually this involves approximate costs and projected, rather than actual, measures of each. Even rough estimates may provide useful insights for planning purposes. Four-box analysis, a variation of cost-effectiveness analysis sometimes used for priority-setting in program planning, is described in Country Study 35.1.

Country Study 35.1 Four-Box Analysis for Program Planning in Malawi

Planning efforts usually generate too many good ideas for the money, human resources, or time available. Therefore, priorities must be set. One of the more practical ways to set program priorities is *cost-impact* or *four-box analysis*.

To do a cost-impact analysis, each major proposed activity is first categorized as high-cost or low-cost (or even no-cost). Each activity is then categorized according to its potential impact as either high-impact or low-impact. High priority is given to high-impact, low-cost activities. Low-impact, high-cost activities are given low priority and are often dropped from the plan. The priority given to the high-impact, high-cost activities depends on funds remaining after the high-impact, low-cost activities have been planned.

In an elaboration of this approach, the Malawi Essential

Drugs Programme, when preparing its 1990–95 workplan, ranked each of eighteen possible areas on four separate scales: current status, necessity for improvement, readiness to act, and cost effectiveness. These four scales were then aggregated into two dimensions: need and feasibility. A composite score as well as the estimated recurrent cost were calculated for each activity.

The accompanying figure illustrates a four-box summary of the priority-setting results from Malawi. The numbers in parentheses indicate the final ranking of the activity. Note that classification under high or low need indicates not absolute need but current status and need for improvement. Feasibility is determined by the additional cost of the activity and readiness to undertake it.

Feasibility	Need High	Need Low
High	Treatment guidelines and drug formulary (1) Inventory control system (2) Financial management for central medical store (3) Pharmacist training (4) Central and regional storage (5) Rational drug use (7)	Distribution decentralization (14) Selection process maintenance (15)
Low	Quality control capacity (6) Development of course for pharmacy technicians (8) Drug inspection system (9) Research on drug use and quantification (10) Drug registration system (11) Patient information/IEC (12)	Local production reassessment (13) Drug procurement improvements (16) Regulation and legislative enforcement (17) Pharmacy assistant training (18)

Source: Adapted from Brasseur 1990.

Political and technical feasibility helps define the likelihood of success. Selecting strategies involves weighing the potential impact or benefits, if successful, against the likelihood of success and the costs of success.

Step 7. Transform Strategies into Action Plans
Once strategies have been selected, the strategic plan should be written down. Generally it should cover the following points as succinctly as possible:

► Mission statement for the organization or program;
► Brief assessment of the current situation: strengths, weaknesses, opportunities, threats;
► Concise description of each goal for the organization;
► Brief summary of each specific strategy for achieving these goals.

Strategic plans do not normally include a great deal of operational detail. Other information, such as the history of past efforts, a listing of options that were considered but rejected, and similar details, is not necessary but may

be included if it would make the plan more understandable or more convincing.

Once the strategic plan has been completed, some form of official endorsement is needed. If all concerned senior officials have been involved in the process and have accepted the plan, a letter of transmittal may be sufficient. In government settings, the plan may need to be presented to a senior ministerial management committee or even to the cabinet. In NGOs and private organizations, strategic plans may need to be endorsed by the governing body or board of directors, which may also have been involved in the planning process.

The benefits of planning begin to be felt only when the plan is implemented. Turning the approved plan into action requires more specific planning, such as a three- or five-year program plan and/or project proposal.

Step 8. Assess Impact and Adjust Strategies
As noted earlier, the true test of any plan is in its implementation. The strategic planning process does not stop

with formulation of the plan or even with its implementation. It continues through ongoing monitoring and periodic evaluation.

Are the strategies being turned into programs and workplans? Are they having the intended impact? If not, does the problem lie with the implementation process? Are different people required? Is more time required? Is the basic goal wrong? Should it be revised? Or are the strategies themselves to blame? A strategy that is good in theory but cannot be implemented under even the best of conditions is not a good strategy.

≡ 35.3 Program Planning

Most planning is done at the program, project, and operational levels. Program planning focuses on clearly defined medium-term objectives within overall long-term goals. A program plan should follow from a strategic plan, national drug policy, or national development plan. Often, however, a program plan follows from historical expectations and assumptions about the role of drug management within the government.

A government essential drugs program, a mission essential drugs service, or any other major pharmaceutical program should have a program plan, regardless of funding sources. A well-formulated plan provides direction and a framework for month-to-month and year-to-year activities and helps coordinate staff, finances, and other resources.

In the context of national essential drugs programs, program plans are often referred to as *pharmaceutical master plans* (WHO/DAP 1993). They provide an overview of the sector and a three- to five-year plan of action and are sometimes called five-year implementation plans.

Program plans are much more specific than strategic plans with respect to objectives, responsibilities, time frame, and usually budget. They are best implemented through detailed annual or semiannual operational workplans (described below).

Program Planning Process

Program planning usually involves a three-stage process. In the *exploration* phase, a planning group is formed, existing long-term goals and strategies are reviewed, and the current situation is assessed. In the *formulation* phase, objectives for the planning period are specified, targets are set for each objective, and resource requirements are determined. And in the *action* phase, the program plan and budget are prepared, implemented, and monitored. Each of these three stages has distinctive operational steps, outlined in Figure 35.4.

Exploration. The first step in program planning is to

Figure 35.4 Program Planning Process

Exploration

Step 1   Establish the planning group.

Step 2   Confirm long-term goals, strategies, and current objectives.

Step 3   Assess the current situation.

Formulation

Step 4   Specify objectives for the planning period.

Step 5   Set targets for each objective.

Step 6   Determine the resources needed for achieving each objective.

Action

Step 7   Prepare the program plan and budget.

Step 8   Implement the plan.

Step 9   Monitor the plan.

establish the planning group, usually the program manager and senior staff. Experienced advisers may help guide the planning process. Representatives of international organizations, donors, and development banks can often provide useful input into the planning process, but they are generally not part of the planning team.

If there is a national drug policy, national development plan, or other form of strategic plan for the pharmaceutical sector, broad objectives have already been developed. Even in the absence of such a plan, most programs have some objectives toward which they have been working. These should be written down and reviewed.

Assessment of the current situation can be rather limited and impressionistic. But whenever possible, assessment of the current situation should be based on monitoring data, indicators, review of progress reports, and other systematic measures described in Chapter 4.

Current problems and constraints can be identified from the systematic assessment. For major problems, a force field analysis (described in Chapter 34) may be useful to identify restraining and driving forces that must be considered if the plan is to achieve its objectives.

Formulation. The next steps are to specify objectives, set targets, and determine resources needed to achieve each objective. As noted above, objectives should be SMART: *s*pecific, *m*easurable, *a*ppropriate, *r*ealistic, and *t*ime-bound.

Figure 35.5 contains an example of a five-year program plan for promoting rational drug use. This plan, which follows from the key elements of a strategic plan outlined in Figure 35.3, illustrates specific objectives that might be included.

As with problem-solving (described in Chapter 34) and

strategic planning (described above), one of the most critical steps in the program planning process is identifying the full range of options. Each option should be analyzed for likely strengths and weaknesses, resource demands, and possible consequences.

Action. Once objectives, priorities, and activities have been established, a draft plan should be prepared, specifying responsibilities, schedules, and budgets, preferably according to activity. Important deadlines should be clearly identified.

First drafts of program plans usually promise too many activities in too short a time for the number of people and amount of money available. For the plan to have any value, it must be realistic. This usually means reducing the number of activities and lengthening the time frame to reflect the amount of staff time and money actually available.

The final step is to implement and monitor the plan, as described in Chapter 34.

Contents of a Program or Project Plan

A program or project plan should include

- a summary of the long-term goal;
- major strategies for achieving the goal;
- specific objectives;
- targets for each objective;
- responsibilities for each activity;
- a schedule for each objective, in chronological order (usually by year);
- a budget for each objective or area of activity.

The written plan usually consists of text and tables. A table showing activities, targets, inputs with budget amounts, and time frame is most useful, as in Figure 35.5.

Although budget figures can be included in the summary table, a separate budget is usually necessary. A program budget should indicate the area of activity (drug supply or rational drug use, for example), the type of expenditure (salary, drug purchases, per diem, and so forth), whether the expenditure is in local or foreign currency, and the likely source of funding. Chapter 42 contains more detailed information on preparing budgets.

In addition to the summary table, some text is necessary to communicate the goal and rationale for the program, to describe specific activities, and to justify the budget.

≡ 35.4 Work Planning

Work planning is the most detailed type of routine planning. A workplan is like a blueprint: it shows each of the smaller steps involved in achieving the larger goal.

Effective managers use workplans to keep efforts focused on planned activities and to coordinate staff efforts. Workplans are not intended to limit staff initiative, but they should help managers and staff say no to unreasonable and unplanned requests and control overly optimistic promises.

A workplan is typically prepared annually to cover a twelve-month period, although some essential drugs programs do operational work planning on a six-month cycle. Compared with program or project plans, workplans should be more specific with respect to outputs, individual responsibilities, precise time frame, and budget requirements.

The steps for preparing an annual workplan—which are similar but not identical to those for preparing a program plan—are:

Step 1. Review long-term goals and existing program plans.
Step 2. Confirm specific objectives for the upcoming year.
Step 3. Set targets for each objective.
Step 4. List major activities for each objective.
Step 5. Prepare an activity-time (Gantt) chart showing the responsibility and timing for each activity.
Step 6. Review or prepare the annual budget.
Step 7. Revise the plan based on available staff, time, and funds.
Step 8. Implement the plan.
Step 9. Monitor the plan.

For each objective and activity, workplans generally specify major tasks involved, measurable outputs, responsibilities for each task, timing (at least to the month), budget, and source of funds for each activity or task.

Under Step 4, it is important to consider what activities are possible for achieving each objective and not be limited to what was done last year.

Step 7 is particularly important. Once Steps 1 through 6 have been completed and there is a draft workplan, the plan must be reviewed carefully and finalized according to available staff, time, and funds. A plan that is unrealistic from the start will quickly lose credibility and have little value as a management tool.

Work Planning Process

Preparation of workplans must involve those who will be implementing them. Because this activity requires a focused effort without interruptions, it is often useful to move out of the office for a day to prepare the workplan. Brainstorming techniques (see Chapter 48) can be useful in generating ideas for specific activities and tasks. In any

Figure 35.5 Five-Year Implementation Plan for Promoting Rational Drug Use

Goal: Rational use—ensure that drugs are rationally prescribed, correctly dispensed, and appropriately used by patients

Objectives/Activities	Output Targets (5 year)	Inputs	Budget ($)	Year 1	Year 2	Year 3	Year 4	Year 5
Selection—maintain an up-to-date list and information on safe, effective, affordable essential drugs.								
Essential drugs list (EDL)—revise and distribute national essential drugs list every 2 years.	2 revisions of EDL	Meeting expenses	2,000	<<——>>				
National formulary manual (NFM)—prepare/revise and distribute national formulary manual at least every 4 years.	First edition of NFM completed and distributed	Meeting expenses, editing services, layout, printing, implementation workshops	32,000		<<——>>			
Prescribing—ensure that drugs are prescribed according to locally recognized standards of care.								
Undergraduate training—ensure that all students are trained in essential drugs concept and rational drug use in basic health curricula (amount of time depends on professional category).	4 curricula designed and implemented (medicine, pharmacy, nursing, paramedical)	Meeting expenses, curriculum materials, books	5,000	<<——>>				
Standard treatment guidelines (STG)—develop/revise and distribute standard treatment manual at least every 4 years.	First edition of STG completed and distributed	Meeting expenses, editing services, layout, printing, implementation workshops	48,000	<<——>>				
Continuing education—provide all clinicians with at least 1 week of in-service training on rational drug use every 3 years.	65% of clinicians trained (1,300 of estimated 2,000)	Workshop costs, short-term training adviser, training materials	42,000		<<——————————>>			>>
Drug information—establish a drug information center in each teaching and provincial hospital.	3 operational drug information centers (3 of 7 hospitals)	Computers, books, software, office materials	21,000			<<———>>	>>	
Self-monitoring—ensure that 70% of health units conduct drug use self-assessment at least once each quarter.	Self-assessment methods developed and implemented at 50% of health units (150 of 300 units)	Short-term adviser, design workshop, implementation workshop, training materials	28,000				<<——>>	>>
Dispensing—ensure that drugs are correctly identified, labeled, and packaged and that patients are clearly instructed on drug use.								
Packaging and labeling—ensure that at least 80% of patients receive drugs in clearly labeled containers or dispensing envelopes.	Packaging and labeling materials provided, sufficient for 80% of patients	Labels, dispensing envelopes	15,000	<<——>>				
Continuing education—ensure that all staff dispensing drugs receive at least 3 days of refresher training every 4 years.	60% of pharmacy staff trained (240 of estimated 400)	Workshop costs, short-term training adviser, training materials	24,000			<<————>>		>>
Patient use—ensure that patients consume drugs as prescribed and do not use drugs in an unsafe manner.								
Undergraduate training—ensure that all students are trained in communications and patient education methods in basic health curricula (amount of time depends on professional category).	Included in prescribing training (see prescribing outputs)	(see above)	(see above)	<<——>>				
Continuing education—include skills for patient education at in-service training workshops.	Included in prescribing continuing education (see prescribing outputs)	(see above)	(see above)		<<———>>			
Patient education materials—ensure that at least 80% of health units have materials for delivering 8 basic drug use messages.	Package of 8 basic drug use messages prepared; package introduced at 50% of health units (150 of 300 units)	Patient survey, short-term communication adviser, materials design, implementation workshop	18,000				<<——>>	>>

case, the tone of meetings should encourage the open exchange of ideas and creative thinking. Sometimes, informal discussions preceding the formal work planning discussion can help staff members reflect on the preceding year, consider the reasons for recent successes and failures, and begin thinking about the next year.

Objectives, targets, activities, and tasks should be consistent with the definitions given earlier in this chapter. Responsibilities for each activity should be listed by unit or office, or sometimes by person or team. The time frame is usually by year or quarter rather than by month.

Generally, workplans should be tied to activity-specific budgets that reflect all required inputs, including staff salaries, drug costs, vehicle costs, and other operating costs. For government programs, routine recurrent costs such as salary and utility expenses may be part of larger divisional budgets and not readily separated. Certainly drug costs and major additional costs should be noted separately.

Activity-Time Chart
At the center of an annual workplan is an activity-time (Gantt) chart, chronogram, or schedule of activities and responsibilities. A Gantt chart provides a clear, concise summary that is invaluable for communicating plans to staff, checking financial and other resource requirements, and monitoring progress.

A Gantt chart groups activities under objectives and usually contains a series of rows for each major activity. Typically, it contains columns for

► the objectives and activities;
► the person or unit responsible for each activity;
► the time period in which the activity will occur.

Output targets or performance indicators for each objective may be listed separately or included as a column of the Gantt chart.

Budgets should be linked to objectives and sometimes to individual activities. Often, budgets are listed in a separate part of the workplan. However, if specific funds and funding sources are associated with each activity, columns in the Gantt chart can specify the amounts and sources of funds.

An example of a Gantt chart for an essential drugs program is shown in Figure 35.6. This example is based on the first year of the program plan shown in Figure 35.5.

Monthly, Weekly, and Daily Workplans
An annual workplan provides major deadlines and a certain level of detail. Individual units and staff members, however, often prepare their own monthly, weekly, or daily schedules or to-do lists. This allows individuals to translate the workplan into short-term tasks and to set priorities to ensure that the most important tasks are being accomplished.

For example, the training officer responsible for the national workshop on undergraduate curriculum listed under "Undergraduate training" in Figure 35.6 may take this activity and prepare a one-page to-do list that contains tasks and target dates for selecting the venue, sending invitations, planning the agenda, obtaining flip charts and other training supplies, and other important tasks. Such lists help spread work out over the available time so that staff are not left with a large number of last-minute tasks before a major event.

Using Workplans to Check Progress
To be an effective management tool, workplans must be readily accessible and frequently reviewed. Wall charts of the workplan and copies taped to desktops are often used.

Workplans should be checked regularly. When specific activities are behind schedule, a decision must be made: reorganize priorities, assign additional staff or provide extra resources to get the activity back on schedule, or accept the delay.

If an annual workplan is well formulated and consistent with long-term program objectives, the performance of a program and its staff can be assessed by the extent to which it adheres to the workplan.

≡ 33.5 Project Planning Methods and Tools
Several planning methods and computer tools exist to help managers. These include methods derived from industrial and engineering management science, methods supported by specific donor requirements, and computer programs for project management.

Management Science Methods
Two commonly used methods from management science are the critical path method (CPM; see Figure 35.7) and project evaluation and review technique (PERT). Although originally formulated as two distinct methods, their similarities are such that they are commonly referred to together as PERT-CPM. The combined method uses a network model to help planners arrange and schedule project activities.

The main steps for PERT-CPM planning are (1) identify all necessary tasks, (2) determine which tasks need to be completed before the next ones are started, (3) estimate the time needed for each task, and (4) combine the information from the first three steps into a diagram of the whole process.

Figure 35.6 Annual Workplan (Gantt Chart), First Year of Five-Year Plan

Goal: Rational use—ensure that drugs are rationally prescribed, correctly dispensed, and appropriately used by patients

Objectives/Activities	Responsibility	Jan	Feb	Mar	Apr	May	Jun	Jul	Aug	Sep	Oct	Nov	Dec
Selection													
Essential drugs list (EDL)—revise and distribute national essential drugs list every 2 years.													
Appoint national drugs and therapeutics committee (NDTC).	Director, medical services		x										
Call for proposals for additions and deletions to EDL.	Chairman, NDTC			x									
Hold NDTC meeting to revise EDL.	NDTC						x						
Prescribing													
Undergraduate training—ensure that all students are trained in essential drugs concept and rational drug use in basic health curricula (amount of time depends on professional category).													
Convene national workshop to outline changes in medical, pharmacy, nursing, paramedical curricula.	Dean, medical school			x									
Organize working groups to prepare detailed core curricula for each health profession.	Individual training institutions				x———>		x						
Support core groups at institutional level to implement curricula changes.	Individual training institutions									————————————>			
Standard treatment guidelines (STG)—develop/revise and distribute standard treatment manual at least every 4 years.													
Appoint committee to coordinate drafting of manual.	Director, medical services	x											
Assign writing responsibilities.	Senior editor/chairperson of editorial committee		x										
Complete draft treatment manual.	Individual authors			x——————————————>					x				
Distribute draft manual for review.	EDP training officer											x	
Continuing education—provide all clinicians with at least 1 week of in-service training on rational drug use every 3 years.													
Do needs assessment (identification of major drug use problems).	Medical school, clinical pharmacology				x								
Design continuing education (CE) programs.	EDP training officer, training consultant					x							
Prepare course materials.	EDP training officer, training consultant						x——>x						
Conduct first CE workshop.	EDP training officer, training consultant									x			
Revise CE program and materials.	EDP training officer, training consultant										x———>x		
Conduct second CE workshop.	EDP training officer and staff												x
Dispensing													
Packaging and labeling—ensure that at least 80% of patients receive drugs in clearly labeled containers or dispensing envelopes.													
Review and revise design of dispensing containers and labels.	Pharmacy school		x										
Include dispensing envelopes and labels in drug tenders.	EDP procurement officer			x									
Prepare circular letter/memorandum to inform dispensing staff.	EDP information officer										x		
Distribute envelopes and labels to health units.	EDP supply officer											x	

The most important benefits of the PERT-CPM method are that it forces managers to estimate realistically the time required for each task or activity and to think carefully about the best sequence of tasks and activities. Full-scale application of the method is most common with complex construction projects, but realistic assessment of time requirements and efficient sequencing of activities should be part of any planning effort.

LogFrame and Related Project Planning Methods

Most donors have a required series of steps that they follow to identify, plan, implement, and monitor projects (see Chapter 43). The logical framework approach (LogFrame or LFA) is one such planning method that has broader applications. The LogFrame approach (NORAD 1990) is used by the U.S. Agency for International Development (USAID), Danida, and several other donors. It begins with an analysis of existing problems and specifies objectives, outputs, activities, inputs, and indicators. LogFrame ensures a logical interrelatedness among project elements, highlights the influence of external factors, and provides a systematic basis for monitoring.

Project Planning Management Software

A number of computer programs based on variations of PERT-CPM and other planning methods can help organize project planning and monitoring. Planning software can be useful for generating charts and schedules of different levels of detail; for determining when too much has been planned for available human or financial resources; for summarizing tasks by objective, unit, or individual; for preparing and monitoring project budgets; and for reporting on project achievements.

In practice, simple spreadsheet programs are the most commonly used software for program planning. The example in Figure 35.5 is from a spreadsheet model in which each category of essential information (such as objective or target) forms a separate column and each task or activity is given a separate row.

Computers are useful for organizing planning information, but they cannot replace clear thinking about project objectives, substitute for personal monitoring of project activities, or make planning decisions.

≡ 35.6 Why Plans Sometimes Fail

Good plans to guide program development and implementation take time and effort. Sometimes, however, plans exist merely on paper: they are made but never actually used. Even well-conceived, well-presented plans can remain unused.

Figure 35.7 CPM Analysis of Plan to Upgrade Central Supply Functions

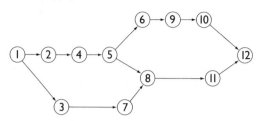

Activity	Activity Description	Time (weeks)	Predecessor Activity
1	Plan to upgrade central drug supply services	6	–
2	Appoint committee to revise essential drugs list	6	1
3	Develop new procurement procedures	8	1
4	Revise essential drugs list, organize by level of care	2	2
5	Quantify drug requirements by level of care	4	4
6	Prepare budget proposal	3	5
7	Prequalify suppliers	12	3
8	Prepare and distribute tender documents	4	5, 7
9	Obtain budget approval	10	6
10	Ensure availability of funds	8	9
11	Complete tendering and place orders	8	8
12	Receive and pay for drugs	12	10, 11

Why do plans sometimes fail to be implemented or, if implemented, fail to achieve their intended objectives? There are many reasons, but some of the more common are

▶ *unrealistic or overly ambitious planning:* Planning must be based on a realistic assessment of the current situation, clear objectives for the future, and a practical assessment of what is possible. Planning, particularly in groups, can sometimes become overly optimistic and idealistic. Planning should be forward thinking but should not confuse hopes and wishes with good judgment about what is possible.

▶ *failure to consider existing commitments:* Plans must be made within the context and constraints of existing commitments. Although there is often the opportunity for great progress, progress takes time. Plans that propose too much in too little time may spread everyone's efforts too thinly to accomplish any of the stated objectives or may compromise the work's quality.

▶ *lack of involvement by the implementers:* Plans are best

made at the levels where they will be carried out. Strategic plans to guide long-term policy must involve policy-makers, medium-term program plans must involve program managers and key program staff, and annual work planning must involve the people whose work is being planned. Without such involvement, plans are likely to lack both the realism and the commitment necessary for effective implementation.

▶ *lack of support:* Success also depends on support from others who are not directly involved in implementation. This may include support from senior staff and officials of ministries (such as treasury) and other governmental bodies, international organizations such as WHO and UNICEF, donors and development banks, local NGOs, and local professional societies. Selective involvement of such individuals in preparing or reviewing a strategic or program plan can lay a good foundation for future support during implementation.

▶ *planning for the wrong reasons:* Some plans are never really meant to be implemented. Examples include plans made only for short-term political gain or to satisfy a condition for receiving a grant or a loan. Whenever possible, however, plans pushed by external needs should also suit the needs of the organization or program. If plans are sometimes made "for appearances only," staff should understand why so that the experience does not undermine staff perceptions of the value of good planning.

▶ *lack of funds:* There is nothing more frustrating than spending considerable time and effort in planning, only to learn that there are insufficient funds to carry out the plan. Whenever possible, planning should be based on a realistic assessment of potential funding sources.

▶ *lack of people or time:* Although plans are made for organizations or programs, they depend on people. Ambitious plans require more people and more capable people. But even a plan that was realistic at the time it was made may fail if key people are transferred or otherwise become unavailable.

▶ *wrong level of planning:* Some managers and staff tend to avoid planning for themselves. They prefer planning for the people below them or making recommendations to the people above them. A fundamental principle of planning, as noted above, is that plans should be developed with the active involvement of those who are central to implementing them.

▶ *poorly presented or overly complicated plans:* Often, the clearest, most useful plans are the shortest plans. For example, an annual workplan for a national essential drugs program may consist of a one-page introduction and statement of objectives, a two-page chart of activities and time frame (Gantt chart), a one-page budget, and one page of text describing the eight major program components. Plans that are poorly organized or overly complex or that provide excessive detail are difficult to understand, let alone implement.

▶ *lack of follow-up and monitoring:* One of the most common management failures is the failure to actually use a plan once it has been prepared. A five-year program plan such as that shown in Figure 35.5 should be reviewed regularly and used to formulate annual workplans. Annual workplans such as that shown in Figure 35.6 should be checked on a weekly or monthly basis. The program's monitoring system (see Chapter 36) should be linked with organizational and program plans. Without this link, the plan loses its value in guiding implementation.

Thus, for plans to be implemented effectively, they must be realistic, they must be developed with input from the people who will implement them, they must have sufficient support, they must have adequate resources, and they must be clearly presented.

≡ 35.7 Progress Review Cycle

Planning represents the beginning of the management cycle. Plans must be implemented, and equally important, implementation must be monitored. When plans are made and implemented, it is important to determine how often progress will be reviewed. The review cycles for strategic plans, program plans, and workplans are different, but they should be linked.

If formal evaluations of progress are carried out (see Chapter 36), they are typically done after two to three years. Such evaluations may focus on long-term strategic plans, program plans, or specific project plans.

Progress toward achievement of the objectives set forth in a program plan or master plan should be reviewed at least annually, whether the plan covers a three-year, five-year, or other period. If a strategic plan exists, progress toward achieving long-term goals is generally reviewed at the same time as the program plan is reviewed.

An annual program review should address the following questions:

▶ What is the progress toward each objective?
▶ What are the implementation problems?
▶ What changes are needed in strategies, objectives, or specific activities?
▶ What activities should be deleted from the plan?
▶ What new activities must be added to achieve the original objectives?

≡ Assessment Guide

Strategic Planning

- ► Does a strategic plan exist for the pharmaceutical sector (for example, a national drug policy or national development plan)? Is it suited to the current political, social, and economic environment? Are its strategies still appropriate and effective?

- ► To what extent did the strategic planning process involve policy-makers and senior staff? Which key stakeholders were identified and consulted?

- ► To what extent did the strategic planning process actively consider new strategic options, such as strategies used elsewhere or suggested by outside experts?

- ► Is the strategic plan written? Does it include a mission statement; a brief assessment of the current situation, including strengths, weaknesses, opportunities, and threats; a concise description of each goal; and a brief summary of each strategy for achieving these goals? Has it been officially endorsed?

- ► Is the strategic plan reflected in program plans and workplans? To what extent are strategies having the intended impact?

Program Planning

- ► If there is an essential drugs program or other major pharmaceutical program, is there a pharmaceutical master plan, five-year implementation plan, or other program plan?

- ► Does each program or project plan include a statement of the goal, strategies, objectives, output targets, responsibilities, schedule, and budget? Does the plan include both text and tables?

- ► Are program plans implemented through annual or semiannual operational workplans?

- ► Have program plans been used in presenting arguments for additional funding?

Work Planning

- ► Are workplans prepared annually?

- ► Do they specify objectives, activities, major tasks, measurable target outputs, individual responsibilities, timing (at least to the month), budget, and source of funds for each activity? Are they realistic in terms of available staff, time, and funds?

- ► Do workplan documents include activity-time (Gantt) charts? Are they used for monitoring?

- ► To what extent are implementing staff involved in the preparation of workplans? Do individual units and staff members prepare, based on the workplan, their own monthly, weekly, or daily schedules or to-do lists?

Planning Tools

- ► What planning methods or computer tools are used to support planning efforts (for example, CPM, PERT, LogFrame, Harvard Project Manager, Timeline)?

Planning as Part of the Management Cycle

- ► Once plans have been established, are they reviewed on a regular basis for implementation progress and problems? Are the review cycles for strategic plans, program plans, and workplans linked?

- ► Have formal assessments or evaluations been done? If so, have the findings and recommendations been incorporated into revised plans?

Progress toward implementation of annual workplans should be formally reviewed at least quarterly, if not monthly. In general, the questions asked during annual progress reviews also apply to quarterly or monthly reviews of workplans. ■

≡ References and Further Readings

★ = *Key readings.*

Baum, W. C. 1982. *Project cycle*. Washington, D.C.: World Bank.

Blanco-Sequeiros, M. 1994. Health projects within the health care system. In *Health and disease in developing countries*, ed. K. A. Lankinen, S. Bergstrom, P. H. Makela, and M. Peltomaa. London: Macmillan.

Brasseur, O. 1990. *Malawi Essential Drugs Programme, final report*. Lilongwe, Malawi: World Health Organization.

Danida (Danish International Development Agency). 1992. *Guidelines for project preparation*. Copenhagen: Danida.

★ Helfenbein, S., S. Seims, and D. Ruhe. 1994. Learning to think strategically. *Family planning manager* 3 (1).

Miller, J., and J. Wolff. 1993. Developing plans and proposals for new initiatives. *Family planning manager* 2 (4).

★ MSH (Management Sciences for Health). 1992a. Developing and using workplans. In *The family planning manager's handbook: Basic skills and tools for managing family planning programs*, ed. J. A. Wolff, L. J. Suttenfield, and S. C. Binzen. West Hartford, Conn.: Kumarian Press.

★ MSH (Management Sciences for Health). 1992b. Planning for the future. In *The family planning manager's handbook: Basic skills and tools for managing family planning programs*, ed. J. A. Wolff, L. J. Suttenfield, and S. C. Binzen. West Hartford, Conn.: Kumarian Press.

NORAD (Norwegian Agency for Development Cooperation). 1990. *The logical framework approach (LFA): Handbook for objectives-oriented project planning*. Oslo: NORAD.

Pegels, C. C., and K. A. Rogers. 1988. *Strategic management of hospitals and health care facilities*. Gaithersburg, Md.: Aspen Publishers.

WHO (World Health Organization). 1984. *Glossary of terms used in the health for all series*. Geneva: WHO.

WHO/DAP (World Health Organization/Action Programme on Essential Drugs). 1993. *Meeting of regional experts on the formulation and implementation of national drug policies and pharmaceutical master plans*. WHO/DAP/93.9. Geneva: WHO/DAP.

| Part I | Part II | Part III | **Part IV** |
| Introduction | Policy and Legal Framework | Drug Management Cycle | **Management Support Systems** |

A Organization and Management ▶
    34 Managing Drug Programs

B Financing and Sustainability
    35 Planning for Drug Management

C Information Management

D Human Resources Management
    36 Monitoring and Evaluation

37 Community Participation

38 Hospital Drug Services

39 Security Management

Chapter 36
Monitoring and Evaluation

≡ Summary

Monitoring and evaluation make up the third step in the management cycle. Monitoring refers to the ongoing review of the degree to which program activities are completed and objectives are being met, to allow for corrective action during program implementation. Monitoring should be an integral part of day-to-day management.

Fully developed monitoring systems, which may be developed in phases, typically consist of a combination of four methods:

1. *Supervisory visits for continual, informal monitoring of workplan implementation and progress toward program plans;*
2. *Routine reporting of selected data through the drug management information system (DMIS);*
3. *Sentinel sites for more detailed reporting when new initiatives or rapid expansion requires more intensive monitoring;*
4. *Special studies whenever an implementation problem or planning question requires specific additional information.*

Management or clinical indicators allow comparison of a program's progress to performance targets and to other programs. Indicators should meet the criteria of clarity, usefulness, measurability, reliability, and validity, as well as acceptance by key stakeholders and consistency of interpretation among stakeholders. For indicators requiring drug-specific information, indicator drugs are usually identified.

To be effective in improving program and staff performance, monitoring requires

- ► *clear communication of plans and targets;*
- ► *regular review and sharing of monitoring results;*
- ► *follow-up to provide feedback and take corrective action.*

Evaluation refers to the periodic analysis of a program's progress toward meeting established objectives and goals. There are three types, which differ in timing and purpose:

1. *Needs assessment (situation analysis, see Chapter 4);*
2. *Formative evaluation (midterm review);*
3. *Summative evaluation (final evaluation).*

Evaluations use data collected through the ongoing monitoring system, supplemented by document review, interviews, additional data collection, and field surveys using standard pharmaceutical assessment indicators.

≡ 36.1 Definitions of Monitoring and Evaluation

Monitoring and evaluation are an integral part of the management cycle, providing a link between planning and implementation. It is important to distinguish between monitoring and evaluation; the terms are frequently used interchangeably, but they should not be.

Monitoring refers to reviewing, on a continuous basis, the degree to which program activities are completed and targets are being met. This allows corrective action to be taken during program implementation.

Evaluation refers to analyzing progress toward meeting established objectives and goals. It provides feedback on whether plans have been met and the reasons for success or failure; it should also provide direction for future plans. Evaluation methods may also be used to carry out a situation analysis or a needs assessment as the first step in a program or planning process.

This chapter is concerned mostly with monitoring, which plays a central role in day-to-day management. Monitoring is closely linked with the drug management information system, described in Chapter 45. Evaluation, which is closely linked with systematic assessment (Chapter 4), is discussed briefly at the end of the chapter.

≡ 36.2 Monitoring Issues

Monitoring is an integral part of day-to-day management in successful drug programs. Systematic monitoring, based on program objectives and linked to specific activities, is essential for improving program performance and achieving long-term program goals. Too often, monitoring is done casually, without a clear plan, without a clear linkage to program objectives and targets, and without any effort to use monitoring results to improve program performance.

Managers of drug programs are concerned with getting the most out of scarce resources. This means making the program as efficient and as effective as possible. Therefore, managers need to generate current, reliable information to be used to make decisions on program performance and operations.

The monitoring system should center on key program activities and objectives. To operate efficiently, it must focus on a small number of specific, clearly formulated monitoring issues that are directly related to performance and are generally taken from program plans, objectives, and targets.

Monitoring is intended to

- ► determine whether activities are being carried out as planned;

▶ measure achievement of targets;
▶ identify implementation problems to initiate corrective action;
▶ identify and reinforce good performance;
▶ identify and strengthen weak performance;
▶ help target supervision to problem areas;
▶ assess whether activities are having their expected effect;
▶ assess long-term trends;
▶ contribute to reviewing and revising program priorities and plans.

Ultimately, monitoring is meant to improve the long-term performance of the program and individual staff members.

≡ 36.3 Monitoring Methods

How are monitoring activities organized, and where does information come from? Monitoring issues can be addressed through a combination of four methods: supervisory visits, routine reporting, sentinel reporting system, and special studies.

Supervisory Visits

Supervisory visits support the performance of individual staff members, provide some on-site, in-service training (see Chapter 47), and represent an important method for informal but direct monitoring of program implementation.

Supervisory visits should reinforce routine reporting requirements. Such visits sometimes involve the collection of information for special studies. Lot quality assurance sampling (LQAS) is one method for quickly obtaining quantitative information during routine visits (WHO/DAP 1993).

Routine Reporting

The core of a monitoring system is routine reporting through the drug management information system (DMIS). The design or revision of a DMIS begins with two basic questions:

1. Who are the users of information from the DMIS?
2. What are their information needs?

A basic DMIS consists of recording-keeping documents, data reporting forms, feedback reports, and procedures that govern the use and flow of information up and down the system. Chapter 45 provides a practical overview and specific advice on the principles of DMIS design. It emphasizes the need to build on existing recording and reporting, involve users in developing the system, use

appropriate data collection methods, integrate the DMIS with other information systems, take advantage of practical analysis methods, and communicate information promptly and clearly.

Depending on the program's objectives, routine reporting focuses on supply, finances, training, quality assurance, drug use, or other areas. Clear presentation of reported information, feedback to those providing the information, and follow-up action contribute to the effectiveness and usefulness of the reporting system. Reports should include both quantitative information and brief descriptions of processes, key problems, and proposed follow-up actions.

The biggest failures in routine reporting systems are overdesign and underimplementation. Collecting too much data usually results in too little analysis. Also, reporting systems that are overly complex result in poor compliance with reporting requirements. Implementing an information system takes time and money. And the more complex the system, the more time and money it takes to make it function.

Therefore, the content of routine reporting systems should be limited to the minimum amount of information that the typical reporting unit can reasonably be expected to provide and that can routinely be analyzed for decision-making and feedback purposes. The simple rule is do not collect what you cannot use.

Sentinel Reporting System

When routine reporting systems are properly collecting only the minimal essential information, a great deal of potentially useful information is routinely *not* collected. To supplement routine reporting, sentinel reporting systems can be useful.

A sentinel reporting system consists of a carefully selected sample of units that are given greater recording and reporting responsibilities. For example, in a country with forty districts, six districts may be selected as sentinel districts. Within each district, a sample of health facilities from each level may be selected. Sentinel reporting differs from routine reporting in the amount of information collected, the frequency or promptness of report submission, and the level of accuracy demanded.

Sentinel reporting is common in disease control programs such as AIDS/HIV prevention, control of diarrheal disease, and treatment of sexually transmitted diseases. Sentinel sites provide a relatively economical means of collecting up-to-date, detailed information on disease incidence, drug resistance patterns, and response to program interventions.

Country Study 36.1 illustrates how a sentinel reporting system has been used to guide the development of the Zimbabwe Essential Drugs Action Programme.

For drug management programs, there are three important questions concerning sentinel reporting: When is it needed? How should sites be selected? What information should be collected?

Need for Sentinel Reporting. A sentinel reporting system is most useful when a system is undergoing rapid or substantial change. Sentinel reporting helps assess the implementation and short-term impact of changes such as

- ► introduction of a major new stock management system;
- ► transition from a central medical stores system to a decentralized system;
- ► introduction or substantial expansion of a user fee program.

Sentinel reporting is particularly important for new or expanded user fee programs in which there are many new record-keeping requirements and many unknowns. Policy-makers and managers can recognize and react more quickly to unexpected or undesirable effects when reliable data on utilization impact, revenue generation, waivers and exemptions, and other key variables are collected and rapidly reported.

The routine reporting system answers only the questions it asks. A sentinel reporting system can be useful to detect unexpected or unintended outcomes.

Recording and reporting formats developed for sentinel sites sometimes prove sufficiently useful and convenient to be incorporated into routine reporting.

Selection of Sentinel Sites. The level and number of health units in a sentinel system depend on the organization of the health and drug management systems, the monitoring objectives, and the overall diversity within the country. If, for example, there is only one central medical store and only a handful of regional stores, they would all be included in sentinel reporting requirements. Generally, at least six units should be included within each level. For example, a sentinel system could include six districts, six district hospitals, and six health centers within each district (thirty-six health centers total). Larger numbers of units are needed in more populous, more organizationally complex, or more diverse countries.

Selection of specific districts, locations within districts, or health facilities is generally purposive, not random. Selection is aimed at achieving diversity rather than statistical representativeness. The selected sites should represent the range of facilities that serve culturally, linguistically, and geographically diverse groups; the distribution of

ministry and nongovernmental facilities; and accessibility.

Staffing levels at indicator sites should be sufficient to handle additional recording and reporting requirements, which may mean extra staff at some sites. Extra incentives are sometimes given for prompt, complete, accurate reporting, although this should be avoided. Prompt feedback of information can be sufficient to motivate staff to respond quickly and reliably. Since cost is a consideration, relatively inaccessible sites are usually excluded, even at the cost of omitting cultural or geographic diversity; however, if these inaccessible sites are particularly likely to suffer drug shortages and delayed delivery, it may be worth the effort to include some of them in the sentinel system.

Information Required from Sentinel Sites. Sentinel sites may differ in the amount of information recorded, the amount of information routinely reported, or the speed at which the information is processed. Additional recording and reporting requirements should be based on the reasons that the sentinel system was established, such as monitoring a new stock management system, assessing transition to a supply agency system, or evaluating the impact of a user fee program.

Most of the principles used in designing a national DMIS apply to sentinel reporting: being selective in deciding which indicators to collect, choosing appropriate data collection methods, and building on existing recording and reporting systems whenever possible. In some instances, it may be appropriate to computerize at sentinel sites or to choose sites that already have computer capability, even if national computerization is not currently foreseen.

Working with Sentinel Sites. Establishing a system of sentinel sites nearly always requires training for key staff at the sites, and frequent supervisory visits, especially in the beginning. Sites may require additional forms, registers, stock records, and other materials.

Finally, a system of sentinel sites is generally maintained for a specified period of time, perhaps for the first several years of a transitional program.

Special Studies

Sometimes managers need to gather information that is not available from routine or sentinel reporting. Examples of topics that may warrant a special study include

- ► names, dosage forms, and values of drugs purchased by individual health units;
- ► average supplier lead times (if not routinely monitored);
- ► names, dosage forms, and value of recently expired drugs;

Country Study 36.1 Sentinel Reporting and Drug Management Indicators in ZEDAP

Baseline Survey. In November 1986, the Zimbabwe Essential Drugs Action Programme (ZEDAP) became operational. Because the drug situation in the country was not known, ZEDAP's first activity was a nationwide survey. The survey was conducted in February 1987, with a representative sample of facilities at all levels. The results indicated severe shortages of essential drugs and supplies, long lead times, lack of standard stock control systems, lack of clinical training materials, and lack of training in drug management. These results served as the basis for the ZEDAP national drug policy and planning workshop in April 1987.

Sentinel Surveillance. To plan supply system improvements, justify budget requirements, and monitor progress, forty-eight sentinel sites were randomly selected from primary, secondary, and tertiary levels. The sentinel surveillance system effectively demonstrated a progressive decline in supply resulting from shortfalls in the semiannual financial allocations. Monthly reports from the facility level were instrumental in convincing the cabinet to assign higher priority to essential drugs and supplies in the government allocation process. Additional funds were set aside for emergency supplies of vital drugs.

The Serial Surveys (1989–93). In 1989, another nationwide survey, using the same sampling method but incorporating large urban areas, was undertaken to assess the progress and impact of the program at its midterm. Indicators and an appropriate instrument were developed, using a participatory process involving managers from districts and provinces, with support from the national essential drugs program and the

World Health Organization Action Programme on Essential Drugs (see the accompanying figure). The same core indicators continue to be used in annual or biennial surveys.

The core indicators assessed the availability of thirty-six indicator drugs and supply items. Implementation of the new national stock control system was checked by using stock management indicators and observing stock-keeping practices. To measure performance of the delivery system for supplies, the intervals at each step and total lead time were noted for the last three orders.

Complementary indicators were incorporated in individual surveys to answer questions relevant at the particular point in the program. For instance, initially, it was important to ascertain whether the new drug list, standard treatment guidelines, and learning materials had reached the target personnel at the primary-level facilities. Later surveys ascertained the number of personnel trained and adherence to the guidelines. The 1993 survey focused on the supply of antitubercular drugs and drug fees.

The data obtained through these monitoring activities were utilized at all levels. District supervisors found the core indicators useful for identifying individual centers that required training support or frequent supervision. The distribution system indicators led to reorganization of the distribution system. The stock control indicators led the ZEDAP team to revise training strategies, shifting from workshop to on-site job training. The indicators and the assessment methods were incorporated into routine supervision and served as the basis for local planning activities.

Indicator	1989	1990	1991	1993
Availability of drugs at rural health centers				
Average availability of 36 indicator drugs (%)	56	80–85	78	64
Stock management				
Stock cards in use (%)	52	78	82	86
Correct stock balance (%)	47	–	72	53
Facilities with expired items (%)	56	39	77	54
Drugs arranged systematically (%)	58	30	89	78
Total lead time				
Monthly orders (days)	71	48	46	46
Drug use				
Prescribing by generic name (%)	85	92	94	92
Average number of drugs per patient	1.4	1.3	1.3	1.6
Antibiotic drugs (%)	22	22	29	30

► reasons for expiration of drugs;

► average percentage of essential drugs available;

► level of patient adherence to prescribed treatment.

Special survey and research methods can be used to obtain this type of information. These methods may involve added expense and may require specialists to design and

carry them out, but many questions can be answered with relatively simple methods. Chapter 41 describes how ABC analysis, lead-time analysis, expiry date analysis, and pipeline analysis can help improve performance and reduce costs.

A manager's role is to identify when additional information is needed and to use experts to help design and conduct these special investigations. Both manager and staff should be involved in the design and implementation of these studies, as well as in the analysis and interpretation of results.

Rapid assessment procedures (RAPs) are often used to assess a specific implementation activity. In-depth interviews, structured observation, focus group discussions, or other qualitative methods (see Chapter 29) are used to explore behavior, attitudes, practices, and causal factors. Another rapid assessment approach is small random sample surveys, which can sometimes be designed, conducted, and analyzed within one month (see MSH/RPM 1995).

≡ 36.4 Designing the Monitoring System

Fully developed monitoring systems typically consist of a combination of the four methods just described. A practical strategy for developing a monitoring system for a drug management program is to:

1. Use *supervisory visits* to carry out continual monitoring of workplan implementation and progress toward program plans. Assessing selected output and performance indicators as part of supervisory visits provides some objectivity and structure.
2. Establish a streamlined *routine reporting system* that regularly and reliably reports only essential management information and provides prompt feedback.
3. Identify *sentinel sites* for more detailed recording and reporting only when new initiatives or rapid expansion requires more intensive monitoring. Their objectives should be clearly identified, and they should be maintained for only as long as they serve a specific purpose.
4. Plan and conduct *special studies* only when a problem or planning question requires information that is not available through either routine reporting or sentinel sites.

Country Study 36.2 describes how these four approaches were combined and how the system evolved for monitoring drug and treatment fees in one East African country.

The principles for designing a monitoring system are to focus on key monitoring questions and indicators, keep data collection to a minimum, develop practical procedures for managing monitoring information, and use information for timely feedback and follow-up action. The KISS concept should be applied: *keep it simple and straightforward* (or *keep it short and simple*).

When time pressures, financial resources, and staff members' inexperience with monitoring methods are limiting factors, *phased development* may make sense, with initial monitoring efforts focused on national issues of

selection and procurement. Medical stores data are often easy to collect. As the program develops, the monitoring system and core indicators can be expanded to cover distribution and drug use.

≡ 36.5 Using Indicators for Monitoring and Evaluation

Systematic monitoring depends on having performance standards or targets. To determine whether adequate progress is being achieved, it is necessary to know what is expected. Indicators help measure changes directly or indirectly and assess the extent to which the targets and objectives of a program are being attained (WHO 1984).

Applications of Indicators

When used to make measurements at one point in time, indicators allow a manager to compare a program's performance with a target level of performance (or to another program's performance) and to identify areas of relative strength and weakness. Applied over time, such indicators can be used to set and monitor performance improvement targets, such as

► monitoring implementation of program plans and workplans;
► evaluating achievement of long-term goals;
► assessing the performance of individual units;
► identifying relative strengths and weaknesses in current policies and systems;
► measuring the impact of new policies or management systems;
► self-monitoring to improve performance;
► demonstrating needs to treasury, donors, or other funders;
► reporting on progress to senior officials, donors, or other interested parties.

By using internationally defined indicators for national drug policy (Brudon-Jakobowicz et al. 1995), drug management (MSH/RPM 1995), and drug use (WHO/DAP 1993), countries can compare their progress with that of other countries.

Five necessary criteria for an indicator are clarity (is easily understood and calculated), usefulness (reflects an important dimension of performance), measurability (can be defined in quantitative or qualitative terms and used within existing constraints on information quality and availability), reliability (permits consistent assessment over time and among different observers), and validity (is a true measure of what it is meant to measure) (Chapter 4). Additional criteria sometimes used to select

Country Study 36.2 Monitoring the Introduction of Drug Fees in Kenya

In 1989, a new user fee program was introduced by the Kenya Ministry of Health (MOH). After early implementation problems, the ministry initiated a program of management improvement and regular fee adjustments. An outpatient drug and treatment fee was introduced in phases, beginning in mid-1992. To assess the impact of the program, in particular the drug treatment fee, a comprehensive monitoring system was implemented in 1991. The system consisted of targeted field supervision, routine reporting, a sentinel system of indicator districts, and special studies.

Targeted Field Supervision. Supervisory staff from the MOH health financing program made regular supervisory visits to each part of the country. Information from routine reporting and other sources was used to identify problem districts and problem facilities. These were visited more often. Gradually, the role of headquarters staff evolved from primary supervision (directly visiting districts and facilities themselves) to secondary supervision: teaching supervisory skills to provincial and district staff by making visits with counterparts.

Routine Reporting. Routine reporting used the financial information system (FIS) and the health information system (HIS). The FIS was developed specifically for the user fee program and consisted of reports from districts and hospitals covering collections, expenditures, insurance claims, exemptions, and bank balances. The existing HIS was adapted to support additional information needs of the user fee system.

Indicator Districts. The routine reporting system was kept to a minimum for reasons of feasibility, cost, and staff availability. Therefore, a system of six indicator districts was developed to provide additional details on the implementation of user fees. Districts were selected to achieve rural-urban and socioeconomic diversity. Specialized information-gathering in the indicator districts included (1) outpatient utilization data from all MOH levels, as well as selected mission and private facilities; (2) rapid household surveys before and after major fee changes to assess care-seeking patterns and knowledge of

fees; (3) outpatient and inpatient surveys to assess patients' perceptions of the fee system and quality changes; and (4) a quality of care checklist to assess the availability of critical patient care inputs.

Special Studies. During implementation, questions arose that could not be answered through either routine reporting or the indicator district system. Special studies were conducted on the planning and expenditure process for the use of revenue; on fee preferences, to assist in expanding the fee schedule; on exemptions, to assist in adjusting exemptions to balance equity and revenue needs; and on revenue losses due to noncollection of inpatient fees.

Uses of Monitoring Information. Supervision and routine reporting information were used to identify districts and facilities that were performing poorly and to strengthen their performance. Supervisory visits corrected misunderstandings of the new management systems. In some cases, staff were intentionally flouting new rules for personal gain, and disciplinary action was taken. Districts and facilities that were performing well were identified and publicly recognized. Data from the indicator districts were used to guide decisions about the type, level, and timing of fee changes. Results from special studies were used to correct management problems and to revise management systems.

Evolution of the Monitoring System. As the new user fee system matured over a five-year period, the nature of the monitoring system evolved. Supervision was decentralized to the provincial and district levels. Routine reporting requirements were simplified to focus on the few critical FIS and HIS reports that most facilities could generate regularly. Indicator districts' data were important to monitor major fee changes, but subsequent fee adjustments were having less and less impact, so little information was being gained from the indicator districts. Efforts were then concentrated primarily on effective local use of targeted supervision and routine reports.

---

drug policy indicators include acceptance by key stakeholders and consistency of interpretation among different stakeholders.

Throughout this manual, the assessment guides provide examples of indicators for specific aspects of drug policy and management, which can be adapted and tested in the context of local monitoring and evaluation plans. The indicators listed in the assessment guides and the examples in this chapter draw on five useful sets of indicators, some of which are described in greater detail in Chapter 4 (Brudon-Jakobowicz et al. 1995; CDHSH 1994; MSH/RPM 1995; WHO/DAP 1993; ZEDAP 1993).

Types of Indicators

Indicators should be tied directly to program plans and annual workplans. One way to view the health management process is that it takes inputs and applies certain

management or clinical processes to create specific service or activity outputs, which have certain immediate outcomes, which lead to a desirable long-term impact on health status. This process is illustrated in Figure 36.1.

Management and clinical indicators can be developed for each point in the health management process. The goals and objectives of an essential drugs program are generally stated in terms of the intended ultimate impact on health status and the more immediate effects on drug availability, drug quality, or drug use needed to achieve this long-term impact. Therefore, indicators for evaluation tend to focus on effects and impact.

In contrast, routine monitoring is concerned with inputs, processes, and outputs associated with specific implementation activities. Consequently, indicators for monitoring focus on financial and tangible inputs; management activities, procedures, training programs, and

Figure 36.1 The Health Management Process and Assessment Points

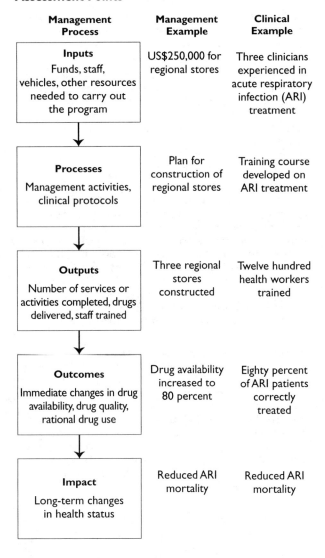

Management Process	Management Example	Clinical Example
Inputs Funds, staff, vehicles, other resources needed to carry out the program	US$250,000 for regional stores	Three clinicians experienced in acute respiratory infection (ARI) treatment
Processes Management activities, clinical protocols	Plan for construction of regional stores	Training course developed on ARI treatment
Outputs Number of services or activities completed, drugs delivered, staff trained	Three regional stores constructed	Twelve hundred health workers trained
Outcomes Immediate changes in drug availability, drug quality, rational drug use	Drug availability increased to 80 percent	Eighty percent of ARI patients correctly treated
Impact Long-term changes in health status	Reduced ARI mortality	Reduced ARI mortality

other process indicators; and numbers of people trained, quantities of drugs delivered, and other output indicators.

Different terms are sometimes used for the concepts illustrated in Figure 36.1. Inputs in the form of financial resources and organizational systems may be called *structural* indicators, *impact* and *outcome* are sometimes used interchangeably, and measures of impact may be called *effects*. Regardless of terminology, the content of the steps in the health management process remains the same.

Selecting Indicators and Setting Performance Targets

Program plans should contain process and output indicators for planned results, such as the training of a specified number of health workers or the production of an essential drug curriculum for medical education. Output targets

usually represent time-limited intermediate progress toward a specific objective: for example, if the objective is to train 75 percent of 2,000 health workers within five years, the first-year output target may be to train 300 health workers (15 percent). Impact indicators measure the attainment of specific levels of achievement. "Achieving 80 percent drug availability at the central, district, and health unit levels" is an example of an impact indicator.

A *performance target* is a desirable and, in principle, attainable standard of performance. For example, the impact indicator may be the percentage of ten indicator drugs in stock, and the performance target may be 80 percent availability at each level for this list of indicator drugs. Performance targets should be set for each indicator.

Performance indicators can be compared against agreed-upon performance standards, over time within the same health unit, among health units of the same level, or across countries. Initially, comparisons among health units may help set realistic performance standards, which can be adjusted upward as the system develops.

The health management process is a useful way to conceptualize indicators. For monitoring purposes, however, it may be more useful to group indicators around specific program areas, strategies, and objectives. Figure 36.2 shows illustrative performance indicators grouped by major program areas related to drug availability.

In selecting indicators, it is important to consider how data will be collected. Some may require information that is readily available at headquarters. Figure 36.2 makes it apparent that some indicators may be routinely available from standard recording and reporting systems (such as percentage of indicator drugs available), whereas other indicators may require a special survey (percentage of drug costs covered by user fees or percentage of health units using stock cards correctly, for example). Some indicators represent annual summary measures (per capita government drug expenditure or percentage by total value of drugs purchased through competitive tender).

Thus, indicators may rely on generally available information from routine reporting, or they may require special surveys or other sources of information. The sources and the cost of collecting and processing these data must be carefully considered in selecting indicators.

It may be useful to distinguish *core performance indicators*, for which data are routinely reported and monitored, from *complementary performance indicators*, for which data may be collected only at sentinel sites or in special studies (see below) or that may be used only for periodic evaluation purposes.

Figure 36.2 Examples of Performance Indicators and Performance Targets

Objective and Performance Indicator	Performance Target
Overall performance	
Central stores: indicator drugs available (unexpired)	90%
District stores: indicator drugs available (unexpired)	90%
Health units: indicator drugs available (unexpired)	90%
Health units: average stockout duration for indicator drugs	10 days
Financing—ensure that financial resources are adequate to meet basic drug needs	
Per capita government drug expenditure	US$1.20
MOH budget allocation for drugs	15%
Actual drug expenditures as % of budgeted allocation for drugs	85%
Drugs costs covered by user fees	60%
Procurement—obtain a regular supply of drugs at favorable prices	
Total value of MOH drugs purchased through competitive tender	95%
Total value of MOH purchases on essential drugs list	98%
Average ratio of unit prices of indicator drugs to international prices	0.9 to 1.1
Average lead time for external suppliers	50 days
Average lead time for local suppliers	20 days
Quality assurance—ensure that procured drugs meet recognized standard of quality and that quality is maintained throughout the distribution chain	
Number of drugs/batches tested out of number of drugs/batches procured	1 out of 4
Number of drugs/batches that failed quality control testing, out of number of drugs/batches tested	0
Central storage—ensure that drugs are properly stored, with minimal expiration and other losses	
Drugs for which stock records and physical counts agree (all drugs)	100%
Average difference between stock records and physical count (all drugs)	Less than 5%
Drugs for which stock records, procurement records, and physical counts agree (indicator drugs)	100%
Value of expired drugs as % of total drug purchases last year	Less than 3%
Delivery—ensure timely delivery of drugs to health units	
Average lead time from CMS to health units, routine monthly orders	30 days
Average lead time from CMS to health units, emergency orders	5 days
Storage at health units—ensure that drugs are properly stored, with minimal expiration or other losses	
Health units using stock cards correctly	75%
Stock records correspond with physical counts	90%
Health units with expired items	25%
Health units practicing FEFO	90%

Potential problems with indicators—failure to take action based on findings, overambitiousness (using too many indicators), failure to focus on key questions, complexity, lack of integration with work planning, failure to build on existing information, and lack of objectivity—are discussed in Section 36.8.

Formulation of Indicators

Indicators may be qualitative or quantitative. Qualitative indicators tend to be yes-or-no questions related to policy and management processes: Is there an official committee for updating the national essential drugs lists? Are drugs procured through competitive tender? Are stock records kept at storage facilities? Is there a standard treatment manual? Qualitative indicators generally reflect structural inputs and procedures that are prerequisites to policy implementation and management performance.

Quantitative indicators allow managers to set specific targets for outputs and performance; they facilitate monitoring the achievement of these targets. Quantitative indicators can be in the form of counts (400 health workers trained), rates (two workshops per year), ratios ($1.10 per tin versus $1.00 per tin = ratio of 1.10), proportions (400 out of 1,200 health workers trained = one-third), or percentages (400/1,200 = 33 percent).

To decide the format for an indicator, it is important to consider the availability of information. Proportions and percentages require that the size of the whole be reliably known; if not, then actual counts may be more useful. For example, if the number of health workers in a district is not precisely known, it is preferable to specify a count (400 health workers trained) rather than a percentage that cannot be verified.

Indicator Drugs

Several of the performance indicators listed in Figure 36.2, mentioned in Chapter 4, or included in chapter assessment guides are based on a list of indicator drugs and relate to drug availability, drug prices, and accuracy of stock records.

Indicator drugs are a small number of representative drugs, which are also known as *tracer* or *index drugs*. Economists use a market basket of common goods and services to measure inflation through the consumer price index. Similarly, the list of indicator drugs is sometimes called a basket of drugs (Brudon-Jakobowicz et al. 1995).

For ease of calculation and consistency of measurement, the number of drugs should be kept small: a list of ten or twenty drugs usually suffices. For calculating rates and percentages, it is convenient to use a number that divides easily into 100 (that is, 10, 20, or 25).

The drugs selected should be on the national essential drugs list or national drug formulary, therapeutically important, widely used, and preferably commonly available internationally for purposes of comparison. In general, drugs with a very high unit cost, such as praziquantel, should be avoided (Brudon-Jakobowicz et al. 1995).

Figure 36.3 provides a list of ten indicator drugs, grouped by therapeutic category of tablet preparations, that should be available at all levels of the health system. Depending on the purpose and uses of the indicators, it may be helpful to distinguish a list of ten core indicator drugs for use at all levels of the health system and a complementary list of ten additional drugs (total list of twenty drugs) for central storage facilities and hospitals.

The complementary list of indicator drugs might include other dosage forms (such as injections and topical preparations) and additional therapeutic categories (cardiovascular drugs and contraceptives, for example). Additional drugs to consider include oral rehydration solutions, procaine penicillin injection, pediatric paracetamol tablets, tetracycline eye ointment, iodine, gentian violet or a local alternative, benzoic acid and salicylic acid ointment, or retinol (vitamin A) (WHO/DAP 1993).

Larger or more diverse lists of indicator drugs may be useful for specific purposes. When first introducing performance indicators and indicator drugs, however, it is probably wise to keep to a core list such as that shown in Figure 36.3.

≡ **36.6 Using the Monitoring System to Improve Performance**

The fundamental purpose of the monitoring system is to improve program and staff performance at all levels, which requires that plans and targets be clearly communi-cated, monitoring results be regularly reviewed and shared, and follow-up action be taken.

Communicating Plans and Targets

Program plans and workplans are sometimes viewed simply as documents for fund-raising or for "the people above." To the contrary, they should be blueprints to guide the day-to-day work of staff at all levels, who need to be aware of the plans and of output and performance targets. Plans and targets should be communicated both in writing and face-to-face: memoranda or circular letters alone are usually insufficient.

Reviewing Progress

A schedule is needed for reviewing progress, with the review period depending on the nature of the plan and the specific indicators. Implementation progress for a five-year program plan, for example, is reviewed at least annually. Key staff meet to systematically assess each objective, each activity, and each output target. For an annual workplan, it is important to review progress each month or at least each quarter.

In a progress review, actual outputs and performance are compared against targets; when there are discrepancies, further discussion is needed. When progress has exceeded expectations, it is worth asking whether there are positive lessons to be learned and whether specific people should be recognized for their work. Figure 36.4 provides an example of a progress review based on the workplan in Figure 35.6.

Figure 36.3 Example of a List of Indicator Drugs

Drug	Form, Dosage
Analgesics/antipyretics	
Acetylsalicylic acid (aspirin)	Tablet, 300 mg
Paracetamol	Tablet, 500 mg
Anthelminthics	
Mebendazole	Chewable tablet, 100 mg
Antibacterials	
Amoxicillin	Tablet, 250 mg
Metronidazole	Tablet, 500 mg
Phenoxymethylpenicillin	Tablet, 250 mg
Sulfamethoxazole + trimethoprim (cotrimoxazole)	Tablet, 400 mg + 80 mg
Antimalarial drugs	
Chloroquine	Tablet, 150 mg base (as phosphate or sulfate)
Gastrointestinal drugs	
Aluminum hydroxide	Tablet, 500 mg
Minerals	
Ferrous salt	Tablet, 60 mg (iron equivalent)

Source: Adapted from Brudon-Jakobowicz et al. 1995.

Figure 36.4 First-Year Progress Review for Promoting Rational Drug Use

Objectives/Activities	Outputs		Expenditures			Comments
	Target	Actual	5-Year Budget	1st-Year Budget	1st-Year Actual	
Selection						
Essential drugs list (EDL)—revise and distribute national essential drugs list at least every 2 years.	Revision of EDL completed	Done	2,000	2,000	2,850	Required additional workshop to finalize
Prescribing						
Undergraduate training—ensure that all students are trained in essential drugs concept and rational drug use in basic health curricula (amount of time depends on professional category).	Curricula designed for medicine, pharmacy, nursing, paramedical training	Initial workshop held, curricula not completed	5,000	5,000	2,670	
Standard treatment guidelines (STG)—develop/ revise and distribute standard treatment manual at least every 4 years.	First edition of STG completed and distributed	Manual completed and printed, not distributed	48,000	48,000	39,860	
Continuing education (CE)—provide all clinicians with at least 1 week of in-service training on rational drug use every 3 years.	65% of clinicians trained (1,300 of estimated 2,000)	Training designed, first workshop held	42,000	42,000	4,830	
Dispensing						
Packaging and labeling—ensure that at least 80% of patients receive drugs in clearly labeled containers or dispensing envelopes.	Packaging and labeling materials provided, sufficient for 80% of patients	Material ordered, not received	15,000	3,000	0	Order placed too late
Patient use						
Undergraduate training—ensure that all students are trained in communications and patient education methods in basic health curricula (amount of time depends on professional category).	Combined with prescribing training	See above	See above	0	0	
Continuing education—include skills for patient education at in-service training workshops.	Combined with prescribing training	See above	See above	0	0	
Total			112,000	100,000	50,210	

When progress is below expectations, it is even more important to ask the reasons:

- ► Were necessary funds, materials, or other inputs lacking?
- ► Were two units unable to communicate their expectations to each other or to coordinate their actions?
- ► Did key staff simply fail to take the plans and performance targets seriously?
- ► Is failure to achieve a specific planned output a reflection of overly ambitious plans?

A well-designed, well-implemented monitoring system can usually provide information on what happened or did not happen. Information about why things happened—or did not happen—may come from the monitoring system or may require management follow-up.

Giving Feedback

No monitoring system is complete without feedback. Giving feedback to individual units or staff members tells them how well the reporting has been done and how useful the information is. Feedback also demonstrates the value and importance of the reports. As such, it represents one of the most powerful tools for motivating staff. Feedback also improves the quality of data by breaking the "bad data cycle" (see Chapter 45).

Direct feedback involves presenting staff with some of the problems and successes brought up in the monitoring or evaluation reports:

- ► Discuss the achievement of specific performance targets.
- ► Identify weak performers for more intensive supervision or training.
- ► Identify and congratulate successful districts and facilities.
- ► Identify policy or program weaknesses and how to strengthen them.

Always check to see whether the information has been used, how it has been used, and what action has been taken.

Taking Action

Effective use of the monitoring system requires prompt follow-up action. There are at least five types of action that a manager can take:

1. *Provide positive feedback* to high-performing units or staff to encourage continued good performance.
2. *Provide corrective feedback* to staff or units that have not met expectations but that should be able to take specific steps to improve their performance; many

problems can be corrected through supervision and retraining.
3. *Reallocate resources* or *reassign staff* to achieve a better fit between the task to be accomplished and the resources or staff available.
4. *Adjust plans and targets* to be more realistic on the basis of actual experience.
5. *Request additional information* to further define a specific performance problem and the reasons for the problem.

Country Study 36.3 illustrates how indicators can be used to improve performance through self-monitoring.

Whatever actions are taken after a progress review, the effects of these actions should be considered at the next progress review.

≡ 36.7 Evaluation

Evaluation is different from monitoring. The word is derived from *value* and means to assess the value of something. Evaluation involves taking a step back to look at the program as a whole, to assess progress toward achieving goals by fulfilling objectives. An evaluation is carried out at a specific time and should have a clear purpose. Whereas monitoring focuses on program *activities*, evaluation focuses primarily on program *objectives*.

Evaluation Questions

Depending on the timing and purpose, evaluations may be of three types (Figure 36.5):

1. Needs assessment (situation analysis);
2. Formative evaluation (midterm review);
3. Summative evaluation (final evaluation).

A needs assessment or situation analysis is meant to appraise the pharmaceutical system or essential drugs program and to identify areas of strength and weakness (see Chapter 4). The purpose is to design a project to address major weaknesses in the system.

Formative and summative evaluations are concerned with answering some or all of the following questions:

- ► Is the program relevant? Are its goals and objectives appropriate to the present circumstances of the country and the pharmaceutical system?
- ► Is the program effective? Is it achieving satisfactory progress toward its stated goals and objectives? What are the reasons for success or failure?
- ► Are monitoring results representative? Do the results from the program's monitoring system reflect the actual situation?

Country Study 36.3 Use of Indicators for Self-Monitoring in Rural Java

The twenty-nine health centers and 109 subcenters of Gunungkidul District in Java, Indonesia, suffer from periodic shortages of drugs, as do other health facilities. These shortages are due to limited resources, increasing patient demand, and overprescribing of injections, antibiotics, and other drugs. To address this problem, the district health team in Gunungkidul undertook a series of activities to improve and control drug use.

The team first surveyed drug use with three prescribing indicators. Results showed extensive polypharmacy (4.2 drugs per case), a high percentage of patients receiving antibiotics (63 percent), and a very high percentage receiving injections (76 percent). The team explored these issues in randomly selected health centers using in-depth interviews, observation, focus group discussions, and questionnaires (see Chapter 29). From this information, a self-monitoring system was developed, pilot-tested, and implemented in all health centers in the district.

Each health center completes a monitoring form each month, based on a survey of thirty cases in each health center and subcenter. Results are discussed locally and forwarded to the District Health Office for review. Data from the four sub-

centers under Widoyo Health Center are compared with those from the previous month (see the accompanying figure). Using this form, health center staff can easily determine whether each indicator has increased or decreased in each facility.

The continuity of the self-monitoring process is guaranteed by

► weekly staff meetings of the district team at which results are discussed;
► monthly district-level meetings for the heads of all health centers;
► regular feedback and occasional supervisory visits to health centers by members of the district team.

After two years, an evaluation showed substantial improvements in all three indicators. Despite these changes in practice, the number of attendances at health centers had remained constant. Interviews with health workers showed improved attitudes toward the use of standard treatments, willingness to improve skills, and increased communication among health workers and the district team.

Local Area Monitoring Form

Health Center: _Widoyo_
Month: _June_   Year: _1994_
No. cases sampled: _30_

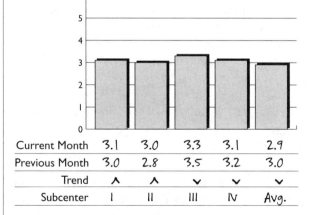

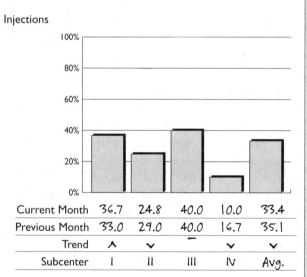

Source: Sunartono and Darminto 1995.

► Is the program efficient? Are the effects of the program being achieved at an acceptable cost compared with alternative approaches to providing the same services?
► Is the program sustainable? Financially and institutionally, can the program continue with present levels of local inputs? If external financial and technical assistance is involved, can the program continue after it has stopped?
► Is the program having the intended impact? Does it appear that the program is achieving or will achieve its intended long-term health care benefits?

Figure 36.5 Types of Evaluation

Evaluation Type	Program/ Project Stage	Purpose
Needs assessment (situation analysis)	Design	Assess current situation Develop program/project plan Acquire baseline for comparison
Formative evaluation (midterm review)	Implementation	Focus on implementation process Assess progress toward goals and objectives Improve program/project implementation
Summative evaluation (final evaluation)	Follow-up	Assess program/project outputs Measure impact of program/ project Demonstrate program/ project impact to donors Recommend future actions

Source: Adapted from García-Núñez 1992.

▶ What future changes should be made? What recommendations can be made for program development, new plans, or project assistance? Are new goals or objectives needed?

In practice, needs assessment, formative evaluation, and summative evaluation sometimes overlap. For example, the final evaluation for one project may also serve as the needs assessment for the next project.

Conducting an Evaluation

Chapter 4 describes three approaches to assessment: self-assessment, limited assessment, and structured assessment. Structured assessment is the most comprehensive but requires the most resources. The choice of assessment approach depends on available financial and human resources, timing, sponsorship, and intended uses of the results.

In the past, most health program and health project evaluations were limited assessments, consisting primarily of interviews, secondary analysis of existing monitoring and other data, and review of available documents. Increasingly, however, evaluations are expected to contain performance data indicating what services and outcomes are resulting from the program. The starting point for an evaluation should be the data collected through the monitoring system, but field surveys using standard pharmaceutical sector assessment indicators (MSH/RPM 1995; WHO/DAP 1993; Brudon-Jakobowicz et al. 1995) will contribute to a much more objective, credible, and useful evaluation.

Evaluation Methods and Tools

An evaluation is much like a research project. The usual considerations of research design apply, including defining the scope and questions for the evaluation, choosing evaluation methods, developing and testing data collection instruments, managing data collection, collating and analyzing data, interpreting results, and presenting the findings.

Methods of obtaining information include document review, key informant interviews, data collection from existing records, and prospective surveys. These methods and the steps involved in a structured assessment are discussed in detail in Chapter 4.

Knowledge, skill, and experience are required to design and execute a credible, comprehensive evaluation. See "References and Further Readings" for several sources that provide practical guidance on evaluation methods.

Who Should Evaluate?

When individuals involved in a program carry out an evaluation, they have the advantage of understanding its aims and design; however, such evaluations can be subjective and may miss important lessons. For this reason, outsiders are frequently asked to perform evaluations. Because they are disinterested, outsiders may be more objective and may bring fresh ideas. Outside evaluators come from local universities, local nongovernmental organizations, international organizations, or organizations in other countries.

There are many advantages to combined insider-outsider evaluations. The outsider, being ignorant of the local situation, can ask the difficult questions, and the insider often knows whether the true answer is being given. It is also useful for the insider to see the program or project through the eyes of the outsider. The outsider benefits because the insider knows where the answers are to be found.

Resources Required

Evaluation is an activity that goes beyond routine monitoring and requires staff, time, and funds to be earmarked for it. In the case of a specific program, money for evaluation should be built into the original proposal. Careful costing should be performed, taking into account all proposed activities.

≡ 36.8 Some Common Pitfalls in Monitoring and Evaluation

Although monitoring and evaluation are two distinct activities, they share certain common pitfalls:

Failure to identify the basic questions: All monitoring and evaluation activities should start with a clear statement of the questions they intend to answer. Without this, there is no focus for information gathering.

Overambitiousness: Collecting too much information is perhaps the most common failing. A basic rule is that more information means greater expense, less accuracy, more time spent managing the data, less time spent interpreting the data and providing feedback, and less time for using the data.

Complexity: Monitoring systems should be as practical and streamlined as possible. Cumbersome systems have often been designed from the top down, with insufficient testing and input from staff involved in generating and using monitoring information.

Lack of integration with planning and implementation: Monitoring and evaluation activities should follow directly from program plans, link closely with ongoing implementation activities, and lead logically into the next round of planning.

Failure to build on existing systems: Existing information systems are never perfect, but considerable resources can be squandered trying to build a separate system instead of building on and strengthening existing systems.

Inadequate resources: Both monitoring and evaluation require considerable financial and human resources. It is generally better to seek additional resources or narrow the scope of assessment rather than try to gather too much information with too few resources.

Lack of objectivity: Management indicators introduce some objectivity into the assessment process; assessments based only on subjective information are less credible and less useful.

Jumping to wrong conclusions: Well-designed monitoring and evaluation systems allow some cross-checking of findings. Taken out of context, individual monitoring reports and evaluation observations can be misleading.

Lack of comparison data: Observations must be compared over time, against agreed-upon performance standards, among health units at the same level, or across countries. Good baseline data against which changes can be compared are especially useful, but to be valid, they must come from the same sources and have the same measures as the follow-up data. If the sources or measures are altered, it is difficult to say whether apparent changes (good or bad) are real or are due to the assessment process.

Other common problems are failure to analyze data promptly, lack of feedback mechanisms to apply results, evaluations that do not gather new information, and monitoring done for the wrong reasons. Inappropriate reasons for monitoring and evaluation include doing the activity because of tradition or donor requirements and using the activity to try to resolve conflicts between donors and recipients or to get information to punish certain staff members (García-Núñez 1992).

Note that monitoring and evaluation are not the same; evaluations and assessments should build on, not substitute for, a routine monitoring system and a reliable DMIS. ■

≡ Assessment Guide

Monitoring Methods and Systems

► Does a program or unit exist to monitor and evaluate pharmaceutical services? Who is responsible for monitoring and evaluation?

► Is monitoring based on program objectives and linked to specific activities? Are these objectives, along with output targets and performance targets, clearly communicated to concerned staff?

► Which of the following methods are used as sources of monitoring information—supervisory visits, routine reporting, sentinel reporting, special studies?

► How often are data collected? How are they used?

► Are monitoring results regularly reviewed and shared? How and with whom? Is feedback provided to concerned staff?

► What actions are taken when problems are detected through monitoring and evaluation?

Indicators

► Have performance indicators been established? If so, how were they established, and who was involved?

Do they include process, output, and impact indicators? Are they both qualitative and quantitative? Have performance targets been set?

► Have indicator drugs been identified for indicators requiring drug-specific information?

Evaluation

► Is progress toward achievement of program goals and objectives periodically assessed through formal evaluation?

► Does the evaluation begin with a clear statement of its basic question? Is this question used as a focus for information-gathering?

► Which of the following methods are used to obtain information—review of existing monitoring reports, additional data collection, document review, interviews, field surveys using standard pharmaceutical assessment indicators?

► How is the evaluation team determined? Does it include insiders and/or outsiders?

≡ References and Further Readings

★ = *Key readings.*

Amondo-Lartson, R., G. J. Ebrahim, H. J. Lovel, and J. P. Ranken. 1984. *District health care.* London: Macmillan.

★ Brudon-Jakobowicz, P., J.-D. Rainhorn, and M. R. Reich. 1995. *Model indicators for monitoring national drug policies.* Geneva: World Health Organization.

CDHSH (Commonwealth Department of Human Services and Health). 1994. *Manual of indicators to measure the effect of initiatives under the Quality Use of Medicine Act of the National Medicinal Drug Policy.* Canberra: Australian Government Publishing Service.

FAO (Food and Agriculture Organization of the United Nations, Regional Office for Asia and the Pacific). 1990. *Participatory monitoring and evaluation: Handbook for training field workers.* Bangkok: Craftsman Press.

Franco, L. M., P. Richardson, J. Reynolds, and N. Kak. 1993. Monitoring and evaluating programmes (user's guide, module 6). In *Primary health care management advancement programme.* Geneva: Aga Khan Foundation.

★ García-Núñez, J. 1992. *Improving family planning evaluation.* West Hartford, Conn.: Kumarian Press.

Hilton, M. 1993. Monitoring and evaluating programmes (facilitator's guide, module 5). In *Primary health care management advancement programme.* Geneva: Aga Khan Foundation.

McMahon, R., E. Barton, and M. Piot. 1992. *On being in charge,* 2d ed. Geneva: World Health Organization.

MSH (Management Sciences for Health). 1992. Improving efficiency and performance indicators (trainer's and participant's guides). In *Managing drug supply training series.* Part 2. *Financing and financial management of drug supply.* Boston: MSH.

★ MSH/RPM (Management Sciences for Health/Rational Pharmaceutical Management Project). 1995. *Rapid pharmaceutical management assessment: An indicator-based approach.* Washington, D.C.: MSH/RPM.

★ Smith, P. G., and R. H. Morrow. 1991. *Methods for field trials of interventions against tropical disease: A toolbox.* New York: Oxford University Press.

Sunartono, Y., and B. Darminto. 1995. From research to action: The Gunungkidul experience. *Essential Drugs Monitor* 20:21–22.

Vaughan, J. P., and R. H. Morrow. 1989. *Manual of epidemiology for district health management.* Geneva: World Health Organization.

WHO (World Health Organization). 1981. *Health programme evaluation: Guiding principles.* Geneva: WHO.

WHO (World Health Organization). 1984. *Glossary of terms used in the health for all series.* Geneva: WHO.

WHO/DAP (World Health Organization/Action Programme on Essential Drugs). 1993. *How to investigate drug use in health facilities: Selected drug use indicators.* WHO/DAP/93.1. Geneva: WHO/DAP.

ZEDAP (Zimbabwe Essential Drugs Action Programme). 1993. *ZEDAP essential drugs survey.* Harare, Zimbabwe: Ministry of Health and Child Welfare, Directorate of Pharmacy.

Part I	Part II	Part III	**Part IV**
Introduction	Policy and Legal Framework	Drug Management Cycle	**Management Support Systems**

A Organization and Management ▶

B Financing and Sustainability

C Information Management

D Human Resources Management

34 Managing Drug Programs

35 Planning for Drug Management

36 Monitoring and Evaluation

37 Community Participation

38 Hospital Drug Services

39 Security Management

Chapter 37
Community Participation

≡ Summary

Community participation in health care is increasing due to the recognized value of locally tailored approaches, as well as the need for increased community financing to supplement government expenditures. Experiences have been many and varied; for example, the Bamako Initiative, which involves communities in the management and financing of basic health services, has been tried in more than thirty countries.

Community participation can involve

▸ *contributing—community members contribute money, labor, or materials;*
▸ *consulting—members are asked for their views and are informed of project plans;*
▸ *controlling—members actively participate in decision-making and in the control of resources.*

When all three levels of participation are present, communities are full partners in providing services.

Full partnership in decision-making means that health development is defined in terms of people's real needs and priorities; community economic, human, and organizational resources are mobilized; and mechanisms are created to increase people's access to information, knowledge, and skills and to help them make their goals and priorities known.

Community participation can support and enhance drug management through

▸ *promotion of appropriate drug use;*
▸ *promotion of preventive health care;*
▸ *cost sharing for pharmaceuticals;*
▸ *management of outreach services;*
▸ *management of facility-based health services.*

Health professionals play a key role in facilitating community participation. They act as motivators; as supporters to the community in establishing strong organizations for community-based activities; as resource persons by establishing links between the community, government agencies, and other organizations; and as trainers, building capacity within the community.

Community participation rarely emerges on its own. It succeeds best within an enabling environment, which includes

▸ *political commitment to the concept of participation;*
▸ *interest in decentralization of health services;*
▸ *existence of a health structure;*
▸ *commitment to developing people's managerial capabilities.*

≡ The failure of traditional top-down development approaches to eradicate poverty and improve the living conditions of the poor has led to increased interest in popular participation in development. Since the 1978 Alma Ata World Conference on Primary Health Care, many governments in developing countries have taken initiatives to expand community participation in the promotion and delivery of basic health services. This expansion represents both a response to the increasing trend toward decentralization and recognition of the value of locally tailored approaches, and an acknowledgment of the need for increasing levels of community financing.

This change is creating a new form of governance for public health systems and altering the relationship between providers and users of health care services. Health professionals are being called upon to adopt new approaches and to work in partnership with communities: in sharing knowledge and skills, in jointly deciding on plans for health care, and in seeking to develop and strengthen the community's capacity to care for itself.

This chapter presents some of the key features of community participation and provides practical guidelines for effective participation of communities in the promotion and delivery of basic health services. The chapter draws on the experiences of many community-based health programs, among them the Bamako Initiative, which has involved communities in the management and financing of basic health services since 1987 (Box 37.1).

There are no clear-cut answers or universally applicable methods in community participation: it varies from one country to another and even from one community to another within the same country, depending on socioeconomic and political contexts. Because communities are not homogeneous, this chapter provides only broad guidelines for increasing community participation. The terms *community, users, consumers,* and *beneficiaries* are used interchangeably.

≡ 37.1 What Does Community Participation Mean?

Although there is a wide consensus on the central role of community participation in primary health care, it is interpreted in many different ways. Community participation is a cumulative process through which beneficiaries develop the managerial and organizational capacity to increase their control over the forces and decisions that affect their lives.

Box 37.1 The Bamako Initiative

The Bamako Initiative was a response to the rapid deterioration of health systems in developing countries during the 1970s and 1980s. Launched in 1987 by African ministers of health at a meeting sponsored by WHO and UNICEF in Bamako, Mali, the initiative had been adopted by more than thirty countries in Africa, Asia, and Latin America by 1994.

The Bamako Initiative aims to ensure affordable essential health services for the majority of the population while containing costs and to restore consumer confidence in the public health system by delegating greater decision-making power to communities to improve the quality of services. Consumers become active partners whose voices count and who foster better health by promoting behavioral change at the household level.

The initiative is based on three assumptions:

1. Governments' ability to make available to the majority of the population a package of affordable and cost-effective essential health services of reasonable quality;
2. The existence of a well-functioning district health system;
3. Active participation of the community in the management of health services and cost sharing.

The strategy is to decentralize decision-making to the district level, reorganize the delivery of primary health care, institute community financing and comanagement of basic health services, and provide a minimum package of essential health services at the level of basic health units. There are four key elements of this strategy:

1. The revitalization of peripheral health care delivery systems, including the network of community health workers who provide outreach services;
2. Strong advocacy for the use of essential generic drugs to ensure access to quality drugs at affordable prices;
3. The sharing of recurrent costs through community financing, with the aim of improving and extending services by generating sufficient income to cover some local operating costs such as essential drug supply, salaries of support staff, incentives for health workers, and investment in community health activities;
4. Community control, including responsibility for the management of local health services. Funds generated by community financing do not revert to the central treasury or health ministry but remain in the community and are controlled by a locally elected health committee.

Bamako Initiative programs have been implemented differently in different countries, and there have been some notable successes. Overall, experiences vary considerably among countries with respect to levels of revenue generation, effect on health care utilization, total cost of program implementation, impact on the poor, and drug availability.

Community participation means that members maintain a strong voice in all issues that affect the well-being of the community at large. It requires genuine community representation in decision-making. The process of community participation can help the poor, in particular, to become better organized and more involved in decisions pertaining to their health.

A community's full partnership in the decision-making process implies

- definition of health development in terms of local needs and priorities;
- mobilization of community economic, human, and organizational resources;
- creation of mechanisms that help people increase their access to information, knowledge, and skills; voice their opinions; and make their goals and priorities known.

Three distinct approaches to community participation exist (Fox 1993):

1. *Contributing:* Community members provide money, labor, or materials for health projects.
2. *Consulting:* Community members are asked for their views and are informed of project plans in order to secure their commitment and contributions to construction, operation, and maintenance.
3. *Controlling:* Community members actively participate in decision-making and in the control of community resources and are engaged in project identification, planning, organization, implementation, monitoring, and evaluation.

Many health professionals have seen community participation as mainly "contributing" to health projects; that is, the community assists the professionals with contributions of labor, materials, or money but only rarely with ideas. In both the contributing and the consulting modes, communities are regarded mainly as beneficiaries of assistance. When communities become controlling as well, the three concepts become synergistic: community members, in partnership with outside development workers, are able to use their heads and their voices—as well as their hands—in the development and operation of facilities and services they can genuinely call their own.

Community participation is thus measured not only by quantifiable project outputs but also by the process of participation:

- Levels of community involvement in needs assessment,

planning, management of resources, implementation of project activities, monitoring, and evaluation;

► People's capacity to manage and organize themselves;

► People's access to new skills, knowledge, and information;

► Level of community organization and solidarity;

► Nature of the relationship between users and providers;

► Level of openness in project management and accountability of health services toward the public being served.

≡ 37.2 Why Promote Community Participation?

It is at the community level that women, men, and children get drinking water; that wastes are controlled to prevent disease; that nutritional deficiencies are identified and actions taken. It is in communities and in households that people choose health care providers, that families make decisions about the use of their resources, that patients decide how to use medicines, and that people determine the number of children they want to have. Therefore, projects aimed at improving access to and use of basic health services, including essential drugs, cannot achieve their objectives and ensure sustainability unless there is a genuine partnership with communities.

Community participation in health is based on the following premises:

► Participation in one's own health care is a basic right to which all people are entitled.

► When health services are linked to local perceptions of needs and are managed with the support of local people, there is more likelihood that they will achieve their objectives and be sustainable.

► By actively participating in project planning and decision-making, people gain confidence in their ability to change their situation and better their health status.

► By solving their own problems, people become more self-reliant and less dependent on outside help.

► Where public health institutions are weak, community participation in management and financing can improve efficiency, increase public accountability, restore users' confidence, mobilize additional resources to complement government resources, and improve the quality of services.

► By encouraging people to become involved, projects can benefit from local skills and resources.

► When people know from the start that a project is theirs, they show a greater sense of responsibility for the

management and maintenance of services and facilities than when projects are controlled by "outsiders."

► The positive experience of planning, implementing, and managing a successful project leads to involvement in other development activities—there is a multiplier effect.

► Health, nutrition, and family planning outcomes can be significantly improved and sustained only when the strengthening of health services, including drug supply, goes hand in hand with community awareness about public health issues and personal health care. Community participation is therefore crucial to promoting healthy lifestyles and better health management at the household and community levels.

≡ 37.3 Community Participation and Drug Management

Community participation can support and enhance improvements in drug management and use in a number of ways:

► Promotion of appropriate drug use;

► Promotion of preventive health care;

► Improvement of drug availability;

► Management of outreach services;

► Management of facility-based health services.

Promotion of Appropriate Drug Use

The inefficient and even unsafe treatment of illnesses through inappropriate drug use is a problem in many settings (see Chapter 28). These problems are caused by irrational drug prescribing practices (such as overprescription) on the part of providers and popular misconceptions, as well as nonadherence to treatment, on the part of patients. Advocacy by organized consumer groups and efforts to improve public access to information are effective ways to address these problems (see Chapter 33).

Consumer education has been shown to improve adherence to recommended drug therapies (see Country Study 37.1). As part of this process, consumers are able to provide feedback to prescribers on the effectiveness of drugs, undesirable side effects, and so on. Such a process is reinforced when personal links have been established between consumers and providers at the community level and when consumers are organized and vocal in demanding quality health services.

When unregulated private markets offer all types of drugs of dubious quality, without prescription, and at exorbitant prices, consumers must be sensitized to the health risks and costs involved. Community health workers, health committees, and networks at the grassroots level can, with increased access to information and technical support from health staff, serve as consumers' advocates for the promotion of reliable sources of local drug procurement and the rational and correct use of drugs.

Consumer education can also help counteract some popular perceptions of what constitutes high-quality health care. For example, patients often think that the more drugs prescribed (especially injectable drugs) the better the treatment. From a medical perspective, however, a single orally administered drug is often the most appropriate therapy. Public education on the futility and the danger of overprescribing and the excessive use of injectable drugs is crucial to improving drug use.

Promotion of Preventive Health Care

Governments and households could save money if efforts were made to promote preventive health care as well as rational drug use. Grassroots community networks can play a crucial role in promoting preventive care and encouraging nondrug therapy at home for minor illnesses.

The process by which health promotion is carried out, including the time and effort that go into developing a community's sense of ownership, is critical to a program's success. In Kenya, for example, as part of an effort to control malaria, Bamako Initiative community health units generated support from the local community to establish a revolving fund for the sale of low-cost, insecticide-impregnated mosquito netting for beds. The demand for bed netting continues to be very high, and community pharmacies are generating significant revenue from their sale. In 1992, the program's community-based information system showed a decrease in malaria cases by as much as 50 percent in some villages since integration of the malaria control program and other preventive health services.

Improvement of Drug Availability

In response to declining public resources for financing pharmaceutical and other recurrent costs, growing numbers of communities are adopting cost-recovery and self-financing schemes in local health centers, dispensaries, and outreach services. The aim is to improve and extend services by generating sufficient income to cover some local operating costs, such as the supply of essential drugs, salaries of some support staff, incentives for health workers, and investment in community health activities.

Community cost-sharing can be based on user fees, prepayment for services, local taxes, and various income-

---

Country Study 37.1 Community Involvement in the Wise Use of Medicines

A community health center in Canada involved members of the target population (those over age sixty-five) in the development of a program to promote the safe use of medicines. During a needs assessment phase, meetings were held with community members to help identify barriers to safe drug use. Concerns expressed included the high number of prescriptions, inadequate information about drug use, problems with packaging and labeling, and high costs. This input led to identification of the program's primary objective: to reduce the incidence of medication misuse in the senior population.

The four strategies of community development, health education, advocacy, and use of mass media were chosen to address the program's objective. Partnerships were built through interagency work groups including program promoters, members of the target community, health professionals and pharmacies, and other community partners to coordinate programming.

Four two-hour sessions were developed to provide information about drug use; these were presented at times and in settings convenient for seniors, often linked with existing gatherings (for example, at community centers, recreation centers, and churches). The sessions were designed to create opportunities for group learning—to promote community members' communication with health professionals, to foster group cohesion and encourage expansion of social supports, and to identify and facilitate the use of community resources.

Community members were trained as cofacilitators for these sessions. They also helped design and distribute flyers promoting the program and reviewed other written materials for readability. Others contributed to the adaptation of materials and communication strategies for outreach to non-English-speaking populations.

---

generating activities. Communities can also help pay health care costs by contributing labor or making direct financial contributions for the improvement and maintenance of health care infrastructure.

Country Study 37.2 illustrates one approach to community-based drug financing. Revolving drug funds are discussed in Chapter 44.

Management of Outreach Services

Over the past twenty years, large numbers of community health workers (CHWs) have been trained in many countries as part of national strategies for primary health care. Although CHW programs have been disappointing in some respects, CHWs have been shown to be an effective means of accelerating and extending the delivery of primary health care when they receive adequate training, are regularly supervised, are provided with adequate

---

Country Study 37.2 Village Drug Cooperatives in Thailand

Since 1977, Thailand has supported primary health care through the training of village health volunteers (VHVs) and village health communicators (VHCs) and the establishment of village drug funds (VDFs). VDFs were introduced as village cooperatives to make inexpensive, good-quality essential drugs readily available.

VDFs were started with a grant of 700 baht (or approximately US$30) from the government. Villagers often raise additional capital through the sale of fund shares. Although most VDFs were established at the initiative of the Ministry of Public Health, about 25 percent have been started by villagers themselves. The private sector (Group of Laemthong Sahakarn Companies, Limited) contributes an additional 700 baht when at least 70 percent of village households participate, and 1,000 baht (approximately US$43) when 80 percent or more participate. Drug funds order their supplies each month from private suppliers and the Government Pharmaceutical Organization, which provides lower-cost generics.

By the mid-1980s, 26,000 of Thailand's approximately 50,000 villages had established drug funds, and in 50 percent of these funds, 70 to 100 percent of households were participating. Each VDF elected a fund management committee from among village leaders, usually including VHVs and VHCs. These fund managers served as accountants, auditors, clerks, and general overseers. Most community funds were selling drugs with a 30 percent markup, and over 85 percent reported making a profit. The majority of funds operated as freestanding VDFs, but up to one-third operated as part of a VDF cum grocery. VDFs cum gro-

ceries made larger profits by selling a broader range of items, including soap, packets of oral rehydration salts, nutritional supplements, and even soft drinks, beer, and cigarettes in some funds. Roughly one in ten VDFs operated within a community center for primary health care. In addition to replenishing drug supplies, some funds provided compensation to members of the management committee and to VHVs and provided returns to shareholders. At peak participation, the number of VDFs had grown to nearly 36,000, covering almost 80 percent of villages.

By 1994, circumstances had changed. A survey found that the proportion of villages with functional VDFs had fallen, perhaps to 50 percent. In most villages, drugs had become widely available through groceries, drugstores, drug peddlers, private clinics, and other sources. VDFs were the source of drugs in only 12 percent of common illness episodes. Freestanding VDFs were having difficulty sustaining their services, whereas VDFs cum groceries had expanded their range of drugs beyond essential drugs in response to community demand. Concerns were also being raised that VHVs and VDFs were not effective in promoting rational drug use.

Thailand's experience suggests that community drug schemes can be established on a large scale provided there is adequate start-up funding, active community participation, a reliable source of essential drugs, and trained VHVs. At the same time, the experience demonstrates that community needs evolve over time. Programs to promote access to drugs and rational drug use must also evolve to meet those needs.

Sources: WHO 1986; WHO/DAP 1995.

---

logistical support, and are linked to established district health systems for technical backup and referral when needed.

CHW responsibilities typically include education on sanitation, nutrition, family planning, child health, and immunizations, in addition to carrying out some minor curative interventions. CHWs can also be valuable in monitoring health in the community and as a referral point between health centers and the community. Country Study 37.3 describes such involvement in Kenya.

Management of Facility-Based Health Services

With the economic crisis of the 1980s, particularly in Africa, infrastructure deteriorated, drugs were often unavailable, and civil servants were unpaid for long periods of time. In response, many governments have begun to involve communities in the management of facility-based health services. Because essential drugs are necessary for integrated, high-quality, cost-effective basic health services, and because people perceive drugs as a quality indicator, drugs have often served as a starting point for community cofinancing and comanagement of facility-based health services.

Locally elected health committees can participate in the day-to-day tasks of managing health facilities by

▸ assisting health staff in developing an appropriate payment mechanism or mechanisms (prepayment scheme, flat rate, or fee for service) and in pricing services, including drugs;

▸ establishing procedures for procuring and managing drugs and other supplies;

▸ determining criteria and developing an administrative system for those who cannot afford to pay or who should be exempt for other reasons;

▸ establishing a system of internal control of receipts and expenditures that ensures financial viability, accountability, and transparency in managing the system;

▸ participating in the day-to-day financial management and bookkeeping and preparing the health center budget;

▸ carrying out stock inventories of pharmaceuticals and other supplies and equipment;

▸ recruiting and managing the support personnel hired with community funds (community pharmacy salespersons, guards, drivers, and so forth).

Country Study 37.3 Community Health Worker Activity in Kenya

In Kenya, within the context of the Bamako Initiative, community health workers (CHWs) are trained to diagnose and treat malaria, diarrhea, worms, conjunctivitis, anemia, scabies, and fever. They are provided with drug kits and log books from the community pharmacy or revolving drug fund, which is managed by a locally elected village health committee (VHC). The CHWs sell drugs at the community level and periodically deposit their proceeds with the VHC treasurer, replenishing their kits from the community pharmacy stock. (Patients are able to purchase some drugs directly from the community pharmacy, which also stocks condoms and mosquito netting.)

In addition to providing basic health care services, CHWs manage a community-based monitoring system that provides essential information for planning health, nutrition, and family planning activities. A joint government of Kenya and UNICEF evaluation confirmed that CHWs' knowledge of disease management and prevention is generally good, with malaria control and treatment being one of the most effective parts of the CHW training course. The evaluation recommended further training in the proper management of drugs and the impregnation of mosquito nets with insecticide.

Kenya Chalk and Board Monitoring System

Activity	Month 1	Month 2	Month 3
Immunization contacts			
Latrines built			
New family planning accepters			
Water sources protected			
Meetings held			
Malaria control			
No. children weighed			
CHWs trained			
Traditional birth attendants trained			

Events	Month 1	Month 2	Month 3
Measles cases			
Diarrhea cases			
Malaria cases			
Worms cases			
Acute respiratory infection cases			
Births in hospital			
Births at home			
Deaths			

Source: UNICEF 1995.

In some countries, health committees have a clear mandate to carry out evaluations of the performance of health staff and, if necessary, file complaints and propose disciplinary measures to district health offices.

Country Study 37.4 describes experiences with community participation within the Bamako Initiative framework.

≡ 37.4 Health Professionals' Contribution to the Process

Health professionals play a key role in facilitating the process of community participation in health, and particularly in drug supply and use:

- ► They act as motivators by drawing out people's untapped skills, experiences, and leadership potential.
- ► They are supporters, helping the community establish strong and appropriate organizations for the planning, implementation, and management of community-based health activities.
- ► They act as resource persons by establishing links between the community, government agencies working in health and health-related areas, and other relevant organizations and services.
- ► They are trainers of community leaders, members of health committees, and community health workers, building on the knowledge and experiences that exist in the community.

To fulfill these roles effectively and to create productive partnerships at the community level, health professionals must be able to

- ► communicate with the community and establish relationships with people;
- ► listen well, and learn from the community;
- ► share skills and experiences with the community;
- ► respect people's ideas, skills, and wisdom;
- ► promote equity in male-female representation and in representation of the various social, economic, and age groups in local decision-making bodies;
- ► be aware of and respect the social practices, traditions, and culture of the community;
- ► foster collaboration with other projects, organizations, and services;
- ► promote a holistic or integrated approach to health development.

≡ 37.5 Facilitating Community Participation in Health Programming

The participatory programming process includes community needs assessment, local decision-making and

Country Study 37.4 The Bamako Initiative in Guinea and Mauritania

Guinea. In 1987, there were only thirty operational health centers in the country, and national immunization coverage was less than 5 percent. In 1993, six years after the launching of the Bamako Initiative, 265 health centers had been established throughout the country using the principles of community cofinancing and comanagement of health services. According to the 1993 national Expanded Programme on Immunization (EPI) coverage survey, the immunization coverage in areas where the initiative was being implemented was 76 percent for the tuberculosis vaccine, 72 percent for DPT (diphtheria, pertussis, tetanus)1/polio 3, 55 percent for DPT/polio, 57 percent for measles, and 70 percent for tetanus (pregnant women). The health system has developed a "bottom-up" planning and monitoring mechanism that enables peripheral health services to effectively assume the responsibilities delegated to them in the framework of the decentralization policy. It is becoming increasingly evident that there is a need to decentralize the monitoring and planning further to the community level, to promote the genuine participation of communities in decision-making and planning. The program has yet to meet this challenge. In this respect, some efforts are being made to establish a community-based information system aimed at involving communities in managing local information on health and nutrition and in identifying appropriate solutions.

Mauritania. The Government of Mauritania adopted the Bamako Initiative in 1988 as the basis for revitalizing the public health system. In addition to improving existing health centers and medical posts, the government developed community basic health units (BHUs) in four experimental areas where villages had previously had no access to health services. The BHU is the most peripheral element of the health pyramid, relying on a community health worker (CHW) and a health committee to carry out basic primary health care activities and ensure community involvement. The system is self-financed by payment of fees for health services, drug replenishment, CHW motivation, and community activities. The contribution of the Ministry of Health includes the initial training of the CHWs, followed by on-the-job training and regular monitoring and technical backup of activities. Results

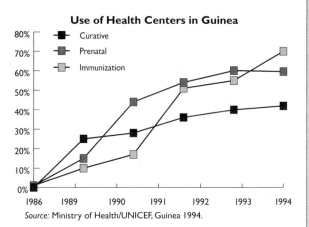

Use of Health Centers in Guinea

Source: Ministry of Health/UNICEF, Guinea 1994.

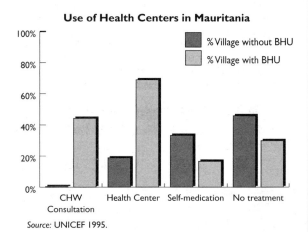

Use of Health Centers in Mauritania

Source: UNICEF 1995.

from nineteen community BHUs for the period 1988 to 1991 show an increase in health services utilization and a reduction in health center referrals by one-third and in self-treatment by one-half.

participatory planning, community organization and leadership, and participatory monitoring. Practical suggestions are given below for each of these phases.

Community Needs Assessment

Needs assessment is the first step in initiating a community-based participatory health project. The purpose is to involve the project beneficiaries in determining their health problems, the causes of those problems, and their primary needs as the basis for planning community activities and for establishing baseline data against which progress can be measured in the future. Areas to be covered, the choice of method, and data analysis issues all need to be considered when planning such an assessment.

Key Areas to Be Covered in Needs Assessment. Community participation at the needs assessment phase is fundamental. When undertaken as a joint exercise, needs assessment can encourage dialog between health professionals and community members, so that accurate and complete information is available to both parties when deciding on appropriate actions.

Community basic health needs: Assessing basic health needs begins with identifying and ranking problems, causes, cost of health care, health-seeking behavior, access to health services, and affordability of health care. Specific needs in relation to problems identified, what the community would like to do to improve its health situation, and community resources that could be mobilized can then be considered.

Community decision-making process and power structures: How does the community work? What are the rules of the group? Who makes them? Who enforces them? How does power depend on sex, age, tribe, kinship, knowledge, money, education? Who makes decisions, and who controls resources at household and community levels? What are the power relations between women and men, between basic service delivery systems and the community, between community and local authorities, between different socioeconomic and political groups? How do people feel about the decisions that affect their lives and the way these decisions are made?

Education and socialization: How do schooling and traditional education influence people's knowledge, attitudes, and behavior in dealing with health issues, in particular their choice of health care provider and their use of drugs?

Beliefs and values: How do beliefs, ideology, or religion affect people's understanding of health and development?

Basic population data: These data include village population, number of households in the village, number of inhabitants living within 5 kilometers of the nearest health facility, and age and sex distribution.

Facilities and infrastructure: What community facilities (schools, churches, temples, markets), clinics, health posts, shops, drugstores, water supplies, street lighting, communications, and transport (such as roads or paths) exist?

Past and ongoing health and health-related projects: Are there past, ongoing, or planned projects or programs of relevance? Achievements, approaches, constraints, resources, organization, and management of activities; services involved; and potential for coordinating efforts all need to be considered.

Methods for Needs Assessment. A community needs assessment is not necessarily a formal investigation. Common sense, creativity, and ingenuity can determine the most appropriate methods, modify existing methods, or suggest new methods.

It is important to start by establishing contacts in the community and identifying key informants who could be useful in providing information and in organizing and facilitating community meetings and group discussions. This can be done in the following ways:

Secondary sources: reviewing data from files, maps, project reports, population census reports, health center records, articles.

Group discussions: holding casual, focused, or deliberately structured discussions at various levels of the community or neighborhood.

Door-to-door visits: conducting structured or informal interviews at a sample of households.

Role playing: helping community members describe their situation and needs by taking different roles.

Participatory mapping and modeling: involving community members in making maps (social, demographic, health, water resources), using the ground, floor, or paper.

Transect walks: systematically walking with informants through an area and observing, asking, listening, discussing; identifying different zones, local technologies, introduced technologies, health-seeking behavior, average distance to nearest health facility, community-felt needs, perceived solutions, opportunities; mapping and diagramming.

Seasonal diagramming: determining, through discussion with community members, seasonal variation in illnesses, health care costs, access to health services, food availability or shortage, economic difficulties and impact on health, and coping mechanisms.

Figure 37.1 provides some tips for participatory mapping. These tips can also be used in other interactions with the community.

Data Analysis. When analyzing the data, bear in mind these key points:

Ranking of health problems and health-seeking behavior: Identify and rank the most important health problems and health-seeking behaviors for each of the major health problems identified; the health care provider (traditional healer, health center, hospital, community health workers, self-treatment); and average cost of treatment.

Wealth ranking: Identify clusters of households according to wealth, including those considered poorest and unable to pay for health care. Identify mechanisms to help the poor.

Analysis of differences: Seek opinions of all groups within the community and analyze differences in opinion by gender, age, social group, economic group, and occupation.

Trend analysis: Compare people's accounts of the past and the present; their reports of how things have changed (how health status has improved or worsened; changes in the size of families, the status of women, level of education, income, food, and nutrition); and the causes of these changes and trends.

Figure 37.1 Tips for Helping in Participatory Mapping

Help people get started by letting them do it themselves.
Be patient. It's *their* map.
Look, listen, and learn.
Facilitate. Don't dominate.
When community members are mapping, modeling, or
 diagramming, *don't* interfere.
Sit back and watch. Or go away!
Keep a permanent (paper) record, including mappers' names,
 to give them credit for their contributions.
If necessary, suggest that sometimes a succession of maps
 works better.

Local Decision-Making and Participatory Planning

Based on the information collected in the needs assessment, community members and health professionals plan together what actions need to be taken, how, when, and with what means.

The planning process should take place in a climate that fosters two-way communication and mutual learning. The steps in participatory planning are shown in Figure 37.2.

Community Organization and Leadership

Certain actions require collective efforts beyond the capacity of individuals, households, and even health committees and community health workers. The creation or strengthening of community organizational capacity is important for empowerment objectives. Creating organizational capacity can be laborious and time-consuming, but it is vital for ensuring the sustainability of community-based projects. The following tips for health professionals and community leaders can facilitate the process of community organization or group formation:

► Identify charismatic community leaders and strengthen their leadership skills.
► Ensure that the people involved are those who are genuinely concerned with community health.
► Clearly define the specific tasks to be performed by each community representative and health service representative.
► Build on existing formal and informal functional grassroots structures that have credibility in the community, to the extent possible. These may include women's groups, youth groups, or religious groups.
► Ensure an equitable representation of women and various socioeconomic groups on village committees.

Participatory Monitoring

Information is an essential tool for local decision-making, and participatory monitoring offers ways to share information. Increasing beneficiaries' capacity to collect information and use it for action is important, since information confers power. By having increased access to information, communities increase their ability to make decisions and gain greater control over their own development.

Participatory monitoring can serve as an educational process, a management tool, and a surveillance system. As an educational process, it increases participants' awareness and understanding of the various factors that affect their health and development in general. As a management tool, it helps measure progress, identify problems, and inform decisions aimed at improving efficiency in the delivery of essential health services, including drugs. Finally, as a surveillance system, participatory monitoring provides community members, health services, and other related services with vital quantitative and qualitative data on the status of community health and nutrition and on consumer behavior. For drug management and use, this information might include data on household expenditures for drugs, sources of procurement, and consumer behavior in the use of drugs.

Some of the methods listed for community needs assessment can also be used for monitoring; for example, the door-to-door survey is essential. The main difference between the two processes is that whereas community needs assessment is usually conducted at the beginning of a project, participatory monitoring is continuous.

When one is developing a community-based monitoring system, the following key issues of participatory monitoring should be considered:

► Village members should be organized around specific tasks: data collection and analysis, presentation of information for community and health service feedback, communication of results, facilitation of the interaction about data issues, and coordination of the participatory planning exercise.
► Staff of health and health-related services should provide continuous technical and methodological backup to the process. Feedback sessions should serve as platforms for maintaining a regular dialog between service users and providers.
► The methodology for gathering and analyzing information should be simple, so that those with little formal education can actively participate. There should be a consensus as to what is the most essential information for action at the community and facility levels.

Figure 37.2 Steps in Participatory Planning

1. Encourage community members to reflect on problems identified through the needs assessment.
2. Facilitate dialog on possible solutions, including pros and cons for each solution.
3. Decide on priority areas that need community action.
4. Set clear and measurable objectives.
5. Establish qualitative and quantitative indicators.
6. Determine resources needed to achieve objectives.
7. Determine the ability and willingness of the community to contribute time, money, and labor; what forms of contribution are needed; and what cost-sharing mechanisms will be put in place.
8. Determine the division of responsibility between the community and health professionals (who will do what).
9. Determine mechanisms for monitoring progress, supervision, and technical backup.
10. Identify training needs for community members and health professionals.
11. Determine mechanisms for ensuring transparency in project management and accountability of health services and community-elected bodies to the public they serve.
12. Determine the frequency of community meetings and the most effective channels for reporting to the community on project activities, including the amount of revenue generated and expenditures.

► It is important to focus on information as a powerful tool for local decision-making and action and not simply on the generation of data.
► Community-based planning and monitoring should be linked to facility-level planning and monitoring. Information at the community level, and the dialog between health staff and users, often generates quantitative and qualitative information that can be vital to improving the performance of health facilities.

≡ 37.6 Creating an Enabling Environment

Community participation rarely emerges on its own. It succeeds best within an enabling environment and with the support of appropriate mechanisms at all levels. Conditions that favor the development of community participation include the following (Oakley 1989):

► Political commitment to community participation in health development and to the general notion of people's participation;
► Interest in the decentralization of health services and the corresponding strengthening of district health sys-

tems that will serve as the basic health unit for community participation;
► Existence of a minimum health structure that can serve as the basis for community participation in health care;
► Development of people's managerial capabilities to take responsibility for a process of participatory health development.

An enabling approach requires training sessions for community representatives and leaders so that they can acquire basic managerial and organizational skills (group formation, leadership), basic financial management skills (budgeting and accounting), communication skills, and methodologies and skills for local information management (data collection, analysis, presentation of information, and feedback).

The process of participation requires technical support from health staff and other development agents. Mechanisms that facilitate putting community participation into practice include

► development of local, community-based structures through which people can participate and hold health services accountable;
► continuous dialog between service providers and community groups—consultation with communities should take place at *all* stages of the process, and health committees should work with other community leaders to find feasible mechanisms for regular interaction;
► better local-level coordination among sectors so that the underlying basis of poor health can be understood;
► support from nongovernmental organizations, which can provide additional resources for health as well as play an important role in promoting community participation;
► supervision by district health offices and other related services.

Finally, community participation in health must be seen as part of the broader network of community participation in development and in all social services. ■

≡ Assessment Guide

Enabling Factors
► Is there political commitment to community participation in health development?
► Is there interest in the decentralization of health services and the corresponding strengthening of district health systems?
► Does a health structure exist?
► Is there a commitment to developing people's managerial capabilities to enable them to take responsibility?

Community Participation Indicators
► Do communities contribute money, labor, or materials to health projects?
► Are community members asked for their views and informed of project plans?
► Do community members actively participate in decisions and in the control of resources?
► What mechanisms exist to increase people's access to information, knowledge, and skills and to help them make their goals and priorities known?
► What organizational structures exist at the community level to facilitate participation?

Community Participation and Drug Management
► Are community health workers used to help extend health care services to peripheral levels?
► Do mechanisms exist for consumers to provide feedback to prescribers on the effectiveness of drugs, undesirable side effects, and so on?
► Does community cost-sharing exist to help cover the costs of health services and drug supply?
► Are communities involved in the management of facility-based health services?

Involvement of Health Professionals
To what extent do health professionals
► establish relationships within the community?
► share skills and experiences with and learn from the community?
► respect people's ideas, skills, and wisdom?
► promote equity in male-female representation and in the representation of various social, economic, and age groups in local decision-making bodies?
► respect the social practices, traditions, and culture of the community?
► foster collaboration with other projects, organizations, and services on behalf of the community?

Community Participation in Program Planning
► Do communities participate in needs assessments?
► Do community members and health professionals plan together what actions need to be taken, how, when, and with what means?
► Are community members involved in monitoring project activities and results?

≡ References and Further Readings

★ = Key readings.

APHA (American Public Health Association). 1983. *Community participation in primary health care.* Washington, D.C: APHA.

Chambers, R. 1992. *Rural appraisal: Rapid, relaxed and participatory.* Discussion paper 311. Sussex, England: University of Sussex Institute of Development Studies.

Dhillon, H. S., and L. Philip. 1994. *Health promotion and community action for health in developing countries.* Geneva: World Health Organization.

Fox, J. 1993. *Rhetoric and reality: A commentary on the UNCHS community development programmes in Ghana, Uganda, and Zambia.* Presented at UNCHS seminar. Copenhagen: United Nations Centre for Human Settlements (Habitat).

Hardon, A., and A. Le Grand. 1993. *Pharmaceuticals in communities: Practices, public health consequences, and intervention strategies.* Bulletin 330. Amsterdam: Royal Tropical Institute.

★ Helfenbein, S., and A. Sayeed. 1994. Increasing community participation in family planning programs. *Family Planning Manager* 3(2):1–18.

Hope, A., and S. Timmel. 1992. *Training for transformation: A handbook for community workers.* 3 vols. Harare, Zimbabwe: Mambo Press.

Jarrett, S., and S. Ofosu-Amaah. 1992. Strengthening health services for MCH in Africa: The first four years of the "Bamako Initiative." *Health Policy and Planning* 7:164–76.

Knippenberg, R., D. Levy-Bruhl, R. Osseni, K. Drame, A. Soucat, and C. Debeugny. 1990. The Bamako Initiative: Primary health care experience. *Children in the Tropics* 184/185:1–94.

★ Korton, David C., ed. 1986. *Community management: Asian experience and perspectives.* West Hartford, Conn.: Kumarian Press.

McPake, B., K. Hanson, and A. Mills. 1993. Community financing of health care in Africa: An evaluation of the Bamako Initiative. *Social Science and Medicine* 36:1383–95.

MSH/FPMD (Management Sciences for Health/Family Planning Management Development). 1994. *Local initiatives program* (brochure). Dhaka, Bangladesh: Ministry of Health and Family Welfare.

Additional information about the Local Initiatives Program and its training and technical assistance services may be obtained from Mr. Abu Sayeed, Program Director, FPMD/ Dhaka, House No. 40/C, Road No. 11, Dhanmondi R/A, Dhaka 1209, Bangladesh.

Newbrander, W., D. Ruhe, M. Hall, and S. Helfenbein. 1994. Working with boards of directors. *Family Planning Manager* 3(5):1–18.

★ Oakley, P. 1989. *Community involvement in health development: An examination of the critical issues.* Geneva: World Health Organization.

★ Rifkin, S. B. 1990. *Community participation in maternal and child health/family planning programmes.* Geneva: World Health Organization.

Rugh, J. 1986. *Self-evaluation: Ideas for participatory evaluation of rural community development projects.* Oklahoma City, Okla.: World Neighbors Publication.

UNICEF (United Nations Children's Fund). 1995. *The Bamako Initiative: Rebuilding health systems.* New York: Bamako Initiative Unit.

WHO (World Health Organization). 1986. *Review of drug programme in Thailand.* Geneva: WHO.

WHO/DAP (World Health Organization/Action Programme on Essential Drugs). 1995. *Implications of community health workers distributing drugs: A case study of Thailand.* WHO/DAP/94.19. Geneva:WHO/DAP.

| Part I | Part II | Part III | **Part IV** |
| Introduction | Policy and Legal Framework | Drug Management Cycle | **Management Support Systems** |

A Organization and Management ▶

B Financing and Sustainability

C Information Management

D Human Resources Management

34 Managing Drug Programs

35 Planning for Drug Management

36 Monitoring and Evaluation

37 Community Participation

38 Hospital Drug Services

39 Security Management

Chapter 38

Hospital Drug Services

≡ Summary

Appropriate drug use in the hospital setting is a multidisciplinary responsibility that includes

- *prescribing by the physician;*
- *preparation and dispensing by the pharmacy department;*
- *medication administration by nurses or other health care professionals;*
- *monitoring the effect of a drug on the patient by all members of the health care team.*

The pharmacy and therapeutics (P&T) committee is responsible for developing policies and procedures to promote rational drug use. Its functions include

- *management of the approved drug list or hospital formulary;*
- *ongoing drug utilization review;*
- *medication error reporting and monitoring.*

Members of the P&T committee should include representatives from the medical, pharmacy, and nursing staffs; hospital administrators; and the quality assurance coordinator. Subcommittees are often formed for in-depth analysis of particular issues.

The pharmacy department, under the direction of a qualified pharmacist, is responsible for the procurement, storage, and distribution of drugs throughout the hospital. Satellite pharmacies in larger hospitals can bring the pharmacist closer to the patient care area.

Drugs may be distributed in bulk, in courses of therapy, or in unit doses. Unit-dose distribution is optimal for patient care but requires initial capital outlay for repackaging equipment and medication cabinets.

Additional mechanisms for inpatient drug management include

- *patient medication profiles, maintained in the pharmacy department;*
- *medication administration records, maintained by nurses;*
- *periodic inspection of drug storage areas;*
- *procedures for strict control of dangerous drugs and controlled substances;*
- *procedures for after-hours pharmacy service.*

Small-scale pharmaceutical production is often not cost effective and should be evaluated by the P&T committee.

The control of narcotics is of particular concern in the hospital setting and requires a systematic approach for the prevention and detection of abuse.

≡ A hospital exists to provide diagnostic and curative services to patients. Drugs are an integral part of patient care. Appropriate use of medications in the hospital is a multidisciplinary responsibility that includes physicians, nurses, pharmacists, administrators, support personnel, and patients. A medical committee, sometimes called the pharmacy and therapeutics (P&T) committee, is responsible for approving policies and procedures and monitoring practices to promote safe and effective drug use. The pharmacy department, under the direction of a qualified pharmacist, should be responsible for controlling the distribution of drugs and promoting their safe use. This is challenging, since drugs are prescribed by physicians, administered by nurses, and stored throughout the hospital.

This chapter covers hospital-specific drug management issues, such as pharmacy department organization and alternative drug distribution systems. Several functions of the P&T committee are discussed, with an emphasis on formulary management. Other important issues relevant to hospital pharmacy services are treated in Chapters 29 and 31, including drug utilization review, adverse drug reaction monitoring, and medication error management.

≡ 38.1 Responsibilities of Hospital Staff

The hospital pharmacist should be an expert on drugs who advises on prescribing, administering, and monitoring, as well as a supply manager who ensures that drugs are available through procurement, storage, distribution, inventory control, and quality assurance. The balance between these two roles varies, depending on the individual's background and the work setting. A pharmacist may assume a prominent clinical role in settings where his or her knowledge of clinical pharmacology and capacity to provide expert advice have earned the acceptance of hospital medical and nursing staff.

The responsibility for establishing policies and procedures related to medications often lies with the P&T committee. Since the drug use process is multidisciplinary, the committee should include representation from all functional areas involved: medical staff, nursing, pharmacy, quality assurance, and hospital administration.

Purchasing and Stock Management

In some hospitals, a separate department manages all hospital purchasing (drugs, medical supplies, equipment, and so forth); this department may be called medical stores or

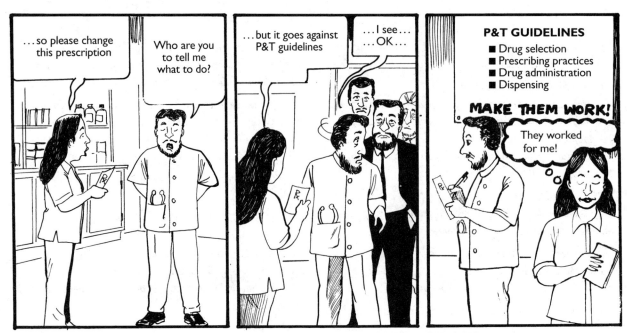

PHARMACY AND THERAPEUTICS GUIDELINES WORK

material management. In such cases, the chief pharmacist prepares an annual budget request for drug purchases and places orders for drugs through the medical stores.

In other situations, the pharmacy department manages drug purchasing directly. No one individual should have total control of drug procurement. A designated committee should review and approve all purchases; this may be a special purchasing committee, or the function may be managed by the P&T committee (see below).

Procedures for procurement and inventory management should be written in a manual that has been approved by hospital administration and the appropriate committees; the procedures for purchasing should follow guidelines provided in Chapters 13 and 15. Stock management procedures in the hospital depend on the size of the hospital and whether there is a warehouse attached to the hospital (see Chapters 23 and 24).

Drug Use

The drug use process can be divided into four components:

1. *Prescribing.* The physician has overall responsibility for the care of the patient, prescribing or ordering medications as part of the treatment plan. The mechanisms to ensure appropriate prescribing within the hospital customarily fall within the purview of the medical staff committees, usually including the P&T committee. The P&T committee may establish protocols or procedures that allow pharmacists or nurses to prescribe within specific guidelines.

2. *Preparation and dispensing.* The pharmacy department, under the direction of a registered pharmacist, is responsible for preparing and dispensing medications. Policies and procedures for these functions should be approved by the P&T committee. The chief pharmacist reports to hospital administration.

3. *Medication administration.* Administering medications is generally the responsibility of the nursing staff. The chief nursing officer oversees all nursing functions. In some cases, physicians may administer drugs such as anesthetic agents. Other health care professionals may administer drugs within the scope of their practice (for example, midwives attending deliveries).

4. *Monitoring the effect of drugs on the patient and ordering appropriate changes in therapy.* Monitoring activities are primarily the responsibility of the physician. However, observation and reporting are required from the person who administered the drug (usually the nurse) and from other members of the health care team involved in the patient's therapy. In some settings, a clinical pharmacist or pharmacologist monitors drug therapy in the hospital and consults on drug therapies that require special expertise to ensure safety and efficacy—for example, aminoglycoside antibiotics, total parenteral nutrition, and anticoagulation.

Government agencies and licensing boards regulate medications through laws and professional practice standards. The laws and regulations usually specify that the chief pharmacist is the person responsible for the control of medications within a hospital, including procurement, storage, and distribution throughout the facility.

Even though the chief pharmacist is responsible for the drug budget and the control of medications in the hospital, he or she does not supervise those who prescribe or administer the drugs. In some hospitals, purchasing, receiving, and storing of drugs are handled by a medical stores department that is not under the supervision of the pharmacist.

These differing responsibilities illustrate the complexity of drug procurement, storage, and use in the hospital. Efforts to improve the system should respect this complexity and include multidisciplinary representation and involvement. Coordination is required at the policy level through the P&T committee; at the management level, beginning with hospital administration; and then through the different branches of the organizational tree.

≡ 38.2 Organization of Hospital Pharmacy Services

In organizing hospital pharmacy services, both the way in which the staff is organized and the physical layout of the building need to be considered.

Personnel

Hospital pharmacy personnel can be divided into three major categories:

1. *Management.* Management includes the chief pharmacist and sometimes deputy chief pharmacists, who are responsible for procurement, distribution, and control of all drugs used within the institution, and for management of personnel within the pharmacy department.
2. *Professional staff.* These professionals are qualified pharmacists who procure, distribute, and control drugs and supervise support staff for these activities. In some facilities, pharmacists provide clinical consulting services and drug information. A job description for a hospital pharmacist appears in Chapter 47.
3. *Support staff.* The support staff category often includes a combination of trained pharmacy technicians, clerical personnel, and messengers.

The smallest hospitals may have only two or three staff members, with the chief pharmacist as the only pharmacist. Larger teaching hospitals that provide extensive drug distribution and clinical services may have over 100 staff members.

The cornerstone for a well-functioning medication system is an up-to-date manual of policies and procedures. Staff should be familiar with the manual and adhere to it.

Physical Organization

The extent of the pharmacy physical facility depends on the size of the hospital and the services provided. A large pharmacy department might have the following sections, within one physical space or in separate locations throughout the hospital:

► administrative offices
► bulk storage
► manufacturing and repackaging
► intravenous solution compounding
► inpatient dispensing
► outpatient dispensing
► drug information resource center
► after-hours pharmacy
► emergency drug storage

Inpatient dispensing is sometimes done from satellite pharmacies throughout the hospital. In larger hospitals, satellite pharmacies are beneficial because they shorten the turnaround time for individual drug orders, especially in distribution systems that dispense drugs packaged for individual patients. Satellites also increase the pharmacist's presence in the patient care area, facilitating interactions with medical staff, nursing staff, and patients, and thus ultimately improving patient care.

Satellite pharmacies reduce the need for ward stocks. However, each satellite requires a certain minimum inventory level of drug products. A system with multiple satellites most likely has a higher total inventory level than a central pharmacy system. The higher inventory and additional personnel costs needed to staff satellite pharmacies may be justified by reductions in drug supply costs (due to wastage) and improvements in patient care. Whether or not there are multiple satellite pharmacies serving inpatients, there are often separate pharmacies serving inpatients and outpatients. Figure 38.1 illustrates how a hospital pharmacy with separate inpatient and outpatient departments is organized in one African country.

≡ 38.3 Hospital Pharmacy and Therapeutics Committee

Most commonly, the committee designated to ensure the safe and effective use of medications in the hospital is the P&T committee. The American Society of Health-System Pharmacists states that "the multiplicity of drugs available and the complexities surrounding their safe and effective use make it necessary for hospitals to have an organized, sound program for maximizing rational drug use. The pharmacy and therapeutics committee, or its equivalent,

Figure 38.1 Multiple-Department Pharmacy System

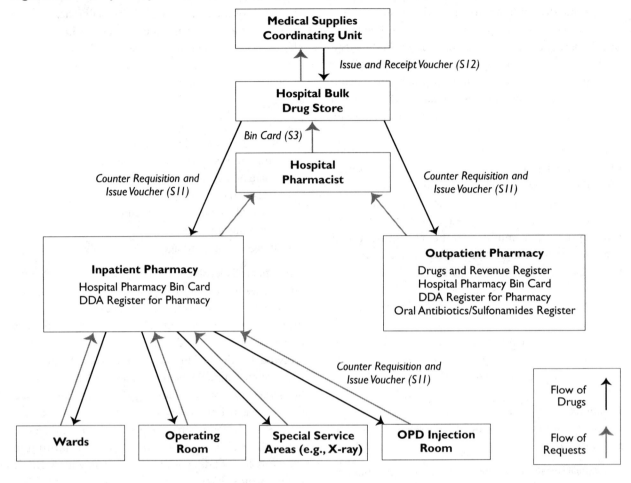

Note: Forms and registers for wards, operating room, special areas, and outpatient department (OPD) injection room are the same as for the central pharmacy system.

DDA = Dangerous Drugs Act.

Source: Ministry of Health, government of Kenya 1994.

is the organizational keystone for this program" (Health-System Pharmacists 1995, 3).

Purpose and Functions

The P&T committee promotes the rational use of medication through the development of relevant policies and procedures for medication selection, procurement, and use and through the education of patients and staff. Country Study 38.1 lists the functions of the P&T committee in a Kenyan hospital.

In some hospitals, the P&T committee becomes overwhelmed with the difficulty of obtaining an adequate supply of drugs. Members are caught up in routine decisions about which drugs to buy, how many, and from whom, rather than focusing on long-term planning, policies, and programs for improving the safe and cost-

effective use of medications. As discussed, in most settings, daily purchasing decisions can be handled by the chief pharmacist, with supervision by the P&T committee or another committee responsible for procurement.

Membership

An effective P&T committee requires that members participate in meetings and assist with other committee activities. Membership should include representation from

- medical staff (including representation from each department);
- pharmacy (the chief pharmacist often serves as the secretary);
- nursing;
- hospital administration;
- quality assurance coordination.

The committee should have broad representation but be sufficiently small and manageable to conduct business efficiently: a membership of eight to fifteen members often fulfills this criterion. The committee may occasionally invite a specialist to make a presentation or provide advice on a particular issue. For example, a cardiologist may attend to advise members regarding a formulary decision on a new cardiac drug. P&T committees often have subcommittees to address particular issues such as antibiotic use, drug use evaluations, or medication errors. Subcommittees can manage specific tasks without consuming a large portion of the P&T committee's meeting time.

Hospital Drug Formulary Management

The hospital drug formulary is the cornerstone of drug management in the hospital, and it should be the principal concern of the P&T committee. The issues related to drug selection for formularies are treated in detail in Chapter 11; the following list provides general guidelines for the hospital setting.

- The formulary list should be limited to conserve resources—it is usually not necessary to stock all drugs on the national formulary.
- Eliminate generic duplication—only one brand or label of each generic drug product should be routinely stocked.
- Select drugs for the formulary based on diseases and conditions treated at the facility.
- Specify drugs of choice for the formulary for common therapeutic indications. Drugs of choice should be selected by comparing efficacy, safety, toxicity, pharmacokinetic properties, bioequivalence, and pharmaceutical and therapeutic equivalence. Cost-effectiveness should be a primary consideration, evaluating alternatives as described in Chapters 3 and 11. Once drugs of choice are selected, they form the basis for standard treatment guidelines and for therapeutic substitution programs (see below).
- Include second-line alternatives to drugs of choice as needed, but minimize therapeutic duplication.
- The hospital formulary should correspond with any national or regional standard treatment guidelines that have been formally approved by the health system.

In addition to the basic formulary process, many hospitals add two additional features—therapeutic substitution and use restrictions for certain drugs in the formulary.

Therapeutic substitution (sometimes called therapeutic interchange) is based on the hospital formulary. The P&T committee provides guidelines for substituting spe-

Country Study 38.1 Functions of a Hospital Pharmacy and Therapeutics Committee in Kenya

Drug Selection and Requirements Planning
- Maintain the hospital formulary list.
- Receive and review management indicators.
- Formulate an annual list of drug requirements.
- Maintain an emergency drug list.
- Approve standard ward stock lists.
- Coordinate drug supply for special programs.

Prescribing Practices and Drug Information
- Standardize prescribing policies and treatment guidelines.
- Undertake drug utilization review studies.
- Oversee antimicrobial sensitivity patterns and infection control.
- Establish antibiotic prophylaxis guidelines.
- Coordinate communications with drug company representatives.

Dispensing and Drug Administration Practices
- Monitor dispensing practices.
- Establish generic and therapeutic substitution guidelines.
- Monitor medication errors and adverse drug reactions.
- Establish automatic stop orders.
- Set limits on dispensing quantities for outpatients.

Source: Ministry of Health, government of Kenya 1994.

cific formulary drugs for specific nonformulary drugs (or a specific category of drugs), usually for specific disease conditions. Whenever a prescription is written for a nonformulary drug that is covered by the therapeutic substitution policy, the designated formulary product is automatically substituted by the pharmacy department (or nurse). Note that this is not generic substitution—the two products are chemically different.

The P&T committee should develop formal written policies specifying which drugs (or categories of drugs) are suitable for automatic therapeutic substitution. These programs usually start with relatively noncontroversial drug categories, such as antacids and vitamins, and progress over time to other therapeutic groups, such as antibiotics and certain cardiac drugs, as physicians become comfortable with the program. Two main arguments are used to justify therapeutic substitution programs. One is that such programs ensure that only the most cost-effective products are routinely used, which has obvious benefits in terms of controlling both actual purchase costs and inventory holding costs (see Chapter 15). In settings where funds are limited, the more limited the list of drugs that are routinely stocked, the more likely it is that all those drugs will always be available. The other justification is that the P&T committee has presumably spent considerable effort selecting drugs that offer the best therapeutic value for the conditions covered by therapeutic substitution. An ancillary benefit is that hospital staff will be more familiar with the proper methods for handling, reconstituting, and administering the formulary products.

Therapeutic substitution is often resisted by staff physicians, but it is now practiced in more than 50 percent of hospitals in the United States (a bastion of physician independence). Note that therapeutic substitution is often practiced informally and unintentionally in hospitals where stockouts are common—if the prescribed drug is out of stock, another must be substituted. Physicians who practice in such situations should be used to the concept.

Normally, there are escape clauses from therapeutic substitution for specific patients. The physician can submit a special form that justifies the use of a specific nonformulary drug for a specific patient (as discussed below).

Use restrictions are most often applied in larger hospitals where there are specialist physicians on staff. Restrictions may apply to certain individual formulary drugs or to certain categories of drugs; the principle is that restricted drugs can be prescribed only by certain specialists or can be used only on certain wards. Such restrictions are generally applied to particularly expensive drugs (such as anticlotting drugs) or particularly toxic drugs (such as cancer chemotherapy); however, some hospitals go further, requiring specialist consultation on many different categories of drugs. Restrictions should be carefully considered; they decrease the use of drugs involved (which may or may not be desirable), increase the demand on specialists (and potentially the cost of services), and increase administrative burdens for nurses and pharmacists who must manage the process.

Methods to promote formulary adherence include:

▶ Review and take action on all nonformulary drug use.
▶ Prohibit use or distribution of samples of nonformulary products.
▶ Establish procedures and approved product lists for therapeutic substitution.
▶ Provide easy access to the formulary list (copies at each drug ordering location and in pocket manuals).
▶ Involve medical staff in all impending formulary decisions.
▶ Advertise and promote formulary changes.

Requests to use nonformulary drugs should be monitored by the P&T committee. If many nonformulary drug requests come from a particular physician, or if there are frequent requests for a particular nonformulary drug, the committee should take action. Actions may include adding the drug to the formulary, educating physicians on the rationale for the nonformulary status of the drug, or banning the drug from use in the hospital. Country Study 38.2 is an example of a procedure for nonformulary drug use in a hospital in the United States.

Drug Utilization Review
Drug utilization review (DUR) is a tool to identify such common problems as inappropriate product selection, incorrect dosing, avoidable adverse drug reactions, and errors in drug dispensing and administration. DUR may then be used to implement action plans for change. DUR is an ongoing, planned, systematic process for monitoring, evaluating, and improving drug use and is an integral part of hospital efforts to ensure quality and cost effectiveness. More appropriate and more effective use of drugs ultimately results in improved patient care and more efficient use of resources.

Chapter 29 provides an overview of the concepts and approaches for investigating drug use. Chapter 31 contains the specific methodologies for developing a hospital DUR program and discusses programs for adverse drug reaction and medication error reporting and monitoring.

≡ 38.4 Inpatient Drug Management
The issues relevant to good dispensing practice—physical facility requirements, good dispensing procedures, course-of-therapy packaging, and skill requirements—presented in Chapter 32 are relevant for hospital pharmacies. Patient education and medication counseling are described in Chapter 33 and are applicable in hospitals. The purchasing and inventory strategies described in Chapter 15 should be applied in the hospital setting.

Drug Distribution Systems
Drug distribution has long been the primary function of hospital pharmacy services.

There are three basic types of drug distribution systems:

1. Bulk ward stock replenishment;
2. Individual drug order system;
3. Unit-dose system.

There are variations of each, and all three systems may be in use in the same facility, depending on the strategy developed. For example, a facility may use the bulk ward

Country Study 38.2 Procedure for the Use of Nonformulary Drugs in a US Hospital

A limited formulary of drugs may not satisfy all individual or unique patient needs. A physician may request use of a nonformulary drug on a one-time (one course of therapy), one-patient basis.

The physician requesting the nonformulary drug or the pharmacist receiving the drug order must fill out the nonformulary drug request form. The pharmacist receiving the request must inform the physician of alternative drugs that may be used. The pharmacist must also indicate how long it will take before the drug will be available. The physician and pharmacist should avoid obtaining the drug by special delivery or borrowing from another hospital if possible.

Nonformulary drugs will be stocked in the nonformulary section of the pharmacy only during the individual patient's course of therapy. The pharmacy will track expenses related to nonformulary drugs and report to the pharmacy and therapeutics committee.

Nonformulary Drug Request Form (For One-Time/One-Patient Use)

Patient: _____ Room #_____ Date:_____

Drug name/strength/dosage form: _____

Current formulary alternatives (suggested by pharmacist):

Why is this agent preferable to the formulary alternatives suggested?

Was this drug request prompted by a manufacturer's representative? ❏ yes ❏ no

Are you requesting permanent addition of the drug to the medication formulary? ❏ yes ❏ no

If so, will you be present at the next pharmacy and therapeutics committee meeting to discuss the advantages of this drug? ❏ yes ❏ no

If accepted, what formulary drugs do you recommend for deletion?

Prescribing doctor:_____

Signature: _____

Figure 38.2 Comparison Matrix for Drug Distribution System

Factor	Bulk Ward Stock	Individual Drug Order	Unit Dose
Material and supply costs	Low	Medium–low	High
Pharmacy labor costs	Low	Medium	High
Nursing labor costs	Medium–low	Low	Low
Pilferage risk	High	Medium	Low
Medication error risk	High	Medium–low	Low

Bulk Ward Stock

In a ward stock system, the pharmacy functions as a warehouse and dispenses bulk containers on requisition without reviewing individual patient drug orders for appropriateness. The main advantage is shorter turnaround time between prescribing and administering the drug. The use of ward stock medications should be minimized, although it is appropriate and desirable for certain situations:

► In emergency departments and operating rooms, drugs are usually required immediately after the physician prescribes them. Unless there is a pharmacy satellite located in these emergency areas, it is not possible to dispense drugs according to individual patient orders. Unfortunately, drugs used in these situations are often expensive, and control is always a challenge for the pharmacy department.
► In life-threatening emergency situations, drugs need to be kept in patient care areas as a time-saving measure.
► High-volume, low-cost drugs can be dispensed from ward stock if there is low risk of medication error.

Individual Drug Order System

The individual drug order system closely resembles dispensing to outpatients: a course of therapy is dispensed according to a written prescription for an individual patient. Compared with ward stock distribution, the advantages are that the pharmacist can review the appropriateness of therapy, a patient-specific medication profile can be maintained, pharmacy charges to patients are facilitated, and closer control of inventory is possible. This system can limit the time intervals for dispensing: for example, an individual supply for three days of therapy is sent initially; if therapy is continued beyond three days, the empty container is returned to the pharmacy to be refilled.

stock system for high-volume, low-cost drugs (aspirin, paracetamol, and antacids) that do not require a high level of control for preventing theft or medication errors. Individual drug order systems or unit doses can be employed for drugs requiring a higher level of control (see Figure 38.2).

Country Study 38.3 Kenya Medication Treatment Record

Purpose. Each inpatient has a medication treatment sheet on which *all* medications prescribed are recorded by the consultant, medical officer, or clinical officer, and on which all drugs administered are recorded by the nursing staff. In addition, individual prescriptions are required for Dangerous Drugs Act (DDA) drugs and specific other drugs designated by the hospital drug and therapeutics committee.

Procedure.

1. At the time of admission, a medication treatment sheet is completed by the clinician with the following information:

   ► Patient's complete name (*all* names must be included to ensure proper identification);

   ► Medication allergies;

   ► Inpatient number;

   ► Ward and bed number;

   ► Age and sex.

2. For easy access during hospitalization, the treatment sheet is kept at the foot or head of the patient's bed with the observation sheet. (Because of this, the diagnosis should *not* be written on the treatment sheet.)

3. All medication orders must be written on the medication treatment sheet by an authorized prescriber (doctor or clinical officer). The order should include the date and time the order was written; the drug name, strength, dose, route of administration, frequency, and duration; a legible official name; and the signature of the prescriber.

4. In addition, for DDA drugs and specific other drugs designated by the hospital drug and therapeutics committee, individual prescriptions are required; entries for DDA drugs must be in red ink.

5. When a drug is administered to a patient, the nurse or clinician administering the drug writes the date and time of administration and signs in the appropriate place on the medication treatment sheet.

6. When an ordered drug cannot be administered for any reason, the nurse writes in the patient's nursing notes the name of the drug, the date, and time the drug was to be administered, and the reason that the drug could not be administered (patient not on ward, unavailability, any other reason).

7. The nursing officer should regularly review medication treatment sheets to ensure that they are being used properly on all wards and that all required information is being recorded.

Source: Ministry of Health, government of Kenya 1994.

Unit-Dose Drug Distribution

The preferred system from a patient care perspective is the unit-dose system, in which there is the lowest possibility for error. Drugs are dispensed in unit-dose packages (each dose is separately packaged) in separate bins or drawers for each patient. Commonly, a twenty-four-hour supply is provided. Drugs returned to the pharmacy can be put back in stock without concern for identity or contamination. This system is efficient but requires a large initial capital outlay for the purchase of repackaging machines and medication cabinets with individual patient drawers. The cost per delivered dose is higher than with bulk packaging, but this may be offset by reduced wastage and easier detection of leakage. Hospitals in some countries have found innovative ways to adapt local technologies to construct their own fixtures and equipment.

Patient Medication Profiles

Patient medication profiles are necessary if hospital pharmacists are to assume responsibility for monitoring inpatient drug therapy. Each profile contains information on the patient's current and recent drug therapy, allergies, diagnosis, height, weight, age, and sex. Pharmacy patient profiles work best in conjunction with unit-dose distribution systems but can be used with the individual drug order system.

A pharmacy profile allows the pharmacist to review all the medications that a patient is taking prior to dispensing the first dose and with each new drug order. Problems with drug therapy, such as allergies, duplicate drug therapy, drug-drug interactions, drug-disease interactions, inappropriate length of therapy, and inappropriate dosing, can be detected and avoided or corrected.

Computerized pharmacy systems display the patient's medication profile on the screen, and the pharmacist edits the screen with each new order. Drug interactions, dosage ranges, and other monitoring functions can be programmed into the computer to assist the pharmacist.

Medication Treatment Record

Also known as the medication administration record (MAR), the medication treatment record helps the nurse schedule treatments for each patient and provides a permanent record of the medications administered. It also allows nurses to review the patient's complete drug regimen and provides a means of conducting audits that compare quantities of drugs dispensed from, and returned to, the pharmacy with quantities administered to the patient. Country Study 38.3 describes the procedure for completing a medication treatment record used in Kenya.

Ministry of Health
Medication Treatment Sheet

MOH 306 Rev.

Patient_____ Allergies _____

Inpatient Ward_____ Age _____

Bed No._____ Sex_____

Name of Institution_____

Note: Use RED pen for DDA. Enter your own signature for every drug given.

TO BE COMPLETED BY CLINICIAN		TO BE COMPLETED BY NURSING STAFF					
			DATES AND SIGNATURE				
DATE	MEDICATIONS	TIME					
		3 AM					
		9 AM					
		3 PM					
		9 PM					
		3 AM					
		9 AM					
		3 PM					
		9 PM					
		3 AM					
		9 AM					
		3 PM					
		9 PM					
		3 AM					
		9 AM					
		3 PM					
		9 PM					
		3 AM					
		9 AM					
		3 PM					
		9 PM					
		3 AM					
		9 AM					
		3 PM					
		9 PM					
		3 AM					
		9 AM					
		3 PM					
		9 PM					
		3 AM					
		9 AM					
		3 PM					
		9 PM					

STAT, PRN, AND PRE-OP MEDICATIONS

TO BE COMPLETED BY CLINICIAN		TO BE COMPLETED BY NURSING STAFF				
			DATES, TIMES, AND SIGNATURE			
DATE	MEDICATIONS					

Source: Ministry of Health, government of Kenya.

Ward and Department Inspections

The pharmacy department should undertake periodic inspections of drug storage areas throughout the hospital to ensure appropriate levels of properly stored drugs, to monitor expiration dates, and to remove unnecessary stock. Figure 38.3 is a sample ward inspection record. When problems are detected in inspections, it is important for pharmacy and nursing staff to develop methods to correct the situation.

Dangerous Drugs and Controlled Substances

Controlled substances require greater attention in the hospital setting than other drugs, just as they do outside the hospital. The various definitions and categories of controlled drugs all relate to abuse and addiction potential.

Procedures specific to the procurement, reception, storage, dispensing, and administration of controlled drugs should establish a readily retrievable trail of accountability for each individual drug unit. The records should document ordering, receiving, dispensing, administration, and wastage. Perpetual inventory records should be used at all storage sites. Controlled substances stored throughout the hospital should be securely double locked within a well-constructed storage area, with the pharmacy department in control of the distribution and duplication of keys.

After-Hours Pharmacy

Although the need for drugs is continuous, many hospitals cannot justify staffing a pharmacy department twenty-four hours a day. If it is necessary to obtain drugs while the pharmacy is closed, either an on-call pharmacist can come in, or a nursing supervisor can dispense drugs. Medication dispensing by nonpharmacists should be limited, however, to preserve the system of checks and balances and to prevent medication errors. To minimize the risk of incorrect dispensing, the following measures can be taken:

► Establish procedures for after-hours pharmacy service.
► Require training or in-house certification of nurses before they undertake dispensing responsibility.
► Prohibit after-hours access to most of the pharmacy. A limited formulary of prepackaged and labeled drugs can be provided in a separate, locked night cabinet.
► Require completion of dispensing records by the nurse and subsequent review by the pharmacist.

≡ 38.5 Small-Scale Hospital Pharmaceutical Production

Drugs produced by the pharmacy must have adequate process and finished-product controls to ensure identity,

Figure 38.3 Sample Ward Inspection Record

Nursing ward:_____ Inspection date:_____

Check each item that complies with standards:
❑ Medication storage area orderly and clean
❑ Internal use/injectable medications separated from disinfectants and toxic medications
❑ Medications properly secured from theft
❑ No unlabeled or mislabeled drugs present
❑ No unauthorized floor stock
❑ No excessive floor stock quantities
❑ Medication refrigerator temperature maintained within limits (see temperature log)
❑ Narcotics properly secured and records complete
❑ Approved emergency drugs in stock
❑ Concentration, date, and time mixed written on reconstituted injectables
❑ Drug formulary list available

Pharmacist's comments on areas of nonadherence to treatment:
_____
_____
_____

Action recommended:
_____
_____
_____

Pharmacist: _____
Nurse in charge: _____

strength, purity, and quality. It is difficult for a hospital pharmacy to accomplish the same cost efficiencies as a drug manufacturer specializing in a particular product line. Most hospitals repackage drugs in smaller unit-dose containers and may prepare specialty items such as creams with special formulations. The P&T committee needs to evaluate the costs and benefits of producing such special preparations as compared with purchasing commercial products. Chapter 19 includes more details on small-scale pharmaceutical production.

≡ 38.6 Controlling Leakage and Drug Abuse

Chapter 39 discusses systematic approaches for detecting, analyzing, and preventing drug losses due to theft, bribery, and fraud. Those approaches are applicable to hospitals and other health facilities.

The control of narcotics is of particular concern in a hospital, since it may be the only type of institution regularly stocking, dispensing, and administering them. Drug addiction among physicians, pharmacists, and nurses is quite common. To avoid drug abuse and prevent leakage:

≡ Assessment Guide

Organization

► Which department and individuals are responsible for ordering drugs and managing inventory?

► What systems are used to manage inventory and procure drugs?

► Apart from the central pharmacy, are there satellite pharmacies? If so, how many?

► How are drugs distributed to wards?

► Is there a hospital formulary? If so, how many items are listed? When was it last updated?

► Is there an after-hours pharmacy? How is this managed?

► Is there a pharmacy and therapeutics committee? If yes, how many meetings were held in the past year? What percentage of members attended? What issues were discussed?

Staffing

► How many pharmacy staff—professional and support—are employed?

► What is the educational level of professional staff?

► What refresher training have the professional pharmacy staff received in the past two years?

► How do the professional pharmacy staff spend their workdays—divided among clinical advice, preparation and dispensing, ward supervision and administration?

Operation

► How many patient admissions were there last year?

► What is the average number of prescriptions per day dispensed by pharmacies to inpatients? To outpatients?

► Among outpatients, what is the average dispensing communication time? What percentage of drugs dispensed are adequately labeled? What is the level of patient understanding?

► How often are ward storage areas inspected?

► Are the medication records accurately filled in?

► How many items are stocked in the central unit, satellite units, and ward stocks?

► How much does the hospital spend annually on pharmaceuticals?

Other Pharmacy Responsibilities

► Are preparations manufactured in the hospital? If so, how many? What quality control measures exist?

► Have drug utilization review activities occurred during the past year? If yes, who reviews the reports?

► Be alert to changes in performance, injuries, and mood swings in workers.

► Ensure double-witness and double-signature procedures for wastage of narcotics.

► Limit access to narcotic storage areas.

► Check patient charts and medication administration records for patterns of consumption; be suspicious if patients receive noticeably more narcotics during a particular shift.

► Ask patients if they received the drugs.

► Use locked boxes or wire cages to ensure security for drugs moved from the pharmacy to the wards.

► Issue individual narcotics boxes to each anesthesiologist daily, and make sure that the box is returned to the pharmacy at the end of the day with a written record of quantities used for each patient.

The same procedures followed for narcotics are sometimes used for antibiotics and other drugs that are easily resold and commonly lost to theft. ■

≡ References and Further Readings

★ = *Key readings.*

General

Eli Lilly and Company. 1994. *Lilly hospital pharmacy survey.* Indianapolis, Ind.: Lilly Corporate Center.

Graham, N. O. 1982. *Quality assurance in hospitals: Strategies for assessment and implementation.* Gaithersburg, Md.: Aspen Publishers.

★ Hassan, W. E. Jr. 1986. *Hospital pharmacy,* 5th ed. Philadelphia: Lea & Febiger.

★ Health-System Pharmacists. 1995. *Practice standards of the American Society of Hospital Pharmacists.* Bethesda, Md.: Health-System Pharmacists.

Joint Commission on Accreditation of Healthcare Organizations. 1995. *Accreditation manual for hospitals* (updated annually). Oakbrook Terrace, Ill.: Joint Commission on Accreditation of Heathcare Organizations.

Sanderson, E. D. 1982. *Hospital purchasing and inventory management.* Gaithersburg, Md.: Aspen Publishers.

Smith, M. C., and T. R. Brown. 1979. *Handbook of institutional pharmacy practice.* Baltimore: Williams & Wilkins.

WHO/DAP (World Health Organization/Action Programme on Essential Drugs). 1993. *How to investigate drug use in health facilities: Selected drug use indicators.* WHO/DAP/93.1. Geneva: WHO/DAP.

★ Williams, R. B., ed. 1985. *Hospital pharmacy management primer.* Bethesda, Md.: Health-System Pharmacists.

Hospital Drug Management Manuals

ASEAN (Association of Southeast Asian Nations). 1989. *Guidelines/manual for good hospital pharmacy practices and management.* Bangkok: ASEAN Technical Cooperation on Pharmaceuticals.

★ Department of Health, Republic of the Philippines (with support from USAID). 1994. *Hospital pharmacy management manual,* 2d ed. Manila: Department of Health.

Ministry of Health, government of Kenya. 1994. *Good management of hospital drugs and medical supplies.* Nairobi: Ministry of Health.

Part I	Part II	Part III	**Part IV**
Introduction	Policy and Legal Framework	Drug Management Cycle	**Management Support Systems**

A Organization and Management ▶

B Financing and Sustainability

C Information Management

D Human Resources Management

34 Managing Drug Programs

35 Planning for Drug Management

36 Monitoring and Evaluation

37 Community Participation

38 Hospital Drug Services

39 Security Management

Chapter 39
Security Management

≡ **Summary**

Security breaches include theft, bribery, and fraud. They can have a substantial, and sometimes disastrous, economic and health impact. A comprehensive security system includes

- *analysis of the sources of security breaches;*
- *determination of methods to improve security;*
- *consideration of costs and savings;*
- *implementation of security measures.*

Security breaches can be found through a combination of informal investigation, independent inventory counts, consumption comparisons, and surveys of drug outlets.

Theft prevention may require

- *providing unique identifiers for all government drug supplies;*
- *attacking the sources of government theft;*
- *closing the outlets for stolen drugs;*
- *improving salaries for staff who handle drugs.*

Controlling bribery requires mechanisms to prevent suppliers from influencing the choice of drugs, purchase quantities, and selection of suppliers.

Fraud control requires close attention to quality assurance procedures and routine stock control procedures. Security measures may be expensive, but they are often very cost effective.

≡ Theft, bribery, and fraud can interfere with the effective functioning of national drug supply systems. In some countries, security breaches can be the single most devastating problem for drug programs. A strong security system can

- minimize shortages;
- minimize abuse or misuse;
- contribute to accurate recordkeeping on drug consumption and disease prevalence;
- ensure that safe and effective drugs are available in authorized outlets at all times.

In one central African country, a hospital pharmacist routinely allowed for losses of 80 to 90 percent on certain drugs when she placed her orders, to ensure that she received enough supplies to treat hospital patients. In an extremely poor Southeast Asian country, losses due to theft are estimated to be more than 30 percent of the total drug supply, despite theoretically strict drug accounting requirements. The government medical store in an East African country is reported to have placed an order for over US$100,000 worth of pharmaceutical cocaine, which vanished from the wharf when it arrived.

There are other examples. In a Central American country, inventory records showed that stock levels of oral ampicillin, antibiotic eye ointment, and dozens of other products were enough for three, five, ten, and up to thirty years, because government buyers received special "commissions" for their purchases. Theft of antibiotics for black market sale and treatment of sexually transmitted diseases (STDs) is common in many countries. Hospitals in the United States have a difficult time controlling staff pilferage, and there have been several incidents in recent years involving theft and resale of significant quantities of public-sector drugs.

Security breaches can and should be tackled. Theft and wastage are caused by a mixture of cultural, political, and economic factors. However, even when bribery and theft are coordinated or condoned at high levels, countries have been able to reduce these activities when a strong commitment has been made by supply system managers.

Improving security involves analyzing the sources of security breaches, developing methods for improving security, and comparing the costs of security measures with the financial and public health costs of inadequate security.

≡ **39.1 Analysis of Security Breaches**

Security breaches include theft, bribery, and fraud, and they can occur at all levels of the drug purchasing and distribution system. Shortages caused by these activities can lead to suffering and death. Figure 39.1 shows the main types of security breaches and the levels at which they occur.

There are three common forms of theft and leakage. Slow, chronic, sustained, small-scale leakage may go unnoticed for a long time; staff with access to the drug storage area are usually responsible for such thefts. Large-scale robbery may involve people both inside and outside the drug supply system. Diversion of a shipment before it reaches its destination may involve people in responsible positions with access to information on the movement of goods.

Some factors that promote theft are

- shortage of essential drugs or high demand for drugs in the private sector;
- poor physical security in stores;
- weak inventory records;
- unlimited access to stores by unauthorized people;
- staff whose salaries are significantly lower than necessary for self-support;

Figure 39.1 Summary of Common Security Breaches

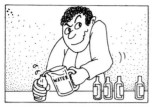

Suppliers (manufacturers, foreign suppliers, importers)
Intentional short packing
Intentional omission of expensive active ingredients
Shipping of products near their expiration date
Dilution and repacking of liquid medications
Delivery of incomplete orders and billing for full amounts

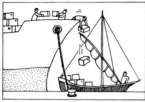

Wharf/Airport
Off-loading of government shipments directly onto vessels bound for nearby
   countries
Petty theft by port workers
Major theft from wharves, customs warehouses, airport fields, and elsewhere

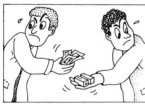

Purchasing Office
Acceptance of bribes in return for purchase of unnecessary types of drugs, purchase
   of excessively large quantities of drugs, or purchase from specific suppliers
Intentional overpurchasing to obtain quantities sufficient for systematic diversion into
   the black market while maintaining legitimate government distribution

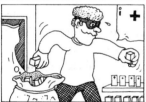

Medical Stores (central, regional, and hospital)
Major theft through breaking and entering
Major systematic theft by employees
Acceptance of bribes from suppliers for intentional overordering of specific items
Intentional underordering by government pharmacists or storekeepers, so that
   shortages will arise, followed by compensatory purchasing from local pharmacists
   who offer illegal "commissions"

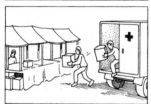

Transportation
Selling of drugs by drivers and at markets along the delivery route
Consumption of preparations containing alcohol by delivery staff, who then refill
   bottles with water
Systematic diversion of large quantities for black market sale
Theft of large quantities by nursing staff for use in their own unofficial private
   practices

In Hospitals
Petty theft by delivery staff, nurses, and doctors for personal and family use
Drinking of spirited preparations by hospital staff, who refill bottles with water
Systematic diversion of large quantities for black market sale
Theft of large quantities by nursing staff for use in their own unofficial private
   practices

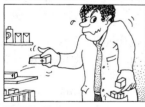

Outpatient Departments
Patients faking illness to obtain drugs for resale
Visits by patients to several clinics to obtain multiple prescriptions for antibiotics,
   analgesics, and other popular resale items
Writing of multiple prescriptions by physicians—to the same person or to false
   names—in return for a share of resulting black market sales

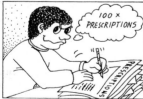

Health Centers/Village Health Workers
Pilfering of health center supplies by government physicians and health workers for
   use in their private practices
Popular black market items overordered from medical stores and diverted by
   physicians, nurses, dispensers, or laborers

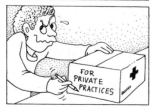

► access by underpaid staff to high-value products;
► inadequate systems for punishing thieves.

Stolen drugs find their way to four major outlets. They may be exported to adjacent countries via legitimate or illegitimate trade routes; sold to local private warehouses, pharmacists, or physicians for subsequent retail sale; sold directly to the public through street vendors; or distributed to family and friends.

≡ 39.2 Systematic Search for Security Breaches

Identifying major security breaches and the places where they usually occur is the first step in controlling them. There are several methods for uncovering theft, bribery, and fraud:

► anonymous, informal information
► unannounced physical inventory counts
► consumption comparisons using inventory records
► survey of suspected sales outlets

Informal channels may be the easiest way to determine whether there is a problem. Pharmacists, physicians, politicians, and other officials often know of, or at least suspect, diversion. Large stocks of unissued and unusable drugs at medical stores, the overnight disappearance of large quantities of drugs, systematic failure of deliveries to reach their final destinations, and frequent shortages at well-supplied facilities indicate a security problem. Responding vigorously to informal reports of diversion can be quite effective.

Unannounced physical inventory counts can uncover security breaches at all levels. The results of a surprise stock count should be compared with drug receipts and issues. It may be sufficient to sample only a selection of facilities at various levels to determine the extent of the problem; certainly, any facilities where problems are suspected should be included in the sample.

Consumption comparisons using inventory records can sometimes be revealing. For example, in one Central American country, theft of significant quantities of medical supplies, equipment, and food was uncovered by comparing the stock issues to each facility with the past consumption patterns at that facility. This suggested that certain hospitals were ordering suspiciously large quantities of supplies. The hospitals and departments involved were then carefully examined, and security breaches were identified. A similar approach has been helpful in other countries.

Surveys of suspected private outlets for black market sales are often effective. When government-purchased drugs can be distinguished by capsule type, batch number, packaging, or some other identifier, a survey of street vendors, pharmacies, and physicians' supplies can identify drugs from government sources.

≡ 39.3 Controlling Theft

Once the major sources of losses have been identified, it is necessary to implement methods to control theft, bribery, and fraud. Theft can be controlled by prevention measures and by closing the outlets for stolen goods.

Inventory Control

Good inventory management and stock control systems are essential for detecting and controlling theft (see Chapter 15). At each level in the supply system, records should indicate how much of each type of drug was received and issued, who received or issued the drugs and verified the amounts, the source of drugs received, and the destination of every issue. Such information provides an audit trail for the purchase, distribution, and consumption of drugs. The records also provide a basis for comparing drug consumption with utilization of services and a starting point for tracing security breaches.

A good information system alone is often not enough, and additional measures are needed.

Unique Identifiers

An individual or firm caught with drugs believed to be stolen may claim that the drugs were purchased. It is difficult to prove theft unless government drugs have unique identifiers, as shown in Figure 39.2. A country can require suppliers to identify government drugs in one or more of the following ways:

► Imprint all containers (bottles, boxes, foil packages) and external packing (cartons, crates) with a unique government seal or monogram.
► Register batch numbers on all immediate containers and external packing and (if purchase quantities are large) agree not to sell products from the same batch to any other buyer in the country or in adjacent countries.
► Emboss tablets and print capsules with a unique government monogram.

Unique identifiers have been introduced in many drug programs. They can, however, increase drug prices significantly, and this has led to the discontinuation of the program in some countries. Whether identifiers should be used depends on the following factors: the types and quantities of drugs purchased, the capacity and willingness of

Figure 39.2 Unique Identifiers

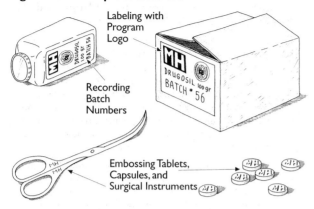

suppliers to provide identifiers, the incremental expense of doing so, the speed with which deliveries are needed, and the source and extent of drug theft.

Imprinting Containers and Packaging. Container imprinting is the most common type of identifier. The immediate container and the external packing are imprinted with the name or initials of the government program, the seal of the government, or some other symbol. In one South American country, individual foil packets as well as external boxes contain the program title, "Medicamentos Básicos," and all are printed with the same color code. In Sri Lanka, all container labels are required to bear the national seal. In Malaysia, containers are labeled as Ministry of Health property.

Imprinted containers can be used to identify stolen drugs only when thieves keep the drugs in their original containers. If large numbers of pills are packaged in plastic-lined containers, it is easy for thieves to remove the inner lining and destroy the identifying imprint. It takes much more time and effort to remove pills from individual foil packets or blister packages.

Container imprinting adds extra time and cost to the packing process. A requirement to imprint all immediate and external containers may delay shipments, increase the price, or completely dissuade some suppliers from bidding. One solution is to require imprinting only for orders that exceed a set minimum quantity or order value.

Batch Number Registration. The use of batch numbers as unique identifiers is less obvious to thieves than imprinted containers. By forbidding contract suppliers to sell products with the same batch numbers anywhere else in West Africa, one West African country was able to identify stolen goods and close several major black market wholesale and retail outlets, recovering thousands of dollars worth of stolen government drugs.

Since the unique batch number requirement does not add time to the manufacturing process, it is less likely to add to the cost or delivery time. However, suppliers may not be willing to restrict sales of a batch unless the requesting supply system purchases all or most of the batch. Thieves who are aware of the system can still remove the label or discard the container. Furthermore, the use of batch numbers as unique identifiers is effective only if the contractual requirement is monitored and enforced.

Tablet Embossing and Capsule Imprinting. Imprinting individual tablets and capsules with the drug program's initials or seal provides the most effective protection against theft for resale in the private sector. However, it is also the option most likely to increase drug prices. Country Study 39.1 gives an example of this practice in Southeast Asia. The embossing and imprinting process is easiest to implement in state-owned factories. With commercial suppliers, there may be increased lead times and large price increases due to the embossing requirement. The pricing gap may decrease if imprinting is required only for large-quantity orders.

Good Management

One principle of theft control is to provide secure storage places with limited access at all points in the distribution system. Country Study 39.2 describes a pilot project for improving inventory control in Sierra Leone.

A second principle is active use of the information system to detect theft and trace the point at which the theft occurred. The best inventory system is useless unless periodic physical stock counts are compared with recorded stock levels.

Although it is probably not possible to design a system that prevents theft at every point in the flow of drugs from port to patient, measures can be implemented to attack the problem at its major sources:

► Reinforce physical storage facilities.
► Introduce systematic and orderly shelving.
► Employ unique product and container identifiers.
► Strengthen inventory control systems at all levels.
► Maintain a perpetual inventory system with regular physical counts.
► Insist on perpetual record checking with discrepancy reporting.
► Concentrate security measures on fast-moving, popular, and expensive items.
► Assign responsibility for security to one person.
► Limit store access to accountable staff only.
► Disallow individual prescription filling from the store.
► Improve staff salaries and working conditions.

Country Study 39.1 Tablet and Capsule Embossing in Southeast Asia

In one successful government pharmaceutical supply program, contracts with suppliers specified that tablets and capsules in quantities over 500,000 units had to be embossed with the Ministry of Health initials. All tablets produced by the government pharmaceutical plant also had to be embossed.

Theft of attractive items such as diazepam, acetaminophen, antibiotics (used extensively for venereal disease), and other drugs was a steady, if small-scale, drain on supplies in major hospitals. Individual ampicillin and tetracycline tablets, which cost the government less than US$.04, were sold for $0.50 to $1.00 each on the black market.

The embossing of tablets did not stop these thefts, but it substantially reduced large-volume theft and subsequent sale to commercial pharmacies and physicians. In one year, losses due to theft during the wharf-clearing and delivery process amounted to 5 to 10 percent. A thorough investigation of pharmacies and doctors' offices in the capital city uncovered several places that dealt in stolen drugs. This led to a rapid reduction in thefts. Without the embossing on the tablets and capsules, it would have been difficult, if not impossible, to prove that the drugs had come from government stores.

Country Study 39.2 Experience in Improved Inventory Control in Sierra Leone

The Sierra Leone Ministry of Health introduced improved security measures as a pilot project in 1986. At the time, the supply system lacked proper storage or inventory control, and essential drugs were in short supply. Over US$1 million worth of drugs had been stolen in 1985. The project's main aims were to enforce accountability, strengthen security, and provide training in store and drug management at central medical stores and selected district, hospital, and peripheral health unit levels.

Improvements were made at the hospital level. First, the hospital store was renovated. Wooden doors were replaced with reinforced double-lock steel doors, windows were fitted with steel bars, and the ceiling was reinforced to prevent access from adjacent rooms. A large lockable shelf was provided for expensive, fast-moving items. All other items were kept in sealed boxes on pallets. A storekeeper was appointed. The hospital pharmacy was cleaned, obsolete items were removed, and shelves and drug cabinets were constructed. The pharmacy was divided into two parts: a mini-store and a dispensing room equipped with a small lockable cabinet. The mini-store supplied the dispensing room. Replenishment was made with a special requisition form only after previous receipts had been accounted for. The dispenser or pharmacist issued drugs by official prescription to patients through a dispensing window. Access to the store was limited to the storekeeper in charge. At the end of the day, the storekeeper, the dispenser, and the cashier audited the day's transactions and tallied the money received against the supplies issued. The money was then deposited in a special revolving drug account that was used to replenish drugs. The strict physical and inventory record control and the weekly perpetual inventory of selected fast-moving drugs improved security.

There were worries, however, about the system's integrity. Several creative methods of pilfering were discovered. In one of the stores, the containers all appeared to be in place when viewed from floor level; when viewed from a height (the supervisor climbed a ladder), empty spaces could be seen where drugs had been removed. It was also discovered that drugs had been removed from their containers and the empty containers replaced on the shelves. After these thefts were discovered, the storekeepers were held responsible. Subsequently, such pilfering techniques were abandoned.

The security system was effective for a few years, but in the early 1990s, the system broke down as major economic and social problems engulfed the country.

Source: Gabriel Daniel, Africare 1994.

When corruption and theft are prevalent in a supply system, extremely low staff salaries are often a contributing factor. Increasing salaries to a level comparable to local private-sector salaries for similar positions is expensive but may be cost effective if losses can be controlled.

Some physical security measures include

- ► improved external and internal lighting;
- ► alarm systems;
- ► watchdogs;
- ► private security agents;
- ► secure fencing;
- ► double locks;
- ► strong, lockable delivery boxes and containers;
- ► closed delivery vans.

Box 39.1 provides a sample of techniques used in various parts of the world. Unfortunately, the comparative effectiveness of the various methods has not been tested and is likely to vary from country to country, depending on the commitment of individuals and on political, cultural, and economic circumstances. Country Study 39.3 describes how Sri Lanka uses strict accounting and audit procedures to minimize opportunities for theft.

Law Enforcement and Closing of Outlets

When the major outlet for stolen goods is black market sale within the country, the incentive to steal is reduced greatly by closing black market outlets. This is more easily done if the outlets can be readily identified and if government drugs carry unique identifiers.

Unfortunately, police may be unwilling or unable to spend time on such activities. To solve this problem, the pharmaceutical section of one Southeast Asian ministry of

Box 39.1 Techniques for Theft Control

Monitor Selected Items
Monitoring should be targeted at those products that are most likely to disappear—those that are fast moving, chronically in short supply, in high demand by consumers, expensive, life-saving, and easy to hide or disguise. A simple way to monitor targeted drugs is:

1. Select a drug that is particularly likely to be pilfered or that may be misused (prescribed inappropriately), for example, tetracycline tablets.
2. Check pharmacy or storeroom inventory records to determine consumption during a specified period. Example: 8,000 tablets were issued during a three-month period.
3. Check medical charts or prescription ledgers and count the number of treatment courses over the same period. Example: 101 adults were dispensed fifty-six tetracycline tablets each.
4. Convert treatment courses to dose units. Example: 5,656 tablets.
5. Compare this figure with the stock issued from the storage area. If there is a significant difference, further investigation and possibly punitive action are warranted.

At the Port
Containerization. If the port is equipped to handle containers, containerization reduces both major and petty theft because containers are physically secure (although entire containers can be stolen).

Rapid Port Clearance. Inadequate and inefficient port-clearing procedures can lead to long delays, providing opportunities for theft if security is weak. Increased efficiency in port clearing reduces theft.

At the Medical Stores
Limited Access. Access to drug storage areas should be limited to the store's staff only. Hospital pharmacies should not be accessible on evenings or weekends or when the pharmacist or dispenser is not present. Limited extra supplies for emergency rooms and wards should be entrusted to medical officers or nurses when the pharmacy is closed. Their distribution should be accounted for and monitored by pharmacy staff.

Secure Locks and Doors. These are essential to good security. Country Study 39.2 describes improvements that can be made.

Unannounced Searches of Medical Stores and Hospital Staff. In some countries, the pharmacist or medical director personally supervises periodic, unannounced searches.

Independent Stock Count. Staff from the central pharmaceutical supply office should visit all major medical stores periodically to perform either a complete or a sampling stock count and an audit of receipt and issue records.

During Transport
Document Verification. A specific staff member should be responsible for checking receipts against the packing slip. A separate invoice should be sent from the issuing store, and the receiving form should be verified against this invoice. This shows where shipments have partially or completely disappeared in transit.

Packing Seals. Shrink-wrapped pallets and tape, wax seals, and wire seals used to close cardboard boxes or other transport containers make tampering obvious.

Strongboxes. When large shipments are made to small numbers of facilities, portable strongboxes or built-in compartments with padlocks should be used. One key should remain at the issuing store and the other at the receiving store.

In Hospitals
Drug Accounting. Ward and outpatient staff should record all drugs received and dispensed. These records should be checked periodically (monthly or bimonthly) against pharmacy issue records.

Issue-Consumption Verification. For dangerous and controlled drugs, and for drugs that are frequently stolen, a consumption report showing the time, date, patient, patient's number, dose, and remaining stock levels should be submitted to the pharmacist with each order for additional stocks.

Presentation of Prescriptions for Ward Issue. For selected expensive or frequently abused drugs, the hospital pharmacy should be provided with a copy of the signed prescription to be filed with the pharmacy before drugs are issued to the ward.

Rotating Stock Containers. Wards can keep a limited number of labeled containers for each drug they stock. When the containers are empty, they must be returned to the pharmacy for replenishment, along with the dispensary record for the drug. The containers allocated for each drug should hold enough stock for several days. Excessive replenishment of stock is cause for suspicion.

Locked Transport Boxes. The pharmacy can issue drugs in wooden or metal boxes with padlocks. Each ward should have its own box. The pharmacist should have a key for all ward boxes, and the head nurse should have the second key for that ward's box.

Upgrading of Transport Staff. In several countries, security has improved when nursing students, dispensers, or nurses, rather than laborers, collect drugs from the pharmacy. When the pharmacy establishes and adheres to an appropriate issuing schedule for wards, it becomes possible for nursing staff to allocate time to collect drugs.

Upgrading of Pharmacy Staff. Gradual replacement of untrained dispensary staff with trained pharmacists and dispensers has been credited with reducing theft in some countries. A combination of more careful screening of individuals, professional socialization, and higher pay may explain this observation.

In Outpatient Departments and Health Centers
Maximum Dispensing Quantities. Setting a maximum quantity prevents patients from altering prescriptions to obtain large amounts of drugs and prevents collaborating physicians from writing excessively large prescriptions.

Recording of Individual Prescriptions. This is recommended to increase the dispenser's accountability.

Dispensing by Physicians and Paramedical Staff. When there is reason to think that health center aides are stealing certain attractive items, the physician and paramedical staff can take responsibility for dispensing these drugs to patients in their examining rooms.

Country Study 39.3 Drug Accounting in Sri Lanka

Government health facilities in Sri Lanka have adopted a detailed drug accounting system to help economize on drug use. This system is also highly effective in reducing theft.

Drug Accounting. At each step where drugs are transferred from one level to the next (for example, divisional stores to institution storeroom), a ledger is kept and complete entries are made for each transaction, including the date, supplier's and receiver's names, and amount issued or received. At the point of dispensing (either to outpatients or on the wards), dispensing records are kept in one of two ways, depending on the type of drug:

► Accountable drugs, which include antibiotics, drugs costing more than US$0.003 per unit, and controlled substances (narcotics), must be accounted for individually. A serial record including the patient's health service number, type of drug, number of units dispensed, and date is kept in a log book. Total amounts recorded in the prescription log must be balanced daily or weekly with stock records.

► Bulk drugs, which consist of all those items not included under accountable drugs, are charged out in bulk to the dispenser, floor nurse, or doctor, usually in units equivalent to container size (for example, 1,000 tablets of aspirin in a tin are recorded as one bulk item). It is not necessary to record individual drug issues for these items.

Auditing. At major institutions, the Ministry of Health (MOH) generally performs an internal audit of drug distribution and dispensing records once a year. Receipts and issues are checked at all levels, including at the dispensary window.

Test Checks. Periodic test checks are conducted by the medical officer in charge, a delegated individual, or, at larger institutions, the chief of nursing. Unannounced, the checker compares the book balance and physical stock for about ten items. The form is prepared in triplicate, with one copy to the medical officer, one to the division's superintendent of health services, and one to the MOH's internal audit department. Ward test checks are done every two weeks, and outpatient dispensary checks are done monthly.

health managed to obtain authority from the police department for its own staff to investigate and prosecute violations, which improved enforcement efforts. Such a solution would not work, however, if theft were coordinated or condoned at the upper levels of the supply system.

When stolen drugs are sold through a multitude of street vendors, closing the outlets may not be feasible, since it is hard to identify and locate them. In these instances, control can be exerted more effectively at the sources of theft rather than at the outlets.

≡ 39.4 Bribery

Illegal payments from suppliers to purchasing officials can occur at all levels and in any country. The supplier may try to use bribery to influence which drugs are bought, the purchase quantities, or which suppliers are selected. A determined supplier can influence decisions in most supply systems. Bribery is made more difficult if separate mechanisms are established for making each of these three decisions, and if all decisions are made by a committee rather than by an individual.

Influencing Choice of Drugs

In Chapter 10, it was noted that the participation of a panel of respected physicians, pharmacists, and public officials often improves the appropriateness of drug selection and makes the process more credible and therefore more acceptable. Another advantage is that it lends greater visibility to the selection process. It is more difficult for a supplier to persuade a whole group to buy an unnecessary type or brand of drug than it is to influence one or two individuals.

Influencing Order Quantities

When inventory control is poor, purchasing officers usually have to estimate rather than calculate the amounts to purchase. If there are no consumption data to compare with these estimates, order quantities can be inflated by bribe-seeking purchasing officers without great risk of detection. In contrast, when inventory control and forecasting are effective and/or when a systematic method of calculation is used to determine order quantities (see Chapters 14 and 15), it becomes much more difficult for the supplier or a purchasing officer to influence the amounts ordered.

Influencing Supplier Selection

Suppliers in many countries attempt to influence the supplier selection decision for a particular order. As discussed in Chapter 16, a transparent tender process and tender awards made by a broad-based committee are the best ways to combat this problem.

≡ 39.5 Fraud

Manufacturers and importers may dilute liquid preparations, omit or reduce the quantity of expensive active ingredients, or short-pack their shipments. Some suppliers may even provide counterfeit or spurious products. This type of fraud can be uncovered by proper quality assurance practices (Chapter 18) and thorough checking of receipts by the receiving clerk at the medical store or pharmacy (Chapters 23 and 24).

Specialists from the Ethiopian Ministry of Health paid visits to selected winners of tenders and found that although many suppliers claimed to meet the criteria for bidding on tenders, they failed to meet even the basic requirements. Their visit to India showed that over 80 percent of forty-five pharmaceutical suppliers to the Ethiopian government medical store failed to meet several basic quality assurance standards.

The supplier should be held accountable both for intentional errors, such as fraud, and for mistakes in formulation or packing. Precise specification of product requirements and rigid enforcement of contracts are essential, as described in Chapter 17.

≡ 39.6 The Cost of Security

In some cases, there are no additional costs specifically attributable to security control. Several methods for preventing security breaches serve a dual purpose, as they are also necessary for the effective procurement and distribution of drugs: establishment of a drug selection committee, quality assurance, inventory control and forecasting, and checking of receipts.

Other security measures are quite costly. It can be expensive to imprint containers, emboss tablets and capsules, hire special security staff, construct secure warehouses and storerooms, and regularly monitor and audit stock records. These expenses must be weighed against the potential savings from reduced theft, bribery, and fraud.

Breaches in security can have substantial medical as well as financial costs. Fraud may have serious and even life-threatening medical consequences if the supplier uses insufficient amounts of active ingredients. Theft raises costs by increasing the volume of drugs that have to be purchased; it also has medical costs resulting from shortages and the use of inappropriate drugs. Bribery and corrupt procurement can be particularly costly. Traditionally, in one South American country, 7 to 10 percent of the procurement value is paid to procurement officials. This adds up to several hundred thousand US dollars each year, because these bribes are added to the drug price. ∎

≡ Assessment Guide

Prevalence of Leaks
- ► Is drug leakage a problem?
- ► What are the annual losses as (1) absolute value and (2) percentage of total annual drug purchases?
- ► Where do leaks occur: at ports, at primary and intermediate stores, at health facilities, during transport?
- ► What types of leaks are experienced in each setting: petty pilferage, major thefts, diversion of shipments, bribery and corruption, supplier fraud? Which are the most significant?

Security Systems
- ► Is there an effective inventory control system?
- ► What systems are used to control theft? Have thefts been detected in the past year? What measures were taken after detection?
- ► What systems are used to control bribery and corruption? Is a committee system used? Has bribery or corruption been detected in the past year? What measures were taken after detection?
- ► Are physical security systems in buildings and vehicles adequate or inadequate?

Theft Detection
- ► How is theft detected: informers, physical inventory count, consumption comparisons, surveys of selected outlets?
- ► Are the police cooperative?
- ► Are junior staff cooperative?
- ► Are senior managers cooperative?

Fraud Detection
- ► What systems are used to control supplier fraud? Has fraud been identified in the past year? What measures were taken after detection?
- ► Are product and packaging specifications adequate?
- ► Do supplier contracts specify penalties in the event of fraud?
- ► How is fraud detected: visits to suppliers, receiving inspections, or assays?
- ► Are there any laws or regulations in place for controlling fraud?

≡ References and Further Readings

Downs, D. E., ed. 1992. *Understanding the freight business,* 4th ed. Egham, Surrey, England: Micor Freight UK.

Parker, D., and W. Newbrander. 1994. Tackling wastage and inefficiency in the health sector (roundtable). *World Health Forum* 15:107–13.

Part I	Part II	Part III	Part IV
Introduction	Policy and Legal Framework	Drug Management Cycle	**Management Support Systems**

Part IV
Management Support Systems

A Organization and Management

B Financing and Sustainability

C Information Management

D Human Resources Management

Section B
Financing and Sustainability

Part I Introduction	Part II Policy and Legal Framework	Part III Drug Management Cycle	**Part IV** **Management Support Systems**	
			A Organization and Management	
			B Financing and Sustainability ▶	**40 Drug Financing** **Strategies**
			C Information Management	
			D Human Resources Management	41 Analyzing and Controlling Drug Expenditures
				42 Financial Planning and Management
				43 Donor Financing
				44 Revolving Drug Funds

Chapter 40
Drug Financing Strategies

≡ Summary

Drugs save lives and improve health, but they are costly, and they are necessary to make effective use of staff and other health resources. Financial sustainability requires a balance among the demand for drugs, the cost of meeting this demand, and available resources. Otherwise, shortages result and quality of care declines.

A drug financing strategy should begin with efforts to make better use of available funds. If improved efficiency in selection, procurement, distribution, and use of drugs does not create the necessary balance, options for increased funding include making the case for greater government funding of drugs, introducing or strengthening user charges or health insurance coverage for drugs, or obtaining donor assistance.

Globally, 60 percent of health care is publicly financed, with the share increasing with national income. For health care and especially for drugs, private spending usually represents a higher share of health financing in lower-income countries. Expansion of private and nongovernmental organization (NGO) health services, including provision of essential drugs, can shift demand away from overstretched public resources. But quality of care and equity must be ensured.

Public financing through national and local government budgets is a major but sometimes inadequate source of financing for drugs. The case for public financing of drugs can be strengthened through better quantification of drug needs, per capita drug budgets, demonstration of the health impact of drugs, recognition of political benefits, improved management, expenditure trend analysis, and comparative expenditure analysis. Efforts should be made to ensure that available public resources are targeted to those most in need.

User charges may exist as government revolving drug funds, community drug schemes, and retail purchase of drugs. Experience indicates that user charges pose many difficulties. Improved drug availability, equity, and efficiency are more likely with local retention and control of revenue, businesslike orientation to financial and supply management, strict measures to ensure accountability, reliable supply of low-cost essential drugs, locally appropriate fee schedules, and adequate protection mechanisms for the poor and other target groups.

Health insurance covers a small but growing portion of the population in most developing countries. Important elements of insurance include risk-sharing and prepayment. Plans vary in the extent of and mechanisms for insurance coverage for drugs. National social insurance schemes, private voluntary insurance, managed care, and community prepayment schemes can increase access to essential drugs. Insurance programs, particularly of the managed care type, have an incentive to encourage cost control and rational drug use.

Voluntary and other local financing can contribute to improving the overall health care and drug financing situation. Donor financing and development loans can help a country develop more efficient drug supply systems and alternative financing approaches. For the poorest countries, some external financing for drugs may be needed to ensure universal access to essential drugs.

Financing mechanisms can be compared in terms of access to drugs, rational drug use, efficiency, equity, sustainability, and administrative requirements. Financial sustainability may require a pluralistic approach in which needs are met through a combination of financing mechanisms.

≡ 40.1 Why Drug Financing Is Important

Financing of pharmaceuticals is a critical issue for several reasons. First, because drugs save lives and improve health, it is important that drug financing ensures access to essential drugs for all segments of the population. Second, drugs are costly. For most ministries of health, drugs represent the largest expenditure after staff salaries. In some countries, up to 80 percent of a household's health-related spending is on drugs. In developing countries, drugs commonly represent from 25 to 50 percent of total public and private health expenditures. Third, inadequate funding for drugs means that expenditures for staff salaries and other health care costs may be used inefficiently or simply wasted.

This chapter considers the factors that determine financial sustainability, sources of health care financing, and strategies to achieve financial sustainability of drug supplies.

≡ 40.2 Balancing the Financial Sustainability Equation

Financial sustainability, as illustrated in Figure 40.1, is achieved only when resources are in balance with costs and are sufficient to support a basic quality of care for a given level of health care demand. If demand for drugs exceeds available resources, the health system is left with only four options:

1. Improve efficiency.
2. Reduce demand.

3. Increase financial resources.

4. Accept a decline in quality of care.

In most settings, it defies economic reality to promise high-quality services and constant availability of essential drugs without also ensuring a high level of efficiency, achieving adequate financing, and controlling demand for drugs (see Figure 40.1).

The same financial sustainability equation applies to NGOs. When demand surpasses available resources, they face the same choices: improve efficiency, control demand, increase financial resources, or accept a decline in quality of care.

For all sectors—public, for-profit private, and not-for-profit private—drug financing should not be approached simply as a question of where do we get the money? It must be approached in terms of methods to improve efficiency and to ensure that demand is appropriate.

Improving Efficiency

Two broad categories of efficiency were defined in Chapter 3: allocative and technical efficiency. *Allocative efficiency* applies to the distribution of services within the population. Spending the majority of a country's drug budget on essential drugs for primary health care, rather than on specialized drugs for national referral hospitals, is likely to save more lives and thereby results in allocative efficiency.

Technical efficiency is achieved if resources are used to produce a given output at the lowest possible cost or to produce greater outputs for the same cost. Drug financing decisions are concerned mostly with technical efficiency, which has two components: therapeutic efficiency (improved selection and use) and operational efficiency (improved management of procurement and distribution).

Efforts to balance the financial sustainability equation should always emphasize finding ways to improve efficiency.

Controlling Demand

Since the demand for health care services may be virtually unlimited, something *always* controls demand. In practice, health systems control demand—by intent or by neglect—through combinations of six possible measures:

1. Increase cost to the patient.

2. Impose rationing or other administrative controls.

3. Provide attractive alternatives.

4. Increase waiting time.

5. Decrease quality of services.

6. Provide targeted education.

Some health services unintentionally control demand through a combination of long waiting times and poor quality (drug shortages, for example). In the worst examples of

Figure 40.1 Financial Sustainability Equation

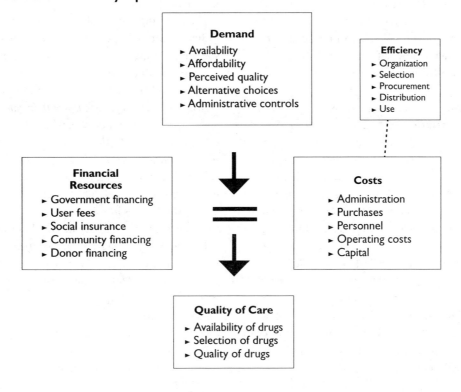

user fee programs, fees are introduced without quality improvements. Not surprisingly, increased cost—added to long waiting times and low quality—further reduces utilization. User fees can both increase financial resources and reduce demand, but measures are needed to ensure access for the poor.

Many government health services operate as if they view private, mission, and other not-for-profit health services as "the competition." Yet overstretched government health services would be better able to care for the neediest members of society if more people with the means to pay sought care outside government health services. If public policy initiatives and program activities resulted in more patients receiving rational, reasonably priced drug therapy through private and other nongovernmental providers, the pressure on government essential drug supplies would be reduced.

Increasing Financial Resources

The components of financial sustainability can be brought into better balance by increasing financial resources. The remainder of this chapter considers ways to maintain or increase financial resources through public financing, user charges, health insurance, community and other voluntary financing, donor financing, and development loans.

≡ 40.3 Health and Drug Financing

Drug financing must be viewed in the overall context of health financing. Funding for the recurrent operating costs and long-term development costs for health services comes from public sources (national and local government budgets, national social health insurance), private sources (direct payment by patients, private health insurance, employers, NGOs), and external development aid.

Health Expenditures among Countries

The relative importance of each funding source varies dramatically among regions and among countries within a region and evolves over time. Regional health expenditure data are shown in Figure 40.2. Country-specific expenditure data are quoted from the World Health Organization (WHO) (Murray and López 1994). Several observations can be made about levels and sources of financing for health.

Health Expenditures Vary Widely among Regions and Countries. Total per capita health expenditures vary tenfold among regions. Among developing countries, annual health expenditures vary from less than US$10 per capita in Tanzania, Zaire, Nepal, and several other countries to over US$100 per capita in several countries in Latin America and the Middle East.

Total Health Spending Depends on Economic Output, but Some Countries Spend More than Others. Health expenditures are directly related to national economic output as measured by gross domestic product (GDP). Developing-country health spending averages about 4 percent of GDP, with little variation among regions. Nevertheless, some developing countries spend relatively less on health (for example, 2.4 percent of GDP for Zaire and 2.1 percent for Vietnam), and others spend more (for example, 6.2 percent for Zimbabwe and 8.6 percent for Nicaragua).

As a Share of the Total, Public-Sector Spending Increases as National Incomes Rise. Globally, health expenditures are about 60 percent public and 40 percent private in origin. Excluding the United States (where private spending is 56 percent of the total spent on health), 75 percent of health costs are publicly supported in established market economies. But in developing countries, private spending is a higher proportion, rising to nearly 65 percent in Zaire and over 75 percent in India.

Developing Countries Devote a Lower Share of Public Spending to Health. Total government spending as a share of GDP is higher among high-income countries (42 percent versus 20 to 30 percent in developing countries). Lower public health spending in developing countries reflects the lower share of health expenditures in the national budget: 10 to 15 percent of government spending in high-income countries is on health, whereas in developing countries the share is less than 8 percent and often less than 5 percent.

The combined result of lower proportional allocations to health and lower overall income is that public-sector spending in Africa and Asia is roughly US$10 per capita, compared with US$56 in the Middle East, US$62 in Latin America, and US$103 among transitional economies.

Insurance Coverage Increases with Income. Median insurance coverage for countries for which data are available is 5 percent in Africa, 6 percent in Asia, 33 percent in Latin America, and over 75 percent in established market economies. In a number of Latin American countries, over 60 percent of the population is covered by health insurance; few countries in Asia reach this level, and most countries in Africa currently have minimal insurance coverage.

Foreign Aid Is a Major Contributor in Certain Regions. Foreign aid accounts for 20 to 30 percent of health expenditures in many African countries and some Asian countries. Private health expenditures in Figure 40.2 include those derived from voluntary, religious, and other NGOs as well as spending by individuals and private companies. NGOs play an important role in the financing and provision of health services in many countries. NGO aid can

Figure 40.2 Health Expenditures by Region, 1990

Region	Health Expenditures			Health Expenditures by Source (% of Total)			Central Government Expenditures				Insurance Coverage (% of Pop. Covered)	
	Total per Capita (US$)	Public Expenditures per Capita (US$)	As % of GDP	Public	Private	Aid Flows	Total as % of GDP Median	No. of Countries	Health as % of Government Expenditures Median	No. of Countries	Median	No. of Countries
Africa (sub-Saharan)	22	10	4.2	43.8	46.6	9.2	30	16	7.0	10	8	15
Asia	25	10	4.6	40.4	57.8	1.7	20	10	4.6	10	10	16
Middle East	97	56	3.5	57.6	42.8	0.7	32	10	4.3	10	15	15
Latin America and Caribbean	103	62	4.0	59.8	38.9	1.2	17	16	6.7	13	35	20
Transitional economies	144	103	3.6	71.2	29.1	0.0	56	5	4.8	5	NA	
Established market economies	1,958	1,196	9.3	61.1	38.9	0.0	42	21	12.4	17	>95	13

Source: Murray and López 1994; WHO 1996.

account for 20 to 30 percent of health expenditures in a number of African and low-income Asian countries; the NGO share can be as high as 50 percent of curative services (Gilson et al. 1994).

Thus, the relative contributions of public and private spending, external aid, and health insurance differ considerably among regions and countries. Level of economic development has a significant influence. But national policy, commitment to health, political and historical factors, and other influences result in substantial differences among countries within the same region and countries at similar levels of development.

Pharmaceutical Expenditures among Countries

Data on pharmaceutical expenditures are much less complete than data on overall health expenditures. Regional pharmaceutical expenditures as of 1990 are shown in Figure 40.3, from which the following observations can be made.

Per Capita Drug Consumption Varies Widely among Regions and Countries. Pharmaceutical expenditures vary greatly among regions. Like total per capita health expenditures, drug expenditures vary up to tenfold among countries within a region.

Spending on Drugs Depends on Economic Output. Spending on drugs is directly related to GDP. Drug consumption as a percentage of GDP shows little variation among regions, ranging from 0.59 percent in Asia to 0.86 percent in Africa (see Figure 40.3). Cameroon, Colombia, France, and the Philippines each spend roughly 1 percent of their GDP on drugs.

Private Spending Represents a Greater Share of Total Spending on Drugs in Developing Countries. Among estab-

lished market economies, private spending on drugs averages one-third of total pharmaceutical spending; two-thirds of pharmaceutical costs are paid through public budgets and social insurance. In contrast, less than half of drug expenditures are publicly funded in developing countries for which estimates are available. In many countries of Latin America and Asia, over three-quarters of pharmaceutical expenditures are privately financed. Exceptions include countries such as Bhutan and Papua New Guinea, where private-sector coverage is low and public supply predominates.

Spending on Drugs Accounts for a Greater Share of Total Health Expenditures in Lower-Income Countries. In most

Figure 40.3 Pharmaceutical Expenditures by Region, 1990

Region	Total Pharmaceutical Expenditures		Private Pharmaceutical Expenditures as % of Total Pharmaceutical Expenditures	
	Per Capita (US$)	As % of GDP	Median	No. of Countries
Africa	8	0.86	68	13
Asia	12	0.59	76	14
Middle East	31	0.74	82–88	4
Latin America and Caribbean	26	0.87	75	23
Transitional economies	19	NA	NA	NA
Developed market economies	137	0.65	33	17

Source: WHO 1996.

high-income countries, pharmaceuticals account for 10 to 15 percent of total health expenditures. In contrast, pharmaceutical expenditures represent 35 percent of total public and private health expenditures in Thailand, 39 percent in Indonesia, 45 percent in China, and 66 percent in Mali (WHO 1996).

Thus, overall spending on drugs is related to economic development. In lower-income countries, however, drugs consume a higher share of total health expenditures. Private expenditures play a major role in overall drug financing.

How much should a country spend on pharmaceuticals? Dumoulin, Kaddar, and Velásquez (1991) have suggested the possible effects of different orders of magnitude for pharmaceutical expenditures:

► Less than $5 per capita per year is unlikely to provide a regular supply of drugs to the entire population.

► An expenditure of $5 to $10 per capita should supply a large part of the population.

► With an expenditure of $10 to $50 per capita, the needs of the entire population should be satisfied.

These figures are based on national averages and allow for a considerable degree of unevenness in access to drugs.

Financing Options for Essential Drugs

Funding options for drugs are essentially the same as those for health care in general: government revenues (national and local); direct payment by patients (fee for service); health insurance (national social insurance or voluntary insurance); community, employer, and other voluntary local financing; donor financing; and development loans (see Figure 40.4 and Country Study 40.1).

Financing arrangements affect the relationships among patients, providers, and the payers or financiers of health services (Figure 40.5). With direct purchase of drugs by consumers, for example, the relationship is primarily between the patient, who is paying for the drugs, and the pharmacy, which is providing the drugs. The government's role is to regulate drug quality and sales outlets.

With managed care, the provider and payer (insurer) are closely linked, if not a single organization. Although this may help control health care costs, it creates a potential conflict of interest between cost control and quality of care. Public supervision as well as competition are important to promote quality of care.

With each financing arrangement, the role of the government is different. Governments must adapt policies as the mix of financing arrangements in the country changes.

Figure 40.4 Funding Mechanisms for Essential Drugs

Public Financing (Government Budgets)
► national government
► local government

User Fees
► public-sector revolving drug funds
► community drug schemes
► direct private drug purchases (out-of-pocket purchases)

Health Insurance (Prepaid Health Schemes)
► social insurance (compulsory health insurance or social security)
► private insurance (indemnity insurance that is voluntary or through an employer)
► managed care (HMOs and other provider-insurer arrangements)
► community health insurance

Voluntary and Other Local Financing
► private voluntary (NGOs)
► voluntary community mechanisms
► cooperatives
► employer-provided health care

Donor Financing
► bilateral grants
► multilateral grants

Development Loans
► World Bank
► regional development banks

≡ 40.4 Public Financing through Government Budgets

Health officials and managers of essential drugs programs argue for increasing expenditures for drugs, sometimes without appreciating the dynamics of public expenditure.

Public financing of drugs can occur through national and local government budgets or compulsory programs such as social security and national social insurance schemes. This discussion focuses on central government funding of drugs; public funding through insurance is covered in Section 40.6 on health insurance.

Determinants of Public Drug Expenditures

Actual public expenditures for drugs are determined by a combination of economic factors, national budget decisions, and internal decisions by health ministries. Major factors include

► national economic output (GDP);
► the share of GDP collected in taxes as revenue for government expenditures (20 to 30 percent in most developing countries);
► the share of government spending devoted to health (3 to 5 percent in most developing countries);
► the relative share of government health spending

Country Study 40.1 Approaches to Drug Financing

Bhutan. Bhutan provides an estimated 90 percent of its pharmaceuticals through the public sector. The Bhutan essential drugs list is regularly updated and in 1995 contained 326 dosage forms categorized by level of use. Although Bhutan received WHO assistance to develop the Bhutan Essential Drugs Program (BEDP), this assistance did not include procurement of essential drugs. Because of its commitment to the health sector, the royal government of Bhutan has funded the largest share of drug expenditures since the inception of the BEDP. For the 1995 fiscal year, public drug expenditures were roughly US$1 per capita, with 70 percent of funding from central government allocations, 20 percent from multilateral sources for specific primary care programs, and 10 percent from bilateral contributions. Drugs for the public sector are purchased through international competitive tenders restricted to qualified suppliers.

European Community. Europe accounts for nearly one-quarter of the world's pharmaceutical consumption. Among most countries of the European Community, pharmaceuticals account for 15 to 20 percent of health expenditures and averaged roughly US$150 per capita in 1990. Two-thirds of pharmaceutical expenditures are funded by public sources, including compulsory health insurance schemes and national health services. In France, for example, over 60 percent of pharmaceuticals are reimbursed through social financing mechanisms. As of 1994, reimbursement was 100 percent for drugs considered irreplaceable and expensive, 35 percent for drugs used for pain and mild disorders, and 65 percent for other prescription drugs. Nearly 10 percent of the population is exempt from co-insurance due to severe disease, disability, or other reasons (Mossialos et al. 1994).

Indonesia. Indonesia has a population of nearly 190 million people (1995) spread over 3,000 islands. Total public and private health expenditures have been estimated at US$9.50 per capita; this figure includes US$3.75 for pharmaceuticals, one-quarter of which comes from public sources. The INPRES (presidential decree)—the central government allocation for drugs—provides nearly two-thirds of the public drug budget. INPRES funds are budgeted on a per capita basis. Each year a per capita allocation is established (US$.50 in 1990). Using official population figures, the per capita amount is used to set provincial and then individual district drug budgets. On a fixed annual schedule, districts are notified of their INPRES budget

for the year and are given an INPRES price list for drugs on the national essential drugs list. Districts place their individual orders, which are then supplied directly to the district warehouses from a combination of public and private sources (see Country Study 6.4). INPRES funds are supplemented by the health insurance scheme for civil servants, which budgets a fixed amount per family insured (US$.80 per family, for example). Some funding for the public drug supply also comes from provincial and district budgets. District-level budgeting and supply arrangements for drugs funded through insurance are similar to those for INPRES drugs. Finally, some drugs are provided through vertical programs and donors; these are supplied through provincial and district stores (WHO/DAP 1989).

Kenya. During the early to mid-1980s, Kenya implemented one of Africa's first essential drugs lists, established a new drug supply system for rural health facilities, and embarked on a program of training in rational drug use. Throughout the 1980s, the program received substantial donor funding for drug procurement, but this support declined during the early 1990s. As of the mid-1990s, drugs for government health facilities are being financed through a combination of central government allocations, donor contributions, and user fees. Government allocations vary by year but are typically less than half of the estimated need of nearly US$1 per capita. Procurement of standard hospital outpatient kits and rural health facility kits has been given first priority by both donors and the government. Government funds are used for kits that are not funded by donors. Up to 40 percent of funds generated locally from user charges and reimbursements from the National Hospital Insurance Fund are used to purchase out-of-stock essential drugs or drugs not provided in the standard kits. Experience indicates that neither central government funds nor user fee revenue alone can eliminate drug shortages. However, projections suggest that drug supply for government facilities could be sustainable with a consistent government expenditure of at least US$.50 per capita for drugs (to subsidize treatment of tuberculosis and sexually transmitted diseases, certain drugs for maternal and child health, high-cost inpatient drugs, and drugs for the poor and certain other target groups), combined with continued improvements in user fee revenue (to recover costs for most common outpatient and inpatient drugs).

---

devoted to recurrent operating expenses versus long-term development;

▶ the relative share of recurrent health expenditures for salaries, drugs, utilities, supplies, and other expenses;

▶ variations in exchange rates, which determine the international purchasing power of local currency allocations;

▶ unexpected fluctuations in the national economy due to devaluations, global changes in commodity prices, political factors, or other events.

Government economic and development policies influence GDP growth and, to an even greater extent, the share

of GDP collected as revenue for government operations. Within the government, resource allocation decisions result from a combination of historical precedent, local political forces, external pressures such as those from donors or development banks, and systematic program planning (see Chapter 3).

Arguments for Expenditures on Essential Drugs

The case for increasing expenditures on essential drugs can be made in the ministry of health or the ministry of finance. Within ministries of health, drugs can account for up to 40 percent of recurrent expenditures but are more

Figure 40.5 Relationships in Health Care Financing

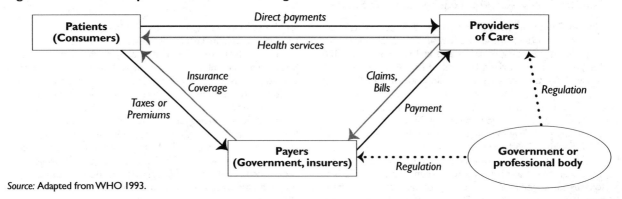

Source: Adapted from WHO 1993.

typically 10 to 20 percent. Drugs are usually second only to staff costs, which typically consume 60 to 90 percent of health budgets.

Obtaining a higher share of the budget for drugs requires changing the balance between staff and nonstaff expenditures or between curative health services that depend on essential drugs and preventive services such as immunization and health education. Managers must be prepared to respond to the argument that, with limited resources, expenditures on preventive services are more cost effective than drug treatment, even at the primary level.

In addition to demands from the health sector, public treasuries are faced with growing demands from education, other social services, industry, agriculture, national development, and defense. Because drugs often constitute such a large and visible share of health expenses, the case for increased expenditure on drugs can sometimes be taken directly to the ministry of finance.

Arguments and approaches that can be used to support central government spending on essential drugs include:

Health impact: As noted in Chapter 1, drugs are a highly cost-effective component of health care. This point is sometimes lost when policy-makers focus on symptomatic drug treatments. The case for drug allocations is strengthened by emphasizing the vital role of drugs in reducing morbidity and mortality from acute respiratory infection (ARI), diarrhea, malaria, tuberculosis, and other common killers. Appropriate treatment of sexually transmitted diseases (STDs) greatly reduces transmission of the AIDS virus, and simple antenatal iron-folate preparations reduce maternal and neonatal morbidity.

Quantification of drug needs: Systematic documentation of specific drug needs has convinced ministries in some countries to increase allocations for essential drugs (see Chapter 14).

Expenditure trend analysis: Budget allocations are typically based on a percentage increase in the budget from the previous year. This may be reasonable for salaries and local currency expenses, but because of the high foreign exchange component for drugs (50 to 100 percent, depending on local production), the last-year-plus approach may lead to a steady decline in purchasing power over time. Appropriate adjustments for both inflation and exchange rates (see Chapter 42) are needed simply to purchase the same quantities of drugs.

Budget gap analysis: Combining quantification of drug needs and expenditure trends reveals any gap between need and historical budgets and expenditures.

Per capita drug budgets: Population size and patient utilization rates for public facilities are major determinants of drug requirements. Per capita drug budgets establish a fixed amount per person per year—for example, US$.50 per capita. Each year, the per capita amount is adjusted for purchasing power (inflation and exchange rate fluctuations), and the total drug budget is calculated by multiplying the adjusted per capita figure by the current population estimate. Country Study 40.1 describes how a per capita drug budget is used in Indonesia.

Impact on utilization: When drugs are out of stock, patient attendance rates drop, reducing the use and impact of all health services.

Political visibility: The public often equates drug availability at government health facilities with quality of services. Drug shortages make for bad press; an adequate supply of drugs makes for good press.

Economic impact: In countries with the potential for local production of essential drugs, adequate public drug expenditures on locally produced drugs provide an important stimulus to the growth of local industry.

Improved management: Central drug supply units sometimes have a history of inefficiency and susceptibility to influence. Restructuring central drug supply services, improving management, and strengthening accounting control can help convince officials to increase government drug allocations.

Comparative expenditure analysis: Measured in absolute or percentage terms, some governments spend much less on essential drugs than others. Relevant regional comparisons by ministry officials and essential drugs program managers may help strengthen the case in countries that are underspending on drugs relative to other countries.

Program managers should carefully consider which of the above approaches, adapted to the local situation, will be most convincing in their own circumstances.

Management of Public Drug Expenditures

Securing an adequate budget for essential drugs is important, but proper financial management is also necessary. Common problems include difficulty gaining access to budgeted amounts, often due to shortfalls in government revenues; inability to spend budgeted amounts as a result of delays in the procurement process; and difficulty obtaining adequate foreign exchange, even if sufficient local funds are available.

Financial planning and management are discussed in Chapter 42. Problems of disbursement of government funds and foreign exchange may be reduced with autonomous central supply agencies (see Chapter 6).

≡ 40.5 Drug Sales and User Fees

The most common form of drug sale is the direct purchase of drugs by consumers from commercial pharmacies, licensed and unlicensed drug sellers, and other retail drug outlets. Excluding high- and middle-income countries with large social or private health insurance coverage, this is the most common source of drugs.

For government, NGO, or community health care programs, user fees for drugs are often part of a revolving drug fund (RDF) or community drug scheme. In an RDF, revenues from drug fees are used to replenish drug supplies. Many different forms of RDFs exist, but the common element is a direct link between fees charged and drugs dispensed. Increasingly, an RDF is simply one component of a comprehensive system of fees for publicly provided health services, which may include fees for outpatient consultation, laboratory investigations, and inpatient care.

In the context of the Bamako Initiative (see Chapter 37), community drug-sale schemes often have broader objectives. These may include health education, provision of preventive services such as immunization, and raising sufficient revenue from drug fees to help finance salaries, medical supplies, or other costs.

Public-sector RDFs and community drug-sale schemes are distinguished from private drug outlets by an emphasis on provision of essential drugs, a concern with affordability, and a direct connection between diagnosis by a health worker and appropriate drug treatment. Proponents of user charges for health care believe that

► substantial revenue can be raised by user fees;
► drug availability and the quality of care are improved;
► equity is promoted because limited public resources can then be targeted to those most in need;
► decentralization is reinforced through local control of resources;
► efficiency is fostered by fees, which reinforce the use of local rather than referral services.

In contrast, opponents of user fees believe that

► net revenue collection is often very low, considering the additional administrative costs of collecting fees;
► drug availability and quality of care often show no improvement;
► user charges replace, rather than supplement, government funding;
► people are dissuaded from seeking essential health care;
► incentives are created for overprescribing.

Considerable experience with RDFs and broader user fee programs provides examples that support both proponents and opponents of user charges. Programs that have implemented high fees with no preparation of the public and little improvement in quality have seen significant decreases in utilization; programs designed with little attention to management and accounting systems have seen substantial abuse and little revenue compared with the cost of fee collection; RDFs established without a reliable source of low-cost drugs have quickly ceased to revolve; and some schemes with drug charges have had problems with overprescribing.

At the same time, most NGOs and many government health services are turning to user charges to help share the cost of services. Chapter 44 provides additional information on RDFs, summaries of countries' experiences, and guidance on designing and implementing RDFs. Factors that are important in the design and implementation of user fee programs include

► local retention and control of revenue;
► continued or increasing levels of government funding for health;

► adequate protection mechanisms to ensure equitable access;

► businesslike orientation to financial management, supply management, and customer relations;

► strict measures to ensure accountability;

► reliable supply of low-cost essential drugs of recognized quality;

► locally appropriate fee schedules;

► phased implementation, beginning at the larger hospitals or selected districts.

In summary, RDFs and community drug schemes are not easy to implement. Many factors can undermine their intended benefits, and large-scale successes in government health services are still limited. Yet sufficient experience has accumulated to suggest that the measures listed above, and described in more detail in Chapter 44, will increase the chance of financial sustainability.

≡ 40.6 Health Insurance

Decisions that affect the availability of health insurance in a country are largely outside the control of national drug policies, essential drugs program managers, and those concerned primarily with pharmaceuticals. As insurance assumes a greater role in many developing countries, however, it is important to understand insurance concepts and to be involved from the beginning in the planning, organization, or regulation of insurance schemes.

Insurance Concepts

The basic purpose of insurance is *risk-sharing*. If an individual suffers serious illness, the cost of treatment can pose a large financial hardship. So individuals find it worthwhile to share the risk through regular payment of insurance premiums to protect themselves from ever having to pay the full cost of a catastrophic illness. Insurance spreads the burden of payment for illness among all the members of the scheme whether they are ill or healthy, poor or not.

In principle, risk-sharing through insurance is most worthwhile when the event insured against is largely unpredictable, infrequent, and costly and unwanted, unplanned, and uncontrollable by the insured. These principles apply most clearly to life, fire, and car insurance.

Applying this traditional view of insurance to medical care presents some difficulties: people can control some aspects of utilization; some services are low cost; some conditions are frequently or continuously experienced (for example, chronic illness); illness is difficult in some cases to define; people sometimes want to incur the haz-

ard (for example, pregnancy); and the presence of insurance increases the use of services. Despite these difficulties, the concept of risk-sharing through insurance has become highly developed in the health sector. Four categories of health insurance can be described:

1. *Social health insurance*: Social security funds, national health insurance funds, and other compulsory systems exist in many countries to provide health insurance for civil servants, people in the formal employment sector, and certain other groups (see Country Study 40.2). Premiums, often deducted directly from salaries or wages, may vary by income to subsidize lower-income members. Services may be provided through government facilities, insurer-operated facilities, or private facilities.

2. *Private health insurance:* Voluntary private indemnity insurance is provided through employers, mutual societies, or cooperatives or directly by companies. Hospital and physician services are usually covered, but there may be limited or no benefits for preventive services, primary care, or outpatient drugs.

3. *Managed care*: An insurance system in which the insurer plays an active role in overseeing the utilization and quality of services is termed managed care. Managed care includes health maintenance organizations (HMOs), preferred provider organizations (PPOs), and managed indemnity insurance. In such arrangements, the insurer directly manages health services or establishes contracts with specific providers. Managed care systems provide necessary health services while attempting to limit unnecessary utilization and minimize the cost increases that often result from regular indemnity insurance.

4. *Community prepaid schemes*: In a number of countries in Asia, Africa, and Latin America, prepayment plans based on insurance concepts have been developed for rural populations, members of cooperatives, and groups in informal employment (see Country Study 40.2).

Insurance systems face several problems that can undermine the potential benefits of prepayment and risk-sharing:

Moral hazard: When members of a health insurance scheme use services more frequently than if they were not insured, it is called moral hazard. Deductibles, copayments, and co-insurance are commonly used to control this problem.

Adverse selection: This term describes the tendency for people at greatest health risk and people with chronic ill-

---

Country Study 40.2 Financing through Health Insurance

Social Insurance in Costa Rica. Created in the early 1940s, the Costa Rican Social Security Fund (CCSS) now provides about 95 percent of hospital services and 85 percent of out-patient consultations. Access is nearly universal, and the health indicators are comparable to those of high-income countries. The CCSS is funded through contributions from employers, employees, and the self-employed; taxes; a hospital lottery; a small contribution from the central government; and income from rent and interest. The CCSS accounts for 80 percent of total health expenditures and provides curative care, individual preventive care such as immunizations, rehabilitation services, and health education. The Ministry of Health is currently focusing on regulation and monitoring.

Pharmaceuticals constitute 10 percent of the CCSS health expenditures. The CCSS formulary, which has existed for several decades, lists 535 drugs and dosage forms and is revised annually. Treatment guidelines, drug utilization studies, and a drug information program are also supported by the CCSS. Drug availability at CCSS pharmacies located in hospitals and outpatient clinics is greater than 90 percent. Formulary drugs are prescribed and dispensed by generic name. Drugs are provided free of charge, and no copayments are required. Nonformulary drugs require prior evaluation and approval by the CCSS Department of Pharmacotherapy, on a case-by-case basis (Normand and Weber 1994).

Community Health Insurance in Guinea Bissau. In Guinea Bissau, a village-level prepayment system—the Abota Scheme—has evolved from community drug financing started in 1980. The prepayment scheme was introduced because of difficulties arising from drug sales and because no monetary economy exists during half the year.

Villagers participate in prepayment for drugs and basic services through an annual contribution made shortly after the harvest, when cash is available. Each village decides on the amount to be collected. If individuals refuse to participate, they must pay for services provided through the fund. The national health system supports the scheme by exempting participants

in the scheme who are referred by their village health workers. A study in one region found an average of 3.5 consultations per person per year and a per capita expenditure of about $.30.

It took four to five years to develop high levels of trust and participation by villagers. Problems with the scheme have included drug shortages at the national level, foreign exchange shortages, and misuse of funds, particularly by supervisors. Nevertheless, the scheme has supported community health services and covers three-quarters of the people in many villages (Charbot et al. 1991).

A Village Insurance Fund in India. For over a decade, Kasturba Hospital in Sevagram, India, has supported community health insurance through village funds. "Premiums" come primarily from sorghum, which is collected annually on a given day by village health workers. Landless laborers and landowners are assessed according to their ability to contribute. Anyone unable to contribute is not included in the scheme the following year. At least 75 percent of the poor community must agree to participate, and in the majority of villages, this requirement has been met.

Contributors receive free primary health care, including treatment of acute illness, immunization, and maternal and child health care. The village fund covers drug costs, other recurrent costs, and payment of the village health worker. Most hospital services are covered for members through a combination of government allocations, village fund revenue, and donations.

At annual village meetings held before sorghum contributions are received, the performance of the system is reviewed, and corrective action is initiated for any problems that are identified. Continuing constraints include persistent demand for tonics and injections (discouraged by village health workers), preventable maternal and neonatal deaths arising from communication and transport constraints, and low community involvement in health activities (Jajoo 1992).

---

nesses to join voluntary insurance programs, whereas the healthiest people, whose premiums should be used to pay the bills of the sicker members, avoid joining. The effect of adverse selection is to raise costs and reduce the risk-sharing effect of insurance.

Skimming: This problem occurs when private insurers use various screening measures to avoid insuring people at greatest health risk. Skimming reduces the equity benefits of insurance by excluding those who are most in need.

Cost escalation: Rising costs can result from improvements in, or greater use of, technology; increased utilization (greater demand due to insurance coverage); and increases in population.

In addition to these problems, insurers, particularly in developing countries, frequently have to deal with misun-

derstanding of the insurance concept by the public and by health providers. Members may think that premiums are like deposits in a savings account: "If I have paid $10 each month in premiums this year, I must be sure to receive $120 worth of health services." This belief leads to unrealistic demands that everyone receive at least as much as he or she has paid in. Insurance is not sustainable in this environment, because there is no risk-sharing. Other members may avoid using their insurance because they believe that they can claim only as much as they have contributed in premiums. Considerable effort may be needed to educate members, the general public, and health providers.

Experienced public and private insurance organizations have developed measures to counter moral hazard, adverse selection, skimming, cost escalation, and lack of familiarity with insurance. Policy-makers, government insurance regulators, and insurers need to work together to implement these measures.

Many countries see the initiation or promotion of one or more insurance schemes as a way to address health financing issues. Yet the complexity of the issues involved is often poorly understood. Ideally, insurance schemes should be designed in the context of an overall health policy and health financing strategy. Issues to address when designing a health insurance scheme include policy objectives, population coverage, benefits to be included (outpatient, inpatient, drugs, and so forth), organization of health services, premium calculation and payment mechanisms, utilization and cost control measures, and administrative arrangements. WHO provides useful guidance for the design of social insurance schemes (Normand and Weber 1994).

Provision of Drug Benefits

Should social health insurance, private health insurance, or community prepaid health care schemes include drugs in their list of benefits? Policy-makers and health officials concerned with financing essential drugs should be prepared to answer this question.

According to the insurance concepts discussed above, drugs might not be a top priority for insurance coverage: common illnesses for which drugs are needed occur frequently, patients and providers may reinforce overprescription and overuse of drugs, and the potential for fraud and abuse is substantial.

However, there are at least three strong arguments for including drugs in insurance schemes. First, drugs are an essential component of modern health care. Second, early treatment of acute illnesses such as malaria, and treatment of chronic illnesses such as diabetes, can reduce costly care for complications and hospitalizations. Third, because drugs make up such a large share of household health costs in many countries, their inclusion in an insurance program will make the program more acceptable and more desirable.

Insurance coverage for outpatient drugs may be provided through private pharmacies, insurer-affiliated pharmacies, in-house pharmacies, or pharmaceutical benefits management schemes. The drug supply mechanism depends in part on whether the insurer functions only as the financier of services or whether, as with managed care, insurance is linked to specific health providers.

When private pharmacies are used, insurers either reimburse members after they have purchased drugs or reimburse the pharmacy directly. This system provides flexibility for the member but has high administrative costs and is open to considerable fraud and abuse. Insurers may require that prescriptions be filled only at specific insurer-affiliated pharmacies that have a contract or working agreement with the insurer. The member's choice is limited, but administrative costs are less, and abuse is easier to control.

Managed care organizations and polyclinics often maintain their own in-house pharmacies. Pharmacy staff may be on salary, or the entire pharmacy service may be contracted out. In either case, the insurer-provider can exert greater control over which drugs are available.

Inpatient drug supplies for insured individuals are usually provided by the hospital as part of routine inpatient care. Drug supply arrangements depend on the hospital's pharmacy services, and billing arrangements depend on the relationship between the hospital and the insurer (large HMOs and social security organizations often operate their own hospitals).

Pharmaceutical benefits management (PBM) schemes contract with insurers to manage pharmacy services. The PBM provider negotiates drug prices with suppliers, sets the formulary of drugs to be used, reviews and adjudicates claims, reviews patterns of utilization by patients and providers, audits the program to prevent fraud and abuse, and implements programs to make drug use more rational. PBM may provide such services through subcontracts with local pharmacies and through mail-order pharmacy services. Although unheard of in most countries, purchase of drugs by mail—especially drugs for chronic diseases—has existed for many years in North America and is widely accepted. Although PBM appears to add another middleman and additional expense, successful PBM schemes reduce costs to insurers.

Cost Control Measures

Well-managed insurance programs—whether public or private, mandatory or voluntary—are always looking for ways to control costs. Controlling the cost of individual services allows an insurance scheme to keep premiums down, expand benefits, or (for commercial insurers) increase profits. Public and private insurance programs control pharmaceutical expenditures through measures related to payment, management, prescribing patterns, and utilization (see Country Study 40.3).

Control of Payment (Can Be Used Separately or in Combination)

► Copayments are payments made by the member, such as a charge of $1 per item for generic drugs and $2 per item for brand-name drugs.

- Co-insurance is a specified percentage to be paid by the member—for example, 25 percent for drugs used in serious and chronic illnesses, 50 percent for most other pharmaceuticals, and 75 percent for symptomatic treatments for minor illnesses.
- A deductible is a specified initial amount the insured must pay before services are covered. It is usually a set amount per quarter or per year.
- Maximum allowable cost (MAC) or maximum reimbursement price (MRP) specifies the highest reimbursement amount for each item to control drug charges, encourage generic substitution, or establish copayment levels.

Control of Prescribing Patterns

- Provider drug budgets encourage providers to work within a total drug budget for a patient population.
- Selective reimbursement of drugs on formulary lists or lists of essential drugs (white lists) encourages compliance. The use of other products or therapeutic categories (black lists), including nonprescription drugs, vitamins, and minerals, can be discouraged by lack of reimbursement.
- Voluntary or mandatory prescribing or dispensing of generic equivalents lowers costs.
- Standard treatment guidelines are recommended to prescribers, especially in managed care programs, for common or high-cost diseases.

Control of Utilization

- Prior authorization by the insurer is sometimes used for all prescriptions but is more common for specific drugs or drug categories.
- Caps on services may be instituted, such as limits on the quantities dispensed, number of items given at one time, frequency of refills, or total expenditures.
- Utilization review identifies overprescription or other forms of inappropriate prescribing or dispensing.

These cost control measures vary in terms of their administrative complexity, effect on access to drugs, impact on rational use of drugs, and acceptability to members and health care providers.

Access to Drugs and Rational Drug Use

Cost control measures must not reduce access to essential drugs, which remain a highly cost-effective element of health care. Yet insurers, particularly those in new programs and low-income countries, are wary of the costs of overuse and fraud. In the extreme, one Latin American

Country Study 40.3 Drug Benefits in Zimbabwe Health Insurance Schemes

Since 1982, Zimbabwe's largest medical aid society has provided a "drug benefit scheme" through which prescription costs are refunded to members wholly or in part. From its inception, the scheme incorporated three cost containment measures: (1) copayment of a flat fee per prescription item (equivalent to the pharmacist's dispensing fee), (2) variable co-insurance based on the therapeutic value (VEN category) of individual items (four categories of drugs vary from 100 percent reimbursement for lifesaving drugs to 100 percent payment by members for over-the-counter drugs), and (3) an annual monetary limit on the value of drug refunds per member.

Member payments are made at the point of dispensing. Pharmacists submit claims to the medical aid society for reimbursement of amounts covered by the drug benefit scheme. The overall savings to the medical aid society from members' payments ranged from 25 to 33 percent of the total retail cost. It is likely that this system also resulted in savings by influencing drug selection and reducing the total number of drugs per consultation.

A "generics policy" has ensured low prices in Zimbabwe's public health services. In contrast, prescribing and dispensing by brand name was the norm in the private sector and meant significantly higher prices. In 1991, prices of brand-name imports escalated; a workshop organized by the Ministry of Health with representatives from professional associations and medical aid societies recommended that reimbursement by medical aid societies be limited to a reference price indexed on generic drug prices.

Lack of low-cost generics delayed implementation of this recommendation until economic reforms in 1993–94 facilitated expansion and greater competition in the private pharmaceutical market. In February 1995, the National Association of Medical Aid Societies instituted a maximum award based on the price of generics, with a forecasted average savings of 40 percent on the brand-name product. Exceptions are made only for patented drugs for which no generic equivalent is yet available. This new system was accompanied by a campaign of information and advocacy, requesting members to insist on generic or to pay the difference, in order to maintain benefits and contain contribution rates.

Source: H. Nazerali.

country in the mid-1990s proposed omitting drugs entirely from its national health insurance scheme.

Unfortunately, those most in need are often the most affected by cost control measures. Experience in developed countries has demonstrated that overly restrictive cost control measures can reduce drug utilization but increase total health care costs through deferred treatment and increases in hospitalization and other costs.

Rational drug use in the context of insurance schemes requires a careful balance between controlling costs and ensuring access to needed drugs. Essential drugs or formulary lists, standard treatment guidelines, prescriber and dispenser training, public and patient education, and other measures described in Chapters 28–33 are relevant to improving drug use in the context of insurance schemes.

≡ 40.7 Voluntary and Other Local Financing

The cost of providing health care, including essential drugs, may be supported by a variety of community, employer, or other local financing sources.

NGOs play a significant role in the health services of some countries. NGOs often attract foreign and local donations of drugs, medical supplies, equipment, and cash. Direct user charges often provide the major share of financing for these services. Essential drug supplies from NGOs may be subsidized by donations of drugs and cash, but markups on drugs are often used to subsidize salaries, immunizations, or other NGO costs.

NGOs that are able to provide significant amounts of health care and remain financially viable help balance the overall national sustainability equation (see Figure 40.1). Thus, as described in Chapter 6, it is in the interest of governments to facilitate NGOs' efforts to provide essential drugs as part of their overall package of services.

Aside from community drug schemes and other Bamako Initiative–type programs, a host of voluntary community mechanisms exists in different countries to help support local health services (see Chapter 37). In some countries, villages maintain sick funds to pay the health costs, including drugs, of the poorest members of the village. Monies come from periodic assessments or special fund-raising events. Aside from structured insurance-like schemes, however, informal community fund-raising has not been able to sustain the supply of drugs for entire communities.

In many countries, some private companies and cooperative societies (coffee growers, for example) provide health care for employees or members by maintaining a company health service, by reimbursing local private health providers ("self-insurance"), or by contributing to private insurance for employees. Companies may also work with local government health facilities, supplementing government funding with company funding for drugs, medical supplies, or other expenses.

Such arrangements also help balance the financial sustainability equation. They should be supported with information about the essential drugs concept, with copies of the national essential drugs list and standard treatment guidelines, and perhaps, on a selective basis, with access to public supply services.

≡ 40.8 Donor Financing and Development Loans

Donor assistance may come from multilateral institutions such as WHO, UNICEF, and development banks; from bilateral arrangements with donor governments; or from charitable organizations, other NGOs, and foundations. Such assistance is typically targeted toward long-term health sector development, often concentrating on specific areas such as primary health care, essential drugs, or immunization. Multilateral and bilateral organizations generally do not support recurrent costs for personnel, regular supplies of essential drugs, and other operating costs. International and local religious organizations and NGOs have supported recurrent costs, but such funding has become more difficult to obtain.

For essential drugs, donor assistance has been used effectively in many countries to provide short- and long-term staff training, to develop and implement national drug policies, to improve storage and transport systems, to improve supply management, to promote rational drug use, to support local production, and to strengthen drug regulatory and quality assurance capacity.

Loans may be used for the long-term development of health care systems, human resources, and physical infrastructure. They may provide working capital to establish a revolving drug fund. But loans generally should not be used to finance the current cost of personnel, drugs, medical supplies, or other routine operating expenses.

In the poorest countries—with minimal foreign exchange earnings, limited cash income among the population, and no local production capacity—combined public and private resources may be insufficient to provide all essential drug needs, even with the best selection, procurement, distribution, and use of drugs. For such countries, outside assistance may be needed to fund some basic essential drug requirements.

Nevertheless, long-term human, financial, and institutional sustainability is an essential consideration in all development projects. Intensive financial support and large teams of advisers may achieve short-term success, but to achieve sustained success, a realistic transition to local staffing and financing must be planned from the outset.

Finally, governments can coordinate assistance from donors by establishing national health and drug policies, by inviting donors to participate in the development of a master plan as a framework for action, and by convening regular donor coordination meetings (see Chapter 43).

≡ 40.9 Comparing Financing Mechanisms

Few health systems rely on a single funding mechanism. Political, economic, and social factors influence options for health financing. But financing mechanisms should meet certain stated policy objectives, and discussions about financing should be informed by a clear understanding of the choices.

Criteria for Evaluating Financing Mechanisms

Access to drugs, rational drug use, efficiency, equity, sustainability, and feasibility are among the most common and important criteria for evaluating funding mechanisms.

Access to drugs: Are the availability and affordability of drugs improved? With user charges, for example, drugs may become more available but less affordable. In the end, are more people receiving the essential drugs they need?

Rational drug use: Does the financing mechanism create incentives for overuse, underuse, or misuse of drugs? Patient demand is high when drugs are free, but provider-induced demand may be high if revenue from drug charges is used for staff salaries. A managed care insurance plan may achieve a uniquely effective balance if it stimulates patient demand by expanding access, uses cost controls to contain demand, and promotes standard treatments by providers.

Efficiency: Does the financing mechanism encourage the maximum output or health benefit from available resources? As noted earlier and in Chapter 3, there are two broad categories of efficiency—allocative and technical. Drug financing decisions often aim to improve technical efficiency related to drug management.

Equity: Who benefits, and who pays for services? Equity in health care means that essential care is provided according to need and financed according to ability to pay. Equity implies universal access (availability and affordability) to basic health services, including drugs, regardless of income level.

Sustainability: Will a reasonable level of funding be maintained over time? Both the amount of revenue generated and the reliability of funding over time are important.

Administrative requirements: What are the administrative and managerial requirements to make the funding mechanism operational? For instance, managing a viable revolving drug fund is many times more demanding than managing a system in which drugs are free. Insurance programs require a host of new administrative arrangements. In contrast, government financing systems are usually well established, and donor administrative requirements, though often tedious, are usually well defined.

Other criteria that may be used to evaluate health financing options include *acceptability, community involvement, flexibility,* and *health impact.* Acceptability refers to the balance of support and resistance from the public, providers, and politicians. With financing mechanisms that meet other criteria, acceptance often grows with experience and understanding. This is typically the case with insurance programs and user charges. Community involvement may be valued for its own sake, but it is often considered with the other criteria because it may contribute to efficiency, equity, and sustainability. Flexibility is the extent to which funds can be used for various purposes. Donor funds tend to have the greatest restrictions, and community financing schemes have greater flexibility. Improved health impact is the ultimate objective of drug financing reforms, but data that directly link funding and impact are scant. Access to essential drugs becomes a more immediate measure of potential impact.

Application of the Criteria for Evaluating Funding Mechanisms

Using these evaluation criteria helps structure the comparison of funding mechanisms. Experience, local circumstances, and degree of subjectivity affect the way individual criteria are applied to financing mechanisms. Figure 40.6 provides an illustrative comparison of funding mechanisms according to the evaluation criteria above. Several overall observations can be made.

Stereotyping and Oversimplification Should Be Avoided. Free government services may appear equitable, unless (as in some countries) political forces result in public drug supplies being concentrated at national and regional referral hospitals in urban areas. User fees for poor rural populations may appear inequitable, but equity is actually improved if a situation of constant shortages requiring private purchase at high prices is replaced by a community drug scheme providing a reliable supply of low-cost drugs. There are national social health insurance programs that provide health benefits in such a way that low-income members are actually subsidizing high-income members. For example, in some countries, social security taxes are imposed only on wages below a certain level, so those with higher earning capacity do not have to pay taxes on much of their income. These wealthier people are often city dwellers who have the greatest access to, and make the most use of, government health services, thereby benefiting disproportionately from the payments of those with lower incomes.

Examples of common misperceptions about access, rational use, efficiency, sustainability, and administrative

Figure 40.6 Comparison of Funding Mechanisms by Evaluation Criteria

Funding Mechanism	Access to Essential Drugs	Appropriate Drug Use	Efficiency	Equity	Sustainability	Administrative Requirements
Public Financing (government budgets)	▲ If budget sufficient and management adequate	▲ With good selection and prescribing	■ No incentive for improvement	▲▼ Depends on who pays taxes and who receives services	▲▼ Depends on economic growth and government revenues	■ No new requirements
User Fees Government revolving drug funds (RDFs)	▲ Access decreases for poor unless exemptions and other protections in place	▲▼ Fees may discourage overuse or lead to underuse; may encourage overprescribing if revenue for staff	▲ Success depends on supply management improvements	▲ Higher-income contribute more; poor benefit if supply improved	▲ With good management, reliable drug supply	▲ Much more demanding than free system
Community drug schemes	▲ Same as RDFs	▲▼ Same as RDFs	▲ Same as RDFs	▲ Local control and targeting support equity	▲ Same as RDFs	▲ Improvements require significant local management capacity
Direct private drug purchases	▲ Primarily benefits urban and higher-income people	▼ Prices create affordability problem, which often leads to inadequate doses	▲ Strong financial incentive	▼ Poor cannot afford essential drugs	▲ For population that can afford drugs	▲▼ Systems exist in private sector
Health Insurance Social	▲ If drug benefits included in benefit package	▲▼ Appropriate use if insurance cost controls in existence; inappropriate use if patients exert pressure on provider for drugs	■ No efficiency incentive	▲ Should be very equitable	▲ Requires good management, adequate premiums	▲ Substantial administrative requirements for new system; requires fraud and abuse controls
Private	▲ Same as social insurance	▲▼ Same as social insurance	▲ Some incentive	▲▼ Increased equity depends on membership	▲ Requires good management, sufficient number of members to maintain sustainability	▲ Same as social insurance
Managed care	▲ Same as social insurance	▲ Often promotes rational use through standard treatments, other measures	▲ Strong incentive	▲▼ Same as private insurance	▲▼ Same as private insurance	▲ Same as social insurance
Community Financing (different mechanisms have different effects)	▲▼	▲▼	▲	▲	▲	▲▼
Donor Financing Bilateral and multilateral grants	▲	▲▼ Similar to public financing	■ Similar to public financing	▲ Usually involves transfer from richer countries	▼ Not sustainable	▲ Reporting
Development requirements loans	▲	▲▼ Same as grants	■ Same as grants	▲▼ Depends on terms and sources of funds for repayment	▼ Not sustainable	▲ Reporting

Key: ▲ = increases; ▼ = decreases; ▲▼ = may increase or decrease; ■ = no change.

requirements could also be cited. The point is that comparison of financing mechanisms should be based on a clear analysis, experience, and the best available information, rather than on untested assumptions or stereotyped thinking.

Evaluation Often Depends on Effectiveness of Implementation. Proponents of revolving drug funds cite their potential for financing a sustainable supply of low-cost drugs. Opponents cite numerous programs that generate minimal revenue with much effort, and examples in which drug charges have led to overprescribing. As noted earlier, the financial performance and health impact of a user fee program are highly dependent on the way in which the program is managed and monitored.

Similarly, insurance programs are complex undertakings. A successful insurance plan must organize the registration of members and dependents, the definition of services covered, accurate projections of payments to set premiums, collection of premiums, handling of claims, payment to providers, utilization review, quality monitoring, and cost control. Bad planning or poor implementation of different elements can result in a program that is inefficient, inequitable, not sustainable, and administratively chaotic.

In short, it is important to distinguish between a financing mechanism that is inappropriate for a given setting and one that might be appropriate but is ineffectively implemented.

Seek Improvement, Not Perfection. Policy-makers sometimes discard a new financing alternative because it has certain limitations, potential inequities, or other undesirable features. The question is not whether a specific financing mechanism meets all criteria—none do. The question is whether it will, on balance, improve the drug financing situation.

Doing nothing about drug financing is often the easiest course for an uncertain policy-maker or a nervous manager. But if financial resources are inadequate, access and quality of care will decline. Analysis of financing mechanisms should aim at identifying actions that will lead to significant improvements, not at finding perfect solutions.

≡ 40.10 Developing a Drug Financing Strategy

Because drug financing is part of health financing, in many countries, complementary financing arrangements are evolving for different health care needs and population groups. Although each financing mechanism has benefits and limitations, the net effect of the pluralist approach is to distribute the burden of health financing across several sectors (see Country Study 40.4).

If essential drug supply is adequate, the challenge for policy-makers and essential drugs program managers is to maintain the funding, drug supply system, and drug use patterns that ensure this adequacy. If the supply of essential drugs is inadequate, efforts should be made to use available funds better through more efficient selection, procurement, distribution, and use of drugs. Efforts to balance public resources and the demand for health care may also include measures to encourage private and NGO health providers.

When efforts to improve therapeutic and operational efficiency and to moderate demand for drugs do not balance the sustainability equation, additional funding is needed. Managers can make the case for greater government funding of drugs, introduce or strengthen user fees for drugs, introduce or expand health insurance coverage for drugs, or seek donor assistance. In each case, efforts should be made to ensure that available public resources are targeted to those most in need.

The challenge for policy-makers, essential drugs program managers, NGO managers, and others concerned with drug financing is to make optimal use of every available source of financing. Success depends on political commitment, adaptation of financing mechanisms to local circumstances, good leadership and management, and modification of financing systems based on experience. Equity of access, quality of drugs, and rational use remain key objectives for any financing strategy. ■

Country Study 40.4 Pluralistic Approach to Health Financing in China

Between 1952 and 1982, China achieved substantial health improvements associated with an emphasis on prevention, community organization, cooperative health financing, and a modest US$5 per capita expenditure. Since the early 1980s, Chinese health policy, following economic policy, has shifted the provision and financing of health care toward a free market system. The result is a pluralistic system of financing in which labor, government employee, and cooperative insurance provide 44 percent of revenue; user fees provide 36 percent; and central, provincial, and local governments provide 20 percent (see Figure A).

The three main types of insurance are

1. **labor insurance** for workers and retirees of state and large collectively owned enterprises and their dependents;

2. **government employee insurance** for government employees, but not their dependents;

3. **cooperative medical insurance** and other prepayment schemes for rural populations. These are remnants and derivations of the cooperative medical programs, which collapsed after economic reforms of the agriculture sector in 1991.

About 50 percent of China's nearly 500 million urban dwellers are covered by one of the first two systems; only 10 percent of the rural population is currently covered by insurance or prepayment schemes.

Government sources account for only about 25 percent of government hospital revenues and 20 percent of health center budgets. Except for drugs and new technologies such as specialized X-rays, the price commission has set prices at less than cost. Hospitals, health centers, and village doctors are allowed a margin of 13 to 15 percent over wholesale prices for Western drugs and 25 percent for traditional herbal medicines. As a result, hospitals and health centers use drug sales to generate extra revenue for salary supplements and other operating costs. Village health stations are staffed by one female and one male village doctor. Although they receive a government stipend for public health work, village doctors derive most of their income from drug sales. Village stations usually stock 100 to 200 commonly used drugs.

Incentives created by these financing changes have reportedly led to overprescribing at hospitals and village stations and the use of more expensive drugs. Prescribing of multiple antibiotics, outpatient intravenous infusions, injections, and various combination drugs is reportedly common. In one study, insured surgical patients had drug costs that were twice those of uninsured patients, with no measurable difference in outcome. Not surprisingly, 45 percent of total health expenditures are for drugs (see Figure B).

China's experience suggests that a pluralistic approach to health financing is possible, but that equity, efficiency, and quality of care may suffer unless there is appropriate regulation, planning, and management. Drug prices must be made more rational to prevent the misuse of drugs, and mechanisms are needed to ensure access for poor, rural, and other needy populations.

Figure A Sources of Health Financing

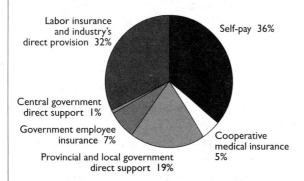

Labor insurance and industry's direct provision 32%
Self-pay 36%
Central government direct support 1%
Government employee insurance 7%
Cooperative medical insurance 5%
Provincial and local government direct support 19%

Figure B Spending by Expense Category

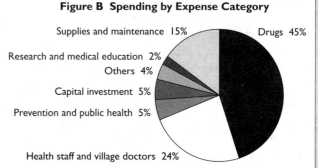

Supplies and maintenance 15%
Drugs 45%
Research and medical education 2%
Others 4%
Capital investment 5%
Prevention and public health 5%
Health staff and village doctors 24%

Sources: Hsiao 1995; Bumgarner 1992.

≡ Assessment Guide

Drug Financing Policy and Needs

- ► Is drug financing included in national health and national drug policy?
- ► Is there a comprehensive estimate of drug financing needs?
- ► Has a formal budget gap analysis been done recently?

National Economic and Health Financing Indicators

- ► What is the per capita GDP?
- ► What is the total national health expenditure (public and private) per capita?
- ► What is the total national health expenditure as a percentage of the GDP?
- ► What are total government expenditures as a percentage of the GDP?
- ► What percentage of total public expenditures do health expenditures represent?
- ► What is the percentage breakdown of health spending by source (public, private, NGO, donor)?

National Drug Financing Indicators

- ► What is the total per capita drug consumption (from all sources)?
- ► What percentage of total health expenditures (from all sources) do drugs represent?
- ► What is the percentage breakdown of drug spending by source (public, private, NGO, donor)?
- ► What percentage of total consumption do imports represent?

Public Drug Financing Indicators

- ► What is the total public expenditure on drugs?
- ► What is the per capita public expenditure on drugs?
- ► What is the percentage breakdown of public health expenditures (personnel, drugs, other)?

Efficiency of Public Drug Expenditures

- ► Allocative efficiency: Is the drug budget appropriately distributed to ensure essential drugs, address priority health problems, and serve groups most in need?
- ► What percentage of the public drug budget is used for national and referral hospitals?

- ► Therapeutic efficiency: Are an essential drugs list and standard treatments used? Is drug use rational?
- ► Operating efficiency: Are procurement and distribution well managed?

User Charges for Drugs (see Chapter 44)

- ► Are user fees charged for drugs and services at government facilities?
- ► Is revenue used as a revolving fund specifically to resupply drugs?
- ► What percentage of government drug expenditures is recovered through user charges?

Health Insurance

- ► What types of health insurance presently exist: compulsory, voluntary, managed care, community?
- ► What percentage of the population is covered by health insurance?
- ► What percentage of those insured have policies that cover drugs?
- ► What methods exist for supply and payment for drug benefits?

Donor Financing (see Chapter 43)

- ► What percentage of total government health expenditures is represented by international assistance?
- ► What is the total value of international aid for drugs?
- ► What are the major sources of donor funding for the pharmaceutical sector?

Effects of Current Drug Financing Arrangements

- ► What is the availability of drugs in the public and private sectors?
- ► How affordable are drugs in the public and private sectors?
- ► How equitable is access to drugs for rural, poor, and medically needy populations?
- ► What are the incentives for rational or irrational drug use?

Note: It is preferable to compare budgets and expenditures in terms of local currency, US dollars, and international dollars. Data for the three most recent years should be used to show expenditure trends. Both budgeted and actual expenditure data should be used. Price basis for drugs should be clarified (producer, wholesale, retail).

≡ Glossary

ABC analysis: Classification of inventory items into three categories (A, B, and C) according to the value of their annual usage, which is useful for analyzing drug consumption and utilization, comparing actual versus planned purchases, justifying procurement budgets, guiding procurement patterns, and setting priorities for stock management.

Accounts payable: Money owed by an organization for goods or services received.

Accounts receivable: Money owed to an organization for goods or services provided.

Accrual basis accounting system: An accounting or budgeting system that records revenue when it is earned, expenses when they are incurred, and the cost of using fixed assets such as buildings or equipment, in contrast to the cash basis accounting system.

Adverse selection: The tendency for people at greatest health risk and those with chronic illnesses to join voluntary insurance programs, whereas the healthiest individuals (whose premiums should be used to pay the bills of the sicker members) avoid joining. The effect is to raise costs and reduce the risk-sharing effect of insurance.

Allocative efficiency: Carrying out the combination of activities that achieves the greatest net benefit.

Analysis of expiry dates: The analysis of stock position versus expiry dates in the supply system inventory to avoid or minimize losses due to wastage.

Asset: Anything of value that helps an organization provide service, for example, cash, land, buildings, equipment, and inventories.

Balance sheet: The financial report that summarizes the value of the assets, liabilities, and reserves of an organization at a specific time.

Bank reconciliation: Comparison of the balance in the bank account according to the bank statement with the balance in the accounting records.

Budget performance report: A report that compares budgeted and actual revenues and expenses.

Capital budget: A plan for the acquisition and financing of fixed or long-term assets.

Cash basis accounting system: The accounting or budgeting system that records revenue only when it is received and expenses only when they are paid, in contrast to the accrual basis accounting system.

Cash flow forecast: A statement prepared from the workplan and budget that projects cash receipts, disbursements, and balances, to help ensure sufficient cash to cover all anticipated financial obligations each month.

Chart of accounts: A listing of all programs, responsibility centers, and categories by which the revenues and expenses will be recorded, with a unique code for each.

Co-insurance: Cost control measure in insurance schemes in which the member pays a specified percentage of the cost—for example, 25 percent for drugs used in serious and chronic illnesses, 50 percent for most other pharmaceuticals, and 75 percent for symptomatic treatment for minor illnesses.

Community drug scheme: A form of revolving drug fund that is managed at the community level and often has broader objectives, such as health education, provision of preventive services, or financing of salaries, medical supplies, or other costs, in addition to the financing of drugs.

Copayment: Cost control measure in insurance schemes in which the member pays a set charge per item received; copayment may be lower for generic drugs, higher for brand-name drugs.

Cost escalation: Rising costs that result from improvements in, or greater use of, technology; increased utilization (greater demand due to insurance coverage); and increases in population.

Current assets: Assets that are typically used or converted into cash within a year, such as cash, drugs, and accounts receivable.

Deductible: Payment of a specified initial amount by an insured person before services are covered; usually a set amount per quarter or per year.

Depreciation: The practice of charging as an annual expense the portion of a long-lasting asset's useful life that is used up each year.

Differential pricing: The setting of different price levels for different types of patients, types of drugs, levels of facility, or other criteria, employed in many revolving drug funds to promote access to services.

Drug stock account: Account maintained as part of an accrual basis accounting system, showing figures for opening and closing balances and drugs received and issued.

Exemption: A release from payment of fees for specific population groups or disease or drug types, employed in many revolving drug fund schemes to promote access to services.

Fixed assets: Assets that have a useful life of longer than one year, such as land, buildings, furniture, and large pieces of equipment.

Fixed costs: Costs that do not vary with the level of service provided or the number of people served—for example, office expenses, insurance, and rent.

Fund balance (or **equity**): In a nonprofit organization, the value of assets less liabilities.

Health insurance: A financing scheme characterized by risk-sharing, in which regular payments of premiums are made by or on behalf of members (the insured). The insurer pays the cost or a set portion of the cost for covered health services.

Income and expense report (also called **income statement** or **profit and loss statement**): The financial report that summarizes income and expenses and cumulative surplus or deficit for the period covered by the report, as compared with the previous year.

International dollars: The relative purchasing power of different currencies based on United Nations comparisons.

Lead-time analysis: The analysis of supplier lead time (interval between decision to order and receipt of stock), to help in selecting the best suppliers for future procurements, and payment lead time (interval between receipt of goods and payment to supplier), to monitor procurement office compliance with contracts.

Liability: Any obligation or debt of an organization owed to suppliers, employees, banks, or other parties.

Managed care: Insurance systems in which the insurer plays an active role in overseeing the utilization and quality of service, for example, through health maintenance organizations (HMOs), preferred provider organizations (PPOs), and managed indemnity insurance.

Maximum allowable cost (MAC) or **maximum reimbursement price (MRP)**: Cost control measure in insurance schemes that specifies the highest amount that will be reimbursed for each pharmaceutical item dispensed.

Moral hazard: Term used to describe what happens when members of a health insurance scheme use services more frequently than if they were not insured.

Operating costs (or **recurrent costs**): The regular expenses of running programs and providing services (as opposed to capital expenses).

Pharmaceutical benefits management (PBM) scheme: Mechanism in which organizations contract with insurers to provide pharmacy services, often through subcontracts with local pharmacies and through mail-order pharmacy services.

Pipeline analysis: Analysis of the logistics system to identify the optimal location and quantities of stock in the distribution network. This serves as the basis for devising more efficient ordering and stock-keeping policies and procedures.

Price comparison analysis: The comparison of a supply system's costs and prices to those of other programs or systems; for example, comparison of procurement prices to those paid by neighboring supply systems or obtainable internationally, or of sales prices to prices in the local private and NGO sectors.

Prior authorization: Cost control measure in insurance schemes in which the insurer retains the right to approve drug use before drugs are dispensed to the patient.

Private health insurance: Voluntary private indemnity insurance provided by private insurance companies through employers, mutual societies, or cooperatives.

Revolving drug fund: A drug sales program in which revenues from drug fees are used to replenish drug supplies.

Social health insurance: Compulsory health insurance provided to civil servants, people in the formal employment sector, and certain other groups through programs such as social security funds, national health insurance funds, and other systems. Premiums are often deducted directly from salaries or wages.

Technical efficiency: Using inputs to achieve the greatest output for a given cost or to achieve a given output at the lowest cost. For drug management, this includes therapeutic efficiency (selection and use) and operational efficiency (management of procurement and distribution).

Therapeutic category analysis: The analysis of expenditures by therapeutic category, for comparison with morbidity patterns and public health priorities, as a means of focusing cost control efforts.

User fees: Charges paid by the users of a service.

Variable costs: Costs that vary according to the level of service provided or number of people served—for example, drug expenditures.

VEN system: A system of categorizing drugs by their public health value (*v*ital, *e*ssential, and *n*onessential), which can be useful in setting purchasing priorities, determining safety stock levels, and directing staff activities.

Waiver: A release from payment of fees based on financial hardship, employed in many revolving drug fund schemes to promote access to services.

≡ References and Further Readings

★ = *Key readings.*

Abel-Smith, B. 1992. Health insurance in developing countries: Lessons from experience. *Health Policy and Planning* 7:215–26.

Ballance, R., J. Pogány, and H. Forstner. 1992. *The world's pharmaceutical industries: An international perspective on innovation, competition and policy*. Prepared for the United Nations Industrial Development Organization (UNIDO). Aldershot, England: Edward Elgar Publishing.

Bumgarner, J. R. 1992. *China: Long-term issues and options in the health transition*. Washington, D.C.: World Bank.

Charbot, J., M. Boal, and A. da Silva. 1991. National community health insurance scheme at village level: The case from Guinea Bissau. *Health Policy and Planning* 6:46–54.

★ Dumoulin, J., M. Kaddar, and G. Velásquez. 1991. *Access to drugs and finance: Basic economic and financial analysis.* WHO/DAP/91.5. Geneva: World Health Organization.

★ Foster, S. 1991. Supply and use of essential drugs in sub-Saharan Africa: Some issues and possible solutions. *Social Science and Medicine* 32:1201–18.

Gilson, L., et al. 1994. The potential of health sector nongovernmental organizations: Policy options. *Health Policy and Planning* 9(1):14–24.

Goodman, H., and Waddington, C. 1993. Financing health care. OXFAM Practical Health Guide no. 8. London: OXFAM.

Hsiao, W. C. L. 1995. The Chinese health care system: Lessons for other nations. *Social Science and Medicine* 41:1047–55.

Jajoo, U. N. 1992. Risk-sharing in rural health care. *World Health Forum* 13:171–75.

Jarrett, S., and S. Ofosu-Amaah. 1992. Strengthening health services for MCH in Africa: The first four years of the Bamako Initiative. *Health Policy and Planning* 7:164–76.

Mossialos, E., C. Ranos, and B. Abel-Smith, eds. 1994. *Cost containment, pricing and financing of pharmaceuticals in the European Community: The policy-makers' view*. Athens: LSE Health and Pharmetrica.

MSH (Management Sciences for Health). 1992. *Financing and financial management of drug supply*. Managing Drug Supply Training Series, part 2. Boston: MSH.

Murray, C. J. L., and D. D. López, eds. 1994. *Global comparative assessments in the health sector: Disease burden, expenditures, and intervention packages*. Geneva: WHO.

★ Normand, C., and A. Weber. 1994. *Social health insurance: A guidebook for planning*. WHO/SHS/94.3. Geneva: World Health Organization.

★ Shaw, R. P., and C. C. Griffin. 1995. *Financing health care in sub-Saharan Africa through user fees and insurance*. Washington, D.C.: World Bank.

Stinson, W. 1982. *Community financing of public health care*. International Health Programs, series 1, no. 4. Washington, D.C.: American Public Health Association.

Vogel, R. J., and B. Stephens. 1989. Availability of pharmaceuticals in sub-Saharan Africa: Roles of the public, private, and church mission sectors. *Social Science and Medicine* 29:479–86.

★ WHO (World Health Organization). 1993. *Evaluation of recent changes in the financing of health services: Report of a WHO study group*. Technical Report Series no. 829. Geneva: WHO.

WHO (World Health Organization). 1996. *Global comparative pharmaceutical expenditures*. Action Programme on Essential Drugs. Geneva: WHO.

WHO/DAP (World Health Organization/Action Programme on Essential Drugs). 1989. *Review of the drug programme in Indonesia: Report of a WHO mission, October 16–November 3, 1989*. DAP 90.11. Geneva: WHO/DAP.

World Bank. 1993. *World development report: Investing in health*. New York: Oxford University Press.

| Part I | Part II | Part III | Part IV |
| Introduction | Policy and Legal Framework | Drug Management Cycle | **Management Support Systems** |

A Organization and Management
B Financing and Sustainability ▶
C Information Management
D Human Resources Management

40 Drug Financing
    Strategies

**41 Analyzing and
    Controlling Drug
    Expenditures**

42 Financial Planning and
    Management

43 Donor Financing

44 Revolving Drug Funds

Chapter 41

Analyzing and Controlling Drug Expenditures

≡ Summary

This chapter focuses on identifying and controlling excess costs in the selection, procurement, distribution, and use of drugs. Several analytical tools are presented that help managers quantify costs and identify areas where costs can be reduced; the information provided is also essential in designing and monitoring interventions to control costs.

The VEN system *categorizes drugs by their relative public health value. It is useful in setting purchasing priorities, determining safety stock levels and drug sales prices, and directing staff activities. The categories in the original system are vital (V), essential (E), and nonessential (N). Some health systems find a two-category system more useful than the three-tiered VEN; for example, the categories might be V and N, differentiating between those drugs that must always be in stock and other drugs.*

ABC value analysis examines the annual consumption of drugs and expenditures for procurement by dividing the drugs consumed into three categories. Class A includes 10 to 20 percent of items, which account for 75 to 80 percent of expenditures. Class B items represent 10 to 20 percent of items and 15 to 20 percent of expenditures. Class C items are 60 to 80 percent of items but only about 5 to 10 percent of expenditures. ABC analysis can be used to

- *measure the degree to which actual consumption reflects public health needs and morbidity;*
- *reduce inventory levels and costs by arranging for more frequent purchase or delivery of smaller quantities of class A items;*
- *seek major cost reductions by finding lower prices on class A items, where savings will be more noticeable;*
- *assign import and inventory control staff, to ensure that large orders of class A items are handled expeditiously.*

Therapeutic category analysis considers the utilization and financial impact of various therapeutic categories of drugs and then compares cost and therapeutic benefit to select the most cost-effective drugs in each major therapeutic category. This can be done to select drugs for a formulary or procurement list.

Price comparison analysis compares drug prices paid by different supply systems, as one measure of procurement efficiency. The analysis can also compare supply system acquisition and selling prices with local private-sector prices to gauge the cost effectiveness of in-house pharmaceutical services and to assess price elasticity for cost recovery.

Total variable cost analysis compiles information on variable costs associated with purchasing and inventory management, to help managers consider options for change in terms of their impact on total variable costs.

Lead-time analysis is a systematic approach to tracking procurement lead times, determining the points at which lead time can be reduced, and adjusting safety stock appropriately. Payment time should also be analyzed (when delayed payment to suppliers is feasible).

Expiry date analysis examines levels of stock on hand and their expiry dates and compares this information with average rates of consumption to assess the likelihood of wastage (and to develop appropriate countermeasures).

Hidden cost analysis examines supplier performance to identify any hidden costs incurred because of problems such as late deliveries and short shipments. Hidden costs may make one supplier considerably more expensive than a competitor that offers a higher unit price but better performance.

≡ 41.1 Tools for Analyzing Costs

The two largest centers of recurrent costs in most public drug supply systems are personnel expenses and drug purchases. Controlling personnel costs usually means reducing staff, which may be politically difficult. However, it may be possible to reform policies so that extra staff are not employed by the drug supply system, where they contribute to lowered productivity and increased losses due to wastage and theft (see Chapter 47).

This chapter concentrates on techniques for analyzing nonpersonnel costs in the drug supply system so that managers can identify major costs, losses, and opportunities for savings. All these techniques have been cited in earlier chapters. Here, the focus is on how to perform each analysis and how to use the results. The techniques considered are

- VEN system
- ABC analysis
- therapeutic category analysis
- price comparison analysis
- total variable cost analysis
- lead-time and payment-time analysis
- expiry date analysis
- hidden cost analysis.

Although it is possible to carry out these analyses manually, it is very time consuming, except in small supply systems that use relatively few drug products. It is much easier to do them with a computer. Expensive computers and customized software are not required—all the analyses in this chapter can be done with commercial spreadsheet software, although therapeutic category analysis is easier with a special-purpose database program.

≡ 41.2 VEN System

The VEN system sets priorities for selection, procurement, and use according to the potential health impact of individual drugs. VEN assigns each drug on the formulary or essential drugs list to one of the following three categories:

V: *vital* drugs are potentially lifesaving, have significant withdrawal side effects (making regular supply mandatory), or are crucial to providing basic health services;

E: *essential* drugs are effective against less severe but nevertheless significant forms of illness but are not absolutely vital to providing basic health care;

N: *nonessential* drugs are used for minor or self-limited illnesses, are of questionable efficacy, or have a comparatively high cost for a marginal therapeutic advantage.

Assignment to the nonessential category does not mean that the drug is no longer on the system's formulary or essential drugs list; in many cases, drugs for minor illnesses are included on the essential drugs list but may be considered a lower priority for procurement than other drugs.

The classification of drugs should not be a one-time exercise. As the national formulary or essential drugs list is updated, and as public health priorities change, the VEN or VN categories should be reviewed and updated. Any new drugs added to the list should be categorized appropriately, and category assignments for older drugs should be reviewed and changed if needed.

The VEN system was developed in Sri Lanka, where it was first applied to importations by the State Pharmaceuticals Corporation. All drugs procured by the corporation were reviewed by a clinical pharmacologist and assigned to one of the three categories. Since the first edition of this book in 1981, the VEN approach has been adapted and used in other countries around the world.

Note that these three categories can be designated differently, as in the following examples from Latin America. In El Salvador, there are three categories in the Cuadro Básico (formulary) for the ministry of health: category 1, essential medicines; category 2, basic medicines; and category 3, complementary medicines. The El Salvador Social Security *Listado Oficial de Medicamentos* also uses categories 1, 2, and 3, with slightly different terminology. The Panama Social Security *Lista Oficial de Medicamentos* uses

categories A, B, and C in a similar manner (not to be confused with the categories in ABC analysis).

Some supply systems may find it difficult to maintain and update the three-tiered VEN system; it may be hard to decide how to classify certain drugs. An alternative is a two-tiered VN system, in which vital drugs are those that should be available at all times, and nonessential drugs, although still on the formulary, are of lower priority and should be purchased only after the need for all V drugs is satisfied.

Either system—two or three categories—will work if the system is maintained; the main objective is an ongoing system to give priority to essential, lifesaving drugs as opposed to expensive nonessential items.

Performing VEN Analysis

Due to its broad implications for procurement and use, classification of drugs into VEN or VN categories is probably best done by a recognized national committee, such as a national formulary committee. The classification should be determined primarily on the basis of the public health impact of individual drugs. Unit prices should be a secondary consideration, and popularity of medications should have minimal influence on the process. Figure 41.1 provides sample guidelines for establishing VEN categories. Examples of drugs classified under this method by the Malawi Essential Drugs Program are given in Figure 41.2.

Figure 41.1 Sample Guidelines for VEN Categories

Characteristic of Drug or Target Condition	Vital	Essential	Nonessential
Occurrence of target condition			
Persons affected (% of population)	Over 5%	1–5%	Less than 1%
Persons treated (number per day at average health center)	Over 5	1–5	Less than 1
Severity of target condition			
Life-threatening	Yes	Occasionally	Rarely
Disabling	Yes	Occasionally	Rarely
Therapeutic effect of drug			
Prevents serious disease	Yes	No	No
Cures serious disease	Yes	Yes	No
Treats minor, self-limited symptoms and conditions	No	Possibly	Yes
Has proven efficacy	Always	Usually	May or may not
Has unproven efficacy	Never	Rarely	May or may not

Figure 41.2 Examples of Drugs Classified by the VEN System

	Vital		Essential		Nonessential	
Criteria	Potentially lifesaving Significant withdrawal side effects Major public health importance		Effective against less severe but nevertheless significant forms of illness		Used for minor or self-limited illnesses Questionable efficacy High cost for marginal therapeutic advantage All these drugs have been deleted from the Malawi Essential Drugs List (1995)	
Health center	Phenobarbitone sodium	tablet, 30 g	Lignocaine HCl	inj, 1%, 25 mL vial	Lignocaine + adrenaline	inj, 1% +1/200,000
	Phenoxymethylpenicillin	tablet, 250 mg	Praziquantel	tablet, 600 mg	Aspirin	tablet, pediatric, 75 mg
	Cotrimoxazole	tablet, 480 mg	Gentian violet	paint, aqueous 0.5%, 500 mL	Suramin sodium	inj, 1 g vial, PFR
	Nystatin	pessaries, 100,000 units	Benzyl benzoate	application, 25%, 100 mL	Nystatin	tablet, 500,000 units
	Pyrimethamine + sulfadioxine	tablet, 25 mg + 500 mg	Magnesium trisilicate complex	tablet, chewable	Amodiaquine	tablet, 200 mg base
	Ferrous sulfate/folic acid	tablet, 200 mg/0.5 mg	Chlorpromazine HCl	tablet, 25 mg	Migril	tablet
	Adrenaline	inj, 1/1,000, 1 mL amp	Aminophylline	tablet, 100 mg	Ferrous sulfate	tablet, 200 mg
	Oral rehydration salts (ORS)	powder, 1 liter (WHO)	Vitamin B complex	tablet	Propranolol HCl	tablet, 10 mg
	Gentamicin	inj 40 mg/mL, 2 mL vial	Aluminum acetate	eardrop, 13%	Magenta	paint, 20 mL
	Condoms with spermicide		Zinc oxide	ointment, 15%	Antisnakebite serum	inj, 10 mL amp
	Measles vaccine, live	inj, 10-dose (5 mL) vial	Mebendazole	tablet, 200 mg	Ergometrine maleate	tablet, 500 mcg
	Ergometrine maleate	inj, 500 mcg/mL, 1 mL amp	Ferrous sulfate	mixture, pediatric, 60 mg/5 mL	Vitamins, multiple	pediatric drops
	Salbutamol sulfate	tablet, 4 mg	Chlorphenramine maleate	tablet, 4 mg	Thymol	mouthwash solution tab
	Vitamin A	capsule, 200,000 IU	Lidocaine + adrenaline	dental cartridge 2% + 1/80,000		
District hospital	Diazepam	inj, 5 mg/mL, 2 mL amp	Diazepam	tablet, 5 mg		
	Atropine sulfate	inj, 600 mcg/mL, 1 mL amp	Paracetamol	tablet, 500 mg		
	Nalidixic acid	tablet, 500 mg	Codeine phosphate	tablet, 15 mg		
	Isoniazid + thiacetazone	tablet, (HT3) 300 mg/ 150 mg	Amoxicillin	elixir, 125 mg/5 mL		
	Digoxin	tablet, 250 mcg	Erythromycin	susp, 125 mg/5 mL		

Source: Malawi Essential Drugs Program.

Applications of VEN Analysis

The major uses of VEN analysis are assigning priorities for drug selection, procurement, and use in a supply system; guiding inventory management activities; and determining appropriate drug prices.

Selection. Vital and essential drugs should be given priority in selection, especially when funds are short.

Procurement. A drug's VEN classification may affect the following:

Order monitoring: Orders for vital and essential drugs should be monitored closely, since shortages in these items require expensive air shipment of supplies.

Safety stock: Safety stocks should be higher for vital and essential items. Inventory savings can be realized by reducing safety stocks of nonessential items.

Order quantities: If funds are short, the VEN system should be used to ensure that enough quantities of vital and essential drugs are bought first.

Supplier selection: Only reliable suppliers should be used for vital and essential drugs. Quality and service for new and unknown suppliers can be tested by awarding them contracts for nonessential drugs.

Use. Review of usage by VEN categories may suggest underuse of vital or essential items or overuse of nonessential items. VEN or VN categories can be compared with ABC analysis and therapeutic category analysis (see following sections) to monitor how well actual use compares with priorities.

Distribution. Use VEN analysis for the following:

Pricing in drug sales programs: Higher prices on popular but marginally useful items such as cough and cold remedies can be used to subsidize immunizations and antibiotics.

Stock control: Special attention should be paid to stock levels of vital and essential items to avoid stockouts.

Assignment of staff: Stock clerks and other inventory control staff who are more experienced or more skilled should be assigned to keep track of vital and essential items.

The application of the VEN system in Malawi is described Country Study 41.1.

Using the VEN System to Guide Purchases

The VEN (or VN) system helps minimize distortions in the drug procurement process and thus maximizes the health impact of available funds. When procurement quantities must be reduced, these steps can be taken:

Step 1. Classify all drugs on the national essential drugs list as

---

Country Study 41.1 Use of VEN in Malawi

In 1994, because of macroeconomic problems, the Ministry of Health (MOH) of Malawi felt the need to further prioritize the drugs on the Malawi National Drugs List (MNDL) for procurement for the public sector. The limited resources allocated made it impossible for the central medical stores (CMS) to ensure the continuous availability of all drugs on the MNDL.

The National Drugs Committee (NDC), the committee responsible for selecting drugs and updating the MNDL, was to review the three-year-old drug list as part of an ongoing review process, and prioritize items on the list using VEN principles. In preparation for the two-day national meeting, all members of the NDC received information on amendments to the MNDL proposed by various health workers in the country (along with scientific evidence backing up the proposals). Members also received a draft protocol for the VEN allocation exercise, clarifying both the rationale for the exercise (continuous availability of the most important drugs) and the proposed therapeutic criteria for allocation to V, E, or N. In addition, they received a list of all drugs on the MNDL by level of use and therapeutic group, with a suggested VEN allocation prepared by the NDC secretariat, with assistance from selected clinicians.

At the start of the meeting, consensus was reached that, in view of the economic circumstances, all items of limited therapeutic benefit (N drugs) should be removed altogether. The VEN system was then used to allocate drugs to V or E according to therapeutic relevance.

Early on during the meeting, it became clear that the VEN criteria had to be reinterpreted in order to reach consensus. For instance, according to the original criteria, aspirin did not qualify as a vital drug. However, the majority of the NDC members believed that, in view of public health implications (aspirin is an antipyretic used as part of malaria treatment and for nonspecific complaints), it should be a V item.

In addition to allocation by therapeutic relevance, all items were allocated by level of use (H, health center; D, district hospital; and C, central hospital) and by expected consumption (A for high- and B for low-consumption drugs).

The NDC agreed with the CMS that the CMS, as a matter of policy, would be responsible for first ensuring the continuous availability of vital high-consumption items (especially HVA items). Procurement of all other drugs would depend on the availability of additional funds and foreign exchange. Low-consumption (especially DEB and CEB) items would not be routinely stocked by the CMS. Clients (hospitals and districts) would be responsible for ordering all B items well in advance (for example, once a year at the beginning of the financial year).

V, E, or N (or V or N): If the funding shortage is temporary, consider options for limiting individual order quantities (and increasing order frequency) for high-turnover V and E drugs, as determined by ABC analysis (see Section 41.3).

Step 2. Reconsider the proposed purchase quantities to make sure they are justified: Check assumptions, order formulas, and the accuracy of calculations. Particular attention should be paid to V and E drugs, since these drugs will be the last eliminated from the list.

Step 3. Try to find additional funds: A clear and well-documented presentation of a system's requirements may result in increased drug budget allocations or additional funds from donors. Introduction of a cost-recovery/cost-sharing system may be an alternative source of additional funds in the long term (see Chapter 44).

Step 4. Remove from the procurement list any N drugs for which there is no clear therapeutic need: Then reassess funds in relation to revised estimates. If there is still a funding gap, proceed to Step 5.

Step 5. Reduce quantities of or eliminate other N items and reassess the estimated procurement cost for remaining items: If requirements still exceed the available budget after all N items are eliminated, proceed to Step 6.

Step 6. Limit therapeutic duplications: If the list of V and E items (or V items in a VN system) contains more than one drug with a similar therapeutic effect, it may be possible to do some tendering by therapeutic subcategory (see Chapters 13 and 16). If certain drugs are usually purchased in more than one strength, it may be possible to limit such duplication and reduce total quantities for the drugs in question. If these sorts of adjustments are not feasible, or if they do not produce the necessary cost reductions, proceed to Step 7.

Step 7. Reduce the quantities of drugs that must be purchased using the "preferential weighting" or "equal misery" approach: With a VN system, this step applies to all remaining drugs on the list. With a VEN system, one option is to purchase the entire quantity of V drugs and allocate remaining funds among E drugs. The alternative is to reduce quantities of both V and E drugs.

The *preferential weighting* strategy protects one or more classes of drugs or one or more classes of facilities. In one variation, the highest-priority classes are exempted from the cuts, and quantities of remaining drugs (or facility estimates) are reduced until the procurement budget balances with estimated purchases. Another option is to reduce quantities for the highest-priority classes less than for the lower-priority classes.

The *equal misery* strategy for reducing quantities is sometimes applied to drugs or facilities. If it is applied to a single list of drugs, all drug quantities are reduced by an equal percentage until the necessary cost reductions are achieved. If equal misery is applied to individual health facility estimates, all health facility estimates are reduced by the same percentage. Equal misery is not recommended for general use in the public drug supply system—in most situations, preference should be given to certain drugs (and sometimes to certain types of health facilities).

≡ 41.3 ABC Analysis

It is well known in inventory management that a relatively small number of items account for most of the value of annual consumption. The analysis of this phenomenon is known as Pareto analysis or, more commonly, ABC analysis.

It is useful in any supply system to analyze consumption patterns and the value of total consumption for all items; it is possible in all but the smallest systems to classify inventory items into three categories (A, B, and C) according to the value of their annual usage. Related tools such as therapeutic category analysis and price comparison analysis build on the basic ABC analysis, and the data for these analyses can be compiled as the ABC analysis is constructed by adding data columns to the spreadsheet.

Applications of ABC Analysis

ABC analysis is an extremely powerful tool, with uses in selection, procurement, management of distribution, and promotion of rational drug use.

Selection. Review of class A drugs may uncover high-usage items for which lower-cost alternatives are available on the formulary or in the marketplace. The ABC analysis also helps managers identify purchases made for items that are not on the formulary or essential drugs list or not approved for use in the supply system. In a West African country in 1993, analyses of consumption in a sample of twenty health facilities showed that three of the facilities (15 percent) continued to use and stock ampicillin suspension regularly, although it had been deleted from the national formulary five years earlier in favor of amoxicillin.

Procurement. ABC analysis can be useful in the following activities:

Determining order frequency: Ordering A items more often and in smaller quantities should lead to a reduction in inventory costs. Note that order frequency and quantity influence supply activities in at least six ways: they (1) determine average inventory (higher order quantity means higher inventory levels); (2) determine procurement workload (higher order quantity means a lower number of orders, and vice versa); (3) determine safety stock (more frequent ordering means less inventory and less safety stock); (4) influence bulk prices (larger orders

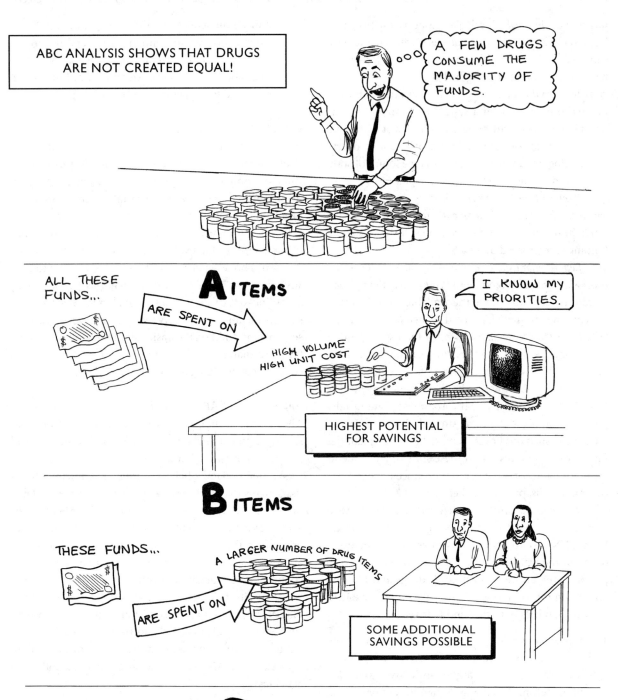
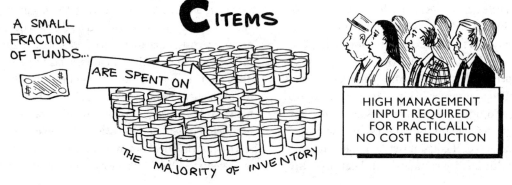

mean more special bulk rates); (5) determine storage space requirements for drugs; and (6) influence the likelihood of losses to expiry (less frequent bulk purchasing may lead to more expired drugs).

Seeking lower-cost sources for A items: The procurement office should concentrate on getting lower prices for A items by looking for cheaper dosage forms or cheaper suppliers. Any price reductions for class A drugs can lead to significant savings.

Monitoring order status: Emphasis should be placed on monitoring the order status of A items, because an unexpected shortage may lead to expensive emergency purchases.

Monitoring procurement priorities: As mentioned earlier (in the VEN discussion), ABC analysis can help monitor procurement patterns in comparison with health system priorities. For example, an ABC analysis of an African state's 1994 procurement showed that the number-one drug in terms of procurement value was antisnakebite serum, and the second was methylated spirit solution. These two items consumed 15 percent of total funds for that state. In another state in the same country, levamisole suspension accounted for 28 percent of the total tender value. This antiworm medicine is no longer listed on the World Health Organization (WHO) *Model List of Essential Drugs*, having been replaced by more cost-effective alternatives.

Comparing actual and planned purchases: ABC analysis can be used to compare actual and planned purchases in a public-sector supply system. For example, in one Latin American ministry of health supply system, the original procurement budget for 1994 specified that 97 items would be purchased through tender at an estimated cost of US$2.5 million. ABC analysis of the year's two tenders showed that 124 items were actually purchased, at a total cost of US$3.36 million. Of the 124 items purchased, 61 (nearly half) did not appear on the procurement plan, and 34 of the drugs that had been on the plan were not purchased. The cost of the unplanned drugs was US$1.17 million. Senior managers were unpleasantly surprised to learn of these discrepancies, and reforms in quantification and procurement procedure were devised for the procurement office.

Distribution and Inventory Management. ABC analysis can affect the following:

Monitoring shelf life: Emphasis should be given to A items to minimize waste due to drugs exceeding their shelf lives.

Delivery schedules: Even when all drugs are ordered only once a year, divided deliveries of A items can lead to increased shelf lives.

Stock count: As discussed in Chapter 15, cyclic stock counts should be guided by ABC analysis, with more frequent counts for A items.

Storage: Improving control for the issuance and storage of A drugs at user points, such as hospitals and health centers, can minimize waste, pilferage, and organized theft of drugs.

Use. Review of high-usage items by health officials, practicing physicians, and other health workers may suggest areas of overuse and underuse.

Performing ABC Analysis

ABC analysis can be applied to total annual consumption, to consumption during a shorter period, or to a particular tender or set of tenders; the basic methodology is the same no matter which data are used. The basic steps are also the same whether the ABC analysis is done manually or by computer, although the process is much easier with a computer.

The process is described in eight steps and illustrated in Figures 41.3-41.5; the example used in the figures comes from a state essential drugs program in West Africa. The figures shown are for part of one tender and do not represent annual drug consumption in the state.

Step 1. List all items purchased or consumed and enter the unit cost: The cost is for one basic unit of an item (column 3 of Figure 41.3). The basic unit should be the same as the issue unit tracked on stock records, except when a smaller basic unit such as a milliliter or gram is needed to incorporate several different bottle, tube, or vial sizes for the same item. See Chapter 46 for a discussion of issue units, basic units, and pack sizes.

Ideally, the actual CIF (cost, insurance, and freight) acquisition unit cost for all items should be used, but this is difficult to track when there have been multiple purchases of an item at different prices. The most accurate alternatives are a weighted average or a first-in/first-out (FIFO) average, as discussed in Chapter 42. In Figure 41.3, the unit cost of one basic unit (tablet) of cotrimoxazole was US$.0098.

Step 2. Enter consumption quantities: Enter the number of basic units consumed or purchased during the period under review. It is important to make sure that the same review period is used for all items to avoid invalid comparisons. Figure 41.3 shows that for cotrimoxazole, 860,000 tablets were purchased.

Step 3. Calculate the value of consumption: Multiply the unit cost by the number of units consumed or purchased to

Figure 41.3 How to Perform an ABC Value Analysis (Steps 1–4)

Product Description	Basic Unit	Unit Tender Price (US$)	Total Units	Value (US$)	% Total Value
Adrenaline HCl 1 mg inj, 1 mL	AMP	.0404	13,000	525	0.16
Ampicillin 125 mg/5 mL powder for susp 100	BOT	.5119	43,970	22,509	6.65
Ascorbic acid 100 mg/5 mL syrup	ML	.0022	1,250,000	2,694	0.80
Benzoin, compound tincture	ML	.0067	532,000	3,582	1.06
Benzyl benzoate 25% lotion	ML	.0051	800,000	4,041	1.19
Benzylpenicillin 1MU inj	AMP	.5276	144,000	75,971	22.44
Calcium gluconate 600 mg	TAB	.0032	995,000	3,171	0.94
Chloramphenicol 1–3% eye oint, 5 gm	TUBE	.7537	3,200	2,412	0.71
Chlorhexidine 5% solution	ML	.0073	2,504,000	18,348	5.42
Chlorhexidine + cetrimide 1.5% + 15% solution	ML	.0064	1,552,000	9,964	2.94
Chloroquine 50 mg base/mL syrup	ML	.0014	5,610,000	7,682	2.27
Chloroxylenol 5% solution	ML	.0034	10,728,000	35,994	10.63
Chlorphenamine maleate 4 mg	TAB	.0009	555,000	498	0.15
Clotrimazole 1% cream, 20 gm	TUBE	.3592	3,300	1,185	0.35
Codeine phosphate 15 mg/5 mL linctus	ML	.0052	490,000	2,530	0.75
Cotrimoxazole 400 mg/80 mg	TAB	.0098	860,000	8,455	2.50
Diethylcarbamazine citrate 50 mg	TAB	.0030	65,000	193	0.06
Dipyrone 500 mg/mL inj, 2 mL	AMP	.0620	13,000	805	0.24
Dipyrone 500 mg/mL inj, 5 mL	AMP	.0898	65,000	5,836	1.72
Erythromycin 250 mg	TAB	.0350	262,000	9,175	2.71
Ferrous salts, equiv to 60 mg iron	TAB	.0007	3,280,000	2,208	0.65
Fortified procaine penicillin, 4 MU inj	VIAL	.3026	100,000	30,259	8.94
Gentamicin sulfate 80 mg inj, 2 mL	AMP	.0628	130,800	8,209	2.43
Hydrocortisone 100 mg inj, 2 mL vial	VIAL	.6387	17,000	10,857	3.21
Hydrogen peroxide 6% solution	ML	.0016	632,000	1,006	0.30
Hyoscine N-butylbromide 10 gm	TAB	.0174	380,000	6,598	1.95
Lidocaine 20 mg/mL inj, 5 mL	AMP	.5574	2,150	1,198	0.35
Metronidazole 200 mg	TAB	.0052	1,080,000	5,576	1.65
Metronidazole 200 mg/5 mL susp	ML	.0055	900,000	4,985	1.47
Multivitamin tab/caps	TAB	.0022	3,395,000	7,622	2.25
Nitrofurantoin 100 mg	TAB	.0055	860,000	4,711	1.39
Oxytocin 10 IU inj, 1 mL	AMP	.2468	14,500	3,578	1.06
Pancuronium 2 mg/mL inj, 2 mL	AMP	.4538	2,600	6,380	1.88
Phenobarbitone 30 mg	TAB	.0025	65,000	160	0.05
Phenobarbitone 60 mg	TAB	.0047	135,000	636	0.19
Piroxicam 20 mg	CAP	.0099	97,000	958	0.28
Prednisolone 8 mg	TAB	.0079	65,000	511	0.15
Propranolol 10 mg	TAB	.0040	15,000	61	0.02
Propranolol 40 mg	TAB	.0067	33,000	222	0.07
Pseudoephedrine 60 mg/triprolidine 2.5 mg	TAB	.0536	100,000	5,360	1.58
Pyramethamine 25 mg/sulfadoxine 500 mg	TAB	.0359	90,000	3,232	0.95
Pyrantel 125 mg/5 mL syrup, 100 mL	BOT	54.4390	160	8,710	2.57
Vitamin B complex	TAB	.0025	1,440,000	3,555	1.05
Water for injection 10 mL	AMP	.0287	220,500	6,336	1.87
Total				338,500	

obtain the total value for each item. In Figure 41.3, column 5 shows that for cotrimoxazole, the total value of purchases was $8,455. Once this is done for each item, add up the total value of all items at the bottom of the column.

Step 4. Calculate the percentage of total value represented by each item: Divide the value of each item by the total value of all items. Enter the results for each item under the heading "percent of total value," as shown in col-

umn 6 of Figure 41.3. At this point, any ABC list will look something like Figure 41.3; in the example, ampicillin suspension (item 2) represented 6.65 percent of total value. (It is useful to carry the percentage to two decimal places, because there may be several items that are close together in value and many that represent less than 1 percent of total value. It is easier to understand the data when these items are clearly differentiated with two decimal places.)

Figure 41.4 How to Perform an ABC Value Analysis (Steps 5–6)

Product Description	Basic Unit	Unit Tender Price (US$)	Total Units	Value (US$)	% Total Value	Cumulated % of Value
Benzylpenicillin 1MU inj	AMP	.5276	144,000	75,971	22.44	22.44
Chloroxylenol 5% solution	ML	.0034	10,728,000	35,994	10.63	33.08
Fortified procaine penicillin, 4 MU inj	VIAL	.3026	100,000	30,259	8.94	42.02
Ampicillin 125 mg/5 mL powder for susp, 100	BOT	.5119	43,970	22,509	6.65	48.67
Chlorhexidine 5% solution	ML	.0073	2,504,000	18,348	5.42	54.09
Hydrocortisone 100 mg inj, 2 mL vial	VIAL	.6387	17,000	10,857	3.21	57.29
Chlorhexidine + cetrimide 1.5% + 15% solution	ML	.0064	1,552,000	9,964	2.94	60.24
Erythromycin 250 mg	TAB	.0350	262,000	9,175	2.71	62.95
Pyrantel 125 mg/5 mL syrup, 100 mL	BOT	54.4390	160	8,710	2.57	65.52
Cotrimoxazole 400 mg/80 mg	TAB	.0098	860,000	8,455	2.50	68.02
Gentamicin sulfate 80 mg inj, 2 mL	AMP	.0628	130,800	8,209	2.43	70.44
Chloroquine 50 mg base/mL syrup	ML	.0014	5,610,000	7,682	2.27	72.71
Multivitamin tab/caps	TAB	.0022	3,395,000	7,622	2.25	74.96
Hyoscine N-butylbromide 10 gm	TAB	.0174	380,000	6,598	1.95	76.91
Pancuronium 2 mg/mL inj, 2 mL	AMP	2.4538	2,600	6,380	1.88	78.80
Water for injection 10 mL	AMP	.0287	220,500	6,336	1.87	80.67
Dipyrone 500 mg/mL inj, 5 mL	AMP	.0898	65,000	5,836	0.24	99.17
Metronidazole 200 mg	TAB	.0052	1,080,000	5,576	1.65	84.04
Pseudoephedrine 60 mg/triprolidine 2.5 mg	TAB	.0536	100,000	5,360	1.58	85.63
Metronidazole 200 mg/5 mL susp	ML	.0055	900,000	4,985	1.47	87.10
Nitrofurantoin 100 mg	TAB	.0055	860,000	4,711	1.39	88.49
Benzyl benzoate 25% lotion	ML	.0051	800,000	4,041	1.19	89.68
Benzoin, compound tincture	ML	.0067	532,000	3,582	1.06	90.74
Oxytocin 10 IU inj, 1 mL	AMP	.2468	14,500	3,578	1.06	91.80
Vitamin B complex	TAB	.0025	1,440,000	3,555	1.05	92.85
Pyramethamine 25 mg/sulfadoxine 500 mg	TAB	.0359	90,000	3,232	0.95	93.80
Calcium gluconate 600 mg	TAB	.0032	995,000	3,171	0.94	94.74
Ascorbic acid 100 mg/5 mL syrup	ML	.0022	1,250,000	2,694	0.80	95.54
Codeine phosphate 15 mg/5 mL linctus	ML	.0052	490,000	2,530	0.75	96.28
Chloramphenicol 1–3% eye oint, 5 gm	TUBE	.7537	3,200	2,412	0.71	97.00
Ferrous salts, equiv to 60 mg iron	TAB	.0007	3,280,000	2,208	0.65	97.65
Lidocaine 20 mg/mL inj, 5 mL	AMP	.5574	2,150	1,198	0.35	98.00
Clotrimazole 1% cream, 20 gm	TUBE	.3592	3,300	1,185	0.35	98.35
Hydrogen peroxide 6% solution	ML	.0016	632,000	1,006	0.30	98.65
Piroxicam 20 mg	CAP	.0099	97,000	958	0.28	98.93
Dipyrone 500 mg/mL inj, 2 mL	AMP	.0620	13,000	805	1.72	82.39
Phenobarbitone 60 mg	TAB	.0047	135,000	636	0.19	99.36
Adrenaline HCl 1 mg inj, 1 mL	AMP	.0404	13,000	525	0.16	99.51
Prednisolone 8 mg	TAB	.0079	65,000	511	0.15	99.66
Chlorphenamine maleate 4 mg	TAB	.0009	555,000	498	0.15	99.81
Propranolol 40 mg	TAB	.0067	33,000	222	0.07	99.88
Diethylcarbamazine citrate 50 mg	TAB	.0030	65,000	193	0.06	99.93
Phenobarbitone 30 mg	TAB	.0025	65,000	160	0.05	99.98
Propranolol 10 mg	TAB	.0040	15,000	61	0.02	100.00
Total				338,500		

Step 5. Rearrange the list: Rank the items in descending order by total value (column 5), starting at the top with the highest value. For example, in Figure 41.3, the highest-value item was benzylpenicillin injection (item 6). This now becomes item 1, chloroxylenol moves to item 2, and so forth. This yields a list that is also ordered by percentage of total value, as in Figure 41.4.

Step 6. Calculate the cumulative percentage of total value for each item: Beginning with the first item at the top, add the percentage in column 6 to that of the item below it in the list (creating column 7). For example, in Figure 41.4, benzylpenicillin injection represented 22.44 percent of total procurement value. Chloroxylenol represented 10.63 percent; the cumulative percentage of the two items was 33.08 percent (rounded) of total procurement value.

Step 7. Choose cut-off points or boundaries for A, B, and C drugs: In general, the following boundaries are used: A

Figure 41.5 How to Perform an ABC Value Analysis (Step 8)

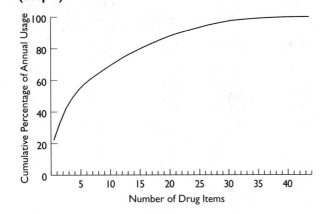

items have the highest annual usage, with 10 to 20 percent of the items usually accounting for 75 to 80 percent of the funds spent. B items represent another 10 to 20 percent of the items that use 15 to 20 percent of the funds, and C items account for 60 to 80 percent of the items but only 5 to 10 percent of the value of annual consumption.

These boundaries are somewhat flexible; for example, class A status might be given to items that cumulatively account for 70 percent of the funds. The decision depends on how volume and value are dispersed among items on the list and how the results of the ABC analysis are going to be used. If class A items are going to be managed more intensively than B and C items, allocation of items to class A must be based on management capacity.

Step 8. Present the results graphically: Plot the percentage of the total cumulative value (column 7) on the vertical or y-axis versus the item number (column 1) on the horizontal or x-axis. Figure 41.5 shows a graph of the sample ABC analysis. The number of items in the drug list influences the slope of the ABC curve. Figure 41.6 shows the results of ABC analysis for a full year's drug consumption in two large supply systems; note the difference in the shape of the curves in comparison to Figure 41.5. In Country I, 25 class A items out of a total of 344 accounted for about 75 percent of the total value. In Country II, which shows a less steep ABC curve, 34 items out of a total of 220 items (15.5 percent) represent nearly 70 percent of the total value. To limit the number of items in class A, a cut-off point was selected that represents a lower proportion of the total value. In general, the steeper the curve, the higher the proportion of the total value that would be included in class A.

≡ 41.4 Therapeutic Category Analysis

Therapeutic category analysis reviews the volume of use and the value of various therapeutic categories and subcategories of drugs. This technique builds on ABC analysis, sorting the ABC list into therapeutic categories (based on the cumulative volume and value of the individual drugs in those categories). Figure 41.7 shows a summary therapeutic category analysis, using data from a Caribbean country. Figure 41.8 provides details on the top three therapeutic categories in Figure 41.7.

Applications of Therapeutic Category Analysis

The applications of therapeutic category analysis are similar to those of ABC analysis. Managers should focus cost control efforts on the therapeutic categories that show the highest consumption and greatest expenditures.

Selection. Therapeutic category analysis can be applied to the following selection activities:

Choosing the most cost-effective products for essential drugs lists and formularies, and finding opportunities for therapeutic substitution: For example, in Figure 41.8, look at the comparison between methyldopa and atenolol. If all hypertensive patients in the sample were converted from methyldopa to atenolol, the health system would save about $17,740—over 7 percent of the total expenditures for drug purchases in this country.

Providing information for pharmacoeconomic analysis: Pharmacoeconomic analysis is the process of comparing cost, therapeutic efficacy, and safety. Two techniques are most commonly used in comparing drug regimens: cost-minimization and cost-effectiveness analysis. Other pharmacoeconomic techniques such as cost-utility and cost-benefit analysis are less appropriate for comparing drug regimens (see Chapter 3). Cost minimization is the simpler of the two techniques—it is used when two therapeutic options are the same in terms of therapeutic benefit and safety but one is less expensive. As discussed in Chapter 3, cost effectiveness is used to compare the costs and benefits of therapeutic alternatives when cost minimization alone is not appropriate. (For more information on pharmacoeconomic analysis, see Bootman et al. 1996 or Freund and Dittus 1992.)

Procurement. As discussed in Chapters 13 and 16, some supply systems tender for certain therapeutic subcategories (for example, first-generation cephalosporins) rather than for individual drugs. A therapeutic category analysis would show managers how many different products in a subcategory are being purchased. If there are

Figure 41.6 Typical ABC Analysis for Two Drug Supply Programs

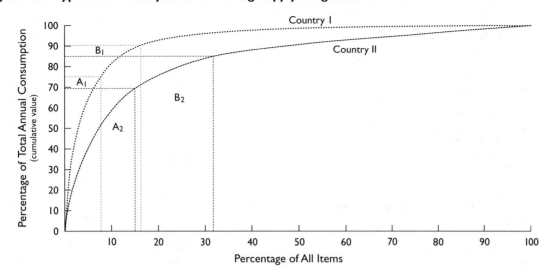

	Country I				Country II			
	ABC Class				ABC Class			
	A	B	C	Total	A	B	C	Total
Number of items	25	34	285	344	34	35	151	220
Percentage of all items	7.3	9.9	82.8	100	15.5	15.9	68.6	100
Value of annual consumption (US$)	11,151,270	2,197,600	1,438,274	14,787,144	6,401,593	1,415,641	1,401,088	9,218,322
Percentage of total annual consumption	75.4	14.9	9.7	100	69.4	15.4	15.2	100

duplications—for example, two oral products are being purchased—tenders could specify only "oral first-generation cephalosporins." Review of Figure 41.8 does not yield obvious candidates for subcategory tendering.

Use. Therapeutic category analysis can help promote rational drug use by:

Identifying potential problems of irrational use: Managers can compare information from the summary (Figure 41.7) and the detailed analysis (Figure 41.8) with known patterns of morbidity, to see how well utilization matches the patterns. For example, in Figure 41.8, note that 3,750 courses of therapy of oral ampicillin were used; the manager might ask how that corresponds with the incidence of diseases that would justify the use of ampicillin. Note that the use of ampicillin was four times greater than the use of oral penicillin (and ampicillin costs twice as much). Are these patterns rational for the situation? There isn't enough information in Figure 41.8 to make that determination, but it might be possible to find out through a small, well-targeted study of prescribing (as described in Chapter 29).

Identifying overprescribing and leakage: Compare the num-

ber of courses of therapy that theoretically should have been provided against patient contact data—for example, are the numbers of diabetic patients treated consistent with the number of courses of therapy?

Performing Therapeutic Category Analysis

Therapeutic category analysis is divided into two phases: the summary analysis and the detailed analysis.

Summary Therapeutic Category Analysis. The summary analysis consists of five steps:

Steps 1–3: Follow the first three steps in ABC analysis (see Section 41.3) to produce a list of drugs, with the volume and value of use calculated for each drug.

Step 4: Add a column and assign each of the drugs to a therapeutic category, as discussed in Chapter 10. The key requirement is a standard formulary coding system. The system can be simple (with relatively broad categories) or complex (with many subcategories). Simple, commonly used coding systems include the WHO *Model List of Essential Drugs* and the American Hospital Formulary Service (AHFS) Pharmacologic and Therapeutic Classification System. More detailed, multilayered

Figure 41.7 Therapeutic Category Analysis Summary

	Formulary Code	Formulary Category	No. of Products	Category Total Cost (US$)	% Total Cost	Cumulative Percentage
1	8.12	Antibacterial/antifungal agents, systemic	30	46,053	19.17	19.17
2	68.20	Antidiabetic agents	5	36,175	15.06	34.23
3	24.08	Hypotensive agents	8	31,006	12.91	47.13
4	40.12	Replacement solution/agents	10	14,834	6.17	53.31
5	84.04	Topical anti-infectives	4	14,302	5.95	59.26
6	40.20	Caloric agents (dextrose solutions)	6	12,480	5.19	64.46
7	28.08	Analgesics/antipyretics	10	11,835	4.93	69.38
8	36.00	Diagnostic strips	1	6,496	2.70	72.09
9	86.00	Antiasthmatic drugs	8	6,195	2.58	74.66
10	4.00	Antihistamines	5	4,892	2.04	76.70
11	38.00	Disinfectants	3	4,846	2.02	78.72
12	28.16	Psychotherapeutic agents (antipsychotic/antidepressant)	14	4,574	1.90	80.62
13	88.28	Multiple vitamins	3	4,318	1.80	82.42
14	20.04	Iron preparations	3	3,207	1.33	83.75
15	56.40	Miscellaneous gastrointestinal drugs	4	3,039	1.26	85.02
16	8.08	Anthelmintics	2	2,663	1.11	86.13
17	92.00	Dispensing envelopes	1	2,643	1.10	87.23
18	68.04	Adrenal hormones	4	2,246	0.93	88.16
19	48.00	Antitussive/antiexpectorant	2	2,240	0.93	89.09
20	56.04	Antacids	2	1,781	0.74	89.84
21	28.04	General anesthetics	3	1,693	0.70	90.54
22	84.05	Topical antifungals	4	1,633	0.68	91.22
23	88.08	Vitamin B preparations	5	1,547	0.64	91.86
24	28.12	Anticonvulsant agents	5	1,465	0.61	92.47
25	92.00	IV administration sets	1	1,300	0.54	93.02
26	12.20	Skeletal muscle relaxants	3	1,283	0.53	93.55
27	52.04	EENT anti-infectives	4	1,283	0.53	94.08
28	40.28	Diuretics	5	1,248	0.52	94.60
29	8.16	Antitubercular agents	5	1,212	0.50	95.11
30	24.04	Cardiotonic and antiarrhythmic agents	6	1,119	0.47	95.57
31	52.08	EENT anti-inflammatory agents	2	1,113	0.46	96.04
32	12.08	Anticholinergic agents	4	925	0.39	96.42
33	56.12	Laxatives	5	886	0.37	96.79
34	84.07	Scabicides/pediculocides	1	765	0.32	97.11
35	76.00	Oxytocics	3	718	0.30	97.41
36	20.12	Anticoagulants and coagulants	2	691	0.29	97.70
37	52.20	Miotics	1	534	0.22	97.92
38	56.22	Antiemetics	3	531	0.22	98.14
39	84.36	Miscellaneous topical preparations	2	515	0.21	98.35
40	72.00	Local anesthetics	6	491	0.20	98.56
41	8.32	Antitrichomonal agents (metronidazole)	3	481	0.20	98.76
42	84.06	Topical anti-inflammatory	2	363	0.15	98.91
43	52.36	EENT miscellaneous	2	358	0.15	99.06
44	28.24	Anxiolytics, sedatives, hypnotics	3	356	0.15	99.21
45	88.12	Vitamin C	1	345	0.14	99.35
46	68.36	Thyroid/antithyroid preparations	2	246	0.10	99.45
47	88.24	Vitamin K-1	1	201	0.08	99.54
48	24.12	Coronary vasodilators	2	189	0.08	99.61
49	12.12	Adrenergic agents	1	188	0.08	99.69
50	64.00	Antidotes/metal antagonists	1	149	0.06	99.75
51	28.10	Narcotic antagonists	1	135	0.06	99.81
52	12.16	Adrenergic blocking agents	1	85	0.04	99.85
53	8.36	Urinary anti-infectives	2	82	0.03	99.88
54	40.08	Alkalinizing agents	1	79	0.03	99.91
55	12.04	Cholinergic agents	1	74	0.03	99.94
56	52.10	Carbonic anhydrase inhibitor	1	63	0.03	99.97
57	40.40	Antigout agents	1	60	0.02	100.00
58	52.24	Mydriatic/cycloplegic	1	12	0.00	100.00
			222	240,241		

Figure 41.8 Therapeutic Category Analysis—Detail with Defined Daily Dose Comparisons

Drug Name	Strength	Basic Unit	Basic Unit Price (US$)	Total Usage Basic Units	Value of Annual Usage (US$)	Defined Daily Dose (No. Comp Units)	Defined Daily Dose Cost (US$)	Standard COT (Days)	Basic Units per COT	Annual No. of COTS	Cost per COT (US$)
Antibacterial/Antifungal Agents, Systemic / $46,053 / 19.2% of total											
Ampicillin	250 mg	Tab	.0351	237,000	8,319	8	.2808	10	80	2962.5	2.81
Ampicillin	500 mg	Tab	.0693	31,500	2,183	4	.2772	10	40	787.5	2.77
Ampicillin sodium inj	500 mg	Amp	.2995	3,120	934	4	1.1980	5	20	156.0	5.99
Ampicillin susp 100 mL	125 mg/5 mL	Bott	.7500	6,951	5,213	0.4	.3000	10	4	1737.8	3.00
Benzathine benzylpenicillin inj	2.4 MU	Amp	.5000	1,848	924	1	.5000	10	5	369.6	2.50
Cephadrine inj	500 mg	Amp	.7500	3,050	2,288	4	3.0000	5	20	152.5	15.00
Cephalexin	250 mg	Tab	.0900	5,200	468	8	.7200	10	80	65.0	7.20
Cephalexin susp 100 mL	125 mg/mL	Bott	1.8000	909	1,636	0.4	.7200	10	4	227.3	7.20
Chloramphenicol	250 mg	Tab	.0300	2,100	63	8	.2400	10	80	26.3	2.40
Chloramphenicol inj	1 gm	Amp	.8000	400	320	3	2.4000	5	15	26.7	12.00
Chloramphenicol susp 100 mL	125 mg/mL	Bott	1.0500	120	126	0.4	.4200	10	4	30.0	4.20
Cloxacillin sodium inj	500 mg	Amp	.2615	2,000	523	4	1.0460	5	20	100.0	5.23
Cloxacillin susp 100 mL	125 mg/5 mL	Bott	1.0000	1,798	1,798	0.4	.4000	10	4	449.5	4.00
Cloxacillin	250 mg	Tab	.0410	9,100	373	8	.3280	10	80	113.8	3.28
Cotrimoxazole IV inj, 5 mL	80/16 mg/mL	Amp	.2000	100	20	5	1.0000	5	25	4.0	5.00
Cotrimoxazole susp 100 mL	200/40 mg/5	Bott	.7500	679	509	0.3	.2250	10	3	226.3	2.25
Cotrimoxazole	400/80 mg	Tab	.0210	75,000	1,575	2	.0420	10	20	3750.0	0.42
Erythromycin susp 100 mL	200 mg/5mL	Bott	1.4600	1,452	2,120	0.25	.3650	10	3	484.0	4.38
Erythromycin	250 mg	Tab	.0419	96,000	4,022	4	.1676	10	40	2400.0	1.68
Gentamicin inj	80 mg	Amp	.1595	5,470	872	3	.4785	5	15	364.7	2.39
Griseofulvin	125 mg	Tab	.0300	3,000	90	4	.1200	10	40	75.0	1.20
Griseofulvin	500 mg	Tab	1.0800	31,000	3,348	1	1.0800	10	10	3100.0	1.08
Nystatin oral susp 60 mL	0.1 MU/mL	Bott	1.1000	494	543	0.25	.2750	10	3	164.7	3.30
Nystatin oral	.5 MU	Tab	.0430	1,100	47	3	.1290	10	30	36.7	1.29
Penicillin G sodium inj	1 MU	Vial	.2575	2,250	579	5.76	1.4832	5	29	77.6	7.47
Penicillin G sodium inj	5 MU	Vial	.5000	1,300	650	1.15	.5760	5	6	216.7	3.00
Penicillin VK susp 100 mL	125 mg/5 mL	Bott	.7500	2,257	1,693	0.4	.3000	10	4	564.3	3.00
Penicillin VK	250 mg	Tab	.0190	72,000	1,368	8	.1520	10	80	900.0	1.52
Procaine penicillin G inj	4.8 mg	Vial	.4157	3,269	1,359	1	.4157	5	5	653.8	2.08
Tetracycline HCl	250 mg	Tab	.0120	174,000	2,088	4	.0480	10	40	4350.0	0.48
Antidiabetic Agents / $36,175 / 15.1% of total											
Chlorpropamide	250 mg	Tab	.0090	336,000	3,021	1.5	.0135	30	45	7466.7	0.40
Glibencamide	5 mg	Tab	.0156	152,000	2,371	2	.0312	30	60	2533.3	0.94
Insulin (soluble) inj, 10 mL	100 IU/mL	Vial	3.9100	385	1,505	0.04	.1564	30	1.2	320.8	4.69
Insulin lente, 10 mL	100 IU/mL	Vial	3.9100	6,568	25,681	0.04	.1564	30	1.2	5473.3	4.69
Insulin lente human inj, 10 mL	100 IU/mL	Vial	6.7100	536	3,597	0.04	.2684	30	1.2	446.7	8.05
Antihypertensive Agents / $31,006 / 12.9% of total											
Atenolol	100 mg	Tab	.0800	29,000	2,320	1	.0800	30	30	966.7	2.40
Hydralazine	50 mg	Tab	.0090	86,000	774	2	.0180	30	60	1433.3	0.54
Hydralazine inj	20 mg/mL	Amp	.9350	410	383	2	1.8700	5	10	41.0	9.35
Methyldopa	500 mg	Tab	.0600	443,500	26,610	4	.2400	30	120	3695.8	7.20
Nifedipine	10 mg	Tab	.0675	7,000	473	3	.2025	30	90	77.8	6.08
Propranolol HCl	40 mg	Tab	.0040	70,000	280	4	.0160	30	120	583.3	0.48
Propranolol	80 mg	Tab	.0060	5,000	30	2	.0120	30	60	83.3	0.36
Reserpine	.25 mg	Tab	.0046	29,500	136	2	.0092	30	60	491.7	0.28

Three category totals: $113,234

schemes are the Anatomical, Therapeutic, Chemical (ATC) System of the Nordic Council on Medicines and the Veterans Administration (VA) Medication Classification System, which is listed in the annual USP–DI, published by the United States Pharmacopeia.

Step 5: Rearrange the list into therapeutic categories, by sorting according to the formulary codes. The values and percentages for the various therapeutic categories are then summed from the results for the individual items in the category, and cumulative percentages are calculated, producing a summary therapeutic category analysis (see steps 4–6 under ABC analysis).

In the summary therapeutic category analysis in Figure 41.7, fifty-eight different therapeutic categories are represented; this country uses the Eastern Caribbean Drug Service formulary coding system (ECDS 1994), which has sixty-nine possible therapeutic categories. The system is based on the AHFS system, with minor modifications.

Note that seven of the categories were responsible for nearly 70 percent of total expenditures. This grouping resembles class A in ABC analysis, and the principle is the same—a relatively small number of therapeutic categories often consume most of the funds in a supply system. To

reduce costs, managers should look first at these high-cost therapeutic categories.

Detailed Therapeutic Category Analysis. The second phase of the analysis focuses on the high-cost categories identified in the summary phase. The goal is to identify possible changes in therapeutic strategy that might prove to be cost effective. This analysis compares the cost for a defined daily dose (DDD) of the drugs (the average daily dose for all patients) and the cost of a defined course of therapy (COT).

This stage of the analysis starts with the detailed list of drugs for important therapeutic categories assembled in phase 1. The list of drugs within the categories can be sorted either alphabetically (which is probably easiest for additional data entry) or by value. Data fields (columns) are added to the list to enter the number of basic units per DDD, the annual usage in DDDs, the cost per DDD, the standard COT in days, the annual number of COTs, and the average cost per COT (see Box 41.1).

Once the standard COT is determined, the final step in constructing the detailed therapeutic category analysis is multiplying the DDD cost by the COT, and dividing the annual number of DDDs by the COT (see Figure 41.8 for examples).

≡ 41.5 Price Comparison Analysis

Acquisition price comparison analysis tells the manager whether the system is getting the maximum benefit from available procurement funds, and if not, how much might be saved with alternative procurement practices. Procurement prices can be compared with prices from other systems, and sales prices can be compared with local private-sector prices. These comparisons can help managers set prices for cost-sharing programs and understand whether it is cost effective to continue with current in-house pharmaceutical services.

Acquisition Price Comparison

Applications. The obvious application of price comparison analysis is to measure procurement performance and to focus efforts on obtaining better prices. The comparison of average tender prices with international prices can be used as a routine indicator of procurement system performance.

The analysis can also identify certain drugs that should be considered for alternative methods of procurement. For example, if a supply system is currently purchasing all drugs from local suppliers, the price comparison analysis may indicate some drugs that could be obtained for a significantly lower price through international tender or even through direct procurement from one of the international nonprofit agencies. Country Study 41.2 shows the results of a 1994 price comparison analysis from one Latin American ministry of health.

Drug Price Comparison Analysis. One potential source for comparative procurement information is a list of prices from a neighboring supply system. Another is the MSH *International Drug Price Indicator Guide* (the book or a software version that allows the user to enter local prices and compare them with the international prices that are already in the system).

Once the comparison prices have been entered for each drug, divide the local price by the comparison price, which calculates the local price as a percentage of the comparison price. Once this has been done, add up all these percentages and divide by the number of drugs to get the average percentage.

A manager can also determine how much overall difference exists for a certain volume of purchases (the weighted average percentage). This is done in a manner similar to the ABC analysis. Total annual values are calculated for each item for both local prices and comparison prices, based on annual consumption. The values at local prices and the values at comparison prices are totaled at the bottom of the respective columns. Then the weighted average percentage is calculated by dividing the total value for all items at local prices by the total value at comparison prices. The weighted average is useful because there may be large differences for individual drugs that skew the simple average comparison.

When using the MSH indicator prices for comparison, it is important to understand that the "average international price" reflects a combination of actual tender prices paid by selected country procurement programs and prices from international nonprofit suppliers such as the United Nations International Packing and Assembling Centre (UNIPAC) and the International Dispensary Association (IDA); it is not a real price. When there is a wide range of prices that make up the average, the average may be much higher or lower than actual prices from any of the individual suppliers or tendering programs listed. If a manager wishes to project savings from alternative procurement methods, it is best to use a *median* individual price from the MSH list for each drug.

The prices being compared must refer to the same year; the drug products being compared must be the same generic products in the same or comparable dosage forms, and the comparison units must be the same. If all these points are not addressed correctly, the price comparison analysis will be invalid.

Comparison of Supply System Prices and Private-Sector Prices

This analysis compares acquisition and selling prices against local private-sector wholesale and retail prices.

Applications. The analysis provides useful information for cost-recovery programs. Note in Figure 41.9 that CMS sales prices at a 30 percent markup were, on average, 82 percent of the private-sector wholesale prices for the same drugs (46 percent of the average retail sales price) and 92 percent of the sales prices from the local Christian Health Association warehouse. This might seem to indicate that CMS could increase prices somewhat. However, this simple comparison is not enough to make a determination, because the key issue is how much services are valued by patients. If public drug services are not valued as highly as private-sector drugs and services, there may be no room at all for price increases. Chapter 44 provides a full discussion of these issues.

The most useful application of this type of analysis is to indicate the cost-effectiveness of in-house pharmaceutical services. If supply system procurement acquisition prices are higher than or nearly as high as the private-sector sales prices, and if it is unlikely that procurement system improvements will be able to significantly reduce acquisition prices, further investigation is warranted—it may be more cost effective to serve public-sector patients through contracts with private pharmacies.

Doing the Analysis. This analysis demands some extra effort to get comparative information. Information on average wholesale and/or retail prices may be available from the local pharmacy association, but if it is not or if it is not reliable, prices in local wholesale and retail outlets can be obtained through a simple survey, focusing on a limited list of essential drugs (see MSH/RPM 1995). If a wide range of prices is obtained in the survey, it may be best to use the simple *median* retail price rather than an average of the prices.

This analysis is set up in the same way as the preceding price comparison analysis, building on the list used for ABC analysis and adding columns of comparative prices from the private sector. If the public supply system is selling drugs from one level to the next or to the public, columns should be provided for both acquisition and selling prices.

Again, a percentage comparison is made, both for individual drugs and an overall average. To show the private-sector price as a percentage of the supply system prices, the retail price is divided by the supply system price. To show the supply system prices as a percentage of the private-sector prices, divide supply system prices by private-sector prices.

Country Study 41.2 Price Comparison Analysis

A price comparison analysis was carried out for a Latin American Ministry of Health (MOH) in the context of a 1994 analysis of public pharmaceutical services. In this analysis, prices from local suppliers were compared with the Eastern Caribbean Drug Service (ECDS) prices, based on information from the MSH *International Drug Price Indicator Guide*. For this particular analysis, ECDS prices rather than average international prices were used because the public-sector procurement volumes were similar in the country and the ECDS for the year in question (about US$2 million each).

The ECDS and the Latin American MOH had sixty-two products in common on their 1994 tenders. The Latin American country received a better price locally than the ECDS did internationally for sixteen of the sixty-two—in some cases, particularly for intravenous fluids, the local price was much better than the international price (largely because shipping costs are a major component of the international price). ECDS international prices were better on forty-six of the sixty-two products. For these forty-six products, the Latin American MOH could have saved about US$250,000 if it had purchased at the same international price received by the ECDS. For four items—hydralazine tablets, amitriptyline tablets, ketamine injection, and multivitamin/minerals tablets—the local price was seven to ten times higher than the ECDS price. On those four items alone, US$37,000 could have been saved by purchasing internationally. The accompanying table shows the format for the price comparison analysis.

Description	Strength	Form	Comp. Unit	Total Units Purchased 2 Tenders	Total US$ at L/A Country Tender Price	Total US$ at ECDS Tender Price	L/A Price as % of ECDS Price
Hydralazine	50 mg	Tablet	Tab	10,000	1,012.58	90.00	1125.1
Ketamine (10 mL)	50 mg/mL	Solution	Amp	4,000	6,484.77	800.00	810.6
Furosemide	40 mg	Tablet	Tab	50,000	1,015.45	275.00	369.3
Bisacodyl	5 mg	Tablet	Tab	30,000	455.63	135.00	337.5
Propranolol	40 mg	Tablet	Tab	150,000	2,384.11	900.00	264.9
Acetazolamide	250 mg	Tablet	Tab	3,000	149.13	66.00	225.9
Methyldopa	500 mg	Tablet	Tab	100,000	11,408.39	5,200.00	219.4
Diazepam	5 mg	Tablet	Tab	200,000	920.97	480.00	191.9
Lidocaine (50 mL)	2% sin epi	Solution	Amp	8,000	11,278.41	6,800.00	165.9
Quinidine sulfate	200 mg	Tablet	Tab	60,000	4,142.52	2,520.00	164.4
Insulin NPH, 10 mL	40 U/mL	Solution	Amp	8,000	29,906.23	18,720.00	159.8
Erythromycin	250 mg	Tablet	Tab	500,000	35,256.07	24,000.00	146.9
Propranolol	80 mg	Tablet	Tab	50,000	796.25	550.00	144.8
Allopurinol	100 mg	Tablet	Tab	15,000	337.75	240.00	140.7
Chloramphenicol	1 gm	Solution	Amp	25,000	25,275.94	18,750.00	134.8
Oral rehydration salts	—	Powder	Packet	200,000	37,086.09	28,800.00	128.8
Oxytocin	10 U/mL	Solution	Amp	25,000	4,415.01	3,487.50	126.6
Benzathine penicillin	2,400.000	Solution	Amp	60,000	33,112.58	28,800.00	115.0
Cotrimoxazole	80 mg+40	Tablet	Tab	2,000,000	39,735.10	35,600.00	111.6
Vitamin B complex	120 mL	Solution	Bot	100,000	43,708.61	40,000.00	109.3
Metronidazole	250 mg	Tablet	Tab	3,000,000	33,112.58	31,500.00	105.1
Cephalexin	500 mg	Capsule	Tab	500,000	79,470.20	79,000.00	100.6
Rifampicin	300 mg	Capsule	Tab	1,600,000	179,938.19	206,400.00	87.2
Gentamicin	80 mg/2 mL	Solution	Amp	200,000	25,518.76	31,720.00	80.5
Halothane	250 mL	Liquid	Bot	2,000	45,934.44	66,000.00	69.6
Dextrose in NaCl, 1 L	5%/0.9% mg	Solution	Amp	110,000	85,724.06	132,000.00	64.9
Cotrimoxazole	240 mg/5	Susp.	Bot	110,000	53,311.26	92,400.00	57.7
Sodium chloride, 1 L	0.9%	Solution	Amp	70,000	43,678.15	112,000.00	39.0
Chloramphenicol	125 mg/5	Susp.	Bot	125,000	71,743.93	245,000.00	29.3
Phenytoin	100 mg	Capsule	Cap	270,000	5,364.24	21,870.00	24.5
					912,677.38	1,234,103.50	

Average Tender Price as % of International Price	195.0%
Standard Deviation—Avg Tender Price/Intl Price	225.1%
Weighted Average %—Tender Price/Intl Price	74.0%

Figure 41.9 illustrates a comparison between CMS prices and local wholesale prices in a West African country in 1993.

≡ 41.6 Total Variable Cost Analysis

Total variable cost was introduced in Chapter 15 as the sum of the drug purchase cost, inventory holding cost, ordering cost, and shortage cost. This analysis compiles the values of these various costs on one data sheet. The compiled data are then reviewed to look for options to reduce the total cost and to perform what-if analysis—examining what happens to inventory holding cost if ordering costs are reduced, and so forth.

Variable costs may be either stable or incremental—if the cost remains the same no matter how many transactions or how much inventory is involved, it is a *stable cost* (sometimes called a fixed cost—see Chapter 42). If the cost increases directly with the number of purchases or volume of inventory, it is an *incremental cost*. In most accounting systems, incremental costs are termed variable costs, but for this analysis, all the costs are variable. The difference between stable and incremental costs is important, because most interventions affect only incremental costs; stable costs remain approximately the same.

Many of the costs discussed in this section are visible, in that they are actual expenditures; others are hidden, in that the costs are not expenditures but represent reductions in available resources. Managers should understand that both visible and hidden costs are real.

Figure 41.10 shows a summary sheet for a total variable cost analysis. In the figure, costs and inventory are shown for an illustrative warehouse and purchasing office in a Latin American country. Inventory and costs are found at all levels of the system; in a supply system with several regional warehouses, the inventory (and associated costs) may be considerably higher in the aggregate at the regional level than at the central warehouse. This is also true for supply systems in which health facilities hold significant quantities of stock. For the most complete picture, total variable costs should be calculated for each significant level of the supply system; however, for simplicity's sake, this example focuses on one central warehouse.

In many supply systems, it is difficult to assemble all this information, but the effort should yield a real understanding of where expenses are concentrated and what sorts of interventions may yield substantial cost savings.

Applications

There are two basic applications for the compiled data on total variable cost: analyzing current costs to find opportunities for cost reduction and modeling the cost impact of potential changes in the supply system.

Analyzing and Controlling Costs. The manager's objective is to identify apparently excessive costs in one or more cost categories, and then to devise strategies to minimize the total variable cost. A review of the compiled data in Figure 41.10 might yield several ideas for reducing costs:

► Reduce the average inventory from the current five months of stock (which would reduce holding costs) by more frequent ordering.

► Reduce the cost of drug purchases through more efficient tendering, potentially adding therapeutic subcategory tendering.

► Cut down on losses.

► Consider whether the number of employees (and salary costs) can be reduced without harming efficiency.

► Cut down on emergency purchases through better stock management.

Meeting any of these objectives would require trade-offs—when one cost component is reduced, another is likely to increase. For example, suppose that a country has the total variable cost profile in Figure 41.10 and uses annual purchasing almost exclusively. It might be possible to reduce the average inventory value by half by changing the purchasing system from an annual system to a combination of annual and biannual tenders (see Figure 15.4 in Chapter 15). There will now be two annual tenders, which will increase the costs related to purchasing.

Using the data from Figure 41.10, drug acquisition costs are projected to be the same. Average inventory value decreases to $2.9 million, with an associated decrease in some incremental holding costs: opportunity cost down to $290,000; losses down to $370,00. This suggests a net savings of $660,000 in holding costs, but what are the likely increased costs? Assuming that the additional tender can be managed by existing staff, the additional purchasing costs should be limited to increases in supplies, communications, and other tendering costs. Assuming that these costs double (in the worst case), the extra incremental purchasing costs would be $117,000, resulting in a net savings of $443,000. Of course, the increases would largely be in visible expenditures, and the decreases would be in hidden costs, but this would be a real net savings to the system.

Modeling the Impact of Alternatives for Change. Suppose that the supply system is considering three options for warehousing and distribution in the future: keeping all services in-house (the current system); a second model in which warehousing is kept in-house, but transport is contracted out; and a third model in which both

Figure 41.9 Price Comparison: CMS 30% Markup Compared with Private-Sector Wholesale and Retail Prices and Christian Health Association (CHA) Prices

Description	Strength	Issue Unit	Projected CMS 30% Markup on 1993 Cost	Wholesale Average Price	CMS Price as % of Avg. Wholesale	Retail Average Price	CMS Price as % of Avg. Retail	CHA May '93 Unit Price	CMS Price as % of CHA
Acetylsalicylic acid	325 mg	Tablet	2.02	2.51	81%	6.43	31%	2.25	90%
Amodiaquine	200 mg	Tablet	25.00	46.14	54%	88.50	28%		
Amoxicillin	25 mg/mL	60 mL bottle	445.90	552.50	81%	725.00	62%	325.00	137%
Amoxicillin	250 mg	Tablet	19.50					20.88	93%
Chloramphenicol	250 mg	Tablet	15.60	18.30	85%	26.25	59%	13.75	113%
Chloroquine	150 mg	Tablet	5.65	8.49	67%	13.57	42%		
Chlorpheniramine	4 mg	Tablet	2.28	3.34	68%	6.88	33%	2.73	83%
Cotrimoxazole	480 mg	Tablet	11.24	12.94	87%	17.50	64%	10.08	112%
Diazepam	5 mg	Tablet	1.09	1.89	57%	4.75	23%	1.75	62%
Ferrous sulfate	60 mg iron	Tablet	1.92	2.08	92%	4.75	40%	1.80	107%
Folic acid + iron	1 mg/60 mg	Tablet	2.05	23.40	9%	32.50	6%		
Frusemide	40 mg	Tablet	2.47	6.13	40%	12.14	20%	4.05	61%
Mebendazole	100 mg	Tablet	3.00	29.93	10%	68.66	4%	9.87	30%
Metronidazole	250 mg	Tablet	5.58	6.99	80%	13.75	41%	6.72	83%
Multivitamin	—	Tablet	3.00	1.79	168%	4.69	64%	2.09	144%
Oral rehydration salts	—	Sachet	37.00	41.25	90%	59.29	62%	44.00	84%
Paracetamol	500 mg	Tablet	3.52	2.97	119%	5.28	67%	2.97	119%
Penicillin procaine	4 MU	Vial	224.00	235.00	95%	350.00	64%		
Penicillin, benzyl	5 MU	Vial	250.00	103.22	242%	166.67	150%		
Reserpine	0.25 mg	Tablet	1.43	3.90	37%	8.57	17%	2.20	65%
Averages—30% CMS Markup as % of other					82%		46%		92%

Figure 41.10 Total Variable Cost Analysis Summary

Cost Category	Total	Incremental	Stable
Drug Acquisition Cost (includes supplier shipping charges and duty)	$14,000,000	$14,000,000	
Inventory Holding Costs			
Average inventory, central warehouse (beginning value plus year-end value, divided by two)	$5,800,000	$5,800,000	
Financial opportunity cost (10% average interest rate)	580,000	580,000	
Losses from inventory:			
Expiry	69,000	69,000	
Spoilage/Wastage	18,000	18,000	
Loss during repacking	200	200	
Short shipments from suppliers	500	500	
Obsolete drugs—no longer used	12,000	12,000	
Unexplained losses	640,000	640,000	
Subtotal	739,700	739,700	
Operating costs—storage and stock management:			
Salaries	665,000		665,000
Space and utilities	117,000		117,000
Communications	4,000		4,000
Supplies	650,000	650,000	
Other direct costs	3,700		3,700
Depreciation	46,900		46,900
Administrative overhead	NA	NA	NA
Subtotal	1,486,600	650,000	836,600
Transport costs—to operating units:			
Salaries	115,000		115,000
Supplies (gas, etc.)	112,000	112,000	
Other direct costs	700	700	
Depreciation	8,100		8,100
Administrative overhead	NA	NA	NA
Subtotal	235,800	112,700	123,100
Total holding cost	3,042,100	2,082,400	959,700
Holding cost as % of average inventory	52%		
% incremental and stable		68%	32%
Purchasing Costs			
Salaries	72,000		72,000
Space and utilities	11,000		11,000
Communications	2,000		2,000
Supplies	70,000		70,000
Other direct costs	400		400
Depreciation	5,000		5,000
Administrative overhead	NA	NA	NA
Subtotal	160,400		160,400
Total additional costs of annual tender	45,000		45,000
Total purchasing cost	205,400		205,400
Shortage Cost (estimate 20% emergency purchases at 20% premium)	560,000	560,000	
Total Variable Cost	$17,807,500	$16,642,400	$1,165,100
% incremental and stable		93%	7%

Note: Data are based on a composite from Latin America and do not represent any specific country.

warehousing and distribution are contracted out. Each of the possible new models implies significant changes in personnel needs and operating costs at the various levels of the supply system. Total variable cost modeling provides a convenient format to ask how the supply system's operating costs would change with each option.

The basic steps in total variable cost modeling are the same, whatever the options being considered. The total variable cost is compiled for the most recent year for which data are available (as illustrated in Figure 41.10), for one or several levels of the supply system, and adjusted for inflation and expected changes in utilization, to estimate the total variable cost with the current system in the year(s) in which change would be implemented. Then, for each of the alternate supply system models, the percentage increase or decrease for each major total variable cost component is estimated and applied to the baseline cost, again adjusting for inflation and changes in utilization in subsequent years.

The resulting models are not exact but do predict the relative cost impact of the alternatives being considered. Sometimes the exercise will identify viable interventions that had not been previously considered. For example, in one Latin American country a total variable cost modeling exercise done in 1996 showed that total variable costs could be reduced by consolidating storage at the regional level and privatizing transport, and that still greater savings could be gained by contracting out for all warehousing and transport (assuming that the system could be managed). However, the models also showed that a far greater savings in total variable cost could result from improved drug selection, if it produced only a 10 percent reduction in drug acquisition costs, than could be achieved even by closing all warehouses and contracting out all storage and distribution functions.

Compiling the Total Variable Cost

The total variable cost is made up of four components, which are compiled in one table:

- ► drug acquisition costs (totally incremental)
- ► inventory holding costs (stable and incremental)
- ► purchasing costs (stable and incremental)
- ► shortage costs (primarily incremental)

Drug Acquisition Costs. This is the net cost of all drug purchases, including shipping and insurance charges from the manufacturer and any duty or customs fees. It is an incremental cost. Data can be obtained from purchasing records, stock records, or supplier invoices.

Inventory Holding Costs. The inventory holding cost has several subcomponents, some of which are incremental and some of which are stable.

The first entry under "Inventory Holding Costs" in Figure 41.10 is the average inventory value (which is used to calculate the percentage of holding costs). The average inventory value is obtained by adding the beginning and ending inventory values for the fiscal year, and dividing by two. The following are the standard components of the inventory holding cost:

Financial opportunity cost: This incremental cost varies with the average inventory value; it is obtained by multiplying the average inventory value by the average interest rate paid on money market accounts in local banks (or sometimes by the average interest rate charged for short-term loans).

Losses from inventory: This is often an incremental cost, in that losses rise as inventory values increase. The amounts may be broken down as shown in Figure 41.10, to the extent that data are available from inventory records. If data are not available, estimate losses as a percentage of the average inventory value, based on local expert opinion.

Operating costs for storage and stock management: These are a mixture of stable and incremental costs. Salaries (which should include benefits), space costs (rent or building depreciation), utilities, communications, other direct costs, and depreciation of equipment are stable costs unless additional staff, space, or equipment is added to manage a growing inventory. When this is done, the added costs are incremental. Supplies are primarily incremental, in that more supplies are used as more stock is stored and distributed. It may be possible in some settings to determine a stable component of the supplies cost. Data should be obtained from financial records or budget books or (if necessary) by estimates from local experts. If administrative overhead is charged as a cost by the supply system, it should be added in the appropriate percentage to operating costs here.

Transport costs to operating units: This includes stable costs (salaries and benefits for transport personnel, depreciation of vehicles) and incremental costs (gasoline, repairs, and travel expenses for transport personnel). Again, if more drivers or vehicles were added to cope with an increased workload, these costs would be incremental.

The total of all these costs is the total inventory holding cost, showing stable and incremental components.

Purchasing Costs. Purchasing costs (sometimes called reordering costs) are the costs associated with managing tenders, placing purchase orders, and receiving goods. Like inventory holding costs, purchasing costs have several components. Salaries (including benefits) should include wages for all staff who are involved in managing tenders, ordering drugs, and receiving them. Note that some staff may be attached to the warehouse rather than the purchasing office, but for this purpose, their costs should be attributed to purchasing. If warehouse staff have multiple responsibilities, including some that are related to purchasing, attribute a portion of their cost to inventory holding and a portion to purchasing. Utilities and space costs include rent, basic communications costs, and all utilities for the purchasing office. Supplies include all forms used in tenders and purchase orders (this might be broken down into stable and incremental components in a perpetual or scheduled purchasing system). Other direct costs include travel costs and maintenance of building and equipment. Depreciation may be calculated on all valuable equipment and on the building if it is owned by the system. Again, if administrative overhead is charged, it should be added using the current percentage. Additional tender costs include costs that are not included in standard purchasing costs but are associated with the quantification, tendering, and adjudication processes, including travel, per diem, and other costs associated with committee meetings.

In a public drug supply system that uses annual or biannual purchasing, most of these purchasing costs can be considered stable, assuming the existence of a procurement office with permanent staff and office space. In a perpetual system, or a scheduled system with periodic orders, the costs of communications and supplies such as forms are incremental with each order placed.

Data on the individual component costs may be available from financial records or budget books; once the individual component costs (actual or estimated) are obtained and recorded, they are summed to produce the total purchasing cost.

Shortage Costs. There are four potential kinds of shortage costs, as discussed in Chapter 15:

► Excess cost of emergency purchases;
► Loss of revenue when clients purchase outside the system;
► Increased morbidity and mortality due to stockouts;
► Loss of goodwill due to erosion of confidence in the system.

Only the first two can be valued for a public drug supply system.

If good procurement records for both regular and emergency purchases are available, the actual cost of emergency purchases can be calculated by recording the difference between the emergency cost and the regular cost per unit or package and multiplying by the quantity purchased for each emergency purchase. If data are not available for all emergency purchases, a sample may be used to estimate the average percentage price difference and the percentage of purchases attributable to emergency purchases (as was done in Figure 41.10).

If the supply system sells drugs from one level to another, it may be possible to obtain itemized data on actual purchases outside the system of items that would normally be purchased inside. An estimate can be made for the value of such purchases based on the breakdown between purchases inside and outside the supply system.

Calculating the Total Variable Cost. The total variable cost is calculated as the sum of the subtotals for each component. In Figure 41.10, the costs total $17.8 million. The major component is drug acquisition, but holding costs and shortage costs are significant factors; purchasing costs are the lowest component. As discussed earlier, the inventory holding costs are mostly incremental, and the purchasing costs are mostly stable.

Once the total variable cost has been compiled, several ratios calculated from total variable cost components can serve as basic indicators for comparing operating efficiency among different parts of the current supply system (or with alternative models). Standard ratios include

► holding cost as a percentage of average inventory, calculated by dividing the total holding cost by the average inventory value, and expressing the result as a percentage. In commercial firms, the inventory holding cost is usually between 25 and 35 percent of average inventory value; in a public drug supply system the percentage may be considerably higher, though it need not be with good inventory management;
► purchasing costs as a percentage of drug acquisition costs, to compare how efficiently the purchasing function is managed;
► average inventory turnover (the total value of drugs purchased and/or distributed, divided by the average inventory value), discussed in Chapter 15;
► personnel costs, space costs, transport costs, other direct operating costs, each as a percentage of total holding costs, showing the relative proportion of total costs attributable to each category;
► total holding cost as a percentage of the value of drugs distributed or the value of receipts, giving an indication of the cost effectiveness of maintaining in-house services as opposed to contracting out some or all aspects of storage and distribution. A variation of this ratio is total variable cost to value of drugs distributed or received.

≡ 41.7 Lead-Time and Payment-Time Analysis

Lead time is defined as the interval between submitting an order and receiving the goods. In many countries, most drugs purchased by the public sector are imported, and lead times are frequently long and variable.

Payment time is defined as the interval between receipt of goods at the warehouse and payment to the supplier. This is of concern in supply systems that have delayed

Figure 41.11 Lead-Time Analysis

Purchase Order	Contract Lead Time	Actual Lead Time	Shipment Days Overdue	Contract Payment Lead Time	Actual Payment Lead Time	Payment Days Overdue
KIT-8001	45	57	12	45	43	0
LUC-8001	45	27	0	45	112	67
LUC-8001	45	119	74	45	20	0
MON-801	45	30	0	45	63	18
VIN-8000	45	21	0	45	96	51

Average lead time		50.8 days	Average pay time		66.8 days
Percentage of orders overdue		50%	% late pay		75%
Average delay when overdue		43 days	Average delay when overdue		45 days

Source: Data come from the Caribbean pooled procurement program.
Note: LUC-8001 was shipped in two partial shipments, one on time, the other not.

payment terms with suppliers; in such systems, monitoring and controlling payment lead time is of paramount importance if the system wishes to continue to pay on delayed terms.

An analysis of lead times and payment times for purchases in 1994 by an international pooled procurement program is presented in Figure 41.11. It shows the variability that occurs in practice and illustrates how to construct a lead-time and payment-time analysis table. Note that the supplier was late in delivering half of this small sample of orders. The average lead time for all shipments was more than fifty days compared with the contractual forty-five days, but the average delay nearly doubled the contract lead time, adding forty-three days on average. In the same figure, the procurement agency paid within the contracted forty-five days for only two of the five shipments. The average payment lead time was sixty-seven days, and for those payments that were overdue, the average was double the contract requirement.

There are two major implications. First, this supplier has a highly variable lead time, and the procurement office needs to either adjust safety stock to cope with the worst case or switch suppliers. Second, there may be little choice if payment lead time is not improved—the supplier may refuse to ship without prior payment. The payment delays may also be affecting the supplier's interest in delivering on time.

When evaluating supplier offers and planning orders and deliveries, it is important that managers use the expected delivery date, based on past performance, rather than the promised delivery date. Many supply systems take the simple average actual lead time from past deliveries and assume that this is the expected lead time. Thus, for the supplier in Figure 41.11, the expected lead time would be fifty-one days (instead of the promised forty-five days). A variation of six days would probably be acceptable in most situations, but two of five shipments were

delayed longer than fifty-one days (much longer in one case). Chapter 15 discusses options for adjusting the simple average lead time to cover substantial variation; one of these methods should be used for this supplier.

≡ **41.8 Analysis of Expiry Dates**

Analysis of expiry dates versus inventory levels is useful for determining how much stock is at risk of wastage. Figure 41.12 shows the results of an expiry date analysis in a Caribbean country.

The analysis is done for each drug by determining the average monthly consumption during the past year (adjusted for periods out of stock), and dividing the quantity in stock by the average monthly consumption to determine the stock position in months. Then the number of months remaining until expiry is calculated.

If the months until expiry are greater than the stock position in months, there should be limited risk of wastage. If the stock position is higher than the months until expiry, there is some risk. Multiply the months until expiration by the average monthly use to get the projected use before expiry; subtract this from the stock on hand to obtain the quantity of stock at risk. The unit acquisition price, multiplied by the quantity at risk, yields the value of stock at risk.

Options to solve the problems identified in this analysis include increasing the use of some of the items at risk by substituting them for other commonly used items (with the consent of prescribers and dispensers). It may be possible to return some of the items to the supplier for credit, or perhaps a barter arrangement can be negotiated with another warehouse or supply system.

In the example from Figure 41.12, it is clear that substantial quantities of stock would have been lost to expiry unless action was taken; the value of the stock at risk was about 2.4 percent of the country's annual drug budget. Note that for cephalexin tablets and injections, action

Figure 41.12 Expiry Date Analysis (Caribbean Country, January 1990)

Name/Strength/Form	Issue Unit	Issue Unit Cost (US$)	Average Monthly Use	Current Stock Position (Units)	Current Stock Position (Months)	Expiry Date	Months Until Expiry	Projected Use	Quantity of Stock at Risk	Value of Stock at Risk
Antacid suspension	500 mL bottle	1.9800	110	2065	18.8	Oct 90	9	990	1,075	$2,128.50
Cephalexin 125 mg/5 mL susp	100 mL bottle	1.8000	4	60	13.5	Jun 90	5	22	38	$68.00
Cephalexin 250 mg	Tablet	.0900	333	8200	24.6	Aug 90	7	2,333	5,867	$528.00
Chlorhexidine gluconate 5% solution	5 L bottle	17.9500	1	45	45.0	Apr 91	15	15	30	$538.50
Chlorpheniramine 2 mg/5 mL elixir	1 L bottle	3.7500	8	140	16.8	Sep 90	8	67	73	$275.00
Codeine linctus	1 L bottle	6.0000	1	58	72.5	Nov 91	22	18	40	$242.40
Dexamethasone inj, 4 mg/mL, 5 mL	5 mL vial	1.4600	17	290	17.4	Feb 90	1	17	273	$399.07
Diazepam inj, 10 mg/2 mL	2 mL ampoule	.1750	150	1300	8.7	Aug 90	7	1,050	250	$43.75
Erythromycin base salts 250 mg	Tablet	.0419	333	6000	18.0	Nov 90	10	3,333	2,667	$111.73
Lidocaine 2% jelly	15 gm tube	2.0700	20	640	32.0	Jun 91	17	340	300	$621.00
Naloxone HCl inj, 0.02 mg/mL, 2 mL	2 mL ampoule	.7500	3	110	44.0	Dec 90	11	28	83	$61.88
Pancuronium bromide inj, 2 mg/mL	2 mL ampoule	1.7500	4	50	12.0	Dec 90	11	46	4	$7.29
Penicillin G benzathine inj, 2.4 MU	Ampoule	.5000	39	1990	50.5	Jun 92	29	1,143	847	$423.46
Penicillin G Na inj, powder, 1 MU	Vial	.2600	33	1000	30.0	May 91	16	533	467	$121.33
Phytomenadione inj, 1 mg/0.6 mL	Ampoule	.1500	83	2000	24.2	Dec 90	11	909	1,091	$163.70
Water for injection, 10 mL	Vial	.1550	117	400	3.4	Apr 90	3	350	50	$7.75
								Total value at risk:		$5,741.35

was needed quickly due to the rapidly approaching expiration date. It was already too late to use up dexamethasone or water for injection. The antacid suspension presented the highest financial risk (nearly half of the total value at risk).

For some of the items at risk, increasing utilization through substitution might be feasible. For example, cephalexin tablets and erythromycin could be substituted for penicillin VK or (for some patients) for ampicillin or cotrimoxazole. Penicillin injection might replace cephalosporins (if they are commonly used). Antacid suspension could replace histamine-2 antagonists in some cases. Substitution would be a less appropriate solution for drugs such as codeine, diazepam, or phytomenadione; probably the best solution for these items (and for most overstocks) would be a barter arrangement with a neighboring supply system.

The real value of expiry date analysis is that, if used regularly, it can help avoid a situation like the one illustrated, by detecting potential problems before they are insoluble.

≡ 41.9 Hidden Cost Analysis

The concept of hidden costs was introduced in Chapters 11 and 12; hidden costs are those costs that occur due to poor supplier performance and are not obvious in the invoice price.

The total cost of purchasing an item from a specific supplier is the sum of the quoted price, any shipping and handling costs, and any hidden costs. In comparing quotations from different suppliers, procurement officers should consider the expected hidden costs for each supplier, based on past performance. One way to do this is to calculate the hidden cost ratio (hidden costs / visible costs). Visible costs are the sum of cost, insurance, and freight (CIF) for all past orders. Hidden costs are

- commissions for local agents;
- plus the cost of late deliveries (including air freight for emergency needs, use of more expensive alternatives, higher cost for emergency replacements, and so forth);
- plus the cost of delivery errors (sum of costs incurred because of short shipments, incorrect drugs shipped, shipments delivered to wrong port, additional port costs because of lack of proper documents, and so forth);
- plus the value of losses due to poor packaging;
- plus the replacement cost of unusable drugs (short shelf lives, disintegrated drugs, and so forth)
- minus the value of cost-saving contributions (deferred payment terms, suggestions for less expensive dosage forms, and so forth).

For example, assume that Supplier A has provided drugs to a supply system at a net CIF cost of US$100,000 (the visible cost). A review of the procurement office's records might show that for these purchases, the following hidden costs were incurred:

- Commission for local agents (3 percent) = $3,000;
- Late deliveries (air freight and higher price for temporary emergency stocks) = $9,000;
- Delivery errors (2 percent average short-packing) = $2,000;
- Losses from poor packaging (not covered by insurance) = $2,500;
- Unusable drugs (replacement cost for tablets that disintegrated in transit; expired products not replaced by supplier) = $5,000;

≡ Assessment Guide

Indicators Related to Analytical Techniques

► Numbers of drugs and value of average consumption for drugs in classes A, B, and C from ABC analysis;

► Value of unplanned purchases (items not on original quantification list) as a percentage of value of total purchases;

► Average supply system acquisition price as a percentage of average international price for indicator drugs;

► Average medical stores sales price as a percentage of local wholesale sales price for indicator drugs—private and NGO sectors;

► Average public-sector pharmacy sales price as a percentage of local retail pharmacy sales price for indicator drugs;

► Ratio of net sales (or value of distributed drugs) to inventory—also called "inventory turnover";

► Operating margin on total sales—the value of total sales, minus the cost of goods sold, divided by the total sales;

► Inventory holding costs as percentage of average inventory value;

► Purchasing costs as percentage of average inventory value;

► Average lead time and payment time for each major supplier;

► Value of drugs at risk of expiry as percentage of inventory value.

Analytical Capacity in Supply System

► Which departments or offices in the supply system are responsible for analyzing recurrent costs and developing cost control strategies?

► What kinds of analyses and reports are produced (and how frequently are they produced)?

► Are computers and spreadsheet software available for analyzing costs in the drug supply system?

► What kinds of software with analytical and reporting capacity, in addition to spreadsheets, are available?

VEN Analysis

► Is there a two- or three-tier system for prioritizing procurement according to public health value (similar to VEN or VN)?

► If there is no formal system, how are priorities determined when there are insufficient funds to purchase all drugs requested?

ABC Analysis

► Has an ABC analysis been done recently of drug consumption or purchases (and if not, does the system have the data and the capacity needed to do this analysis)?

► How do usage and expenditures compare with health priorities?

► How is information from ABC analysis used to improve purchasing and inventory management?

Therapeutic Category Analysis

► Have there been recent efforts to analyze consumption and expenditures by therapeutic category (and if so, how is the information used)?

► How are the merits of one drug product compared with those of other products in drug selection and procurement?

► Does the purchasing office sometimes tender by therapeutic category or subcategory rather than for specific drugs?

Price Comparison Analysis

► What sources of data are available for price comparison analysis? (See also price comparison indicators above.)

Total Variable Cost Analysis

► Availability of expenditure reports or budget estimates of operating costs in warehouses and purchasing offices.

► Value of accounts receivable from patients and from other facilities.

► Value of bad-debt write-offs.

► Value of total purchases and total sales (or value of drugs distributed).

► Value of cost of goods sold (or distributed).

► Beginning and ending inventory value for the fiscal year for major warehouses and health facilities, and average inventory value.

- ► Inventory shrinkage: the sum of beginning inventory value plus purchases, minus the sum of cost of goods sold plus ending inventory value.
- ► Value of any donations received or stock returns from clients.
- ► Value of operating costs—stable and incremental—for stock management functions (ideally at each major level of the system).
- ► Value of expired and/or wasted stock removed during the year and any such stock remaining.
- ► Value of operating costs associated with drug transport.
- ► Value of operating costs—stable and incremental—for purchasing functions.
- ► Value of incremental costs associated with managing tenders.
- ► Value of incremental costs of emergency purchases to cover shortages.

- ► Value of lower-level purchases outside supply system (for centralized procurement systems).

Lead-Time and Payment-Time Analysis
- ► How are lead times and payment times tracked and used by the purchasing office?

Expiry Date Analysis
- ► How does the supply system track expiration dates? Are reports prepared on the expiry status of drugs in stock?
- ► What is done about stock that will likely expire before it can be used?

Hidden Cost Analysis
- ► Are hidden costs calculated for regular suppliers to the supply system, and if not, are records adequate to compile the information?

- ► Cost-saving contributions (discount achieved because of Supplier A's suggestion of alternative dosage forms for a few common items) = $1,500.

Based on this experience with Supplier A, the procurement office calculates the hidden cost ratio of 23 percent, derived from ($3,000 + $9,000 + $2,000 + $2,500 +$5,000 - $1,500) / $100,000. This information can then be used to project total costs of later orders for comparison with competing suppliers. A hidden cost ratio of 23 percent for Supplier A means that the total cost for the drug supply system will be about $1.23 for every $1.00 quoted by Supplier A for a product. If Supplier A quotes a CIF price of $100 for an item, the total expected cost would be $123. If Supplier B quotes a CIF price of $110 but Supplier B has an estimated hidden cost ratio of only 5 percent, the expected total cost ($115) would make Supplier B the most cost-effective choice.

It is rarely possible to be precise with hidden cost estimates, but criteria for reviewing supplier performance might include hidden costs as one aspect of comparison. If there are large differences in hidden cost ratios between two suppliers, based on past performance, this might be a deciding factor in the choice. As discussed in Chapter 16, if hidden costs are to be considered in evaluating supplier offers, this should be clearly specified in procurement evaluation criteria and in tender documents. ∎

≡ References and Further Readings

★ = *Key readings.*

★ Bootman, J. L., R. J. Townsend, and W. F. McGhan. 1996. *Principles of pharmacoeconomics*, 2d ed. Cincinnati, Ohio: Harvey Whitney Books Company.
★ Creese, A., and D. Parker. 1994. *Cost analysis in primary health care.* Geneva: World Health Organization.
Dear, A. 1990. *Inventory management demystified.* London: Chapman and Hall.
ECDS (Eastern Caribbean Drug Service). 1994. *Regional formulary and therapeutics manual*, 4th ed. Castries, St. Lucia: ECDS.
Freund, D. A., and Dittus, R. S. 1992. Principles of pharmacoeconomic analysis of drug therapy. *PharmacoEconomics* 1:20–32.
MSH (Management Sciences for Health). 1992. Systematic cost reduction. In *Managing drug supply training series.* Part 1. *Policy issues in managing drug supply.* Boston: MSH.
MSH (Management Sciences for Health). 1995. *International drug price indicator guide* (updated annually). Boston: MSH.
★ MSH/RPM (Management Sciences for Health/Rational Pharmaceutical Management Project). 1995. *Rapid pharmaceutical management assessment: An indicator-based approach.* Washington, D.C.: MSH/RPM.
MSH/RPM (Management Sciences for Health/Rational Pharmaceutical Management Project). 1996. *Prescription analysis software system—user's manual.* Washington, D.C.: MSH/RPM.
WHO Collaborating Centre for Drug Statistics Methodology. 1996. *Anatomical therapeutic chemical (ATC) classification index.* Oslo: WHO.

Part I	Part II	Part III	Part IV
Introduction	Policy and Legal Framework	Drug Management Cycle	**Management Support Systems**

A Organization and Management

B Financial and Sustainability ▶

C Information Management

D Human Resources Management

40 Drug Financing Strategies

41 Analyzing and Controlling Drug Expenditures

42 Financial Planning and Management

43 Donor Financing

44 Revolving Drug Funds

Chapter 42
Financial Planning and Management

≡ Summary

Effective financial planning and management are vital for the successful generation, safekeeping, and use of funds to achieve program objectives.

Government budgeting and accounting systems operate on a cash basis, recording a transaction only when cash is involved. Private-sector or semi-autonomous government programs, including many revolving drug funds (RDFs), use an accrual system, which also records noncash transactions such as drugs issued. Public-sector managers can complement government accounting systems with elements of an accrual system to support more effective and efficient program management.

Long-range financial plans include projections of both funding and expenditures for the next several years and thus facilitate the long-range planning of health services. For an RDF, a long-range plan can project the point in the future when revenues from drug sales will be sufficient to cover drug program expenses. The realization of projected revenues depends on the development and implementation of detailed drug pricing strategies.

The first-year figures from a "rolling" long-range plan provide the basis for an annual budget, which is used to plan and control spending for the current year. Whereas government budgets may be based on fixed funding, an RDF budget is flexible, with the level of expenditure dependent on sales revenue. A cash flow forecast helps ensure the availability of sufficient cash to cover anticipated obligations each month. Cost analysis is used to measure program efficiency and to help set prices.

Principles for effective financial control include

- ▸ *dividing duties among different individuals;*
- ▸ *regulating transactions through the use of written procedures;*
- ▸ *recording and monitoring all transactions.*

The accounting system should produce the following standard reports on a monthly and annual basis:

- ▸ *budget performance report;*
- ▸ *income and expense report;*
- ▸ *balance sheet;*
- ▸ *summary of accounts payable and receivable.*

≡ Government allocations continue to be a major source of financing for drug supply in many countries. Although public expenditure decisions are usually made in ministries of finance and of planning (see Chapter 3), program managers can often lobby for more funding for their programs and activities. They are better able to do so if they understand the issues involved in public-sector resource allocation, can argue effectively for greater investments in health, and can demonstrate responsible and efficient use of existing resources.

With public financing of drug supply, managers of drug programs are responsible for ensuring that resources are used in the best way possible to achieve program objectives. Financial management is a vital aspect of this. Managers need to plan, control, and monitor the generation, safekeeping, and use of funds, and they must be able to provide proper financial reports to government authorities and donors. This chapter provides a working knowledge of the necessary financial management concepts and skills.

Drug programs generally define their objectives in terms of services provided. However, financial objectives are becoming increasingly important as programs try to maintain or expand services, often in the face of reduced funding. Programs need to seek increased government and donor funding, generate additional revenues from cost sharing, and be efficient and cost effective in the provision of services. To achieve these objectives, program managers must be able to

- ▸ prepare long-range plans to project the need for services, devise the most cost-effective way to provide them, outline the resources needed, and help secure government and donor funding;
- ▸ set sales prices that are affordable, competitive, and meet program cost-sharing goals (discussed in Chapter 44);
- ▸ prepare and use budgets to plan and contain expenses;
- ▸ prepare cash flow forecasts to ensure the availability of cash to cover anticipated financial obligations;
- ▸ analyze costs to assess cost effectiveness and monitor efficiency;
- ▸ control and manage the collection, safekeeping, and spending of funds;
- ▸ keep proper accounting records and prepare reports for management, government, and donors.

Public-sector financial management systems, as traditionally designed, are often less than ideal for managing drug programs. This is especially true with regard to the collection of sales revenue, which is often a new feature in government ministries. Under such circumstances, managers of government programs may need to develop and use complementary systems to help them manage their resources effectively.

This chapter describes both how to get the best use from existing government financial management systems and how to develop complementary procedures. If all these procedures are used, the resulting system should provide a good basis for effective financial management. The sample budgets and reports shown are based on the hypothetical case of a government drug program that is beginning to sell and account for drugs, as in an autonomous revolving drug fund (see Chapter 44). These examples are interrelated, and the figures can therefore be followed from one to another.

≡ 42.1 Getting the Best from a Government Financial System

In recent years, many government departments have begun to follow the private sector in terms of demonstrating "value for money" through the effective and efficient use of resources. However, they have often been hampered by the limitations of budgeting and accounting systems designed only to control spending.

Government drug programs generally suffer from the same problem: the accounting system keeps track of expenditures for drug procurement, but it does not record the value of drugs distributed or lost. The main problem is usually that the government accounting system operates on a *cash basis*, recording a transaction only when cash is received or spent. Under such a system, drugs purchased on credit are not recorded in the accounting records until payment is made, and drug issues are not recorded at all if cash is not received. A cash-based system does not record donated drugs or equipment, drugs issued free of charge, drug losses, purchases and sales on credit, accounts receivable, accounts payable, and depreciation, and there is no accounting record of the stock of drugs. Without such information, it is almost impossible to manage a program properly.

A private-sector program, or a semi-autonomous government program such as a revolving drug fund (RDF), is more likely to use an *accrual-basis* accounting system. Such a system records all transactions at the time they are made. For example, a purchase of drugs on credit is recorded when the drugs are received, increasing the balance in the drug stock account and creating a liability to the supplier. When the supplier is paid, the liability is canceled and the cash balance is reduced. All noncash transactions, such as

donations of drugs, depreciation, and stock write-offs, are also recorded.

Figure 42.1 compares a traditional government budget (cash basis) and an RDF budget (accrual basis). The two budgets are based on the same events, except that the RDF budget includes noncash transactions. The government budget for 1992 shows drug purchases of US$230,000 as an input to the system, but no figure for services delivered as an output. The RDF budget, however, shows the projected cost of drugs issued ($250,000) as a measure of program output; the $230,000 of drug purchases are recorded in a separate *drug stock account*.

Unlike the government budget, the RDF budget also takes into account the value of donated drugs received, the cost of expired or lost drugs, and depreciation on fixed assets. In the government cash budget, for example, operating income is shown as $260,000 (based on a government allocation of $135,000 plus projected sales revenue of $125,000), which will be used to purchase $230,000 of drugs and to pay expenses of $30,000. Total operating income in the RDF budget, however, includes the government allocation of $135,000 (shown as a grant) and sales revenue of $125,000, plus $50,000 in donated drugs, for a total of $310,000; this operating income will be used to distribute $250,000 of drugs (cost of drugs issued), cover stock losses of $12,500 (cost of expired drugs), pay operating expenses of $30,000, fund depreciation of $10,000, and generate an operating surplus (income less expenses) of $7,500. The assets that represent that surplus and the reserve of $10,000 for depreciation appear as an increase of $17,500 in drug stock from the previous year (see closing balance in the drug stock account in Figure 42.1).

Note also that the format of the RDF budget provides more useful management information by grouping categories: for example, showing the deficit made from buying and selling the drugs in the drug account. In both the government and the RDF formats, the actual income and expenses for the previous year are shown next to the budget figures for comparison.

When possible, an accrual basis should always be used. However, if a cash basis must be used because of government rules, elements of an accrual system should be used to complement the government accounting figures and provide more complete information. Priority should be given to those elements that, when adjusted, would have the greatest impact on the overall figures. The most important element is generally the maintenance of complete accounts for drug transactions.

In order to track drug transactions on an accrual basis,

Figure 42.1 Comparison of Traditional Government and RDF Budgets

CENTRAL MEDICAL STORES Traditional Government Budget (Cash Basis)	Actual 1991	Budget 1992
RECURRENT BUDGET		
EXPENDITURES		
Salaries	18,000	19,000
Vehicle operations	2,500	2,700
Other transport	1,500	1,600
Packaging and labeling	3,000	3,300
Utilities	2,000	2,200
Office supplies	1,000	1,200
Drug purchases	160,000	230,000
GROSS EXPENDITURES	188,000	260,000
APPROPRIATIONS IN AID		
Sales revenue	0	125,000
NET EXPENDITURES	188,000	135,000
(Government allocation)		
CAPITAL BUDGET		
Equipment	5,000	10,000

CENTRAL MEDICAL STORES Revolving Drug Fund (Accrual Basis)	Actual 1991	Budget 1992
OPERATING BUDGET		
INCOME FROM GRANTS		
Grants	188,000	135,000
Donated drugs	98,000	50,000
Total grants (A)	286,000	185,000
DRUG ACCOUNT		
Sales revenue	0	125,000
Less cost of drugs issued	240,000	250,000
	(240,000)	(125,000)
Less cost of expired drugs, etc.	15,000	12,500
Surplus/deficit on drug account (B)	(255,000)	(137,500)
EXPENSES		
Salaries	18,000	19,000
Vehicle operations	2,500	2,700
Other transport	1,500	1,600
Packaging and labeling	3,000	3,300
Utilities	2,000	2,200
Office supplies	1,000	1,200
Total operating expenditures	28,000	30,000
Depreciation	0	10,000
Total expenses (C)	28,000	40,000
INCOME LESS EXPENSES (A+B−C)	3,000	7,500
CAPITAL BUDGET		
Equipment	5,000	10,000
PATIENT VOLUME	520,000	500,000

DRUG STOCK ACCOUNT	1991	1992
Opening balance	85,000	88,000
Purchases	160,000	230,000
Donations	98,000	50,000
	343,000	368,000
Less cost of issues	240,000	250,000
Less drug losses	15,000	12,500
Closing balance	88,000	105,500

accounts should be opened for stock, accounts payable, and accounts receivable. This double-entry system reflects each transaction in two accounts. The drug stock account starts with the stock balance, and all subsequent drug transactions are reflected in the account, so that at any given time, the balance reflects the value of stock on hand. Drugs bought on credit increase the stock balance in the stock account and create a liability in accounts payable.

Drugs received as donations (valued at the equivalent local cost) increase the stock in the stock account and are credited to a donations-in-kind account. The cost of lost, damaged, or expired drugs reduces the stock in the stock account and is debited to a drug losses account. The cost of drugs issued or sold reduces the stock balance in the stock account and is debited to a cost-of-drugs-issued or cost-of-sales account. All transactions are valued at the purchase cost, and the balance in the stock account therefore equals the cost of stock on hand.

The cost of drugs issued can be calculated by recording the cost of each drug at the time of issue, but this usually requires a computerized inventory system. However, the figure can be calculated manually by adding the cost of drugs purchased and donated to the cost of the opening drug stock and deducting the cost of the closing drug stock. Provided that the same method is used to value both opening and closing stocks, the resulting figure represents the cost of drugs used plus the cost of expired, missing, and damaged drugs.

The other adjustments that can be made to produce an accrual-based report from a government account relate to depreciation and operating expenses. However, since a government usually replaces fixed assets through capital budgets, it is probably not worth making this adjustment unless the program will have to replace assets from self-generated resources in the future. Also, it may not be worthwhile to bring operating expenses such as salaries or electricity onto an accrual basis if the amounts are relatively small and the expenses are paid on a regular basis.

The remaining sections of this chapter describe other elements of good financial management that should be in place, whether a program is governmental or autonomous. Some of these elements relate to the planning and management of sales revenues, which apply only to those programs that currently sell drugs or plan to in the future.

≡ 42.2 Long-Range Financial Planning

It is important to have a long-range view of both program objectives and activities and the resources needed to carry them out. A long-range plan must include a realistic financial plan showing what funding is anticipated and how it will be spent. Without this, unachievable objectives may be set. A long-range plan might cover five years and should be a "rolling" plan—updated each year for a new five-year period beginning with the current year. The plan is broken down to show what activities will be carried out each year and the estimated funding and expenditures for each year. Program planning and financial planning are inseparable, and both program and financial managers must be involved in the development of the financial plan.

A long-range plan is just as necessary for a grant-funded government drug program as it is for an RDF. With a grant-funded program, it is an attempt to plan services based on estimated levels of fixed funding and, at the same time, to justify additional funding. With an RDF, it is a plan for both revenue generation and services, with each

being completely dependent on the other. Often a program is a mixture of grant and revenue funding. For example, administration could be covered by a grant, whereas the purchase of drugs is funded from revenue.

In summary, long-range financial planning is important because it results in

► an assessment of resources required for necessary services;
► a review of the financial feasibility of plans and a determination of whether more funds will be needed or activities will have to be reduced;
► a plan for long-term resource generation and investment;
► greater ability to seek funding successfully;
► prioritization of essential program activities;
► a plan to obtain resources when they are needed;
► a tool that can be used to set periodic programmatic and financial benchmarks.

Figure 42.2 shows an example of a long-range financial plan for a grant-funded government drug program that is to be converted to a revenue-funded RDF over a three-year period. The layout of the plan serves both types of program equally well. Note that the plan shows the forecasted levels of patients to be served, the likely inflation rate, and average patient cost and price, which makes it easier to see what is being projected. All long-range financial plans must build in a factor for annual inflation, as this example does. For expenditures on imported goods, changes in exchange rates over time must be considered as well. Box 42.1 gives further details on adjusting for price levels and exchange rates.

The long-range financial plan in Figure 42.2 projects that sustainability will be reached in 1994. In that year, sales revenue exceeds total expenses for the first time. Another way to look at it is that the increased drug price (25 percent over cost) is enough to generate a trading surplus of $73,205, which is more than the total nondrug expenses of $60,100. Although surpluses of income over expenses are projected in previous years, they are due to grants and donations rather than to drug sales.

≡ 42.3 Setting Drug Sales Prices

Although the process of long-range financial planning includes projection of total revenues from drug sales, it is only through the development and implementation of detailed pricing strategies that these revenues will be realized.

Building on the long-range plan shown in Figure 42.2, Figure 42.3 presents an example of price setting to achieve

Figure 42.2 Five-Year Financial Plan

CENTRAL MEDICAL STORES REVOLVING DRUG FUND
Five-Year Financial Plan 1992–96

	Actual 1991	Planned 1992	Planned 1993	Planned 1994	Planned 1995	Planned 1996
OPERATING PLAN						
INCOME FROM GRANTS						
Grants	188,000	135,000	50,000	0	0	0
Donated drugs	98,000	50,000	50,000	50,000	30,000	20,000
Total grants (A)	286,000	185,000	100,000	50,000	30,000	20,000
DRUG ACCOUNT						
Sales revenue[a]	0	125,000	302,500	457,531	553,613	669,872
Less cost of drugs issued[b]	240,000	250,000	302,500	366,025	442,890	535,897
	(240,000)	(125,000)	0	91,506	110,723	133,975
Less cost of expired drugs etc.[c]	15,000	12,500	15,125	18,301	22,145	26,795
Surplus/deficit on drug account (B)	255,000	(137,500)	(15,125)	73,205	88,578	107,180
EXPENSES						
Operating expenses[d]	28,000	30,000	41,000	45,100	49,610	54,571
Depreciation	0	10,000	12,000	15,000	15,000	16,000
Total expenses (C)	28,000	40,000	53,000	60,100	64,610	70,571
INCOME LESS EXPENSES (A+B–C)	3,000	7,500	31,875	63,105	53,968	56,608
CAPITAL PLAN						
ACQUISITIONS						
Equipment	5,000	10,000	5,000	2,000	3,000	10,000
Vehicles				15,000		
Buildings					100,000	
TOTAL	5,000	10,000	5,000	17,000	103,000	10,000
FUNDING						
Government	5,000	10,000				
Donors					100,000	
Reserves			5,000	17,000	3,000	10,000
TOTAL	5,000	10,000	5,000	17,000	103,000	10,000
Patient volume[e]	520,000	500,000	550,000	605,000	665,500	732,050
Avg. drug cost per patient visit/day	0.46	0.50	0.55	0.61	0.67	0.73
Avg. price per patient visit/day	0.00	0.25	0.55	0.76	0.83	0.92
ASSUMPTIONS						
Increase in patient volume			10%	10%	10%	10%
Inflation rate		10%	10%	10%	10%	10%
Price as a % of drug cost	0%	50%	100%	125%	125%	125%

PROJECTED REVENUES, 1992–96

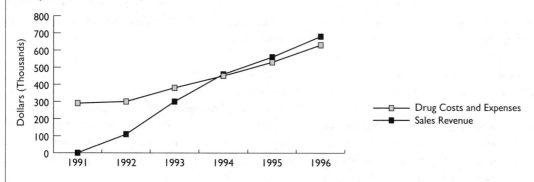

[a] Drugs will be sold from 1/1/92 with 50% recovery of drug purchase price in the first year.
[b] Drug cost is expected to increase with inflation and patient volume.
[c] Cost of drugs expired or lost is estimated at 5% of cost of drugs issued.
[d] Includes additional $8,000 for administering cost recovery from 1993.
[e] Patient volume is the total of outpatient visits and inpatient bed days.

Box 42.1 Adjusting for Price Levels and Exchange Rates

Any comparison of money amounts at different points in time requires consideration of the possible effect of inflation and/or changes in the exchange rate. Such situations include budgeting and forecasting future expenditure needs, pricing in revolving drug funds, and analyzing expenditure trends.

Inflation

Inflation can arise when the cost of imported goods rises due to rising world prices or exchange rate depreciation. Inflation also arises when the growth in a country's expenditure or consumption of goods and services exceeds the growth in its supply or production of goods and services.

Changes in the price level make the comparison of expenditures in different years more complicated: the purchasing power of a given budget depends on the price level during that year. Expenditures that are not adjusted to account for changes in the price level are called *nominal* or *current-price* expenditures; when they are adjusted to reflect changes in the price level, they are called *real* or *constant-price* expenditures. To compare expenditures in different years, they can be translated into the same "price units" using a gross domestic product (GDP) deflator series, which is usually available from the ministry of economic planning or other central government agency. In these series, one year is chosen as the base year, and other years are expressed as values relative to the base year.

The accompanying figure shows the evolution of health expenditures in Kenya over time, in both current prices and constant prices. Using current prices, expenditures appear to increase from 1988 to 1993. However, when expenditures are translated into constant dollars, in this case using 1990 as the base year, it becomes clear that the real value of expenditures has actually fallen from KSh. 3,000 million in 1988–89 to KSh. 1,800 million in 1993–94.

Health Expenditures, Kenya, 1988–94 (Current and Constant Prices)

Exchange Rates

The exchange rate is the price of foreign currency that equalizes the balance of payments. It is the price at which the inflow of foreign currency from exports and foreign aid is equal to the demand for foreign currency to purchase imports. The exchange rate may be fixed (determined by the government) or flexible (determined in foreign exchange markets).

Changes in the exchange rate over time can make expenditure projections more complicated when a significant proportion of total expenditures is on imported goods (such as drugs). This is often the case in countries undergoing structural adjustment, where the exchange rate may be experiencing large, somewhat unpredictable changes. In these circumstances, it is often useful to separate the local currency and foreign currency items in the budget, so that the foreign currency costs can be updated more easily in response to new information. The ministry of health or planning may be able to provide assistance in making projections about the exchange rate.

---

the drug sales revenue of $457,531 projected for 1994. The example is simplified—including only four drugs and two geographic regions—but it shows how prices can be set based on drug cost. The example is for 1994, the year in which sales revenue is projected to exceed total expenses in the five-year plan. In this analysis, the 1994 net sales revenue of $457,531 is shown under (3) Summary Forecast. Anticipating a total volume of social discounts or waivers valued at $24,157, the gross sales revenue is projected at $481,688.

Projected purchase costs for each drug, and estimates for stock losses and overhead expenses, lead to the establishment of the drugs' full cost. Drug sales prices are then determined, based on these costs, with various markups added and adjustments made to achieve a program's social as well as financial objectives. The adjustments for social discounts and regional equity would take into account willingness and ability to pay. With the availabil-

ity of drug use estimates by region, revenue contributions by drug and by region can be calculated. Price adjustments are then made as needed to ensure that the sum of revenue contributions will equal the overall projected sales revenue. Pricing for RDFs is discussed in more detail in Chapter 44.

≡ 42.4 Budgeting

In addition to a long-range financial plan, it is necessary to have a detailed budget to plan and control spending for the current year. An annual budget should be based on the first-year figures from the current rolling long-range financial plan and should reflect the activities programmed for the year.

The budgeting process must begin well before the start of the year, because it takes time for budgets to be approved. This is especially so with government budgets, where there is a predetermined schedule for submitting a draft budget

Figure 42.3 1994 Price Structure and Forecast

CENTRAL MEDICAL STORES REVOLVING DRUG FUND
1994 Price Structure and Forecast

(1) PRICE STRUCTURE

	Drug 1	Drug 2	Drug 3	Drug 4
A Purchase price[a]	1.00	2.00	3.00	4.00
B Inward freight, duty, etc.[b]	0.05	0.00	0.15	0.20
C Direct cost	1.05	2.00	3.15	4.20
D Stock losses[c] (C x 5.00%)	0.05	0.10	0.16	0.21
E Overhead expenses[c] (C x 16.42%)	0.17	0.33	0.52	0.69
F Full cost	1.27	2.43	3.83	5.10
G Stock replenishment reserve[c] (C x 2.00%)	0.02	0.04	0.06	0.08
H Profit[c, d] (C x 1.61%)	0.02	0.03	0.05	0.07
I Standard price	1.31	2.50	3.94	5.25
J Drug use policy adjustment[e]	0.13	-0.25	0.43	-0.42
K Adjusted price	1.44	2.25	4.37	4.83
L Markup to cover social discount[f] (C x 6.60%)	0.07	0.13	0.21	0.28
	1.51	2.38	4.58	5.11
Regional equity adjustment				
Adjusted regional price, Region 1[g]	1.21	1.91	3.66	4.09
Adjusted regional price, Region 2[g]	1.66	2.62	5.04	5.62

(2) FORECASTED REVENUE BY DRUG AND BY REGION

	Drug 1	Drug 2	Drug 3	Drug 4	Total
Sales volume					
Expected number of units sold, Region 1	14,070	12,665	12,665	9,999	49,399
Expected number of units sold, Region 2	28,144	25,335	25,335	20,001	98,815
Expected number of units sold, total	42,214	38,000	38,000	30,000	148,214
Revenue contribution by drug					
Cost of drugs issued	42,214	76,000	114,000	120,000	352,214
Inward freight, duty, etc.	2,111	0	5,700	6,000	13,811
Direct cost	44,325	76,000	119,700	126,000	366,025
Stock losses	2,216	3,800	5,985	6,300	18,301
Overhead expenses	7,278	12,479	19,654	20,689	60,100
Total cost	53,819	92,279	145,339	152,989	444,426
Stock replacement reserve	886	1,520	2,394	2,520	7,320
Profit	713	1,222	1,925	2,026	5,886
Net sales revenue	55,418	95,021	149,658	157,535	457,632
Drug use policy adjustment	5,542	(9,502)	16,462	(12,603)	(101)
	60,960	85,519	166,120	144,932	457,531
Markup to cover social discount	2,925	5,016	7,900	8,316	24,157
Gross sales revenue	63,885	90,535	174,020	153,248	481,688
Regional equity adjustment					
Adjusted sales revenue, Region 1	17,034	24,140	46,401	40,862	128,437
Adjusted sales revenue, Region 2	46,852	66,396	127,621	112,387	353,256
Total	63,886	90,536	174,022	153,249	481,693

(3) SUMMARY FORECAST

	% of Cost	Income & Exps
Sales revenue		481,688
Less social discounts	6.60%	24,157
Net sales revenue		457,531
Cost of drugs issued		366,025
		91,506
Less: stock losses	5.00%	18,301
Gross profit		73,205
Less: overhead expenses	16.42%	60,100
Operating profit	3.58%	13,105
Less: stock replacement reserve	2.00%	7,320
Net profit		5,785

Notes: In a decentralized program, the field programs would use the sales price of the central program as the purchase price for their program. The other costs added to the transfer price would be those incurred at the field level. If reserves are managed at the central level for the whole program, they would not also be maintained at field levels.

[a] Use the price of the most recent purchase.

[b] Drug 2 is manufactured locally. Freight and duty costs for other drugs were estimated as a percentage.

[c] All other costs and markups for reserves are allocated as a percentage of direct costs, based on the annual budget.

[d] A nonprofit organization would not have a profit markup but would have markups for building necessary reserves to cover a bad year or a disaster (such as major stock damage), assuming insurance is not available.

[e] This adjustment relates to a cross-subsidy from nonessential drugs (here drugs 2 and 4 are essential).

[f] An average of 5 percent of services are provided free over both regions. The higher level of social discounts in Region 1 is not borne by only the full payers in that region.

[g] This cross-subsidy is from the richer Region 2 to the poorer Region 1. Region 2 is assumed to have twice the volume of sales of each drug of Region 1.

to the ministry of health, from which it is forwarded to the ministry of finance. If the budgeting is decentralized, the process will take longer and will have to start earlier.

The budget should show funding sources as well as expenses. A grant-funded government budget is a fixed budget, where funding is known and the objective is to make sure that expenditures do not exceed the funding level. If any income comes from sales revenue, the budget is flexible, since the level of expenditure will depend on the level of income.

Budget Detail

All the resources to be obtained should be shown in the budget. Additional resources that are to be donated should be included so that the budget shows the total resources needed to carry out planned activities. Refer to the example of an RDF budget in Figure 42.1. Separate budgets are prepared for operating (recurrent) funds and capital (development) funds.

The operating budget covers the cost of all items consumed during the year, including salaries, allowances, drugs, transport, travel, postage, telephone, office supplies, heat, electricity, water, and office rent. Any donated items such as drugs or office supplies should be shown and identified as relating to a specific funding source. When assets are to be replaced from sales revenue, depreciation should be included as an expense.

The capital budget must show all land and buildings to be bought or built, as well as vehicles and equipment to be purchased. All assets that have a long life (over one year) and a significant value should be included. The definitions of life and value should be in accordance with government regulations or with current accounting standards, if not covered by regulations. A donated item, such as a vehicle, should be shown in the capital budget and related to a specific funding source.

Budgeting Method

In government programs, although budgets are prepared according to program needs, the amount approved generally follows a historical basis: that is, the previous year's budget is adjusted by a percentage to reflect the expected change in overall government funding and, to some degree, shifting program priorities. Resource allocation decisions may also be affected by political and other external forces, as discussed in Chapter 3.

Unless there is other funding from donors or sales, the main purpose of budget preparation is to try to obtain the level of funding needed to provide services. Once the amount of funding is decided, the job of the manager is to use it to achieve approved program objectives in the most cost-effective way. This is not easy when the distribution among line items is inefficient and cannot be changed.

In programs that have some autonomy and that have funding from donors or from sales, the budget is prepared more as a planning tool, with a relationship among program activities, expenditures, and income. For example, in the 1992 RDF budget shown in Figure 42.1, the ability to purchase and distribute $250,000 worth of drugs depends on the ability to recover half the cost in sales revenue. Once the budget is approved, the manager has certain autonomy to reduce or increase expenditures, depending on funding levels, or to shift funds among line items to achieve maximum efficiency.

Whichever type of budget is used, the preparation involves identifying, quantifying, and costing the resources needed; determining the level of available funding; and adjusting expenditures to the expected level of funding.

Identify, Quantify, and Cost the Resources Needed. Each activity in the workplan must be examined, and the staff time, supplies, and equipment needed to carry it out must be quantified. For example, the manager of a central medical store must decide how many staff are needed to properly handle and record the drugs, what types of equipment (such as forklifts or computers) are needed, what it takes to run them, and what supplies are needed. (See the discussion of quantification of drug needs in Chapter 14.) When the quantity of each resource is determined, the cost can be estimated. If some of the resources are to be purchased long after preparing the budget, a percentage for inflation should be added to the current price.

Determine the Level of Available Funding. Funding may include government allocations, donor grants, and sales revenues. It is important to show each funding source separately and to show the relationship between any earmarked funding source and the expenditures to which it relates. It should be recognized that not all the government funding may materialize—sometimes only salaries are maintained at the budgeted level. The budget should be prepared as if the whole government allocation will be provided, but managers should anticipate that some funds may not arrive.

In the case of revenue generated from sales, it is important to be conservative when preparing estimates, since there is a risk that such revenues might not be forthcoming (for instance, due to collection problems). Sales revenues depend on the forecasted volume of sales for each drug and the price. From this must be deducted the sales value of drugs to be provided free (either to the poor or for exempt services) and any estimated losses, such as for leakage, deterioration, or expiration.

Adjust Expenditures to the Expected Level of Funding. This adjustment is cyclical. Activities are originally determined in accordance with needs and with an optimistic view of funding. As the actual level of funding becomes clear, if it is less than hoped, activities are reduced or made less costly. It is useful to set priorities among the activities so that it is clear in advance which activities will be cut if funding is lacking.

The budget must always show the basis for each line item. For example: Fuel for transporting drugs—$8,000 (4 vehicles at 20,000 miles per year, 10 miles per gallon, $1 per gallon). A budget that clearly relates financial estimates to activities is easier to justify, and this can help managers obtain the required funding. The RDF budget example in Figure 42.1 shows the number of patients to be served, which is useful. It could also show type of patient (children), disease (malaria), and geographical areas to be covered.

≡ 42.5 Cash Planning

Even though there may be sufficient funds in the budget, there may be times when there is not enough cash to pay the bills, especially if funding is irregular or large payments must be made (such as for a bulk purchase of drugs). A cash flow forecast helps ensure sufficient cash to cover all anticipated financial obligations each month. An example of a cash flow forecast is given in Figure 42.4.

The cash flow forecast should be prepared from the workplan and budget. The process is simple: start with the anticipated cash balance (cash in hand and at the bank) and add receipts and deduct payments in the months when they are expected to fall. In the example, it is expected that grants will be received periodically, in January, April, July, October, and December. Sales revenue is expected to vary only slightly each month. A loan of $50,000 will be available in January. Capital purchases, receipts, and payments relating to accounts receivable and payable should be included in the cash flow forecast, but those items that do not result in cash receipts or payments (depreciation, stock losses) can be omitted.

If the balance at the end of any month is negative, there will be insufficient funds that month. When that happens, either activities or funding schedules will have to be changed or credit will have to be obtained. If there is a significant surplus, it may be desirable to put it into a deposit account at the bank to earn interest, but risks should not be taken to earn higher interest rates.

Where an additional sales markup is being charged on drugs to cover replacement cost, it is wise to put the additional funds generated into a separate bank account so that they will be available when the time comes to replace the drugs. Likewise, the depreciation fund can be put into a separate bank account as a special reserve. Payments to such special reserve accounts should be treated as cash payments in the cash flow forecast so that they are not perceived as available to cover operating costs. In the month when they will be used to replace drugs or a fixed asset, the funds should be shown as incoming revenue.

Failure to predict cash flow accurately can result in cash shortages, which can mean problems with paying salaries (resulting in demoralization of staff), replenishing drug stocks, keeping vehicles operational, or replacing equipment. Any one of these can prevent a program from achieving its objectives.

≡ 42.6 Costing

Cost analysis is an important management tool, as it allows managers to measure the efficiency of their programs. Efficiency can be understood as getting the most output for a given quantity of resources (for example, purchasing more drugs with a constant budget), or achieving a given level of output at minimum cost (such as treating a bacterial infection at lowest cost). Efficiency concepts are discussed in more detail in Chapter 3. By determining the cost of each unit of output (which in a drug supply system is the cost of drugs), managers can compare the efficiency of their programs over time or with other organizations. Cost figures can also be used to estimate the financial impact of serving different patient volumes, different patient types, or different disease types and to set prices.

The starting place in establishing costs is the original purchase price of each drug. This varies over time, depending on the supplier, the date of purchase, the unit of purchase, and the volume. The costing method depends on the purpose of the exercise: an average cost can be used for comparisons, and the cost of the most recent purchase should be used for setting a sales price. If there are significant transport costs for imported drugs, they should be added to the purchase cost of the particular drugs supplied.

Other costs, including the transport charges for in-country distribution, are best allocated in total, particularly if the cost information is used to set prices. To add high transport costs to the cost of drugs sent to remote places is not equitable, especially since the patients in those areas are often poorer.

If the total operating costs of the drug supply system come to 10 percent of the total cost of the drugs distributed, the cost of each drug is its purchase price plus its

Figure 42.4 Cash Flow Forecast

CENTRAL MEDICAL STORES REVOLVING DRUG FUND
Cash Flow Forecast 1992

	Cash Budget 1992	Monthly Allocation											
		Jan	Feb	Mar	Apr	May	Jun	Jul	Aug	Sep	Oct	Nov	Dec
RECEIPTS													
Grants	145,000	33,750			33,750			33,750			33,750		
Sales revenue	125,000	10,000	10,250	10,500	10,500	10,750	11,000	10,750	10,500	10,500	10,000	10,250	10,000
Loan	50,000	50,000											
Total receipts	320,000	93,750	10,250	10,500	44,250	10,750	11,000	44,500	10,500	10,500	43,750	10,250	20,000
PAYMENTS													
Drug purchases	230,000	57,500			57,500			57,500			57,500		
Salaries	19,000	1,583	1,583	1,584	1,583	1,583	1,584	1,583	1,583	1,584	1,583	1,583	1,584
Vehicle operations	2,700	225	225	225	225	225	225	225	225	225	225	225	225
Other transport	1,600	134	133	133	134	133	133	134	133	133	134	133	133
Packaging and labeling	3,300	275	275	275	275	275	275	275	275	275	275	275	275
Utilities	2,200	183	184	183	183	184	183	183	184	183	183	184	183
Office supplies	1,200	100	100	100	100	100	100	100	100	100	100	100	100
Total payments	260,000	60,000	2,500	2,500	60,000	2,500	2,500	60,000	2,500	2,500	60,000	2,500	2,500
Receipts less payments	60,000	33,750	7,750	8,000	-15,750	8,250	8,500	-15,500	8,000	8,000	-16,250	7,750	17,500
Less capital expenditures	10,000			4,000									6,000
Net cash flow	50,000	33,750	7,750	4,000	-15,750	8,250	8,500	-15,500	8,000	8,000	-16,250	7,750	11,500
Add opening cash balance	0	0	33,750	41,500	45,500	29,750	38,000	46,500	31,000	39,000	47,000	30,750	38,500
Closing cash balance	50,000	33,750	41,500	45,500	29,750	38,000	46,500	31,000	39,000	47,000	30,750	38,500	50,000
Patient volume	500,000	40,000	41,000	42,000	42,000	43,000	44,000	43,000	42,000	42,000	40,000	41,000	40,000

in-country transport costs (for imported drugs) plus 10 percent. A charge for depreciation should be included in the cost.

If drugs are being repackaged, the cost of these procedures may be attributed to the specific drugs as direct costs. However, if the overall costs are low (say, less than 20 percent of the total drug costs), it may not be worthwhile to allocate them to individual drugs, since such costing can be complicated and lengthy. Donated resources should be included at the equivalent local cost so that the full cost of each drug is calculated. For costing to work properly, the accounting system should be on an accrual basis, or all bills must be paid promptly; otherwise, cost calculations will not be accurate.

Using the figures for 1991 from Figure 42.2, it is possible to do a simple cost exercise. The total costs for that year were $240,000 for drugs issued, $15,000 for drugs lost, and $28,000 for operating expenses. These two expenses represent an additional 6.25 percent and 11.67 percent on top of the cost of drugs issued. If a drug cost $1.00 to purchase, it would be necessary to add 6.25 percent (6 cents) to cover drug losses and 11.67 percent (12 cents) to cover operating expenses. The total cost, or full historical cost, for the drug would therefore be $1.18.

The above example shows certain costs to be direct and others indirect. Direct costs are those that can be attributed directly to the items being costed (for instance, the purchase price of the drug). Indirect costs are those that cannot be attributed directly, such as drug losses and general operating expenses. The easiest way to allocate these indirect costs is to treat them as percentage additions to the direct cost of each drug, as in the example.

Costs are often divided into fixed (stable) and variable (incremental) costs. Rent of a warehouse would be fixed, since it would not vary with the quantity of drugs held. Packing materials would be variable, since they vary directly with the quantity of drugs issued. This division between fixed and variable costs is useful when determining the break-even point (the production or service volume at which sales revenue equals expenses). Figure 42.5 shows a graph of the revenue and expenses with different patient levels, using 1994 prices and expenses from the general example. The sales price must be enough to cover the fixed and variable costs, as well as the need for reserves, at the expected volume of sales. In the figure, this is achieved with a volume of about 500,000 patients.

≡ 42.7 Controlling and Managing Resources
Good financial controls and a sound accounting system are the basis for effective financial management. Although

Figure 42.5 Break-Even Analysis: 1994 Prices for Different Volumes

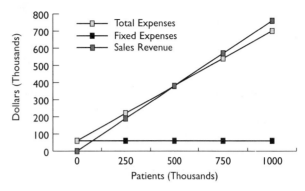

Sales revenue	0	190,000	380,000	570,000	760,000
Cost of drugs issued	0	152,500	305,000	457,500	610,000
Cost of expired drugs	0	7,625	15,250	22,875	30,500
Variable expenses	0	160,125	320,250	480,375	640,500
Operating expenses (fixed expenses)	60,100	60,100	60,100	60,100	60,100
Total expenses	60,100	220,225	380,350	540,475	700,600
Number of patients	0	250,000	500,000	750,000	1,000,000

Note: Break-even point is where number of patients is approximately 500,000.

financial managers and accountants are responsible for establishing and maintaining the control and accounting systems, the general manager must know enough about the system to supervise staff and to detect any problems.

Standardized financial controls and accounting procedures help ensure that resources are generated and used properly and that a complete and accurate financial picture of operations and assets and liabilities can be obtained. See Figure 42.6 for a financial control checklist.

The three main principles of an effective financial control system are:

1. Divide duties among individuals so that no one person can control all phases of a transaction. For example:
   ▸ Tasks of requesting payment, authorizing payment, and issuing checks should each be carried out by a different person.
   ▸ The person who prepares a bank reconciliation should not handle or record receipts or payments.
2. Use financial control procedures to regulate transactions. For example:

Figure 42.6 Manager's Checklist for Good Financial Control

Controlling Receipts
- ❏ Issue prenumbered receipts for all cash received.
- ❏ Keep all original receipts and copies of canceled checks.
- ❏ Control all receipt books in use and in stock, and lock up all unused receipt books.
- ❏ Keep all cash and checks received separate from other funds. Do not use them as a source for payments, and bank them promptly.
- ❏ Reconcile the bank balance every month.
- ❏ Use a register to record all checks received.
- ❏ Do not cash personal checks from petty cash.
- ❏ Use a register to record all donations of supplies or fixed assets, showing the value.

Controlling Assets
- ❏ Maintain up-to-date inventory records and reconcile balances each month with the accounting records.
- ❏ Physically check a sample of inventory balances each month.
- ❏ Maintain a fixed assets register.
- ❏ Keep up-to-date maintenance and inspection records.
- ❏ Put permanent identification marks on all equipment.
- ❏ Protect against loss or theft of assets with appropriate security and insurance.
- ❏ Keep usage records for equipment and vehicles (for example, log books)
- ❏ Monitor advances and accounts receivable and make sure that they are cleared within a prescribed period.
- ❏ Place cash reserves in low-risk, interest-earning investments (such as bank savings accounts).

Controlling Expenditures
- ❏ Establish detailed procurement procedures.
- ❏ Obtain written bids or quotes for all purchases above a specified limit and file them with the purchase order.
- ❏ Use a local purchase order for all local purchases.
- ❏ Check that goods and services purchased are received and recorded (drugs must be entered in inventory records).
- ❏ Check that the quality, quantity, and price of goods or services received correspond to purchase specifications.
- ❏ Make all payments for goods or services by check.
- ❏ Require supporting documentation for all purchases.
- ❏ Make sure that all expenditures are genuine, reasonable, and in line with program plans and budgets.
- ❏ Check the proposed expenditure against the budget and ensure that the budget is up-to-date regarding donor contributions and sales revenue.
- ❏ Check that funds are available.
- ❏ Check that the petty cash balance is maintained at the agreed level of imprest.

Controlling Liabilities
- ❏ Keep accounts payable to a minimum.
- ❏ Maintain control over suppliers' invoices, know what supplies have been paid for and when they will be delivered, and monitor date of receipt.

- ▶ Issue preprinted, serially numbered receipts for all inflows of cash.
- ▶ Deposit all cash receipts in the bank and make deposits promptly.

3. Use the accounting system to record and monitor all transactions and assets. For example:
- ▶ Record all issues of drugs in the accounting records and have the value of stocks form part of the accounting system.
- ▶ Produce monthly income and expenditure statements from the accounting system and review the figures for stocks, sales, and waivers.

Usually, government systems have extensive approval procedures before funds can be spent. However, managers still need to ensure that the funds have been spent wisely and well. The first step is to have a strict approval process for expenditures. This means keeping good records of uncommitted fund balances for each line item (with separate amounts for each donor, if necessary) and approving expenditures only after ensuring that they are within the budget. If the spending follows the current budget and the budget has been regularly reviewed so that it is in line with program needs, the use of the funds can be approved.

It is also important to review prices paid for services or products to ensure that the best price and quality were obtained, and to check that the services or products were actually received. For example, before paying a bill for painting a storeroom, the manager should visit the storeroom to see whether a good job was done. Before paying for a batch of drugs, the manager should go to the store and see whether they are on the shelves and in the stock records. Checking a few of the items purchased should be sufficient.

To avoid spending all the available budget during the first few months, a monthly spending limit may be established, and any expenditure in excess of that would require special approval. Since the expenditure budget is based on a particular level of funding, it is vital to update the budget if any significant variation in funding is expected (anything over 5 percent would be significant). For example, if a donor that was going to provide 10 percent of the drug supply can now provide only 5 percent, the budget needs to be revised. If additional funding is generated, the expenditure budget can be increased accordingly.

The accounting and reporting system must provide fast, accurate information in terms of funds received and expenditures made so that budget adjustments can be made promptly. It is essential to produce a budget report every month. This report shows the budgeted and actual figures for each revenue and expense category for the

Figure 42.7 Budget Report

CENTRAL MEDICAL STORES REVOLVING DRUG FUND
Operating Budget Report March 1992

	Budget 1992	Budget Year to Date	Budget Month	Actual Year to Date	Actual Month	Variance Year to Date
INCOME FROM GRANTS						
Grants	135,000	33,750	0	33,000	0	(750)
Donated drugs	50,000	12,500	4,167	15,000	5,000	2,500
Total grants	185,000	46,250	4,167	48,000	5,000	1,750
DRUG ACCOUNT						
Sales revenue	125,000	31,250	10,417	30,000	9,000	(1,250)
Less cost of drugs dispensed	250,000	62,500	20,833	64,000	21,000	(1,500)
	(125,000)	(31,250)	(10,416)	(34,000)	(12,000)	(2,750)
Less cost of expired drugs, etc.	12,500	3,125	1,042	3,500	1,500	(375)
Surplus/deficit on drug account	(137,500)	(34,375)	(11,458)	(37,500)	(13,500)	(3,125)
EXPENSES						
Salaries	19,000	4,750	1,583	4,800	1,600	(50)
Vehicle operations	2,700	675	225	700	240	(25)
Other transport	1,600	400	133	390	120	10
Packaging and labeling	3,300	825	275	800	300	25
Utilities	2,200	550	183	600	150	(50)
Office supplies	1,200	300	100	296	110	4
Total operating expenditures	30,000	7,500	2,499	7,586	2,520	(86)
Depreciation	10,000	2,500	833	2,500	833	0
Total expenses	40,000	10,000	3,332	10,086	3,353	(86)
Income less expenses	7,500	1,875	(10,623)	414	(11,853)	(1,461)
Patient volume	500,000	41,667	125,000	40,997	123,489	(1,511)

month and for the year to date and gives the variance between the year-to-date budget and the year-to-date actual figures. Negative variances must be investigated and appropriate action taken. A sample budget report is shown in Figure 42.7.

Cash and bank movements and balances should be reviewed daily to make sure that receipts and payments are as expected and that there are sufficient funds to meet obligations. A statement should be obtained from the cashier each morning showing the opening balance, cash received by source, payments made, closing balance for the previous day, and payments due that day.

It is also important to have an annual external audit, which helps ensure that controls are operating properly and that transactions are being properly recorded. This should be an institutional audit that covers both donor funds and the organization's own funds. Separate audits of individual donor funding should be discouraged, since they do not provide a complete picture and take up exces-

sive amounts of management time. Instead, managers should attempt to persuade donors to share the cost of the institutional audit.

≡ 42.8 Accounting and Reporting

An autonomous drug program can normally establish its own accounting and reporting procedures. However, a government program usually has to follow uniform accounting procedures. As described in Section 42.1, government accounting systems generally do not provide adequate information on transactions or assets and do not allow performance to be measured. In order to satisfy management needs, supplementary records need to be kept and additional reports produced. The following books are usually necessary for a complete system:

▶ Cash-received book showing the date and source of receipt (such as donor, government, or sales point) and when and where the cash was deposited;

- Cash-paid book showing payee, purpose, funding source, and bank account;
- Petty cash book for small cash payments;
- Accounts receivable ledger with accounts for people who owe money to the organization;
- Accounts payable ledger with accounts for people who are owed money by the organization;
- Journals showing purchases and sales made on credit, transfers between accounts, and donations in kind;
- General ledger with income, expense, asset, and liability accounts;
- Salary book showing details of staff salaries and allowances;
- Inventory records showing the quantity and cost of all drugs received, issued, and on hand by type of drug;
- Fixed assets register showing the quantity and cost of all fixed assets bought, sold, and on hand.

The chart of accounts, which sets out the accounts structure, lists all accounts with a unique code for each. The code is used primarily to identify the type of asset, liability, revenue, or expense (for example, bank account, drug sales, or salaries), but it can also be used to identify a responsibility center (such as a regional distribution center) or donor fund (such as a tuberculosis program). For the accounting system to provide the control and information required, the accounts must be structured appropriately. For example, in order to readily produce a report showing expenses for each regional center, each expense item must be coded by regional center and posted to a separate account.

Transactions must be recorded and processed promptly and accurately. For example, if all drug issue records are not up-to-date in the accounting books, it will be impossible to reconcile the inventory balances in the accounting department with those shown on the warehouse stock cards.

The accounting system should produce a number of basic reports that provide all the information needed to review financial progress and status. In particular, the reports should indicate clearly if the program is

- meeting its financial objectives—for example, generating a surplus;
- operating efficiently and effectively;
- looking after its assets;
- generating and using resources properly;
- meeting donor requirements.

Reports should be produced both monthly and annually. The most common standard reports are as follows:

Budget performance report: This monthly report compares budgeted and actual revenue and expenses (see Figure 42.7).

Income and expense report: This report, produced monthly and annually, shows all income and expenses to date and the cumulative surplus or deficit (Figure 42.8). For comparative purposes, figures for the previous year and the current year budget are shown. A key figure to help analyze the results is the deficit or surplus on drugs as a percentage of the cost of drugs issued or cost of sales. This figure shows the extent to which drug costs are being recovered. For the 1992 figures shown in Figure 42.8, the deficit of $138,000 represents 57 percent of the cost of drugs issued ($242,000). This means that 43 percent of the cost of drugs is being recovered, taking into account stock losses. In Figure 42.2, the projected surplus of $73,205 for 1994 represents 20 percent of the $366,025 for drugs issued. These percentages are a measure of effective pricing, revenue collection efficiency, and control over stock losses.

Balance sheet: This report, produced monthly and annually, shows the condition of the program at one point in time. It has the balances at the end of the period for all assets, liabilities, reserves, and fund balances (Figure 42.9). Some key ratios are used to help managers analyze the situation. The ability of the program to meet its current liabilities in the short term is measured by comparing the cash balance with the accounts payable (in 1992, this would be $16,095 compared with $1,000). The same measure in the medium term compares the total current assets with the total current liabilities ($140,095 compared with $1,000 in the same example). When assessing the ability of a program to meet its liabilities, it is vital to be sure that the amounts for drug stock and accounts receivable are realistic—that is, that they will result in cash income that can be used to meet those liabilities.

Drug stock account: It is important to prepare a summary of the drug stock account as an attachment to the income and expense report (see Figure 42.8). This summary shows the total figures for drugs received and issued and opening and closing balances, and it provides a picture of the movements on that account. If a computerized accounting program is used, it should be possible to produce a similar report for each drug, which is useful for measuring sales frequency and months of stock on hand. Chapters 41 and 15 discuss a number of analyses that can help managers understand and control inventory costs.

Accounts payable and receivable: These additional reports support the figures shown in the balance sheet and

Figure 42.8 Income and Expense Report

CENTRAL MEDICAL STORES
REVOLVING DRUG FUND
Income and Expense Statement 1992

	Actual 1991	Budget 1992	Actual 1992
INCOME FROM GRANTS			
Grants	188,000	135,000	130,000
Donated drugs	98,000	50,000	50,000
Total grants	286,000	185,000	180,000
DRUG ACCOUNT			
Sales revenue	0	125,000	120,000
Less cost of drugs issued[a]	240,000	250,000	242,000
	(240,000)	(125,000)	(122,000)
Less cost of expired drugs, etc.	15,000	12,500	16,000
Surplus/deficit on drugs	(255,000)	(137,500)	(138,000)
EXPENSES			
Salaries	18,000	19,000	20,000
Vehicle operations	2,500	2,700	2,876
Other transport	1,500	1,600	1,745
Packaging and labeling	3,000	3,300	2,908
Utilities	2,000	2,200	2,190
Office supplies	1,000	1,200	1,186
Total operating expenditures	28,000	30,000	30,905
Depreciation	0	10,000	10,000
Total expenses	28,000	40,000	40,905
Total income less expenses	3,000	7,500	1,095
Patient volume	520,000	500,000	490,346

[a] DRUG STOCK ACCOUNT

	Actual 1991	Actual 1992
Opening stock	85,000	88,000
Purchases	160,000	230,000
Donations received	98,000	50,000
	343,000	368,000
Less cost of drugs dispensed	240,000	242,000
	103,000	126,000
Less cost of drugs expired, etc.	15,000	16,000
Closing stock	88,000	110,000

Figure 42.9 Balance Sheet

CENTRAL MEDICAL STORES
REVOLVING DRUG FUND
Balance Sheet December 31, 1992

	12/31/91	12/31/92
ASSETS		
Fixed assets[a]		
Equipment		
Cost	40,000	50,000
Depreciation	0	10,000
	40,000	40,000
Current assets		
Drug stock	88,000	110,000
Cash	0	16,095
Accounts receivable	0	14,000
	88,000	140,095
Total assets	128,000	180,095
LIABILITIES AND CAPITAL		
Long-term liabilities		
Loan	0	50,000
Current liabilities		
Accounts payable	0	1,000
Capital		
Balance at beginning of year	0	128,000
Accounting adjustment	128,000	0
Donated assets	0	0
Surplus during year	0	1,095
Closing balance	128,000	129,095
Total liabilities and capital	128,000	180,095

[a] FIXED ASSETS

Equipment	Cost	Depreciation
Balance as of 1/1/92	40,000	0
Additions	10,000	0
Disposals	0	0
Annual charge	0	10,000
Balance as of 12/31/92	50,000	10,000

show the balance for each debtor and creditor, with a breakdown of the balance by month of origin.

Certain reports, such as the income and expense report, can be prepared for different responsibility centers, such as regional distribution centers. If there are different funding agencies that require separate reports, the reports can be prepared by funding source, provided that this is built into the account structure. Producing reports by responsibility center or funding source is easy if the accounting system is computerized. However, with a manual accounting system, the accounts can be set up in only one way—by responsibility center or by funding source. The decision should be based on the relative importance of each kind of analysis and the ease of extracting information from the accounting system. For example, if regional sales are of interest, these data can be extracted from the monthly regional reports.

Where a drug sales program is in place, it is important to record and report revenue lost due to drugs distributed

---

Box 42.2 Three Methods of Accounting for Drugs Issued

FIFO (first in/first out). Issues are charged out at the purchase cost of the earliest batch in stock. This method charges less to cost of sales and values stock higher.

LIFO (last in/first out). Issues are charged out at the purchase price of the latest batch in stock. This method charges more to cost of sales and values stock lower.

AVG (average). Issues are charged at the average price of the items in stock; the average is updated every time a new purchase is made. This puts the same value on issues and stocks.

LIFO is the most conservative method, because it puts the lowest value on stocks and the highest value on issues. The average method is somewhat conservative, and the FIFO method is the least conservative. With both FIFO and LIFO, record keeping is more complicated, because it is necessary to keep track of how much balance remains from each purchase, and issues may have to be charged out at two or more prices.

Example of the Effect of Three Methods of Accounting for Drugs Issued

	# Units	Unit Price	FIFO	LIFO	AVG	Avg. Unit Cost[a]
Bought January 1	100	$1	$100	$100	$100	
Bought February 1	100	$2	$200	$200	$200	
Balance February 1	200		$300	$300	$300	$1.50
Issued February 22[b]	120		$140	$220	$180	
Balance February 28	80		$160	$80	$120	
Bought March 1	100	$3	$300	$300	$300	
Balance March 1	180		$460	$380	$420	$2.33
Issued March 26	80		$160	$240	$186	
Balance March 31	100		$300	$140	$234	

[a] Average unit cost changes with new purchase.
[b] The figures for the February 22 issues are calculated as follows:
- ► FIFO—100 units at $1 and 20 units at $2;
- ► LIFO—100 units at $2 and 20 units at $1;
- ► AVG—120 units at the average unit cost of $1.50 (total cost of $300 divided by total quantity purchased of 200).

---

free of charge. Waivers for sales to the poor and for exemptions for special age groups or other categories should be recorded using special receipts. These sales should be authorized by the manager. They should be put into the books as sales and debited to a special account for free issues. They will then appear as an expense in the income and expense report.

In order to measure a program's output in terms of drugs issued or the surplus or deficit from drug sales, it is necessary to record the cost of drugs issued. This is an accounting transfer from the drug stock account to a cost-of-issues account. The drugs issued are valued at the cost of purchase—that is, at the same value at which they went into the drug stock account.

When quantities of a drug in stock have been bought at different prices, there are different ways to value the quantity issued and, at the same time, the value of stock on hand. See Box 42.2 for a comparison of the three common methods. It is important to remember that the accounting method used determines how much surplus or deficit is shown in the income and expense report and how much stock value is shown in the balance sheet. The most

important thing is to be consistent—the same method should be used each year.

It is recommended that the average method be used, since it is the easiest to understand. Calculating the average cost is simple: the financial balance in the stock account is simply divided by the number of units on hand. The average cost is updated every time a new purchase is made. Issues are then charged out at the average cost of the items in stock.

Where there is high inflation or large exchange fluctuations, and a computerized accounting program is used, it may be useful to keep stock records in a stable foreign currency. Local currency records must still be kept, however.

In an autonomous RDF, it is extremely important to generate sufficient revenue to replace stocks. This is best done through creation of a reserve for the purchase of replacement stocks. For example, if it is expected that the replacement cost will be 20 percent above the current cost, an extra 20 percent markup should be added to drug sales prices, and an amount equivalent to that 20 percent for all sales for the month should be added to the reserve set aside to replace the drugs (see Section 42.3 and Chapter 44). ■

≡ Assessment Guide

Current Drug Budget and Expenditures

► What is the Ministry of Health's (MOH) per capita budget or expenditures on pharmaceuticals, in US dollars?

► What was the value of the public drug budget spent per capita in the last year, out of the average value of the same budget during the past three years?

► How much of the public drug budget was spent, out of the public drug budget allocated?

► During the last fiscal year, how much did CMS spend on fuel for drug transport, maintenance, administration, other expendables, hired labor, warehouse space cost (rent, telephone, utilities), or other costs (describe)?

Accounting System

► Is the drug program's accounting system on a cash basis or an accrual basis?

► Do accounts exist for stock? What accounting method is used to value drug stocks and issues—FIFO, LIFO, or average costing?

► Are records kept on the value of donated drugs? The cost of expired or lost drugs? Depreciation of fixed assets?

► Are records maintained for accounts payable? Accounts receivable?

► Does a chart of accounts exist?

Financial Planning, Budgeting, and Cash Planning

► Is there a long-range financial plan projecting both funding and expenditures for the next five years, and maintained on a rolling basis? Is a factor for inflation built into the plan?

► If drug sales are anticipated, have pricing strategies been determined? Does the plan project the point at which revenues will cover expenses?

► Which offices are responsible for developing and approving budgets? (List steps and persons or offices responsible.) What information is used in developing budget requests?

► What information and supporting documents are submitted with budget requests?

► How does the MOH access budgeted funds for routine procurement—scheduled allocation or access whenever needed?

► What approvals are required for expenditures?

► How does the MOH access funds for emergency procurement?

► What is the average lead time for MOH approval of procurement allocation (for both routine and emergency procurements) and for approval of foreign exchange allocation?

► How does the MOH access foreign exchange for procurement?

► Is the annual budget based on the first-year figures from the long-range financial plan? Are there separate operating and capital budgets?

► Does the budget relate financial estimates to activities in terms of number of patients to be served, types of patients, diseases, and/or geographical areas to be covered?

► Has a cash flow forecast been developed to support the budget?

Costing

► Are the costs of in-country transportation, repackaging, drug losses, and other operating expenses included in total drug costs?

► Are analyses performed with regard to the cost of serving different patient volumes, different patient types, or different disease types?

► For an RDF, has a break-even point been projected?

► What method is used to value inventory?

Financial Control and Reporting

► Are duties divided among individuals so that no one person can control all phases of a transaction?

► Are preprinted, serially numbered receipts issued for all inflows of cash? Are cash receipts deposited promptly?

► Is there a budget approval process, by which expenditures are approved only after ensuring that funds are available?

► Is the budget revised when funding is greater or less than anticipated?

► Is a budget report produced every month, showing budgeted and actual figures and variances for each revenue and expense category?

► Are income and expense reports, balance sheets, summaries of the drug stock account, and reports on accounts payable and receivable prepared monthly and annually?

► Is an annual institutional audit performed by external auditors?

≡ References and Further Readings

★ = *Key readings.*

★ Creese, A., and D. Parker. 1994. *Cost analysis in primary health care. A training manual for programme managers.* Geneva: World Health Organization.

★ Garner, C. W. 1991. *Accounting and budgeting in public and non-profit organizations.* San Francisco: Jossey-Bass.

★ Glynn, J. J. 1993. *Public sector financial control and accounting,* 2d ed. Oxford: Blackwell Publishers.

Goodman, H., and C. Waddington. 1993. *Financing health care.* OXFAM Practical Health Guide no. 8. London: Oxfam.

Herkimer, A. G. Jr. 1986. *Understanding hospital financial management,* 2d ed. Rockville, Md.: Aspen Publishers.

★ Herkimer, A. G. Jr. 1989. *Understanding health care accounting.* Rockville, Md.: Aspen Publishers.

★ MSH (Management Sciences for Health). 1991. Managing your finances. In *The family planning manager's handbook: Basic skills for managing family planning programs.* Boston: MSH.

MSH (Management Sciences for Health). 1992. Financial planning (trainer's and participant's guides. In *Managing drug supply training series.* Part 2. *Financing and financial management of drug supply.* Boston: MSH.

Reynolds, J. 1993. Cost analysis (user's guide, module 8). In *Primary health care management advancement programme.* Geneva: Aga Khan Foundation.

Vian, T. 1993. Analyzing costs for management decisions. *Family Planning Manager* 2(2):1–18.

WHO (World Health Organization). 1994. *Cost analysis in primary health care: A training manual for programme managers.* Geneva: WHO.

| Part I | Part II | Part III | **Part IV** |
| Introduction | Policy and Legal Framework | Drug Management Cycle | **Management Support Systems** |

A Organization and Management

B Financing and Sustainability ▶ 40 Drug Financing
Strategies

C Information Management

D Human Resources Management 41 Analyzing and
Controlling Drug
Expenditures

42 Financial Planning and
Management

43 Donor Financing

44 Revolving Drug Funds

Chapter 43
Donor Financing

≡ Summary

International assistance to support health and pharmaceutical projects is available from bilateral agencies, multilateral institutions such as development banks and United Nations agencies, and nongovernmental organizations and foundations. The types of assistance available include

- *financial assistance (loans or grants)*
- *commodities*
- *technical expertise*
- *study tours and fellowships*
- *research funding*

Finance ministries, rather than health ministries, generally play a leadership role in negotiating assistance agreements; nevertheless, health ministries can

- *increase political visibility for the health sector;*
- *identify health priorities;*
- *prepare project proposals;*
- *obtain government support for the presentation of proposals to donor agencies.*

Proposals must increasingly satisfy donors' concerns about consistency with government policies, government commitment, health care reform, project impact, and sustainability.

Many donors follow a two-stage proposal process, requiring submission and approval of a project profile, followed by a more detailed project document. Project documents are often developed through the logical framework approach and include

- *project goals (development objective)*
- *project purpose (immediate objective)*
- *outputs*
- *activities*
- *inputs and resources*

Private foundations tend to follow more flexible procedures for reviewing grant proposals and overseeing grant-funded projects. Most donors require periodic progress reports and evaluation.

It is common to contract with outside professionals for expert advice at various stages of a project. The selection process tends to be highly structured for long-term consultants, who will serve for two years or longer, and more informal for short-term consultants. Carefully chosen consultants can provide impartial input that allows implementation of new or controversial initiatives.

Ministries of health can facilitate donor coordination and collaboration by developing and communicating national policies and programs, by inviting donors to participate in the development of a master plan as a framework for action, and by hosting regular donor coordination meetings.

≡ 43.1 The Role of Donors in Development

Demand for health services exceeds available resources in developed or developing nations. Working with restricted budgets, governments are forced to establish priorities. Even after making these difficult decisions, health officials often find that they still lack the funding required for implementing some priority programs.

It is in such situations that international development assistance, also called external cooperation, can provide funds and technical expertise to complement national efforts. Equally important, this assistance can serve as a catalyst for major health system reforms that would otherwise be difficult to accomplish. Policy-makers and managers can benefit their health initiatives and programs by understanding where to obtain such assistance, the criteria that must be met, and the ongoing commitments that must be fulfilled to establish and maintain fruitful relationships with donor and funding agencies.

Health is expected to become an increasingly important component of programs and projects supported by donor funds. International health agencies, such as the World Health Organization (WHO) and the United Nations Children's Fund (UNICEF), have long insisted that health is not only a product of development but also an important component of, and contributor to, the development process. Development banks and donor agencies agree that investment in basic health services is an investment in development.

Health programs and projects supported by external assistance will continue to include activities related to pharmaceuticals that range from the straightforward (procurement of drugs for a specific program, such as malaria control) to the complex (reorganization of the public-sector supply system). The funding for these activities is expected to grow in parallel with the growth in overall funding for health projects.

≡ 43.2 Sources of International Assistance for Health

Government agencies and private institutions in the industrialized nations provide financial and technical resources to developing countries through bilateral agencies, multilateral institutions such as development banks and United Nations agencies, and nongovernmental organizations (NGOs) and foundations. Cooperation can also be provided directly on a government-to-government basis. Government donations and concession loans that include at least a 25 percent nonreimbursable component (in effect, a 25 percent donation) are referred to as official development assistance (ODA), and they are the major source of external funding for projects in the developing world. (This is not to be confused with the British Overseas Development Administration, also referred to as ODA.)

In 1991, ODA from eighteen member countries of the Organization for Economic Cooperation and Development (OECD) was about US$56 billion, representing an average of one-third of 1 percent of their gross national products, which was below the 0.7 percent goal proposed by the OECD. Denmark, Sweden, Norway, and the Netherlands, however, reached or exceeded this goal. Figure 43.1 lists the major international donors involved in health.

According to the World Bank, development funds for the health sector reached $4.8 billion in 1990, of which $4 billion was from ODA and $0.8 billion from NGOs and foundations, amounting to about $1 per person in developing countries. Figure 43.2 summarizes the flow of these resources.

The trend is for development assistance in health to be provided through multilateral channels. The number of World Bank projects in health, population, and nutrition increased from eight in 1987–89 to twenty-one in 1990–92. The World Bank has become the largest single source of external assistance for essential drugs and other pharmaceutical products and is expected to spend $300 to $500 million for those projects during the 1990s.

The NGOs providing international assistance range from well-known foundations such as Rockefeller and Kellogg to small church-related agencies. The procedures these agencies follow tend to be less stringent than those of bilateral and multilateral agencies. In addition, they give great weight in the approval process to an affinity of purpose or ideology between donor and recipient organizations, as well as to whether they have an established, positive ongoing relationship.

Although development funds have traditionally been provided to recipient governments, an alternative mechanism is to target funds directly to NGOs, particularly community-based NGOs. This mechanism, which has gained increasing acceptance as a way to ensure that resources reach target populations at the local level, tends to be favored by NGOs and foundations in developed countries. The official bilateral and multilateral agencies are more reluctant to become directly involved in small projects due to the high costs of reviewing, supervising, and evaluating such initiatives.

≡ 43.3 Types of Assistance

The types of assistance offered (and the conditions attached) can vary widely:

- financial assistance (loans or grants)
- commodities
- technical expertise
- study tours and fellowships
- research funding

In negotiating development assistance of any type, governments are advised to ensure that the assistance supports their national health priorities rather than diverts attention from them.

Financial Assistance

Loans issued by the World Bank or its regional counterparts, such as the Asian, African, or Inter-American Development Banks, are an increasing source of financial assistance in the health sector. Loans are also provided on a government-to-government basis as part of bilateral agreements that, in turn, reflect political commitments. Such loans are much more favorable than those from commercial banks: interest rates are lower, repayment schedules are adjusted to a country's financial capabilities, and there is frequently a nonreimbursable grant component.

Since these loans become part of the national debt and must be repaid by future government administrations, they should be accepted only after thorough study of the costs and benefits. In general, loans should be used for investment—for the development of infrastructure and national capability—and not to cover recurrent health expenditures or to pay for consumables, such as drugs. In addition, a bank's internal procedures may raise the real cost of the loan (for example, by including the total cost of preproject planning expenses, as well as the time and travel of bank representatives and consultants, which can be substantial).

Grants, which do not require repayment, are a much sought after source of assistance. There are costs to the recipients, however, and some of them are not always obvious. For example, a grant can include a requirement that the recipient demonstrate commitment to the work by the assignment of counterpart resources (staff and infrastructure) to complement those of the grant. Such commitments can siphon away scarce resources from

Figure 43.1 Major International Donors Involved in Health

Bilateral Donors

Country	Acronym	Agency Name, City
Australia	AIDAB	Australian International Development Assistance Bureau
Austria	—	Federal Ministry of Foreign Affairs, Department of Development Aid, Vienna
Belgium	BADC	Belgian Administration for Development Cooperation, Brussels
Canada	CIDA	Canadian International Development Agency, Hull, Quebec
Denmark	Danida	Danish International Development Agency, Ministry of Foreign Affairs, Copenhagen
Finland	FINNIDA	Finnish International Development Agency, Ministry for Foreign Affairs of Finland, Helsinki
France	—	Ministère de la Coopération et du Développement, Paris
Germany	BMZ	Federal Ministry for Economic Cooperation, Bonn
	GTZ	German Agency for Technical Cooperation, Eschborn
Italy	DGCS	Department for Development Cooperation, Ministry of Foreign Affairs, Rome
Japan	JICA	Japan International Cooperation Agency, Tokyo
Netherlands	DGIS	Directorate-General for International Cooperation, Ministry of Foreign Affairs, The Hague
New Zealand	—	Ministry of Foreign Affairs, Wellington
Norway	NORAD	Ministry of Development Cooperation, Oslo
Sweden	SIDA	Swedish International Development Authority, Stockholm
Switzerland	DDA	Direction de la Coopération au Développement et de l'Aide Humanitaire, Département Fédéral des Affaires Etrangères, Bern
United Kingdom	ODA	Overseas Development Administration, London
United States	USAID	U.S. Agency for International Development, U.S. Department of State, Washington, D.C.

Key United Nations Agencies and Multilateral Donors

Acronym	Organization
ADB	Asian Development Bank
ADB	African Development Bank
CEC	Commission of European Communities, Brussels
IADB	Inter-American Development Bank
IBRD	International Bank for Reconstruction and Development (World Bank)
UNDP	United Nations Development Programme
UNFPA	United Nations Population Fund
UNICEF	United Nations Children's Fund
UNIDO	United Nations Industrial Development Organization
WHO	World Health Organization

other, more important health programs. National priorities can become distorted if disproportionate attention is given to an issue simply because it is the fashionable "cause of the year" and can attract grant money or loans.

Commodities

Funds are often made available for the purchase of commodities such as drugs, medical supplies, laboratory reagents, equipment, or computers. The conditions for commodity purchase should be subject to negotiation to ensure not only that price and quality are acceptable but also that the commodities meet country needs and do not lead to an unacceptable level of dependence on a foreign source. Pharmaceutical products should correspond to those on the national list of essential drugs and should be labeled in a language understood in the country (see Chapter 20).

Only as a last resort should loans be used to buy pharmaceuticals. This essential, recurring expenditure should be within the national financial capacity.

Some assistance agreements limit the provision of critical supplies to periods of economic crisis or emergencies caused by natural disasters. The guidelines for donations included in Chapter 20 are relevant not only for donated commodities but also for those purchased through grants or loans.

Technical Expertise

Donors can provide funds to obtain the managerial or technical expertise required for project execution, both short term (for example, two weeks to set up a laboratory instrument and to train staff in its use) or long term (for example, management of a four-year project). The work must be carried out with in-country counterparts to trans-

Figure 43.2 Disbursements of External Assistance for the Health Sector, 1990

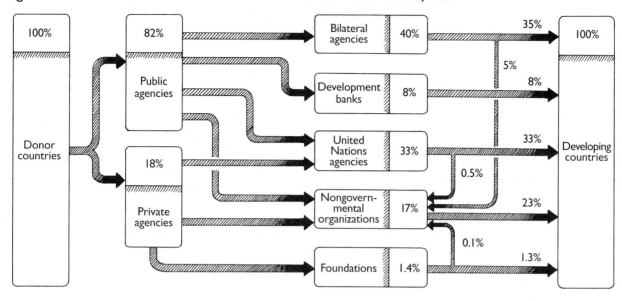

fer technical competence to the recipient country and not perpetuate a relationship of dependence.

Study Tours and Fellowships

Study tours, fellowships, and other forms of training are important investments in a country's professional capacity and are attractive to the individuals who benefit directly. Such opportunities can provide a powerful incentive to improve job performance, particularly for officials and employees receiving low government salaries. Arrangements should be in place, however, to ensure that individuals who have benefited from this assistance return to share their knowledge and skills with fellow workers, and that they remain in their jobs for a sufficient length of time to justify the investment.

Research Funds

Funds are increasingly available for operational research and evaluation. This is in recognition of the fact that a project's chances of success are enhanced by a clear understanding of the environment in which the project is to take place, by ongoing monitoring during project implementation, and by an impact evaluation after completion. Well-designed research proposals may be a prerequisite for funding approval.

≡ 43.4 Negotiating Assistance for the Health Sector

There is intense competition within countries for development assistance funds. Donor policies determine not only which countries will be selected but also what sectors and programs will be supported. These policies change with world events, the state of the donor country's economy, the relationship between donor and recipient countries, and the political parties in power and their respective ideologies. Governments interested in external assistance must become acquainted with each donor's policies, priorities, and procedures.

Although recipient countries generally cannot influence donors' broad priorities, actions at the national level can increase the share of assistance assigned to health. A ministry of health (MOH) can be proactive, for example, in designating a particular unit to mobilize external resources. This responsibility would include determining the availability of international technical and financial resources and understanding the criteria that must be met to obtain them.

Information describing the level, duration, and type of assistance available, as well as the timing for presentation of proposals, is generally available at the country level through development banks, embassies, and offices of United Nations agencies. A useful source of general information is *International Cooperation in Health: Agency Profiles* (WHO/PAHO 1992).

The MOH does not usually play a leadership role in dealing with donor governments or development banks and must represent its interests to the ministries of planning, external relations, and finance, which are likely to carry out the negotiations. Specifically, the MOH should

► increase political visibility for the health sector;
► identify health priorities;

▶ prepare project proposals;
▶ obtain government support for the presentation of proposals to donor agencies.

Achieving political visibility is the major challenge for health authorities. They must convince government policy-makers that health conditions have a direct impact on national well-being and stability and that adequate health coverage contributes to social equity and economic development. The acknowledgment of health-sector objectives in the national development plan allows for the inclusion of health care projects in the portfolio approved by the planning ministry.

Health-sector priorities should be based on the needs and resources of the population. Ministry officials then use these priorities to identify projects that can benefit from external assistance. In this way, external resources not only are channeled to priority areas in health but also are consistent with, and complement, national development policies.

Donor agencies are likely to limit financial support to program areas that have been explicitly mentioned in the national plans. If governments do not define their priorities for external cooperation, donor agencies may apply their funds according to their own policies and priorities. Thus, it is fundamental that national priorities be made known to the parties involved, to discourage funding of independent and isolated activities that do not complement country efforts.

Health authorities should take the initiative to approach appropriate donor agencies regarding their interest in supporting specific program areas, such as essential drugs. Even at an early stage, a donor appreciates receiving a written proposal, however preliminary and general it may be, to determine if there is sufficient interest to proceed further. The planning ministry should be kept informed of any contacts and progress achieved.

≡ 43.5 Securing Donor Interest

As demand for assistance funds increases, donor agencies have become more selective about the project proposals they will consider. Proposals must meet general criteria regarding government policies and commitment, private-sector involvement, impact, and sustainability in order to satisfy the concerns of donors.

The conditions for assistance may require recipient governments to take steps toward reforming or even restructuring the health sector. Where pharmaceuticals are concerned, this may mean profound changes in how the drug supply is managed; it may require, for example, moving from a centralized government agency that handles all aspects of procurement, warehousing, and distribution to a system that limits central government involvement to coordination and supervision and delegates operational aspects to provincial and local levels or to the private sector.

Government Policies

Project proposals must be consistent with the priorities of the recipient country. Drug projects should refer to official policies in this area, particularly if there is a national drug policy and action plan to improve the availability of essential drugs and to promote the rational use of drugs.

Government Commitment

The commitment of the recipient government to the objectives of the proposal should be reflected in its assignment of staff, space, and equipment to these objectives. The external contribution is generally intended to complement the counterpart contribution, not the other way around.

Health Care Reform

Extensive health system reforms are under way in many countries. Their aim is to restructure the organization, financing, and provision of health services to achieve greater equity, efficiency, and quality using available resources. This often includes stimulation of competition and greater involvement by the private sector. Donors may require that pharmaceutical reforms be undertaken as part of health care reform. Thus, representatives of the health professionals' associations and of the local pharmaceutical industry may be included in the formulation of a project and identification of strategies for its implementation. Private-sector involvement in drug supply is discussed in Chapter 6.

Impact

The expected impact of a project should be explicitly stated in the proposal; donors are wary of projects that simply propose to do more of what is already being done. They are interested in supporting initiatives that will noticeably change the status quo at the policy-making and/or operational levels. How will the project improve existing conditions? Will it result in an integrated and intersectoral program that will be more cost effective than the present one? Although the impact of a single project may be difficult to quantify, an effort should be made to explain its expected impact.

Sustainability

Donors are increasingly interested in the sustainability of their investments. Even at the proposal stage, they want assurance that achievements will not disappear once external funding has ended. There have been numerous examples of project funds being used unwisely to support unusually high salaries or luxurious offices; when the funding for these salaries and offices ends, so does the interest in activities launched.

To prevent this backlash, project activities should be designed to be carried out as much as possible within the normal structures and working environment. Also, arrangements should be in place before the project ends to institutionalize the project's achievements, that is, to provide the funds for the staff, infrastructure, and supplies required to continue the activities started. Special attention is required in projects that include the purchase of essential drugs as a central element: in these cases, financial mechanisms must be installed to ensure that the drugs continue to be available once external aid has ended.

≡ 43.6 Project Formulation Documents

Many donors follow a two-stage proposal process for new projects, requiring submission and approval of a project profile, followed by a more detailed project document. Donors may be willing to assist in the preparation of these documents, or governments may request assistance through local offices of WHO, UNICEF, or UNDP.

The Project Profile

The project profile should contain sufficient information for preliminary discussion and decision-making. It should describe and reflect broad agreement within the government regarding the problem to be solved, the proposed solution, and the estimated cost. According to the *Standardized Format for PAHO Project Documents and Profiles* (WHO/PAHO 1993), the minimum requirement at the project profile stage is that the problem analysis, goal, purpose, and strategy be well presented; other elements should be at least outlined, and a skeleton budget should be included. A model table of contents based on the PAHO guidelines is shown in Figure 43.3.

It is critical that all parties that may be affected or involved in the project be included in early planning discussions to avoid the sense that a particular project belongs to a specific official or unit. Such an attitude discourages the participation of other individuals or institutions and limits the coordination required to ensure that project goals are pursued in an appropriate manner.

The project profile is submitted for review to the donor agency. Months may go by before a response is received. The response, even if highly positive, almost always contains recommendations for changes or additions to ensure

Figure 43.3 Model Table of Contents: Project Profile

Cover

I. Profile data
  1. Development problems to be addressed by the project
  2. Relevance of project to host country health policy and priorities
  3. Project goal (development objective)
  4. Project purpose (immediate objective)
  5. Project strategy
  6. Description summary
  7. Concerned parties
  8. Project area and target group (beneficiaries)
  9. Present situation and end-of-project situation
  10. Special considerations
  11. Other donors or programs in the same field
  12. Assumptions and risks (also called "external factors")
  13. Skeleton budget
  14. Recurrent cost implications (sustainability)
  15. Host country commitment
  16. Uncovered issues and possible need for further studies

II. Annexes (as required)

that the proposal complies with donor requirements, some of which, at first sight, may not seem relevant. The recommendations, however, should *not* be overlooked. More likely than not, they reflect a political decision of the donor country that any project to be funded must address certain issues of national or global interest. The issues vary according to the source of funds, but common ones include environmental protection, the role of women, alleviation of poverty, and human rights.

Once the donor institution is satisfied that its concerns will be addressed in the project and confirms its support, the complex work involved in preparing the project document begins.

The Project Document

The project document is more detailed than the profile because it is intended to guide project implementation and to serve as the reference for monitoring and evaluation. It often serves as the legal basis for the commitments assumed by the donor and recipient.

Donor agencies usually require that the project design be systematic and comprehensive; many favor the logical framework approach (LFA), which is described in Box 43.1. The LFA, or LogFrame, uses a hierarchy of key elements to design the project (see also Chapter 35):

► project goals (development objective)
► project purpose (immediate objective)
► outputs
► activities
► inputs and resources

Box 43.1 The Logical Framework Approach

Most donors follow a prescribed series of steps to identify, plan, implement, and monitor projects. The logical framework approach (LogFrame or LFA) is one methodology used by USAID, Danida, NORAD, CIDA, and others.

LogFrame planning is most effective when it is undertaken in the context of a workshop held in the project area that is attended by representatives of all involved parties and led by a facilitator experienced in the LogFrame method. The planning process begins with a step-by-step analysis of existing problems and of the groups and institutions affected. Objectives or desirable conditions are then formulated. Possible options or project components are identified, and their viability is assessed in relation to agreed-upon criteria (for example, total cost, benefits to priority groups, probability of achieving objectives, social risks), leading to the selection of one project strategy.

The output of such a planning process using LogFrame is a project design, which serves as a point of reference throughout the life of the project. The project design, or project matrix, contains these key elements:

Target groups: Identification of the project's intended beneficiaries, defined according to geographical area, activity, economic situation, needs, access to social services, gender, age, social status, and other relevant categories.
Development objective: Anticipated long-term objective toward which the project will contribute.
Immediate objective: Intended effect of the project on the direct beneficiaries.
Outputs: Results that can be guaranteed by the project as a consequence of its activities, the combined impact of which should be sufficient to achieve the immediate objective.
Activities: Actions necessary to transform given inputs into planned outputs within a specified period of time.
Inputs: The "raw materials" necessary to produce the intended outputs—for example, funds, personnel, materials, services.
External factors: Situations, events, conditions, or decisions that are necessary for project success but are largely or completely beyond the control of project management.
Indicators: Specification of the performance standards to be reached to achieve the objectives; basis for monitoring and evaluation.

LogFrame ensures a logical interrelatedness among project elements, highlights the influence of external factors, and provides a systematic basis for monitoring. As a standardized approach to planning, LogFrame also facilitates common understanding and better communication among governments, donor agencies, decision-makers, and managers.

Limitations arise from adhering to LogFrame too rigidly. Regular project reviews can provide opportunities to re-evaluate and adjust key elements as circumstances change. LogFrame should be supplemented with other tools such as cost-benefit analysis and impact analysis, as appropriate. The full benefits of LogFrame can be achieved only through systematic training of all parties involved.

Source: Adapted from NORAD 1990.

Annex 43.1 contains an annotated format for the project document.

Like the project profile, the project document is submitted to the funding agency for review. Once donor comments and recommendations have been received and responded to satisfactorily by the recipient, donor approval of the project follows. Disbursement of funds for each project year is approved after submission of an annual workplan, which should include an introduction, specific objectives and strategies, planned activities, and a budget.

≡ 43.7 Donor Participation in Project Implementation

The days are long gone when donors limited their participation to disbursing project funds according to an agreed-upon budget. Donors often want to participate actively at all stages of a project. There is a greater insistence on well-designed projects, and donors are willing to assist by providing guidelines and training or working jointly with local officials.

A donor may also express interest in having the project contract the services of professionals from the donor country or purchase essential drugs or equipment from donor-country suppliers. These issues should be discussed openly, and the agreements reached should be clearly reflected in the project document.

Scheduled annual, midterm, and final project evaluations provide a formal occasion for the donor to examine in detail the progress of the project according to the objectives in the original document. However, there are many other opportunities during the project for the donor and project manager to interact. Many donor agencies have permanent missions in recipient countries, with staff who develop direct working relationships with local institutions. Finally, periodic visits by officials from donor headquarters or regional offices offer an opportunity to obtain firsthand information on government policies and priorities and to assess whether these remain consistent with the objectives of the projects being funded.

≡ 43.8 Obtaining Grants from Private Foundations

Private foundations are an important source of international assistance, primarily for NGOs whose philosophies, missions, and values correspond with those of the donors. Foundations' procedures for reviewing and approving grant proposals and for overseeing grant-funded projects tend to be considerably more flexible than those of bilateral and multilateral agencies. Nonetheless, four important steps should be followed.

Step 1. Identification of Potential Foundations

Funding groups and directories identify foundations of potential interest, describe the interests and funding priorities of individual foundations, and provide broad guidelines and criteria for application.

Step 2. Targeting of Selected Foundations

It is useful to review annual reports of the foundations under consideration for information about their programs, geographic areas of interest, monetary range of grants, and proposal guidelines. This review can help grant seekers develop a list of foundations whose funding criteria fit their interests.

The development of foundation proposals takes time, persistence, and the cultivation of personal relationships: introduction to foundation staff, discussion of mutual areas of interest with program officers, and making a case for support, all before a proposal is formally submitted.

Step 3. Proposal Development

A foundation proposal should generally include the following key elements and be limited to ten pages:

▶ Description of the organization;
▶ Problem to be addressed;
▶ Proposed solution;
▶ Statement of objectives and methodology;
▶ Plan for project management;
▶ Evaluation plan;
▶ Budget.

A cover letter summarizes the proposal and provides a strategic link between the proposal and the foundation's mission and interests. In addition, the letter makes a specific request for funding the proposed activities.

Step 4. Proposal Submission and Follow-Up

Foundations do not generally have deadlines for submission of proposals but review them on a rolling basis. Staff look at the proposal whenever it is received to determine its compatibility with the foundation's current interests and priorities, its technical merit, and the financial and management capacity of the submitting organization.

If a proposal is deemed appropriate, it is reviewed by the board of trustees for final consideration and approval. Meetings of the board are usually scheduled quarterly. The review process can take up to six months to complete.

When an award is made, the foundation presents a payment and reporting schedule to the grantee. Grant funds are restricted to those activities outlined in the proposal. At the end of each grant period, a narrative and a financial report on the specific use of funds are usually required.

≡ 43.9 Use of Local and International Advisers

Regardless of funding source, expert advice can be required at various stages of a project, such as design, implementation, specialized problem-solving, and external evaluation. If the donor or recipient does not have the required expertise available in-house, it is common to contract outside professionals. In some cases, the donor may require the use of an external consultant, to ensure that the appropriate technical expertise is applied and to provide a degree of independence from local political pressures. Recipients, whether governments or NGOs, may seek outside consultants who are respected for their technical or managerial competence and can provide impartial input to overcome the objections of special-interest groups and support new or controversial initiatives.

Clear and early identification of what is expected from a consultant is crucial. This is done with clear terms of reference that define what is to be produced, a specific time frame, and supervision and reporting responsibilities.

Consultants' qualifications should also be spelled out. For a specific, highly technical, and short-term assignment, such as training government inspectors in good manufacturing practices, five years of experience as an inspector in a well-established regulatory agency, plus knowledge of the local language, may be sufficient. A consultant who will be managing a four-year project to develop a national essential drugs program should have extensive experience in similar projects internationally; counterparts in the host country will benefit from the consultant's experience in other parts of the world.

The process of selecting a consultant can vary from an informal interview for a short-term employee to a highly structured process for a project manager or specialist who will serve for one year or longer. In the latter case, the donor, the host government, and any participating agencies often work together to advertise the search and ensure the prompt review of applications by a selection committee. Although a formal process may take six months or longer, it provides legitimacy and authority to those selected for key project posts.

The selection of consultants for specific short-term assignments (for example, advising warehouse staff on good storage practices) should be carried out in a much shorter time. This can be achieved with the cooperation of international and bilateral organizations such as WHO,

UNICEF, USAID, and Danida; they have rosters of specialized consultants who have worked with them and for whom they can provide references.

Government-to-government requests for expert assistance are also common and are promoted by international agencies through technical cooperation among countries (TCAC) projects. The expert provided is not a consultant per se but a professional who does the same job in his or her own country. Under a TCAC project, the host government covers travel and local expenses, and the cooperating government continues to pay the official's salary.

Joint consultancies with an international and a local consultant should be considered. They combine the advantages of the international consultant's insights from similar projects in other parts of the world and the local consultant's knowledge of the environment and local contacts. A positive side effect is the mutual transfer of knowledge, allowing both consultants to further their professional development.

Tensions between international consultants and local staff are not uncommon. The reasons are rarely technical; rather, local staff may resent the fact that an international consultant is a donor-imposed requirement, is highly paid, or conveys a paternalistic attitude. These problems can be overcome by a dedicated and qualified consultant who identifies with the objectives of the project, includes local personnel in all aspects of its implementation, and is willing to share knowledge. Regardless of the quality of a consultant, however, the government or the NGO should always see the consultant's recommendations as advice that may be accepted or rejected in light of the country's best interests.

≡ 43.10   Progress Reports and Evaluations

Donors' demands may increase as the project progresses, since the funding officials need to know whether their investment is resulting in the positive changes envisioned in the project plan. Toward this end, they may request a semiannual status report and an annual report accompanied by a financial statement. Reports provide the project manager with an opportunity to describe the project's achievements, problems encountered and actions taken to overcome them, and any discrepancies between the original workplan and actual implementation. Any potential changes in project objectives should be discussed and approved in advance by the funding agency.

Project evaluation provides a structured environment for donor-recipient interaction, whether carried out midway through the project or as a final exercise. The mission of the evaluation team, which includes donor representatives, is to determine whether planned objectives were achieved and the reasons for successes and failures. The project document serves as the basic guide in this work, and the value of having developed clear objectives, clarified the assumptions and risks, and selected manageable indicators becomes evident. (See Chapter 4 for a more detailed discussion of indicators for pharmaceutical sector assessment.)

Before the evaluation team arrives, the project manager should prepare a summary of major project accomplishments; the more specific it is, the better. Arrangements should be made for evaluators to visit sites where project activities have taken place. Presentations on the results achieved should be made by those directly responsible for the activity or, better yet, by those benefiting from it.

It is in the project manager's interest to provide the evaluation team with information about achievements as well as difficulties that were overcome. The government's commitment to the project should also be highlighted, in part by quantifying the administrative support and space provided and the staff and resources assigned. The most convincing evidence is documented changes in government policies that would lead to institutionalization of the goals pursued by the project.

A favorable evaluation facilitates future discussion with the donor agency regarding extension of the present project or preparation of new initiatives. However, successful completion of the original project should not lead a recipient country to assume that continuing funding is assured and that an expanded or new project can be launched. A major goal of donor agencies is to promote greater self-reliance, and after a certain period of external support, donors expect recipients to absorb the costs for consolidating and expanding the gains achieved under the project. Donor's priorities also change, often for reasons that may have little or nothing to do with the recipient country. This further emphasizes the importance of staying up-to-date regarding what sectors and program areas are priorities for international development assistance.

≡ 43.11   Donor Coordination and Collaboration

Donor assistance can be critical to a country's ability to deliver high-priority health services. Therefore, it is vital that this assistance be used efficiently. Too often, donor-supported projects are developed and negotiated independently, resulting in overlap in some program areas and continuing gaps in others.

Donor coordination has been a problem, but fortunately, it is improving. At the international level, donors

≡ Assessment Guide

Sources and Types of Assistance

► Describe current development assistance received from international sources. Is the assistance provided on a government-to-government basis or through bilateral agencies, multilateral institutions, or NGOs and foundations?

► Does the international assistance support national health priorities and programs? To what extent is it useful in catalyzing health system reforms that would otherwise be difficult to accomplish?

► What types of international assistance are provided—for example, funds (loans or grants), commodities, technical assistance, fellowships?

► When loans are provided, are they used for investment purposes rather than to cover recurrent health expenditures?

► When the assistance is provided in the form of commodities, are purchase terms negotiated to ensure appropriate products, price, and quality?

Ministry of Health Involvement

► Have health-sector priorities been clearly articulated to support national development policies?

► Does the MOH take an active role in identifying sources and types of assistance and representing its interests to the ministries of planning, external relations, and finance, which are likely to carry out negotiations with donors?

► Does the MOH facilitate the cooperation of multiple donors by communicating national policies and programs, inviting donors to participate in the development of a master plan, hosting regular donor coordination meetings, or giving periodic progress reports to donors?

Project Development

► Are project proposals written in a way that is consistent with government policies, specifically the national drug policy (if one exists)?

► Is government commitment reflected in the assignment of staff, space, and equipment to project objectives?

► Do project proposals include plans for evaluating impact and sustainability and other issues of concern to donor agencies?

► Does each proposal include a description of the problem to be addressed? Are project goals, purposes, and strategies clearly stated? Are outputs, activities, and inputs specified?

► Are all involved parties included in project planning?

► Are external consultants employed in project design, implementation, or evaluation to provide specific technical expertise and independence from local political pressures?

---

are developing their broad priorities with consideration of the priorities of others. At the country level, they are meeting more often to exchange information and even to explore possibilities for joint efforts.

WHO distinguishes between coordination, the integration of various inputs into a cohesive whole, and collaboration, the agreement of parties to work together toward a common goal. A third element, cooperation, includes both collaboration and coordination (WHO/DAP 1995). A fourth element, communication, facilitates—or, by its absence, may prevent—the other three.

Ministries of health are in a powerful position to influence donor cooperation. Although they may be motivated by a desire to reduce duplication of effort, they may also find an important opportunity to build support and momentum for health program priorities such as essential drugs programs. As Country Study 43.1 illustrates, the MOH can facilitate donor cooperation by taking the lead: developing and communicating national policies and programs, inviting donors to participate in the development of a master plan as a framework for action, hosting regular donor coordination meetings, and giving periodic progress reports to donors using performance indicators. Country Study 43.2 demonstrates a failure of initiative and coordination. ∎

Country Study 43.1 Donor Coordination in Ethiopia

In the early 1990s, Ethiopia was receiving donor support from several bilateral and multilateral agencies to strengthen its pharmaceutical sector, which had been weakened by years of civil war. These donor-assisted activities included a Bamako Initiative project and a national essential drugs project (EDP). Other donors routed their assistance through NGOs such as the Ethiopian Red Cross Society. Donor cooperation was weak, and after the withdrawal of the main donor, the EDP suddenly came to a stop.

After the end of civil war in 1991, donors and the new transitional government of Ethiopia agreed to jointly revitalize the health services. Since the availability of essential drugs was seen as a key factor, donors and the MOH agreed to add a pharmaceutical component to the Ethiopian Recovery and Reconstruction Programme (ERRP) to provide essential drugs and medical supplies for relief efforts. All donors agreed that the joint program would be coordinated by the MOH, assisted by a small consulting company.

Contributing to this success were monthly meetings of the donors' health advisers and representatives of the MOH. After one year of emergency drug supplies, they recognized the need to shift from relief efforts toward the development of sustainable programs for drug supply. To begin this process, the MOH, with the assistance of ERRP consultants, convened a roundtable with donors in May 1993. This meeting resulted in the formation of a team composed of MOH and donor representatives, who drafted a master plan for a comprehensive Ethiopian national drugs program (ENDP).

At a second donor meeting in February 1994, efforts began in earnest to coordinate support to the entire pharmaceutical sector. The existing projects of several donor organizations were integrated into the ENDP master plan.

With WHO guidance, the MOH developed a plan of collaboration to focus program efforts in priority areas during a transitional period, while awaiting further donor commitment and funding. Other donors provided extra drug supplies to cover this bridging phase from the emergency program to a sustainable system.

Although donors and the MOH agreed on most technical points, consensus could not be reached on all points in the master plan. The MOH pharmacy department took the initiative and presented its own version of the ENDP master plan to all donors through the Ministry of External Economic Cooperation.

The master plan provided the basis for further discussion and development of plans by the MOH and the donors. Although donor coordination and collaboration have improved dramatically, more efforts are needed to transform these concepts into reality.

Source: Adapted from WHO/DAP 1995.

Country Study 43.2 Lack of Donor Coordination in a West African Country

A West African country suffered from a lack of coherent drug policies, resulting in the near absence of affordable essential drugs in its health facilities. The MOH tried twice to break this deadlock by starting a procurement agency for essential drugs, but these institutions failed to achieve their objectives. Drug prices remained too high, procurement procedures were unnecessarily bureaucratic, and the selection of drugs was poor.

Several donors had assisted the MOH over the years, but in an uncoordinated fashion. One UN agency tried to introduce a vertical essential drugs program (EDP), but the sudden withdrawal of funds by a bilateral donor ended the program in 1989. An evaluation of this program by another UN agency identified key problems as the lack of a national drug policy (NDP), absence of several key elements of an EDP, absence of training in rational use, and nonsystematic collection of data.

Many bilateral donors were actually supporting the country with drugs, but coordination was poor. The MOH strategy was to ask individual donors to support the pharmaceutical services in certain provinces. Probably due to weak central policies, the MOH allowed each donor to set up its own system. There was little exchange of information experiences among the various provinces and donors, leading to duplication of effort and incompatible systems.

In June 1991, a meeting of five UN agencies criticized the MOH for the lack of an effective NDP and the near absence of essential drugs under generic names. One bilateral donor tried to assist the MOH pharmacy department in technical aspects of regulation. After some years, however, it also switched its attention to one region.

A large UN agency and a multilateral donor pressed for the creation of another essential drugs procurement agency (the third in ten years) and provided the funds for its set-up. Although the MOH organized some drug policy workshops, and another UN agency assisted with the development of an NDP, no clear policy decisions were made. Another bilateral donor sent a large team of consultants to study its possible role in the drug field; the team wrote a comprehensive description of the problems and proposed the development of a five-year pharmaceutical master plan by all parties, linked to an NDP. Expectations for a jointly coordinated effort increased. However, the MOH and other donors were even more confused when this particular donor deferred its decision for at least a year. Some donors pressed for further development of a national drug procurement agency, and others insisted that an NDP be developed first. Meanwhile, one donor left the country. The MOH still lacks the funds and expertise to develop a comprehensive NDP and five-year pharmaceutical master plan. The sudden devaluation of the regional currency has increased local interest in generic essential drugs and has also resulted in a flow of drug aid. It remains to be seen whether this will result in a sustainable development of an NDP based on the essential drugs concept.

Unfortunately, this case shows the low efficiency of uncoordinated donor activities in the absence of MOH commitment.

≡ References and Further Readings

★ = *Key readings.*

Baum, W. C. 1982. *Project cycle.* Washington, D.C.: World Bank.

Blanco-Sequeiros, M. 1994. Health projects within the health care system. In *Health and disease in developing countries*, ed. K. S. Lankinen, S. Bergstrom, P. H. Makela, and M. Peltomaa. London: Macmillan.

Danida (Danish International Development Agency). 1992. *Guidelines for project preparation.* Copenhagen: Danida.

Dowling, M. A. C. 1989. *Raising funds for health programmes.* HMD/89.4. Geneva: World Health Organization.

★ Hodson, H. V., ed. 1991. *The international foundation directory*, 5th ed. London: Europa Publications, Ltd. (18 Bedford Square, London WC1B 3JN, England).

IDRC/WHO (International Development Research Centre/World Health Organization). 1991. *Health systems research training series.* Vol. 2, part 1. *Proposal development and fieldwork*, ed. C. M. Varkevisser, I. Pathmanathan, and A. Brownlee. Ottawa: IDRC.

Jankowski, K., ed. 1996. *Directory of international corporate giving in America and abroad.* Rockville, Md.: Taft Group (835 Penobscot Bldg., Detroit, Mich. 48226).

★ Janovsky, K. E. 1987. *Project formulation and proposal writing.* WHO/EDUC/87.187. Geneva: World Health Organization.

Kaijage, F. J., ed. 1993. *Management consulting in Africa: Utilizing local expertise.* West Hartford, Conn.: Kumarian Press.

Kubr, M. 1994. *How to select and use consultants: A client's guide.* Geneva: International Labour Organization.

NORAD (Norwegian Agency for Development Cooperation). 1990. *The logical framework approach: Handbook for objectives-oriented project planning.* Oslo: NORAD.

Olson, S., and M. M. Feczko, eds. 1993. *The foundation directory*, 15th ed. New York: Foundation Center (79 Fifth Avenue, New York, N.Y. 10003-3076).

UNDP (United Nations Development Programme). 1988. *Programme and project manual.* New York: UNDP.

WHO/DAP (World Health Organization/Action Programme on Essential Drugs). 1995. *Collaboration and coordination in national drug policy development.* WHO/DAP/MAC(7)/95.7. Geneva: WHO/DAP.

★ WHO/PAHO (World Health Organization/Pan American Health Organization). 1988. *Funding for health projects: A guide to American private foundations.* Washington, D.C.: WHO/PAHO.

★ WHO/PAHO (World Health Organization/Pan American Health Organization). 1992. *International cooperation in health: Agency profiles.* Washington, D.C.: WHO/PAHO.

WHO/PAHO (World Health Organization/Pan American Health Organization). 1993. *Standardized format for PAHO project documents and profiles.* OPS.DEC.93.02. Washington, D.C.: WHO/PAHO.

World Bank. 1993. *World development report: Investing in health.* New York: Oxford University Press.

Annex 43.1 Standardized Annotated Format for Project Document

[Cover]

Date prepared: _____

Country: _____

Project number: _____

Proposed title: _____

Estimated duration: _____

Tentative cost:

    Estimated external donor contribution: _____

    Estimated counterpart costs: _____

Person responsible for preparation of project profile:

    _____

    Position: _____

I. Logical Framework (project matrix, one to two pages)

II. Executive Summary (This should not exceed two pages. It should include information on the project, its purpose, strategy, and cost. It is also recommended that it include references to the national context as well as its perspectives for sustainability once external cooperation ceases.)

III. Project Data

1. **Context:** brief explanation of the major characteristics of the development setting, including the main characteristics of the health sector, host country development strategies, prior ongoing assistance (including that in the negotiation phase), socioeconomic and political conditions, and institutional framework (such as responsible ministry and/or government institutions, local bodies, NGOs, interagency agreements).

2. **Project justification:** reasons for undertaking the project and for its design, including problem to be addressed, expected end-of-project situation; target group or beneficiaries, project strategy and implementation arrangements, special considerations, host government support capacity, coordinating arrangements, and reasons for assistance from donor.

3. **Project goal (development objective):** the long-term development aim at the sectoral or subsectoral level that this project, along with other efforts, is meant to help attain.

4. **Project purpose (immediate objective):** a statement of what the project itself is expected to achieve, described as a desired end result, including specification of time, place, quantity, and beneficiaries.

5. **Outputs:** the tangible products that should be produced by the project, such as systems developed or persons trained, described in concrete and verifiable terms.

6. **Activities:** the substantive tasks that will be carried out under the project to produce the specified outputs.

7. **Inputs and resources:** the raw materials of the project, such as equipment, supplies, personnel, fellowships, and the timing of each for budget purposes; detailed specifications such as technical requirements, job descriptions for expatriate advisers, and training programs are presented in annexes.

8. **Assumptions and risks:** a description of those conditions outside the immediate control or influence of the project that are necessary for the achievement of project objectives, and those that may arise to delay or prevent such achievement; measures envisaged for responding to the latter should be included.

9. **Indicators and means of verification:** measures that will demonstrate achievement of project objectives and outputs and that serve as the basis for monitoring; such measures contain the time period, region, target group, and quantity and quality; the data or evidence needed for this measurement and where it will be found should be described.

10. **Prior obligations and prerequisites:** specification of any host government actions that are a precondition for assistance, such as budget modification, ad hoc regulations, or legislation.

11. **Organization and administration:** description of the organization responsible for project implementation, including its steering and management committees; the division of authority and responsibility within the organization or between different implementing agencies; and the main administrative procedures to be observed.

12. **Organizational and financial sustainability:** an assessment of the commitment and capacity of the responsible organization to mobilize the required resources for sustaining the results of the project once assistance is withdrawn.

13. **Project monitoring, reporting, and evaluation:** description of the mechanisms for monitoring, report preparation and review, and evaluation, and the parties responsible for each.

14. **Budget and finance:** budget presented by component (for example, equipment, personnel) and by activity and divided into investment cost and recurrent costs; annual recurrent cost implications for the host country beyond the project period should also be included.

15. **Financial reporting and auditing:** description of accounting, financial reporting, and auditing procedures to be applied, including frequency, institutions involved, responsibility, and feedback mechanisms; specification of arrangements made to ensure proper data collection.

16. **Project implementation plan:** the framework within which the project will be implemented, including a time frame for project inputs and activities, the sequence of activities, and the timing for transfer of funds.

IV. Annexes (as required)

Sources: Based on standardized *Project Formulation Framework* of UNDP, the *Project Proposal Document* of Danida, and WHO/PAHO 1993.

Part I Introduction	Part II Policy and Legal Framework	Part III Drug Management Cycle	**Part IV** **Management Support Systems**
			A Organization and Management
			B Financing and Sustainability ▶
			C Information Management
			D Human Resources Management

40 Drug Financing Strategies

41 Analyzing and Controlling Drug Expenditures

42 Financial Planning and Management

43 Donor Financing

44 Revolving Drug Funds

Chapter 44
Revolving Drug Funds

≡ Summary

Many governments, nongovernmental organizations (NGOs), and community health programs have implemented user fees to fund or partially fund the cost of drugs or other health services. Many different forms of revolving drug funds (RDFs) exist. Their common element is that fees are charged for drugs dispensed. In the context of the Bamako Initiative, community drug schemes often have cost-recovery objectives and include the financing of health education, immunization, and other aspects of primary health care.

Supporters assert that RDFs can raise substantial revenue; improve drug availability and quality of care; promote equity by making drugs more accessible to the poor, while charging those who can afford to pay; reinforce decentralization through local control of resources; and encourage efficiency in drug management and drug use. Others caution that collection costs may exceed revenue collected; there may be no improvement in drug availability and other quality measures; user charges are a form of "sick tax" that substitutes for public spending; people are dissuaded from seeking essential health care; and incentives are created for overprescribing.

Planning and implementing an RDF require simultaneous commitment to public health goals and sound business management. A number of steps are involved:

Feasibility: Determine whether the concept of an RDF is politically acceptable, economically viable, and realistic in terms of managerial requirements.

Organizational structure and legal status: Decide which RDF functions will be centralized and which decentralized. Seek government or legal endorsement for such issues as retention of revenue at the facility or district level. Community involvement is often essential for the acceptability, credibility, and accountability of RDFs.

Pricing and exemptions: Establish policies that ensure access to services and also maintain the financial integrity of the RDF. Determine fee collection mechanisms as well as fee levels. Consider willingness to pay and cost data in setting drug prices.

Financial planning: Ascertain initial capitalization requirements and recurrent costs. The availability of government and donor subsidies helps determine the RDF's cost-recovery objectives.

Supply management: Consider management requirements, since weaknesses in any area can threaten the RDF's service performance and financial viability.

Public communications: Tailor target audiences, messages, and media to each stage of RDF implementation.

Monitoring and supervision: Put in place recording, reporting, supervisory, and other measures to monitor impact on patients, financial performance, drug availability, and drug use.

Establishing and sustaining RDFs have been difficult in practice. Improved drug availability, equity, and efficiency are more likely with local control and retention of revenue; reliable supply of low-cost essential drugs; locally appropriate fee schedules; protection mechanisms to ensure equitable access; continued or increased levels of government funding for health; businesslike orientation to personnel, financial management, and supply management; strict measures to ensure accountability; and implementation in phases or through a well-conceived pilot approach.

Examples of successful large national RDFs are few. Revenues are often much less than expected. Equity of access often decreases. Reliable drug supply, management, accountability, and rational drug use are challenges for any RDF. Countries and programs that implement RDFs should do so with a full understanding of the problems other programs have faced and the solutions that have succeeded elsewhere.

≡ Revolving drug funds (RDFs) are difficult to implement. Examples of successful large-scale public RDFs are limited. Revenues are often much less than expected. Utilization of health services and, therefore, equity of access often decrease. Accountability, management, reliable drug supply, and rational drug use are challenges.

At the same time, many countries providing "free" health services have found that public resources are insufficient to meet rising costs and increasing demand. When funds are limited, provision of essential drugs is among the first components of health care to suffer: drugs short-

ages become common even when selection, procurement, distribution, and use are efficient and rational.

Cost sharing through drug fees is one of several drug financing strategies described in Chapter 40. This chapter is concerned with programs in which drug fees are used to finance essential drugs at the national level, at the district level, at individual institutions such as teaching and referral hospitals, or through community drug schemes.

Drug fees may be simply one component of a broader program of user fees. Although such programs may not think of themselves as RDFs, this chapter should be useful for any program involved in setting drug fees and using the revenue to resupply drugs.

≡ 44.1 The Revolving Fund Concept

Why Establish RDFs?

In an RDF, a sum of money (contributed by the government, donors, or the community) is used to purchase an initial stock of essential and commonly used drugs to be sold, ideally at a price sufficient to replace the stock of drugs and ensure a continuous supply (see Figure 44.1). Reasons usually given for establishing an RDF are:

► Essential drugs are a critical component of effective preventive and curative care.
► The increased availability of drugs is perceived as a real improvement in the quality of care.
► Drugs are tangible, and most patients are willing to pay for them.
► The public spends significant amounts of money for pharmaceuticals from the private sector, often buying inadequate quantities at high prices. Drugs supplied through an RDF are generally more affordable.
► Patients may attach greater value to drugs for which they have paid. A potential result is improved patient adherence to treatment.
► RDFs linked to essential drugs programs offer the potential for increasing the efficiency of drug services as well as generating additional revenue.
► Increased price awareness by prescribers and patients may result in improved use of drugs.

Although the primary objective of private pharmacies is to maximize *profit*, the objective of RDFs is to maximize *access*. If current public financing is sufficient to ensure universal access to essential drugs without charge, then drug fees are unnecessary. If current financing is inadequate, an RDF provides supplementary resources to make low-cost essential drugs more accessible. If the alternative for low-income and geographically isolated populations is paying high prices and traveling long distances to buy drugs in the private market, an RDF may make drugs more accessible.

Experiences with RDFs

There are numerous examples of experiences with user fee programs and, in particular, with RDFs (see the country studies and "References and Further Readings"). From these experiences, proponents of user charges suggest that

► substantial revenue can be raised by user fees, which adds to central allocations;

► drug availability and quality of care are improved with the additional revenue;
► equity is promoted because limited public funds can be targeted to the most needy, while the rest pay;
► decentralization is reinforced through local control of resources;
► efficiency is fostered through lower fees at first-level facilities to reinforce the referral system and higher fees at higher-level hospitals to reduce the disproportionately large expenditures typically made on drug supply for referral hospitals.

Not all governments or health financing experts favor user fees for drugs. Opponents observe that

► collection costs may exceed revenue collected when the full cost of developing the system and all additional administrative costs are considered;
► there may be no improvement in drug availability and other quality measures (as has occurred in some user fee programs);
► user charges may become a form of "sick tax," substituting for rather than supplementing central allocations;
► people, particularly the poor and other target groups, are dissuaded from seeking essential health care;
► incentives for overprescribing are created if revenue is used to support staff salaries.

Two decades of experience with RDFs and user fees for services demonstrate the need for thoughtful design, careful implementation associated with quality improvement, and good management. Programs that have implemented large fees with no preparation of the public and little improvement in quality have seen significant decreases in utilization; programs designed with little attention to management and accounting systems have resulted in abuse and generated little revenue compared with the cost of fee collection; programs that have not reinvested revenues to improve quality have resulted in a decline in public confidence and utilization; RDFs without a reliable source of low-cost drugs have quickly ceased to revolve; and some schemes with drug charges have led to overprescribing.

At the same time, drug supply and utilization of health services have increased where there has been strong leadership, revenues have maintained a steady supply of drugs, financial and drug management systems are sound, fee levels and exemptions have protected target groups, and accountability has been good. Country Study 44.1 describes one promising RDF.

Figure 44.1 The RDF Cycle

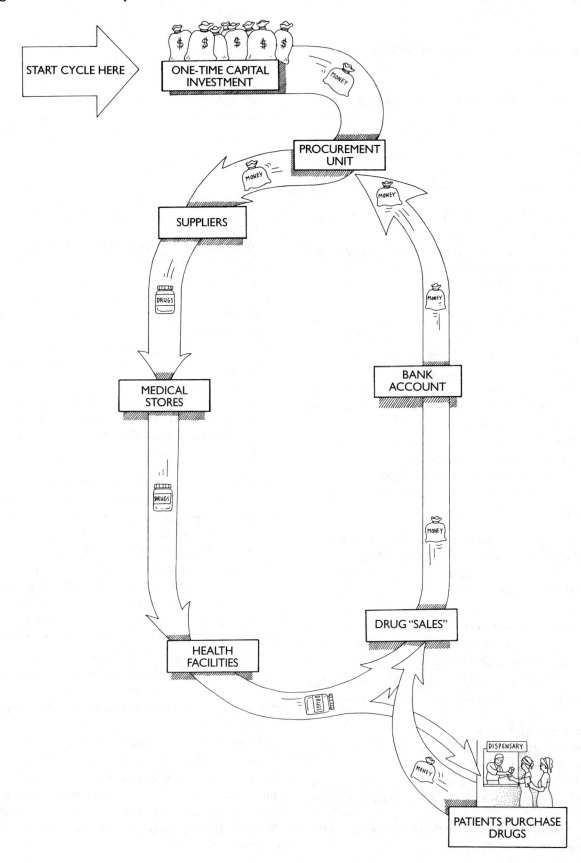

START CYCLE HERE

ONE-TIME CAPITAL INVESTMENT

PROCUREMENT UNIT

SUPPLIERS

MEDICAL STORES

BANK ACCOUNT

HEALTH FACILITIES

DRUG "SALES"

PATIENTS PURCHASE DRUGS

DISPENSARY

Country Study 44.1 Impact of an RDF on Equity of Access and Financial Performance in Cameroon

Between 1989 and 1992, the Cameroon national budget decreased by 30 percent, health spending declined from 5.2 percent to 4.4 percent of the national budget, and drugs were no longer funded from the budget. Utilization of public health services declined, staff remained mostly idle, and patients were left to buy drugs at high prices on the private market. Faced with this situation, the Ministry of Health (MOH), with donor assistance, introduced RDFs, beginning in 1991 with two provinces.

Private Nonprofit Health Fund. A Provincial Solidarity Fund for the Promotion of Health (PHF) was established in each province as a private nonprofit association. Participating villages elect members to local and district health fund committees (HFCs), which send delegates to the PHF general assembly. The PHF and HFC hire managers, accountants, and clerks on private-sector terms; oversee payment of staff bonuses based on annual performance indicators; manage health area bank accounts; and ensure that private-sector accounting and audit procedures are followed. The PHF manager makes regular health facility visits to supervise drug deliveries, inventory management, fee collection, and accounting practices (see the accompanying figure).

Continuing Public-Sector Role. Existing legal structures were changed to accommodate the PHF. Provincial health officers, pharmacists, and other professionals continue to provide technical supervision. The MOH funds all personnel costs for health staff, but only 15 percent of nonsalary operating costs is funded from the MOH budget, with the rest funded from the PHF.

Drug Supply Sources. PHFs have purchased drugs in bulk from the Centre d'Importation et d'Approvisionnement en Médicaments Essentiels (CIAME), a local nonprofit international drug procurement service, but they also have the right to buy drugs internationally. CIAME costs are less than half of private-sector costs due to the use of generic drugs and bulk packaging and the exemption from the import duties placed on brand-name drugs. The CIAME warehouse maintains sufficient stocks of most items to fill PHF orders within weeks. Drug fees are set well below private-sector retail prices.

Financial Performance. Cost-recovery levels rose from 22 percent of nonsalary costs in the first year of the PHF to 62 percent in the third year. By the third year, drug fee revenue was sufficient to cover all drug costs, including procurement, distribution, supervision, and financial management. The PHF was also generating sufficient funds to pay local cold-chain expenses and some other local costs. Twenty percent of PHF expenditures was for salaries and performance bonuses for PHF operations. PHF revenue was also used to support training and supervision in standard treatments and rational drug use.

Facility Utilization. Phased introduction provided a natural way to assess the impact of changes through household surveys, observations at health facilities, and monitoring of utilization data. Use of health centers increased significantly for people in PHF areas compared with those in which PHFs had not been implemented.

Equity of Access. The probability of the poorest quintile seeking care increased in PHF areas at a rate greater than that of the rest of the population. This is contrary to previous studies, which generally found that the poorest are most hurt by user fees. Before the PHF, travel and time costs involved in seeking alternative sources of care were high. When drugs became available at local health centers, the fees paid represented an effective reduction in the price of care. Since the poor are most responsive to price changes, they appear to be benefiting more than others from local availability of high-quality drugs.

In this setting, user fee revenue was able to increase drug supply and health care utilization through a combination of public-sector and private nonprofit efforts. The approach included a reliable source of low-cost, high-quality drugs (CIAME), a private-sector approach to accountability and financial management, phased implementation, and locally acceptable fees.

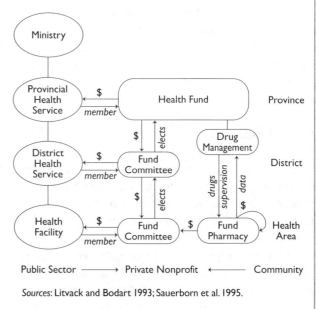

Sources: Litvack and Bodart 1993; Sauerborn et al. 1995.

Steps for Planning and Implementing an RDF

The planning and implementation of a successful RDF requires simultaneous commitment to public health goals and sound business management principles. Each of the following steps requires careful attention:

- Carry out a situation analysis and feasibility assessment.
- Prepare a financial plan that considers cost-recovery objectives, capitalization requirements, and long-term financial needs.
- Determine the organizational structure, staffing, and legal status of the RDF.
- Develop an implementation plan.
- Determine pricing and exemption policies.
- Develop the necessary systems for drug management and financial management.

Figure 44.2 Cost-Recovery Potential Determined by Patients and Costs, Not by Policy

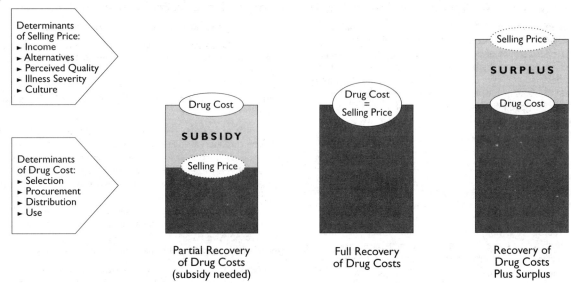

▶ Prepare public communications for RDF introduction.

▶ Monitor impact and adjust the program accordingly.

≡ 44.2 Situation Analysis and Feasibility Assessment

Governments considering whether to introduce cost recovery must address questions of political, economic, and managerial feasibility, given local circumstances (see Figure 44.2).

Political Issues

Three political issues are key to establishing an RDF: acceptance of the user fee concept, local retention of fee revenue, and political and administrative decentralization.

Acceptance of User Fees. Although many believe strongly in the concept of universal access to health care, a policy of free drugs is worth little if drugs are unavailable. When RDFs have been proposed in settings where drugs at health facilities have been scarce, public reaction has generally been positive. And when an RDF has resulted in a noticeable increase in the availability of drugs, public acceptance has been much greater than government officials anticipated. Conversely, if people have experienced a steady supply of drugs provided free of charge by the government, they are more likely to oppose any introduction of fees. In this setting, the need for an RDF should be carefully considered.

Local Retention of Fee Revenue. The "law of the treasury" often requires that revenues earned by any arm of government be remitted to the central government. RDFs will not revolve, however, unless the facilities that collect drug

fees can retain this revenue to replenish their drug supplies. Reinvestment of revenues in the collecting facility also promotes a sense of community ownership, which further protects and strengthens the RDF. Facilities in a pilot project area are often permitted to retain revenues, but replication on a broader scale requires permanent changes in government policy.

Political and Administrative Decentralization. The question of local involvement and autonomy can be politically sensitive. Successful RDFs often involve community participation and supervision, which ensures financial sustainability and greater community interest in the local health facility. Local empowerment must be accepted and supported by higher levels of government (which must give department or provincial authorities the authority and flexibility to design policies appropriate for their areas).

Economic Issues

Can sufficient funds be recovered to justify the effort required to make an RDF successful? The answer to this question depends on national and local economic strength, patients' ability and willingness to pay, "competition" from other sources of supply, the availability of capital, policies on exemptions and subsidies, and the program's overall ability to balance public health and economic objectives. All these issues should be carefully considered. Household and patient surveys that ask people about their choice of health services and health care expenditures can reveal a great deal about both willingness and ability to pay for health treatment.

Economic feasibility is also influenced by the level at

which fees are introduced. Should RDF implementation be top-down, starting first in hospitals, or bottom-up, beginning in the community? There are advantages and disadvantages to each approach.

Despite the many concerns relating to economic feasibility, health service utilization and equity may actually *improve* with drug fees: in Cameroon, the establishment of an RDF led to significantly higher rates of utilization, and the poorest people benefited most from the local availability of effective drugs (see Country Study 44.1). A brief explanation of the economic underpinnings of this observation may be illuminating. Although opponents to cost sharing often speak about the increase in cost, purchasing drugs locally often avoids the high travel and time costs of seeking care elsewhere and reduces total expenditures for an episode of illness. The key lesson is that price must be examined from the perspective of the patient.

Managerial Issues

Given the human and physical infrastructure, can a cost-recovery system be made to operate? Accountability, a businesslike orientation, supply management capacity, and human resources capacity are especially critical when an RDF is initiated at the community level, because management systems and capacity may need to be developed.

Demonstrated commitment by the government (and often by the donor) is essential. Is support available to help maintain the fund until self-sufficiency is reached?

≡ 44.3 Financial Planning

RDF financial planning involves defining the cost-recovery objective, the role of government and external funding, capitalization requirements, and foreign exchange issues. Since the goal of an RDF is to maintain steady drug supply while serving as many people as possible, careful analysis of both recurrent costs and regular government and donor contributions is necessary. Drug sales must make up the difference between these two. Many countries that are eager to commence cost-recovery programs fail to do a careful financial analysis prior to embarking on such programs. As a result, a well-intentioned RDF may quickly decapitalize; some revenues are raised, but there is not necessarily a direct relationship between revenues and stock replacement.

Cost-Recovery Objective

The cost-recovery objective for an RDF may be set by policy, but the actual level of cost recovery depends on the response of patients to drug fees, the number of exemptions, collection efficiency, and other factors. Although some programs attempt to cover all primary health care costs through user fees, many countries have found it extremely difficult to recover full costs on a large scale.

Cost-Recovery Alternatives. The level of cost recovery reflects the relationship between the total operating costs and the total revenues collected. Possible cost-recovery objectives include

- partial recovery of drug costs, which requires continued subsidy from government or other sources;
- full recovery of drug costs;
- full recovery of drug costs plus some local operating costs;
- full recovery of all drug costs and local operating costs.

A tension between public health and financial objectives is inherent in the RDF concept. Since RDF fees are intended to increase the availability of essential drugs at the local level, they must not serve as financial barriers to people receiving needed services. The RDF must improve total access to service, not decrease it. Yet the fees must be high enough to ensure replenishment of supplies and financial sustainability of the RDF.

Establishing a realistic cost-recovery objective depends on striking a balance among operating costs, revenue collection, and government and other funding.

Operating Costs. Drug costs should be calculated based on the full replacement cost of drugs. This cost includes the original purchase price (with insurance and freight), price increases due to inflation and currency fluctuations, and the cost of losses due to expiration, spoilage, and pilferage. Other recurrent costs include management of the procurement office, transportation, storage at various levels, and perhaps repackaging or other costs. In addition to drug costs, local operating costs include health workers' salaries, fuel for vehicles, consumable items such as dressings, cold-chain costs, and utilities (see Chapter 42).

Revenue Collection. Revenue collection in RDFs is determined by patients' willingness to pay, exemption rates, and collection efficiency; it is often far below target levels.

The price at which most patients will buy drugs at a government health facility—a reflection of their willingness to pay—depends on several factors:

- Household income, which can vary dramatically by season, especially in rural areas;
- The availability and cost of alternative sources of drugs and health care (the "competition");
- Perceived quality of the drugs and associated health care services;

▶ The severity of the illness;

▶ Cultural factors, such as the priority given to health care for men, women, and children.

Basing RDF prices only on actual costs sometimes leads to a dramatic and dangerous decline in health facility utilization. Because of differences in access, perceived quality, and usual quantities of drugs purchased, direct comparison with private-sector prices can be misleading. Estimates of willingness to pay can be made using the techniques described in Section 44.6 on pricing.

Exemption rates are another major determinant of actual revenue collections. In cost-recovery programs with broad exemption criteria, over 50 percent of patients do not pay; a high level of cost recovery is difficult, if not impossible, in such circumstances. Exemption criteria, administrative arrangements, and mechanisms for financing exemptions are considered later in this chapter.

Finally, total revenue reflects collection efficiency: what share of expected revenues is actually collected? When the number of patients treated, quantity of drugs dispensed, drug prices, and exemption rates are considered, how much money should have been, and how much money actually was, collected? It is not unusual to find that actual collections are less than two-thirds—sometimes as little as one-third—of expectations.

Reasons for collection inefficiency include simple laxity in implementing fees, unofficial ("backdoor") exemptions, and pilferage of drugs and cash. A high collection rate depends on sound drug management systems, well-developed financial management and accountability measures, regular monitoring and supervision, and, when necessary, vigorous use of disciplinary and legal measures. Collection inefficiency is a major threat to RDFs.

Role of Government and External Funding

Government and external funding is often necessary to plan and implement an RDF and to cover the cost of exemptions, subsidize high-cost drugs, and fund other health system costs not financed through user fees.

Maintaining Government Funding. If continued government funding for drugs is needed, how can it be secured? What strategies can ensure that RDF revenue supplements, rather than substitutes for, central treasury allocations?

The simple but vague promise of "continued funding at present levels" may be difficult to monitor and enforce in practice. Trends in government revenues, allocations among ministries and within the ministry of health, local inflation, and foreign exchange fluctuations (which usually have a major impact on drug purchasing power) all

make it difficult to interpret increases or decreases in drug budgets.

At least three strategies exist: (1) maintain an annual per capita drug budget (as in Indonesia, Country Study 40.1), (2) establish a budgeting formula and an agreed-upon list of groups of patients or treatments for public support (for example, children, antenatal supplements, tuberculosis treatment), or (3) exclude RDF revenue entirely from all national or local budget information and expenditure analysis.

The last approach has been implemented in one East African country by showing user fee revenue as a nominal amount in official budget figures and excluding it from historical comparisons and budget analyses. The result has been that rising user fee and insurance revenue has had no measurable impact on central government allocations for health.

Funding from Donors and Development Loans. Grants and development loans can be instrumental in planning and implementing an RDF. This category of funding may include financing of start-up capital, development costs, and price subsidies during the first few years of operation. However, such funding should not be relied on for long-term subsidy, because it puts the RDF's financial sustainability at risk.

In an RDF, donated drugs should normally be sold through health facilities at regular RDF prices and revenues used to support health services, as determined by the community. Distributing donated drugs without charge creates confusion for health staff and patients. An exception would be drugs provided to support programs such as leprosy or tuberculosis control, which are often included in the list of exempt health conditions.

Start-Up Financing

Starting or expanding a revolving drug fund requires working capital, support for the development of management systems, and sometimes partial subsidy of drug costs.

Capitalization Requirements. Capitalization has to do with filling the RDF pipeline from central warehouses through peripheral drug stores, with appropriate inventories at each level, before drug sales begin. Only when the pipeline is filled is the RDF able to revolve. Gaps in the pipeline mean missed deliveries from one level to the next and eventual stockouts at the point of service delivery.

Seed stock for RDF capitalization may be provided by the central government or by an external donor, or it may be contributed at the local level by the community. Pipeline calculations for an RDF are illustrated in Box 44.1. The pipeline is affected by inventory management decisions

Box 44.1 Pipeline Calculations for Capitalizing an RDF

A revolving drug fund must have sufficient *working capital* (drugs and cash) to start revolving and keep revolving. Working capital depends on the amount of drugs and cash in the pipeline. The length of the pipeline is measured in numbers of months. It is determined by the number of levels in the distribution system, the safety stock at each level, and the average working stock (which depends on the delivery interval—see Chapter 15). The diameter of the pipeline is determined by the final outflow—the total value of drugs dispensed per month.

The following example illustrates a pipeline calculation for establishing an RDF to serve a network of 210 community pharmacies. It includes a central supply agency, district stores, and the community pharmacies.

The pipeline for the proposed drug sales program begins with the disbursement of funds for procurement and ends at the point where funds are collected and made available for purchasing replenishment supplies. The pipeline can be broken down into a number of segments, described in the next column and illustrated in the accompanying diagram.

Average Monthly Sales. The number of low-, medium-, and high-volume community pharmacies and the average monthly sale per pharmacy are estimated in the table on the next page.

Capital Requirements. With an average pipeline length of sixteen months and an average consumption for all 210 pharmacies of $65,000 per month, total capital requirements would be:

$$16 \times \$65,000 = \$1,040,000$$

Sources of Capital and Possible Cost Savings. Working capital can be supplied from various sources: the purchase pipeline and safety stock could be financed by donations, the working stock for central and district levels by government allocations, and the community pharmacy funds from community fund-raising efforts. Improved procurement payment terms, more rapid flow of drugs through the system (faster turnover), and more efficient bank transfers could shorten the pipeline and reduce capitalization costs.

Cash and Drugs in the Pipeline	Months

Purchase pipeline. In this example, it is assumed that roughly 50 percent of drugs will be purchased from international sources and 50 percent from local sources. For international purchases, an average of 6 months will elapse between the provision of a letter of credit and the receipt of the pharmaceuticals at the central supply agency. For domestic purchases, payment will be made upon receipt. Therefore, the average purchase pipeline will be three months.   3

Central supply agency safety stock. A three-month safety stock will be maintained at the central supply agency.   3

Central supply agency working stock. The supply agency will tender once a year but will receive deliveries every four months. This implies a maximum working stock of four months and an average working stock of two months.   2

District safety stock. The district medical stores of the supply agency will maintain a two-month safety stock.   2

District working stock. The district medical stores will receive shipments from the central supply agency every two months, implying a maximum working stock of two months and an average working stock of one month.   1

Community pharmacy safety stock. The community pharmacies will maintain a one-month safety stock.   1

Community pharmacy working stock. The community pharmacies will be resupplied once a month, implying a maximum working stock of one month and an average working stock of half a month.   0.5

Community pharmacy cash on hand. The community pharmacies will use their revenues once a month when they purchase their resupplies from the district medical stores. On average, these funds will have been held half a month by the community pharmacies.   0.5

District to center cash transfer. Money received by the district medical stores will be deposited within the week at the local branch of the national bank. On average, it will take one month for this money to be credited to the account of the supply agency.   1

Cash on hand. In general, purchases made by the supply agency will represent one-third of its annual turnover. As a result, money will sit in the agency's central account up to four months, or an average of two months, before being used to effect a purchase.   2

Total Pipeline = 16

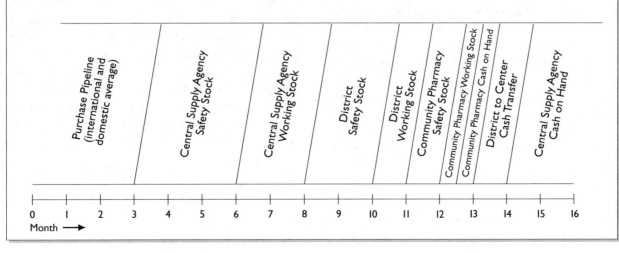

> **Box 44.1 Number and Average Monthly Sales of Community Pharmacies (cont.)**
>
> | | Low Volume | Medium Volume | High Volume | Total |
> |---|---|---|---|---|
> | Number of community pharmacies | 150 | 50 | 10 | 210 |
> | Average number of patients per month per pharmacy | 500 | 1,250 | 2,500 | – |
> | Average cost per drug item | $.20 | $.20 | $.20 | – |
> | Average items per patient | 2 | 2 | 2 | – |
> | Average monthly sales per pharmacy | $200 | $500 | $1,000 | – |
> | Total monthly sales (drug cost) | $30,000 | $25,000 | $10,000 | $65,000 |

(Chapter 15), distribution system design (Chapter 21), and cost-saving measures related to pipeline management (Chapter 41).

Overcapitalizing RDFs wastes money, but RDFs that are undercapitalized quickly break down. This occurs when fees are collected from drug sales, but funds are inadequate to replenish drug stocks. When revenues intended for drug purchases are inadequate to purchase all necessary drugs, funds may be used for emergency purchases of small quantities at higher-than-expected prices or to pay other expenses, further decapitalizing the fund.

Development and Implementation of Management Systems. Support may be needed to develop drug and financial management systems and for training, community orientation, monitoring, and other implementation activities.

Price Subsidies. Lower prices and broader exemptions may be needed at the beginning to gain acceptance for the system. The total development cost of an RDF, therefore, may need to include funds to partially subsidize prices for the first few years.

Foreign Exchange

Foreign exchange is an extremely important issue that requires support and cooperation from government groups outside the health sector. Where local currency is not freely convertible and the demand for foreign exchange exceeds supply, government commitment is required to provide the foreign exchange necessary to replenish drug supply on a regular basis. This issue can be problematic, since RDFs are designed by health policy-makers, and foreign exchange allocations are made outside the health sector, often by the ministry of finance, central bank, or national planning ministry. Coordination among different arms of government is difficult, but it is essential to ensure the sustainability of supply.

Liberalization of foreign exchange markets has greatly improved the situation in many countries. Even where governments continue to allocate foreign exchange for government ministries, it may be possible for an RDF to obtain a waiver to obtain foreign exchange on the open market.

≡ 44.4 Organizational Issues

Organizational issues for RDFs include their structure, drug supply system, need for a multidisciplinary team, community involvement, and legal issues.

Organizational Structure

RDFs can be managed through a highly centralized structure, a decentralized approach, or a mixed approach in which different functions are managed at different levels. Centralized systems have the potential advantages of a standardized drug list, bulk purchasing, and national uniformity in pricing policies. However, decentralized price setting, determination of exemption policies, and adjustments in the drug list may make an RDF more responsive to local circumstances.

In practice, many RDFs combine the two. For example, procurement may be centralized, and policies with regard to prices and exemptions may be determined locally. Or the central government may provide training and supervision, with all other management systems, including procurement and distribution, decentralized, as in Zaire. Country Study 44.2 illustrates some of the variety that exists in RDF organizational design and management structure. Country Study 44.1 illustrates a system that mixes private nonprofit management of the RDF with public delivery of services. Country Study 37.2 describes the organization of village drug schemes in Thailand.

The important issue is to identify the key requirements for RDF implementation and to clarify where responsibility lies for each. Major routine functions include

- ▶ product selection (review and revision of the essential drugs list);
- ▶ procurement and distribution;
- ▶ price setting;
- ▶ determination of exemption policies;

Country Study 44.2 RDFs in Three Countries

Benin. The Benin Central Purchasing Office was established in 1991 as a single national supply and sales structure for essential drugs and medical supplies. Health facilities in the public and private nonprofit sectors purchase drugs directly from the Central Office; there are no regional depots. Purchases are made with cash only; no credit is extended to customers. This cash is then used to procure additional supplies. This RDF has been supported by Benin's community financing policy, which allows health units to replenish their funds at the community level and thus maintain their purchasing capacity. The Central Office follows private-sector management practices: recruitment of a small number of competent staff, clearly defined procedures for financial and inventory management, and continuing supervision by an independent management committee and an audit office (see Country Study 6.2).

Ethiopia. The Ethiopian Red Cross Society, in collaboration with the Danish Red Cross, WHO, and the Ministry of Health, has established thirteen pharmacies, one drug shop, and four satellite centers in thirteen administrative regions of the country. A coordination unit at headquarters procures drugs through international tendering; maintains central medical stores; distributes supplies along with price lists; and oversees the staffing, management, and collection of fees in all pharmacies. Aided by computerized records, headquarters also oversees stock management—moving supplies that are nearing expiry from overstocked facilities to understocked ones—and monitors the financial status of each pharmacy. The Ethiopian Red Cross Society RDF offers no exemptions; existing MOH facilities and private pharmacies offer alternative sources of supply. Participating pharmacies in the RDF sell essential drugs at an established markup over CIF (cost, insurance, and freight) cost. A fixed percentage of the markup is intended to cover headquarters operating costs, and the remainder to cover the pharmacy's own operating costs. Any surplus is to be returned to the community to support public health activities of the community's choosing. In the first year of operation, RDF pharmacies covered all costs to reach a break-even point after approximately eight months. Replenishment of supply at the headquarters level is threatened, however, due to currency devaluation.

Zaire. The health system in Zaire is highly decentralized, and the 306 health zones (each covering 80,000 to 100,000 people) have the autonomy to design their own health delivery and financing systems. The central government provides training, supervision, and minimal financial support while emphasizing community financing. Each zone has a different organizational structure that is manifested in various payment schemes, procurement processes, and levels of overall efficiency. Health or development committees identify needs, develop budgets, determine indigent care policies, and determine how to raise the necessary funds. Most zones centralize the procurement of drugs for their health centers, usually purchasing from a pharmaceutical depot at the subregional level that operates on an RDF basis. Zones in subregions without depots must procure from other sources, such as wholesale suppliers, if near a city, or the private sector; they are at higher risk of not maintaining adequate stock. Decentralized health zones with autonomy over the delivery and financing of their health care have established various cost-recovery schemes in response to different circumstances. Staff salaries are dependent on revenues as an incentive for careful management of fee collection. Health centers have recovered, on average, nearly 80 percent of their operating costs.

► audit and financial oversight;
► local representation and oversight.

Drug Supply System

RDF survival depends on a regular supply of low-cost, high-quality drugs; if procurement and distribution are not reliable, the RDF will quickly stop functioning. RDFs may be established as part of a major effort to revitalize government drug supply systems, including central medical stores (CMS), or in conjunction with the establishment of an autonomous drug supply agency.

RDFs may also be supplied through a direct delivery system, in which tenders establish the supplier and price for each item and drugs are delivered directly by suppliers to districts and major facilities. Finally, drugs may be supplied through a prime vendor system, in which the government establishes a contract with a single private distributor (the prime vendor) as well as separate contracts with drug suppliers. The prime vendor manages drug distribution by receiving drugs from the suppliers and distributing them to districts and major facilities.

Drug supply strategies—including the CMS system, autonomous agencies, direct delivery, and prime vendors—are described in detail in Chapter 6. Because a reliable supply of drugs is essential to the success of RDFs, decision-makers and managers involved in planning or implementing RDFs must carefully consider the best drug supply strategy.

Multidisciplinary Team

Just as an immunization program needs staff specialized in cold-chain maintenance, epidemiology, and community mobilization, RDFs need staff specialized in certain areas. In addition to staff with clinical and pharmacy training, RDFs need staff with skills in economics, business, and accounting. Such skills are often found in other ministries and in the nongovernmental sector. Recruitment of some specialized staff may be needed.

Community Involvement

Community involvement can be essential for the acceptability, credibility, and accountability of RDFs. Informal involvement may include advising on program development and the collection and use of revenue and participating in public awareness campaigns. Formal involvement may include participation in generating start-up funds, setting fees, determining who receives exemptions, ensuring accountability, and monitoring the use of revenues.

Involvement of community leaders and provision of information to the public are particularly important at the outset, when user charges are just being introduced or when there are major program changes. Chapter 37 discusses community participation in greater detail.

Legal Aspects

Government-run RDFs and broader user fee programs often involve policies and actions that are not strictly legal under current law or whose legal status is unclear. Examples include the policy that user fee revenue will add to, not replace, central government allocations; retention of revenue at the facility or district level; opening of local bank accounts; carrying forward of unspent funds to the next fiscal year (as opposed to returning funds to the treasury); and independent external audits of RDF financial accounts and stocks.

Depending on local conventions and the policy or action involved, official endorsement may require various combinations of ministry circulars, legal notices, cabinet approval, acts of parliament, and presidential decrees (executive orders). Generally, the more cumbersome the method (such as an act of parliament), the harder it is to reverse. This can provide a degree of protection from future political whim. Therefore, if there are some principles that are vital to the success of the RDF (such as local retention of fees or additivity to treasury allocations), it may be worth the effort to have these principles endorsed through legal notice or even an act of parliament.

≡ 44.5 Implementation Planning

Implementation planning involves decisions about bottom-up versus top-down implementation, phasing and pilot testing, and development of RDF procedures.

Bottom-Up versus Top-Down Implementation

Bottom-up versus top-down development of user charges is both a policy question and an implementation question. It is rarely feasible to introduce fees at all levels at the same time. Therefore, should fees be introduced first at the hospital level or at the community level?

Arguments favoring starting at the top include the following (Griffin 1988; Blakney et al. 1989):

Equity: Higher-level facilities generally serve populations that are better able to pay for services and have access to other health providers.

Reinforcement of referral system: Introducing charges at higher levels encourages the use of cost-effective lower-level services.

Revenue potential: Higher-level facilities provide large volumes of more costly drugs and other services.

Administrative capacity: Senior managers, drug management staff, accountants, and other necessary staff may be better equipped to undertake the additional administrative burden.

Impact evaluation: It is easier to monitor the health care and financial impact of user fees at a smaller number of more accessible facilities.

Arguments favoring starting at the level of the community or primary care facilities include:

Demand: Communities are actively interested in ensuring a regular supply of essential drugs.

Lack of alternatives: Rural populations often have fewer choices in health care; if the government or community cannot provide drugs, they may go without.

Support for prevention: Increasing drug availability at the primary health care level also attracts people for essential preventive services.

Community involvement: A bottom-up approach provides greater opportunity for community involvement. Also, government or donor start-up funds may be supplemented by community contributions.

The relative strength of the case for bottom-up versus top-down implementation varies with local circumstances. Too often, however, the choice is strongly influenced by local political pressures or donor interests rather than by the merits of each approach.

Experience and careful monitoring can help determine the viability of an RDF at each level. The cost of establishing and maintaining user fees at the lowest level may be greater than the revenue collected.

Phasing and Pilot Testing

Most countries find it unworkable to implement an RDF at all levels and in all parts of the country at the same time. Success depends on developing and testing fees, drug supply procedures, and financial management systems. This is best done through pilot testing or phased implementation.

Pilot testing an RDF in one province or one district before it is implemented nationally enables systems to be developed and monitored under close supervision. In countries such as Nepal, Nigeria, and Liberia, different approaches to RDFs in different parts of the country allowed cross-fertilization of experience.

Pilot tests can be misleading, however, if they are conducted only in more accessible, better organized areas; if they are conducted with much more intensive technical and financial support than could be expected with national implementation; or if they result in systems suitable to the pilot area but less suitable to other parts of the country.

Phased implementation, beginning at the higher levels of the system, offers the advantage of firmly establishing effective drug supply, financial management, pricing, exemption, and accountability systems at each level before proceeding to the next level. A phased approach can help build public acceptance, test and revise fee structures, develop management capacity, and train staff over a reasonable period of time.

With phased implementation, the high-level facilities in each area serve as training and demonstration centers for the next level: provincial hospitals establish their systems, then become training sites for district hospitals; district hospitals develop their systems and become training sites for health centers; health centers become training sites for health posts or community health workers. Following the management development approach described in Country Study 34.1, it may take six to eighteen months to develop, implement, and reinforce RDF management systems at each level.

With either a pilot or a phased approach, an RDF cannot expand any faster than the capacity of the supply system to provide a steady supply of essential drugs.

Development of RDF Procedures
An essential aspect of any approach is the development of procedures for drug and financial management. Normally, a procedure manual or set of manuals should be developed. Shorter versions of these manuals, including one-page checklists, can be prepared to address the information needs of specific levels and functions.

≡ 44.6 Pricing and Equity of Access
RDF pricing and exemption policies are critical for ensuring that patients in need of essential drugs and medical supplies receive them and that the RDF does not decapitalize. These two requirements pull in opposite directions, creating a constant tension. And prices, as well as the accompanying policies with regard to exemptions, are the mechanism by which the necessary balance is achieved.

Pricing Strategies
Pricing for RDFs involves two related questions: what type of drug fees should be charged, and what should the level of fees be?

Type of Drug Fee. Alternatives include course-of-therapy fee, prescription fee, item fee, multilevel item fee (price bands), and variable item fee (see Figure 44.3). These mechanisms can be compared with respect to the following criteria:

Impact on prescribing practices: Does the fee create incentives for prescribing more drugs or fewer drugs, higher-cost or lower-cost drugs?

Impact on patients: Is the fee likely to dissuade patients from buying needed drugs, or does it create incentives for patients to use drugs more cost effectively? Will patients feel that they have paid a fair price?

Ease of collection and accounting: How easy is it for health staff to calculate the required payment, to make change, and to keep accurate payment records?

Balancing drug costs and revenue: How closely do the fees received for individual drugs balance the actual cost of drugs dispensed? Is it easy for fund managers to ensure that the collected funds are sufficient to resupply the drugs dispensed?

The impact of fees on prescribing practices is not shown in Figure 44.3 because it depends on whether health staff salaries or bonuses depend on revenue derived from drug fees. Like private practitioners, government and community health care providers are likely to prescribe more drugs and more costly drugs if their income depends on drug sales.

Course-of-therapy fees, multilevel item fees, and variable item fees can all differ for individual drugs. In such instances, the fees charged to patients can be based on the actual cost of the drug, an assessment of the health impact of the drug, or a combination of these factors. Pricing can be based on the VEN system (see Chapter 41): for example, the equivalent of \$.10 per item for vital drugs, \$.20 per item for essential drugs, and \$.30 per item for nonessential drugs. With this approach, vital drugs may be sold at prices lower than their replacement cost.

With the variable item fee, the price can be based on a fixed percentage markup over cost, a variable percentage markup, actual cost plus a fixed dispensing fee, or another formula (see the discussion of retail margins in Chapter 6). For example, higher-cost drugs or drugs with a greater health impact may have a lower markup.

It is important to consider ease of collection and accountability, because administrative and accountability problems are major constraints on the success of RDFs.

Figure 44.3 Comparison of Types of Drug Fees

Type of Fee	Example	Impact on Patients[a]	Ease of Collection and Accounting[b]	Balancing Drug Costs and Revenue[c]
Course-of-therapy fee Fixed fee for diagnosis based on standard treatment	$.20 for one episode of malaria treatment $.30 for one episode of pneumonia $1.00 for one month of hypertension treatment	► Promotion of standard treatments ► No incentive to overuse or underuse drugs	+++	0
Prescription fee Standard drug fee per visit	$.40 per visit (regardless of number, amount, or type of drugs)	► Patient pressure for more drugs ► No incentive for cost consciousness	+++	0
Item fee Standard fee per drug	$.20 per item (regardless of amount or type of drugs)	► Patient pressure for high-cost drugs ► Incentive to use fewer drugs	++	+
Multilevel item fee Three to five levels or price bands	Fee based on drug category: A $.10 per item B $.20 per item C $.30 per item	► Preference to buy low-cost drugs ► Incentive to use fewer drugs	+	++
Variable item fee Variable fee per drug, based on type or cost of drug	Drug cost plus 20% for all items	► Preference to buy low-cost drugs ► Incentive to use fewer drugs ► More cost consciousness	0	+++

Source: Adapted from MSH 1992.
[a] Drug prescribing is influenced by whether the prescriber's salary depends on drug revenues (see text).
[b] +++ = easiest for collection and accounting.
[c] +++ = easiest to balance drug costs and revenues.

Unfortunately, course-of-therapy and prescription fees—which are the easiest to implement and are in some respects the most equitable—make it difficult to ensure that revenues collected are sufficient to pay for drugs dispensed.

One approach is to begin with fees that are easy to implement and then move to more complex but financially sustaining fees as the program evolves. More complex fees require more staff training and more sophisticated accounting systems, which can be implemented over time. Country Study 44.3 describes how this evolution occurred in Nepal and its effect on the utilization of health services, prescribing patterns, and cost per patient.

Level of Drug Fee. What level of fee is appropriate? With an item fee, for example, should the fee be the equivalent of $.10 per item, $.15 per item, or $.20 per item? If the system is introduced first at rural hospitals, prices can be set on the low side, and patient response can be monitored. Prices can be adjusted accordingly during the first year or two, before moving to the next level.

For RDFs, as in business, there are two basic approaches to price setting: the willingness-to-pay or market approach, and the cost-based or accounting approach. Pricing decisions should draw on information from both approaches.

In the *willingness-to-pay approach*, price levels can be set by using any feasible combination of the four methods used by private companies:

1. *Consumer opinion:* Survey questionnaires and/or focus groups ask community members what they would be willing to pay for specific services.
2. *Expert opinion:* The most efficient way to set prices is by asking someone who really knows the "product" and the population. The expert must have firsthand knowledge of the population being served and how people value drugs. Ministry officials and essential drugs program managers are usually not expert at price setting.
3. *Comparative pricing:* It is useful to survey private facilities, mission hospitals, retail pharmacies, patent medicine sellers, and other nongovernmental providers to find out their drug charges. However, results must be interpreted in light of differences in income level and perceived value of services.
4. *Test pricing:* Companies sometimes use early experience in a small area to establish national prices; the response to initial prices can be used to adjust subsequent prices.

In the *cost-based approach*, prices are established according to the cost-recovery objectives. Because RDF revenues are used to purchase replacement stocks, a factor for inflation and anticipated stock losses must be built into the calculation of sales price. Some programs include a factor for "stock replacement reserve" and "general reserves," and any program offering exemptions must adjust for them (see Chapter 42). In the cost-based approach to pricing, the markup percentage must also be determined. Many programs use a fixed percentage, with the more expensive drugs thus producing higher revenues. Other programs use variable markups.

In determining pricing strategies, it must be remembered that the sustainability of the RDF depends on covering some or all of the costs of the system. (What that portion is, and exactly which costs are to be covered, may vary.) The objective is not to maximize profits but to maximize service delivery at a certain basic quality level. Willingness to pay is usually as important as cost data in determining drug prices. For example, before the RDF is introduced, estimated sales prices for all drug items should be compared with those of similar drugs sold by the private sector. If, after accounting for the replacement costs of drugs and exemptions, RDF prices are higher than private-sector prices, the whole RDF strategy must be reconsidered.

Pricing decisions must be made in full recognition of the tension between cost-recovery objectives and social policies regarding access to care. At the same time, administrative requirements for collecting fees must be considered. Most experiences in pharmaceutical cost recovery suggest that when equity-oriented exemption policies and administrative realities are considered, it is often a struggle simply to recover the full replacement cost of drugs and delivery. Cost-recovery potential is determined ultimately by patients' willingness and ability to pay for drugs, and not by a policy that mandates a specified markup (see Figure 44.2).

Financial sustainability of RDFs depends on keeping drug fees in line with changes in the cost of drugs. During periods of high local inflation and foreign exchange fluctuation, frequent price adjustments may be required. Fee increases may present a short-term hardship to patients, but unless it is certain that the government or a donor will finance the shortfall, such increases are imperative for the survival of the RDF.

Ensuring Equity of Access

Protection mechanisms—a safety net—are needed to ensure continued access to essential drugs for the poor, the medically needy, and other target groups.

Many programs would like to establish generous exemption policies. But if the RDF is to be viable over the long run, the revenues collected, along with budget subsidies, must be sufficient to purchase replacement drug stocks.

As illustrated in Figure 44.4, calculation of the anticipated cost of exemptions leads to determination of the "base" for

---

Country Study 44.3 Comparison of Prescription Fee and Item Fee in Nepal

The Britain Nepal Medical Trust (BNMT) started its first cost-sharing drug scheme in rural Nepal in 1980. Patients at health posts were charged a prescription fee of 5 rupees (about US$.17), regardless of the number of drugs. The fee represented 43 percent of the actual drug cost. Since patients felt cheated if they received cheap drugs or few drugs, the scheme was criticized for encouraging overprescribing.

A new scheme introduced by the BNMT in 1990 charged an item fee, using two price bands (NRs. 1 and 3, US$.03 and $.10). The prices were calculated to approximate the charge used in the prescription scheme, assuming the observed average of 2.5 items per prescription. The original fee of NRs. 5 per prescription was roughly one-third of the average charge in local shops.

Introduction of the item fee scheme was associated with a rise in average daily attendances at health posts from nine to thirty-two patients a day, a 240 percent increase over the corresponding period in the previous year. No similar rise was seen in health posts that continued with a prescription fee. The item fee scheme also encouraged the prescribing of fewer drugs (1.8 versus 2.4 in the prescription fee scheme), at lower overall cost. Fewer antibiotics were prescribed (33 percent versus 54 percent in the prescription fee scheme). The fewer drugs prescribed made the item fee scheme 24 percent cheaper to run on a per patient basis. However, the rise in attendance meant that the absolute level of subsidy required (that is, cost of additional drugs not covered by the patient fees) was higher.

The itemized charge system in the item fee scheme was found to involve more administrative work at the health post level; this may be the main threat to the scheme's long-term viability.

Source: Fryatt et al. 1994.

---

cost recovery: the total costs that must be recovered to ensure that the RDF does not decapitalize. Assessment of total costs to be recovered and government subsidies available determines cost-recovery targets (that is, what percentage of total costs must be recovered from paying patients). This, in turn, suggests various pricing strategies.

As Figure 44.4 shows, the lower the pharmaceutical subsidy provided by the government, the greater the burden of generous exemption policies on the local community. Because of this burden, local communities should contribute to the discussion on establishing exemption policies.

Types of Protection Mechanisms. Exemption from payment, partial exemption (sliding scale), and differential prices are the most common protection mechanisms. Differential pricing is the setting of different price levels by type of patients, level of the health system, or type of drugs. Fee levels may be higher for adults than for children.

Figure 44.4 Impact of Multiple Exemptions on the Cost-Recovery Base of an RDF

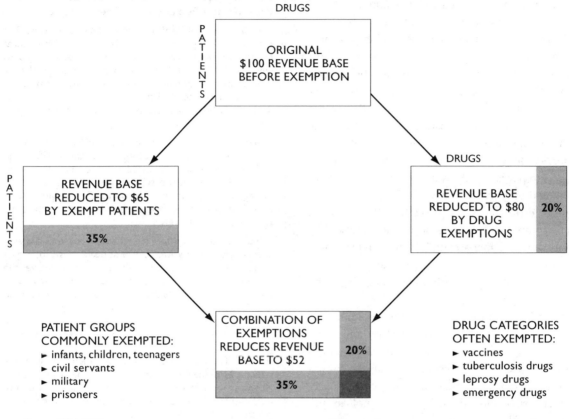

Source: MSH 1992.

Note: Reduce the patients to 65% of original and the drugs to 80% of original, which leaves a revenue base of .80 × .65 = .52 of $100 = $52.

Drug and service fees also may be graduated by level of care, with referral hospitals charging the highest fee for a given drug or service, district hospitals charging lower fees, health centers charging even lower fees, and community health workers charging the lowest fees. In addition to reinforcing referral patterns, this approach seeks to improve equity by making drugs more affordable through community health workers and lower-level health facilities. Differential pricing by the VEN classification helps make the most essential drugs available at the lowest prices.

The type of fee may also provide some protection. Registration or consultation fees paid before seeing a clinician may dissuade people from seeking needed care, even if they would have been exempt from payment. But when drug fees are in effect, the most acutely ill patients will have been identified before the issue of payment arises.

Exemption Criteria. Criteria used to grant full or partial exemptions fall into three main categories:

1. *Poverty*: people below a certain income or standard of living;

2. *Personal factors*: children (usually those under five), the elderly, the disabled, prisoners, and some categories of students;

3. *Health conditions*: pregnancy, to encourage proper antenatal care; communicable diseases such as tuberculosis, AIDS, and sexually transmitted diseases (STDs), to encourage treatment or control spread.

For political reasons, user fee programs sometimes begin with broad exemptions that include civil servants, teachers, members of the military, war veterans, older children, and other groups that are able to pay and for which there are no equity or public health arguments for exemption. Financial sustainability depends on narrowing the list of exemptions as the RDF gains acceptance and as systems develop to target those truly in need.

Administering Exemptions. The practicalities of administering exemptions often present the greatest barrier to ensuring equity in RDFs. Procedures should be administratively feasible, exempt the correct groups, and prevent abuse by those who do not meet exemption criteria.

Exemptions and differential pricing based on objective

Country Study 44.4 Approaches to Exemptions in User Fee Programs

Belize. The indigent are fully exempt, and a sliding scale (variable percentage exemption) is applied to emergency patients, patients with specific illnesses, and lower-level civil servants. Health facility clerks base means testing (assessment of income) on self-declared household income or occupation, with little verification. Exemptions are granted inconsistently by clerks, who are reluctant to question patients firmly and often grant exemptions to relatives and friends.

Ethiopia. Households below a certain income, tuberculosis patients, and leprosy patients receive full exemption through local authorities. In rural hospitals, 20 to 60 percent of outpatients and 7 to 40 percent of inpatients are exempt. In Addis Ababa hospitals, 10 percent of outpatients and 30 to 35 percent of inpatients are exempt.

Jamaica. The poor, women with high-risk pregnancies, and patients with chronic conditions receive full or partial exemptions. Social service committees of the local council administer a means test for allocating food stamps. The same results are used by the MOH. Between 17 and 30 percent of the population is exempt.

Kenya. There are two types of release from payment: discretionary waivers based on income, and automatic exemptions based on the patient being underage, being a civil servant, having an exempt illness (tuberculosis, STD), receiving a preventive service (family planning, antenatal care), or meeting other specified criteria. At hospitals, granting a waiver is a two-step process: one person recommends the waiver (usually the clinician seeing the patient), and a second person authorizes the waiver (usually the medical superintendent). Various forms and checklists were tried, but none proved more practical than staff judgment. A numbered waiver authorization form is used

for accountability purposes. A 1993 analysis found that over 50 percent of outpatients were exempt by this process. To gain political and public acceptance, the exemption age had been increased to fifteen years, and civil servants were exempt. But by 1994, after user fees were widely accepted, the exemption age was reduced to five years and the civil servant exemption was removed. Efforts were also made to remove other exemptions that had no public health or economic rationale.

Niger. At Niamey National Hospital, civil servants and military personnel pay 20 percent of the fee, children under five years pay 25 percent, and children aged six to twelve years pay 50. Indigents, infectious disease patients, and psychiatric patients are fully exempt. Eligibility is based on income, determined by hospital social workers and based on occupation and appearance. Outpatient exemptions are mostly for civil servants. In practice, the nonexempt have lower median income than the exempt. Exemptions based on kinship and friendship occur.

Philippines. Payment follows a sliding scale based on category of patient and level of service: class A pays full cost; class B, 50 percent; class C, what they can; and class D, nothing. Patients are interviewed by medical social workers. In 1985, 72 percent of patients in sixty district hospitals were classified as indigent.

Zaire. Exemptions are provided to indigents, a category that is defined in most health zones to include the old, the very poor, the very sick, and, in some zones, children. Government employees were provided free drugs in most zones in the past, but no longer. In general, 10 percent of patients have been exempted from fees.

Sources: Gilson et al. 1995; Collins et al. 1996.

criteria such as pregnancy, age, or diagnosis are easier to implement than more subjective criteria. Even verification of age can be difficult, however. Exempting children under age five (who are usually known to the staff of well-child clinics) is easier to enforce than exempting children under age fifteen (who may be difficult to distinguish from young adults).

Although policy-makers usually agree that the poor should be exempt, defining who is poor is difficult, particularly in noncash economies. Measures used to assess poverty level include type of employment, household income (cash and noncash), household expenditures (for example, total cash and noncash expenditures during the last month), and wealth (housing, land, livestock, and other personal holdings).

Verifying poverty or other exemption criteria may not be difficult in a local dispensary where patients are well known to staff. But in a busy, less personal health center or hospital outpatient department, it can be quite difficult. Country Study 44.4 illustrates different approaches to waiver systems.

Financing the Cost of Exemptions

An effective system of exemptions and other protection mechanisms is essential to ensure equity of access. Unless someone pays the cost of these exemptions, however, an RDF will soon cease to revolve. Exemptions can be financed through any combination of

- central government recurrent budget allocations;
- higher markups on drugs for patients who can pay;
- community contributions;
- local or external donors.

A certain level of government financial support is usually necessary to ensure equitable access for the poor and other target groups; otherwise, prices for paying patients must be increased to cover the cost of exemptions. In practice, using higher markups for paying patients to finance exempt patients usually fails, unless the proportion of exempt patients is low and collection efficiency is high. In community drug schemes, village health committees sometimes maintain "poor funds" to pay for those who cannot afford drug fees.

Finally, exemptions may be financed by local or external donors, but few are willing to provide long-term subsidies. In some cases, however, donors support exemptions through in-kind contributions (drugs for acute respiratory infection, diarrheal disease, or nutritional support), with the understanding that treatment will be dispensed without charge if the patient meets established exemption criteria. As discussed in Chapter 20, country program managers and policy-makers, rather than donors, should decide how donations will be handled in cost recovery.

≡ 44.7   Management of Drugs and Money

RDFs face much more demanding management requirements than free systems. The concepts of *service performance* and *cost control* must pervade the management of RDFs.

Drug Supply Management

Selection, procurement, quality assurance, distribution, management information, and drug use are all handled somewhat differently in the context of an RDF.

Selection. The essential drugs list for the RDF (its "product line") must be based on essential drugs selection criteria (see Chapter 10). But provider perspectives and patient preferences must also be considered. For example, if there are two drugs that are therapeutically equivalent and similar in price, the more popular ("sellable") one should normally be purchased. Supply of high-cost, low-volume drugs with limited health impact is probably best left to the private sector, since such drugs can tie up working capital and result in losses to expiry.

Procurement. Regardless of the level at which procurement is managed, there must be a reliable source for the purchase of resupplies. Turning to local distributors or private pharmacies to cover delayed shipments from normal sources often raises costs beyond what can be recovered through sales. Even if the RDF is managed by a government entity (as opposed to a parastatal or private organization), the procurement cycle must be freed from the treasury cycle to ensure that drugs can be bought when needed and tenders are not automatically canceled between fiscal years. Procurement must ensure maximum bulk discounts (such as one-year competitive contracts) while controlling inventory holding costs (for example, by arranging three or four deliveries per year of high-volume items).

Quality Assurance. Quality assurance procedures must ensure both the reality and the appearance of quality. For example, dispensing containers should protect the drug, but their appearance may also influence whether patients feel that they have paid a fair price for the drug inside.

Distribution and Inventory Control. Distribution must be through a "pull" system, based on actual demand. Inventory records must be accurate to ensure the purchase of correct quantities. Underestimates result in lost sales and gaps in health service for clients, and overestimates can lead to costly expirations. Transport arrangements must ensure steady supply.

Management Information. Give-away systems can sometimes afford not to know what happens to drugs after they are distributed, but RDFs need good information on which products are in demand and which ones are not. Information on stockouts is needed from facilities, since inventory records at distribution depots may not fully reflect undersupply problems.

Rational Use. If health workers benefit directly from drug sales, there must be monitoring to ensure that workers are not irrationally catering to patient demands (for more injections, for example) or overprescribing. Prescribers and dispensers must ensure that poorer patients, who cannot afford to buy everything prescribed, know which are the necessary, curative drugs (for example, chloroquine for malaria) and which are the optional, symptomatic drugs (such as paracetamol). Dispensing staff must guard against patients buying subtherapeutic quantities of all drugs prescribed, rather than therapeutic quantities of only the curative drugs.

Financial Management and Accountability

Traditional accounting systems for governments and not-for-profit organizations are designed primarily to account for funds spent. RDFs require systems that ensure reliable collection of fees, safekeeping of revenue, and proper expenditure of revenue.

Systems and Procedures. Standard procedures must be implemented for fee collection, stock control and valuation, reporting, banking, auditing, and control of expenditures. Potential sources of theft, fraud, and abuse must be monitored to minimize losses.

Examples of accountability problems include clerks who charge patients the full fee but record only half the fee and pocket the difference; dispensing staff who give a patient ten tablets, record having issued twenty tablets, and keep the difference; accounting staff who record and deposit less than the full amount collected; and procurement staff who authorize payment to suppliers for drugs never received and share the payment with the supplier.

Chapter 42 describes procedures and systems for financial management and accounting in the context of RDFs. In government-operated RDFs, procedures must be consistent with the law. It is therefore important that government accounting officials review and endorse RDF accounting procedures.

Enforcement. Even the best-designed systems for financial management and accountability require enforcement. At each level, regular supervision should focus on areas of potential abuse. Disciplinary procedures provide a range of possible responses, from warnings through dismissal, depending on the severity and frequency of the offense. RDF managers should be prepared to invoke disciplinary procedures and to bring criminal charges when necessary. Government procedures on misuse of public funds must be visibly and vigorously applied to ensure full collection and proper expenditure of revenue. Well-publicized prosecution of one prominent offender can be a highly effective method for improving overall adherence to procedures.

≡ 44.8 Preparing Health Staff, Patients, and the Public

Introducing or expanding an RDF requires building support from health staff, patients, and the public through orientation programs, training, and good communication.

Orientation and Training for Health Staff

For RDFs at the national, institutional, or community level, it is important to orient senior officials to the objectives and organization of the program. Even if most such officials will have no direct program responsibility, their work may be indirectly affected and, in practice, their support (formal or informal) may be needed.

Training should consider the information needs of pharmacy, drug management, accounting, and other staff directly involved in the RDF, as well as the needs of health workers and unskilled staff whose cooperation is needed. Training should focus on new knowledge, skills, and attitudes needed by each group. In addition, all staff should receive basic orientation that will enable them to correctly inform patients and the community about the RDF.

Communications for the Public and Patients

Public and patient acceptance is vital for the implementation and further development of RDFs. A communications strategy should systematically address the following issues:

Target audiences: Target groups include national leaders, community leaders, local opinion leaders (who may be different from official community leaders), health workers, patients currently attending facilities, and the general public.

Opinion survey: A "market survey" using questionnaires, in-depth interviews, and/or focus group discussions can help assess how high-priority target groups might respond to fees, and how much pricing elasticity may exist.

Messages: It is important to build on the positive aspects of user fees, without making promises that cannot be kept. Clarifying exemptions, such as for maternal and child health, is good public relations and good public health. If the RDF fees are for drugs only, promote this: "The doctor is still free." Community participation and management, if appropriate, can be important concepts to convey.

Media and methods: Choice of media for communication depends on local availability and practices. Print media, radio, television, and local meetings are all appropriate options. In countries such as Nigeria, Kenya, and the Philippines, where newspapers have good coverage, stories of small successes can be distributed regularly as press releases at low cost to the program (through print media, radio, local meetings).

Once the preceding issues have been addressed, an effective communication plan can be developed to support the implementation plan for the RDF. Chapter 33 is aimed primarily at public and patient communications for improved drug use, but it provides useful information for preparing an RDF communication plan.

≡ 44.9 Monitoring and Supervision

Regular monitoring and supervision are essential to assess the impact of RDFs on patients and financial performance. Supervisory visits should focus on patients' responses to user fees, implementation of exemption procedures, drug availability, and key aspects of the collection and accounting system. A supervision checklist can help ensure that critical functions are reviewed. Routine reporting systems must be adapted to handle financial and drug supply information, as well as health care information.

Visits should be targeted to facilities whose reports indicate poor performance or for which routine reports are not available. An RDF in the Caribbean uses routine reports to classify community pharmacies as red, yellow, or green and to direct supervision efforts accordingly. In East Africa, a national cost-sharing program uses routine reports similarly, to classify districts for the purpose of targeted supervision.

With new RDFs, major new fees, or other major changes, supervisory visits should be as frequent as possible. Sentinel sites and special studies may be needed to guide the development of the program and to assess its impact. Chapter 36

Country Study 44.5 User Fees and RDFs in Africa: Mixed Performance and Variable Impact

Since the mid-1980s, increasing demand for health services, growing population, and economic constraints have led an increasing number of countries to introduce or intensify efforts to supplement public budgets with revenue from user charges. A survey of thirty-seven anglophone, francophone, and lusophone countries in sub-Saharan Africa demonstrates the promise and limitations of user fees as of the early 1990s.

Extent of User Fees. National systems of user charges exist in twenty-five of the thirty-seven countries. All but two of the remaining twelve countries had user fee projects in some areas or plans for national fees. Improved drug supply was the primary or a major aim of cost recovery for two-thirds of the countries. The Bamako Initiative approach to strengthening primary health care and community drug schemes (see Chapter 37) was being implemented in parts of twenty-eight countries.

Structure of User Fees. In the majority of the countries, a specific drug fee was being charged, often in addition to registration fees, visit fees, daily bed fees (for inpatients), or other fees. The type of drug fee varied across the full range of alternatives described in Figure 44.3. Most countries provide some form of exemption for the poor. Countries were evenly divided in assigning responsibility for eligibility determination to the community or to health staff; in only a few countries was this a shared responsibility.

Revenue Generation. Overall cost recovery from user fees has been quite low, usually less than 10 percent of total recurrent expenditures. Revenue generation is often higher when funds are used to pay for drugs. Recovery of drug costs is reported to be over 80 percent in some programs in five of the countries. Although average markups for individual drugs sometimes exceed 100 percent, these markups are offset by exemptions, drug losses, inflation, and other factors.

Health Service Utilization and Quality of Care. Health service utilization frequently declined with the introduction of user fees, dramatically so in some countries. The decline sometimes persisted, but utilization often recovered over time. Drug availability, the most frequently cited quality-of-care indicator, was reported to have improved in sixteen countries that introduced or expanded user fees. In countries in which drug availability increased, utilization tended to increase. Large, persistent decreases in utilization were reported most frequently when user fees were introduced with no improvement in drug availability.

User fees have been widely implemented in sub-Saharan Africa. From this study, it appears possible to increase drug availability and health care utilization when user fee revenue is used to resupply drugs. But drug fees rarely cover the cost of all drugs, and virtually no large-scale program has been able generate sufficient funds to cover all nonsalary costs, let alone salary costs (the largest part of most health budgets). Fee structures, management systems, local retention of revenue, community involvement, and availability of low-cost drugs are all factors that influence the operation of user fee programs. The impact of user fees must also be assessed in light of overall health financing reforms, the effects on the poorest segments of the population, and the effects on rational drug use.

Source: Adapted from Nolan and Turbat 1995.

describes these and other relevant aspects of monitoring (Country Study 36.2 describes monitoring for the introduction of drug fees in Kenya), and Chapter 45 discusses information system design. Key issues for RDF monitoring appear in the assessment guide at the end of this chapter.

Decapitalization must be avoided, as it quickly leads to failure and loss of community confidence. Each health center operating an RDF should be visited every month or two to ensure that procedures are being followed and that the RDF will not become decapitalized.

If possible, a formal evaluation should be planned within the first three years of a new program to assess its overall impact, equity, sustainability, efficiency, and long-term prospects. Chapters 4 and 36 describe methods for such an evaluation.

≡ **44.10 Common Pitfalls and Lessons from RDFs**

Although the concept of RDFs is simple, the successful establishment and long-term sustainability of such schemes have been fraught with difficulty. Often the monies collected are insufficient to replenish the original stocks, and the fund soon becomes depleted. An important factor in RDF failure is a resistance to thinking of the fund in business terms. A lack of careful economic and financial analysis in planning the fund, or weaknesses in financial management or in management of the supply system, can lead to failure. Country Study 44.5 describes the situations of user fees and revolving drug funds in thirty-seven countries of sub-Saharan Africa as of the early 1990s.

Common Pitfalls

Specific causes for RDF decapitalization include (see Figure 44.5)

- unanticipated increases in procurement cost due to inflation or changes in exchange rates;
- underestimation of the capitalization costs of the supply system;
- rapid program expansion for which additional capital funds are not made available;
- unanticipated losses of drugs through theft, deterioration, or expiry;
- high operating costs that exceed budget amounts;
- prices set too low for intended level of cost recovery;
- too many exemptions that are not subsidized;
- funds tied up in the national banking system or ministry accounting systems;
- delays in collecting subsidies and other payments from government agencies;

Figure 44.5 Cycle of Terrors

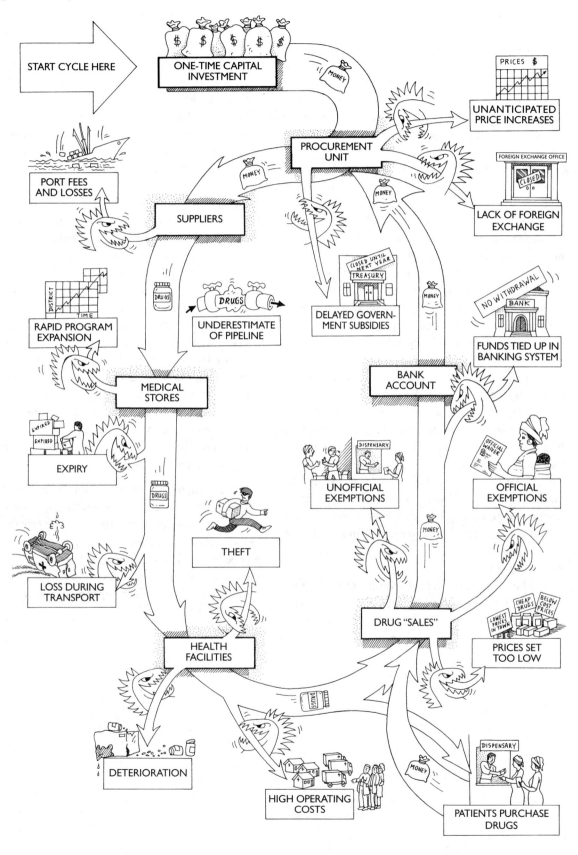

► foreign exchange limitations that restrict international purchases for resupply.

Guidelines from RDF Experiences

There are no guaranteed strategies for designing and implementing an RDF. However, experience with RDFs suggests some guidelines that may increase the chance that an RDF will improve drug availability, ensure equity of access, and promote greater efficiency.

Local control and retention of revenue: Keeping the money locally creates an incentive for revenue collection and promotes the use of revenue to improve quality. When fees are remitted to a general government account, there is little incentive to collect fees and virtually no visible improvement in the supply of drugs or the quality of care. Community supervision of an RDF is important to ensure its proper management and accountability.

Reliable supply of low-cost essential drugs: RDFs require a dependable supply system. Some governments have established independent drug supply services specifically to supply RDFs.

Locally appropriate fee schedules: The types and levels of charges cannot be determined simply as a matter of policy. Pricing decisions must consider both the cost of drugs (and services) and the demonstrated willingness to pay. Fees must be adjusted regularly to reflect increases in real costs.

Protection mechanisms to ensure equitable access: Exemptions, partial exemptions, and other protection mechanisms are necessary to ensure that patients are not denied essential services. Lower fees or free services at the lowest levels of health care encourage patients to use local facilities first.

Continued or increasing levels of government funding for health: Government allocations are still needed for preventive services and to subsidize the poor and other tar-

get groups. Collection of user fees should not lead to a reduction of government allocations.

Businesslike orientation: Personnel management, financial management, supply management, and "customer relations" systems provide built-in checks and balances. Qualified staff must be explicitly assigned to RDF activities. District and facility managers must set collection targets, monitor performance against targets, and take corrective action. Active community involvement is important for the acceptability, credibility, and accountability of RDFs. Public communications should explain the program and ensure that charges and protection mechanisms are understood.

Strict measures to ensure accountability: In addition to systems for the control of drugs and revenues, dependable monitoring (often with local community involvement) is important: spot checks, periodic independent audits, and vigorous use of legal and disciplinary mechanisms when abuses are uncovered. Systems that fail to respond effectively to theft of drugs are unlikely to fare any better when cash starts disappearing. Government procedures on the misuse of public funds must be visibly and vigorously applied to ensure full collection and proper expenditure of revenue.

Planned implementation: Phased implementation or a well-conceived pilot approach can help build public acceptance and develop management capacity before the system expands to cover the entire country.

Implementation of RDFs depends on a host of issues and, ultimately, on good management. Government and, in many cases, donor commitment is necessary for several years to ensure that sustainable organizational arrangements, financial management, and drug supply management systems are in place. The success of an RDF lies in the details of planning and implementation. ■

≡ Assessment Guide

Policy, Organization, and Implementation

► Are key functions related to pricing, exemptions, supervision, and other aspects of drug management and financial management clearly assigned and effectively performed?

► Are central, district, facility, and community roles clearly and appropriately identified and communicated to all concerned?

► Are policy or legal clarifications needed with regard to exemptions, local retention of revenue, or banking and accounting procedures?

► Are policy-makers oriented, have health staff been trained, and has the public been adequately informed about the RDF?

Drug Management and Financial Management Systems

► Does the RDF have a reliable source of drugs through the CMS, an autonomous supply agency, or some other drug supply mechanism?

► What types of drug fees are used: course-of-therapy fee, prescription fee, item fee, multilevel item fee, variable item fee? Should the type of fee be revised to create incentives for more rational use of drugs or to improve accountability?

► Are fee levels set on the basis of drug costs, assessment of ability to pay, or a combination of the two factors?

► Is there a system for regular supervision at each level and a supervision checklist?

► Are revenues, expenditures, stock levels, and other measures reported and reviewed on at least a quarterly basis?

► Are financial management systems backed up by administrative and legal actions to ensure accountability?

Impact on Patients and Households

► Is the number of patients decreasing, or are people being dissuaded from seeking necessary care?

► What is the impact of drug fees on the poorest households? Is access increasing or decreasing? Are expenditures on other household essentials such as food being affected?

► What are the expected and actual percentages of patients exempted from payment? Do specific exemption criteria exist, and are they implemented as intended to ensure equity of access?

► Is the availability of essential drugs, and therefore the quality of care, increasing?

► Are drugs being rationally prescribed and bought? Is there overprescribing or underprescribing by health staff? Overpurchasing or underpurchasing by patients?

Financial Performance

► What costs were intended to be covered by drug fees: a portion of drug costs, full drug costs, or drug costs plus a surplus to cover other recurrent costs?

► What percentage of the cost-recovery objective is being achieved?

► What percentage of MOH drug expenditures is funded by user fees? What level of continued government funding has been planned, and what level is actually being provided?

► How is the cost of exemptions, different prices, and other protection mechanisms being funded? Can protection mechanisms be sustained to ensure access to the poor and other target groups?

► Is the current level of capitalization sufficient to ensure a steady supply of drugs?

Note: This assessment guide assumes that an RDF exists. Section 44.2 discusses feasibility assessment when an RDF does not exist.

≡ References and Further Readings

★ = Key readings.

Blakney, R. B., J. I. Litvack, and J. D. Quick. 1989. *Financing primary health care: Experiences in pharmaceutical cost recovery.* Boston: Management Sciences for Health/PRITECH.

Collins, D., J. D. Quick, S. N. Musau, D. Kraushaar, and I. M. Hussein. 1996. The fall and rise of cost sharing in Kenya: The impact of phased implementation. *Health Policy and Planning* 11:52–63.

Creese, A. L. 1991. User charges for health care: A review of recent experience. *Health Policy and Planning* 6:309–19.

★ Creese, A., and J. Kutzin. 1995. *Lessons from cost-recovery in health.* Forum on health sector reform. Discussion paper no. 2. Geneva: World Health Organization.

★ Cross, P. N., M. A. Huff, J. D. Quick, and J. A. Bates. 1986. Revolving drug funds: Conducting business in the public sector. *Social Science and Medicine* 22:335–43.

Day, L. M. 1993a. *Designing a family planning user fee system: A handbook for program managers.* Washington, D.C.: Service Expansion and Technical Support (SEATS) Project.

Day, L. M. 1993b. *User fees for sustainable family planning services.* Washington, D.C.: Service Expansion and Technical Support (SEATS) Project.

Dunlop, D., and D. Capin. 1992. *Economic and policy choices of pharmaceuticals in developing countries.* Washington, D.C.: World Bank.

★ Foster, S., and N. Drager. 1988. How community drug sales schemes may succeed. *World Health Forum* 9:200–206.

Fryatt, R. J., P. Rai, S. P. Crowley, and Y. B. Gurung. 1994. Community financing of drug supplies in rural Nepal: Evaluating a "fee per item" drug scheme. *Health Policy and Planning* 9:193–203.

Gilson, L., S. Russell, and K. Buse. 1995. The political economy of user fees with targeting: Developing equitable health financing policy. *Journal of International Development* 7:369–401.

Griffin, C. C. 1988. *User charges for health care in principle and in practice.* Economic Development Institute seminar paper 37. Washington, D.C.: World Bank.

Litvack, J., and C. Bodart. 1993. User fees plus quality equals improved access: Results of a field experiment in Cameroon. *Social Science and Medicine* 37:369–83.

Litvack, J. I., D. S. Shepard, and J. D. Quick. 1989. Setting the price of essential drugs: Necessity and affordability. *Lancet* 8659:376–79.

★ McPake, B. 1993. User charges for health services in developing countries: A review of the economic literature. *Social Science and Medicine* 36:1397–1405.

McPake, B., K. Hanson, and A. Mills. 1993. Community financing of health care in Africa: An evaluation of the Bamako Initiative. *Social Science and Medicine* 36:1383–95.

MSH (Management Sciences for Health). 1992. *Managing drug supply training series.* Part 2. *Financing and financial management of drug supply.* Boston: MSH.

Musau, S. 1992. Charging fees for family planning services. *Family Planning Manager* 1(3):1–12.

Nolan, B., and V. Turbat. 1995. Cost recovery in public health services in sub-Saharan Africa. EDI technical materials. Washington, D.C.: World Bank.

Sauerborn, R., C. Bodart, and R. O. Essomba. 1995. Recovery of recurrent health service costs through provincial health funds in Cameroon. *Social Science and Medicine* 40:1731–39.

Shaw, R. P., and C. C. Griffin. 1995. *Financing health care in sub-Saharan Africa through user fees and insurance.* Washington, D.C.: World Bank.

Waddington, C., and A. Panza. 1991. Ten questions to ask about revolving drug funds. *Tropical Doctor* 21:50–53.

| Part I | Part II | Part III | **Part IV** |
| Introduction | Policy and Legal Framework | Drug Management Cycle | **Management Support Systems** |

A Organization and Management
B Financing and Sustainability
C Information Management
D Human Resources
   Management

Section C
Information Management

| Part I | Part II | Part III | Part IV |
| Introduction | Policy and Legal Framework | Drug Management Cycle | **Management Support Systems** |

Part IV — Management Support Systems

A Organization and Management
B Financing and Sustainability
C Information Management ▶
D Human Resources Management

45 **Drug Management Information Systems**

46 Computers in Drug Management

Chapter 45

Drug Management Information Systems

☰ Summary

The planning process for a new or revised drug supply system should include a drug management information system (DMIS). The DMIS is an organized system for collecting, processing, reporting, and using information for decision-making. Information for each subsystem is collected by means of

- *record-keeping documents, a combination of registers, ledgers, and filing systems, which typically are not circulated;*
- *data reporting forms, such as periodic status reports, which transmit data to other departments or levels for use in making management decisions;*
- *feedback reports, also called analytical reports, which are usually provided to the units that collected the data.*

Design or revision of a DMIS should be based on the information needs of users at each level and should build on existing forms, reports, and procedures. Any newly designed forms should be field-tested with staff who will use them.

Other issues to consider include

- *selection of performance indicators (discussed in Chapter 36);*
- *integration of the DMIS with other data collection systems;*
- *computerization at appropriate levels.*

A successful DMIS requires effective use of the data generated. This includes

- *data processing to reduce large amounts of data to a manageable number of key indicators, often in summary tables;*
- *presentation of information in graphic form to simplify interpretation;*
- *interpretation of information to identify trends and potential problems;*
- *action in response to both positive and negative results.*

☰ 45.1 Importance of a Drug Management Information System

Coordinating the elements of a drug supply system requires accurate and timely information. Because a drug supply system uses many forms and other documents, managers often feel as if they are buried under mountains of data. They are unable to analyze and use many of these data for improved decision-making. Many factors affect the usability of these data, including their quality and quantity (for example, missing or incomplete data or too much data to analyze effectively). Hence, many managers find themselves making decisions based not on information but on intuition.

This chapter focuses on the practical aspects of organizing and managing a routine drug management information system (DMIS). It should be read in conjunction with Chapters 36 and 41. Chapter 36 puts information management into the broader context of monitoring and evaluating program performance against long-term goals and objectives and against medium-term workplans and targets. Chapter 41 presents a variety of tools for analyzing data produced by the DMIS.

Functions of a Drug Management Information System

An effective DMIS is able to synthesize the large volume of data generated by drug management operations. It then reduces the data to information for use in planning activities, estimating demand, allocating resources, and monitoring and evaluating drug management operations. This information is often in the form of a few key indicators. Indicators should be targeted for staff at all levels so that they can monitor both their own performance and that of the units for which they are responsible.

Another important function of a DMIS is to improve accountability. Much of the recording and reporting in a DMIS is intended to create a paper audit trail for products as they enter or leave a drug supply system.

Data and Information

It is necessary to understand the distinction between data and information to appreciate how a management information system functions. *Data* represent real-world observations. Data, in and of themselves, often have little value and take on meaning only after they are sorted, tabulated, and processed into a more usable format. *Information* is a meaningful aggregation of data that can be evaluated for a specific use. In other words, information is processed data that contains sufficient context to make it meaningful. The tools in Chapter 41 are intended primarily to aggregate data into useful information.

For example, data from a health center reveal that 3,000 chloroquine tablets were distributed last month. Is this consumption level abnormal? It would be difficult to answer this question without analysis. The data can be converted to information by comparing the 3,000 tablets distributed with the number distributed the previous month, say 1,000. This interpretation could then be expressed as a 300 percent increase in chloroquine distribution.

In a DMIS, data are routinely collected on a common set of *indicators*, usually expressed as proportions or rates. These indicators measure performance toward objectives.

The Information Systems Pyramid

It is helpful to see information systems as a pyramid (Figure 45.1). At the base of the pyramid are operational information systems. These include subsystems—procurement, distribution, financial management, drug use—that handle data at the transaction level. Every item that moves in and out of inventory must be tracked, and decisions must be made about how much to supply to a health facility, when to reorder, and how much to bill. This level is characterized by a high volume of data that must be recorded and processed, usually daily.

The next level of the pyramid is formed by management information systems (MIS). These typically provide summaries of operational data on a periodic basis (for example, monthly or quarterly) to help managers of specific departments monitor the performance of their units. Annual reports often summarize information on key indicators from many different operational subsystems, such as procurement, personnel, financial management, or stock control (see the sample report format in Annex 45.1). Information provided by the MIS helps managers answer questions such as:

- ► How do expenditures compare with the budget in the central medical stores?
- ► How effective is the inventory control system in eliminating stockouts and cutting stock losses?
- ► What is the delivery performance over the last period?
- ► Are the trends generally favorable, or are indicators worsening?

The highest level of the information systems pyramid is the executive information system (EIS). This system further summarizes management information for use in strategic planning and policy-making. An EIS typically generates programwide information on how effective the organization is in accomplishing its mission. Systems at this level track a very limited number of indicators routinely. They provide users with the tools, such as total variable cost analysis and price comparison analysis (see Chapter 41), to perform periodic queries on data at every information system level, either to investigate the causes

Figure 45.1 The Information Systems Pyramid

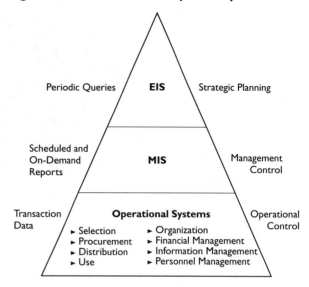

of problems or to perform "what-if" analyses to test the impact of changes in strategy. Some of the strategic questions that an EIS can help answer include:

- ► Should the transport and delivery function be contracted out?
- ► Could savings be obtained by combining orders with those of another large buyer?
- ► Which districts are the best served?
- ► Would targeting underserved areas with more marketing and training be worthwhile?

In practice, many organizations group the EIS and MIS together and refer to them collectively as an MIS.

≡ 45.2 Meeting Information Needs of Users at All Levels

Staff at every level use information to make decisions that affect the overall functioning of a drug supply system. For example, a storekeeper can monitor the temperature chart on a vaccine refrigerator and save thousands of dollars' worth of vaccine from spoiling when the refrigerator begins to malfunction. The chief pharmacist may be unaware that large quantities of a drug are due to expire in the warehouse. But if the pharmacist had information about expiration dates and could match this with data on the stock levels in health facilities, drugs could be dispatched to facilities that are running low, thereby averting waste of money and drugs.

A good DMIS alerts staff to problems and triggers critical actions from all levels. Usually, this means that there is

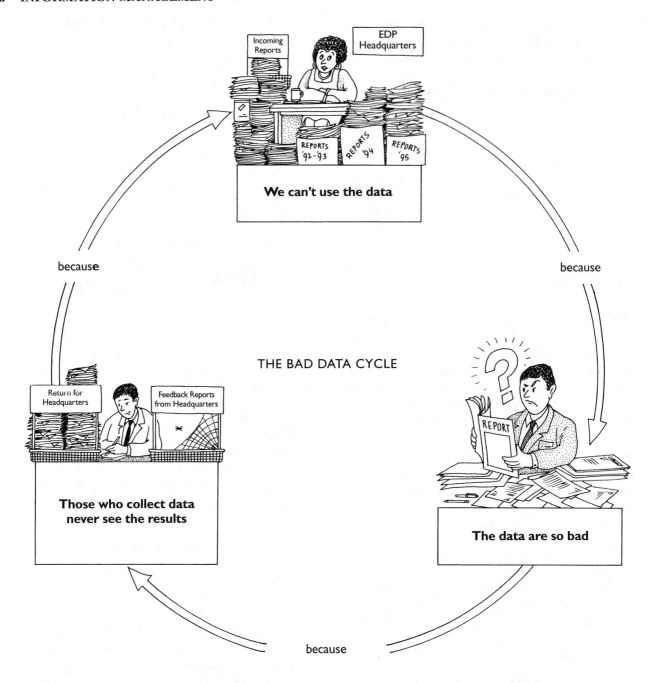

THE BAD DATA CYCLE

not a strict separation between data collectors and information users. Analysis and use of data are encouraged at every level. Figure 45.2 summarizes key information users and some of their most important information needs for each level of the system.

≡ 45.3 Typical Components of a Drug Management Information System
The operational systems level of a DMIS can be examined further using the analogy of the information systems pyramid. This level typically contains four subsystems: selec-

tion, procurement, distribution, and use. Information is necessary within each of these subsystems to manage finances, drug stocks, and personnel efficiently.

The documents that form the basis of the information system can be grouped into three areas: record-keeping documents, data reporting forms, and feedback reports.

Record-Keeping Documents
A combination of registers, ledgers, and filing systems is used to maintain data about the activities of a specific organizational unit. Normally, records stay in one place

Figure 45.2 Information Users and Information Needs

Level and Function	Users	Information Needs
National		
Selection	National essential drugs committee	Morbidity patterns Standard treatment strategies
Procurement	Procurement unit	Drug utilization rates Lead times Supplier performance Prices Funds available for procurement
Drug use education	Training unit	Number of staff trained in essential drugs use Number of public education messages developed and campaigns conducted
Financial management	Finance unit	Operating costs Revenues Value of inventory Stock turnover rates Stock fund growth or loss
Provincial/District		
Warehousing	Medical stores manager	Drug utilization rates Maximum and minimum stock levels Lead times for requisitions from national level Shelf life Warehouse maintenance and equipment needs Stock losses
Distribution	Logistics manager	Distribution schedules Vehicle utilization records Maintenance and fuel costs
Facility		
Use	Medical director, pharmacist	Prescription patterns Patient adherence Drug availability Patient load
Inventory control	Storekeeper	Maximum and minimum stock levels Lead times for requisitions Prices Drug utilization rates Shelf life Cold storage temperature variations

and are not circulated to other departments or levels. An efficient record-keeping system enables its users to quickly retrieve information about activities and simplifies the job of aggregating data for reporting purposes.

Data Reporting Forms

Forms for reporting data differ from the records described above because they are designed for transmission to other parts of an organization. Copies of forms filed at various points in the distribution network help form the audit trail for tracing the flow of drugs and funds. These forms typically include requisition/issue vouchers to document stock transfers and periodic status reports, such as monthly or annual reports (see Annex 45.1). Status reports can be descriptive and principally qualitative forms, or they can be standardized quantitative forms

designed to transmit data on specific indicators to others. Individual health facilities report to district offices. These, in turn, report to provincial offices, which report to the central office to project future drug needs, revise budgets, and assess drug utilization.

Feedback Reports

Analytical reports are produced from data reported by other units. These feedback reports have two main purposes: to address issues highlighted by status reports, and to analyze how each reporting unit has performed relative to other similar units. The reports are usually fed back to the units that first collected and provided the data. Experience has shown that regular and useful feedback is one of the best ways to improve data quality and reporting compliance. Once staff see that their data are

Figure 45.3 Flow of Documents in a Basic Supply System DMIS

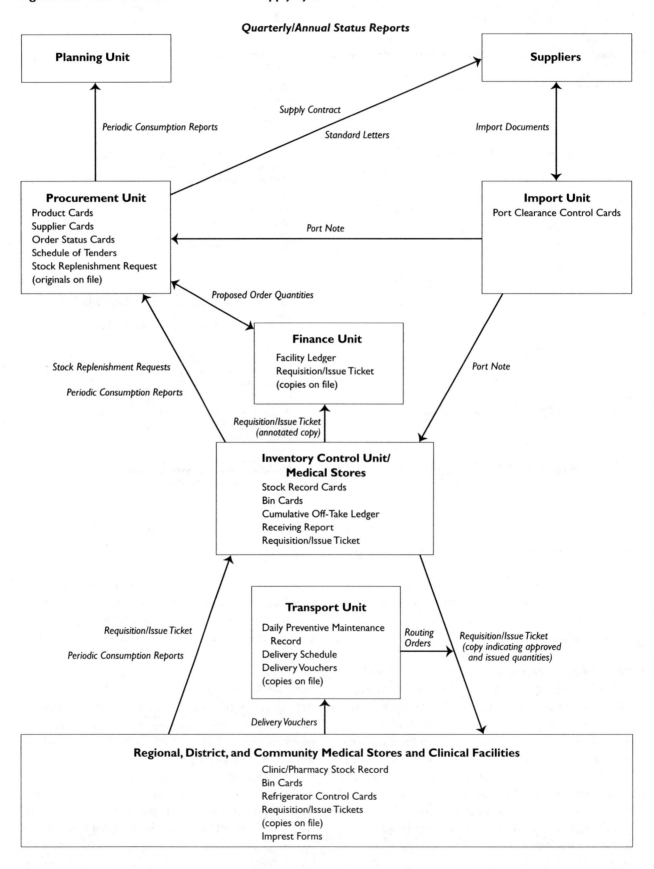

Figure 45.4 Forms and Records for a Basic Supply System DMIS

	Originated/ Maintained by
Forms	
Supply contract—statement of the terms of supply, usually publicized with the call for offers, specifying exact drug requirements, dosage forms, quality standards, labeling and packaging, delivery date, and other supply details	Procurement unit
Standard letters—form letters used in correspondence with suppliers to provide and obtain information regarding outstanding orders	Procurement unit
Import documents—used to confirm the supply contract, guarantee payment, and certify the quantity and quality of shipment contents, and to provide other types of trade information	Procurement, supplier, shipper, banks
Port note—notification from import unit to procurement and medical stores that a specific shipment has arrived and has been cleared from port	Import unit
Receiving report—notification to inventory control that a specific shipment has been received; indicates damages, short shipments, and other problems	Medical stores
Requisition/issue ticket—request for specific quantities of standard items from medical stores; amended by inventory control if stocks are low; filled by medical stores; copies provide audit trail; return copy is packing slip	Medical stores, health facilities
Stock replenishment request—request to procurement to begin the procurement cycle for specific items; sent at reorder level or reorder interval	Inventory control
Proposed order quantities—proposed order quantities for a single procurement cycle; finance unit estimates cost and adjusts if needs exceed available funds	Procurement
Routing order—delivery order for drivers; provides a record of vehicle movements, indicates the order of deliveries (planned to minimize travel)	Transport unit
Delivery voucher—signed receipt indicating that a specific shipment of drugs has been delivered intact	Medical stores, health facilities
Imprest forms—simplified supply requisitions for use by smaller clinical facilities and individual health workers	Health centers and workers
Records	
Product cards—product specifications and supplier history for each item; used to prepare bid specifications and select suppliers	Procurement unit
Supplier cards—record of experiences with individual suppliers, including delivery record, adherence to contract, drug and packaging quality, and other performance factors; used in supplier selection	Procurement unit
Order status cards—used to monitor the status of outstanding orders to reduce lead times, supplier defaults, and port delays	Procurement unit
Schedules of tenders—summaries of offers from each supplier on each product in a tender purchase	Procurement unit
Port clearance control cards—used for a manual control system to monitor port-clearing activities and thereby shorten port delays	Import unit
Stock record cards—cards or a ledger used to record stock balances, issues, receipts, and outstanding orders; essential in inventory decisions such as when and how much to order	Medical stores, health facilities
Bin cards—similar to stock record cards but kept in medical stores with the physical stock to record supply movement in and out of the stores	Medical stores
Facility ledger, cumulative off-take ledger—records indicating the quantity and cost of drugs issued to individual facilities; used for budgeting, billing, and/or estimating future needs	Finance unit, inventory control
Daily preventive maintenance record—checklist of daily vehicle maintenance activities used to promote preventive maintenance	Transport unit
Delivery schedule—monthly timetable for requisitions and deliveries; prepared for maximum staff and vehicle efficiency	Transport unit
Refrigerator control cards—temperature and maintenance log to ensure proper cold-chain storage	Clinical facilities
Reports	
Quarterly and annual status reports—to national level	
Feedback reports—from national level to warehouse/facilities	

being used, they become much more conscientious about data collection.

A good information system also includes procedures to govern the use and flow of information up and down the drug supply network. These procedures typically include details about how to collect data for the various documents, the authorizations needed, the schedule for preparation, and to whom the documents should be sent. Figures 45.3 and 45.4 illustrate the flow of documents in a basic DMIS.

If parts of the information system are computerized, clear guidelines must exist for the entry, maintenance, and archiving of data, as well as for the preparation and distribution of standard feedback reports. In addition, procedures are often needed for conducting periodic analyses and sharing data among different levels of the organization.

Data collection methods can take various forms in a DMIS. Although routine collection of data from all levels and facilities for monthly, quarterly, or annual reports is most common, sample surveys, rapid assessment techniques, and sentinel reporting systems are also important (see Chapter 36). In many cases, these collection methods provide data that are more reliable for decision support.

≡ 45.4 Steps in Designing or Revising a Drug Management Information System

When a new drug supply program is started or an old program is revised, the basic planning should include establishing a complete information system. All necessary forms should be available, and all staff should be trained to use these forms before drugs start moving through the system. Without this preparation, recording of drug consumption and forecasting of drug needs quickly breaks down. The principal steps in designing or revising a DMIS are shown in Figure 45.5.

A DMIS should be based on the information needs of the users at each level. To the extent possible, it should build on existing forms, reports, and procedures. Adding as few new elements as possible and removing unnecessary forms and reports will simplify the system and increase the chances that information will be recorded and reported. In some cases, it may be necessary to develop worksheets to facilitate the collation of data from records into summary report forms.

Procedures and training to help users perform simple data analysis and presentation of key trends within their own units before reporting to higher levels can help avoid problems caused by feedback loop delays. For example, a storekeeper may wish to maintain a graph of the average number of days out of stock of selected products to see if stock control is improving or getting worse.

It is essential to field-test any newly designed records and report forms with staff from the units that will eventually use the new system. Staff at actual work sites can almost always suggest better ways to do things, as well as point out places where the new forms or procedures are unclear. Computerized procedures and feedback report formats should also be field-tested and revised. Chapter 46 contains more information about computerization.

≡ 45.5 Key Issues in Designing or Revising a Drug Management Information System

Many issues need to be considered to ensure the success and sustainability of the DMIS.

Involve users in design and pilot testing: The feasibility and usefulness of a DMIS increase with user involvement. In addition, users should be trained to manage its evolution.

Be selective in choosing indicators: To save time and money, use proxy indicators when they make data collection more efficient and are likely to be accurate. For example, although it would be useful to know the average number of days each drug is out of stock, it may be more practical to report the number of drugs out of stock at a particular moment. Chapter 4 introduces the concept of performance indicators, and Chapter 36 discusses their use in monitoring. In general, indicators should be selected in areas such as selection, procurement efficiency, product and service quality, distribution efficiency (stockouts, overstocks), rational use, financial management, human resources management (training activities, for example), and reporting compliance with the DMIS.

Strive for representativeness, not comprehensiveness: Representativeness can be achieved by using sentinel data collection systems or sampling methodologies either to select subsets of facilities to survey or to monitor lot quality to focus on the best- and worst-performing service units (see Chapter 36.)

Choose appropriate data collection methods: When possible, use available data sources and rapid assessment methods to collect information on drug use at the health service and household levels. Use supervisors to gather observational data, complete checklists, and provide immediate feedback and support to staff. Finally, use sentinel systems to generate higher-quality but fewer data from a subset of health facilities (see Chapter 36).

Common errors at different points in the recording and reporting process are noted in Figure 45.6, which

Figure 45.5 Steps in Designing or Revising a DMIS

1. Identify information users.
2. Identify information needs for each user, including selected indicators (see Chapter 36).
3. Review existing record-keeping and reporting procedures.
4. Match existing information with information needs to identify overlaps, gaps, and items that can be deleted.
5. Draft record-keeping and reporting procedures to fill the gaps.
6. Develop procedures to help users do simple data analysis and presentation of key trends.
7. Field-test any newly designed records and report forms.
8. Make modifications to record-keeping and reporting forms based on field-test results.
9. Prepare detailed instruction manual.
10. Develop procedures for preparing feedback reports and computerize them, if appropriate.
11. Train information users at all levels in data collection, reporting procedures, and use of information.
12. If the DMIS is computerized, provide training for staff in general computer use and specific applications.
13. Monitor the system's implementation, including the quality and regularity of reporting.
14. Adapt the records, report forms, and software as information needs evolve.

Figure 45.6 Improving Recording and Reporting Accuracy

Kinds of Problems	Sources of Problems	Possible Solutions
Errors in recording	There are too many data items on a single page	Limit number of data items per page
		Use checklists wherever possible
	Data items are not clearly labeled	Label data items in large letters
	There are no instructions for data entry	Provide instructions for each data entry
	Data need to be recopied several times on different forms	Use carbons if multiple copies are necessary
Errors in deciphering	Entries are illegible	Use checklist to avoid illegible handwriting
	Data entries are abbreviated because of insufficient entry space	Leave sufficient space to avoid abbreviations
Errors in tabulating	Columns are too long	Add summary lines in long columns
	There are too many columns on a single page	Limit number of columns to five columns per page
	There is no place to tally page summaries	Add a sheet for page summaries

also describes common sources of problems and possible solutions.

Integrate the DMIS with other data collection systems: System integration is particularly important in the health sector when information about service delivery is being collected. Health workers are often overburdened by multiple or vertical reporting systems for immunizations, family planning, disease control programs, and so on. When this is the case, try to collect data through existing reporting systems or other means, such as medical record reviews and sample surveys, rather than introducing additional routine reports.

One important factor for computerization is the adoption of standard coding systems for drugs, health facilities, diseases, and geographic areas. In addition, it is often necessary to develop standard data file structures to promote compatibility among different software programs in use (see Chapter 46).

Develop practical analysis methods to facilitate data interpretation and use: Staff should be taught the graphic techniques described below for use with two to four key indicators and utilize them to monitor their own performance. Worksheets can help staff aggregate data and calculate indicators manually from existing records.

Computerize at appropriate levels: It is critical to achieve the right mix of computer and manual systems and to ensure that they are fully integrated so that units that do not have computers can produce their reports manually. Keep in mind the adage, If you can do it by hand, the

computer might make it more efficient, but if you can't, the computer is likely to make it worse. Decisions about computerization (see Chapter 46) should take into account

▶ local resources to support computer hardware and software installation, maintenance, and training;
▶ volume of data to be processed (the data entry bottlenecks often associated with highly centralized computer systems can be avoided by decentralizing—one researcher's rule of thumb is that it is not worth entering a survey on the computer if there are fewer than 200 records);
▶ complexity of analysis required.

Ensure that information is communicated effectively: Key decisions need to be made about what, how, and with what frequency data will be communicated to higher levels. Do all data need to be transmitted and analyzed at a higher level, or only summary data? Do raw data need to be reviewed by line managers before being submitted for analysis, or can line managers rely on analyzed feedback from a central information clearinghouse? For computerized systems, can some data be entered in

Figure 45.7 DMIS Information Stages

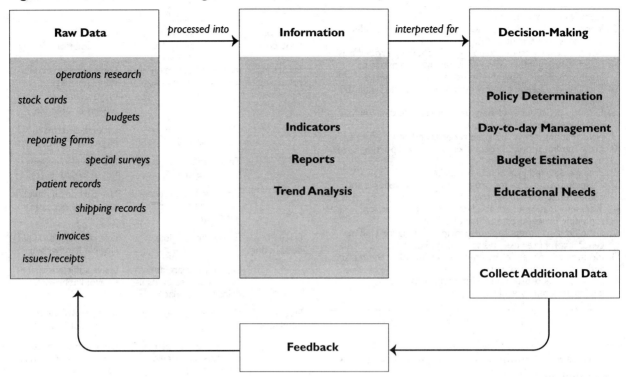

decentralized computer centers and transmitted in batches, using either disks or modems? Can parts of the system be designed for on-line use from remote locations? However data are transmitted, careful attention must be paid to setting up and monitoring reporting schedules so that timely information can be produced.

≡ 45.6 Implementing a Drug Management Information System

Implementation of DMIS changes should be more successful with proper field testing, phased implementation, flexibility, and adequate training. Field testing should involve not only the well-performing sites but, more importantly, the average or worse-performing sites.

A phased approach may be useful. Develop modules that can be applied and tested as they are completed, rather than developing the entire system from start to finish before the users ever see it.

Flexibility is also important. Build in flexibility to change reporting formats, data entry screens, and feedback reports. Staff need to adapt a DMIS and perform ad hoc analyses as information needs evolve.

Finally, staff at all levels need sufficient training for their role in the information system, which may include design and development of an MIS, data collection, computerized data processing, and use of data.

≡ 45.7 From Information to Action

The most fundamental element of a successful DMIS is the effective use of the data generated by the system. Figure 45.7 illustrates the process of transforming data into information and interpreting them for use in decision-making. The key steps are processing data, presenting information, interpreting information, and taking action.

Processing Data

Data processing can take many forms, ranging from simple data aggregation by district, calculation of averages, or trend analysis over time to the use of sophisticated statistical techniques such as analysis of variance. The objective here is to reduce large amounts of data to a manageable amount, often using summary tables. It is important to remember that a computer is not necessary for data processing. Tally sheets can be developed to help users gather data from many sources and to compute totals, counts, and averages.

Presenting Information

Some people have difficulty interpreting information presented in tables. Simple techniques for graphing tabular data can help simplify interpretation. A computer spreadsheet or graphics program can make this both easier and elegant. Some common graph types are

Figure 45.8 Graph Styles

Bar Graph

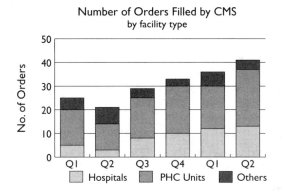

Number of Orders Filled by CMS
by facility type

Pie Chart

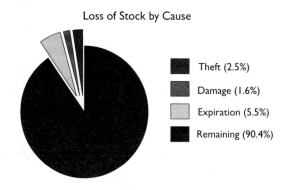

Loss of Stock by Cause

Theft (2.5%)
Damage (1.6%)
Expiration (5.5%)
Remaining (90.4%)

Line Graph

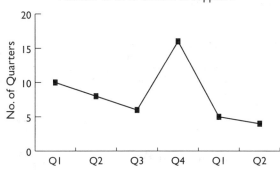

Number of CMS Orders to Suppliers

Map

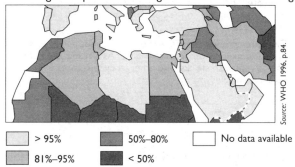

Percentage of Population with Regular Access to Essential Drugs

> 95%   50%–80%   No data available
81%–95%   < 50%

► bar graphs: comparison of values for different items or for the same item at different physical locations;
► line graphs: presentation of trends over time for continuous variables;
► pie charts: demonstration of the relationships among the parts of a whole;
► maps: demonstration of the geographic distribution of indicators.

Figure 45.8 illustrates some common graph styles and their key uses.

Interpreting Information
Interpreting the information is often the most interesting part of using data. Listed below are a number of points to consider in this process.

Are the Data Correct? If the sources (registers, for example) were reviewed again, would the same figures result? Were the calculations made correctly?

Do Any of the Figures Seem Improbable? In absolute terms—without making any calculations—do any numbers seem odd? Do expenditures seem too high or too

low? Are there too many priority drugs out of stock? Are too few orders from facilities being filled? Does the number of emergency purchases seem too high? (Small variations from month to month may be insignificant and should be disregarded.)

How Do the Figures Compare with Previous Figures? Is there a trend toward improvement even though the figures may not seem good in absolute terms? For example, even though there is some revolving drug fund decapitalization, is it less than last year? Using a simple graph or a wall chart can help identify such trends.

How Do the Figures for Different Geographic Areas Compare? Are some districts more successful than others? Do some need extra help building up their clientele or re-evaluating procurement or quantification methods? Does more targeted training, education, and communication work need to be done for staff or clients?

What Might Be the Causes of Problems Identified in Reports? Could external factors (such as clients' economic problems or seasonal variations) be responsible for problems? What could their internal causes be (for example, poor estimation of drug requirements or delays in processing

---

Box 45.1 Example of Information Interpretation and Use

Year	Essential Drugs Program (EDP) Price	World Price	World Price Index
1992	3,600	3,000	120%
1993	3,300	3,100	106%
1994	3,800	3,050	125%
1995	2,800	3,000	93%

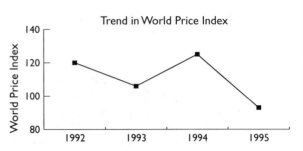

Observation: The difference between the price that the EDP has been paying for its drugs and the world price has been decreasing steadily, except in 1994.

Possible Interpretations	Possible Actions
An increasing proportion of central medical stores drugs are being purchased in bulk competitive tenders.	The overall trend is very positive. Ensure that procurement officers are congratulated for a job well done.
A greater share of the priority drugs are now manufactured within the country, so the costs of transport and clearance are decreasing.	Continue to focus on identifying local manufacturers to bid for large orders.
The jump in price in 1994 was due to serious delays in the arrival of major international orders. As a result, the EDP had to replenish stocks with emergency purchases from local pharmacies.	Get more information about why the large procurement was delayed. If it was due to vendor performance, look for a different vendor. If it was due to poor planning within the EDP, set earlier deadlines or order more stock so that the pipeline can be shortened.

---

orders or clearing items through the ports)? Use a table similar to the one in Box 45.1 to list possible interpretations of the information on key indicators.

Taking Action

Based on interpretations of the information, possible courses of action can be listed for each scenario.

Discuss Reports with Colleagues. When reports are first prepared, discuss them in a staff meeting. Others may offer useful insights into why specific indicators are getting better or worse, and they may have helpful suggestions about changes that could be made.

Provide Feedback. When reports are sent from other units, simple feedback can be given, such as acknowledging receipt of the report and providing a response on any issues that require action. Better yet, a routine mechanism can be developed to provide some analysis of data on key indicators in reports received from all reporting units. This should help people compare their performance with that of other units. Automating the preparation of feedback reports is an important use for computers in a DMIS.

For Each Interpretation, Identify Possible Actions. Note that action should not be limited to dealing with problems; it is also important to focus on the positive results seen. If one quarter had especially good results, see what can be learned from staff about what went right and try to replicate it (see Box 45.1).

Gather More Data. If reports indicate that a problem might exist, confirmation can be obtained through a survey or a special supervisory visit.

Correct the Problem. Many problems can be corrected through supervision and retraining. But there may be situations in which sanctions and disciplinary action are required—the survival of the program may depend on it. ∎

≡ Assessment Guide

Information System Design

► Does the overall plan for the drug supply program include an information management plan?

► Does the information management plan support strategic, program, and work planning needs? Does it support monitoring and evaluation for assessing the implementation of these plans?

► Have key information users been identified at all levels? Have their needs for information related to management decisions been specified?

► Are data reporting forms, such as periodic status reports, designed to be easily completed from existing registers, ledgers, and filing systems?

► Have key indicators been defined? Are their uses understood by staff at all levels?

► Is there at least one indicator for each key area of activity?

► Is the DMIS integrated with other information systems? If not, how much duplication of data is there between systems?

► If computerized systems exist, are they integrated with manual systems?

Data Collection, Reporting, and Use

► Are data collection methods appropriate for the types of data being collected?

► How long does it take staff to fill in the reporting forms each month, quarter, and year? Can these times be reduced?

► Are report forms standardized? Are instructions available for filling them in?

► Are there any overlaps in the data being reported at different intervals? Are any types of data collected that are never used?

► Do staff use any data to complete report forms before sending the forms on to higher levels?

► Are feedback reports provided routinely to the units that collected the data? Do they incorporate graphic as well as tabular information?

► Is there a schedule for report preparation, data transmission, and feedback reporting?

► Is the information generated by the DMIS used for management decisions?

≡ References and Further Readings

★ = *Key readings.*

Bertrand, W. E. 1989. Information as a primary health care intervention: The impact of new technology on improving health for all. *Information technology for development* 4:741–49.

Millar, M. 1993. Assessing information needs (facilitator's guide, module 1). In *Primary health care management advancement programme*. Geneva: Aga Khan Foundation.

MSH (Management Sciences for Health). 1991. Managing and using information. In *The family planning manager's handbook: Basic skills and tools for managing family planning programs*, ed. J. A. Wolff, L. J. Suttenfield, and S. C. Binzen. West Hartford, Conn.: Kumarian Press.

MSH (Management Sciences for Health). 1992. Drug supply management information strategies and systems. In *Managing drug supply training series. Part 3. Supply management*. Boston: MSH.

★ Reynolds, J. 1993. Assessing information needs (user's guide, module 1). In *Primary health care management advancement programme*. Geneva: Aga Khan Foundation.

★ Timmons, R., and M. Egboh. 1992. Using service data: Tools for taking action. *Family Planning Manager* 1(2):1–12.

WHO (World Health Organization). 1993. *Guidelines for the development of health management information systems*. Manila: WHO Regional Office for the Western Pacific.

★ WHO (World Health Organization). 1996. *World health report*. Geneva: WHO.

Wilson, R. G., E. E. Echols, J. H. Bryant, and A. Abrantes, eds. 1989. *Management information systems and microcomputers in primary health care*. Geneva: Aga Khan Foundation.

Annex 45.1 Example of Annual EDP Status Report

A. Identification

1. Year of report	
2. EDP office name	
3. State	

B. Staffing positions in EDP units

Location	No. Approved	No. Filled	No. Transferred
a. EDP office			
b. CMS			
c. Total			

C. Procurement

	Number	Value
1. Contracts awarded this year:		
a. Competitive tender		
b. Restricted tender		
c. Others		
d. Total contracts awarded		
2a. Contracts awarded to local manufacturers		
2b. Percent of total procurements (2a/1d) x 100		%
3. World price index for selected priority drugs		%

D. Training

Workshop Course Type	Number Held	Total Days	No. of Participants		
			Professional	Paraprofessional	Other
1. Rational procurement					
2. Stores management					
3. Quality assurance					
4. Financial management					
5. MIS/computers					
6. Rational use					
7. Information, education, and communication					
8. Training of trainers					

E. Inventory control (from inventory audit report)

1. Average lead time for filling stock requisitions from district stores and health facilities (days)		
2. Total value of stock at end of year inventory		
3. Stock lost due to:	Value	% of Total
a. Expiration		
b. Damage		
c. Theft		

F. Comments

G. Signatures

CMS manager	Date
Financial accountant	Date
EDP project manager	Date

H. Local supplier performance for deliveries completed this year

Name of Local Supplier	No. of Deliveries Completed	Total Value	Value of Rejected Drugs	Avg. Lead Time	Avg. Delay of Deliveries
Average lead time for local suppliers (sum of avg. lead times/no. of local suppliers)					

I. Foreign supplier performance for deliveries completed this year

Name of Foreign Supplier	No. of Deliveries Completed	Total Value	Value of Rejected Drugs	Avg. Lead Time	Avg. Delay of Deliveries
Average lead time for foreign suppliers (sum of avg. lead times/no. of foreign suppliers)					

J. Financial management

1. Expense summary	Amount	% of Total
a. Stock procurement		%
b. Transport costs		%
c. Workshops and IE&C		%
d. Fellowships and ext. training		%
e. Supplies and equipment		%
f. Maintenance and repairs		%
g. Other expenses		%
Total expenses		100%
2. Income summary		
a. Sales of CMS stock		%
b. Other income		%
Total income		100%

3. Financial data	
a. Total value of stock issues (from J2a)	
b. Total operating costs (1b+1c+1d+1e+1f)	
c. Total value of stock at end of year (from E2)	
d. Value of prepaid pipeline orders	
e. Other debts	
f. Stock fund value at end of previous year	

4. Financial indicators	
a. Operating costs as % of sales ((3b/3a) x 100)	
b. Number of stock turns (3a/((3c+3f)/2))	
c. Stock fund value at end of last year (3c+3d−3e)	
d. Stock fund growth ((4c−3f)/3f x 100)	

Part I Introduction	Part II Policy and Legal Framework	Part III Drug Management Cycle	**Part IV** **Management Support Systems**

A Organization and Management
B Financing and Sustainability
C Information Management ▶   45 Drug Management
Information Systems
D Human Resources Management

**46 Computers in
Drug Management**

Chapter 46

Computers in Drug Management

≡ Summary

Users should first define what functions or tasks computers will be used for, identify appropriate software for those functions, and then select hardware that is capable of using the software efficiently.

A computerization process is easier when

► *efficient manual procedures exist;*
► *staff are capable of, and interested in, learning to use computers;*
► *funds have been allocated for training, maintenance, and equipment upgrades;*
► *there is a reliable power supply.*

Drug management programs should usually begin with basic word-processing and spreadsheet applications. This allows users to gain experience and develop support systems for supplies, repairs, and security. Specialized drug management programs are often used for quantification of drug requirements, procurement, inventory management, or drug use analysis.

Drug information is increasingly available through electronic communications systems. Many drug supply systems have, or will soon have, access to Internet communications. Two main options are available: E-mail and World Wide Web browsers. Use of the Internet for international communications has become increasingly important.

Central to most drug management applications is a drug master file, including drug name, strength, dosage form,

and therapeutic category. A coding system with a unique identifier for each drug product must be developed.

Microcomputers, also known as personal computers or PCs, can be used in all aspects of the drug management cycle. Hardware refers to the computer's electronic and mechanical parts, which include

► *a microprocessor chip;*
► *memory chips (RAM, for random-access memory);*
► *input devices (keyboard, floppy disk drive, mouse, scanner);*
► *storage devices (hard disk drive, floppy disk, CD-ROM, magnetic tape);*
► *output and peripheral devices (monitor, printer, modem, network card, speakers).*

Software refers to instructions that can be understood and executed by the computer. Categories include

► *the operating system, which coordinates and directs information for the microprocessor;*
► *general-purpose software, such as word-processing, spreadsheets, and database management software;*
► *special-purpose software, such as presentation graphics, project management, and accounting software;*
► *utility programs, such as antivirus, file backup, and data recovery programs;*
► *specialized drug management software, often a custom-programmed database application.*

≡ Since their introduction in the late 1970s, microcomputers have revolutionized many aspects of drug management. The technology is evolving very rapidly, and applications that were unthinkable in small computers five years ago are now common. Worldwide communications networks use computers to access services that were formerly confined to universities and government agencies.

When used effectively, computer systems save money, promote efficiency, and improve the quality of services. However, poorly conceived or implemented computer systems waste money, decrease efficiency, and distract attention from other management improvements.

This chapter introduces the uses of computers in drug management and examines special issues in computerizing drug management information. It also discusses specifications for computer applications in drug management, considerations for hardware selection, and requirements for maintaining and supporting computers. Preparing

data for computerization is discussed, along with coding systems and definitions of units. This chapter focuses on personal computers because they are the most widely used by essential drugs programs. It is beyond the scope of this chapter to instruct users in particular software programs or to make recommendations for the purchase of a specific piece of hardware or software.

The question today is often not whether but rather how and how much to computerize. What is even more important, however, is how to computerize efficiently. This chapter provides guidelines to help decision-makers computerize their operations effectively.

≡ 46.1 Uses of Computers in Drug Management

Computers can be used in all aspects of the drug management cycle, from selection to use. They are capable of manipulating text and numbers and producing correspondence, newsletters, forms, reports, tables, graphs, and charts. Using communication devices, users can exchange or share this information with other computers at the same site via a local area network (LAN) or with computers anywhere in the world. Figure 46.1 summarizes some of the many current computer applications for drug management.

≡ 46.2 When and How to Computerize

Computer technology changes very quickly, with machines continually becoming faster, more capable, and less expensive. The benefits of computers in managing drugs depend on the choice of tools, the commitment to using the tools, and the ability to overcome the hurdles involved in incorporating computers into the organization. There is no standard formula for successful computerization in drug management, but rather a mix of elements; the right mix can yield great benefits.

Benefits and Limitations of Computerization

Some of the benefits of computerization are to

- simplify and speed up complex tasks;
- increase accuracy by checking spelling, calculations, and data integrity;
- update and access information quickly;
- automate repetitive tasks;
- provide management information for decision-making;
- allow organizations to expand the volume and scope of operations;
- streamline administrative processes;
- generate timely reports without repeated efforts in compiling data.

However, computers still have limitations. They cannot assume responsibilities, make decisions, define problems, set objectives, improve the basic data available, or make a person more organized. They cannot fulfill needs if appropriate hardware and software are not chosen, and they are not a one-time expense: funds are required for upgrades, training, and support over time for both hardware and software.

Conditions in an organization that support computerization include

- efficient existing manual procedures;
- other departments that have computerized successfully;
- staff capable of, and interested in, operating computers;
- a reliable power supply;
- adequate funds to support maintenance, training, and equipment upgrades.

Figure 46.1 Computer Applications for Drug Management

Area of Activity	Uses
Project planning	▶ Workplans ▶ Simulation programs ▶ Annual reports
Selection	▶ Essential drugs list preparation ▶ Literature searches
Requirements planning	▶ Quantification of drug needs ▶ ABC analysis ▶ Weight and volume analysis of kits
Financing	▶ Budget management ▶ Drug sales monitoring ▶ Accounting ▶ Financial analysis
Procurement	▶ Tender document preparation ▶ Tender monitoring ▶ Bid analysis ▶ Purchase orders and receiving reports ▶ Monitoring of order status
Inventory control	▶ Monitoring of stock positions ▶ Monitoring of expiry dates ▶ Prediction of reorder dates and quantities ▶ Invoicing
Transport	▶ Vehicle routing and scheduling ▶ Weight and volume calculation ▶ Transport voucher preparation
Drug registration and control	▶ Database of registration data ▶ Adverse reaction reporting ▶ Drug recalls
Drug information	▶ Formulary preparation ▶ Literature searches ▶ Mass data storage (CD-ROM) ▶ Drug bulletin production ▶ Training material preparation
Rational use	▶ Formulary ▶ Standard treatment schedule ▶ Calculation of WHO drug use indicators ▶ Survey analysis ▶ Training (simulation games)
Personnel management	▶ Training software ▶ Personnel records ▶ Supervision monitoring ▶ Payroll calculations
Health statistics	▶ Population data ▶ Morbidity data ▶ Mortality data
Utilization	▶ Health care coverage calculations ▶ Drug consumption analysis
Presentation	▶ Graphs and charts ▶ Overhead transparencies for training
Communication	▶ Fax ▶ Electronic mail ▶ Mailing

Figure 46.2 Key Steps in the Computerization Process

1. Identify the tasks or the system to be computerized with a detailed analysis of needs versus current systems.

2. Survey the environment and consider integrating with other systems to the extent feasible. (What software and hardware are being used by other departments? Is there an institutional computer policy? What equipment is already available?)

3. Evaluate the staff situation (actual versus needed).

4. Select software before hardware.

5. Identify whether the software needed is available in the local language and to which original version it is equivalent (non-English-language versions are sometimes not as current as English versions).

6. Ensure the availability of supplies and maintenance.

7. Select the hardware and software suppliers that provide the most support.

8. Plan progressive implementation (one step at a time) and involve current and future users in the design and implementation process.

Conditions that can impede computerization include

- hardware or software not suited to the task;
- not enough trained operators;
- lack of a maintenance plan;
- lack of reliable power (voltage surges ruin computers and databases);
- inadequate supply of diskettes, paper, or print ribbons;
- unsuitable physical environment (exposure to dust, heat, or magnets, which can damage hardware and software).

Starting the Computerization Process

Begin with the basic questions: What will the computer be used for? Who will use it? Where will it be used? What is the budget for equipment, software, and maintenance? What special functions may be required? Will there be a need to share data? Will a network be necessary? The key steps are listed in Figure 46.2.

In computerization, users should walk before they try to run. Trying to do everything at once increases failure rates, so organizations often computerize in phases (see Figure 46.3). This enables computer operators to handle increasingly demanding tasks, permits support systems for supplies and repairs to develop, and allows security systems to be put in place to protect against electrical damage, computer viruses, theft, and other hazards.

Perhaps most important, computerization in phases allows users to develop a clearer concept of what computers can do, what kind of information they want from the computerized system, and which modifications are needed in reporting and management systems to obtain this information. It is crucial to plan computerization carefully so that there is a smooth implementation with a minimum

Figure 46.3 Illustrative Phases in Computerization

Phase I: Convenience Computing
This includes tasks that could be done with a typewriter and calculator but are easier on the computer. If the computer "goes down" (temporarily stops working), the work can still be done. Examples:
- word processing
- simple databases (for example, an address list)
- simple budgets

Phase II: Periodic Analyses and Special Activities
These tasks would be extremely difficult to do by hand but could be delayed for a few days or weeks if the computer were down. Examples:
- quantification exercises
- complex project budgets
- survey analysis

Phase III: Essential Daily Activities
These tasks involve large volumes of data handled daily or almost daily. If the computer went down, the work would be seriously impaired. Examples:
- inventory control
- accounting
- drug registration

---

of interruption and dislocation in the work. Country Study 46.1 provides some examples of good and bad computerization experiences.

Computer Software: Options and Guidelines

Because of the competitive nature of the market, software packages, like hardware, are becoming cheaper. They are also becoming more powerful, and upgraded versions appear regularly. Upgrades may mean that the software packages require upgraded hardware resources (such as hard disk space, microprocessor power, and memory) to run effectively. This is the main argument for choosing software before hardware and for including hardware upgrades in the budget.

Computer magazines are a valuable source of comparison articles on software and hardware. "Aftermarket" software books published by companies such as Cyber or Que are often easier to use than the manual provided by the company.

Three broad categories of computer software are useful in drug management: general-purpose, special-purpose, and utility programs.

General-Purpose Software

General-purpose software programs (such as word processing, desktop publishing, spreadsheets, and commercial database programs) perform routine daily activities or periodic analyses. The most important factor in choosing general-purpose software is access to local support. Some questions to consider are: Which package is the most

Country Study 46.1
Sample Computerization Experiences

Poor Planning. The central medical store (CMS) in a sub-Saharan African country was computerized as part of a program to strengthen the computer capacity of the Ministry of Health. Unfortunately, the firm chosen to do the work did not realize that two previous attempts at computerization had failed due to internal organizational issues that had little to do with computers. The firm repeated many of the previous mistakes, because it believed that the introduction of technology could establish organizational systems and controls, and it did not examine the organization's existing structure.

An ambitious plan to computerize inventory and financial accounts within three months was devised. What resulted was hardware that could not be serviced locally and inadequate training of staff. Only a few poorly attended meetings were held with CMS management, and for many reasons, the data entered into the software were never accurate or up-to-date.

After nine months, the main CMS computer was stolen. No data backup had been made for over three months because there were no diskettes available. The last four months of data were lost, and no one thought that the system should be revived. No maintenance budget had been set aside for recurring costs such as printer ribbons, diskettes, and systems maintenance, and the computers were being used only for word processing.

Computer Integration Issues. In a rapidly developing South Asian country, problems have occurred in the integration and transfer of data. Many departments have computerized, and there is overlapping data collection and processing, because responsibilities have not been clearly defined. In addition, incompatible software packages have been used; coding of key data, such as locations and drug names, has not been consistent; and data linking has been very difficult. Many of the problems could have been avoided by clear definitions of responsibilities, a software policy, and a common coding system for key data.

Well-Planned Computerization. A Southeast Asian country has undertaken the process of computerizing slowly. Initially, data on drug consumption, procurement, supply, and health statistics were collected manually. Computers were first used to enter these data into a spreadsheet program. Although this worked well initially, the amount of data to be processed eventually overloaded the system, and the decision was made to upgrade it. Appropriate software and a systems developer were carefully selected. Training of local staff by expatriate staff was very successful and is still important for maintenance of the system. Computerization has helped provide useful management data for consumption analysis, drug procurement and supply, and reallocation of supplies among health facilities. A computerized registration system is planned. Computerization has been relatively successful in this country because a step-by-step approach was used, starting from manual systems and developing the system with end-users to meet their information needs.

Figure 46.4 Desirable Features of Standard Commercial Software

- ❏ Easy menu-driven installation
- ❏ General and context-sensitive on-line help
- ❏ On-screen menus
- ❏ Mouse capability
- ❏ WYSIWYG mode (what you see is what you get: displays the information on-screen as it will be printed)
- ❏ On-screen or manual-based tutorial
- ❏ Import and export of data between various similar standard packages (for example, exchange of data between two different database formats)
- ❏ Import and export of data between software applications developed by the same software company (such as between a spreadsheet and a database program)
- ❏ Extensive use of function keys or key combinations to speed up various tasks and data entry
- ❏ Multiple print fonts for quality output
- ❏ Comprehensive manual with concrete examples
- ❏ In-country or international telephone or fax support (free for a limited period, extendable by contract)
- ❏ Network or multiuser compatibility

common locally? Is local training available? What software is in use in other local offices with which the program interacts? Standard features of "user-friendly" commercial software packages are listed in Figure 46.4.

Word Processing. Word-processing programs are replacing the typewriter. For most offices, 80 percent of computing time is spent on word processing. It is usually the easiest task to learn, because the input and output are obvious even to a novice. It is therefore a good way to get acquainted with computers. These programs are mainly used for correspondence and for producing reports, mass mailings, and documents. Features such as graphics capabilities, spelling checkers, search-and-replace functions, and generators for tables of contents make documents easier to produce.

Desktop Publishing. This software has word-processor features but is more powerful in handling graphics, large documents, and production of camera-ready copy to be used by a printer for newsletters, bulletins, training materials, or even books.

Spreadsheet. A spreadsheet is a worksheet made of horizontal and vertical lines that define a matrix of rows and columns. It is modeled after an accountant's ledger, and data are entered in cells identified by coordinates in the matrix. Any type of data (text or numbers) can be entered in these cells, and sophisticated calculations and analyses (such as those discussed in Chapter 41) can be performed.

A major advantage of spreadsheets is their ability to revise totals, percentages, and other calculations immediately after any number or set of numbers is changed, allowing experimentation with "what if" alternatives. They can be linked together to allow consolidation of accounts and can produce graphics and charts of the data entered.

In drug management, spreadsheets are used for budgeting, financial analysis, quantification of drug requirements, ABC analysis, price comparisons, pricing models, and creating or revising national essential drugs lists, as discussed in other chapters.

Database. A database file is like an electronic filing cabinet. Data (characters, numbers, dates, formulas, or memos) are stored in fields. The combination of fields forms a record, and the records constitute a database file. Database software can store and manipulate large amounts of data quickly. Databases are used in many business applications, where they allow users to

- ► sort data in any order using multiple sorting keys;
- ► establish relationships between databases and generate sophisticated consolidated reports;
- ► quickly retrieve data according to specific criteria;
- ► develop complex applications using powerful programming languages;
- ► import and export data.

In drug management, databases are used in data-intensive tasks such as inventory control, procurement, tender management, detailed analyses of prescriptions, accounting, and drug registration. Databases are superior to spreadsheets for this type of application because they store more data in smaller files with less need for duplicating entries. Their structure permits easy data manipulation for access and reporting, and they can be designed to check the data entered for consistency with previously entered data. A relational database is particularly useful in drug management because it allows multiple records for the same basic item (good for inventory management, tender analysis, or drug use analysis). An example of a relational database is shown in Figure 46.5. Note how a common field links separate records in the database, limiting the need for duplication of data entry and facilitating data retrieval and reporting.

Software Suite. The Windows operating system has given IBM-compatible computers a user interface similar to that of the Apple-Macintosh and has promoted the development of software "suites" that package word-processing, spreadsheet, database, graphics, and communication programs as one product. These individual programs are combined in one software package and are designed to allow easy exchange of information among the different programs. In some cases, however, the packaged programs are not as powerful as individual stand-alone software.

Special-Purpose Commercial Software
Drug management systems often need special-purpose commercial software packages, such as presentation graphics, project management, statistical, accounting, bibliographic, and communications programs.

Presentation Graphics. A simple graph often has more visual impact than a complex table, so presentation graphics packages can be useful for preparing effective and attractive reports, funding proposals, overhead transparencies, and slides.

Project Management. Project management software organizes and tracks project tasks to be accomplished according to a defined schedule and shows potential conflicts in the use of resources. Budgeting information can also be included.

Statistical. Although spreadsheets and databases have standard statistical functions, it is sometimes preferable to use a dedicated statistical package. Epi Info, developed and distributed at cost by the World Health Organization (WHO) and the Centers for Disease Control and Prevention (CDC), integrates basic word-processing, data entry, statistical, and database functions. It is particularly useful for processing survey data and tabulating data stored in standard database programs.

Accounting. Accounting programs are available with a wide range of capabilities. Basic bookkeeping can be done with spreadsheets, but a dedicated accounting package is often more appropriate. Selection depends on local factors: What can the bookkeeper use? What does a donor use? What support is available? What bookkeeping technique is used? Is the accounting format compatible with local regulations? Increasingly, reputable local accounting firms can advise which accounting programs are most suitable for an organization.

Bibliographic. Bibliographic software greatly facilitates storing, searching for, retrieving, and manipulating bibliographic information on books, journals, training materials, and government and project documents. This kind of software requires staff to keep the database up-to-date.

Communications. Communications software, initially designed to send and receive files via fax or modem, is evolving rapidly to electronic mail and access to on-line services. See "Electronic Communications and Drug Information" below for more applications.

Utility Programs
Programs called utilities help manage and maintain computers and stored data. Common utilities include antivirus, file management, file backup, file exchange, data recovery, data compression, and network software.

Figure 46.5 Example of Relational Database Structure for Inventory Control

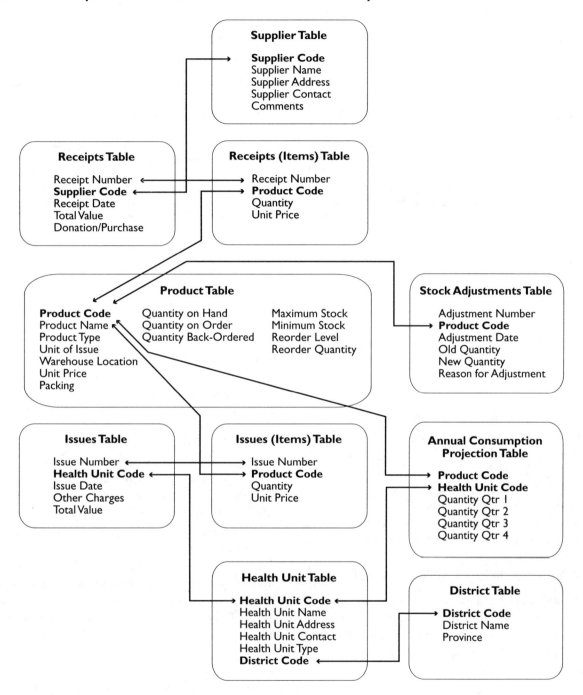

Because operating systems now include many of the commonly needed utilities, it is best to become thoroughly familiar with the capabilities of a particular operating system before buying a separate utility.

A current antivirus program is absolutely vital for computer units that handle essential day-to-day functions such as inventory control, drug registration, accounting, or maintenance of national health statistics. It is also essential for any system that receives data from outside sources, including branch offices within the country.

Custom Software

Development of custom-built software, such as an inventory program, is a complex and time-consuming task. Although the idea of custom-built software is attractive, purchasing software that has already been written and

Figure 46.6 Computer Hardware Specifications

Hardware	Indicator	Significance
Hard drive	Megabyte (MB)	The number of megabytes describes the storage capacity of the hard drive— how much data and software it can contain. One megabyte equals one million letters or numbers.
Processor chip	Chip type, with speed in megahertz (MHz)	The chip type and speed determine how quickly the computer can make calculations, run software, and function.
RAM (random-access memory)	Megabyte (MB)	The amount of RAM in a system determines how many tasks the computer can run at once and how complicated a program it can handle.
Monitor	Type, dot pitch	The type of monitor dictates the complexity of images and colors it can display. The dot pitch controls the sharpness of the image on the screen, with a lower dot pitch causing less eyestrain.
Printer	Characters per second (CPS), pages per minute (PPM), dots per inch (DPI)	Dot matrix printers are judged in CPS, and laser printers in PPM. Both are important when producing large amounts of output. Printer quality is measured in DPI and is important when producing high-quality output.
Modem	Baud	The baud rate is how much information a modem can send in a second and controls how long it takes to send a file over a telephone line.
CD-ROM drive	Speed	The speed of a CD-ROM drive describes how quickly it can access and read information from a CD-ROM.

tested by others is usually preferable, unless a suitable program cannot be found. If new software does need to be developed, it is important to approach this task in a step-by-step fashion:

- ► Define the system requirements.
- ► Choose the software and tools for developing the custom program.
- ► Design a system.
- ► Develop and program the system.
- ► Test and debug the system.
- ► Implement the system through data entry and training.
- ► Develop system documentation and a complete users' manual.
- ► Provide system support, revision, and upgrades.

Frequently, lack of time, money, or expertise results in unusable software. Developing custom software always takes longer than expected and may go over budget. Users should explore all alternatives carefully before choosing to develop software themselves.

Computer Hardware: Options and Guidelines

The size and speed of computer hardware are changing so quickly that it is impossible to give specific recommendations as to what a user should buy. When purchasing computers and peripheral devices such as printers, the important issues are processing, storage, memory, and output capacities. Always buy the most powerful equipment that the budget will allow, especially if it will be a few years before a new computer can be purchased.

Hardware is improving so rapidly that it is best not to buy a computer until shortly before it will be used. Delaying a purchase for even a month can mean a lower price or greater capabilities for the same price. Figure 46.6 describes different types of computer hardware. In general, bigger numbers are better for the indicators listed.

≡ 46.3 Specialized Software for Drug Management and Control

Pharmaceutical systems that successfully computerize usually begin with basic word-processing and spreadsheet applications and then seek specialized applications for inventory management, procurement, drug regulation, or drug use analysis. This section provides an overview of types of specialized software for various tasks and guidelines to consider when evaluating alternatives. Examples of specific types of programs are given, and others are listed in the references at the end of the chapter.

Quantification of Drug Requirements

Quantification of drug requirements (see Chapter 14) is complex, and a computer can greatly speed up the process. Spreadsheets can be used if there are not too many data. Worksheets can be set up to forecast requirements using consumption data; formulas can be entered into the spreadsheet for estimates based on different scenarios. Spreadsheets can be linked, or a single spreadsheet can be divided into sections (one to record the morbidity profile, one to organize the standard treatments, and one to summarize drug requirements within therapeutic categories). Linking spreadsheets requires an advanced level of proficiency in using spreadsheets.

Database software for forecasting has been developed by Management Sciences for Health (MSH). Users enter consumption data (past and forecasted use) in one module, and morbidity data (number of expected cases for each age range and for each health problem) in another module. Once standard treatments are defined, the software generates a table that compares the drugs needed using both consumption and morbidity methods. Predefined reports also present either budget forecasting or ABC analysis by product or therapeutic category.

Basic Data Analysis and Production of Formulary Manuals

Basic commercial software can be used for many drug management purposes, such as data analysis and publication of formulary and therapeutics manuals.

Data Analysis. Spreadsheets are ideal tools for the development of a drug list, because they allow easy manipulation of both text and numbers. It is very easy to create a spreadsheet listing drugs and data on price, consumption, lead time, and formulary category. Formulas can then be added to perform various analyses, such as ABC analysis, price comparison analysis, and therapeutic category analysis (see Chapter 41).

Formulary Manuals. A word-processing program can be used to develop a formulary manual with treatment guidelines. A desktop publishing program can produce documents ready for printing (see Chapter 11 for a discussion of layout and printing considerations).

Procurement and Inventory Management

Spreadsheets can automate aspects of procurement and inventory management, but they are not ideal for processing large amounts of data. Database software is more appropriate. Unless activities are limited to either procurement or inventory management alone, using the same database program for procurement, inventory management, and accounting is preferable, because these activities are interconnected.

Inventory management is often part of a commercial accounting software package, but it typically focuses on accounting and lacks features specific to drug management, such as the ability to track multiple products for the same code number, or to track items by lot number and expiry date.

Database programs have been developed by MSH and others specifically to manage procurement and inventory control in public pharmaceutical systems (see Annex

Figure 46.7 Checklist for Selecting or Creating Procurement and Inventory Management Software

General Features of Procurement and Inventory Software

❏ Restricts user access to a particular module with password protection
❏ Allows multiple users
❏ Handles various currency formats
❏ Uses various pricing options
❏ Automates backup routines
❏ Generates custom reports
❏ Checks data integrity (for example, it is impossible to enter a letter or other character if a number is expected, and vice versa)
❏ Links with a full accounting package
❏ Exports data, such as to a spreadsheet for specific analysis

Specific Features of Procurement Software

❏ Manages simultaneous tenders
❏ Generates all tender documents
❏ Manages bids and purchase orders in multiple currencies
❏ Compares bids using a common unit regardless of pack size variation
❏ Generates contracts and purchase orders for suppliers
❏ Monitors order status and payments
❏ Monitors supplier performance (lead time, contract price versus invoiced price)
❏ Generates receiving reports
❏ Updates inventory databases

Specific Features of Inventory Software

❏ Tracks monthly consumption
❏ Keeps track of stockout periods
❏ Calculates average monthly consumption, taking into consideration past consumption and stockout periods
❏ Calculates minimum and maximum stock levels
❏ Calculates optimum reorder level, taking into consideration minimum stock, actual stock balance, lead time, procurement and forecasting periods, and outstanding orders, as well as user-defined maximum and minimum stock levels
❏ Monitors expiry dates by lot
❏ Generates picking lists by location
❏ Manages distribution according to expiry date and/or location
❏ Monitors clients' consumption and budget
❏ Allows multiple purchase and selling prices, as well as the possibility to enter discounts, surcharges, and taxes
❏ Generates audit report

46.1). Figure 46.7 provides a checklist of features that should be included in procurement and inventory management software. Figure 46.8 lists standard reports that should be produced by such software. Country Studies 46.2 and 46.3 illustrate how inventory management and procurement software has been used to improve public-sector drug management.

Figure 46.8 Standard Reports for Procurement and Inventory Software

Procurement and inventory management software should generate standard reports to support decision making, such as the following.

Inventory Reports
Stock status report: lists all products in the product master file, including product code and description, unit of measure, quantity in stock, quantity on order, quantity reserved, quantity available.
Reorder report: lists all products that are below the reorder level, with reorder quantity.
Overstock report: lists all products exceeding the maximum level.
Inventory valuation report: lists the current value of the inventory, based on the chosen valuation method (LIFO, FIFO, average).

Order Reports
Open order report: lists orders from customers that have been entered and not yet shipped.
Back order report: lists all unshipped back orders.
Order history report: reports on all orders (shipped and non-shipped) on file.

Product Reports
Catalog report and price list: lists all products in the product master file. Can contain pricing information and be used as a price list.
Product history report: lists by stock item total quantities and sales values for each fiscal period.

Sales Analysis and Forecasting Reports
Customer analysis report: lists sales made to each customer in a specified period.
Ranked customer analysis report: same as above, but ranked by sales volume, with cumulative percentages.

Functional Lists/Outputs Printed by the System
List of "picking tickets"
List of delivery notes/invoices
List of stock count sheets

Multilocation Reports
(if using a system that tracks stock in multiple locations)
Transfer advice report: a reorder advice report that lists products that are over the maximum or under the reorder level. This makes it possible to determine if a product that is unavailable or understocked in one location is available in another location.

Financial Reports
(if linked to financial information)
Credit hold orders report: orders that are on hold because the customer is over the credit limit.
Debtors and creditors report: lists of those who owe and are owed money.

Tender Reports
Bid evaluation report: for each product in a tender, lists all suppliers that offered bids, with information on the supplier (country, delivery time) and on the quoted product (unit cost, quoted unit price, bid converted to base currency, manufacturer, quality of sample, and any other details).
Supplier performance report: lists, for a given supplier, details of all previous quotations, orders, and deliveries, including both a comparison between date promised and date delivered and the condition of products.
Product quotation record: for each product, lists previous bids, with details of the supplier and the quoted prices. If an order was made, this is indicated with supply timeliness and quality information.
Database listings: lists suppliers and products. The supplier listings are also available as mailing labels and for mail-merging into a word-processed letter.

Hospital Pharmacy Management Software

Specialized hospital pharmacy software can support various aspects of a hospital pharmacy (Chapter 38), including

- patient medication profile
- records of intravenous therapy
- management of total parenteral nutrition
- unit-dose management
- medication administration record
- order entry and inventory management
- drug interaction checking
- allergy checking
- food and drug interactions
- duplicate therapy checking
- lab value monitoring
- outpatient prescriptions
- patient billing

Hospital pharmacy software can also be included in hospital management software. The *Hospital Software Sourcebook* (McKenzie 1993) provides information on a variety of commercial hospital pharmacy software packages available in the United States, with a summary of software features, prices, and conditions of availability.

Accounting and Financial Management

Most public-sector supply systems are bound by government accounting regulations, which differ from country to country. Commercial accounting software is widely available but may require modification to correspond with local regulations. If a specialized drug management program is used for inventory control, it is important that the inventory software and the accounting software be modified to communicate with each other.

Learning how to perform basic spreadsheet analysis is a must for the modern essential drugs program manager. Spreadsheets can be used for both simple and sophisticated analyses of program finances. See Chapter 41 for examples.

Drug Use Analysis

Simple analyses of drug use patterns can be done with spreadsheets and commercial database software. Commercial software is available for analyzing data on drug use from large databases. These software programs are usually fairly expensive (thousands of US dollars per installation). PASS (Prescription Analysis Software System) was developed by MSH specifically for drug use analysis in public-sector systems. The software provides reports on basic drug use indicators, such as the percentage of injectables or generic drugs prescribed, and allows comparisons of

Country Study 46.2 INVEC-2

INVEC-2 is a relational database program for inventory control and management. It maintains a perpetual inventory record of all medical store items and tracks purchases and receipts from suppliers, as well as issues to health facilities. The program is designed to handle the specific requirements of pharmaceuticals and can manage stock by lot number. INVEC-2 can process multiple tenders simultaneously and includes forecasting capabilities. This user-friendly program also tracks consumption and recommends reorder quantities based on several variables. It produces over thirty standard reports.

The software can be single user or multiuser and can track stock levels at consuming facilities, as well as payments and bank account transactions. All the functions work together, so when issues are made, orders are placed, and drugs are received, INVEC-2 automatically updates the stock level of the drugs, the transaction history of the health facility, and all financial records, including accounts payable and receivable. INVEC-2 is the second version of the program and is available in English and Spanish. The first version of INVEC was installed in Nigeria, Belize, Senegal, Rwanda, and the eastern Caribbean. INVEC-2 is installed in the eastern Caribbean, Mexico, and Zimbabwe.

In the Caribbean, it is in use in the central medical stores (CMS) of St. Vincent and the Grenadines, St. Lucia, Grenada, and Dominica. The CMS of these islands manage up to 2,000 items each, ranging from pharmaceuticals to medical supplies to mops.

In Mexico, the Spanish version of INVEC-2 is installed in eighteen sites in Mexico City. It is being used in two warehouses and sixteen urban health districts by the Mexican Social Security Administration. All these locations manage both pharmaceuticals and medical supplies.

INVEC-2 is installed in four sites in Zimbabwe. There is a multiuser installation in Harare, which performs centralized procurement for the regional medical stores. The program is also used in three regional stores for inventory management and local purchases.

INVEC and INVEC-2 were developed by the Drug Management Program of MSH.

Country Study 46.3 ECPRO-2

ECPRO-2 is a tender and procurement management software program. The program evolved, over several years, from a simple D-base program to a sophisticated multiuser database management system. It is used by the Eastern Caribbean Drug Service (ECDS) in management of the entire tender cycle and provides accounting information to manage revolving drug funds that are used to finance procurement for eight countries.

ECPRO-2 compiles forecasting data from the countries and generates requests for bids and other tender documents. After the bids are entered, the program analyzes them and generates the adjudication documents. When the tender board decisions are entered, ECPRO-2 can produce a list of awards for each supplier. The program is used to track countries' purchase orders and payments to suppliers. In addition, it monitors suppliers' compliance with contract terms, such as lead times and pricing.

The program has enabled ECDS, a relatively small organization, to function effectively and efficiently as a procurement agency for over five years, with no outside support. ECPRO-2 allows it to make all purchases centrally and distribute supplies directly from the suppliers to the islands. ECPRO-2 was developed by the Drug Management Program of MSH.

drug use patterns by facility, prescriber, region, and drug category.

Drug Registration

Drug registration software can help the drug regulatory authority track the hundreds or thousands of registered products. Registration data can be tracked in a manual card system, sorted by product name or company, but it is very time-consuming to retrieve data needed for specific purposes. Database programs can automate this procedure, retrieving records meeting specific criteria almost instantaneously. SIAMED, a drug registration software program, is available from WHO/DMP. Computers can

greatly facilitate drug registration by improving access to information, but they do not provide the enforcement capacity essential to give registration meaningful impact. A legal framework for drug registration and a flexible and efficiently functioning drug regulatory authority are prerequisites to successful computerization of drug registration. Figure 46.9 presents the features needed in drug registration software; Country Study 46.4 discusses computerization of drug registration in Peru.

≡ 46.4 Electronic Communications and Drug Information

Communications and drug information are discussed together because drug information is increasingly available through electronic communication systems.

Electronic Communications

Although computers have long been used by universities and industry for communications, document services and the ability to share data became readily available to the average computer user in the early 1990s. Computers are powerful and relatively cheap communication tools. Computer-based communication is possible through electronic mail (E-mail), the World Wide Web, computer-to-computer modem connection, or fax (facsimile).

If a good telephone line is available, computers equipped with a fax-modem can send and receive fax messages or

Figure 46.9 Features of Registration Software

Names and Identifications

- ► Registration of products by vendor and manufacturer;
- ► Identification by international nonproprietary name (INN) and brand name;
- ► Identification of alternative generic names (US Adopted Name [USAN], British Approved Name [BAN]);
- ► Cross-indexing between generic and brand names, active ingredients, and authorized vendors and manufacturers;
- ► Records of imports and foreign exchange applications and authorizations related to products, vendors, and manufacturers.*

Pharmacological Information

- ► Pharmacopeial standards applicable to product;
- ► Identification of active and inactive ingredients;
- ► Patent status, local and international.

International Information

- ► Country of origin;
- ► Product status and regulatory action in other countries;
- ► Variable handling of applications from suppliers based in the registering country.

Quality Assurance

- ► Certification by regulatory agency in country of origin (WHO certification scheme);
- ► Dates and results of quality tests and assays;
- ► Summary of results of clinical trials;
- ► Summary of manufacturer's documentation of efficacy and safety;
- ► Good manufacturing practices inspection results;
- ► Registration and licensing of wholesale suppliers, licensed pharmacies, and other licensed drug outlets.*

Administrative Tracking

- ► Duration of license, dates of approval and renewal (or denial);
- ► Dates of receipt and action on registration;
- ► Dates and results of agency hearings and regulatory actions regarding products, vendors, and manufacturers;
- ► Postmarketing tracking, including reports on adverse reactions and product quality complaints;
- ► Variable length of authorization for marketing;*
- ► Records of price agreements and price control categories and decisions (as applicable).*

Optional feature.

complete documents in just a few seconds. Modern word-processing software can send fax messages directly from the computer. The transmission speed and quality depend on the quality of the telephone line, but error protection protocols can help ensure the integrity of the transmitted data.

The fastest-growing computer-based communications medium is the Internet. A growing number of countries have local connections to the Internet, which can send any data (including E-mail messages or computer files) for

---

Country Study 46.4 Computerizing CONAMAD, Peru's Drug Regulatory Authority

Peru introduced drug registration in 1961, and by 1986, data on 4,200 products were stored in a manual card index system. The data were sorted according to brand name and a locally developed pharmacological classification system of 220 groups. Finding all products with a certain active ingredient was a time-consuming activity: all 4,200 cards had to be screened individually.

The Peruvian authorities' desire to implement a new national drug policy made quick and easy access to these data mandatory. The decision was made to computerize the manual card system, and the necessary computer hardware and a short-term expert were chosen to develop the software with drug regulatory agency (DRA) staff and Ministry of Health (MOH) programmers.

A needs analysis was done, and a computer with locally available hardware support and maintenance was selected. An uninterruptible power supply and a tape backup were added to protect the equipment and data. A database software program popular at the time, dBASE III+, was chosen, because it was already known to programmers in the DRA. The MOH was already using the same database software for a national drug price control program and a Pan American Health Organization program to exchange and control prices of imported raw materials.

A custom program, PERUDIS, was developed by the consultant and the local staff during four visits over a two-month period. The pharmacists and administrative staff who had described the specifications tested the menu-driven program and gave constant feedback on flaws and possible expansions.

Standardized reports can be made using the menu, including lists of all products containing a particular ingredient, lists of products that must be reregistered, and lists of products from a certain manufacturer. The program also has different levels of password-controlled access and safeguards built in to protect the integrity of the data.

Entry and cleaning of data on 4,200 products took nine months. The system became operational by the end of October 1987. Since 1989, MOH programmers have adapted the system to local needs and rewritten it for use in the local area network of the MOH.

Some of the main lessons learned were the importance of allowing ample time for computerization, computerizing only properly functioning manual systems, developing software in close cooperation with users, and planning carefully to ensure that the right classification and coding systems are selected.

In 1989, the PERUDIS software was rewritten in English and installed as ZIMDIS in Zimbabwe. In 1991, WHO took over the further development of DRA software, and the program is now called SIAMED. It is available free of charge for national DRAs from the WHO Division of Drug Management and Policies in Geneva.

Drug Information

Traditional sources of drug information are journals and textbooks such as those listed in Chapter 30. However, maintaining an up-to-date library of texts and journals is costly, and information is not easily accessed.

Computers can greatly facilitate access to drug information. For example, MEDLINE, a nonprofit service of the US National Library of Medicine, provides access to more than six million articles from 3,000 medical journals. The more commonly used and readily available computer databases for drug information are listed and discussed in more detail in Chapter 30.

CD-ROM is relatively inexpensive technology that can store about 680 megabytes of data on one compact disk. A subset of MEDLINE can be obtained on CD-ROM disks, which can be read and printed by computers equipped with a CD-ROM drive.

Through powerful indexing routines and huge storage capacity, CD-ROMs permit very fast access to drug information. Books such as *Martindale: The Extra Pharmacopoeia*, the *British National Formulary*, Meyler's *Side Effects of Drugs*, *Physicians' Desk Reference*, and *USP Drug Information* are already available in CD-ROM format. CD-ROMs with drug information or advice for poisoning are used in many pharmacies and drug information centers in industrialized countries, and use is spreading quickly around the world as computers become more widely available.

≡ 46.5 Building a Drug Master File in a Database

This section describes essential concepts for building the main reference file in a database (that is, the drug master file).

Drug Master File

Common to nearly all forms of database management is a master file, which includes features for drug management such as drug name, strength, dosage form, and therapeutic category. For procurement and inventory control systems, the drug master file usually has supplementary information on cost and pack size. The full description of a product can be split into database fields to sort and classify the data (see Figure 46.5).

Figure 46.10 briefly describes the information commonly contained in a basic drug master file. The development of this file should be carefully planned around several issues, including product coding systems, definition of units, and identification of supplier-specific products.

only a fraction of the cost of a telephone connection. Once the connection is available, Internet use is relatively inexpensive, especially for universities and governments. Instead of a telephone number, the Internet uses character-based E-mail addresses (for example, dmp@msh-dc.org for the MSH Drug Management Program). The two basic user approaches to the Internet are via standard E-mail software (either stand-alone or part of a commercial service such as Compuserve) and via browser software to access the World Wide Web. As of 1996, access to the Web is not available in all countries but is increasing exponentially. Popular browser software programs such as Netscape Navigator and Microsoft Explorer contain both E-mail and Web capacity. New versions are released regularly and can be obtained by downloading them from the Internet. Box 46.1 contains information about HealthNet, a low-cost international network that may be of assistance.

In recent years, discussion groups have formed to exchange information via the Internet. For example, E-DRUG is a discussion group that uses regular E-mail to exchange information on essential drugs management issues. PharmWeb is a World Wide Web site that offers information on worldwide pharmacy and pharmaceutical management issues and organizations. PharmWeb links the user to various Web sites maintained by organizations active in the field. See Annex 46.1 for contact information for E-DRUG and PharmWeb.

Figure 46.10 Standard Information in a Master Drug Data File

Description	Example	Explanation
Product code	AMP250C	Each entry in the drug data file must have a unique code. (See text for discussion of coding options.)
Generic name	Ampicillin	The official international nonproprietary name (INN) is generally preferred. The WHO *Model List of Essential Drugs*, which is regularly updated, uses the INN.
Strength	250 mg	The International System of Units (SI), with related SI abbreviations, should be used. "Strength" can be split into "strength number" (250, for example) and "strength unit" (such as mg), but this often creates unnecessary confusion and coding difficulties.
Route of administration	PO	Standard abbreviations should be used. For example, PO = per os (oral), IV = intravenous, TOP = topical.
Dosage form	CAP	Standard abbreviations should be used. For example, CAP = capsule, TAB = tablet.
Issue unit	CAP	The smallest unit by which a drug can be conveniently distributed. (See text for further explanation.)
Defined daily dosage (DDD)	4	The usual total daily therapeutic dosage for an adult. In computer systems, this is best defined in terms of issue unit per DDD.
DDD unit	gm	The unit in which the DDD is measured.
National essential drugs list (EDL)/formulary status	Y	Is the drug listed in the national EDL or formulary? Y = yes, N = no.
Therapeutic class	44:29	It is useful to categorize drugs by therapeutic or pharmacologic class. Several systems exist, including the ATC, BNF, AFHS, and PAHO systems, and that used for the WHO *Model List of Essential Drugs*. (See Chapter 30 for further discussion of therapeutic category systems.)
Prescription status	POM	Status for retail sales. For example, POM = prescription-only medicine, OTC = over-the-counter.
Level of care	A	National EDLs may categorize drugs according to level of care. For example, A = all levels, B = all levels except dispensary, and so forth.
ABC classification	A	Classification of a drug as A, B, or C according to the volume consumed and unit cost. (See Chapter 41 for discussion of ABC analysis.)
VEN classification	V	Classification of a drug as V, E, or N, according to its therapeutic value as vital, essential, or nonessential. (See Chapter 41 for discussion of the VEN system.)
WHO status	M	Is the drug on the WHO *Model List of Essential Drugs*? This can be listed as Y (yes) or N (no). It can also be listed as M (main), C (complementary), E (therapeutically equivalent), or N (not on the list).

Drug Master File Code

A computer program must be able to identify each drug product quickly and without confusion. Once a coding system has been chosen, it must be maintained without ambiguity, or duplication will occur. There are many options for coding systems. The simplest system is the "dummy" code, which has no intrinsic meaning—for example, 12345 is assigned to the first item entered in the list, 12346 for the second, and so on. With this system, the only question is how many digits are needed; the key point is that the code should be unique. In most systems, a five-digit code is sufficient for many years. If there is a large number of different items, a six-digit code might be prudent.

A more complex option is an "information-bearing" code, in which each digit has significance—for example, ampicillin 500 mg capsules might be coded as AMP500C.

In some countries, formal information-bearing codes have been developed at the national level for drug products. An example is the nine-digit National Drug Code in the United States, in which the first four digits signify the manufacturer or labeler, the next three digits show the product, and the last two show the package size.

There are arguments favoring both of these coding options, as well as others. Data entry errors are reduced with more complex coding schemes, but the time required to enter data may be greater. An information-bearing coding scheme takes more time to develop and maintain than a simple numeric code for products. Note that a separate coding scheme will be needed for therapeutic categories, as shown in Figure 46.10. Several international coding systems for drug categories are discussed in Chapter 10.

Figure 46.11 Units in Drug Management

Code	Description	Strength	Form	Issue Unit — Comp. Units per Issue Unit	Comp. Unit	Pack Size — Issue Units per Pack Size	Issue Unit	Min. Order — Pack Size Units per Min. Order	Pack Size	Pack Size Cost	Min. Order Cost	Cost per Issue Unit	Cost per Comp. Unit
AMP250T	Ampicillin	250 mg	Tab	1	Tab	1,000	Tab	5	Bottle	34.00	170.00	0.0340 per tab	0.0340 per tab
PIL2OD	Pilocarpine	2%	Drops	15	mL	12	Dropper	1	Box	17.52	17.52	1.4600 per dropper	0.0973 per mL
BNT0T	Bacitracin + neomycin	USP	Oint	3.5	gm	100	Tube	1	Box	100.00	100.00	1.0000 per tube	0.2857 per gm
NACL09I	Sodium chloride	0.9%	Inj	1,000	mL	12	Vial	10	Box	1.56	15.60	0.1300 per vial	0.0001 per mL
AMP500I	Ampicillin	500 mg	Inj	1	Vial	100	Vial	1	Box	30.00	30.00	0.3000 per vial	0.3000 per vial
PEN5MI	Penicillin	2 MU	Inj	1	Vial	12	Vial	6	Box	6.00	36.00	0.5000 per vial	0.5000 per vial
COD0S	Codeine	USP	Syrup	500	mL	1	Bottle	6	Box	7.00	42.00	7.0000 per bottle	0.0140 per mL
SAL200S	Salbutamol	100 mcg per dose	Inh	200	Doses	1	Inhaler	100	Box	2.70	270.00	2.7000 per inhaler	0.0135 per dose
COND0L	Condom	—	Disp	1	Condom	100	Condom	10	Box	1.50	15.00	0.0150 per condom	0.0150 per condom
BIS10S	Bisacodyl	10 mg	Supp	1	Supp	12	Supp	10	Box	10.00	100.00	0.8333 per supp	0.8333 per supp
AL90L	Alcohol	95%	Liq	1	Liter	210	Liter	1	Drum	100.00	100.00	0.4762 per liter	0.4762 per liter
JEL0J	Jelly, lubricating	BP	Jel	142	gm	12	Tubes	1	Box	100.00	100.00	8.3333 per tube	0.0587 per gm
GLOV7D	Glove	7	Disp	2	Glove	50	Pair	1	Box	100.00	100.00	2.0000 per pair	1.0000 per glove
NED21G	Needle	21 g	Disp	1	Needle	100	Needle	10	Box	10.00	100.00	0.1000 per needle	0.1000 per needle

Health Problem Coding

Health problem information must be coded for diagnosis-specific drug use analysis and morbidity quantification of drug requirements. The accepted standard is the WHO *International Classification of Diseases* (ICD-10), a hierarchical classification based on major and minor disease categories, which is available on diskette. Most information systems are now based on the ICD system, although local adaptations often result in different groupings of individual health problems.

Definition of Units

When computerizing drug systems, considerable confusion can arise over the definition of units. For example, in the preliminary quantification exercise for a large essential drugs project, requirements for benzyl benzoate (a topical preparation for skin infestations) were calculated in milliliters, whereas the essential drugs list specified liters. This led to a 1,000-fold error that increased estimated drug requirements by US$1 million.

Defining the basic unit, issue unit, defined daily dose unit, pack size, and minimum order can help avoid major mistakes.

Basic or Comparison Unit. The basic unit is the smallest unit in which a drug can be conveniently dispensed or administered. It is also used to compare prices of different sized bottles or vials. The total number of basic or comparison units is equal to one issue unit. For example, 100 tablets make up one bottle, with the tablet as the basic unit and the bottle as the issue unit.

Issue Unit. The issue unit is used to count and distribute the stock. It allows the comparison of items of different pack sizes but the same issue unit. The total number of issue units per pack is equal to one pack size.

Pack Size. In procurement, the pack size is used to request bids. Suppliers usually give the product cost for a pack size.

See Figure 46.11 for more examples of units. Individual computer systems may handle these concepts differently, but managers of drug programs must be thoroughly familiar with the problems of defining drug units. Unambiguous local definitions must be established, and everyone involved in recording, entering, verifying, or using the computer data must be trained to use these definitions.

≡ 46.6 Maintenance and Support Requirements

Using computers, like any electronic tool, requires access to reputable repair services and supplies. Even more important, however, is a reliable, adequately trained staff.

Staff Recruitment and Training

Discussions about starting computerization often focus only on software and hardware, but computers are useless without competent staff to run them. Recruitment and training are key to maintaining good computer services, particularly when day-to-day operations such as inventory management and accounting are to be computerized.

Experienced typists interested in learning new skills can be recruited for word-processing and data entry tasks. Computer courses are now available in many countries. The cost of courses should be built into computerization budgets, along with sufficient funds each year to train new staff and retrain old staff in new software.

When specialized drug management programs are installed by outside organizations, they must provide adequate training that is spread out over time so that staff can raise their own questions as they become familiar with the new system.

At least two people need to be familiar with each specific computer program and operation so that sickness, annual leave, or job changes will not bring the computer unit to a halt.

Protecting Data

Data in a computer are stored on magnetic media, such as a hard disk or floppy diskette. Unfortunately, magnetic storage media can lose data, so other precautions must be taken. The computer, along with all data on the hard drive, might be stolen or could be harmed by dust or high-voltage electrical spikes.

Data can also be damaged by a computer virus when programs or data are exchanged via diskettes. This risk increases when illegally copied (pirated) software is used. A virus can result in anything from harmless messages appearing unexpectedly on the computer screen to complete loss of data on the hard drive. To avoid getting a computer virus, accept diskettes only from users who take precautions against viruses, use virus checker software that automatically scans the computer's hard drive every day, and check floppy diskettes. Regular updates of virus checker programs are needed because new viruses are created continually.

Floppy diskettes can be damaged by magnetic fields (from loudspeakers, telephones, and metal detectors), and by moisture, particles, and dust. Thus, having only one copy of data is risky, and the importance of making backup copies cannot be overemphasized. Basic rules for maintaining backups are:

- Make at least one backup copy of all important work when it is created.
- Back up routine work daily with separate sets of diskettes or tapes used in rotation for extra security, especially for large databases such as inventory control systems.

Figure 46.12 Lessons for Successful Computerization

- Assess what software is needed before choosing hardware.
- Ensure software and hardware compatibility.
- Secure local support for hardware and software.
- Have a well-functioning manual system.
- Provide adequate staff training and involve staff in the computerization process.
- Computerize in phases, allowing sufficient time for each step.
- Establish and enforce strict procedures for data and equipment protection, using backups, virus checkers, restricted access, surge suppressors, and so on.
- Set aside adequate funds in each year's budget for hardware and software maintenance, supplies, and staff training.
- Plan and budget for timely hardware and software upgrades.

- Ideally, store backups off-site to guard them from fire or theft. Consider saving and archiving an entire set of data at the end of each month or quarter.

Access to computers should be restricted to authorized staff; most computer operating systems and software can be protected with passwords, which are required to enter the system (and which allow managers to track use of the computer).

Maintaining Computers

Computers are adversely affected by humidity, static electricity, extreme temperatures, dust, cigarette smoke, and food or liquid spilled on the keyboards. In addition, continuous display of the same screen can cause an image to "burn into" the screen, where it will always appear as a shadow. Computers are also vulnerable to frequent switching on and off, sudden physical movements while the hard disk is running, misuse by untrained staff, and unprofessional repair attempts. To protect computers:

- Make sure that a reliable firm (or government department) is under contract to support hardware and software.
- Train all operators in proper computer handling.
- Protect the computer room with air-conditioning—if possible—against excess heat, humidity, and dust.
- Do not eat or drink near the computer or smoke in the computing room.
- Protect keyboard, monitor, and computer with covers.
- Do not set the brightness of the monitor too high (make the room a bit darker, if needed) and use a "screen saver" (which changes the screen display regularly after a certain period of inactivity).
- Always use spike/surge protectors (for computer, printer, and fax) and an uninterruptible power supply.

≡ Assessment Guide

Use of Computers in Drug Management

► In which phases of drug management will computerization be most useful: drug selection and formulary development, registration, quantification of drug requirements, procurement, inventory control, prescription analysis, other areas?

► Does a drug master file exist? Has a coding system been developed to uniquely identify drug products? Is the ICD or other coding system used to identify health problems?

Readiness for Computerization or Expansion

► Are computers currently used for producing correspondence, newsletters, reports? Preparation of tables, graphs, charts? Budgets and other spreadsheet applications? Electronic communications?

► Do good manual systems exist for drug management functions?

► Are staff capable of and interested in learning to operate computers?

► Are resources available for staff training? Supplies such as diskettes, paper, and print ribbons? Computer support and periodic upgrades, as needed?

Computerization Planning

► Have needs been identified and the specific tasks, functions, and systems to be computerized carefully analyzed?

► Has appropriate software been identified, for example, for word processing, spreadsheets, database management, and/or special functions such as presentation graphics, project management, accounting, or electronic communications?

► Is training available for each software package? Are manuals or other instruction books available?

► Have hardware specifications been defined in terms of operating system, microprocessor speed, available RAM, storage capacity, monitor, printer, modem, uninterruptible power supply? Is this hardware capable of running the software identified?

► Has the computerization process been planned in phases, so that experience with computer applications will develop in parallel with broad systems development?

► Have procedures been developed for data and equipment protection, such as restricted access, use of an uninterruptible power supply and surge suppressors, virus checking, backing up data files, and storing backups off-site?

Hardware and Software Support and Maintenance

► Is there a firm in the country or area that sells software and provides support? Does this firm provide training in use of the software?

► Is there a firm in the country or area that sells and maintains computer hardware?

► Is there a government agency or department that can provide support services to the supply system?

Car batteries with an inverter or a separate fuel generator may also provide safe electrical power.

► Move the computer only when it is switched off.

► Use reliable maintenance and repair services.

≡ 46.7 Lessons for Successful Computerization in Drug Management

Successful computerization in drug management can greatly increase an organization's efficiency, productivity, and capabilities, but it must be carefully planned. It is easy to make expensive mistakes through a lack of knowledge or forethought, thereby hindering rather than helping a project. Following the list in Figure 46.12, and considering the issues raised earlier in this chapter, will help a manager avoid or prevent such mistakes. The information presented in this chapter should enable a manager to ask the right questions and effectively plan the computerization of an organization. ∎

≡ Glossary

Apple: Company that made one of the first personal microcomputers. It now makes the Macintosh and Power Macintosh lines of computers.

Backup: An extra copy of software or data, normally kept on file in case the original program is damaged or lost.

Baud: A measure of the speed at which data travels (normally between a computer and a peripheral).

Bit: A binary digit (1 or 0).

Bug: A flaw or problem in a software program.

Byte: A sequence of bits that represents a single character. In most small computers, a byte is eight bits.

CD-ROM (compact disk read-only memory): A medium for storing large amounts of data that can be accessed quickly and selectively using a CD-ROM drive. CD-ROMs are less vulnerable to damage than diskettes.

Chip: A generic term for an integrated circuit, a single package holding thousands of microscopic electronic components. The processor of a computer is one.

CPU (central processing unit): The "brain" of the computer, which directs and processes input and output.

Data: Numerical or verbal representations of facts that are processed to produce information.

Database: A collection of related data that can be retrieved and manipulated by a computer.

Debug: To go through a program to remove mistakes.

Density (double, high): Describes how much information can be stored on a storage medium.

Disk: A round piece of magnetic-coated material used to store data.

Disk drive: Part of a computer that reads data from, or writes data to, a disk.

Diskette: Small, removable disk with a layer of magnetic material that can store information. Also called a "floppy." The usual sizes are 3.5 inches and 5.25 inches in diameter.

Dot matrix printer: A printer that produces lower-quality output than a laser printer. The twenty-four-pin printers produce better-quality print than the nine-pin varieties. This type of printer is the best type for printing on multiple kinds of paper.

Downtime: Any period when a computer is not available or not working.

Field: In a database, the basic column unit, in which the same type of information appears.

File: An organized collection of bytes stored on disk, maintained by the operating system, and referenced by name.

Hard disk: A nonremovable, fast-spinning, rigid piece of equipment made of stainless steel with a magnetic layer, which stores huge amounts of data inside a computer.

Hardware: The physical equipment of a computer system, such as the computer, monitor, and printer. Useless without software.

IBM-compatible: Description of a computer that is functionally identical to the microcomputers standardized by International Business Machines.

Inkjet printer: A type of printer with print quality between that of a dot matrix printer and a laser printer.

Laptop/notebook: Small computer that incorporates the CPU, monitor, and keyboard in one unit and can run on batteries. A notebook computer is smaller than a laptop.

Laser printer: A type of printer that uses laser technology to produce very high print quality.

Mainframe: Big, powerful, expensive computer, usually used by universities and the military. Usually not necessary for managing drug supplies.

Memory: Circuitry and devices that hold the bits the computer can access. Examples are RAM (random-access memory) and ROM (read-only memory).

Minicomputer: Smaller than a mainframe but still too big or costly for an individual; may be useful for storing large amounts of data in a central medical store.

Modem: An electronic device that allows computer equipment to send and receive information through telephone lines.

Monitor: A TV-like display used with most computers to show the information being input and output.

Motherboard: The board containing the computer's circuitry, onto which all other parts of the CPU are attached.

Mouse: A small, mobile manual device that controls movement of the cursor and selection of the function on a computer display.

MS-DOS (Microsoft Disk Operating System): The most widely used operating system; usually has a version number.

Network: An interconnected system of computers. The components do not have to be physically close to one another—they can be connected by telephone or data lines.

Operating system: Software that oversees the overall operation of a computer system. It enables other software to communicate with the hardware and must be present for the computer to function.

Peripherals: Equipment (usually hardware) that is external to the computer itself. Examples are tape drives and speakers.

Power spikes/surges: Major fluctuations in electrical current that can disrupt the computer's internal operation and damage hardware.

Printer: A device to produce hard-copy output.

RAM (random-access memory): The main type of memory used in microcomputers, also known as read/write memory because data in RAM can be easily changed.

Record: One entry, or row, in a database.

ROM (read-only memory): Memory where information is permanently stored and cannot be altered. This form of memory is also random access.

Scanner: A piece of hardware that reads information from text or images and converts it into digital form for a computer to use.

Server: The main computer on a network; provides storage and processing capabilities for client computers.

Software: Programs or segments of programs.

Spreadsheet: A program for calculating and linking numbers.

Virus: An undesirable program that displays bizarre messages on the screen or printer or destroys data on the computer. Transferred mainly by sharing diskettes without testing them first with antivirus software.

Sources: Berge et al. 1986; Computer Associates 1992.

≡ References and Further Readings

Ankrapp, B., and Di Lama, S. 1996. *HealthCare software source-book*. Gaithersburg, Md.: Aspen.

Berge, N., M. D. Ingle, and M. Hamilton. 1986. *Microcomputers in development: A manager's guide*. West Hartford, Conn.: Kumarian Press.

Brown, M. 1996. *Using Netscape 3*. Indianapolis, Ind.: Que Corp.

Burch, J. G., and G. Grudnitski. 1989. *Information systems: Theory and practice*. New York: John Wiley and Sons.

Computer Associates. 1992. *CA-Clipper programming and utilities guide for DOS, version 5.2*. Islandia, N.Y.: Computer Associates International.

D'Emanuele, A. 1996. The communications revolution. *International Pharmacy Journal* 10(4):129–34.

Knorr, E., ed. 1995. *The PC bible*, 2d ed. Berkeley, Ca.: Peachpit Press.

Management Sciences for Health (MSH). Using electronic communications in family planning. *Family Planning Manager* 5(2):1–30 and supplement, A primer for accessing and using electronic communications technology, 1–13.

Omara, M., and G. Routledge. 1996. *Using your PC*, 2d ed. Indianapolis, Ind.: Que Corp.

Richardson, P. 1993. Computers (manager's guide). In *Primary health care management advancement programme*. Geneva: Aga Khan Foundation (PO Box 6179, CH-1211, Geneva 6, Switzerland).

Coding Systems

Gouveia, W. A. 1972. A mnemonic drug coding system. *American Journal of Hospital Pharmacy* 29:248–49.

International Classification of Diseases (ICD-10-CM). 1995. Books or tape. Geneva: World Health Organization.

International nonproprietary names (INN) for pharmaceutical substances. 1988. Cumulative list no. 7. Regularly updated. Geneva: World Health Organization. (INN names on diskette available in SIAMED or from WHO/DMP.)

McEvoy, G., ed. 1995. *AHFS: American Hospital Formulary Service drug information*. Bethesda, Md.: American Society of Health-System Pharmacists.

NLN Newsletter (about ATC/DDD methodologies, training, and so forth). Nordic Council on Medicines and WHO Collaborating Center for Drug Statistics Methodology, PO Box 100 Veivet, N-0518 Oslo 5, Norway.

PAHO (Pan American Health Organization). PAHO drug classification system. PAHO/HSS Washington, D.C.: PAHO.

WHO Collaborating Centre for Drug Statistics Methodology. 1993a. *Guidelines for ATC classification*, 4th ed. Oslo. Nordic Council on Medicines and WHO Collaborating Center for Drug Statistics Methodology (PO Box 100 Veivet, N-0518 Oslo 5, Norway). ATC codes also available on diskette/tape.

WHO Collaborating Centre for Drug Statistics Methodology. 1993b. *Guidelines for DDD*, 2d ed. Oslo: WHO.

Annex 46.1 Drug-Related Computer Applications

Computer Applications

Drug Interaction Program. 1991. *The medical letter.* Updated regularly.

Epi Info 6.0 integrated software. 1994. WHO/CDC.

INTDIS. ADR search software and manual. 1994. WHO Collaborating Center for International Drug Monitoring.

MEDLINE. Database of medical literature, accessible on-line through Datastar, Dialog, or NLM. CD-ROM version through Silver Platter. Contact MEDLARS Management Section Service Desk at 800-638-8480 for Grateful Med search engine information from the US Department of Health and Human Services.

MSH (Management Sciences for Health). Software programs developed by MSH, with free manuals available.

CLM. Commodities and Logistics Management software program. 1994.

ECPRO-2. Tendering and procurement software program. 1995.

INVEC-2. Inventory and tender management program and manual. 1995.

PASS. Prescription Analysis Software System. 1995.

PASS and the drug price guide are freestanding programs, available on request; the other programs require trained installation assistance but are available in demonstration copies. Contact the MSH Drug Management Program at 1655 N. Ft. Myer Dr., Suite 920, Arlington, Va. 22209, US, or E-mail to dmp@msh-dc.org.

MSH/INRUD (Management Sciences for Health/International Network for Rational Use of Drugs). 1994. *Drug use bibliography.* Brochure or software (using Reference Manager software). Updated regularly.

Pharmaceutical Society. *British national formulary* (BNF). Updated every six months. Paperback or CD-ROM.

QUANTED. Drug quantification software and user manual. 1989. WHO/DAP.

SIAMED. Software and draft user manual for the WHO model software package for drug regulatory authorities. 1994. WHO/DMP Geneva and PAHO/HSS Washington.

SUMA. Supply management project software for use in disaster relief efforts. 1995. PAHO.

SWEDIS. Comprehensive drug management software with modules for drug registration, inventory control, procurement, E-mail (DISNET), and so on. Pharmasoft Swedis AB, PO Box 1237, S-75142 Uppsala, Sweden.

Internet Contacts

E-DRUG

Worldwide ongoing E-mail conference. To subscribe, send E-mail to: majordomo@usa.healthnet.org. Leave the subject line blank. Your message should read: "Subscribe e-drug [your E-mail address]."

HealthNet

John J. Mullaney
Executive Director
SatelLife
1360 Soldiers Field Rd.
Boston, Mass. 02135
Muriel Hodges, Project Manager
mhodges@usa.healthnet.org
Tel.: 617-789-5455, ext. 104; fax: 617-789-4771
To view the Web site: http://www.healthnet.org
To send E-mail via the Internet: info@usa.healthnet.org

Management Sciences for Health

Drug Management Program
To view the Web site: http://www.msh.org
To send E-mail via the Internet: dmp@msh-dc.org

PharmWeb

World Wide Web site with pharmacy-related information and links to other sites maintained by organizations active in drug management. To view the Web site: http://www.pharmweb.net. To send E-mail via the Internet: pharmweb-admin@man.ac.uk.

World Health Organization

Action Programme on Essential Drugs
Information on DAP's political and administrative components, including its mandate, management approach, and worldwide projects, and on its technical components and services. These include national drug policies, indicators, drug information and documentation, rational drug use, training courses, and publications, including the *Essential Drugs Monitor.* To view the Web site: http://www.who.ch; choose DAP under WHO PROGRAMMES. Selected documents and publications can easily be downloaded from the DAP Web page. To send E-mail via the Internet: dapmail@who.ch (there is an E-mail link from the WHO Web page as well).

Drug Management and Policies
Information on drug regulatory affairs, national drug regulatory authorities, safety, and quality control. Many publications can be downloaded or ordered from the WHO Publications Sales department. To view the Web site: http://www.who.ch; select DMP under WHO PROGRAMMES. To send E-mail via the Internet: dmpmail@who.ch (there is an E-mail link from the WHO Web page as well).

Part I	Part II	Part III	Part IV
Introduction	Policy and Legal Framework	Drug Management Cycle	**Management Support Systems**
			A Organization and Management
			B Financing and Sustainability
			C Information Management
			D Human Resources Management

Section D

Human Resources Management

| Part I | Part II | Part III | Part IV |
| Introduction | Policy and Legal Framework | Drug Management Cycle | **Management Support Systems** |

A Organization and Management
B Financing and Sustainability
C Information Management

D Human Resources Management ▶ **47 Personnel Management**

48 Designing and Implementing Training Programs

Chapter 47
Personnel Management

≡ Summary

Managing people is an important and challenging task for any manager. Different leadership styles—directive, consulting, or avoiding—may be required in different situations. Multiple channels of communication may be used.

There are several ways to select staff to fill positions within an organization. Although norm-based staffing is commonly used, workload-based staffing is generally more effective. Job descriptions are required for each position, and new employees require orientation and training.

Employees are motivated by many factors that can be affected by management. Supervision should be supportive and requires various skills to be effective. A range of supervisory methods is available. Conflict resolution is an inevitable part of personnel management, with various styles for use in different situations. An effective manager also delegates authority and responsibility carefully. Conducting effective meetings and managing time are other skills that a manager requires.

Good management is to organization what health is to the body—the smooth functioning of all its parts. It highlights priorities, adapts services to needs and changing situations, makes the most of limited resources, improves the standard and quality of services, and maintains high staff morale.

—McMahon et al. 1992, 3

≡ Management was described in Chapter 34 as the process of using human, financial, and other resources to achieve results. Important aspects of planning, implementation, monitoring, and evaluation were considered in Chapters 34, 35, and 36. Several of these aspects, including work planning, relate directly to personnel management and should be kept in mind. This chapter focuses on specific skills required for managing people.

≡ 47.1 Leadership Styles

Being a manager means being a leader, in one sense or another. Three leadership styles can be clearly distinguished: directing, consulting, avoiding. These styles define the way in which managers interact with their staff to formulate plans, make decisions, and solve problems.

A *directing manager* recognizes that a problem needs attention, decides what to do about it, and communicates that decision to the staff group. This management style involves giving orders and expecting compliance.

When a *consulting manager* notices a problem, he or she first makes sure that the staff are aware of the situation and then engages them in a discussion about alternative courses of action and ideas for possible solutions.

An *avoiding manager* takes a passive, "leave-them-alone" approach. Problems are left to work themselves out. The manager has spotted a problem but chooses to do nothing about it. There are occasions when avoidance might be the best policy—for example, when a problem is so trivial that it is not worth spending time on, or when taking action might only inflame an otherwise contained situation.

Most people say that they prefer to be in groups led by a consulting-style manager. This is not surprising, given the way control is exercised and the manner in which the "climate" is set in both groups. Figure 47.1 compares the ways meetings tend to be conducted with directing versus consulting managers.

Although staff may prefer a consulting manager, in many countries, directing managers predominate. The reasons, no doubt, depend on many factors:

► Lack of exposure to more modern approaches to management—this is especially true of older managers;
► Prevalence of more directive models of leadership within family and social groups;
► Lack of confidence in personal ability and a resultant fear of being shown up in open discussion.

People may also believe that efficiency can come only with a brusque and uncompromising style of leadership. However, it is important to follow the first rule of management: *you can never manage an organization alone.* For this reason, the consulting style is often the most effective.

The objectives of most organizations can be met only through combined efforts. The staff will be more motivated to work together if they are led by a manager who is not afraid to ask for their opinions and is ready to accept and use their ideas. A work group becomes a team if manager and staff

► communicate openly
► share information
► discuss and agree on strategies
► set targets
► have tea or coffee together

In doing these things, a manager will convert a work group into a team.

Figure 47.1 Different Management Styles in the Conduct of Meetings

	Directing Manager	Consulting Manager
Control	► By controlling the behavior of the members, the leader operates as if he or she owns the group. ► Leader uses conventional committee procedures to keep order. ► Decisions are usually made by the leader after minimal consultation.	► Staff can influence the direction the meeting takes. ► Staff are encouraged to express ideas and conduct business in a flexible manner. ► Decisions are made collectively as often as possible.
Climate	► Leader tries to suppress expression of feelings and views that might differ from his or hers. ► All conflict is avoided. ► Behavior the leader regards as disruptive is handled outside the group.	► Members are not discouraged from expressing feelings and opinions. ► Conflicts with the leader's views are accepted. ► Problems among group members are faced within the group.

≡ 47.2 Channels of Communication

The previous section implies that effective managers have good communication skills, but no set formula will work every time. Five main channels used in interpersonal communication are set out, with their positive and negative aspects, in Figure 47.2.

Choosing the Channel

The key factor in communication is deciding which of the five channels should be used in any given situation. Two basic skills help in communicating with others: the ability to use all five channels and the sensitivity to choose the most appropriate channel on any particular occasion. Relating this communication model to the analysis of leadership styles, it is clear that the directing style relies mainly on the first channel (controlling), whereas the consulting style uses all the channels at different times, as appropriate.

Nonverbal Communication

Effective communicators have the ability to alternate among the five channels like nimble telephone switchboard operators. However, unlike using the telephone, where only the voice is important, interpersonal communication involves both words and body language. Therefore, a good manager must be aware of factors such as posture, gestures, and facial expressions.

Improving Communication

A manager can improve communication with staff in a number of ways:

Clarify ideas before attempting to communicate them: Good communication depends on clear thinking. Think about how best to express the idea and what format to use (for example, a formal circular, an informal memo, or a talk), and try to assess its likely impact.

Follow up on any communication: Good communication depends on feedback. Ask questions and encourage reactions.

Be a good listener: Good communication also depends on good listening. Careful attention to what people say helps one know what is best to say to them.

The rest of this chapter addresses some of the main functions of personnel management—staff selection, motivation, supervision, and meetings—in light of what has been said about leadership and communication.

≡ 47.3 Choosing Staff

Determining the staffing requirements of a drug program means taking into account factors such as the size of the program and its goals, location, and place within the agency of which it is a part. Three interrelated questions can be used for an initial determination of staffing requirements:

1. What is the scope of the services to be offered in relation to the selection, procurement, distribution, and use of pharmaceuticals?
2. What different types of workers are required at each level of the system?
3. What is the optimal number of employees needed to deliver these services in the most efficient and effective manner?

There can be considerable variation in administrative arrangements, even within one agency or government. For example, drug selection and use may fall under the purview of the ministry of health, whereas procurement and distribution may be handled by a different ministry responsible for supplies. There are also many options in linkages with drug supply sources. If pharmaceutical

Figure 47.2 Comparison of Communication Channels

Channel	Examples	Positive Aspects	Negative Aspects
Controlling—used when telling someone what to do, giving an order, or making a criticism	"Do it this way." "No, not that way, silly!"	Can provide necessary direction	Can result in inflexible dictating
Caring—used when expressing concern for someone's welfare	"How are you today, Aziz?" "Don't worry—it will be OK."	Can be nurturing	May become unasked-for smothering
Computing—used when giving, processing, or exchanging information; when reasoning, measuring, calculating; when thinking as opposed to feeling	"If we allow too many exemptions, the revolving drug fund will collapse." "On average, how many patients attend this health center per day?"	Necessary calculations may provide an objective viewpoint	May come across as thoughtless lack of feeling or compassion
Complying—used in "editing" what we say; when conforming to the wishes of another person; when adapting our behavior in light of the likely reactions of the other person	"Would you mind if I ...?" "I'm sorry, I won't do it again."	May be polite accommodation	May be undignified subservience
Expressing—used when spontaneously expressing feelings of pleasure or pain; having fun, expressing humor, sharing a joke	"Great—that was really great!" "Ouch!"	Displays honest emotions	May result in selfishness and egotistical behavior

procurement and distribution are provided directly by a government agency, then all jobs may be performed by government staff. If the central procurement office is limited to negotiating with commercial suppliers for direct delivery to health facilities, then most of the importation, bulk inventory control, and bulk storage occur within the private sector.

No matter how the organizational structure and contractual arrangements are defined, all the tasks and related jobs must be performed if the drug supply system is to operate reliably and expeditiously. An organizational chart describing the relationships among different staff positions is very useful.

Calculating and justifying the number of drug management staff needed can be difficult. The *norms approach*, which specifies a standard staffing level, or norm, for each staff cadre, quickly breaks down in practice. For example, a norm that says that each regional store needs three supplies officers will result in overstaffing at small regional stores and understaffing at busier stores.

The *workload approach* to staffing is based on the activities, volume of work (workload), and activity standards for each type of staff at each level. This is known as the WISN, or workload indicator of staffing need, approach (Shipp 1993).

Country Study 47.1 illustrates the workload standards set for hospital pharmacy staff in Kenya. In this example, the work of pharmacy staff was found to consist of three main activities: supplying inpatient wards, dispensing to outpatients, and operating the sterile preparation unit. Standards set for each of these activities (ninety outpatients per day per pharmacy staff member, for example)

make it possible to calculate the number of staff needed for each facility.

The WISN method is generally a much more realistic approach for determining staffing needs than the norms approach. Because it is based on actual workload, results from the WISN method are more readily explained and defended.

≡ 47.4 Job Descriptions

One of the most important functions of a drug supplies manager is to ensure that the tasks of the organization are distributed equitably. This involves matching the jobs that need to be done with the skills and abilities of the individuals who make up the workforce. Each position should have a written job description and a summary of duties and responsibilities.

Job descriptions are important management tools. They are helpful in

▶ determining job qualifications, because the tasks to be performed in a particular job determine the necessary skills and experience;

▶ orienting new employees, because the written job description explains basic duties to new employees;

▶ establishing performance expectations and supervising staff.

Format for a Job Description

There is no fixed format for job descriptions, but most have five distinct sections:

Job title: The title gives only the briefest information

needed to identify the job, for example, "director of pharmaceutical services" or "chief supplies officer."

Job summary: A brief paragraph summarizing the main responsibilities of the job.

Duties and responsibilities: The core of the job description is a detailed description of the work to be performed, task by task. It should include the following information:

- Nature of the tasks involved;
- How the tasks are to be carried out;
- Frequency and scheduling of tasks;
- Expected percentage of time to be taken up by each main task;
- Reporting requirements.

Qualifications: A statement of the qualifications and requirements necessary for satisfactory job performance, including education, experience, knowledge, skills, and abilities.

Reporting relationship: The person's supervisor should be listed. Also, it is useful to add a chart that indicates the structure of the organization, particularly if it shows reporting relationships.

An example of a job description for a chief supplies officer is presented in Figure 47.3.

Developing a Job Description

When a job description is outdated or nonexistent, the situation can be remedied by compiling and analyzing information, writing a job description, assigning time allocations, and obtaining agreement on the job description.

Compile Information. There are several ways to obtain the information needed to build a job description:

- Questionnaire about key aspects of the job, completed by the employee;
- Observing and interviewing the employee while various tasks are being performed;
- Group interview when a number of employees perform the same job;
- Daily record of work done, kept by the employee in the form of a log or diary.

Analyze Information. Identify the major tasks and related clusters of minor ones. Review each cluster to ensure that it accurately represents the tasks to be performed. Arrange the main tasks and related minor ones in a logical sequence, to give a clear overview of the job.

Write the Job Description. Group together activities related to one duty, such as planning, budgeting, or supervising. In writing the descriptive statements, use active

Country Study 47.1 Pharmacy Personnel Planning in Kenya

Most pharmacies in Kenya operate with inadequate numbers of pharmacists and pharmaceutical technologists. Workload-based indicators of staffing needs developed by the ministry provide the following staffing guidelines:

- Eight inpatient wards per day can be served by one pharmacy staff member.
- Ninety outpatients per day can be served by one pharmacy staff member.
- Two hundred outpatients can be served by one clerk. (Clerks are essential for maintaining the required user fee records.)

In addition, a sterile preparation unit that produces 100 bottles of 500 mL per day needs two trained subordinate staff and a cleaner. Aside from the supervising hospital pharmacist, the unit needs one permanent pharmaceutical technologist.

Source: Ministry of Health, government of Kenya 1994.

verbs and be concise. Try to avoid any ambiguity or vagueness. If someone is responsible for signing the drug supplies order, state "signs the drug supply order" rather than "approves the drug supplies order."

Each statement should describe one functional element of the job and be able to stand by itself. Normally, duties should be arranged from the most to the least time-consuming, or in order of importance.

Assign Time Allocations. Estimate the percentage of time required for each main task. Work with multiples of 5 percent and check that the total time allocated adds up to 100 percent.

Obtain Agreement. It is good management practice for the immediate supervisor to review the job description with the employee to ensure that the listed duties and responsibilities are mutually understood and accepted. To formalize this process, there should be space for the signatures of both the supervisor and the employee.

Orientation and Training

Every organization has its own culture, a set of goals and expectations, policies and procedures, and norms and standards. Sometimes these are not made explicit, and a written job description alone can never convey all the nuances of a job. It is only one tool in the broader process of orientation and training.

New managers especially need to become familiar with the organization they have joined. There are three essential steps to accomplish this:

1. Explore the new work environment. This means getting acquainted with staff members (both senior and

Figure 47.3 Sample Job Description for a Chief Pharmaceutical Supplies Officer

JOB DESCRIPTION

JOB TITLE: Chief pharmaceutical supplies officer, Pharmaceutical Services, Ministry of Health

JOB SUMMARY: Responsible for the overall operation of the central medical stores unit: ordering and distributing drugs, medical supplies, and other related products; supervising stock control; providing technical inputs to the national drug formulary committee and tender board; and preparing reports on all aspects of the operation of the service.

DUTIES AND RESPONSIBILITIES:

(% of time)

60%   1. Provide drugs, medical supplies, and other products to all government health institutions by
- estimating requirements for drug and nondrug products;
- supervising preparation of drug orders;
- monitoring distribution of drugs and other supplies;
- preparing monthly, quarterly, and annual reports on the status of the service.

20%   2. Supervise the control of drugs and other supplies to ensure continuous availability by
- maintaining an up-to-date inventory control system;
- continually evaluating the logistics management system;
- implementing stock management guidelines and procedures;
- liaising with a drug testing laboratory to monitor drug quality.

10%   3. Provide technical inputs to management, as well as other agencies involved in monitoring the supply of drugs and other products, by
- functioning as a standing representative of the central traders' committee;
- serving as a member of the national formulary committee;
- providing technical information to these committees as required.

10%   4. Administer the dangerous drug component of the pharmaceutical supplies program by
- issuing import certificates covering dangerous drugs;
- ordering, distributing, and monitoring psychotropic and narcotic drugs for government institutions;
- preparing monthly, quarterly, and annual reports on the use of these drugs.

QUALIFICATIONS:

Education:
- pharmacy degree;
- certificate in management.

Knowledge and experience required:
- pharmaceutical principles and practices;
- drug supplies management;
- sources of supply for medical and nonmedical drugs;
- procedures for the estimation and importation of narcotic drugs.

Abilities required:
- forecasting drug supply requirements;
- coordinating drug supply services;
- monitoring the quality of the work of others;
- using computers.

Working conditions:
- work is performed at the central medical stores department.

REPORTING RELATIONSHIP: Responsible to the director of pharmaceutical services

SIGNATURES:

Incumbent _____ Date _____

Director of pharmaceutical services _____ Date _____

junior) as well as the physical location of job sites, outreach services, and training facilities.

2. Review the mission and strategy of the organization. This involves acquiring a sound understanding of the long- and short-term goals of the enterprise; its structure and general mode of operation; and the roles, responsibilities, and functions of the individual members of the workforce.

3. Identify training needs and opportunities. Managers need to do this for themselves as well as for their subordinates.

Before questioning others, good managers need to ask the following questions of themselves:

▶ Do I have a job description?

▶ Have I discussed it with my supervisor?

▶ Am I clear about the objectives of the organization? Can I explain them to others?

▶ How does my department relate to other departments? Can I explain how they relate to mine?

▶ What resources do I have at my disposal to achieve the organizational objectives? Consider buildings, facilities, transport, utilities, medical supplies, finances, and personnel.

▶ Do I have a staff development plan and a personal development plan?

Chapter 48 explores orientation and training in greater detail.

Staff Procedures Handbook

The regulations and rules governing work should be gathered together in a staff handbook that is regularly updated and includes information on

▶ organizational purpose and objectives;

▶ organizational structure;

▶ activities;

▶ address and telephone lists;

▶ safety and health policies;

▶ personnel classifications;

▶ hours of work;

▶ personnel policies, including recruitment, performance planning, and review of records;

▶ ethical standards;

▶ grievance, disciplinary, and termination policies;

▶ salary policies, including overtime;

▶ vacation, holidays, and other leaves;

▶ pension and insurance benefits;

▶ administrative procedures, including communication, travel, procurement, and parking.

Producing a handbook takes time and effort, but it is useful for both supervisors and staff to know the policies and procedures of the organization, and the handbook may be essential backup when disputes arise.

≡ 47.5 Motivating Staff

If staff members were asked to brainstorm on all the factors that affect their attitudes about work, the resulting "pressure map" might look something like Figure 47.4. If staff are then asked to say whether each of these pressures is positive or negative, they are likely to find more negatives than positives on the chart. Most will feel that they are poorly paid and are expected to handle heavy workloads with limited resources. Because advancement frequently depends on formal educational qualifications or on "affiliations" rather than on the quality of work done, many may feel that they have low promotion prospects. Supervision is often constrained by lack of transport and other resources. If a staff member has extensive family responsibilities, there will be a temptation to look outside the job for opportunities to increase income. In such circumstances, it may be difficult to motivate staff.

Many of these factors are not within the control of individual managers. Some of these problems relate to a general lack of funds for running health services; other obstacles cannot easily be overcome within the constraints of typical budgeting and civil service procedures. Figure 47.5 outlines a variety of staff motivation factors.

Conventional motivational approaches in the private sector often rely on reward schemes, improved working conditions, or competition for promotions and pay increases. These approaches are not easy to apply to public health workers. Consequently, emphasis must be placed on an "internalized" approach to factors other than money and privileges that can motivate people, even those who are poorly paid.

To motivate workers within public-sector agencies, managers must depend a great deal on their skills as communicators and supervisors. Managers need to be

▶ enthusiastic about and dedicated to their work, which they manifest in words and deeds;

▶ sensitive to the pressures experienced by individual staff members;

▶ able to communicate openly using all five communication channels mentioned previously;

▶ willing, whenever possible and appropriate, to involve staff in making decisions, especially about matters directly affecting their own work;

Figure 47.4 Staff Pressure Map

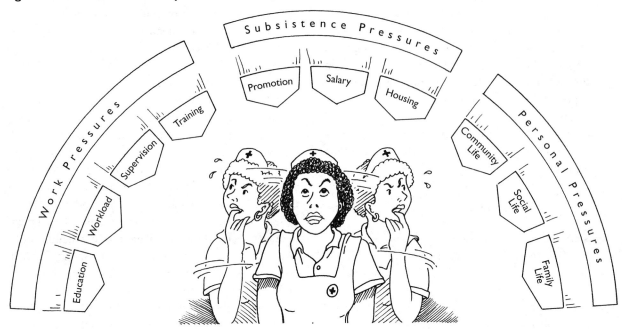

▶ ready to acknowledge good performance as well as firmly committed to pointing out bad performance.

Staff respond positively when they are given interesting and challenging work assignments by supervisors who are themselves clearly working hard toward fulfilling the organization's objectives.

☰ 47.6 Supervising Staff

Splitting the word *supervision* into its two parts reveals some interesting facts about the meaning of the word. The basic meaning of *super* is "over"; the basic meaning of *vision* is "sight." Putting these two together again, *supervision* can be seen simply as "oversight." But *super* can also mean "excellent," and *vision* can mean "foresight." In this sense of the term, supervision is about quality and planning. A supervisor becomes someone with the experience and skill to guide the work of others.

These two contrasting meanings mirror the distinction made at the beginning of this chapter between the directing and consulting styles of management. Supervision can focus on either discipline or development.

Qualities of Supervision

Several characteristics are likely to define supervisors who are concerned about the developmental as well as the disciplinary aspects of supervision. These supervisors are

▶ knowledgeable and enthusiastic about the jobs they are supervising;

▶ sensitive to staff members' needs and feelings;

▶ capable of supporting and guiding without harassment;

▶ skilled in communication—good listeners, approachable, and open-minded about ideas that conflict with their own;

▶ ready to praise good work and quick to support their staff;

▶ able to preserve harmony within the team and workforce by minimizing personal jealousies and conflicts;

▶ able to organize effectively and mobilize staff;

▶ able to allow staff to complete assigned duties without interference;

▶ willing to delegate tasks;

▶ scrupulous in making regular supervisory visits and punctual in keeping appointments;

▶ capable of appraising staff without bias and writing reports on the basis of work performance rather than hearsay or favoritism.

Tools for Supervision

One major aspect of supervision is knowing what to look for. There are a number of control mechanisms that can be of great help.

Work Schedule. A work schedule is an outline of the major activities that a staff member is expected to do and the days and times when various tasks are to be carried out. A district pharmacist, for example, could develop a work schedule that sets out the days and times to fill prescriptions at the pharmacy, conduct school education activities, maintain records, and prepare requisitions and reports.

Daily Log or Diary. A daily log or diary is a rich source of information on the use of time, provided that it is kept in sufficient detail.

Budgets and Expense Records. A budget is a specific, itemized plan. A budget and expenditure review can provide a useful means of keeping track of a project or work program.

Appraisal Reports. Appraisal reports inform those at higher levels about individual staff performance. They usually focus on

► nature of the work carried out;
► assessment of how well the work was done;
► description of skills involved in carrying out tasks;
► comments on commitment, punctuality, and interpersonal relations.

Unfortunately, appraisal reports, which are supposed to be used in determining promotability, tend to be treated as confidential. Often they are not even accessible to the staff member concerned. Ideally, supervisors should be able to use these reports to provide regular performance feedback to staff.

Exit Interviews. When a staff member leaves a position for any reason, it is useful for the supervisor to interview the person. On this occasion, frank opinions may be voiced, as the individual has nothing to lose. The supervisor may acquire new knowledge about other workers and managers and may also receive suggestions about how the working practices or environment could be improved.

Feedback Skills

Another aspect of supervision from which everyone can benefit is informed discussions about work performance. Good managers try to provide feedback as a regular feature of the work experience. Done well, it both enhances individual performance and improves teamwork.

When giving feedback, consider the following prescriptions:

► Deal only with what is known for certain.
► Describe actual behavior ("You did not attend the last two meetings") rather than making judgmental comments ("You are irresponsible").
► Start with positive feedback before giving negative feedback.
► Do not exaggerate.
► Listen as well as talk.

Figure 47.5 Staff Motivation Factors

Monetary Incentives
► Higher base salaries;
► Ensured promotion opportunities;
► Housing, hardship, and other allowances (continue or increase);
► Retirement benefits (continue or increase);
► Salary based on individual productivity;
► Bonuses tied to preventive services;
► Share of user fee revenue to encourage specific performance improvements;
► Salary supplements.

Nonmonetary Incentives
► Attractive postings;
► Reduced work hours for same salary;
► Provision of all supplies needed to work;
► Local control over spending user fee revenue;
► Training opportunities (local or overseas);
► Good management (people feel good about doing good work);
► Effective supervision;
► Local autonomy to reduce staff, increase salaries;
► Admitting privileges on amenity wards.

Disincentives
► Unsupportive management;
► Failure of management to involve staff in decisions;
► Civil service tenure;
► Nepotism;
► "Godfather" phenomenon.

Techniques found to be successful in prompting discussion of problem areas include:

► Ask open rather than closed questions, avoiding those that can be answered with a simple yes or no. ("What is your experience of this matter?")
► Present possible scenarios that encourage concrete descriptions. ("If you were faced with such a problem, how would you tackle it?")
► Rephrase the speaker's words. ("You are saying that you feel that you are not trusted, because you are not allowed to handle the finances for the workshops—am I right?")
► Acknowledge the other person's feelings. ("You seem to be very worried about this matter—am I right?")
► Concentrate on what is being implied as well as what is being said. People are much more willing to talk if they are convinced that they are really being heard.

Clearly, such techniques go well beyond simple criticism or interrogation.

The One Minute Manager

The essential staff supervision skills discussed above are summarized in the concept of the *one minute manager* (Blanchard and Johnson 1982), consisting of three elements: one minute goals, one minute praisings, and one minute reprimands.

One minute goals (or one minute goal setting) involve stating very briefly what is expected, verbally or in writing. Important goals for an individual can be written down in less than one minute on one piece of paper, to establish mutual expectations. The important thing is to clearly communicate to the staff member what is expected.

One minute praisings involve agreeing with staff about what is expected in advance (one minute goal setting), then praising them immediately when they perform accordingly. According to *The One Minute Manager*, one of the most effective ways to motivate people is to "catch them doing something right." That is, give staff positive feedback when they perform well or have achieved a specific objective. The feedback should be immediate and brief and indicate specifically what they did right. Depending on the culture, a handshake or touch on the shoulder may reinforce the message.

One minute reprimands are necessary when staff have done something wrong or failed to meet expectations. Effective reprimands require skill, and they consist of two parts. First, the manager tells the person directly and specifically what was done wrong and how he or she feels about it. Then, after a brief pause, the manager reminds the person that although his or her performance in this situation has been unsatisfactory, his or her work is valued, and better work is anticipated in the future. To be most effective, the reprimand should be given in private, should be brief, should not personalize the poor performance, and should end with a positive, forward-looking message.

The essence of the one minute manager, therefore, is to establish clear expectations ("You will be responsible for organizing the supply management workshop"); to provide prompt and specific positive feedback ("You did an excellent job organizing last week's workshop"); and, when necessary, to provide prompt and specific negative feedback ("You really did a poor job organizing last week's workshop. I know you can do better next time").

≡ 47.7 Disciplining Staff

A good manager should not shirk the responsibility of disciplining staff when necessary. However, in a drug supply program within a ministry of health, there may be little a manager can do beyond submitting a report recommending disciplinary action to higher levels. Measures such as indictment, suspension, transfer, or dismissal are normally outside the powers of a program manager. Nevertheless, it is important to maintain fairness and dig-

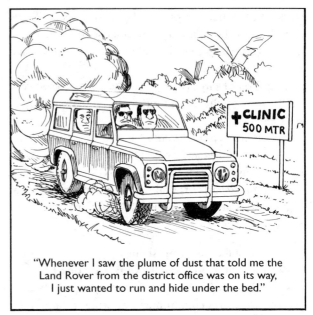

"Whenever I saw the plume of dust that told me the Land Rover from the district office was on its way, I just wanted to run and hide under the bed."

SUPERVISION SHOULD BE POSITIVE AND SUPPORTIVE, NOT FEARED.

nity in coping with situations that might lead to making disciplinary recommendations. The following guidelines are suggested:

► If it is necessary to take disciplinary action (whether a verbal warning, a written warning, or a report to higher authorities), the action should be immediate. Discipline that follows soon after the offense is more likely to be associated with the offense itself than with the manager. A delayed action can lead to resentment and a lack of trust.

► There should be advance warning. Unexpected discipline is usually regarded as unfair. Staff are more likely to understand and accept the need for disciplinary action if they are given a clear presentation of the rules, followed by a warning that disciplinary measures will be taken if the rules are infringed.

► Discipline should be consistent. If it is imposed differently under the same conditions, staff will be confused or frustrated, and the manager will quickly lose their respect.

► Discipline should be impartial. It should be clear that a particular behavior is being challenged and not the personality of the individual staff member.

Of course, it is always better to deal with problematic situations before they become crises that call for formal disciplinary procedures. If someone is making mistakes, a good manager takes that person aside for a talk. Criticizing someone's behavior is perhaps one of the most difficult tasks a manager faces. The challenge is to remain objective and avoid blaming. This means that the manager must

► present the perceived problem clearly;
► ask for the other person's point of view and listen when it is given;
► avoid expressing anger or frustration and remain calm and firm;
► focus on possible solutions rather than harping on mistakes;
► discuss ways to resolve the issue and how such problems might be avoided in the future.

≡ 47.8 Handling Conflict
Conflicts can occur when employees feel that their needs are not being met or their concerns are being ignored. Conflicts inevitably occur in the struggle to secure adequate resources for effective drug supply systems. This section reviews conflict resolution strategies that harmonize with the consultative, participatory approaches emphasized in this chapter.

Two forces determine how conflicts play out:

1. *Assertiveness*: the extent to which a person attempts to satisfy his or her own needs;
2. *Cooperation*: the extent to which a person attempts to satisfy the needs of others.

There are a number of styles by which individuals or groups manage conflict, but each can be understood as an interplay between these two driving forces. Figure 47.6 illustrates five styles of conflict resolution (Williams 1983a).

The two dimensions of assertiveness and cooperation define a model that provides a framework for describing various styles of conflict management and for assessing their relative strengths and weaknesses.

Competing Style
The competing style involves maximum assertiveness and minimum cooperation. Competitors try to satisfy their own needs at the expense of other parties, using whatever powers are at their disposal. They try to gain power through direct confrontation or manipulation. A competitive style is not necessarily bad; it depends on the circumstances. In situations in which life is threatened (an outbreak of cholera, for example), a manager might need to take quick and decisive action, even if it means riding roughshod over those who challenge his or her policies.

Strengths. A competitive strategy might be appropriate when

► quick, decisive action is vital;
► an unpopular decision needs to be made;
► there is no doubt about what is the right course of action;
► defensive measures are urgently required.

Weaknesses. A competitive strategy can lead to

► lost opportunities for collaboration or compromise;
► degeneration into stubborn opposition.

Accommodating Style
Accommodation is at the opposite pole from competition; it is characterized by unassertive and totally cooperative behavior. It means putting the other party's needs above one's own.

Strengths. Accommodation is an appropriate strategy when

► the other party is clearly in the right;
► preserving harmony is the most important consideration;
► gaining goodwill is the most important outcome.

Weaknesses. Too much accommodation can lead to

► reduced influence, respect, and recognition (someone who earns the label "accommodator" will always be expected to give in);
► people taking advantage of a perceived weakness.

Avoiding Style
Avoiding is characterized by zero assertiveness and zero cooperation—it means choosing not to engage. The avoider evades the issue, withdraws from the discussion, and never bothers to press for a resolution. Avoiding can sometimes be employed effectively as an interim strategy.

Strengths. Avoidance may be appropriate when

► discussions become overheated and a cooling-off period is advisable;
► a conflict should be delayed until more information is gathered or a closer analysis can be made;
► the issue is relatively unimportant;
► there is not enough time to come to a resolution;
► the issue is identified as only a symptom of a substantial and extensive problem that needs to be dealt with later.

Weaknesses. An inappropriate use of avoidance procedures can lead to

► communication breakdown, as when staff "left in the dark" stop taking initiatives;

Figure 47.6 Conflict Resolution Model

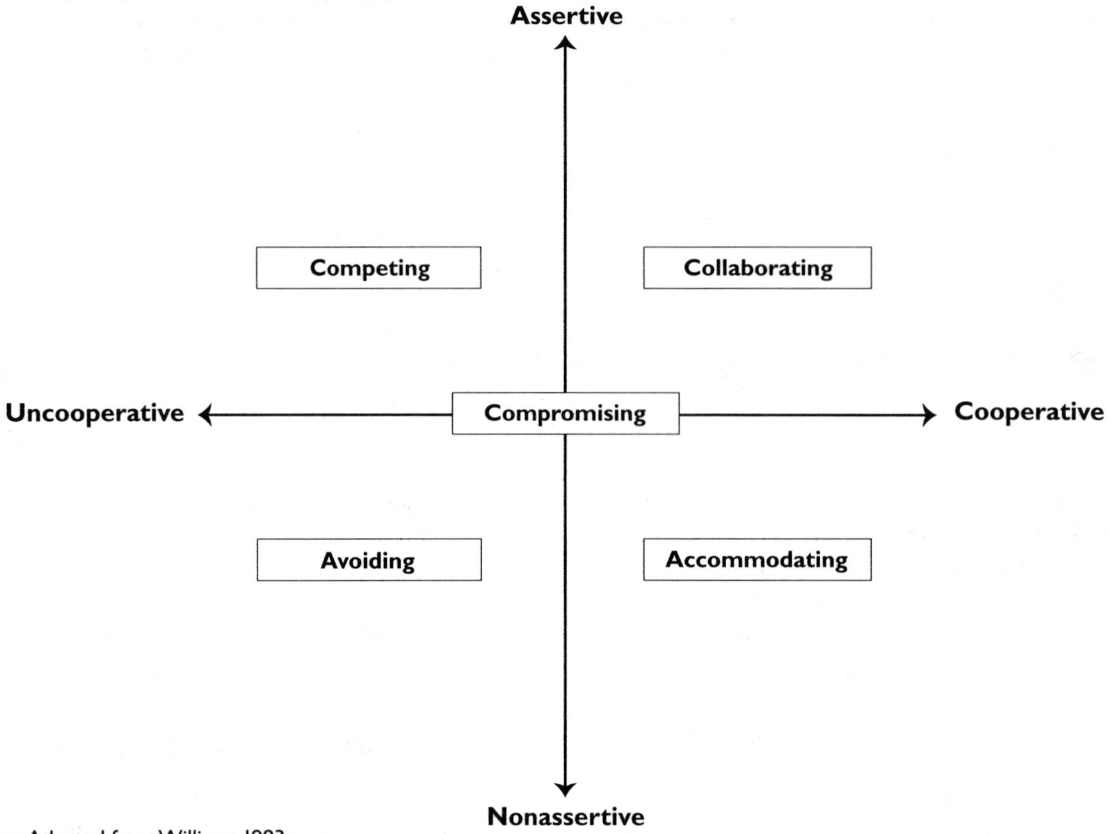

Source: Adapted from Williams 1983a.

► reduced effectiveness, as decisions are made by default;
► conflicts persisting and then flaring up later.

Collaborating Style

In the collaborating style, there is a maximum use of both assertiveness and cooperation. Those using this style seek to satisfy the needs of all parties concerned. Collaboration is the best way to develop consensus solutions to problems and achieve a commitment to those solutions. Neither side feels that it has lost out in any way, so this is an ideal management style.

Strengths. The collaborating style is most effectively used when

► the needs and concerns of the parties are sufficiently important to warrant the time and energy it takes to collaborate properly;
► all parties agree to combine resources and efforts for a more effective outcome.

Weaknesses. This is the most time-consuming and energy-sapping style. It can result in

► relatively unimportant matters getting too much attention;
► the establishment of cumbersome procedures, which may lead to frustrating delays in making decisions and taking action.

Compromising Style

Compromise is an intermediate strategy, midway between competition and collaboration, avoidance and accommodation. The objective is to find a solution that partly satisfies both parties. It is a style characterized by the well-known phrase "splitting the difference."

Strengths. Compromise solutions are appropriate when

► the parties are strongly committed to mutually exclusive goals, and it is clear that no solution will be wholly satisfactory to both of them;
► the goals of both parties are important but not worth the effort needed for collaboration;
► temporary solutions are sought for complex issues because the time for decision-making is short.

Weaknesses. If compromises are made too readily or casually:

► important principles may be disregarded;

► the value of the enterprise may be diminished.

In conflict situations, the best approach to take depends on the circumstances. A good manager is in command of all the channels of communication, is sensitive to the needs of the situation, and can select the correct approach. Unfortunately, what tends to happen is that individual managers and groups become locked into one preferred style of conflict management and use it in almost every situation.

Collaboration and compromise are the styles that match the consulting, all-channels-open, problem-solving management approaches explored in this chapter.

≡ 47.9 Delegation

Effective delegation enables managers to become much more productive and, therefore, more successful. Unfortunately, many managers have never learned how to delegate effectively. A sure sign of trust between manager and staff is the manager's willingness to delegate responsibilities. If delegation happens consistently and properly, the effectiveness of a team can be greatly enhanced.

Delegation is more than simply assigning tasks to subordinates. Delegation skills involve the following steps:

1. *Select the right person for the job.* Delegation works well only when the person to whom work is being delegated is capable of handling the task. Delegating to the wrong person invites failure.

2. *Clearly specify the assignment being delegated.* Unless the assignment is clear, the staff member may do too much or too little.

3. *Define the level of authority being delegated.* Is the staff member being asked to investigate a problem and then report back to the manager for a decision and action? Is the staff member to investigate, see the manager for a decision, and then act? Or is the staff member to investigate, decide, and act—informing the manager afterward? Both manager and staff member risk anger or frustration if the level of authority is not made clear.

4. *Inform concerned parties.* Unless other staff are informed of what assignments have been delegated to whom, they may feel that a staff member's actions are inappropriate. They may think that the staff member is trying to take over the manager's job rather than acting on the manager's behalf.

5. *Monitor, don't meddle.* Once an assignment has been delegated, it is important to monitor progress. It may be necessary to advise the staff member of possible problems. But if the manager intrudes, short-circuits, undercuts, goes around, or otherwise meddles in the assignment, the staff member will lose interest in doing a good job. Accepting that the assignment will probably be done differently from the way the manager would have done it is part of delegating. Different is not necessarily worse. Staff often have more time or other insights that allow them to do the task better than the manager would have.

6. *Complete the delegation neatly.* Once the assignment has been completed, the manager should be briefed by the staff member. Necessary follow-up actions should be identified. Most importantly, the staff member should receive positive feedback if the assignment went well and clear, direct negative feedback if the assignment did not turn out well. Specific corrective action should be suggested.

When these basic steps are not followed, the result is often confusion, poor decision-making, mistrust, and frustration. Managers are afraid to delegate because "the staff will mess it up," and staff are afraid to take the initiative because "the boss will tell me I messed up."

Directing managers have trouble delegating because they do not like to give up control. Avoiding managers have trouble delegating because they do not provide clear guidance and feedback. Consulting managers generally do the best job of delegating.

Delegation has three main benefits. First, it provides subordinates with the opportunity to accumulate valuable experience and develop new skills. Second, delegation prevents managers from being overworked, a condition that can cause delays in decision-making. Finally, delegation frees senior managers to concentrate on long-term planning activities.

≡ 47.10 Conducting Meetings

Properly run meetings can be vital to the effectiveness of an organization: they are forums for gathering information, reviewing progress, discussing ideas, planning actions, and resolving conflicts. Improperly run meetings can be a colossal waste of time.

It is time for a meeting if

► an issue affecting the work team needs to be clarified;

► there are concerns that should be shared with a group;

► the group needs to be involved in a problem-solving and decision-making activity;

► a group has asked for a meeting.

762 HUMAN RESOURCES MANAGEMENT

It is not time for a meeting if
▶ the decisions have already been made;
▶ the calendar says that a meeting is due but there are no urgent matters to discuss.

Conditions for Effective Meetings

However informal and lively the interaction, effective meetings are usually the result of careful planning. The following are some of the most important factors that contribute to a meeting's success:

Purpose: The objectives of the meeting should be clear to all participants.

Preparation: The members should be knowledgeable about the topics under discussion. It is often necessary to circulate relevant papers beforehand.

Control: The chairperson should be *in* authority but not *the* authority; responsible for the conduct of the meeting but not the only decision-maker in the group.

Size: The group should be small enough for everyone to make a contribution, unless the meeting is merely a gathering for dispensing information.

Setting: The seating should be arranged so that everyone has eye contact with everyone else.

Atmosphere: The climate should be such that participants feel free to offer ideas and to challenge and be challenged.

Summary: The meeting should end with a statement of what has been achieved.

Record: It is important to take accurate minutes of the meetings so that efficient monitoring can take place and those responsible for arranged actions can be held accountable.

Time: The meeting should begin on time and last for a predetermined length of time.

Skills of Chairing

The success of meetings depends on the kind of control exercised by the chairperson. Some of the main techniques used to facilitate open and purposeful discussion and decision-making are:

Initiate: Start by ensuring that all members know the objectives and agenda of the meeting.

Seek opinions: Invite participation by bringing members in when it is known that they will have something to contribute.

Clarify: Rephrase or illustrate points so that they can be understood by all members.

Steer: Bring the discussion back on track when it veers off course.

Summarize: Pull together the ideas that have been expressed and sum up the conclusions that have been reached.

Keep time: End the meeting on time.

Finally, the conclusions of most meetings can be encapsulated in a brief plan of action, recording what is to be done, by whom, and by when.

≡ 47.11 Managing Time

Staff time and personal time are resources that need to be managed. Time wasting diverts a manager from important tasks. The most frequent time wasters include

▶ lack of objectives;
▶ failure to set priorities;
▶ absence of deadlines;
▶ unnecessary or badly structured meetings;
▶ visitors arriving without appointments;
▶ telephone interruptions;
▶ too little or too much information;
▶ attempts to do too much in too little time;
▶ overemphasis on easier, more routine work at the expense of harder tasks;
▶ long breaks and social chat;
▶ inability to say no.

To avoid wasting time, the following techniques may be useful:

▶ Clarify objectives by writing them down.
▶ Set one major objective each day and accomplish it.
▶ Keep a log of how days are spent, and review it.
▶ Reserve the best time of the workday to concentrate on the most important task.
▶ Stay quiet when a conversation is not going anywhere, and the other person will soon stop talking.
▶ Take work to a quiet place—the unoccupied office of someone on leave, a nearby library, or home—when an assignment must be finished.

Time is one resource that, when lost, is lost forever. A manager who makes good use of time is investing well in his or her own future as well as the future of the program. ■

≡ Assessment Guide

Structure

► Does an organizational chart of staffing positions and relationships exist? When was it last revised?

► Do job descriptions for these positions exist? When were they last revised? Does each staff member have a copy of his or her job description?

► What orientation and initial training are given to newly appointed staff?

► Is there a staff procedures handbook? Is it regularly updated?

► Have any senior staff members received training in personnel management?

Function

► What training has occurred in the past five years for staff in personnel management? What training is planned?

► What formal communication channels exist to convey information from senior to junior workers and in the reverse direction?

► What supervisory systems exist? In particular, are there regular performance appraisal meetings with written records?

► Are there exit interviews with departing employees? Are written records kept?

► What disciplinary procedures exist? How often have the formal methods been used in the past year?

► Do staff meetings have an agenda? Are minutes kept of the meetings? Do the meetings begin and end on time?

≡ References and Further Readings

★ = Key readings.

★ Amondo-Lartson, R., G. Ebrahim, H. Lovel, and J. Ranken. 1984. District health care: Challenges for planning, organization, and evaluation in developing countries. London: Macmillan.

Benavente, J., and C. Madden. 1993. Improving supervision: A team approach. Family Planning Manager 2(5):1–18.

Blanchard, K., and S. Johnson. 1982. The one minute manager. New York: Berkley Books.

★ Kolehmainen-Aitken, R.-L., and P. Shipp. 1990. Indicators of staffing need: Assessing health staffing and equity in Papua New Guinea. Health Policy and Planning 5:167–76.

Longest, B. Jr. 1980. Management practices for health professionals, 2d ed. London: Preston Editions.

★ McMahon, R., E. Barton, and M. Piot. 1992. On being in charge: A guide to management in primary health care, 2d ed. Geneva: World Health Organization.

Ministry of Health, Government of Kenya. 1994. Good management of hospital drugs and supplies manual. Nairobi: MOH.

★ Ministry of Health, Government of Zimbabwe. 1991. Human relations at work. Section E, part 1 of Zimbabwe medical stores handbook. Harare: MOH.

MSH (Management Sciences for Health). 1991. Staffing your program and supervising and supporting your staff. In The family planning manager's handbook: Basic skills and tools for managing family planning programs, ed. J. A. Wolff, L. J. Suttenfield, and S. C. Binzen. West Hartford, Conn.: Kumarian Press.

Noel, M. W., and J. L. Bootman, eds. 1986. Human resources management in pharmacy practice. Gaithersburg, Md.: Aspen Publishers.

Pedler, M., J. Burgoyne, and T. Boydell. 1986. A manager's guide to self-development, 2d ed. New York: McGraw-Hill.

Shipp, P. J. 1993. Guidelines for developing and using workload indicators of staffing need. Geneva: World Health Organization.

WHO (World Health Organization). 1988. The role of the pharmacist in the health care system. Geneva: WHO.

Williams, R. B. 1983a. Conflict resolution. Gainesville, Tenn.: Health Professionals Advancement Institute.

Williams, R. B. 1983b. Effective delegation. Gainesville, Tenn.: Health Professionals Advancement Institute.

Williams, R. B. 1985. Hospital pharmacy management primer. Bethesda, Md.: American Society of Hospital Pharmacists.

| Part I | Part II | Part III | Part IV |
| Introduction | Policy and Legal Framework | Drug Management Cycle | Management Support Systems |

A Organization and Management
B Financing and Sustainability
C Information Management

D Human Resources Management ▶

47 Personnel Management

48 Designing and Implementing Training Programs

Chapter 48

Designing and Implementing Training Programs

≡ Summary

Training is any planned activity to transfer or modify knowledge, skills, and attitudes through learning experiences. Continual training of personnel is required, because without it, work performance tends to decline, and a number of competencies are forgotten. Changing circumstances and new approaches and technologies demand new skills and attitudes. However, training cannot solve structural, organizational, or policy problems within an organization.

An assessment of training needs is normally carried out before any training is done. It involves

- ► *observing workers performing normal duties;*
- ► *interviewing workers and others;*
- ► *studying routine reports or performance reviews, along with job descriptions.*

A training program is then designed to improve the performance of a particular task or tasks, taking into account the educational levels of the personnel and the time and resources available for training. Options range from short courses to long-term placements in academic institutions, either in the country or region or overseas. All options must be weighed against the immediate operational needs of the essential drugs program, as there may not be enough personnel to run facilities when people go for training.

Once the subject areas have been chosen, the mix of learning methods to achieve maximum effectiveness depends on the audience and the experience of the trainer. Methods that can be used include lecture, discussion, case study, role playing, group exercise, brainstorming, demonstration, and worksheet. If there are no published training materials, the trainer must develop both trainers' and participants' guides. Audiovisual aids must also be developed and properly used to stimulate and sustain interest.

Evaluation of the training is carried out during the course and at its conclusion. Whenever possible, the trainer should keep in touch with participants after they return to their work situations to assess the appropriateness and effectiveness of the training.

≡ In some countries, there are no continuing education programs; therefore, many health workers lack access to new ideas and approaches that can improve their work performance. Well-designed training programs can fill this need.

Training is broadly defined as any planned activity to transfer and modify knowledge, attitudes, and skills through learning experiences. Training should be based on competencies: the abilities required to do work to the standards expected. Therefore, training should result in changes in work behavior that lead to an improved, efficiently functioning essential drugs system. At the same time, it must be recognized that training alone is unlikely to change overall supply system performance unless the environment and supervisory systems support change (see Chapter 34).

Learning requires active involvement of learners. Different people learn in different ways—some are visual, some verbal, and some learn only by doing. Therefore, combining training opportunities and training techniques is usually more effective than using only one approach. The training can be formal or informal, academic or applied, and in public agencies or private institutions.

Finally, training is a dynamic process. The improved performance, changed attitudes, and new skills acquired must be maintained by continuing education and on-the-job training.

≡ 48.1 Training Objectives

The training of personnel in drug management has four major objectives:

1. To increase knowledge about the special needs of pharmaceutical systems;
2. To change attitudes about the importance of drug management, thus improving the environment for change;
3. To improve skills in the specific tasks to be completed for efficient functioning of the drug supply system;
4. To improve work behavior, so that people function better at assigned activities and fulfill their potential.

Training needs to be directed at three levels of personnel:

1. Policy-makers, who are responsible for creating the environment needed for improved drug management;
2. Mid-level managers, who are responsible for planning and supervising activities required in the management and use of drugs;
3. Line personnel, who are responsible for carrying out the work of drug management.

A thorough needs assessment should occur before training is undertaken.

An essential drugs program (EDP) alone is not in a position to handle the training objectives for policy-makers and mid-level managers. Many of these objectives are best handled by general management training. However, it is still possible and necessary to reorient this group through information exchanges, reports, and occasional seminars on drug policies and issues. The EDP should concentrate on training for operations-level personnel, who often lack the basic knowledge and skills necessary to be effective at their jobs.

Finally, training alone will not result in significantly improved performance unless it is linked to the changes in policy, organizational structure, procedures, and resource allocations discussed in previous chapters. Country Study 48.1 gives an example of integrating training into overall program changes in one pharmaceutical supply system.

≡ 48.2 Conducting a Needs Assessment

A training needs assessment is an appraisal of the knowledge, skills, and attitudes of personnel to help plan a training program that will enable them to carry out the operations of the drug supply system more effectively. Training will be effective only if all areas of the pharmaceutical supply system are assessed frankly and carefully.

Management may request staff training when performance in a specific area is inadequate or declining. When new technologies, such as computers, are introduced, training is needed to assist staff in adapting to the new work environment.

Methods for assessing training needs are outlined below. The optimal method depends on the goals of the assessment and the level of the individuals being assessed.

Observing a worker perform routine duties reveals both strengths and weaknesses, but it must be recognized that behavior may be influenced by the presence of an observer. For example, a clinical worker examining a patient is likely to be more thorough than usual if someone is watching. Specific training needs can be determined more clearly by using well-established indicators, such as those described in Chapter 36, and observation methods such as those described in Chapter 29.

Interviews with supervisors, administrators, users of services, and workers can help determine what skills need to be taught or improved. If workers fear reprisals from management, reassurances about confidentiality of information will be necessary to obtain good data. In some situations, a training needs analysis can be done by conducting a group interview, in which the staff are invited to identify competencies in terms of knowledge, attitudes, and skills. Staff rate themselves on a graph in relation to each of the chosen competencies. Exit interviews with workers leaving their jobs can also be useful. Finally, inter-

Country Study 48.1 Human Resources Development in Asia

Bhutan. Bhutan has had an active essential drugs program since 1987. In 1991, a detailed review of staffing requirements was undertaken, together with the development of a pharmacy staff plan. Seven national pharmacists and forty-five pharmacy technicians were required. In 1991, four pharmacists were chosen to undergo training in India. Following academic training, the pharmacists were attached to established and well-run hospital pharmacies in India and Nepal for an additional year at the expense of the government of Bhutan. Upon their return to Bhutan, the pharmacists undertook a two-year rotation through different departments paired with expatriate pharmacists. In addition, they took short courses in drug supply management, quality control, and drug legislation and regulatory control.

The pharmacy technician training course was also expanded to include six students per year to reach the target of forty-five technicians by 1995 and fifty-five by 2000.

Myanmar. The essential drugs program in Myanmar has undertaken pilot activities in nine townships. The program has supported refresher courses with community cost-sharing projects as well as courses for doctors in public service and for ships' captains. In addition, the program manager has undertaken on-the-job training as part of supervising the nine pilot projects. Publications on estimating drug requirements, store management systems, and standard treatment schedules, as well as a newsletter, have been produced and distributed. This work has been undertaken in collaboration with the Myanmar Medical Association.

Source: WHO reports.

views with users of the services can help in assessing levels of satisfaction.

Analyses of job and task descriptions may reveal special training needs. Self-administered, anonymous questionnaires for both managers and workers can also be valuable.

Several types of reports are useful assessment tools:

▶ Organizational reports, for an overview of the performance of the organization and personnel;

▶ External evaluation or appraisal reports, for an outsider's view of the organization and its training needs (and performance);

▶ Annual or semiannual performance reviews.

≡ 48.3 Developing a Comprehensive Training Program

A training program is a schedule of activities showing training goals, objectives, subject areas, methods, trainers, trainees, and locations. A good training program focuses on performance problems, such as long delays in getting drugs from suppliers to the main stores, or delays in distributing drugs from mid-level stores to user units. Figure 48.1 shows how the training program proceeds from a problem, through needs assessment, training, and evaluation, to a change in behavior that results in better performance.

The key elements of a training program are learning units, courses, and practical experiences. A learning unit teaches individuals to perform a specific task. Courses are usually less task-specific and are conducted for a group of people away from their jobs. Practical experiences are needed to supplement training units and courses.

Implementing a Training Program

There are two basic approaches to implementing a training program. One approach is centered on the trainer, who controls learning contents and experiences. The other approach is centered on the learner, with the trainer acting as a guide and providing resources. This approach assumes that people are able and willing to learn if they are given the proper materials in an atmosphere that is conducive to learning. This is the preferred method, because it is participatory, learners' experiences are shared, and participants have more freedom to learn at their own speed.

Strategies

Training strategies must be appropriate to the educational level of personnel and to the resources available in the country, feasible in terms of the amount of time and travel involved, and relevant to the job. In some countries, governments often place officials in jobs that require a higher degree of technical capacity than they possess. In such cases, managers and trainers need to work together to close the gap between requirements and ability.

Training programs must consider the resources available. For example, an individual working in a central medical store that uses a simple card system for inventory control should be trained in the operation of that system rather than a computerized system that may never be installed.

Training programs must be feasible. It is important to recognize that governments may not be able to allow a senior official to take an extended training leave, regardless of potential long-term benefits. It may not be possible for some officials to be absent for more than one week.

Training can be short, lasting one to four weeks, or it can extend over three to twenty-four months. Preservice training is conducted at established institutions. In-service training is offered either as part of a planned staff development program or after an assessment of deficiencies has determined what training is needed at the workplace.

Figure 48.1 The Training Process for Improved Performance

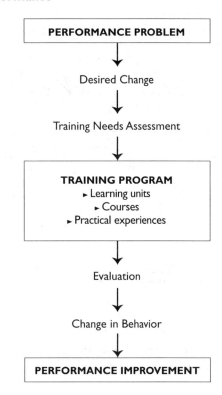

The decision about the kind of training program to use depends on the issues raised in Figure 48.2, as well as the criteria of appropriateness, feasibility, and relevance. The training program is likely to include a combination of long- and short-term training, observation trips, conferences and seminars, and in-country counterpart training.

Long-Term Training. Long-term training is often in an institution of higher learning (sometimes in overseas institutions). Such training, whether in academic or nonacademic settings, is most useful for highly technical areas such as research and development of new drugs, quality assurance, local production, or improved manufacturing practices. The provision of fellowships for doctors, pharmacists, industrial engineers, and other technical professionals is most appropriate here.

This approach is limited because it is not the specific duty of an EDP to provide basic training, and most programs cannot afford to have top personnel away for a long time. If personnel fail to return, the costs for training new personnel can be high.

Short-Term Training. Short-term training is usually conducted over a period of one to three months in academic or nonacademic settings. To work effectively, the trainee needs to be separated from everyday work responsibilities.

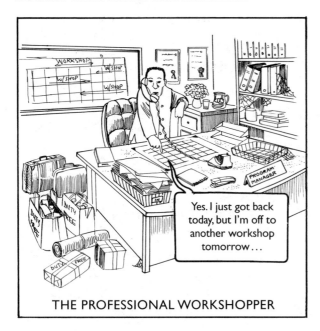

THE PROFESSIONAL WORKSHOPPER

Figure 48.2 Issues to Consider When Designing Training Programs

Audience
► trainers to be trained
► senior government officials
► administrators in government ministries
► line personnel

Mode
► preservice training
► on-site job training, counterpart training
► classroom (off-site, in-service training)
► tours, observational trips
► workshops and seminars
► courses (short or long term)

Length
► seminar (two weeks or less)
► short-term course (one to three months)
► long-term course (six to twenty-four months)

Location
► developing country
  – local college or university
  – national management institute (where one exists)
  – international sponsor (for example, WHO, UNICEF, USAID, Danida, SIDA)
► developed country
  – industry
  – university
  – independent private group
  – government agency

Funding Source
► government
► private organizations
► donor agencies
  – private charity, such as a church group
  – industry
  – university

This approach is appropriate for most training needs in drug management, especially for top- and middle-level personnel. Prerequisites for effective short-term training include

► a sufficient supply of people with initial background training;
► courses available in the language of the participants;
► course design that uses training modules to allow for flexible curricula to meet the needs of target groups;
► intensive, practical training so that a good mix of information and skills is gained in a short time;
► adequate follow-up of graduates, including provision of continuing education programs, to ensure that they continue to function effectively.

In addition to training the target groups outlined in Figure 48.3, this type of program is suitable for the training of trainers who will return to their jobs and train others in the techniques and skills they have learned. Thus, short-term training should also include pedagogical and leadership skills and provide some institution-building capacities. Annex 48.1 provides further information on workshop logistics and evaluation.

A number of institutions have developed training materials and can provide training at the regional or international level. Some private nongovernmental institutions in the United States, such as Management Sciences for Health (MSH), and semigovernmental institutions such as the Eastern and Southern African Management Institute (ESAMI) in Arusha, Tanzania, offer training in individual countries. In addition, some institutions are beginning to develop regional training centers in management, but these are not necessarily oriented toward public health programs.

Observation Trips. Countries that do not have formal training programs but have successfully implemented EDPs can offer useful and practical examples for personnel from other countries. In addition, some multinational and national pharmaceutical manufacturers have regional or local warehouses, manufacturing plants, and laboratories that are good sites for visits. Observation trips work best when combined with short-term training, to reinforce in a practical way the skills learned; they can benefit both the visitors and the institution visited. This is especially true if the trainer accompanies the trainees.

Conferences and Seminars. Standardized curricula prepared by an international institution can be used to present regional conferences and seminars. This approach works well for focusing on particular components, such as drug distribution or use. It is also an effective way to promote

Figure 48.3 Subject Areas, Training Needs, and Target Groups

Subject Area	Training Needs	Target Groups
Selection	Essential drugs lists Public formulary Sources of information Safety and efficacy Cost comparisons Levels of use Hospital formularies National drug policy	Policy- and decision-makers in: Ministry of health (MOH); Ministry of finance (MOF); other ministries Service providers: doctors; nurses Auxiliary personnel Pharmacists/dispensers
Procurement	Quantification of drug needs Procurement cycle Forecasting Purchasing methods Scheduling of purchases Terms of payment Selection of suppliers Payment mechanisms Organization of procurement services Quality assurance Make-or-buy decisions Shipment specifications	Division of planning, MOH Division of finance, MOH Division of administration or purchasing, MOH MOF Central procurement service (if it exists) Central laboratories, MOH Drug regulatory bodies Senior MOH/MOF officials for policy decisions (such as make-or-buy)
Distribution	Logistics cycle Information system Port clearing Warehouse operations Packaging/repackaging Transportation Security	Division of planning, MOH Division of administration, MOH Operations personnel in: port; warehouses (central, regional, and district) Transportation
Use	Promotion of appropriate therapy Training of health workers Dispensing practices Patient education Information systems Patient adherence Rational drug use indicators	Program directors Program supervisors Doctors Nurses Pharmacists Dispensers Auxiliary and community health workers Patients and clients

longer training programs, information-sharing among developing country personnel, desire for improvement, and general sensitization of policy-makers to the importance of drug management.

In-Country Counterpart Training. An outside consultant with expertise in an aspect of pharmaceutical management, such as computerized inventory, can train counterparts by working on site for a period of weeks or months. Short-term consultancies work best when they are focused on a specific activity (for example, a drug

packaging process or the development of an operations manual). Longer periods (from two to four years) are required for overall systems renovation. Meaningful improvements in pharmaceutical logistics systems can be made using long-term, on-site consultants. The major limitations are

expense: international agencies characteristically spend US$7,000 to $10,000 a month to support an in-country consultant;

lack of regional effect: only the individual country benefits, although participants in a program could train others;

lack of appropriate institution building: the host country may not be able to continue innovations after the departure of the consultant.

Assistance for the Design and Implementation of Training Courses

The skills involved in designing and implementing a training program can be learned by observing good trainers and paying attention to how they use different methods. In addition, most large EDPs should have a minimum of one or two staff members who have formal training in training methods and the design of training programs. Training-of-trainers courses are frequently offered by local, regional, or international training institutes.

Another valuable resource for the training program is the practical experience of organizations and institutions in the pharmaceutical supply process. Among these are international organizations, governmental and nongovernmental organizations, universities, developing country institutions, and programs already operating in developing countries.

However, with few exceptions, these organizations have made service rather than training their highest priority. Training programs have usually been established on an ad hoc basis to fulfill a specific need rather than in a systematic and comprehensive way. But some programs address specific areas for a particular level in the supply system or for multiple levels in a vertical disease control program (see Country Study 48.2).

Annex 48.2 lists organizations that have practical experience in the design and/or implementation of training programs. These organizations are invaluable resources for the development of many types of training programs.

≡ 48.4 Selecting Subject Areas and Setting Learning Objectives

A training needs assessment should indicate which subject area, topic, or target group should be given priority, as

Country Study 48.2 A New Approach to Training Medical Stores Staff

The Zimbabwe medical stores, with support from Danida (Danish International Development Agency), devised a scheme for offering the medical stores staff courses that could be taken either by correspondence or at national schools and colleges. With the help of a local college, interested persons were tested on their level of knowledge and then offered a chance to take courses in a limited number of subjects, including literacy, English, mathematics, accounting, and science. Although 140 of the 210 staff members showed interest, 110 staff members actually began studies, with 20 taking adult literacy classes, 30 taking the primary school exams, about 40 taking specified high school subjects, and the rest, who were already well educated, taking courses in purchasing and supply, accounting, and business. Typing and computer training were also popular. This program has continued, with a total of 60 people studying at any one time under the scheme. The total cost for this group is less than sending 1 person overseas for three months.

It is a matter of great satisfaction for management, and even more for the employees, that employees have learned to read and write, thereby broadening their horizons and giving them opportunities to take on jobs with more responsibility. It is hard to measure the degree of personal satisfaction felt by a worker who is suddenly able to read his children's report cards.

Loss of employees who take training and then defect to other institutions is surprisingly low, and only a few have left for this reason. Instead, they tend to follow up their training with further training, such as high school subjects or a higher degree in accountancy. Employees are aware that this kind of educational opportunity is not easily obtainable elsewhere and are satisfied to put their newfound knowledge to use within the organization.

Not all students have the time or proper circumstances to finish their studies. There is a 40 percent dropout rate, as social factors make it difficult for some workers to study.

The scheme has been evaluated as a success, in terms of both the retention rate of workers at all levels and their positive experiences in the organization, with increased competence often leading to promotion. The organization benefits from its employees' augmented qualifications, experience, and loyalty.

Source: Zimbabwe Essential Drugs Action Programme 1994.

shown in Figure 48.3. In many countries, some subject areas require more attention than others, but certain basics must be provided: the selection process needs to be well managed and participatory; procurement officers need training in efficient purchasing methods and quantification of drug needs; distribution—proper storage, efficient transportation, and security of drugs—is a continuing concern; and use is becoming a major focus of many EDPs.

In addition to these basic drug management skills, staff in essential drugs and related health programs will benefit from training in other areas, including

- general management;
- financial management, budgeting, and accounting;
- computer systems and information management;
- training program development and management;
- training materials development;
- public communications;
- personnel planning and management;
- program planning, monitoring, and evaluation;
- proposal development and writing.

EDPs and other drug supply systems often run into difficulty not because they lack technical expertise but because they lack critical management skills. Thus, when considering subject areas, it is important to think broadly about what skills are most needed to improve the performance of the organization.

≡ **48.5 Learning Methods**

A variety of learning experiences can be used in training, including

lecture: a direct talk with or without learning aids but without group participation;

discussion: a method in which the participants learn from one another with little or no facilitator involvement;

case study: a real situation is presented in a brief paper or presentation, then analyzed by participants;

role playing: participants act out the roles of those represented in a given situation;

group exercise: a number of participants undertake an activity together, followed by a critical analysis of the process involved;

brainstorming: members of a small or large group are encouraged to contribute any suggestion that comes into their heads on a given subject, initially with no criticism, but later with a sifting and assessment of all ideas (because brainstorming is such a versatile but sometimes misunderstood method, it is described in detail in Box 48.1);

demonstration: the facilitator shows learners how and what should be done while explaining why, when, and where an action is done; participants then perform the action;

worksheet: a step-by-step approach to identifying problems or solutions through written questions or problems, with space provided for answers.

The uses, advantages, disadvantages, and trainers' role

Box 48.1 Brainstorming: A Versatile Technique for Training, Planning, and Problem-Solving

Brainstorming is a group technique that is useful in training situations. It also helps work groups be more creative in decision-making and problem-solving. The basic process is easy. The facilitator writes the topic or questions on a flip chart, whiteboard, or blackboard. Group members are asked to call out their ideas in short phrases that can be written down readily. To keep the discussion moving, a tight time limit is usually set—typically, five to ten minutes. The facilitator should be prepared to stimulate brainstorming with a few examples or prompting questions.

The creativity of brainstorming is enhanced by giving the group the following short set of guidelines before starting:

No idea is a bad idea: No matter how odd, unconventional, or silly an idea may seem, no idea should be ignored.

No discussion of ideas is allowed: Discussion of ideas can come later. Grimaces, groans, and other nonverbal judgments discourage creative thinking and should also be avoided.

Everybody is encouraged to contribute: The facilitator should try to get everyone to make at least one suggestion.

Go for quantity: This encourages the maximum contribution and discourages people from screening out potentially good ideas before suggesting them.

Build on other people's ideas: Although discussion of ideas is discouraged, generating new ideas from those already suggested is fine.

After the brainstorming session, ideas are usually typed up, organized in some way, and brought back to the group for discussion.

Although brainstorming can generate many creative ideas, it is not always successful. Some people may be discouraged from contributing, and there may be inhibitions about raising certain ideas. Brainstorming can also be dominated by certain individuals or get stuck on one part of the topic. Sticking to the above guidelines will help. In addition, methods to make brainstorming more productive include:

► Prepare a broad range of prompts that can be used to direct the group's thinking into new areas if suggestions are getting stuck in one area.
► Begin by asking each person to brainstorm individually for a few minutes and write down ideas.
► Divide the group into several smaller groups to brainstorm on the same topic. Then compile and discuss the topics in a larger group.
► Limit the number of suggestions by an individual group member. Generally, this degree of directness should be reserved for situations in which one group member dominates the brainstorming session.
► If brainstorming covers several topics, use separate pages or boards for each major topic.

for each of these methods are summarized in Figure 48.4. Some of the methods are more suitable for adult participatory training, and others work well in formal academic settings (such as lectures or seminars). Most

people learn better in an active rather than a passive fashion. A combination of methods is likely to be more effective than the exclusive use of one method.

Sequencing Topics

Sequencing means arranging topics in a logical order during training. In doing this, bear in mind that most people prefer to learn in easy and progressive stages. Adults, especially experienced trainees, usually prefer to start with an overview of the whole course before concentrating on particulars. The best approach is to sequence topics to build on previously completed content and learning experiences.

Developing Teaching Materials

Training materials may not be available for the kind of in-service training that would best suit a particular EDP. Many countries, however, have developed their own teaching materials using a number of approaches. These materials can be requested and used as is or adapted to suit specific needs. Materials from international sources are listed in Annex 48.2.

Manuals

Many countries have good manuals that are not being used effectively by their health workers, often because the workers were not involved or consulted in developing the manuals. A better approach is to ask knowledgeable persons to write on one or two topics; circulate drafts among selected end-users; and develop the final version in a workshop involving end-users, the authors, and EDP officers. This approach creates a sense of ownership (see Chapter 11), which leads to increased use of the materials developed.

The topics can be compiled under one cover or distributed as a series of individual modules, as occurred in Zimbabwe (see Country Study 48.3).

Trainers' and Participants' Guides

Training materials should include guides for both trainers and participants, as well as audiovisual aids. It may be possible to obtain some of these materials from established programs. Typical contents of trainers' and participants' guides are outlined in Figure 48.5. Both provide structured but adaptable notes and exercises for each unit. The participants' guide should contain the technical content for the unit, including definitions of all essential terms and concepts. The trainers' guide should provide guidance on how the session should be taught.

Figure 48.4 Comparison of Training Methods

Method	Useful for	Advantages	Disadvantages	Trainers' Role
Lecture	Passing on information and facts Giving specific information related to occupation, job, or task	Allows much material to be passed on in a short time Handles a large number of participants Permits lecturer to be in full control	Learner is passive Not everything said is remembered Little feedback to lecturer	Provide information Answer questions
Discussion	Stimulating interest and thought Generating possible solutions to problems Consolidating other types of learning Developing consensus	Stimulates learners' interest Involves learners actively	Time-consuming Requires learners to have facts about the topic Needs to be well controlled to have value Can be dominated by a few active persons	Establish small groups early in course Help groups select moderators and rapporteur Clearly specify tasks for each group Assign time limits for each task and enforce them
Case study	Problem-solving Attitude change Building analytical skills	Involves learners actively Allows sharing of learners' experiences with others Stimulates ideas and discussions of concrete subject	Time-consuming to prepare Not easy to validate Discussion may focus on different areas than those intended by trainer	Carefully prepare or read case and relevant material Ask provocative questions to provide key issues for discussion Guide discussion to achieve analysis, possible solution, recommendations for action
Role playing	Developing interactive knowledge and modifying attitudes Introducing humor and liveliness into training	Stimulates interest Is fun Is active Uses participants' experiences	Time-consuming to prepare Observers may be passive Some key points may not be addressed Those engaged in role playing may learn more than observers	Choose a suitable story to illustrate key points Debrief (discuss insights gained from role playing)
Group exercise	Team building Developing interactive skills Studying group dynamics	Facilitates high participation of motivated learners	Trainers' skills required to guide the exercise Takes time for group to work in harmony	Prepare carefully to ensure that everything is organized
Brainstorming	Stimulating creative thinking Generating possible solutions Consolidating past learning Providing diversion	Promotes active participation of learners Uses learners' experiences and ideas	Time-consuming Some learners may be passive Requires high trainers' skills	Record suggestions Reorganize into groups Lead discussion at end
Demonstration	Showing correct procedures and required standards	Stimulates a lot of interest Can be used for large groups	Takes effort to produce Good viewing by learners is difficult in a large group	Arrange for demonstration materials in advance Do demonstration alone to ensure that everything works Observe participant demonstrations Correct mistakes promptly Encourage slow learners
Worksheet	Quantitative exercises requiring calculations Working out solutions for issues of case studies	Helps learners relate their general learning to some specific area of their work	Time-consuming Difficult to prepare	Prepare a worksheet based on real situations to show difficulties and successes Guide the learners but leave most responsibility with participants

Audiovisual Aids

Audiovisual aids are useful because they stimulate the trainee and help reinforce the ideas presented. However, poor visual aids can confuse participants.

Commonly used visual aids include posters, wall charts, chalkboards, flip charts, overhead projections, and slides. Records and tapes are common audio aids. Videotapes and films are good audiovisual aids, but their expense often makes them impractical.

In developing visual aids, the following points should be kept in mind:

► Use only one idea per visual aid to avoid crowding.
► Use large letters and clear drawings.
► Allow plenty of time for preparing the visual aids and time for obtaining and testing the equipment.

Country Study 48.3 A Participatory Approach to Developing Training Materials in Zimbabwe

When the Zimbabwe Essential Drugs Action Programme (ZEDAP) was initiated in 1986, an early task was the development of training and resource materials related to drug use and drug management.

An initial national survey identified the crucial topics and existing materials. Fifteen topics were identified, and knowledgeable authors were invited to produce a first draft covering "the minimum necessary information for a first-level health worker." These drafts were reviewed in a series of week-long review and field-test meetings. The reviewers were invited from all districts of the country and from all cadres. Most reviewers were nurses or nurse tutors, although some review groups also included a doctor and a pharmacist or pharmacy technician.

The reviewers were divided into three groups and used a Delphi method, in which each group reviewed the work of the other groups. The revisions were made quickly, and a draft suitable for field testing was developed. The reviewers took the draft to three rural facilities, where the materials were field-tested. Based on this experience, a second draft was produced and circulated to all reviewers and training schools. Based on the comments received, a final version was produced using desktop publishing technology.

The materials were then used in a series of provincial or district training workshops to retrain all health workers within a two-year period. The reviewers of the materials acted as facilitators for these workshops.

In addition to the training and reference manuals, an essential drugs list and standard treatment guidelines (EDLIZ) has been produced based on the original materials.

The major advantage of this approach has been the widespread acceptance of the materials by health workers due to the extensive consultation that took place during their preparation.

This ZEDAP approach was successfully used in Malawi in the 1990s.

Source: Laing and Ruredzo 1989.

Figure 48.5 Outline of Trainers' and Participants' Guides for Workshops

Trainers' Guides
- Summary
  - learning objectives and content of the unit
  - preparations that the trainer must make
  - supplementary reading material
- Unit outline and session plan
  - prerequisites for participation in the session
  - components of the session and the estimated time
  - visual aids to be used
- Teaching notes
  - technical background
  - instructions for activities
- Visual aids (which can be copied onto transparencies or redrawn on flip charts)

Participants' Guides
- Session guide
  - learning objectives and content of the unit
  - basic information the participant must have before attending the session
  - additional reading materials
- Session notes (containing basic technical information, including definitions of essential terms)
- Session activities (with worksheets and instructions)

should take into account the nature of the target group or audience (Who are they? Are they senior or line managers?) and their level of knowledge and skill (Have participants been trained in the subject to be presented or related subjects?).

Preparation

Time used in preparation is time well spent. On average, the amount of time spent preparing the first presentation of a course or training session equals three times that spent presenting it. So a one-week course would require three weeks of preparation. After looking up information and consulting manuals and books that are relevant to the subject, the trainer chooses appropriate learning methods and puts together a session plan. He or she takes steps to acquire or prepare appropriate participants' guides and audiovisual aids well in advance. If possible, the trainer should rehearse the presentation before colleagues, keeping in mind issues of time and clarity.

Presentation

The trainer should always come to the training venue and the session early to check out the room, the seating arrangements, and the audiovisual equipment (Figure 48.6). A friendly chat with participants before the session creates a more comfortable environment.

Formal introductions should take place at the beginning of the first session. One way to do this is to ask pairs of participants to interview each other; then each presents

- Test the materials in a rehearsal before the session, preferably in front of critical colleagues.

In showing visual aids, the trainer should take care to

- check the visual aids and equipment a few minutes before the session begins;
- always face the audience, without obstructing their view, and use a pointer;
- switch off the equipment during discussions.

≡ 48.6 Training and Presentation Skills

A trainer is expected to be knowledgeable, possess excellent communication skills, and be able to communicate at the level of the participants. To be effective, the trainer

Figure 48.6 Seating Arrangements for Various Training Applications

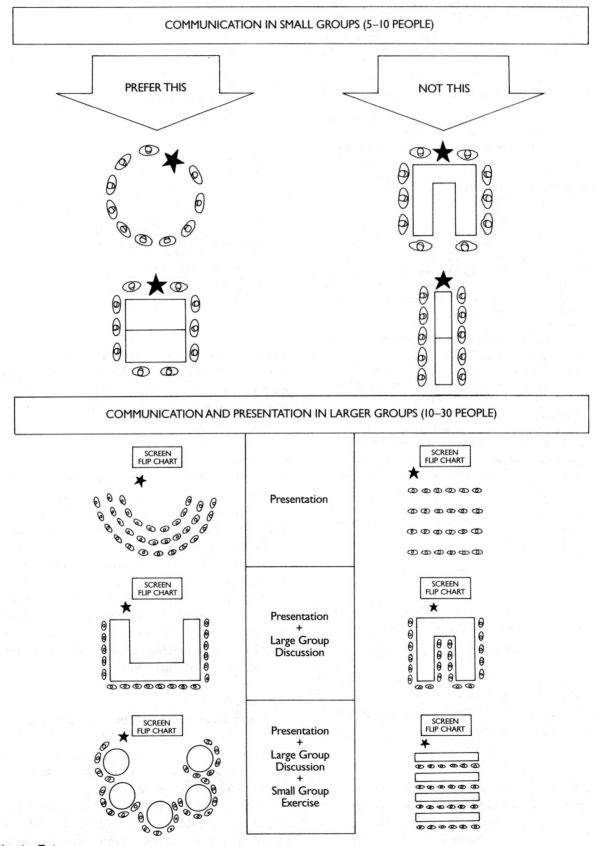

Key: ★ = Trainer or presenter.
Source: Adapted from McMahon et al. 1992.

≡ Assessment Guide

Training Programs

- Was a needs assessment conducted before the training programs were developed?
- What training programs have been held?
- How many people of each target group have been trained? What percentage is that of the total target number?
- What methods were used for the training?
- What were the evaluation results for knowledge change? Participant assessments? Work performance change?
- How much money has been spent on training activities (if possible, compare budget to actual expenditures)? What percentage of the overall program budget is this?

Sites and Institutions

- Which institutions provide training for staff working in the pharmaceutical sector?

- Over the past two years, where has training occurred? For whom?

Trainers

- At each of the institutions identified, how many trainers are there?
- How many of these people have been formally trained as trainers?
- In the courses undertaken, what were the evaluation ratings of the trainers?

Materials

- What training materials were used for the training courses?
- Where and how were the materials developed? When were they last updated?
- How widely available are the training materials?
- Do the training materials correspond with current policies?

---

the other to the group or records the information on a wall chart for all to see.

The actual session should begin with the trainer presenting the objectives of the course or session and summarizing its main points. These main points are then expanded using the chosen learning methods. At the end of the session, the trainer should always summarize the discussion, making sure to allow time for questions and clarification.

Trainers' Personal Style

Personal appearance and style can make a difference in keeping participants' interest during a session. The trainer should maintain eye contact with the group and make sure that his or her voice is clear and can be heard by everybody. When interest appears to be flagging, the trainer needs to be flexible and willing to change the schedule, perhaps by introducing a role play or arranging a short field visit. A

good story or joke can also help revive interest. In a session in which participants are divided into small groups, having the trainer move from group to group stimulates interest. During a long course, it is important to allocate time for dinners and other social activities.

Assessment

Assessing the performance and progress of the participants is one of the trainer's key roles. These assessments should be done as formative evaluations while the course is in progress and as cumulative evaluations after it is over. In training, formative assessment is important, because the aim of the course is to improve performance, not to grade the participants. The trainer can help them learn more quickly and more completely by providing them with constructive criticism during the course. The trainer can also use the feedback from evaluations to adjust the content and methods of the training to meet participants' needs better. ∎

≡ References and Further Readings

★ = *Key readings.*

General

CPA (Commonwealth Pharmaceutical Association), COL CPA (Commonwealth Pharmaceutical Association), COL (Commonwealth of Learning), and WHO/DAP (World Health Organization/Action Programme on Essential Drugs). 1995. *The management of drug supplies: A distant learning course.* London: CPA, COL, and WHO/DAP.

★ Guilbert, J. J. 1992. *Educational handbook for health personnel,* 6th ed. WHO Offset Series no. 35. Geneva: World Health Organization.

Hubley, J. 1993. *Communicating health: An action guide to health education and health promotion.* London: Macmillan.

Kanfer, F. H., and A. P. Goldstein. 1986. *Helping people change: A textbook of methods.* New York: Pergamon Press.

★ Laing, R., and R. Ruredzo. 1989. The essential drugs programme in Zimbabwe: New approaches to training. *Health Policy and Planning* 4:229–34.

★ McMahon, R., E. Barton, and M. Piot. 1992. *On being in charge: A guide to management in primary health care,* 2d ed. Geneva: World Health Organization.

MSH (Management Sciences for Health). 1991. Training for effective performance. In *The family planning manager's handbook: Basic skills and tools for managing family planning programs,* ed. J. A. Wolff, L. J. Suttenfield, and S. C. Binzen. West Hartford, Conn.: Kumarian Press.

★ MSH (Management Sciences for Health). 1992. *Managing drug supply training series.* Boston: MSH.

Oshang, A., D. Benbouzid, and J. J. Guilbert. 1993. *Educational handbook for nutrition teachers: How to increase your skills and make it easier for students to learn.* Geneva: World Health Organization.

PAHO (Pan American Health Organization) Regional Program of Development in Health Services. 1992. *Training material concerning the supply system in institutions of the health sector: Modules for self learning.* Washington, D.C.: PAHO.

Pike, R. W. 1990. *Creative training techniques handbook: Tips, tactics, and how-tos for delivering effective training.* Minneapolis, Minn.: Lakewood Books.

Rees, F. 1991. *How to lead work teams: Facilitation skills.* San Diego, Calif.: Pfeiffer and Company.

Werner, D., and B. Bower. 1983. *Helping health workers learn.* New Delhi: Voluntary Health Association of India.

WHO (World Health Organization). 1990. *Systems of continuing education: Priority to district health personnel.* Technical Report Series no. 803. Geneva: WHO.

Audiovisual Aids

WHO/DAP maintains a list of audiovisual aids that is regularly updated in their *Selected Annotated Bibliography on Essential Drugs.* WHO/DAP can also supply videos of country programs that can be used for training programs. Address: WHO/DAP, CH-1211 Geneva 27, Switzerland

Teaching Aids at Low Cost (TALC) also supplies books and slides for teaching. It has a slide set on essential drugs that can serve as introductory material. Address: PO Box 49, St. Albans, Herts. AL1 4AX, England.

Annex 48.1 Workshop Logistics

Workshop and Support Checklist

Advance Planning

❏ Content, topics, session
❏ Participant list
❏ Short-term consultant(s) and facilitator(s)
❏ Budget, including materials, travel, accommodations
❏ Venue: reservations, deposit, other concerns
❏ Invitations to participants and follow-up phone calls

Workshop Material

❏ Ruled writing pads, pens, pencils with erasers
❏ Document binders
❏ Flip charts and pens
❏ Blank overhead transparencies and pens
❏ Masking tape and transparent tape
❏ Stapler and staples
❏ Hole punch
❏ Photocopying paper
❏ Computer paper, printer ribbon, blank diskettes, multiplug adapter
❏ Letterhead stationery and envelopes
❏ Paper clips, scissors, Post-it pads, rubber bands, White-out, glue
❏ Calculator
❏ Name badges

Workshop Support Responsibility

❏ Logistics: supervision of conference site, meals, breaks, and accommodations
❏ Finances: payment of cash food allowances, paperwork, and reimbursement for transportation expenses
❏ Secretary for word processing
❏ Vehicle and driver
❏ Messenger and photocopier

Workshop Support Facilities

❏ Telephone access (incoming and outgoing) for facilitators
❏ On-site photocopy machine (with toner and paper) for low-volume copies
❏ Photocopy service site for high-volume copies
❏ Computer and printer
❏ Overhead projector, extra bulb, extension cord of adequate length
❏ 35 mm slide projector and projector screen

Set-up of Main Meeting Room

❏ Opening session and plenary sessions: horseshoe versus classroom style seating with extra chairs
❏ Break room or area
❏ Groups of approximately equal size
❏ Overhead and slide projector check: screen that all participants can see, projector proper distance and angle from screen, sufficiently long electric cord, extra bulb

❏ Transparencies and pens
❏ Flip charts and pens available for plenary and small groups

Daily Preparation of Meeting Room

❏ Projectors: position, cord, spare bulb, transparencies, pens
❏ Blackboard or whiteboard: cleaner, pens
❏ Flip charts: location, paper, pens

Workshop Administration Checklist

❏ Upon arrival at the training site, make sure that the conference room is arranged properly and note any changes that need to be made. Find out if there are additional rooms available for small group discussions. Set up a registration desk near the entrance and a working table where appropriate. Arrange the handouts on a separate table where they are readily accessible.

❏ Set up the projector and test it. Make sure that the projection screen can be seen easily by all participants.

❏ Put the writing pads, pens, and programs into the document binders and place them on the tables.

❏ Inform the management of the site about all the practical arrangements.

❏ Put up a sign board at reception displaying the location of the conference room and registration time.

❏ Using the list of participants, write the name tags and spread them out on the registration desk so that the participants can collect them as they register. This can be done either the evening before or in the morning before registration begins.

❏ Give a copy of the program to the management so that they know when to serve tea or coffee and meals.

❏ During the introductory session, make administrative announcements: when allowances will be paid (night-out allowances are normally paid at the end of day one; reimbursements for travel expenses are normally paid at the break on the last day, upon presentation of receipts as documentation).

❏ As soon as the last person has registered, type out the participant list and start preparing the receipts for participants to sign when receiving allowances. Use a duplicate receipt book with a carbon. Mark the receipt number against the participant's name on the list to make paying easier.

❏ Type out a separate list for reimbursing the transport expenses and make out payment receipts. Fuel and other travel receipts can be collected on day one when paying out allowances.

❏ Give a copy of the participant list to hotel management, indicating the participants who are not staying at the site so that they know how many extra teas and lunches to charge for. Also, give management the names of the people who are settling their own bills (facilitators, secretaries) so that they will not be included in the main bill.

❏ On the last day, have the hotel management prepare the detailed bill and check it against the participant list.

Annex 48.2 Sources of Assistance for Training Programs to Improve Pharmaceutical Logistics

The following organizations and institutions offer training in selected activities relevant to the pharmaceutical supply process. This listing is not exhaustive, nor is it an endorsement of individual training programs. For details, these organizations should be contacted directly.

This listing is arranged with international organizations listed first, followed by national and private organizations and institutions. Also included is a list of short courses on drug policy, drug management, rational drug use, and related subjects.

International Organizations

World Health Organization (WHO), 1211 Geneva 27, Switzerland

Action Programme on Essential Drugs (DAP)

An operational arm of WHO. Assists member states in the development and implementation of drug policies, the supply of essential drugs of good quality at the lowest possible cost, and the development of training in the rational use of drugs.
Telephone: 41 22 791 21 11; fax: 41 22 791 41 67.

Division of Drug Management and Policies (DMP)

Participates in regional and national training courses for drug regulators. Works closely with WHO collaborating centers on drug regulation and quality assurance and control. Upon request from drug regulatory authorities, coordinates training in such centers. Provides training in drug registration and computerization of drug regulatory data, as well as good manufacturing practices (GMPs), analytical control, and preparation of chemical reference substances. Fosters visits to regulatory authorities in developed countries and coordinates training in drug quality control and GMPs offered by the International Federation of Pharmaceutical Manufacturers Associations.
Telephone: 41 22 791 36 61; fax: 41 22 791 07 46.

Expanded Programme on Immunization (EPI)

Has developed modular course materials in cold-chain logistics for procurement and importation managers, storage and distribution managers, and field-level users. Provides training workshops in practical exercises, group activities, and case studies.

United Nations Children's Fund (UNICEF), Supply Division, 866 United Nations Plaza, Sixth Floor—Room A-6114, New York, N.Y. 10017, US

Offers training at UNIPAC (the UNICEF Supply Division International Packing and Assembly Centre in Copenhagen) in the methodology of inventory control, stock rotation, and quality assurance in warehouse receiving. Training is arranged on an individual basis, usually for personnel involved with UNICEF projects, but occasionally for non-UNICEF agencies and individuals under special agreement. Other training is sometimes arranged on the assessment of priority pharmaceutical needs, vehicle maintenance, and the production of oral rehydration salts according to WHO standards.

United Nations Development Programme (UNDP), Division of Information, One United Nations Plaza, New York, N.Y. 10017, US

Sponsors training in the quality control of vaccines in conjunction with the WHO EPI. Training programs are designed in collaboration with the health authorities of developing countries.

United Nations Industrial Development Organization (UNIDO), Pharmaceutical Industries Unit, Chemical Industries Section, Industrial Operations Division, Vienna International Centre, PO Box 300, A-1400, Vienna, Austria

Offers seminars and training in pharmaceutical production and technology transfer. Promotes technical cooperation among developing countries.

United Nations Institute for Training and Research (UNI-TAR), United Nations, New York, N.Y. 10017, US

Conducts seminars in procurement and warehousing, although not specific to pharmaceuticals.

Asian Productivity Organization, Aoyama Dai-Ichi Mansions, 4-14 Akasaka 8-Chome, Minato-Ku, Tokyo 107, Japan

Short-term training in production management and project feasibility studies. Available only to members of the Asian Productivity Organization. Course work in English. Fellowships available.

International Federation of Pharmaceutical Manufacturers Associations (IFPMA), 67 Rue St.-Jean, 1201 Geneva, Switzerland

Has offered training in quality control to employees of governmental control laboratories and governmental pharmaceutical inspection services in the developing world. Training tailored to individual needs. Candidates for training are nominated through WHO.

National and Private Organizations and Institutions

Management Sciences for Health (MSH), 165 Allandale Road, Boston, Mass. 02130, US. Telephone: (617) 524-7799; fax: (617) 524-2825.

Drug Management Program, 1655 North Fort Myer Drive, Suite 920, Arlington, Va. 22209. Telephone: (703) 524-6575; fax: (703) 524-7898; Internet: dmp@msh-dc.org.
Management Training, 400 Centre Street, Newton, Mass. 02158. Telephone: (617) 527-9202; fax: (617) 965-2208.

Offers short-term courses in English, French, and Spanish on rational drug use and other aspects of pharmaceutical management and on other topics, including health financing, health and family planning program management, management information systems, and management of training programs. Over the past fourteen years, more than a thousand health professionals from sixty countries have participated in MSH courses in the United States and other countries.

Robert Gordon University, School of Pharmacy, Course Tutor (EDM/RDU), Schoolhill, Aberdeen AB9 1FR, Scotland, UK. Telephone: 224-626559; fax: 224-262500.

WHO collaborating center. Offers a short course for health care professionals involved in the management of pharmaceuticals and a course to improve the level of effectiveness in the management of drugs as a health care resource and improve the rational use of drugs.

Center for International Health, Boston University, 53 Bay State Road, Boston, Mass. 02115-2101, US. Telephone: (617) 353-4524; fax: (617) 353-6330; Internet: CIH@bu.edu.

Offers short courses, including drug policy and management courses, that can be sequenced to complete the master's of public administration degree.

National and Private Organizations and Institutions (cont.)

University of Groningen, Faculty of Medicine, Department of Clinical Pharmacology, 9713 BZ Groningen, The Netherlands. Telephone: 31 50 632812; fax: 31 50 632809.

WHO collaborating center. Offers summer courses in problem-based pharmacotherapy teaching for clinical and clinical pharmacology teachers.

Eastern and Southern Africa Management Institute (ESAMI), PO Box 3030, Arusha, Tanzania

A regional institution. Provides a full schedule of practical short-term courses on a wide variety of general management and health management topics. Brings people from different countries to share and exchange experiences in a regional context. Takes its services to client institutions through tailor-made interventions using its knowledge of the region. Annually undertakes more than 100 short-term programs involving over 3,000 participants. Serves participants from other English-speaking African countries and from countries outside Africa, in addition to its nineteen member countries in the region.

Mahidol University, Dean, Faculty of Pharmacy, Sri Ayuthaya Road, Bangkok 10400, Thailand. Telephone: (66-02) 246-1188-93; fax: (66-02) 247-4696.

Offers short courses on pharmaceutical management, including utilization of essential drugs, GMP training, and pharmaceutical economics.

Istituto de Ricerche Farmacologiche Mario Negri, Via Eritrea 62, 20157 Milan, Italy

Provides teaching activities in laboratory technician training programs and specialized courses for graduates wishing to pursue careers in research. Trainees receive fellowships through the institute; 15 percent of fellowships go to foreign scientists. Participants acquire knowledge on site and work with research scientists from different countries.

Kampsax International, PO Box 1143, 112 Stamholmen, DK-2650, Hvidovre, Denmark

Offers training in public administration; health, sanitation, and socioeconomic aspects of water supply; and geographical information systems. Training is in English; bilingual manuals can be prepared, if required.

State University of Ghent, Ghent, Belgium

Six-week courses in pharmaceutical technology: production techniques (manufacturing of tablets and capsules, granulation, and direct compression methods, preparation of ampoules and perfusion solution, ointments); sterilization procedures; formulation of intramuscular drugs; planning for production of antibiotics, sulfonamides, antiseptics. Offered in English or French.

Catholic University of Leuven, Universiteitskal, Oude Markt 13, 3,000 Leuven, Belgium

Has offered courses in supply management, with funding from WHO.

About the Editors

Jonathan D. Quick, a family physician who is now the director of the Action Programme on Essential Drugs at WHO/Geneva, edited the first edition of *Managing Drug Supply.* From 1984 to 1989, Dr. Quick directed MSH's Drug Management Program. He later worked for MSH in Peshawar, Pakistan, with the Afghanistan Cross-Border Health Project, and in Nairobi with the Kenya Health Care Financing Project.

James R. Rankin has directed the MSH Drug Management Program since 1989. He also directed the USAID-funded Rational Pharmaceutical Management Project from 1992 to 1995 and, previously, the Eastern Caribbean Regional Pharmaceuticals Management Project. He spent a decade providing pharmaceutical consulting services to state and federal health systems in the United States while managing pharmaceutical services for Presbyterian Medical Services in New Mexico. He served on the Executive Committee of Revision for the US Pharmacopeia between 1980 and 1990 and has been a member of the USP Panel on International Health since 1990.

Richard O. Laing, a Zimbabwean physician, is the associate director of the Center for International Health at Boston University. He served as a senior staff associate and training coordinator of the Drug Management Program of MSH and coordinated the International Network for the Rational Use of Drugs from 1989 to 1994. He previously served with the Zimbabwe Ministry of Health as director of health manpower training and as provincial medical director. He is a member of the USP Panel on International Health.

Ronald W. O'Connor has served as president of MSH and as a member of its Board of Directors since MSH was founded in 1971. In addition, Dr. O'Connor directed MSH health development projects over two decades in Afghan-istan and the Learning for Life Project in the United States, and he has consulted for health and family planning programs worldwide for thirty years. An editor of the first edition of *Managing Drug Supply* and two books on health care in Afghanistan, Dr. O'Connor is a graduate of Yale University, the College of Physicians and Surgeons at Columbia University, the Harvard School of Public Health, and the Sloan School of Management at the Massachusetts Institute of Technology.

Hans V. Hogerzeil coordinates activities on rational drug use and country programs in East Africa, Indonesia, and Thailand for WHO/DAP in Geneva. Previously a mission doctor in rural India and Ghana, he has authored many publications on distribution systems, essential drugs in emergency situations, drug stability in tropical climates, and teaching of rational prescribing.

M. N. G. Dukes, a physician and attorney, is a former director of the Euro Health Group in Copenhagen. He previously held the positions of professor at the University of Groningen, the Netherlands, and head of the Pharmaceuticals Programme, WHO/EURO, from 1982 to 1990. From 1972 to 1982, he was the medical director of the Netherlands Drug Approval Agency. He has edited, among other books, *Meyler's Side Effects of Drugs* and *Drugs and Money.*

Andrew Garnett is an architect with Levitt Bernstein Associates in London. He was formerly a consultant on health planning for Feilden Battersby Health Systems Analysts, and he served as Senior Architect in the Ministry of Health of Gongola State, Nigeria, from 1977 to 1979. He specializes in primary health care logistics, space planning, and the preparation and design of management guidelines. Mr. Garnett has carried out recent consultancies in these areas for Danida, UNICEF, and WHO. ∎

Authors by Chapter

This list shows the contributors to each chapter. Contributors are listed alphabetically, not in relation to the proportion of material they contributed. Several chapters retain a substantial portion of the text from the first edition of this book. For those chapters, the authors from the earlier edition are listed last and denoted by an asterisk.

1. *Toward Sustainable Supply and Rational Use of Drugs*
   M. N. G. Dukes (Euro Health Group)
   Jonathan D. Quick (MSH)

2. *Historical and Institutional Perspectives*
   M. N. G. Dukes (Euro Health Group)
   Ronald W. O'Connor (MSH)

3. *Economics for Drug Management*
   Kara Hanson (Harvard School of Public Health)
   David Henry (University of Newcastle)
   Jonathan D. Quick (MSH)
   Germán Velásquez (WHO/DAP)

4. *Pharmaceutical Supply System Assessment*
   James R. Rankin (MSH)

5. *National Drug Policies*
   Pascale Brudon (WHO/DAP)
   M. N. G. Dukes (Euro Health Group)

6. *Drug Supply Strategies*
   Jonathan D. Quick (MSH)
   James R. Rankin (MSH)
   Germán Velásquez (WHO/DAP)

7. *Pharmaceutical Legislation and Regulation*
   M. N. G. Dukes (Euro Health Group)
   Marcelo Vernengo (Universidad de Belgrano)
   Robert L. Watt

8. *Legal Aspects of Drug Management*
   M. N. G. Dukes (Euro Health Group)

9. *Pharmaceutical Production Policy*
   John Holley (Integral Development Associates)
   Paul J. N. Lamberts (Deventer Hospital Pharmacy)
   Ronald W. O'Connor (MSH)
   Robert L. Watt

10. *Managing Drug Selection*
    Hans V. Hogerzeil (WHO/DAP)

11. *Treatment Guidelines and Formulary Manuals*
    Chris Forshaw (WHO, Malawi Essential Drugs
      Programme)
    Hans V. Hogerzeil (WHO/DAP)

12. *Essential Medical Supplies and Equipment*
    Hans V. Hogerzeil (WHO/DAP)
    Kirsten Myhr (University of Trondheim)

13. *Managing Procurement*
    Jonathan D. Quick (MSH)
    James R. Rankin (MSH)

14. *Quantifying Drug Requirements*
    Chris B. Olson (MSH)
    James R. Rankin (MSH)

15. *Inventory Management*
    James R. Rankin (MSH)
    *Vimal S. Dias (MSH)
    *Jonathan D. Quick (MSH)

16. *Managing the Tender Process*
    Johan van Haperen (Danida)
    James R. Rankin (MSH)

17. *Contracting for Drugs and Services*
    Elvira Beracochea (MSH)
    Sherita Gregoire (Goodwill, Dominica)
    *Vimal S. Dias (MSH)
    *Jonathan D. Quick (MSH)

18. *Quality Assurance for Drug Procurement*
    David Lee (MSH)
    *Jonathan D. Quick (MSH)

19. *Small-Scale Local Production*
    Paul J. N. Lamberts (Deventer Hospital Pharmacy)
    Robert L. Watt

20. *Drug Donations*
    Christel Albert
    Hans V. Hogerzeil (WHO/DAP)

21. *Managing Distribution*
    Anthony Battersby (Feilden Battersby Health Systems
      Analysts)
    Andrew Garnett (Feilden Battersby Health Systems
      Analysts)
    *James Bates (MSH)

22. *Importation and Port Clearing*
Vimal S. Dias (MSH)
John Ellery (Greenshields Cowie)
Hilary Vaughan (Crown Agents)

23. *Medical Stores Management*
Anthony Battersby (Feilden Battersby Health Systems Analysts)
Vimal S. Dias (MSH)
Andrew Garnett (Feilden Battersby Health Systems Analysts)
Jean-Pierre Sallet (MSH)
John C. Turnbull

24. *Drug Management for Health Facilities*
Richard O. Laing (MSH)
Hanif S. Nazerali

25. *Planning and Building Storage Facilities*
Jan F. Dik (Euro Health Group)
Therese Edera-Piech (Design Development, Nairobi)
Andrew Garnett (Feilden Battersby Health Systems Analysts)

26. *Transport Management*
Anthony Battersby (Feilden Battersby Health Systems Analysts)
Andrew Garnett (Feilden Battersby Health Systems Analysts)

27. *Kit System Management*
Miguel M. de Clerck (Médecins sans Frontières)
Jean-Pierre de Lamalle (Médecins sans Frontières)
Myriam Henkens (Médecins sans Frontières)
Hans V. Hogerzeil (WHO/DAP)
Ignacio J. Packer (Médecins sans Frontières)

28. *Managing for Rational Drug Use*
Richard O. Laing (MSH)
Budiono Santoso (Gadjah Mada University)

29. *Investigating Drug Use*
Dennis Ross-Degnan (Harvard University)

30. *Drug and Therapeutics Information*
Keith W. Johnson (US Pharmacopeia)
O. M. J. Kasilo (University of Zimbabwe Medical School)

31. *Promoting Rational Prescribing*
Richard O. Laing (MSH)
David Ofori-Adjei (University of Ghana Medical School)
Chris B. Olson (MSH)
Budiono Santoso (Gadjah Mada University)

32. *Ensuring Good Dispensing Practices*
Paul D. Spivey (Robert Gordon University)

33. *Encouraging Appropriate Drug Use by the Public and Patients*
Daphne A. Fresle (WHO/DAP)

34. *Managing Drug Programs*
Jonathan D. Quick (MSH)

35. *Planning for Drug Management*
Jonathan D. Quick (MSH)
*James Bates (MSH)
*A. Frederick Hartman

36. *Monitoring and Evaluation*
Agnes B. Guyon (UNICEF)
Jonathan D. Quick (MSH)

37. *Community Participation*
Aida Girma (Bamako Initiative Project, UNICEF)

38. *Hospital Drug Services*
Chris B. Olson (MSH)
Anthony Savelli (MSH)

39. *Security Management*
Gabriel Daniel (Africare)
*Jonathan D. Quick (MSH)

40. *Drug Financing Strategies*
William Newbrander (MSH)
Jonathan D. Quick (MSH)
Catriona Waddington (Overseas Development Administration)

41. *Analyzing and Controlling Drug Expenditures*
Peter J. Graaff (Malawi Essential Drugs Programme, WHO)
James R. Rankin (MSH)
*Vimal S. Dias (MSH)
*Jonathan D. Quick (MSH)

42. *Financial Planning and Management*
David H. Collins (MSH)

43. *Donor Financing*
Enrique Fefer (PAHO)
Margaret Hume (MSH)
Irene Klinger (PAHO)

44. *Revolving Drug Funds*
Margaret Hume (MSH)
Jennie I. Litvack (World Bank)
Jonathan D. Quick (MSH)

45. *Drug Management Information Systems*
David R. Wilson (MSH)

46. *Computers in Drug Management*
Wilbert Bannenberg
Paul Krystall (Data Dynamics)
Julie E. McFadyen (MSH)
Jonathan D. Quick (MSH)
James R. Rankin (MSH)
Jean-Pierre Sallet (MSH)

47. *Personnel Management*
Carl F. Browne (Ministry of Health and the Environment, St. Vincent and the Grenadines)
John Fox (Intermedia)

48. *Designing and Implementing Training Programs*
Sam Muziki (WHO/DAP)
*A. Frederick Hartman

Reviewers

G. Angila, Nairobi
D. Arhinful, Centre for Tropical Clinical Pharmacology and Therapeutics, Accra, Ghana
P. Auxila, MSH, Boston, Mass.
S. Bennett, London School of Hygiene and Tropical Medicine, London
Bimo, Yayasan Indonesia Sejahtera, Jakarta
R. Blakney, Haven of Hope Hospital, Hong Kong
D. Brahams, London
D. Broun, World Bank, Washington, D.C.
F. Burnett, Eastern Caribbean Drug Service, Castries, St. Lucia
T. Bwire, Ministry of Health, Nairobi
P. Carlevaro, UNICEF, New York
R. Chaudhury, National Institute of Immunology, New Delhi
R. Christensen, Danida, Copenhagen
S. Clein, Department of Health, Papua New Guinea
B. Corbé, Médecins sans Frontières, Brussels
M. Couper, WHO, Geneva
W. van Damme, Prince Leopold Institute of Tropical Medicine, Antwerp
H. den Besten, International Dispensary Association, Amsterdam
V. Diwan, Karolinska Institute, Stockholm
D. Dunlop, World Bank, Washington, D.C.
A. E. Elmendorf, World Bank, Washington, D.C.
M. Everard, WHO/EMRO, Alexandria
J. Fink, University of Kentucky, Lexington, Ky.
E. H. Froese, Seattle, Wash.
L. Gilson, London School of Hygiene and Tropical Medicine, London
C. Griffin, World Bank, Washington, D.C.
H. Haak, Indonesia
A. Hardon, University of Amsterdam, Amsterdam
M. Helling-Borda, WHO/DAP, Geneva
N. Heltzer, Prison Health Services, Dover, Del.
A. Herxheimer, UK Cochrane Center, Oxford
J. Hetzke, WHO/DAP, Geneva
C. Hodgkin, Health Action International, Amsterdam
S. Holand, WHO/DAP, Geneva
P. Itumbi Njue, PHC Coordinator, Nairobi
F. Iyun, University of Ibadan, Nigeria
D. C. Jayasuriya, UNDP, New Delhi
K. de Joncheere, PAHO/WHO, Brazil
K. K. Kafle, Tribhuvan University, Kathmandu
Q. Kintanar, Department of Health, Manila
R. Kinuka, Uganda Red Cross Society, Kampala

J. M. Kioko, Ministry of Health, Nairobi
G. Kodzwa, UNICEF/Mozambique
E. Lauridsen, Euro Health Group, Copenhagen
R. Lunt, Geneva
A. F. B. Mabadeje, University of Lagos, Nigeria
J. McKim, Patan Hospital, Kathmandu
B. McPake, UNICEF, New York
B. Melgaard, Danida/Bhutan
M. Miralles, MSH, Arlington, Va.
Mission for Essential Drugs staff pharmacists, Nairobi
E. Molosiwa, Scottish Livingstone Hospital, Molepolole, Botswana
C. Morlock, Santa Fe, N.M.
M. Munck, Zimbabwe Essential Drugs Programme, Harare
S. Musau, Carr, Stanyer, Gitau & Co., Nairobi
J. Muschell, WHO/DAP, Geneva
O. F. Nielsen, Danida, Nicaragua
S. Nightingale, US Food and Drug Administration, Rockville, Md.
E. Nordberg, Karolinska Institute, Stockholm
S. Odongo, Kenya Essential Drugs Programme, Nairobi
E. Ombaka, Christian Medical Commission, Geneva
P. Petit, Danida/Tanzania
V. Reggi, WHO, Geneva
M. Reich, Harvard School of Public Health, Boston, Mass.
L. Salako, Nigerian Institute of Medical Research, Lagos
P. Saunders, OXFAM, London
J. B. Seltzer, MSH, Boston, Mass.
R. Skinner, ECHO, Surrey, England
A. Smith, University of Newcastle, Australia
M. Soakai, Ministry of Health, Tonga
M. Stegeman, Dutch Ministry of Foreign Affairs, Gravenhage, The Netherlands
G. Sterky, Karolinska Institute, Stockholm
S. Suryawati, Gadjah Mada University, Yogyakarta
M. Tan, Health Action International, Manila
M. Thuo, University of Nairobi, Nairobi
B. Timmons, MSH, Boston, Mass.
G. Tomson, Karolinska Institute, Stockholm
A. N. Tukura, CHANPHARM, Nigeria
G. Weeda, Government Medical Stores, Harare
A. Wehrli, WHO, Geneva
R. Wilson, Aga Khan Foundation, Geneva
F. Winnubst, Eindhoven, The Netherlands
E. Wondemagengnehu, WHO, Geneva
J. Zijp, Medical Supplies Department, United Mission to Nepal, Kathmandu

Index

Biological testing, 282
Bits (binary digits), defined, 744
Black market drugs: local agents and, 238; private outlets for, 598, 600; procurement offices and, 597; in Southeast Asia, 600; theft and, 596; in West Africa, 599
Block contracts, 268
Block-stacked pallets, 353
Boats, 395
Bottom-up implementation, 698
Bottom-up planning, 539
Box trailer units, 395–96
Brainstorming, 770, 771, 772; force field analysis and, 527, 528; in strategic planning, 542; in work planning, 545
Brand-name drugs (*see also* Counterfeit drugs): doctor choice of, 82; donations of, 307; former dominance of, 10; generic-name bidding and, 168; inefficient choice of, 33; marketing of, 261; medical education and, 472; in national formularies, 146; prices of, 126; research-based manufacture of, 240
Branded generics: defined, 136
Brazil, 85
Break-even analysis, 665
Bribery *see* Corruption
Briefs (programs) *see* Programs (project briefs)
Britain *see* United Kingdom
British Medical Association, 91
British National Formulary (organization), 457
British National Formulary (publication), 1, 127–28, 139; arrangement of, 133; in CD-ROM format, 739; chapter introductions of, 145; national formulary committees and, 145; Nepalese use of, 458
British Overseas Development Administration, 675
British Pharmacopoeia, 156, 243, 261, 272
Browser software, 739
Budget performance reports, 666–67, 668; defined, 626
Budgets (*see also* Service-level projection of budget requirements), 660–63; assessment of, 43; capital, 626, 658, 662; computer hardware in, 730; contractor payments and, 264; donor projects and, 680; estimation of, 186–87; evaluation of, 622; forecasting software for, 735; of hospital stores, 584; indicators for, 47; insurer cost control and, 619; limitations of, 656; managerial approaches to, 222–23; nonlisted drugs and, 134–35; prescriber participation in, 476–77; procurement efficiency and, 178–79; program plans and, 537, 545; for public education, 502; public financing through, 178; RDF implementation and, 694; in "real" terms, 29; reductions for, 191; reports on, 45, 211; service contracts and, 268; for storage construction, 384; supervision and, 757; total procurement costs and, 196, 201; updating of, 666; use studies and, 438; workplans and, 547
Buffer stock *see* Safety stock
Bugs (computers): defined, 744
Building contractors, 382, 389, 391
Building contracts, 388–89, 391
Building laws, 384, 388
Building manuals, 390
Buildings (*see also* Commercial buildings; Storage buildings), 294
Bulk purchases, 170; ABC analysis and, 633, 635; cash flow and, 663; defined, 181; by RDFs, 704
Bulk storage, 367
Bulk ward stock system, 374, 585, 588–89

Bulletins (*see also* Journals), 453; comparative reviews in, 133; in DICs, 457; formularies and, 144, 145; prescribers and, 471; production of, 458–59; sample issue of, 460
Bureau of Pharmaceutical Laboratories (Malaysia), 283
Bureaucratic inertia, 527
Burkina Faso, 306
Business law, 102–5, 107
Bytes: defined, 744

Calls for offers, 243; defined, 181
Cambodia, 62, 417
Cameroon, 61, 461, 611, 691, 693
Canada, 95, 104, 504, 505, 573
Canadian International Development Agency, 680
Capital, working, 694, 695
Capital budgets, 626, 658, 662
Capital costs, 29, 35, 384, 461
Capital equipment (*see also* Depreciation), 151, 153, 296, 397
Capital financing, 76, 461, 694–96, 706
Capitation-based reimbursement, 478
Capsules: analysis of, 282; counting of, 488, 493; cross-contamination of, 485; imprinting of, 598, 599, 600; inspection of, 346; local production of, 298; packing of, 262, 488, 491, 492
Car batteries, 743
Card files: defined, 332
Career development (logistics personnel), 358
Caribbean area (*see also* Eastern Caribbean Drug Service): average inventories in, 228; category-based tendering in, 169; consumption-based quantification in, 193, 194; estimated-quantity contracts in, 236; expiry-date analysis in, 651; INVEC-2 in, 737; lead-time analysis for, 650; RDF reports in, 705; regional laboratories in, 94; therapeutic category analysis in, 638
Caribbean Community, 171
Caribbean Regional Drug Testing Laboratory, 172, 283
Carrying costs (*see also* Holding costs), 402
Cartels, 31
Cartons, 262, 403, 415
Case records, 438–39
Case study method, 770, 772
Cash basis accounting system, 656, 657; defined, 626
Cash books, 667–68
Cash deposits, 666
Cash donations, 310
Cash flow, 335, 695
Cash flow forecasts, 663, 664; defined, 626
Catheters, 160
Catholic and Protestant Medical Bureau (Uganda), 74
Catholic Secretariat (Kenya), 86
Catholic University of Leuven, 779
Causal forecasting, 221
CD-ROM drives, 734, 739
CD-ROMs, 457, 504, 739; defined, 744
Center for International Health (Boston University), 778
Central America, 502–3, 596, 598
Central banks, 179, 261
Central Drugs Laboratory (India), 93
Central governments: CMS system and, 78; essential drug expenditures of, 614–15; funding by, 612, 694, 698, 703; patents and, 104; resource allocation by, 27; revenues of, 692; social welfare perspective on, 28

About Management Sciences for Health, Euro Health Group, and the WHO Action Programme on Essential Drugs

Management Sciences for Health (MSH) is a private, nonprofit corporation dedicated to closing the gap between what is known about public health problems and what is done to solve them. Since its founding in 1971, MSH has collaborated with health decision-makers throughout the world to improve the quality of health and population services and to make these services available and affordable for all.

During its twenty-five-year history, MSH has assisted public- and private-sector health and population programs in over 100 countries. MSH has provided technical assistance, conducted training, carried out applied research, and developed systems for use in health program management. Its technical and management staff from 36 nations is based in Boston, Massachusetts, Washington, D.C., and field offices throughout the world.

Through the Drug Management Program (DMP), MSH helps organizations and governments maximize the availability and therapeutic benefits of drugs while minimizing their costs through technical assistance, applied research, and training courses in developing countries (in collaboration with local and regional institutions) and in the United States.

MSH coordinates the International Network for Rational Use of Drugs (INRUD), which works to improve drug prescribing and use. MSH has developed both manual and computerized drug management information systems, including a half-dozen software packages used around the world. MSH is the publisher of the first edition of this textbook, the annual *International Drug Price Indicator Guide*, the multivolume *Managing Drug Supply Training Series*, and the manual *Rapid Pharmaceutical Management: An Indicator-Based Approach*.

In collaboration with the United States Pharmacopeia, MSH manages the Rational Pharmaceutical Management (RPM) Project, a worldwide cooperative agreement supported by the US Agency for International Development.

RPM provides technical assistance in assessing pharmaceutical systems, computerizing drug management, improving drug procurement and logistics, expanding drug information resources, and promoting rational drug use.

The **Euro Health Group (EHG)**, an affiliate of MSH, is a technical assistance organization based in Copenhagen. It works in Africa, Asia, Central America, and Eastern Europe, with support from donors that include the International Red Cross, the Commission of European Communities, the Danish International Development Agency and other European bilateral agencies, the World Bank, and regional development banks. EHG services focus on drug management and other health-related areas, including nutrition and family planning.

In 1981, **WHO's Action Programme on Essential Drugs (DAP)** was established to support countries' efforts to achieve equitable access to essential drugs and to ensure the quality, safety, efficacy, and rational use of drugs. DAP assists countries in the development and implementation of national drug policies and essential drugs programs. In addition to this direct support, DAP plays a leadership, coordination, and advocacy role in promoting the essential drugs concept by preparing technical guidelines and manuals, publishing the *Essential Drugs Monitor*, developing training programs, and facilitating cooperation among countries.

Many of the items cited in the "References and Further Readings" sections of this manual are WHO publications covering the development of national drug policies, appropriate use of essential drugs, estimation of drug requirements, investigation of drug use at health facilities and in the community, teaching of good prescribing practices, and sizing of medical stores. DAP also undertakes and promotes operational research aimed at expanding existing knowledge about the most effective and economical means of selecting, procuring, distributing, and rationally using drugs. ∎

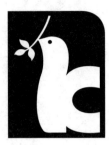 Kumarian Press is dedicated to publishing and distributing books and other media that will have a positive social and economic impact on the lives of peoples living in "Third World" conditions no matter where they live.

**As well as books on International Health,
Kumarian Press also publishes books
on the Environment,
International Development,
Nongovernmental Organizations,
Government, Gender and Development**

To receive a complimentary catalog, request writer's guidelines, or to order books call or write:

Kumarian Press, Inc.
14 Oakwood Avenue
West Hartford, CT 06119-2127
USA

Inquiries: 860-233-5895
Fax: 860-233-6072
Order toll free: 800-289-2664

e-mail: kpbooks@aol.com